MEDICAL-SURGICAL

# NURSING CARE PLANNING GUIDES

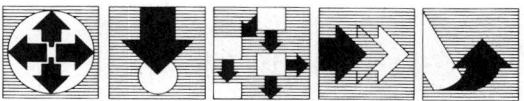

THIRD EDITION

**Susan Puderbaugh Ulrich, RN, MSN**
Nurse Educator and Consultant
Lane Community College
Eugene, Oregon

**Suzanne Weyland Canale, RN, MSN**
Nurse Educator and Consultant
Lane Community College
Eugene, Oregon

**Sharon Andrea Wendell, RN, MSN**
Nurse Educator, Consultant, and
Oncology Nurse Clinician
Lane Community College
Eugene, Oregon

**W.B. Saunders Company**
*A Division of Harcourt Brace & Company*
Philadelphia London Toronto Montreal Sydney Tokyo

**W.B. SAUNDERS COMPANY**

*A Division of*
*Harcourt, Brace & Company*

The Curtis Center
Independence Square West
Philadelphia, PA 19106

Drug therapies and medical and nursing treatments change as new information is revealed through research in the basic and clinical sciences. The authors have exerted every effort in making this book current, accurate, and consistent with accepted standards at the time it is published. The authors, editors, and publisher are not responsible for errors or omissions or for consequences arising from application of information in the book, and they make no warranty, expressed or implied, concerning the book's content. The reader should implement any practice described in this book according to professional standards of care taking into account the individual circumstances of each patient and each situation. Readers should always check product information such as package inserts for new information and changes about dosage and contraindications before administering any medication. They should be particularly cautious when using new, experimental, or infrequently prescribed drugs.

**Library of Congress Cataloging-in-Publication Data**

Ulrich, Susan Puderbaugh.
Medical-surgical nursing care planning guides / Susan Puderbaugh Ulrich, Suzanne Weyland Canale, Sharon Andrea Wendell. — 3rd ed.
p. cm.
Rev. ed. of: Nursing care planning guides / by Susan Puderbaugh Ulrich, Suzanne Weyland Canale, Sharon Andrea Wendell. 2nd ed. 1990.
Includes bibliographical references and index.
ISBN 0-7216-5198-4
1. Nursing—Planning. 2. Nursing care plans. I. Ulrich, Susan Puderbaugh. Nursing care planning guides. II. Canale, Suzanne Weyland. III. Wendell, Sharon Andrea. IV. Title.
[DNLM: 1. Nursing Care—handbooks. 2. Nursing Diagnosis——handbooks. WY 39 U45m 1994]
RT49.U47 1994
610.73—dc20
DNLM/DLC 93-32872

Medical-Surgical Nursing Care Planning Guides ISBN 0-7216-5198-4



Printed in United States of America

Last digit is the print number: 9 8 7 6 5 4 3 2

# Preface

*Medical-Surgical Nursing Care Planning Guides* is a comprehensive reference to guide the planning of holistic nursing care for hospitalized adults with commonly recurring medical-surgical conditions. It has been updated to include current nursing diagnoses and advances in nursing and medical science. The nursing care plans in this book provide a basic standard of care that must be individualized according to each client's history, current physiological and psychological status, medical orders, and specific response to treatment.

With increasing specialization by health care professionals, client care is easily fragmented, making it difficult to see the interrelationships that are the basis of high quality nursing care. These care plans integrate the various aspects of nursing care to assist the student and practitioner in seeing those interrelationships. Each care plan utilizes the nursing process, includes nursing and collaborative diagnoses, and reflects a format commonly used in health care settings and educational institutions.

There are a total of 61 standardized nursing care plans included in this book. Unit I replaces the Introduction in the second edition and has been modified to assist the student and practitioner to more effectively utilize the care plans to meet the individual client's needs. The unit includes specific guidelines for adapting the care plans and uses a case study format to demonstrate the actual selection of pertinent diagnostic labels and the individualization of etiology statements, desired outcomes, and nursing actions.

A new addition to the book (Unit II) addresses 24 of the most commonly used nursing diagnoses in the acute care setting. The primary purposes of this unit are twofold: to provide the reader with a rationale for each action and to provide guidelines for documentation that meet professional, accreditation, and legal standards. The definition of the label and a desired client outcome are also included for each diagnosis. This unit will also facilitate the planning of individualized care for the client with a medical-surgical condition that is not addressed in this text.

Unit III focuses on care of the elderly client and the biopsychosocial changes that occur with aging. The care plan is directed toward the client who is hospitalized for management of a medical-surgical condition but it can easily be used to plan care for the elderly client in a variety of health care settings. Units IV to VII include care plans that provide standardized information regarding conditions or treatment modalities. The standardized care plans in Unit IV on Preoperative and Postoperative Care should be used in conjunction with each surgical care plan in the text. The care plans on Immobility and Terminal Care (Units V and VI) are applicable to a wide range of conditions and should be utilized whenever appropriate. The care plans in Unit VII cover treatment modalities for neoplastic disorders and are referred to when appropriate in the care plans on neoplastic diseases. Each of the standardized care plans in these units can also be used in planning care for a client with a condition not covered in this text. When care plans in Units IV to VII are to be used with a care plan in Units VIII to XIX, the authors indicate this at the beginning of the plan by the phrase **Use in conjunction with** or **Refer to.**

Units VIII to XIX are divided according to body systems. Care plans within each unit deal with conditions that are frequently seen in an acute care setting. Each care plan includes a comprehensive list of appropriate nursing and collaborative diagnoses with client outcomes and actions that facilitate the achievement of each outcome. Each care plan is organized as follows:

### INTRODUCTION

The introduction provides the reader with an overview of the condition including a basic definition and discussion of the pathophysiological mechanisms involved and/or a description of the surgical procedure or selected treatment modality. This overview is not intended to be a substitute for the information provided in medical-surgical nursing texts or other references but rather a quick refresher or a starting point for additional research. Within this section the reader will also find the focus of the care plan (highlighted in bold print) and the overall goals of care.

### DIAGNOSTIC TESTS

Diagnostic tests included in this section are those commonly performed either prior to or during hospitalization to confirm the presence of a disease process or the need for the surgical procedure or treatment modality.

### DISCHARGE CRITERIA

This section includes criteria that serve as a guide for determining the client's readiness for discharge from the acute care setting. Recognizing that client education is a vital aspect of health care, the authors use these discharge criteria as the basis for the detailed teaching plans that are included at the end of each care plan.

### NURSING AND COLLABORATIVE DIAGNOSES

The nursing and collaborative diagnoses describe the actual or high-risk health problems that a client with a particular condition may experience. The nursing diagnoses were selected from those approved by the North American Nursing Diagnosis Association (NANDA) through 1992. In a few instances the authors have included nursing diagnoses that are not currently on the NANDA list. These diagnostic labels are usually noted in the text by an asterisk (*) and an explanatory footnote. Nursing diagnoses that are not unique to a particular condition but that may be relevant for a client (e.g. spiritual distress) have not consistently been included but should be considered when individualizing each care plan. Collaborative diagnoses have been included to incorporate potential complications and electrolyte imbalances for which there are no established nursing diagnostic labels. With the exception of "knowledge deficit," each nursing and collaborative diagnosis includes a specific etiological statement. An etiology for the "knowledge deficit" diagnosis was not included because of the numerous individual variables that affect the teaching-learning process. In order to provide consistency in the care plans, the nursing and collaborative diagnoses statements have usually been listed in the same order in all the care plans. No attempt has been made to prioritize the diagnoses. Priorities will need to be established by the student and practitioner based on current client assessments and needs.

## DESIRED OUTCOMES

The desired outcomes for the nursing and collaborative diagnoses provide specific, measurable criteria for evaluating client progress and identifying when goals of care have been met. These outcomes identify a favorable status that can be achieved or maintained by the implementation of the identified nursing actions. The outcome criteria for the nursing diagnoses are based on the defining characteristics approved by NANDA. Target dates for the desired outcomes have not been included since these are determined by the client's current status.

## NURSING ACTIONS AND SELECTED PURPOSES/RATIONALES

Included in this section are nursing actions that are appropriate for assisting the client to achieve the desired outcomes. The actions include detailed assessments that are based on the defining characteristics for the label as defined by NANDA. These assessments assist the user to determine if the nursing or collaborative diagnosis is an actual problem or if the client is at high risk for developing it. The nursing interventions are specific and realistic yet global enough to allow for regional and multidisciplinary variations in standards of care. The selected purposes or rationales, which appear in italics, have been included to clarify actions that may not be fundamental nursing knowledge. The actions included for the nursing diagnosis "Knowledge deficit" utilize terminology that most clients can understand.

• • •

NANDA approved nursing diagnoses are listed alphabetically on the inside front cover of this edition to facilitate individualization of the standardized care plans included in the text. The index allows the reader to easily locate specific care plans and nursing and collaborative diagnoses. It also allows the reader to utilize the text in planning care for the client with a medical or surgical condition not addressed in this edition.

Ultimately, the value of a systematic approach to individualized client care is measured by its effect on the quality of care provided to the client. The authors hope that the third edition of this book will assist with the integration of the numerous aspects of client care, facilitate critical thinking and implementation of the nursing process, and provide both the student and the practitioner with a guide for planning and implementing high-quality client care.

# Acknowledgments

To our numerous readers who shared their expertise.
To our students who are a continual source of inspiration.
To our friends for their support and encouragement.
Most importantly, to our families for their love, patience, and encouragement:

Joe and Christopher Canale
Curt, Shannon, and Chad Ulrich
Steve and Traci Wendell

**THIRD EDITION REVIEWERS**

Batterden, Roxanne Aubol, R.N., M.S., CCRN, Nurse Educator, The Johns Hopkins Hospital, Baltimore, Maryland
Bean, Cheryl A., D.S.N., R.N., C.S., OCN, School of Nursing, Indiana University, Indianapolis, Indiana
Bellarts, Stella, Ed.D., R.N., M.N., Assistant Professor of Nursing, University of Portland, Portland, Oregon
Calamaro, Christina J., M.S.N., CRNP, Children's Hospital of Philadelphia, Philadelphia, Pennsylvania
Cantley, Mary, R.N., M.S.N., Department of Nursing, Anderson University, Anderson, Indiana
Cappelli, Rosemary, M.A., School of Nursing, Trenton State College, Trenton, New Jersey
Chappell, Susan M., R.N., M.S.N., C.D.E., The University of Texas at Arlington, Arlington, Texas
Chimielewski, Chris, R.N., M.S., CNN, Hospital of the University of Pennsylvania, Philadelphia, Pennsylvania
Ciribassi, Bonnie, R.N., CCRN, MBA, Director, Critical Care, John C. Lincoln Hospital, Phoenix, Arizona
Crooks, Laura K., R.N., M.S.N., Allegheny General Hospital, Pittsburgh, Pennsylvania
David, Linda, R.N., CPAN, Yale New Haven Hospital, New Haven, Connecticut
Denman-Treinen, Angela, R.N., B.S.N., OCN, Kenneth Norris Comprehensive Cancer Center, University of Southern California, Los Angeles, California
Dickson, Gail W., R.N., C.S., Ed.D., College of Nursing, University of South Carolina, Columbia, South Carolina
Higgins, Bonnie, R.N., M.S.N., Associate Professor, Medical-Surgical Coordinator, Tarrant County Junior College, Fort Worth, Texas
Jackson, Janet E., M.S., R.N., Bradley University, Peoria, Illinois
Jacobson, Ann Fuhry, M.S., R.N., University of Texas at Arlington, Arlington, Texas
Janek, Ann Marie, M.S.N., R.N., ONC, The Medical Center, Beaver, Pennsylvania
Jones-Dickson, Charlie, Ed.D., R.N., School of Nursing, University of Alabama, Birmingham, Alabama
Leek, Connie, M.S.N., R.N., C., OCN, City of Hope National Medical Center, Duarte, California
Makrevis, Celeste S., R.N., M.S.N., CCRN, Cardiovascular Clinical Nurse Specialist, Kaiser Foundation Hospital, San Francisco, California
McDonald, Maureen, M.S., R.N., C., C.N.A., C.S., School of Nursing, Brockton Hospital, Faculty and Clinical Nurse Specialist, Medical Nursing, Boston City Hospital, Boston, Massachusetts
McLeod, Margaret Elaine, M.S.N., R.N., C.S., C.D.E., Veterans Administration Medical Center, Nashville, Tennessee
Mooney, Nancy E., M.A., R.N., ONC, New York University, New York, New York
Moye, Carol Eve, R.N., B.S.N., ONC, Orthopaedic Nurse Management Consultants, Albuquerque, New Mexico
O'Neill, Mary S., R.N., M.S.N., West Georgia College, Carrollton, Georgia
Price, Holly J., R.N., C., M.S.N., Assistant Director, School of Nursing, Providence Hospital, Sandusky, Ohio
Robinson, Adela E., R.N., M.N., CCRN, St. Joseph Medical Center, Burbank, California
Rogers, Willetta H., R.N., M.S.N., Department of Nursing Science, Lincoln University, Jefferson City, Missouri
Roush, Deborah L., R.N., M.S.N., School of Nursing, Valdosta State College, Valdosta, Georgia
Rumsey, Kimberly A., R.N., M.S.N., OCN, The University of Texas M.D. Anderson Cancer Center, Houston, Texas
Sampel, Mary E., M.S.N., R.N., Associate Professor, School of Nursing, St. Louis University, St. Louis, Missouri

Schuster, Sally E., M.S.N., R.N., Assistant Professor, Gannon University, Erie, Pennsylvania, and Hamet Medical Center, Erie, Pennsylvania

Smith, Gloria A. Hinderer, M.S., R.N., CRRN, C.S., Rush–Presbyterian–St. Luke's Medical Center, Chicago, Illinois

Taylor, Carol A., R.N., M.S.N., Assistant Professor, School of Nursing, Duquesne University, Pittsburgh, Pennsylvania

Vontz, Marilyn, R.N., B.S., M.S.N., M.A., Nurse Educator, School of Nursing, Bryan Memorial Hospital, Lincoln, Nebraska

Whitney, Stuart L., M.S., R.N., Lecturer, The University of Vermont, Burlington, Vermont

# Contents

UNIT

# I

# *Individualizing a Standardized Care Plan*

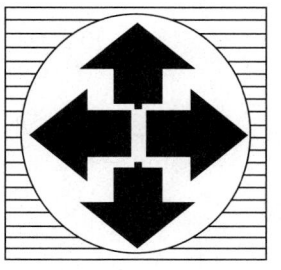

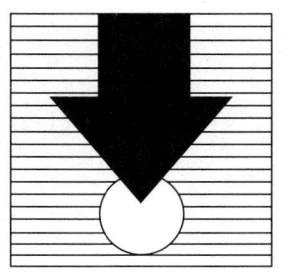

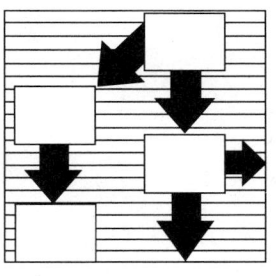

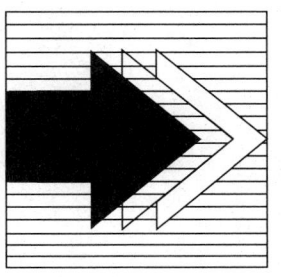

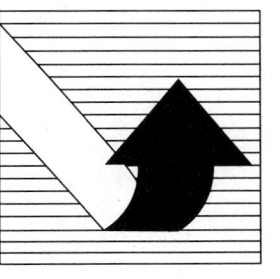

## ❖ Steps in Individualizing a Standardized Care Plan

Planning nursing care is an exciting challenge and a rewarding experience when one sees positive results because of his/her efforts. However, planning care that is individualized and comprehensive can be a tedious process because of lack of time and adequate resources. This book is intended to facilitate the process by providing nursing care plans to be used in the care of adult clients with common recurring medical-surgical conditions. Within each care plan is a list of possible diagnoses with related etiological factors, desired outcomes with measurable behavioral criteria, and a list of appropriate nursing actions with selected purposes or rationales. Safe, comprehensive care can be planned in a minimal amount of time with this book.

To be most effective, the standardized nursing care plan must be adapted to the client's individual needs. A process for planning individualized client care follows:

1. read the admission sheet and the medication administration record of the assigned client
2. review the history, current diagnostic test results, nurses' notes for the last 48 hours, physician's progress notes, and current consultations
3. interview the client and complete a physical assessment using the tool provided by your nursing school or clinical facility
4. highlight abnormal data obtained
5. read about the client's diagnosis in a current medical-surgical nursing text
6. select the appropriate standardized care plan(s) from this text
7. select the nursing and collaborative diagnoses within the plan(s) appropriate for your client; choose from among the etiological factors those that are relevant and modify them as appropriate
8. set priorities for the nursing/collaborative diagnoses using a system such as Maslow's hierarchy of needs
9. modify the desired outcomes so that they are measurable and realistic for your client; establish appropriate target dates
10. select from the list of nursing actions those that are relevant to the client's care; add to or modify the actions to meet the needs of your particular client; include medications, treatments, client preferences, and actions that will facilitate the achievement of the desired client outcomes.

The following situation is used to illustrate how these standardized nursing care plans can be used by the student and the practitioner in planning individualized client care:

> Mary G. is a 50-year-old woman who has been hospitalized in the terminal stages of cancer of the lung. She has been bedridden for the past 3 weeks because of severe bone pain due to metastatic lesions. She has four children ranging in age from 13 to 19 years. Both Mary and her husband have been trying to prepare the children for her death. They have no other family members living nearby.

**1. Read the admission sheet and the medication administration record of the assigned client.**

It is determined that Mary is a 50-year-old married woman. Her religious preference is Protestant. Her diagnosis is *stage IV cancer of the lung.* She *needs assistance with all activities of daily living* and is *receiving morphine sulfate, 15 mg q2h, for pain relief.* She is also receiving *Dialose, 1 capsule/day; Phenergan, 25 mg IM q6h prn; and milk of magnesia, 30 ml p.o. every evening.*

**2. Review the history, current diagnostic test results, nurses' notes for the last 48 hours, physician's progress notes, and current consultations.**

From the history it is determined that Mary had a *lobectomy 3 years ago* and experienced *disease recurrence 1 year ago.* She was treated with chemotherapeutic drugs until 3 months ago when she elected to stop treatment. She has *metastasis to the spine, ribs, and pelvis* and has been *bedridden for the last 3 weeks.* The progress notes indicate that Mary's *condition is steadily deteriorating* and the goal of care is to keep her comfortable.

Diagnostic test results reveal that Mary's *RBC, Hb, Hct, and serum protein levels are decreased.*

The nurses' notes reveal that Mary *needs assistance with all activities.* She is able to feed herself but is only *consuming 10% of her meals.* She *has not had a bowel movement for 6 days.* Mary is voiding adequate amounts and her intake and output are balanced. She has been *crying frequently* and *states that neither she nor her husband is ready for her death.*

3. **Interview the client and complete a physical assessment using the tool provided by your nursing school or clinical facility.**

   The interview and physical assessment reveal that Mary has *persistent reddened areas on her left hip and coccyx; diminished breath sounds in the bases; shallow respirations of 24/minute; crackles [rales] in both lungs; and a cough that is productive of yellow, foul-smelling sputum.* She has *hypoactive bowel sounds and a firm, distended abdomen* and states that she usually has a bowel movement every other day after breakfast. Mary is alert and oriented and able to move all extremities. She *complains of pain in her back, rib, and pelvic area.*

4. **Highlight abnormal data obtained.**

   Abnormal data for Mary is designated in italics in steps 1 through 3.

5. **Read about the client's diagnosis in a current medical-surgical nursing text.**

   Review cancer of the lung and care of the terminally ill client and the immobile client.

6. **Select the appropriate standardized care plan(s) from this text.**

   Based on the physician's statement that Mary has been admitted for pain control and terminal care and will have no further palliative treatment, it is determined that the appropriate care plans for Mary are Cancer of the Lung, Terminal Care, and Immobility.

7. **Select the nursing and collaborative diagnoses within the plan(s) appropriate for your client. Choose from among the etiological factors those that are relevant and modify them as appropriate.**

   It is determined that there are numerous diagnoses and etiological factors from the care plans on Cancer of the Lung, Terminal Care, and Immobility that are appropriate. Examples of some of these nursing diagnoses follow. The etiological factors have been modified to reflect Mary's situation.

   a. **Ineffective breathing pattern** related to fear and anxiety; pain; respiratory depressant effects of morphine sulfate; and impaired lung/chest wall expansion associated with recumbent positioning, weakness, and abdominal distention.
   b. **Ineffective airway clearance** related to:
      1. excessive mucus production associated with inflammation of lung tissue resulting from the disease process;
      2. stasis of secretions associated with decreased activity and weak cough effort;
      3. airway obstruction associated with presence of tumor.
   c. **Pain: back, rib, and pelvic** related to bone metastasis.
   d. **Constipation** related to:
      1. diminished defecation reflex associated with suppression of urge to defecate because of increased back and pelvic pain when attempting to use bedpan and decreased gravity filling of lower rectum resulting from horizontal positioning;
      2. decreased ability to respond to urge to defecate associated with weakened abdominal muscles and impaired physical mobility;
      3. decreased gastrointestinal motility associated with decreased activity, use of morphine sulfate, and increased sympathetic nervous system activity that occurs with anxiety and pain;
      4. decreased intake of fluids and foods high in fiber associated with anorexia.
   e. **Grieving** related to loss of control over her life and usual body processes, changes in body image, loss of significant others, and imminent death.

The process for individualization of etiologies is demonstrated below using the nursing diagnosis of **Constipation** as a prototype. Note that some or parts of the etiological statements from the standardized nursing care plan are omitted if they do not apply to this case study.

| **STANDARDIZED** | **INDIVIDUALIZED** |
|---|---|
| *(etiologies from Care Plan on Immobility)* | |
| **Constipation** related to: | **Constipation** related to: |
| a. diminished defecation reflex associated with: | a. diminished defecation reflex associated with: |
| 1. suppression of the urge to defecate because of reluctance to use bedpan | 1. suppression of the urge to defecate because of increased back and pelvic pain when attempting to use bedpan |
| 2. decreased gravity filling of lower rectum resulting from horizontal positioning | 2. decreased gravity filling of lower rectum resulting from horizontal positioning |
| b. weakened abdominal muscles associated with generalized loss of muscle tone resulting from prolonged immobility | b. weakened abdominal muscles associated with generalized loss of muscle tone resulting from prolonged immobility |
| c. decreased gastrointestinal motility associated with decreased activity and the increased sympathetic nervous system activity that occurs with anxiety. | c. decreased gastrointestinal motility associated with decreased activity and the increased sympathetic nervous system activity that occurs with anxiety and pain. |
| *(etiologies from Care Plan on Terminal Care)* | |
| a. diminished defecation reflex associated with decreased neural responses in terminal state and decreased gravity filling of lower rectum resulting from horizontal positioning | a. diminished defecation reflex associated with decreased gravity filling of lower rectum resulting from horizontal positioning |
| b. decreased ability to respond to the urge to defecate associated with weakened abdominal muscles, impaired physical mobility, and decreased level of consciousness | b. decreased ability to respond to the urge to defecate associated with weakened abdominal muscles and impaired physical mobility |
| c. decreased gastrointestinal motility associated with decreased activity, increased sympathetic nervous system activity resulting from anxiety, and use of some medications (e.g. opiates, antacids containing aluminum or calcium) | c. decreased gastrointestinal motility associated with decreased activity, use of morphine sulfate, and increased sympathetic nervous system activity resulting from anxiety and pain |
| d. decreased intake of fluid and foods high in fiber associated with anorexia, dysphagia, and difficulty feeding self | d. decreased intake of fluid and foods high in fiber associated with anorexia |
| e. decreased peristalsis and loss of bowel tone associated with long-term use of laxatives. | e. omit—not applicable. |

**8. Set priorities for the nursing/collaborative diagnoses using a system such as Maslow's hierarchy of needs.**

Because Mary is terminally ill, the top four priorities are:
1. Pain: back, rib, and pelvic
2. Grieving

3. Ineffective airway clearance
4. Constipation

**9. Modify the desired outcomes so that they are measurable and realistic for your client. Establish appropriate target dates.**

The process for individualization of a desired outcome is demonstrated below using the nursing diagnosis of **Constipation** as a prototype.

| STANDARDIZED | INDIVIDUALIZED |
|---|---|
| *(outcome from Care Plan on Immobility)* | |
| The client will not experience constipation as evidenced by:<br>a. usual frequency of bowel movements<br>b. passage of soft, formed stool<br>c. absence of headache, anorexia, abdominal distention and pain, rectal pressure, and straining at stool. | Mary will have resolution of constipation as evidenced by:<br>a. passing a soft, formed stool at least every other day<br>b. absence of headache, increased anorexia and abdominal distention, abdominal pain, rectal pressure, and straining at stool. |
| *(outcome from Care Plan on Terminal Care)* | |
| The client will maintain a bowel routine that provides optimal comfort. | Same as above. |

**10. Select from the list of nursing actions those that are relevant to the client's care. Add to or modify the actions to meet the needs of your particular client. Include medications, treatments, client preferences, and actions that will facilitate the achievement of the desired client outcomes.**

The process for individualization of nursing actions is demonstrated below using the nursing diagnosis of **Constipation** as a prototype.

| STANDARDIZED | INDIVIDUALIZED |
|---|---|
| *(actions from Care Plan on Immobility)* | |
| a. Ascertain client's usual bowel elimination habits. | a. Omit—bowel habits already known. |
| b. Assess for signs and symptoms of constipation (e.g. decrease in frequency of stools; passage of hard, formed stools; headache; anorexia; abdominal distention and pain; feeling of fullness or pressure in rectum; straining at stool). | b. Assess Mary every shift for signs and symptoms of continuing constipation (e.g. absence of bowel movement; passage of hard, formed stool; headache; increased anorexia and abdominal distention; abdominal pain; feeling of fullness or pressure in rectum; straining at stool). |
| c. Assess bowel sounds. Report a pattern of decreasing bowel sounds. | c. Assess bowel sounds. Report a pattern of decreasing bowel sounds. |
| d. Implement measures to prevent constipation: | d. Implement measures to relieve Mary's constipation: |
| 1. encourage client to defecate whenever the urge is felt | 1. encourage Mary to defecate whenever the urge is felt |
| 2. place client in high Fowler's position for bowel movements unless contraindicated; provide privacy and adequate ventilation | 2. place Mary on bedpan in high Fowler's position 30 minutes after breakfast; provide privacy |
| 3. encourage client to relax during attempts to defecate *in order to promote relaxation of* | 3. encourage relaxation during defecation attempts by turning on radio |

| STANDARDIZED | INDIVIDUALIZED* |
|---|---|
| *(actions from Care Plan on Immobility)*—**cont'd** | |
| *the pelvic floor musculature and the external anal sphincter* | |
| 4. instruct client to increase intake of foods high in fiber (e.g. nuts, bran, whole-grain breads and cereals, raw fruits and vegetables, dried fruits) unless contraindicated | 4. offer bran cereal and fresh fruit for breakfast; encourage Mary to select foods high in fiber for lunch and dinner |
| 5. instruct client to maintain a minimum fluid intake of 2500 ml/day unless contraindicated | 5. encourage Mary to increase her fluid intake; offer 200 ml of apple juice, orange juice, or water every hour while she is awake |
| 6. encourage client to drink warm liquids upon arising in the morning *in order to initiate the gastrocolic and duodenocolic reflexes and stimulate peristalsis* | 6. offer hot tea with breakfast |
| 7. encourage client to perform isometric abdominal strengthening exercises unless contraindicated | 7. omit—not applicable for terminally ill client |
| 8. increase activity as allowed | 8. omit—not applicable |
| 9. administer laxatives, stool softeners, and/or enemas if ordered. | 9. administer milk of magnesia, 30 ml p.o. each evening and Dialose, 1 capsule p.o. each morning; consult physician about increasing dose of Dialose if constipation persists. |
| e. Check for impaction if client has not had a bowel movement in 3 days, if he/she is passing liquid stool, or if other signs and symptoms of constipation are present. Administer oil retention and/or cleansing enemas as ordered followed by digital removal of stool if necessary. | e. Check for impaction since Mary has not had a bowel movement for 6 days and other signs and symptoms of constipation are present. Consult physician for an order for oil retention and/or cleansing enemas. Remove stool digitally if necessary. |

| STANDARDIZED | INDIVIDUALIZED |
|---|---|
| *(actions from Care Plan on Terminal Care)* | |
| a. Establish a routine time for defecation based on client's usual bowel elimination pattern. | a. Place Mary in high Fowler's position on bedpan 30 minutes after breakfast. |
| b. Perform actions to reduce fear and anxiety (see Nursing Diagnosis 18 [p. 176]). | b. Perform actions to reduce fear and anxiety (a few individualized actions from Nursing Diagnosis 18 in Care Plan on Terminal Care would be included here). |
| c. Assist client to toilet or bedside commode or place in high Fowler's position on bedpan for bowel movements unless contraindicated. | c. See action a. |
| d. Assist with titration of laxative agents (e.g. combination of a | d. Administer Dialose, 1 capsule p.o. each morning and milk of |

*The italicized information from the standardized action is a purpose or rationale and is omitted here. It should be placed in the rationale column of an individualized care plan.

| STANDARDIZED | INDIVIDUALIZED |
|---|---|
| *(actions from Care Plan on Terminal Care)—**cont'd*** | |
| stool softener and bulk-forming agent or lubricant with a peristaltic stimulant). | magnesia, 30 ml p.o. each evening. |
| e. If client is taking antacids containing aluminum or calcium, consult physician about alternating them with antacids containing magnesium. | e. Omit—not applicable. |

**Individualized care plan for Mary for the nursing diagnosis of Constipation:**

| DATA | NURSING DIAGNOSIS | DESIRED OUTCOME | NURSING ACTIONS |
|---|---|---|---|
| States has not had bowel movement for 6 days<br>Bowel sounds hypoactive<br>Physician's order: milk of magnesia, 30 ml each evening prn—taking every evening; Dialose, 1 capsule p.o. every morning<br>Abdomen firm and distended<br>Bedridden for 3 weeks<br>Consuming only 10% of meals<br>States usually has bowel movement q.o.d. after breakfast<br>Activity—bed rest; requires assistance with all activities<br>Receiving morphine sulfate every 2 hours | Constipation related to:<br>a. diminished defecation reflex associated with suppression of urge to defecate because of increased back and pelvic pain when attempting to use bedpan and decreased gravity filling of lower rectum resulting from horizontal positioning;<br>b. decreased ability to respond to urge to defecate associated with weakened abdominal muscles and impaired physical mobility;<br>c. decreased gastrointestinal motility associated with decreased activity, use of morphine sulfate, and increased sympathetic nervous system activity that occurs with anxiety and pain;<br>d. decreased intake of fluids and foods high in fiber associated with anorexia. | Mary will have resolution of constipation as evidenced by:<br>a. passing a soft, formed stool at least every other day<br>b. absence of headache, increased anorexia and abdominal distention, abdominal pain, rectal pressure, and straining at stool. | 1. Assess Mary every shift for signs and symptoms of continuing constipation (e.g. absence of a bowel movement; passage of hard, formed stool; headache; increased anorexia and abdominal distention; abdominal pain; feeling of fullness or pressure in rectum; straining at stool).<br>2. Assess bowel sounds. Report a pattern of decreasing bowel sounds.<br>3. Implement measures to relieve Mary's constipation:<br>a. encourage Mary to defecate whenever the urge is felt<br>b. place Mary on bedpan in high Fowler's position 30 minutes after breakfast; provide privacy<br>c. encourage relaxation during defecation attempts by turning on radio<br>d. offer bran cereal and fresh fruit for breakfast; encourage Mary to select foods high in fiber for lunch and dinner<br>e. encourage Mary to increase her |

**Individualized care plan for Mary for the nursing diagnosis of Constipation—*cont'd:***

| DATA | NURSING DIAGNOSIS | DESIRED OUTCOME | NURSING ACTIONS |
|---|---|---|---|
| | | | fluid intake; offer 200 ml of apple juice, orange juice, or water every hour while she is awake<br>f. offer hot tea with breakfast<br>g. administer milk of magnesia, 30 ml p.o. each evening and Dialose, 1 capsule p.o. each morning; consult physician about increasing dose of Dialose if constipation persists<br>h. perform actions to reduce fear and anxiety (e.g. allow family to spend time with her, control discomfort).<br>4. Check for impaction since Mary has not had a bowel movement for 6 days and other signs and symptoms of constipation are present. Consult physician for an order for an oil retention and/or cleansing enemas. Remove stool digitally if necessary. |

UNIT

# II

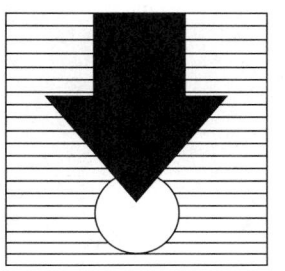

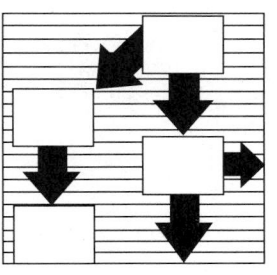

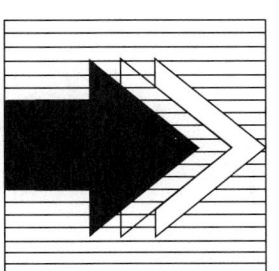

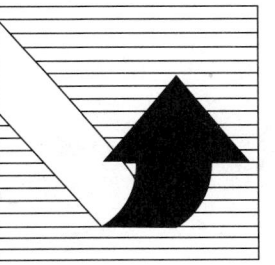

# *Actions, Rationales, and Documentation for Selected Nursing Diagnoses*

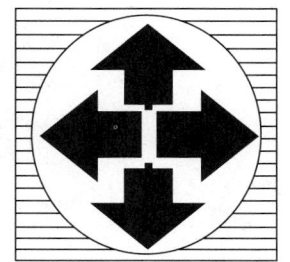

## ❖ Nursing Diagnosis: *Activity Intolerance*

### Definition

A state in which an individual has insufficient physiological or psychological energy to endure or complete required or desired daily activities.

### Desired Outcome

The client will demonstrate an increased tolerance for activity as evidenced by:
a. verbalization of feeling less fatigued and weak
b. ability to perform activities of daily living without exertional dyspnea, chest pain, diaphoresis, dizziness, and significant change in vital signs.

### Documentation

a. Activity level
b. Physiological responses to activity
c. Statements of weakness and fatigue
d. Therapeutic interventions
e. Client teaching

| NURSING ACTIONS | RATIONALES |
|---|---|
| **Assessments** | |
| 1. Assess for signs and symptoms of activity intolerance:<br>a. statements of fatigue and weakness<br>b. exertional dyspnea, chest pain, diaphoresis, or dizziness<br>c. abnormal heart rate response to activity (e.g. increase in rate of 20 beats/minute above resting rate, decrease in rate, rate not returning to preactivity level within 3 minutes after stopping activity, change from regular to irregular rate)<br>d. decreased systolic B/P or a significant increase (10-15 mm Hg) in systolic or diastolic pressure with activity. | 1. Early recognition of signs and symptoms of activity intolerance allows for prompt intervention. |
| **Prevention/Treatment** | |
| 2. Implement measures to promote rest and/or conserve energy (e.g. maintain prescribed activity restrictions, minimize environmental activity and noise, provide uninterrupted rest periods, assist with care, limit the number of visitors). | 2. Rest and activities that conserve energy result in a lower metabolic rate and subsequent reduction in the rate of oxygen utilization. This results in more available oxygen and improved activity tolerance. |
| 3. Implement measures to increase cardiac output (e.g. administer positive inotropic agents as ordered, elevate head of bed, discourage smoking) if decreased cardiac output is contributing to client's activity intolerance. | 3. Sufficient cardiac output is necessary to maintain adequate tissue perfusion and oxygenation, which are both essential for normal activity tolerance. |

| NURSING ACTIONS | RATIONALES |
|---|---|
| **Prevention/Treatment—*cont'd*** | |
| 4. Implement measures to reduce fever if present (e.g. administer tepid sponge bath, administer antipyretics as ordered). | 4. An elevated temperature increases the metabolic rate with subsequent depletion of available energy and a decrease in ability to tolerate activity. |
| 5. Discourage smoking and excessive intake of beverages high in caffeine such as coffee, tea, and colas. | 5. Both nicotine and excessive caffeine intake increase cardiac workload and myocardial oxygen utilization, thereby decreasing the amount of oxygen available for energy production. |
| 6. Maintain oxygen therapy as ordered. | 6. An oxygen deficiency results in anaerobic metabolism, which is less efficient than the aerobic mechanism of energy supply. Supplemental oxygen helps restore the more efficient aerobic metabolism, thereby improving energy levels and activity tolerance. |
| 7. Implement measures to improve respiratory status (e.g. encourage use of incentive spirometer; elevate head of bed; assist with turning, coughing, and deep breathing) if ineffective breathing pattern, airway clearance, or gas exchange is contributing to client's activity intolerance. | 7. Altered respiratory function can lead to inadequate gas exchange and tissue oxygenation, which results in decreased activity tolerance. |
| 8. Implement measures to maintain an adequate nutritional status (e.g. provide a diet high in essential nutrients, provide dietary supplements as indicated). | 8. Adequate nutrition is essential for normal metabolism (the process by which nutrients are transformed into energy). |
| 9. Administer vitamins and minerals as ordered. | 9. Vitamins serve as catalysts in energy production and many minerals are essential for normal metabolism. |
| 10. Implement measures to treat anemia if present (e.g. administer prescribed iron, folic acid, and/or vitamin $B_{12}$; administer whole blood or packed red cells as ordered). | 10. Anemia reduces the oxygen-carrying capacity of RBCs. Resolution of anemia increases oxygen availability to the cells with subsequent increased energy production and improved activity tolerance. |
| 11. Increase client's activity gradually as allowed and tolerated. | 11. A gradual increase in activity helps prevent a sudden increase in cardiac workload and myocardial oxygen consumption and the subsequent imbalance between oxygen supply and demand. |
| 12. Instruct client to report a decreased tolerance for activity and to stop any activity that causes chest pain, shortness of breath, dizziness, or extreme fatigue or weakness. | 12. These symptoms indicate that activity has been increased beyond a therapeutic level. Stopping activity when this occurs helps prevent excessive demands on the heart. |

| NURSING ACTIONS | RATIONALES |
|---|---|
| **Prevention/Treatment—*cont'd*** | |
| 13. Consult physician if signs and symptoms of activity intolerance persist or worsen. | 13. Notifying the physician allows for modification of treatment plan. |

## ❖ Nursing Diagnosis: *Airway Clearance, Ineffective*

### Definition

A state in which an individual is unable to clear secretions or obstructions from the respiratory tract to maintain airway patency.

### Desired Outcome

The client will maintain clear, open airways as evidenced by:
a. normal breath sounds
b. normal rate and depth of respirations
c. absence of dyspnea
d. absence of cyanosis.

### Documentation

a. Breath sounds
b. Rate, depth, and ease of respirations
c. Presence of cyanosis
d. Effectiveness of cough efforts
e. Description of sputum
f. Therapeutic interventions
g. Client teaching

| NURSING ACTIONS | RATIONALES |
|---|---|
| **Assessments** | |
| 1. Assess for and report signs and symptoms of ineffective airway clearance (e.g. abnormal breath sounds; rapid, shallow respirations; dyspnea; cyanosis). | 1. Early recognition and reporting of signs and symptoms of ineffective airway clearance allow for prompt intervention. |
| **Prevention/Treatment** | |
| 2. Implement measures to decrease pain if present (e.g. splint chest or abdominal incision with pillow when coughing and deep breathing, administer prescribed analgesics 30 minutes before planned activity). | 2. Pain often interferes with a client's willingness to move, cough, and deep breathe. Pain reduction enables the client to increase activity and cough and deep breathe more effectively. |
| 3. Instruct and assist client to turn, deep breathe, and cough or "huff" every 1-2 hours. | 3. Turning mobilizes secretions. Deep breathing dilates the airways, loosens secretions, and stimulates coughing. Coughing or "huffing" (a forced exhalation technique) mobilizes secretions and facilitates their removal from the respiratory tract. |
| 4. Increase activity as allowed and tolerated. | 4. Activity mobilizes secretions and stimulates deep breathing, which dilates the airways, loosens secretions, and stimulates coughing. |
| 5. Implement measures to liquefy tenacious secretions (e.g. maintain fluid intake of 2500 ml/day, humidify inspired air). | 5. Liquefying tenacious secretions facilitates mobilization and expectoration of secretions. |

| NURSING ACTIONS | RATIONALES |
|---|---|
| **Prevention/Treatment—*cont'd*** | |
| 6. Assist with administration of diluent and mucolytic agents via nebulizer or IPPB treatment as ordered. | 6. Diluents and mucolytics are mucokinetic agents that thin hyperviscous secretions. Thinner secretions are easier to mobilize and remove from the respiratory tract. |
| 7. Assist with or perform postural drainage, percussion, and vibration if ordered. | 7. Postural drainage, percussion, and vibration are chest physiotherapy techniques that facilitate mobilization and removal of pulmonary secretions. Percussion and vibration loosen secretions and postural drainage promotes their removal by gravity flow. |
| 8. Perform suctioning if needed. | 8. Suctioning removes mucus from the respiratory tract. It also stimulates coughing, which helps mobilize secretions and clear airways. |
| 9. Administer expectorants if ordered. | 9. Expectorants stimulate the production of mucus, which ultimately decreases the viscosity of secretions and facilitates their mobilization and removal from the respiratory tract. |
| 10. Discourage smoking. | 10. Smoke causes bronchoconstriction, increases mucus production, and impairs ciliary function. This results in narrowed airways and stasis of pulmonary secretions. |
| 11. Protect client from exposure to irritants such as smoke, flowers, and perfume. | 11. Smoke, flowers, and/or perfume may act as respiratory irritants. The bronchospasm and increased mucus production that can occur narrow the airways and result in less effective airway clearance. |
| 12. Reinforce correct use of incentive spirometer and assist with IPPB treatments if ordered. | 12. Incentive spirometer use and IPPB treatments enhance airway clearance by promoting bronchodilation, loosening secretions, and stimulating a cough. |
| 13. Administer the following medications if ordered:<br>a. methylxanthines (e.g. theophylline)<br>b. sympathomimetics (e.g. epinephrine, isoetharine)<br>c. corticosteroids (e.g. methylprednisolone, prednisone). | 13. These medications improve bronchial airflow and promote more effective airway clearance. Methylxanthines and sympathomimetics increase cAMP, which promotes bronchodilation. Corticosteroids reduce airway inflammation and decrease bronchial hyperreactivity. |
| 14. Administer central nervous system depressants judiciously. | 14. Central nervous system depressants can depress the cough reflex, which results in stasis of secretions. |

**NURSING ACTIONS** / **RATIONALES**

**Prevention/Treatment—*cont'd***

15. Consult physician if signs and symptoms of ineffective airway clearance persist or signs and symptoms of impaired gas exchange (e.g. restlessness, irritability, confusion, decreased $Pa_{O_2}$ and increased $Pa_{CO_2}$ levels) are present.

    *Rationale:* 15. Notifying the physician allows for modification of the treatment plan.

## ❖ Nursing Diagnosis: *Anxiety*

### Definition

A vague, uneasy feeling whose source is often nonspecific or unknown to the individual.

### Desired Outcome

The client will experience a reduction in anxiety as evidenced by:

a. verbalization of feeling less anxious
b. usual sleep pattern
c. relaxed facial expression and body movements
d. stable vital signs
e. usual perceptual ability and interactions with others.

### Documentation

a. Signs and symptoms of anxiety
b. Client's perception of precipitating factors
c. Therapeutic interventions
d. Effectiveness of interventions
e. Client/family teaching

**NURSING ACTIONS** / **RATIONALES**

**Assessments**

1. Assess client for signs and symptoms of anxiety (e.g. verbalization of concerns, insomnia, tenseness, tremors, irritability, restlessness, diaphoresis, tachypnea, tachycardia, elevated B/P, facial pallor or flushing, narrowed perceptual field, withdrawal, noncompliance with treatment plan).

    *Rationale:* 1. Early recognition of signs and symptoms of anxiety allows for prompt intervention. Be aware that each level of anxiety (mild, moderate, severe, panic) requires specific kinds of nursing intervention.

**Prevention/Treatment**

2. Encourage verbalization of feelings and concerns and provide feedback.

    *Rationale:* 2. Verbalization of feelings and concerns helps the client focus on factors that may be causing anxiety. Providing feedback helps the client clarify and validate his/her feelings and concerns and identify techniques that can reduce anxiety.

3. Assist client to identify specific stressors and ways to cope with them.

    *Rationale:* 3. Identification of specific stressors is necessary so that coping strategies can be identified and implemented before anxiety escalates.

4. Orient client to hospital environment, equipment, and routines.

    *Rationale:* 4. Familiarity with the environment and usual routines reduces the client's

| NURSING ACTIONS<br>Prevention/Treatment—*cont'd* | RATIONALES |
|---|---|
| | anxiety about the unknown, provides a sense of security, and increases his/her sense of control, which all help to decrease anxiety. |
| 5. Introduce staff who will be participating in the client's care. If possible, maintain consistency in staff assigned to his/her care. | 5. Introduction of the staff familiarizes the client with those people who will be working with him/her, which provides a sense of comfort with the environment. Consistency in staff assignment provides the client with a feeling of stability, which reduces the anxiety that typically occurs with change. |
| 6. Assure client that staff members are nearby. Respond to call signal as soon as possible. | 6. Close contact and a prompt response to requests provides a sense of security and facilitates the development of trust, which help to reduce feelings of anxiety. |
| 7. Maintain a calm, supportive, confident manner when interacting with client. | 7. A sense of calmness and confidence conveys to the client that someone is in control of the situation, which helps to reduce feelings of anxiety. |
| 8. Reinforce physician's explanations and clarify misconceptions the client has about the diagnostic tests, disease condition, treatment plan, surgical procedure, and/or prognosis. | 8. Factual information and an awareness of what to expect help to decrease the anxiety that arises from uncertainty. |
| 9. Implement measures to reduce respiratory distress if present (e.g. elevate head of bed, encourage client to breathe deeply and more slowly, administer oxygen as ordered). | 9. Respiratory distress is often a manifestation of anxiety; it also may induce anxiety. Improvement of respiratory status facilitates relaxation, which inhibits the escalation of anxiety. |
| 10. Implement measures to reduce pain if present (e.g. administer prescribed analgesics, instruct and assist with relaxation techniques). | 10. Pain creates anxiety for most clients because it is perceived as a threat to his/her well-being. Pain also causes sympathetic nervous system stimulation with subsequent feelings of tenseness and increased anxiety. |
| 11. Provide a calm, restful environment. | 11. A calm, restful environment allows the client to relax and promotes increased feelings of security, which reduce anxiety. |
| 12. Instruct client in relaxation techniques and encourage participation in diversional activities. | 12. Relaxation techniques reduce muscle tension and other physiological effects of anxiety. Activities that the client enjoys provide a means of distraction, which may minimize feelings of anxiety. |

| NURSING ACTIONS | RATIONALES |
|---|---|
| **Prevention/Treatment—*cont'd*** | |
| 13. Arrange for a visit from clergy if client desires. | 13. Religion is a source of comfort and security for many people. Interaction with clergy can help reduce client's feeling of anxiety. |
| 14. Initiate a financial and/or social service referral if indicated. | 14. Concerns about financial matters can be a source of great anxiety. Assistance with resolution of these concerns helps to allay anxiety. |
| 15. Encourage significant others to project a caring, concerned attitude without obvious anxiousness. | 15. Anxiety is easily transferable from one person to another. If significant others project a caring, concerned attitude without obvious anxiousness, they convey empathy and a sense of reassurance and security, which help reduce the client's anxiety. |
| 16. Administer antianxiety agents if ordered. | 16. Benzodiazepines, the drugs of choice to treat anxiety, are thought to affect the limbic system by augmenting gamma-aminobutyric acid (GABA) activity. |
| 17. Include significant others in orientation and teaching sessions and encourage their continued support of the client. | 17. Significant others can reinforce information given if anxiety has reduced the client's ability to concentrate on, recall, and learn information. In addition, the presence of significant others provides the client with a sense of support, which helps reduce anxiety. |
| 18. Provide information based on current needs of client and significant others at a level they can understand. Encourage questions and clarification of information provided. | 18. Providing the client and significant others with information they are not ready to process or unable to understand tends to increase anxiety. Being able to ask questions and clarify information helps reduce anxiety that arises from uncertainty and not clearly understanding information presented. |
| 19. Consult physician if above actions fail to control anxiety. | 19. Notifying the physician allows for modification of the treatment plan. |

## ❖ Nursing Diagnosis: *Aspiration, High Risk for*

### Definition

The state in which an individual is at risk for entry of gastrointestinal secretions, oropharyngeal secretions, or solids or fluids into tracheobronchial passages.

### Desired Outcome

The client will not aspirate secretions or foods/fluids as evidenced by:
a. clear breath sounds
b. resonant percussion note over lungs
c. absence of cough, tachypnea, and dyspnea.

### Documentation

a. Breath sounds
b. Percussion note over lungs
c. Respiratory rate and effort
d. Presence of cough
e. Pulse rate
f. Color of tracheal aspirate
g. Therapeutic interventions
h. Client teaching

### NURSING ACTIONS / RATIONALES

#### Assessments

1. Assess for and report signs and symptoms of aspiration of secretions or foods/fluids (e.g. rhonchi, dull percussion note over affected lung area, cough, tachypnea, dyspnea, tachycardia, presence of tube feeding in tracheal aspirate).

   *Rationale:* 1. Early recognition and reporting of signs and symptoms of aspiration allow for prompt intervention.

2. If client is receiving tube feedings, add food coloring to the solution.

   *Rationale:* 2. The addition of food coloring helps differentiate the tube feeding solution from respiratory secretions, which allows for early recognition of aspiration and prompt intervention.

3. Assist with studies that show if aspiration is occurring during swallowing (e.g. videofluoroscopy) if ordered.

   *Rationale:* 3. Aspiration of food/fluid during the swallowing process is evident on studies such as videofluoroscopy. Knowing when aspiration occurs during the swallowing process aids in the development of an individualized plan of care to prevent further aspiration.

4. Monitor chest x-ray results. Report findings of pulmonary infiltrate.

   *Rationale:* 4. Evidence of pulmonary infiltrate on chest x-ray results can indicate that aspiration has occurred.

#### Prevention

5. Implement the following measures to prevent aspiration if client has a depressed or absent gag reflex, severe dysphagia, and/or is not alert:

   *Rationale:* 5. The risk for aspiration of oral secretions and foods/fluids is high when mechanisms to protect the client's airway (e.g. gag reflex, swallowing reflex) are impaired or he/she has structural or neurological impairments that allow oral secretions and foods/fluids to pass from the pharynx to the larynx rather than from the pharynx through the esophagus.

| NURSING ACTIONS | RATIONALES |
|---|---|
| **Prevention—*cont'd*** | |
| a. withhold oral foods/fluids | a. Withholding oral foods/fluids eliminates the possibility of aspiration of same. |
| b. place client in a side-lying position | b. Placing the client in a side-lying position allows oral secretions to accumulate in the mouth (where they can be expectorated or removed by suctioning) rather than flow into the pharynx, where they can be aspirated. |
| c. perform oral hygiene and/or oropharyngeal suctioning as often as needed to remove excess secretions. | c. Removing excess secretions and debris from the mouth and pharynx prevents them from entering the larynx and being aspirated. |
| 6. Implement measures to prevent vomiting (e.g. eliminate noxious sights and odors, administer antiemetics as ordered). | 6. When client vomits, the gastric contents travel up the esophagus, through the pharynx, and into the mouth. While vomitus is in the pharynx, it is possible for it to flow through the larynx into the lungs. |
| 7. If client is receiving tube feedings, check tube placement before each feeding or on a routine basis if tube feeding is continuous. | 7. Verification of feeding tube placement ensures that the liquid feeding goes into the alimentary tract rather than into the lungs. |
| 8. Implement measures to prevent the accumulation of gastric secretions and foods/fluids in the stomach and thereby reduce the risk of regurgitation (e.g. maintain gastric decompression as ordered, provide small meals rather than large ones, do not administer gastric tube feedings if the residual exceeds specified amount [usually 75-100 ml], maintain client in high Fowler's position for at least 30 minutes after meals and tube feedings, administer upper gastrointestinal stimulants as ordered). | 8. As gastric secretions or foods/fluids accumulate in the stomach, upward pressure is placed on the esophageal sphincters. If the pressure increases significantly and/or the client has incompetent esophageal sphincters, regurgitation can occur. Contents that move up through the esophagus into the pharynx can spill into the larynx, resulting in aspiration. |
| 9. Implement measures to prevent aspiration when client is eating and drinking: | 9. When the client is eating and drinking, he/she is at high risk for aspiration before the swallowing reflex is triggered (the larynx and pharynx are at rest and the airway is open at this time), during swallowing if the larynx does not close completely as the bolus of food/fluid passes from the back of the mouth through the pharynx, and after swallowing when the larynx opens again. |

| NURSING ACTIONS<br>**Prevention—*cont'd*** | RATIONALES |
|---|---|
| a. perform actions to improve swallowing if indicated (e.g. select foods/fluids appropriate to client's swallowing ability, reinforce exercises to strengthen and develop muscles used in swallowing) | a. Improving the client's ability to swallow helps ensure that foods/fluids do not enter the larynx when he/she is eating and drinking. |
| b. place client in high Fowler's position | b. This position uses gravity to facilitate movement of the bolus of food/fluid through the pharynx into the esophagus. Once the bolus reaches the esophagus, the risk for aspiration is greatly reduced. |
| c. if the client has a delayed swallowing reflex, instruct him/her to tilt head forward when eating and drinking (devices such as a nose-cup [cup with half circle cut out of side held uppermost] help the client maintain this position while drinking) | c. Tilting the head forward widens the valleculae (wedge-shaped spaces formed between the base of the tongue and the epiglottis). This position increases the chance that the bolus will rest in the valleculae while the swallowing reflex is being triggered rather than having it fall into the larynx. |
| d. instruct client to avoid laughing or talking when swallowing | d. Normally, when the swallowing reflex is triggered, the folds of the larynx that form its three valves (the epiglottis and epiglottic folds, the false vocal folds, and the true vocal folds) contract so that aspiration does not occur as the bolus of food/fluid passes from the back of the mouth through the pharynx. When the client talks and laughs, air is forced through the trachea and the larynx opens. Instructing the client to avoid talking and laughing when swallowing reduces the risk of having his/her airway open when the bolus is in the pharynx. |
| e. encourage client to concentrate on eating and drinking and allow ample time for meals and snacks | e. If the client becomes distracted when eating or drinking and/or eats or drinks too quickly, swallowing and breathing attempts can become uncoordinated. This results in the larynx being open when the food/fluid is in the pharynx, which greatly increases the risk for aspiration. |

**NURSING ACTIONS**

**Prevention—*cont'd***

f. instruct client to cough twice or clear his/her throat after swallowing if indicated.

**RATIONALES**

f. If the client has a swallowing impairment such as decreased pharyngeal peristalsis, residual material can remain in the pharyngeal recesses after the swallowing reflex has occurred. Coughing or clearing his/her throat after swallowing helps propel the residual matter upward, where it can be expectorated or used to trigger another swallowing reflex, rather than having it remain in the pharynx, where it could spill over into the larynx and be aspirated.

10. Instruct and assist client to perform oral hygiene after meals.

10. If the client has impaired tongue movement, he/she is often unable to sweep the mouth effectively to remove food particles that remain after eating. Performing oral hygiene after meals removes these particles so that they do not fall into the pharynx, where they can enter the larynx and be aspirated.

## ❖ Nursing Diagnosis: *Breathing Pattern, Ineffective*

### Definition

The state in which an individual's inhalation and/or exhalation pattern does not enable adequate pulmonary inflation or emptying.

### Desired Outcome

The client will maintain an effective breathing pattern as evidenced by:
a. normal rate and depth of respirations
b. absence of dyspnea
c. blood gases within normal range.

### Documentation

a. Rate and depth of respirations
b. Use of accessory muscles for breathing
c. Oximetry results
d. Therapeutic interventions
e. Client teaching

**NURSING ACTIONS**

**Assessments**

1. Assess for signs and symptoms of an ineffective breathing pattern (e.g. shallow respirations, tachypnea, dyspnea, use of accessory muscles when breathing).
2. Monitor for and report abnormal blood gases.

**RATIONALES**

1. Early recognition of signs and symptoms of an ineffective breathing pattern allows for prompt intervention.
2. Blood gases measure $PaO_2$, $PaCO_2$, $SaO_2$, and pH. They provide information about ventilatory function and are an

| NURSING ACTIONS | RATIONALES |
| --- | --- |
| **Assessments—*cont'd*** | |
| | important indicator of the effectiveness of the client's breathing pattern. |
| 3. Monitor for and report significant changes in oximetry results. | 3. Oximetry is a noninvasive method of measuring $SaO_2$. The results provide a guide for evaluating respiratory status and the effectiveness of treatment. |
| **Prevention/Treatment** | |
| 4. Implement measures to reduce chest or upper abdominal pain if present (e.g. splint incision with pillow during coughing and deep breathing, administer prescribed analgesics 30 minutes before planned activity). | 4. A client with chest or upper abdominal pain often guards respiratory efforts and breathes shallowly in an attempt to prevent additional discomfort. Pain reduction enables the client to breathe more deeply. |
| 5. If client has abdominal pain or an abdominal incision, instruct him/her to bend knees while coughing and deep breathing. | 5. With knees bent, tension on the abdominal muscles is reduced and the abdominal discomfort that occurs with coughing and deep breathing is lessened. |
| 6. Implement measures to decrease fear and anxiety (e.g. assure client that breathing deeply will not dislodge tubes or cause incision to break open, interact with client in a confident manner). | 6. Fear and anxiety may cause a client to breathe shallowly or hyperventilate. Fear and anxiety also stimulate the sympathetic nervous system, which results in an increased demand for oxygen with compensatory hyperventilation. |
| 7. Implement measures to increase strength and activity tolerance if client is weak and fatigued (e.g. provide uninterrupted rest periods, maintain optimal nutrition). | 7. An increase in strength and activity tolerance enables the client to breathe more deeply and participate in activities to improve breathing pattern. |
| 8. Place client in a semi- to high Fowler's position unless contraindicated. Position with pillows to prevent slumping. | 8. A semi- to high Fowler's position allows for maximum diaphragmatic excursion and lung expansion. Maintenance of proper body alignment and prevention of slumping are essential because slumping causes the abdominal contents to be pushed up against the diaphragm and restrict lung expansion. |
| 9. Assist client to turn from side to side at least every 2 hours while in bed. | 9. Compression of the thorax and subsequent limited chest wall and lung expansion occur when the client lies in one position. Turning from side to side allows for increased expansion of the uppermost lung. |
| 10. Instruct client to deep breathe or use incentive spirometer at least every 2 hours. | 10. Deep breathing and use of an incentive spirometer promote maximum inhalation and lung expansion. |

| NURSING ACTIONS | RATIONALES |
|---|---|
| **Prevention/Treatment—*cont'd*** | |
| 11. Assist with IPPB treatments as ordered. | 11. IPPB treatments deliver air or oxygen into the lungs at a positive pressure, thereby enhancing maximum lung inflation. |
| 12. Instruct client in and assist with diaphragmatic (abdominal) and pursed-lip breathing techniques if appropriate. NOTE: Diaphragmatic breathing is most often indicated for clients who have had thoracic surgery or clients who have chronic obstructive pulmonary disease (COPD) or certain neuromuscular conditions that may cause fixation or weakening of the diaphragm. Pursed-lip breathing is encouraged primarily for clients with COPD. | 12. Diaphragmatic breathing is performed to strengthen the diaphragm and the abdominal muscles that help move the diaphragm. This helps the client breathe more efficiently and regain optimal lung function. Pursed-lip breathing prolongs exhalation and promotes greater alveolar emptying. |
| 13. Instruct client to breathe slowly if he/she is hyperventilating. | 13. Hyperventilation is an ineffective breathing pattern that can eventually lead to respiratory alkalosis. The client can often slow breathing rate if he/she concentrates on doing so. |
| 14. Instruct clients at risk for abdominal distention to avoid intake of large meals, carbonated beverages, and gas-forming foods (e.g. beans, cauliflower, cabbage, onions). | 14. The accumulation of large amounts of food and gas in the gastrointestinal tract causes gastric distention, which may put pressure on the diaphragm and thereby impair lung expansion. |
| 15. Instruct client in and assist with apical and/or basal expansion exercises if appropriate (may be indicated for clients with painful respiratory conditions or clients who have had thoracic or abdominal surgery). | 15. Apical and basal exercises improve expansion of apical and/or basal areas of the lung by having the client focus on selectively expanding these areas of the chest. |
| 16. Increase activity as allowed and tolerated. | 16. During activity, especially ambulation, the client takes deeper breaths, thus increasing lung expansion. |
| 17. Administer central nervous system depressants judiciously. Hold medication and consult physician if respiratory rate is less than 12/minute. | 17. Central nervous system depressants can cause depression of the respiratory center in the brainstem, which results in a reduction of all phases of respiratory activity (rate, minute volume, and tidal exchange). |
| 18. Consult physician if ineffective breathing pattern continues or signs and symptoms of impaired gas exchange (e.g. restlessness, irritability, confusion, decreased $PaO_2$ and increased $PaCO_2$ levels) are present. | 18. Notifying the physician allows for modification of treatment plan. |

## ❖ Nursing Diagnosis: *Cardiac Output, Decreased*

### Definition

A state in which the blood pumped by an individual's heart is sufficiently reduced that it is inadequate to meet the needs of the body's tissues.

#### Desired Outcome

The client will maintain adequate cardiac output as evidenced by:
a. B/P within normal range for client
b. apical pulse regular and between 60-100 beats/minute
c. absence of gallop rhythms
d. absence of fatigue and weakness
e. unlabored respirations at 14-20/minute
f. normal breath sounds
g. usual mental status
h. absence of vertigo and syncope
i. palpable peripheral pulses
j. skin warm, dry, and usual color
k. capillary refill time less than 3 seconds
l. balanced intake and output
m. absence of peripheral edema and jugular vein distention
n. hemodynamic measurements such as cardiac output (CO), pulmonary artery pressure (PAP), pulmonary capillary wedge pressure (PCWP), and central venous pressure (CVP) within normal range.

#### Documentation

a. Vital signs
b. Heart sounds
c. Activity tolerance
d. Breath sounds
e. Ease of respirations
f. Mental status
g. Peripheral pulses
h. Capillary refill time
i. Skin color and temperature
j. Intake and output
k. Presence of edema
l. Presence of jugular vein distention
m. Hemodynamic measurements
n. Therapeutic interventions
o. Client teaching

#### NURSING ACTIONS

#### Assessments

1. Assess for and report signs and symptoms of decreased cardiac output:
   a. variations in B/P (may be increased because of compensatory vasoconstriction; may be decreased when compensatory mechanisms and pump fail)
   b. arrhythmias
   c. presence of gallop rhythm
   d. fatigue and weakness
   e. dyspnea, tachypnea
   f. crackles (rales)
   g. restlessness, change in mental status
   h. vertigo, syncope
   i. diminished or absent peripheral pulses
   j. cool, clammy skin
   k. pallor, mottling, or cyanosis of skin
   l. capillary refill time greater than 3 seconds

#### RATIONALES

1. Early recognition and reporting of signs and symptoms of decreased cardiac output allow for prompt intervention.

| NURSING ACTIONS | RATIONALES |
|---|---|
| **Assessments—*cont'd*** | |
| m. oliguria<br>n. peripheral edema<br>o. jugular vein distention (JVD)<br>p. hemodynamic changes such as decreased CO and increased PAP, PCWP, and CVP (use internal jugular vein pulsation method to estimate CVP if monitoring device not present). | |
| 2. Monitor ECG readings and report significant abnormalities. | 2. ECG readings provide data regarding functioning of the heart's electrical conduction system. Altered conduction can cause arrhythmias, which decrease cardiac output. |
| 3. Monitor chest x-ray results. Report findings of cardiomegaly, pleural effusion, or pulmonary edema. | 3. Chest x-ray films provide data regarding size of the heart and fluid accumulation in the pleural space, pulmonary interstitium, and alveoli. The presence of cardiomegaly, pleural effusion, and/or pulmonary edema can contribute to or be caused by decreased cardiac output. |
| **Prevention/Treatment** | |
| 4. Implement measures to reduce cardiac workload: | 4. The work of the heart is determined by the amount of blood pumped (preload) and the pressure the ventricle pumps against (afterload). Reduction of cardiac workload reduces the work that the compromised heart must perform in order to pump an adequate amount of blood. This results in increased cardiac output. |
| a. place client in a semi- to high Fowler's position | a. Elevation of client's upper body reduces cardiac workload by:<br>1. decreasing venous return from the periphery and subsequently reducing preload<br>2. reducing venous pooling in the lungs and subsequently lowering pulmonary vascular congestion and resistance<br>3. lowering the diaphragm, which enhances ventilation, thereby increasing oxygen availability. |
| b. instruct client to avoid activities that create a Valsalva response (e.g. straining to have a bowel movement, holding breath while moving) | b. When a Valsalva maneuver is performed, cardiac output falls as intrathoracic pressure rises and venous return declines. When the client exhales, venous return suddenly increases as |

| NURSING ACTIONS<br>**Prevention/Treatment—*cont'd*** | RATIONALES |
|---|---|
| | intrathoracic pressure falls. This results in a marked increase in cardiac workload. |
| c. perform actions to promote physical and emotional rest (e.g. maintain a calm, quiet environment; limit the number of visitors; maintain activity restrictions) | c. Physical rest reduces cardiac workload by lowering the body's oxygen requirements. Reducing stress and promoting emotional rest prevent unnecessary sympathetic nervous system stimulation and the subsequent increase in heart rate and blood pressure. |
| d. perform actions to promote adequate tissue oxygenation (e.g. maintain oxygen therapy as ordered, encourage deep breathing exercises and use of incentive spirometer) | d. When tissue oxygenation is adequate, the heart does not need to work as hard to supply oxygen to the tissues and more oxygen is available for myocardial use. |
| e. discourage smoking | e. Nicotine stimulates catecholamine output, which increases heart rate and causes vasoconstriction and subsequently increases cardiac workload. Smoking also reduces oxygen availability because hemoglobin has a greater affinity for the carbon monoxide in smoke than for oxygen. This increases cardiac workload as the heart tries to compensate for the reduced oxygen levels. |
| f. discourage excessive intake of beverages high in caffeine such as coffee, tea, and colas | f. Excessive caffeine can increase cardiac workload by increasing the force of myocardial contractions and heart rate. |
| g. perform actions to prevent or treat fluid volume excess (e.g. maintain prescribed fluid and dietary sodium restrictions, administer diuretics as ordered) | g. Fluid volume excess increases cardiac workload by increasing vascular volume, which increases preload and afterload. |
| h. increase activity gradually as allowed and tolerated. | h. A gradual increase in activity prevents a sudden increase in cardiac workload. Activity also strengthens the myocardium. |
| 5. Administer the following medications if ordered: | |
| a. positive inotropic agents (e.g. digitalis preparations, dobutamine, dopamine, amrinone) | 5. a. Positive inotropic agents increase cardiac output by improving myocardial contractility. |
| b. nitrates (e.g. nitroglycerin) | b. Nitrates cause generalized vasodilation with the greatest effect being on venous resistance. This decreases preload and, to a certain |

| NURSING ACTIONS<br>**Prevention/Treatment—*cont'd*** | RATIONALES |
|---|---|
| | extent, afterload, thereby reducing cardiac workload. |
| c. balanced vasodilators (e.g. nitroprusside) | c. Balanced vasodilators have arteriolar and venous dilating effects. This results in decreased afterload and preload and an overall reduction in cardiac workload. |
| d. arterial vasodilators (e.g. hydralazine, minoxidil) | d. Arterial vasodilators reduce cardiac workload by decreasing afterload. |
| e. alpha-adrenergic inhibitors (e.g. prazosin, terazosin) | e. Alpha-adrenergic inhibitors reduce cardiac workload by decreasing total peripheral vascular resistance, thereby decreasing preload and afterload. |
| f. angiotensin-converting enzyme (ACE) inhibitors (e.g. captopril, enalapril, lisinopril) | f. ACE inhibitors block the formation of angiotensin II, which results in a decrease in total peripheral vascular resistance and decreased aldosterone output. These effects reduce cardiac workload by decreasing preload, afterload, and sodium and water retention. |
| g. beta-adrenergic blocking agents (e.g. propranolol, acebutolol, metoprolol, timolol, atenolol, nadolol, pindolol) | g. Beta-adrenergic blockers reduce cardiac workload by competing with beta-adrenergic agonists for available receptor sites, thus blocking sympathetic stimulation of the heart. |
| h. anticholinergic agents (e.g. atropine) and sympathomimetics (e.g. isoproteronol) | h. Anticholinergic and sympathomimetic agents have positive chronotropic effects and increase cardiac output by increasing heart rate. |
| i. antiarrhythmics (e.g. quinidine, flecainide, lidocaine, disopyramide, procainamide, amiodarone) | i. Antiarrhythmics improve cardiac output by correcting conduction abnormalities. By improving conduction and slowing and/or decreasing irregularity of the heart rate, the diastolic filling time is prolonged, resulting in an increased stroke volume. |
| j. calcium channel blocking agents (e.g. nifedepine, verapamil, diltiazem, nicardipine). | j. Calcium channel blockers dilate the coronary arteries, thus improving coronary blood flow and myocardial oxygen supply. They also reduce cardiac workload by dilating peripheral vessels, which decreases afterload. Some calcium channel blockers (primarily verapamil) also act to slow the heart rate. |

| NURSING ACTIONS | RATIONALES |
|---|---|
| **Prevention/Treatment—*cont'd*** | |
| 6. Consult physician if signs and symptoms of decreased cardiac output persist or worsen. | 6. Notifying the physician allows for modification of treatment plan. |

## ❖ Nursing Diagnosis: *Constipation*

### Definition

A state in which an individual experiences a change in normal bowel habits characterized by a decrease in frequency and/or passage of hard, dry stools.

### Desired Outcome

The client will maintain usual bowel elimination pattern as evidenced by:
a. usual frequency of bowel movements
b. passage of soft, formed stool
c. absence of headache, anorexia, abdominal distention and pain, feeling of rectal fullness or pressure, and straining at stool.

### Documentation

a. Occurrence of last bowel movement
b. Characteristics of stool
c. Presence of signs and symptoms of constipation
d. Bowel sounds
e. Therapeutic interventions
f. Client teaching

| NURSING ACTIONS | RATIONALES |
|---|---|
| **Assessments** | |
| 1. Ascertain client's usual bowel elimination habits. | 1. Knowledge of the client's usual bowel elimination habits is essential in determining if constipation is present because the frequency of defecation varies among individuals. |
| 2. Assess for signs and symptoms of constipation (e.g. decrease in frequency of stools; passage of hard, formed stools; headache; anorexia; abdominal distention and pain; feeling of fullness or pressure in rectum; straining at stool). | 2. Early recognition of signs and symptoms of constipation allows for prompt intervention. |
| 3. Assess bowel sounds. Report a pattern of decreasing bowel sounds. | 3. Bowel sounds are produced by peristaltic activity. A pattern of decreasing bowel sounds indicates a decrease in bowel motility, which can result from or lead to constipation. |
| **Prevention/Treatment** | |
| 4. Encourage client to defecate whenever the urge is felt. | 4. The urge to defecate occurs when feces move into the rectum, thus initiating the defecation reflex. When the client responds to this urge within minutes, defecation usually occurs without difficulty. If the urge to defecate is suppressed by contracting the external anal sphincter for several minutes, the defecation reflex stops and does not occur again until additional feces enter the |

**NURSING ACTIONS** / **RATIONALES**

**Prevention/Treatment—*cont'd***

(Rationale continued) rectum. Continued or prolonged inhibition of the defecation reflex results in a progressive decrease in its effectiveness.

5. Assist client to toilet or bedside commode or place in high Fowler's position on bedpan for bowel movements unless contraindicated.

   Rationale: A sitting or high Fowler's position promotes the expulsion of stool by:
   a. taking advantage of gravity
   b. causing relaxation of pelvic muscles and contraction of abdominal muscles with subsequent straightening of the anorectal angle.

6. Provide privacy and adequate ventilation during client's attempts to have a bowel movement.

   Rationale: A lack of privacy and adequate ventilation during bowel movement attempts can cause anxiety for the client, which results in stimulation of the sympathetic nervous system and subsequent inhibition of peristalsis. Anxiety can also cause contraction of the pelvic muscles and external anal sphincter. Embarrassment can result in a reluctance to respond to the urge to defecate. All of these factors contribute to constipation.

7. Encourage client to relax during attempts to defecate.

   Rationale: When a client is feeling calm during defecation attempts, he/she is better able to relax the pelvic floor musculature and the external anal sphincter, thus facilitating the passage of stool.

8. Instruct client to increase intake of foods high in fiber (e.g. nuts, bran, whole-grain breads and cereals, raw fruits and vegetables) unless contraindicated.

   Rationale: Foods high in fiber provide bulk to the fecal mass, which keeps the stool soft because of the ability of fiber to absorb water. Soft, bulky stool passes through the intestine more rapidly, reducing the amount of water absorbed from it by the large intestine, and subsequently preventing the formation of hard, dry stool that is difficult to expel. In the rectal area, the presence of bulky stool causes distention of the rectal wall, which triggers the defecation reflex.

9. Instruct client to maintain a minimum fluid intake of 2500 ml/day unless contraindicated.

   Rationale: If fluid intake is inadequate for normal body processes, more fluid than usual is absorbed from the intestinal contents as they pass through the colon. This results in hard, dry stool, which is difficult to evacuate.

10. Encourage client to drink warm liquids upon arising in the morning.

    Rationale: Drinking warm liquids stimulates the gastrocolic and duodenocolic reflexes, resulting

| NURSING ACTIONS<br>**Prevention/Treatment—*cont'd*** | RATIONALES |
|---|---|
| | in increased peristalsis. These reflexes are the strongest when a person eats or drinks following a period of fasting. |
| 11. Increase activity as allowed and tolerated. | 11. Activity stimulates peristalsis, which facilitates the passage of stool through the intestines. |
| 12. Encourage client to perform isometric abdominal strengthening exercises unless contraindicated. | 12. The normal defecation process depends on adequate abdominal muscle tone and strength, which are necessary to raise intraabdominal pressure enough to promote defecation. |
| 13. Encourage the use of nonnarcotic rather than narcotic analgesics when possible for pain management. | 13. Narcotic analgesics inhibit peristalsis, which delays transit of intestinal contents. This delay also results in increased absorption of fluid from the fecal mass with the subsequent formation of hard, dry stool. |
| 14. Administer laxatives and stool softeners if ordered. | 14. Laxatives facilitate the evacuation of stool by softening the stool, stimulating peristalsis, and/or increasing fecal bulk. Stool softeners draw fat and water into the fecal mass, thus softening the stool and making it easier to expel. |
| 15. Administer cleansing and/or oil retention enemas if ordered. | 15. A cleansing enema stimulates peristalsis and promotes defecation by irritating the sigmoid colon and rectal wall and/or distending the lower bowel with a large volume of fluid. An oil retention enema facilitates defecation by lubricating the rectum and lower bowel and softening the fecal mass. |
| 16. Perform digital stimulation of the anal sphincter if indicated. | 16. Digital stimulation of the anal sphincter stimulates the defecation reflex. |
| 17. Check for impaction if the client has not had a bowel movement in 3 days, if he/she is passing liquid stool, or if other signs and symptoms of constipation are present. Digitally remove stool if necessary. | 17. An impaction prohibits the normal passage of feces. Digital removal of an impacted fecal mass may be necessary before normal passage of stool can occur. |
| 18. Consult physician if signs and symptoms of constipation persist. | 18. Notifying the physician allows for modification of treatment plan. |

## ❖ Nursing Diagnosis: *Coping, Ineffective Individual*

### Definition

Impairment of adaptive behaviors and problem-solving abilities of a person in meeting life's demands and roles.

### Desired Outcome

The client will demonstrate the use of effective coping skills as evidenced by:
a. verbalization of ability to cope
b. use of appropriate problem-solving techniques
c. willingness to participate in treatment plan and meet basic needs
d. absence of destructive behavior toward self and others
e. appropriate use of defense mechanisms
f. recognition and use of available support systems.

### Documentation

a. Client statements related to coping ability
b. Ability to meet basic needs and problem solve
c. Factors inhibiting successful coping ability
d. Current coping strategies used
e. Inappropriate behavior
f. Support systems available and/or used
g. Therapeutic interventions
h. Client/family teaching

| NURSING ACTIONS | RATIONALES |
|---|---|
| **Assessments** | |
| 1. Assess for and report signs and symptoms of ineffective individual coping (e.g. verbalization of inability to cope; inability to ask for help, problem solve, or meet basic needs; destructive behavior toward self or others; inappropriate use of defense mechanisms; inability to meet role expectations). | 1. Early recognition and reporting of signs and symptoms of ineffective individual coping allow for prompt intervention. |
| 2. Assess client's perception of current situation including precipitating factors and effectiveness of coping mechanisms. | 2. The client's perception of the situation is the major determinant of his/her response. An awareness of the situation from the client's point of view helps the nurse develop interventions that will facilitate coping. |
| **Prevention/Treatment** | |
| 3. Allow time for client to adjust psychologically to his/her situation. | 3. Time is necessary for cognitive appraisal of the situation and development of effective coping strategies. |
| 4. Assist client to recognize and manage inappropriate denial if it is present. | 4. Denial is a major defense mechanism used to deal with illness, particularly when the client is unable to deal with the realities of his/her situation or is grieving. If denial persists or is inappropriate, it inhibits the client's ability to cope. |
| 5. Implement measures to reduce fear and anxiety (e.g. encourage verbalization about | 5. Fear and anxiety inhibit clarity of thought and problem solving and the subsequent |

**NURSING ACTIONS**

**Prevention/Treatment—*cont'd***

the situation, instruct in relaxation techniques, administer antianxiety agents as ordered).

**RATIONALES**

development of effective coping techniques.

6. Implement measures to reduce discomfort (e.g. administer prescribed analgesics, encourage use of relaxation techniques).
   - 6. The presence of discomfort, particularly if it continues, can reduce the client's ability to effectively identify and use coping strategies.
7. Encourage verbalization about current situation and ways comparable situations have been handled in the past.
   - 7. Verbalization assists the client to reflect on the situation he/she is dealing with and to develop coping strategies based on previous successful experiences.
8. Assist client to identify personal strengths and resources that can be used to facilitate coping with the current situation.
   - 8. The development of effective coping strategies is dependent on the client's ability to recognize and use personal strengths and resources.
9. Demonstrate acceptance of client and create an atmosphere of trust and support. Set limits on inappropriate behavior.
   - 9. An environment where acceptance, trust, and support exist is essential for the client to feel free to express his/her true feelings and concerns and subsequently begin to cope with his/her situation. Limits need to be set on inappropriate behavior because it inhibits the development of adaptive coping strategies.
10. Arrange for a visit with another individual who has successfully adjusted to a similar situation.
    - 10. Contact with another individual who has experienced and successfully adjusted to a similar situation provides the client with support and insight into ways to effectively cope with his/her situation.
11. Include client in planning of care, encourage maximum participation in treatment plan, and allow choices when possible.
    - 11. Active participation in the planning of care allows the client to maintain a sense of control. This enhances his/her self-esteem and subsequent ability to cope.
12. Instruct client in effective problem-solving techniques (e.g. accurate identification of stressors, determination of various options to solve problem).
    - 12. Effective problem-solving skills are essential to the development of useful coping strategies because they enable the client to identify the problem clearly and select and implement viable options for solving it.
13. Assist client to maintain usual daily routines whenever possible.
    - 13. The ability to maintain usual daily routines enhances the client's feelings of control and hopefulness about being able to resume his/her life as it was before the situation being experienced.
14. Assist client as he/she starts to plan for necessary life-style and role changes after discharge.
    - 14. The setting of appropriate priorities and realistic goals is necessary if the client is to

| NURSING ACTIONS | RATIONALES |
|---|---|
| **Prevention/Treatment—*cont'd*** | |
| Help client to identify priorities and attainable goals. | cope effectively with the changes being experienced. |
| 15. Assist client and significant others to identify ways that personal and family goals can be adjusted rather than abandoned. | 15. Adjustment rather than abandonment of personal and family goals reduces the feeling of loss and increases the probability of positive adaptation to the situation being experienced. |
| 16. Assist client, through methods such as role playing, to practice coping strategies. | 16. Practicing coping strategies in a safe environment helps the client to integrate these skills so that they are more easily implemented when the need arises. |
| 17. Assist client to identify and use available support systems. Provide information about available community resources that can assist client and significant others in coping with the situation at hand. | 17. Social support provides a sense of acceptance and reduces the feelings of aloneness, which are often experienced in a crisis situation. Community resources are usually able to provide both information and psychological support for the client and significant others and subsequently facilitate the development and success of coping strategies. |
| 18. Encourage client to share with significant others the kind of support that would be most beneficial (e.g. listening, inspiring hope, providing reassurance and accurate information). | 18. Techniques or behaviors that facilitate one's coping ability vary from person to person and need to be clearly communicated to significant others in order to maximize their support. |
| 19. Assess for and support behaviors suggesting positive adaptation to changes experienced (e.g. participation in treatment plan and self-care activities, communication of the ability to cope, use of effective problem-solving strategies). | 19. Positive reinforcement of effective coping strategies increases the likelihood of continued use and enhancement of these strategies. |
| 20. Consult physician about psychological and vocational rehabilitation counseling if appropriate. Initiate a referral if necessary. | 20. If client is unable to cope effectively and/or is unable to pursue his/her vocation, additional counseling may be necessary. Consulting with physician and making referrals can help the client to meet his/her needs and cope effectively. |

## ❖ Nursing Diagnosis: *Diarrhea*

### Definition

A state in which an individual experiences a change in normal bowel habits characterized by the frequent passage of loose, fluid, unformed stools.

| Desired Outcome | Documentation |
|---|---|
| The client will have fewer bowel movements and more formed stool. | a. Frequency of defecation<br>b. Characteristics of stool |

**Desired Outcome—*cont'd***

**Documentation—*cont'd***

c. Complaints of abdominal pain and cramping
d. Presence of bowel sounds
e. Therapeutic interventions
f. Client teaching

| NURSING ACTIONS | RATIONALES |
|---|---|
| **Assessments** | |
| 1. Ascertain client's usual bowel elimination habits. | 1. Knowledge of the client's usual bowel elimination habits helps determine the severity of the diarrhea. |
| 2. Assess for and report signs and symptoms of diarrhea (e.g. frequent, loose stools; urgency; abdominal pain and cramping). | 2. Early recognition and reporting of signs and symptoms of diarrhea allow for prompt intervention. |
| 3. Assess bowel sounds regularly. Report an increase in frequency of bowel sounds. | 3. Bowel sounds are produced by peristaltic activity. An increase in frequency of bowel sounds indicates an increase in bowel motility, which can lead to decreased absorption of water from the intestinal contents and subsequent frequent liquid stools. |
| **Prevention/Treatment** | |
| 4. Restrict oral intake if ordered. | 4. The ingestion of food stimulates the gastrocolic and duodenocolic reflexes, resulting in increased peristaltic activity. If client is having diarrhea, restriction of oral intake helps reduce bowel activity. |
| 5. When oral intake is allowed, gradually progress from fluids to small meals. | 5. Gradual introduction of small amounts of fluid and then food helps prevent a sudden increase in peristalsis and subsequent diarrhea. |
| 6. Instruct client to avoid the following foods/fluids: a. gas producers (e.g. cabbage, beans, onions, cauliflower) | 6. a. Gas exerts pressure on the walls of the colon, which results in stimulation of the colonic nerves and subsequent increased peristalsis. |
| b. those that are spicy or extremely hot or cold | b. Spicy foods can irritate the bowel, which results in increased peristalsis and excessive mucus secretion with subsequent increased liquidity of intestinal contents. Extremes in temperature of ingested foods/fluids can also stimulate peristalsis. |
| c. those high in lactose (e.g. milk, milk products) | c. Diarrhea may temporarily deplete the gastrointestinal enzymes necessary for the digestion of lactose. The undigested lactose draws water into the intestinal lumen and produces an |

**NURSING ACTIONS** | **RATIONALES**

**Prevention/Treatment—*cont'd***

osmotic type of diarrhea. The lactose also serves as a base for bacterial fermentation in the colon. The lactic and fatty acids produced by this fermentation process irritate the colon with a subsequent increase in bowel motility and diarrhea.

d. those high in sorbitol (e.g. apple juice, peaches, sugarless gum, dietetic foods) and fructose (e.g. apple juice)

d. Sorbitol and fructose are not well absorbed by many people and tend to draw water into the intestine, which induces an osmotic type of diarrhea.

e. those high in fiber (e.g. whole-grain cereals, raw fruits and vegetables).

e. Fibrous foods may mechanically irritate the bowel and stimulate peristalsis.

7. Implement measures to reduce fear and anxiety (e.g. provide client teaching, interact with client in a calm manner, administer prescribed antianxiety agents).

7. Extreme fear and anxiety can cause excessive stimulation of the parasympathetic nervous system, which results in increased peristalsis and excessive mucus secretion in the distal colon and subsequent diarrhea.

8. Encourage client to rest.

8. Physical activity stimulates peristalsis.

9. Discourage smoking.

9. Nicotine excites the sympathetic and the parasympathetic postganglionic neurons simultaneously with a predominant parasympathetic effect in the gastrointestinal tract. This results in increased peristalsis and relaxation of sphincters, promoting an increased propulsion of feces through the gastrointestinal tract.

10. Implement measures to remove fecal impaction if present (e.g. digital removal of stool, oil retention enema).

10. A fecal impaction causes a mechanical obstruction of the bowel. The area proximal to the obstruction secretes excessive mucus and fluid in an attempt to lubricate the fecal mass and move it toward the anus. This mucus and fluid leaks around the bowel mass, resulting in diarrhea.

11. Administer the following antidiarrheal agents if ordered:

a. opiate or opiate-like substances (e.g. loperamide, diphenoxylate hydrochloride)

11.a. Opiates inhibit the propulsive contractions of the intestine and stimulate the segmental activity that mixes intestinal contents. This results in a reduction of gastrointestinal motility and a more formed stool.

**NURSING ACTIONS**

**Prevention/Treatment—*cont'd***

b. bulk-forming agents (e.g. methylcellulose, psyllium hydrophilic mucilloid, calcium polycarbophil)
c. intestinal flora modifiers (e.g. *Lactobacillus acidophilus*, Lactinex, Bacid).

12. Consult physician if diarrhea persists.

**RATIONALES**

b. Bulk-forming agents absorb water in the bowel, which results in a more formed stool.
c. Intestinal flora modifiers may be used to promote recolonization of normal intestinal flora in clients who have diarrhea associated with antimicrobial therapy.

12. Notifying physician allows for modification of the treatment plan.

## ❖ Nursing Diagnosis: *Fluid Volume Deficit*

### Definition

The state in which an individual experiences vascular, cellular, or intracellular dehydration.

### Desired Outcome

The client will not experience a fluid volume deficit as evidenced by:
a. normal skin turgor
b. moist mucous membranes
c. stable weight
d. B/P and pulse within normal range for client and stable with position change
e. small vein filling time less than 3-5 seconds
f. BUN and Hct within normal range
g. balanced intake and output
h. urine specific gravity within normal range.

### Documentation

a. Vital signs
b. Condition of skin and mucous membranes
c. Weight
d. Small vein filling time
e. Intake and output
f. Presence of nausea, vomiting, or other contributing factors
g. Intravenous fluid therapy
h. Client teaching

**NURSING ACTIONS**

**Assessments**

1. Assess for and report signs and symptoms of fluid volume deficit:
   a. decreased skin turgor
   b. dry mucous membranes, thirst
   c. sudden weight loss of 2% or greater
   d. low B/P and/or postural hypotension
   e. weak, rapid pulse
   f. delayed small vein filling time (longer than 3-5 seconds)
   g. elevated BUN and Hct
   h. decreased urine output with a change in specific gravity (the specific gravity will usually be increased with an

**RATIONALES**

1. Early recognition and reporting of signs and symptoms of fluid volume deficit allow for prompt intervention.

| NURSING ACTIONS | RATIONALES |
|---|---|
| **Assessments—*cont'd*** | |
| actual fluid volume deficit but may be decreased depending on the cause of the deficit). | |
| **Prevention/Treatment** | |
| 2. Implement measures to reduce nausea and vomiting if present (e.g. administer antiemetics as ordered, instruct client to ingest foods/fluids slowly, eliminate noxious sights and odors). | 2. Nausea often causes the client to have a decreased fluid intake. Vomiting results in excessive loss of fluid. |
| 3. Implement measures to control diarrhea if present (e.g. administer antidiarrheal agents as ordered, discourage intake of foods that are spicy and foods high in fiber, discourage smoking). | 3. Diarrhea results in excessive loss of gastrointestinal fluid. |
| 4. Implement measures to improve oral intake unless contraindicated (e.g. consider client's dietary preferences, eliminate noxious sights and odors, allow adequate time for meals and snacks). | 4. An increase in the amount of oral fluid intake helps ensure adequate hydration. |
| 5. Maintain a fluid intake of at least 2500 ml/day unless contraindicated. If oral intake is inadequate, maintain intravenous fluid therapy as ordered. | 5. Adequate fluid intake needs to be provided in order to replace losses and/or ensure adequate hydration. |
| 6. Consult physician if signs and symptoms of fluid volume deficit persist or worsen. | 6. Notifying the physician allows for modification of treatment plan. |

## ❖ Nursing Diagnosis: *Fluid Volume Excess*

### Definition

The state in which an individual experiences increased fluid retention and edema.

### Desired Outcome

The client will not experience fluid volume excess as evidenced by:

a. stable weight
b. B/P within normal range for client
c. absence of $S_3$ heart sound
d. balanced intake and output
e. usual mental status
f. normal breath sounds
g. BUN and Hct within normal range
h. urine specific gravity within normal range
i. absence of dyspnea, orthopnea, peripheral edema, and distended neck veins
j. small vein emptying time less than 3-5 seconds
k. CVP within normal range.

### Documentation

a. Blood pressure
b. Weight
c. Heart sounds
d. Intake and output
e. Mental status
f. Breath sounds, ease of respirations
g. Presence of edema and jugular vein distention
h. Small vein emptying time
i. CVP readings
j. Therapeutic interventions
k. Client teaching

| NURSING ACTIONS | RATIONALES |
| --- | --- |
| **Assessments** | |
| 1. Assess for and report signs and symptoms of fluid volume excess:<br>a. weight gain<br>b. elevated B/P (B/P may not be elevated if fluid has shifted out of vascular space)<br>c. presence of an $S_3$ heart sound<br>d. intake greater than output<br>e. change in mental status<br>f. crackles (rales), diminished or absent breath sounds<br>g. decreased BUN and Hct<br>h. decreased urine specific gravity<br>i. dyspnea, orthopnea<br>j. peripheral edema<br>k. distended neck veins<br>l. delayed small vein emptying time (longer than 3-5 seconds)<br>m. elevated CVP. | 1. Early recognition and reporting of signs and symptoms of fluid volume excess allow for prompt intervention. |
| 2. Monitor chest x-ray results. Report findings of pulmonary vascular congestion, pleural effusion, or pulmonary edema. | 2. Chest x-ray films provide data about pulmonary vascular status and fluid accumulation in the pleural space, pulmonary interstitium, and alveoli. |
| **Prevention/Treatment** | |
| 3. Maintain fluid restrictions as ordered. | 3. Fluid restriction helps to reduce total body water and prevent the accumulation of excess fluid. |
| 4. Restrict sodium intake as ordered. | 4. When blood filters through the kidneys, the majority of sodium ions are reabsorbed by the renal tubules. Water is attracted to sodium and is also reabsorbed. Restriction of sodium intake reduces the amount of sodium that passes through and is reabsorbed by the kidney. This results in decreased retention of water. |
| 5. Encourage client to rest periodically in a recumbent position if tolerated. | 5. Lying flat promotes venous return, which results in lower venous hydrostatic pressure with subsequent reshifting of fluid from the interstitial space into the vascular space. The increase in vascular volume improves renal blood flow and promotes diuresis. A recumbent position also results in decreased activation of the renin-angiotensin-aldosterone mechanism with a subsequent reduction in sodium and water retention. |
| 6. Administer diuretics if ordered. | 6. Most diuretics inhibit sodium reabsorption in the renal |

**NURSING ACTIONS** | **RATIONALES**

**Prevention/Treatment—*cont'd***

tubules. This results in decreased water reabsorption and subsequent excretion of excess fluid.

7. Consult physician if signs and symptoms of fluid volume excess persist or worsen.

7. Notifying the physician allows for modification of treatment plan.

## ❖ Nursing Diagnosis: *Gas Exchange, Impaired*

### Definition

The state in which the individual experiences a decreased passage of oxygen and/or carbon dioxide between the alveoli of the lungs and the vascular system.

### Desired Outcome

The client will experience adequate $O_2/CO_2$ exchange as evidenced by:
a. usual mental status
b. unlabored respirations at 14-20/minute
c. blood gases within normal range.

### Documentation

a. Respiratory rate
b. Difficulty breathing
c. Mental status
d. Oximetry results
e. Route and rate of oxygen administration
f. Therapeutic interventions
g. Client teaching

**NURSING ACTIONS** | **RATIONALES**

**Assessments**

1. Assess for and report signs and symptoms of impaired gas exchange:
   a. restlessness, irritability
   b. confusion, somnolence
   c. tachypnea, dyspnea
   d. decreased $PaO_2$ and increased $PaCO_2$.

1. Early recognition and reporting of signs and symptoms of impaired gas exchange allow for prompt intervention.

2. Monitor for and report significant changes in oximetry results.

2. Oximetry is a noninvasive method of measuring $SaO_2$. The results provide a guide for evaluating respiratory status and the effectiveness of treatment.

**Prevention/Treatment**

3. Place client in a semi- to high Fowler's position unless contraindicated. Position with pillows to prevent slumping. If client is experiencing dyspnea or orthopnea, position overbed table so he/she can lean on it if desired.

3. These positions allow for increased diaphragmatic excursion and maximum lung expansion, which help to fully aerate the lungs and enhance $O_2/CO_2$ exchange.

4. Instruct and assist client to turn, deep breathe, and cough or "huff" at least every 2 hours.

4. Turning from side to side mobilizes secretions and allows for increased expansion of the uppermost lung. Deep breathing dilates the airways, loosens secretions, stimulates coughing, and promotes maximum lung expansion. Coughing or "huffing" (a forced exhalation technique)

**NURSING ACTIONS**

**Prevention/Treatment—*cont'd***

**RATIONALES**

mobilizes secretions and facilitates their removal from the respiratory tract. These actions promote optimal lung aeration and $O_2/CO_2$ exchange.

5. Reinforce correct use of incentive spirometer at least every 2 hours.

5. Incentive spirometer use promotes deep breathing, which improves lung expansion and helps clear airways by loosening secretions and stimulating a cough. These actions help to aerate the lungs and enhance $O_2/CO_2$ exchange.

6. Implement measures to facilitate removal of pulmonary secretions (e.g. suction, postural drainage, percussion, vibration) if ordered.

6. Excessive secretions and/or client's inability to clear secretions from the respiratory tract lead to stasis of secretions, which can impair $O_2/CO_2$ exchange. Suction and chest physiotherapy may be necessary to facilitate removal of pulmonary secretions and thereby promote adequate gas exchange.

7. Assist with IPPB treatments as ordered.

7. IPPB treatments deliver air or oxygen into the lungs at a positive pressure, thereby enhancing maximum lung inflation, aeration, and gas exchange.

8. Maintain oxygen therapy as ordered.

8. Supplemental oxygen increases the amount of oxygen available for gas exchange.

9. Maintain activity restrictions as ordered. Increase activity gradually as allowed and tolerated.

9. Activity restrictions promote rest, which lowers the body's oxygen requirements and thus increases the amount of oxygen available for gas exchange. A gradual increase in activity prevents a sudden increase in oxygen demand and helps to mobilize secretions and improve lung expansion.

10. Discourage smoking.

10. Smoking impairs gas exchange because it:
    a. reduces effective airway clearance by causing bronchoconstriction, increasing mucus production, and impairing ciliary function
    b. decreases oxygen availability (hemoglobin binds with the carbon monoxide in smoke rather than with oxygen)
    c. causes vasoconstriction and subsequently reduces pulmonary blood flow.

11. Administer central nervous system depressants judiciously. Hold medication and consult

11. Central nervous system depressants cause depression of the respiratory center and

| NURSING ACTIONS | RATIONALES |
|---|---|
| **Prevention/Treatment—*cont'd*** | |
| physician if respiratory rate is less than 12/minute. | cough reflex. This can result in hypoventilation and stasis of secretions with subsequent impaired gas exchange. |
| 12. Consult physician if signs and symptoms of impaired gas exchange persist or worsen. | 12. Notifying the physician allows for modification of treatment plan. |

## ❖ Nursing Diagnosis: *Grieving*

This diagnostic label includes anticipatory grieving and grieving following the actual loss.

### Definition

The state or a response of physical or psychological suffering that precedes or follows an actual or perceived loss of something valued.

### Desired Outcome

The client will demonstrate beginning progression through the grieving process as evidenced by:
a. verbalization of feelings about the loss
b. expression of grief
c. participation in treatment plan and self-care activities
d. use of available support systems.

### Documentation

a. Signs and symptoms of grieving
b. Client's perception of loss
c. Strengths demonstrated in coping with loss
d. Support systems used
e. Client/family teaching

| NURSING ACTIONS | RATIONALES |
|---|---|
| **Assessments** | |
| 1. Assess for signs and symptoms of grieving (e.g. change in eating habits, inability to concentrate, insomnia, anger, noncompliance, withdrawal from significant others, denial of loss). | 1. Assessment of signs and symptoms of grieving helps the nurse determine the phase of grieving the client is experiencing. This knowledge aids in the development of effective strategies that can assist the client to progress through the phases of grieving. |
| 2. Assess for factors that may hinder and facilitate client's acknowledgment of the loss. (Grieving is affected by factors such as previous experience with loss, developmental stage, support systems, spiritual and cultural background, health status, and significance of the loss.) | 2. In order for grief work to begin, the client needs to acknowledge the loss. An awareness of factors that may hinder and facilitate this acknowledgment assists the nurse to develop effective strategies to accomplish this goal. |
| **Prevention/Treatment** | |
| 3. Assist client to acknowledge the loss experienced (e.g. encourage conversation about the loss including how or why it occurred and its impact on | 3. The client needs to acknowledge the loss in order for grief work to begin. Adaptive denial is a protective defense mechanism that |

| NURSING ACTIONS | RATIONALES |
|---|---|
| **Prevention/Treatment—*cont'd*** | |
| his/her future). Gently correct misconceptions. | commonly occurs during the initial period following a loss. It allows the client time to mobilize resources that facilitate effective coping and keeps him/her from being overwhelmed by the loss. If denial continues, however, it impedes the progression of grief work. |
| 4. Discuss the grieving process and assist client to accept the phases of grieving as an expected response to an actual and/or anticipated loss. | 4. An awareness of the feelings and behaviors commonly associated with each phase of the grieving process assists the client to accept his/her responses to the loss. |
| 5. Allow time for client to progress through the phases of grieving (phases vary among theorists but progress from shock and alarm to acceptance). | 5. Grieving is a process that occurs in a sequence of phases or stages that progress over time. Some phases may not be experienced by the client and some may overlap or recur. The amount of time necessary to reach resolution of grief is very individual, may take months to years, and must be allowed to occur in order to reduce the risk for dysfunctional grieving. |
| 6. Provide an atmosphere of care and concern (e.g. provide privacy, be available and nonjudgmental, display empathy and respect). | 6. A supportive, nonthreatening environment provides the basis for a constructive, therapeutic relationship. This allows the client to express his/her feelings of grief and work toward its resolution. |
| 7. Implement measures to promote trust (e.g. answer questions honestly, provide requested information). | 7. A feeling of trust in the caregiver promotes the development of a therapeutic nurse/client relationship in which the client can feel free to verbalize his/her feelings. This facilitates the progression of grief work. |
| 8. Encourage the verbal expression of anger and sadness about the loss experienced. Recognize displacement of anger and assist client to see the actual cause of angry feelings and resentment. Establish limits on abusive behavior if demonstrated. | 8. The verbal expression of feelings of anger and sadness facilitates movement toward resolution of grief. Displacement of angry feelings needs to be acknowledged so that grieving can progress but should not be allowed to interfere with the therapeutic process. |
| 9. Encourage client to express his/her feelings in whatever ways are comfortable (e.g. writing, drawing, conversation). | 9. Expression of feelings in whatever ways are comfortable for the client helps him/her integrate both the positive and negative aspects of the loss and move toward its acceptance. |

| NURSING ACTIONS | RATIONALES |
|---|---|
| **Prevention/Treatment—*cont'd*** | |
| 10. Assist client to identify personal strengths that have helped him/her to cope in previous situations of loss. | 10. The identification of personal strengths that have been helpful in previous situations of loss helps the client develop appropriate coping techniques to deal with the current loss. This facilitates progression through the grieving process. |
| 11. Support behaviors suggesting successful grief work (e.g. verbalizing feelings about loss, focusing on ways to adapt to loss, learning needed skills, developing or renewing relationships). | 11. Positive feedback about behaviors that suggest successful grief work reinforces those behaviors and promotes positive adaptation to loss. |
| 12. Explain the phases of the grieving process to significant others. Encourage their support and understanding. | 12. When significant others are knowledgeable about the phases of the grieving process, they are more likely to understand and accept the client's behavior and assist him/her to move toward resolution of grief. |
| 13. Facilitate communication between the client and significant others. | 13. A client's loss and/or response to the loss will affect his/her significant others. Communication between them may need to be facilitated so that successful grief work occurs. |
| 14. Provide information about counseling services and support groups that might assist client in working through grief. | 14. Counseling and support groups can assist the client in working through grief by:<br>a. providing insight into his/her responses to the loss<br>b. decreasing the feelings of aloneness and isolation that frequently accompany a loss<br>c. helping to identify methods or skills he/she can use to cope with the loss. |
| 15. Arrange for a visit from clergy if desired by client. | 15. Spiritual support can be a source of strength and solace to the client and can facilitate resolution of grief. |
| 16. Consult physician if signs of dysfunctional grieving (e.g. persistent denial of losses, excessive anger or sadness, hysteria, suicidal behaviors) occur. | 16. Notifying the physician allows for modification of the treatment plan. |

# ❖ Nursing Diagnosis: *Infection, High Risk for*

### Definition

The state in which an individual is at increased risk for being invaded by pathogenic organisms.

**Desired Outcome**

The client will remain free of infection as evidenced by:
a. absence of fever and chills
b. pulse within normal limits
c. normal breath sounds
d. voiding clear urine without complaints of frequency, urgency, and burning
e. absence of heat, pain, redness, swelling, and unusual drainage in any area
f. WBC and differential counts within normal range for client
g. negative results of cultured specimens.

**Documentation**

a. Temperature
b. Pulse rate
c. Breath sounds
d. Characteristics of urine, sputum, and wound drainage
e. Evidence of inflammation in any area
f. Evidence of unusual drainage in any area
g. Therapeutic interventions
h. Client/family teaching

| NURSING ACTIONS | RATIONALES |
|---|---|
| **Assessments** | |
| 1. Assess for and report signs and symptoms of infection:<br>a. elevated temperature<br>b. chills<br>c. increased pulse<br>d. abnormal breath sounds<br>e. cloudy, foul-smelling urine<br>f. complaints of frequency, urgency, or burning when urinating<br>g. presence of WBCs, bacteria, and/or nitrites in urine<br>h. heat, pain, redness, swelling, or unusual drainage in any area<br>i. elevated WBC count and/or significant change in differential. | 1. Early recognition and reporting of signs and symptoms of infection allow for prompt intervention. |
| 2. Obtain specimens (e.g. urine, vaginal, mouth, sputum, blood) for culture as ordered. | 2. Cultures are done to identify the specific organism(s) causing the infection. Culture results provide the physician with information necessary to determine the most effective treatment. |
| **Prevention/Treatment** | |
| 3. Maintain a fluid intake of at least 2500 ml/day unless contraindicated. | 3. Adequate hydration helps prevent infection by:<br>a. maintaining adequate blood flow and nutrient supply to the tissues<br>b. maintaining sufficient urine volume, which reduces urinary stasis and subsequent colonization of pathogens in the urinary tract |

| NURSING ACTIONS<br>Prevention/Treatment—*cont'd* | RATIONALES |
|---|---|
| | c. liquefying respiratory secretions, which facilitates removal of secretions. |
| 4. Use good handwashing technique and encourage client to do the same. | 4. Good handwashing removes transient bacteria, which reduces the risk of transmission of microorganisms. |
| 5. Maintain meticulous aseptic technique during invasive procedures (e.g. catheterizations, venous and arterial punctures, injections, tracheal suctioning, wound care). | 5. Maintenance of aseptic technique during invasive procedures reduces the possibility of introducing pathogens into the body. |
| 6. Change equipment, tubings, and solutions used for intravenous infusions and procedures such as irrigations, wound care, and tube feedings according to hospital policy. | 6. The longer that equipment, tubings, and solutions are in use, the greater the chance of colonization of microorganisms, which could then be introduced into the body. |
| 7. Rotate intravenous insertion sites according to hospital policy. | 7. Intravenous insertion sites need to be changed routinely in order to reduce persistent irritation of one area of a vein wall and the resultant colonization of microorganisms at that site. |
| 8. Protect client from others with infections. | 8. Protecting the client from others with infections reduces his/her risk of exogenous infection. |
| 9. Implement measures to maintain healthy, intact skin (e.g. keep skin lubricated, clean, and dry; instruct or assist client to turn every 2 hours; keep bed linens dry and wrinkle-free). | 9. Healthy, intact skin provides a physical barrier against microorganisms. The skin is also slightly acidic because of the fatty acids contained in the sebum. The acidity helps inhibit the growth of microorganisms. |
| 10. Implement measures to reduce stress (e.g. reduce fear, anxiety, and pain; help client identify and use effective coping mechanisms). | 10. Stress causes an increased secretion of cortisol. Cortisol inhibits the immune response, which increases the client's susceptibility to infection. |
| 11. Maintain an optimal nutritional status. Administer vitamins and minerals as ordered. | 11. Adequate nutrition is needed to maintain normal function of the immune system. Inadequate intake of protein and some vitamins and minerals can cause atrophy of lymphoid tissue and can depress T and/or B lymphocyte function, resulting in an increased susceptibility to infection. |
| 12. Instruct and assist client to perform good perineal care at least every shift and after each bowel movement. | 12. The perineal area contains a large number of organisms. Routine cleansing of the area reduces the risk of colonization of the organisms and |

| NURSING ACTIONS<br>**Prevention/Treatment—*cont'd*** | RATIONALES |
|---|---|
| | subsequent perineal, urinary tract, and/or vaginal infection. |
| 13. Instruct and assist client to perform good oral hygiene as often as needed. | 13. The oral cavity contains a large number of organisms. Good oral hygiene reduces the risk of colonization of the organisms and subsequent oral cavity infection and/or pneumonia (can occur if pathogens are aspirated). |
| 14. Maintain patency of wound drain(s) and change dressings as often as needed. | 14. Wound drainage contains many pathogens that multiply in a warm, moist, dark environment. Maintaining patency of wound drains and keeping dressings clean and dry prevent the accumulation and stasis of drainage and the subsequent risk for colonization of these microorganisms. |
| 15. Implement measures to prevent urinary retention (e.g. instruct client to urinate when the urge is felt, promote relaxation during voiding attempts, administer bethanechol as ordered). | 15. Urinary retention increases the client's risk of urinary tract infection by:<br>a. causing small tears in the bladder mucosa as a result of bladder distention<br>b. compromising bladder mucosal integrity as a result of reduced blood flow in the bladder wall (as the intravesicular pressure increases, it puts pressure on the blood vessels in the wall of the bladder)<br>c. increasing the number of microorganisms in the urine (stagnant urine is conducive to the growth of microorganisms). |
| 16. Implement measures to prevent stasis of respiratory secretions (e.g. assist client to turn, cough, and deep breathe; increase activity as allowed and tolerated). | 16. Respiratory secretions provide a good medium for growth of microorganisms. By preventing stasis, there is less chance of colonization and a decreased risk for development of respiratory tract infection. |
| 17. Administer antimicrobials as ordered. | 17. Most antimicrobials disrupt cell wall synthesis, which halts the growth of or kills microorganisms. |

## ❖ Nursing Diagnosis: *Nutrition, Altered: Less Than Body Requirements*

### Definition

The state in which an individual experiences an intake of nutrients insufficient to meet metabolic needs.

#### Desired Outcome

The client will maintain an adequate nutritional status as evidenced by:
a. weight within normal range for client's age, height, and body frame
b. normal BUN and serum albumin, Hct, Hb, transferrin, and lymphocyte levels
c. triceps skinfold thickness within normal range
d. usual strength and activity tolerance
e. healthy oral mucous membrane.

#### Documentation

a. Weight
b. Triceps skinfold thickness
c. Activity tolerance
d. Condition of oral mucous membrane
e. Type of diet and amount consumed
f. Therapeutic interventions
g. Client/family teaching

| NURSING ACTIONS | RATIONALES |
|---|---|
| **Assessments** | |
| 1. Assess for and report signs and symptoms of malnutrition:<br>a. weight below normal for client's age, height, and body frame<br>b. abnormal BUN and low serum albumin, Hct, Hb, transferrin, and lymphocyte levels<br>c. triceps skinfold thickness less than normal<br>d. weakness and fatigue<br>e. stomatitis. | 1. Early recognition and reporting of signs and symptoms of malnutrition allow for prompt intervention. |
| 2. Monitor percentage of meals and snacks client consumes. Report a pattern of inadequate intake. | 2. An awareness of the amount of food/fluid the client consumes alerts the nurse to deficits in nutritional intake. Reporting an inadequate intake allows for prompt intervention. |
| **Prevention/Treatment** | |
| 3. Implement measures to relieve nausea and vomiting if present (e.g. administer antiemetics as ordered, eliminate noxious sights and odors). | 3. Nausea decreases the client's desire for and/or ability to consume needed nutrients. Vomiting results in an actual loss of nutrients. |
| 4. Implement measures to control diarrhea if present (e.g. administer antidiarrheal agents as ordered, discourage intake of spicy foods and foods high in fiber). | 4. The increased intestinal motility and/or irritation and inflammation of the intestinal mucosa that occur with or cause diarrhea decrease the absorption of nutrients in the bowel. In addition, diarrhea results in an actual loss of nutrients. |
| 5. Implement measures to reduce pain, fear, and anxiety if present. | 5. Pain, fear, and anxiety are stressors that stimulate the sympathetic nervous system, |

| NURSING ACTIONS<br>Prevention/Treatment—*cont'd* | RATIONALES |
|---|---|
| | which subsequently increases the basal metabolic rate and the breakdown of glycogen into glucose. This results in an increased utilization of nutrients. The slowed gastrointestinal motility that can also occur with sympathetic nervous system stimulation causes early satiety, which decreases oral intake and further compromises the client's nutritional status. |
| 6. Implement measures to improve oral intake: | 6. The client is more likely to achieve or maintain a good nutritional status if he/she has a good oral intake. |
| a. perform actions to relieve gastrointestinal distention if present (e.g. encourage and assist client with frequent position changes and ambulation unless contraindicated, administer gastrointestinal stimulants as ordered) | a. Distention of the gastrointestinal tract (especially the stomach and duodenum) stimulates the vagus nerve and subsequently the satiety center located in the ventromedial area of the hypothalamus. When the satiety center is stimulated, the feeding center in the ventrolateral area of the hypothalamus is inhibited. This results in a reduction in the client's appetite and a subsequent decrease in oral intake. |
| b. increase activity as allowed and tolerated | b. Activity usually promotes a general feeling of well-being, which can result in improved appetite. |
| c. maintain a clean environment and a relaxed, pleasant atmosphere | c. Noxious sights and odors can inhibit the feeding center in the hypothalamus. Removing the unpleasant stimuli helps to prevent this from occurring. In addition, maintaining a relaxed, pleasant atmosphere reduces the client's stress and promotes a feeling of well-being, which tends to improve appetite and oral intake. |
| d. encourage a rest period before meals if indicated | d. The physical activity of eating requires some expenditure of energy. If the client is fatigued, he/she is less likely to continue eating. |
| e. provide oral hygiene before meals | e. Good oral hygiene freshens the mouth by moistening the oral mucous membrane and removing unpleasant tastes. This can improve the taste of foods/fluids, which |

| NURSING ACTIONS<br>Prevention/Treatment—*cont'd* | RATIONALES |
|---|---|
| | helps stimulate appetite and increase oral intake. |
| f. serve small portions of foods/fluids that are appealing to the client; adhere to personal and cultural (e.g. religious, ethnic) preferences whenever possible | f. Foods/fluids that appeal to the client's senses (especially sight and smell) and are in accordance with his/her personal and cultural preferences are most likely to stimulate the feeding center and promote interest in eating. Serving small portions of foods/fluids rather than large ones reduces the risk of gastric distention and subsequent stimulation of the satiety center and loss of appetite. Small portions are also less likely to discourage or overwhelm an anorexic client. |
| g. encourage significant others to bring in client's favorite foods unless contraindicated and eat with him/her if client desires | g. A client's favorite foods/fluids tend to stimulate his/her appetite more than institutional foods/fluids. The presence of significant others during meals helps create a familiar social environment that can stimulate appetite and improve oral intake. |
| h. if client is experiencing dyspnea, place him/her in a high Fowler's position and provide supplemental oxygen therapy during meals if indicated | h. Because a person cannot swallow and breathe at the same time, relief of the client's dyspnea increases the likelihood of his/her maintaining a good oral intake. In addition, relieving dyspnea decreases the client's anxiety about and preoccupation with breathing efforts and increases his/her ability to focus on eating and drinking. |
| i. perform actions to compensate for taste alterations if present (e.g. add extra sweeteners to foods unless contraindicated, encourage client to experiment with different flavorings and seasonings, provide alternative sources of protein if meats such as beef or pork taste bitter or rancid, administer zinc as ordered) | i. Foods/fluids that have little or no flavor or an unusual taste are not likely to stimulate the feeding center. Enhancing the taste of foods/fluids and providing nutritious alternatives to those that taste unusual to the client help to stimulate his/her appetite and improve oral intake. |
| j. allow adequate time for meals; reheat foods/fluids if necessary | j. If the client feels rushed during meals, he/she tends to become anxious, lose his/ |

| NURSING ACTIONS<br>Prevention/Treatment—*cont'd* | RATIONALES |
|---|---|
| | her appetite, and stop eating. Appetite is also suppressed if foods/fluids normally served hot or warm become cold and do not appeal to the client. |
| k. limit fluid intake with meals unless it has a high nutritional value. | k. When the stomach becomes distended, its volume receptors stimulate the satiety center in the hypothalamus and the client reduces his/her oral intake. Drinking liquids with meals distends the stomach and may cause satiety before an adequate amount of food is consumed. |
| 7. Ensure that meals are well balanced and high in essential nutrients. Offer dietary supplements between meals if indicated. | 7. The client must consume a diet that is well balanced and high in essential nutrients in order to meet his/her nutritional needs. Dietary supplements are often needed between meals to help the client accomplish this. |
| 8. Administer vitamins and minerals if ordered. | 8. Vitamins and minerals are nutritional substances that the body needs to maintain metabolic functioning. The source of most vitamins and all minerals is exogenous. If the client's dietary intake does not provide adequate amounts of them, oral and/or parenteral supplements may be necessary. |
| 9. Allow the client to assist in the selection of foods/fluids that meet nutritional needs. Obtain a dietary consult if necessary. | 9. The client who is actively involved in menu planning is more likely to comply with the diet plan. In addition, the involvement increases his/her sense of control, which promotes a feeling of well-being and can lead to an increased oral intake. A dietitian is best able to ensure that the foods/fluids selected will meet the client's nutritional needs. |
| 10. Perform a 72-hour calorie count if ordered. Report totals to dietitian and physician. | 10. A calorie count provides information about the caloric and nutritional value of the foods/fluids the client consumes. The information obtained helps the dietitian and physician determine if alternative methods of nutritional support are needed. |
| 11. Consult physician about alternative methods of providing nutrition (e.g. parenteral nutrition, tube feedings) if client does not consume enough food or fluids to meet nutritional needs. | 11. If the client's oral intake is inadequate, an alternative method of providing nutrients needs to be implemented. |

## ❖ Nursing Diagnosis: *Oral Mucous Membrane, Altered*

### Definition

The state in which an individual experiences disruptions in the tissue layers of the oral cavity.

**Desired Outcome**

The client will maintain a healthy oral cavity as evidenced by:
a. absence of inflammation and discomfort
b. pink, moist, intact mucosa.

**Documentation**

a. Client complaints of oral dryness and/or discomfort
b. Condition of oral mucous membrane
c. Presence of oral lesions
d. Therapeutic interventions
e. Client teaching

**NURSING ACTIONS** / **RATIONALES**

**Assessments**

1. Assess client for signs and symptoms of altered oral mucous membrane (e.g. complaints of oral dryness and discomfort, inflamed and/or ulcerated oral mucosa).
   - Rationale: Early recognition of signs and symptoms of altered oral mucous membrane allows for prompt intervention.
2. Culture oral lesions as ordered. Report positive results.
   - Rationale: A positive culture reveals the organisms present in a lesion and provides direction for the treatment plan.

**Prevention/Treatment**

3. Instruct and assist client to perform good oral hygiene after meals and as often as needed.
   - Rationale: Good oral hygiene helps maintain health of the oral mucous membrane by reducing the number of bacteria in the mouth, which subsequently decreases the risk of infection. Brushing the teeth removes debris and plaque that can irritate the gums. Brushing also stimulates circulation to gum tissue, which increases the supply of nutrients to the cells and facilitates the removal of waste products of metabolism.
4. Use a soft bristle brush, sponge-tipped applicator, or low-pressure power spray for oral hygiene if indicated.
   - Rationale: These devices are useful for removing debris from client's mouth without causing pain and trauma to the oral mucous membrane.
5. Avoid use of products such as lemon-glycerin swabs and commercial mouthwashes containing alcohol.
   - Rationale: Lemon-glycerin swabs have a drying and irritating effect on the oral mucous membrane, which predisposes the membrane to cracking and subsequent breakdown. The use of these swabs may also increase the acidity in the mouth, which reduces the buffering capacity of saliva and creates an environment conducive to growth of some pathogens. The alcohol in

| NURSING ACTIONS<br>Prevention/Treatment—*cont'd* | RATIONALES |
|---|---|
| | some commercial mouthwashes has a drying effect and acts as an irritant to the oral mucous membrane. |
| 6. Encourage client to rinse mouth frequently with water or dilute mouthwash. | 6. During periods of illness, salivary flow may be reduced as a result of effects of certain medications and/or fluid volume deficit. Rinsing the mouth frequently helps alleviate dryness, promotes comfort, and reduces the possibility of cracking and breakdown of the oral mucosa. |
| 7. Lubricate client's lips frequently. | 7. Lubricating the client's lips prevents them from becoming dry and cracked. |
| 8. Encourage client to breathe through nose rather than mouth. | 8. Air inspired through the nose is humidified by the layer of mucus that coats the lining of the nasal cavity. Air inspired through the mouth lacks this moisture and is drying to the oral mucous membrane. |
| 9. Encourage client not to smoke. | 9. Smoke is a chemical irritant to the oral mucosa. |
| 10. Encourage a fluid intake of at least 2500 ml/day unless contraindicated. | 10. Adequate hydration is necessary to keep the oral mucosa moist, which reduces the risk of cracking and breakdown. |
| 11. Encourage client to chew gum or suck on sour, hard candy if allowed. | 11. Chewing gum or sucking on sour hard candy stimulates salivation. This alleviates dryness of the oral mucosa and helps reduce the risk of cracking and breakdown. |
| 12. Offer hot tea with lemon or warm lemonade at regular intervals unless contraindicated. | 12. Lemon stimulates salivation, which helps alleviate dryness of the oral mucosa and reduces the risk of breakdown. The warmth of the fluid promotes vasodilation, which improves the blood flow and supply of nutrients to the oral mucosa. |
| 13. Encourage client to use artificial saliva if indicated. | 13. Artificial saliva lubricates the oral mucous membrane in the absence of normal salivary flow. This helps reduce dryness and the subsequent risk of cracking and breakdown. |
| 14. Assist client to select foods of moderate temperature and those that are soft and bland. | 14. Foods that are extremely hot or cold, hard, spicy, and/or acidic may result in thermal, mechanical, or chemical trauma to the oral mucosa. |
| 15. Encourage client to maintain an adequate nutritional status. | 15. The oral mucous membrane has a very high rate of cellular turnover and an adequate nutritional status is necessary to maintain its health. |

**NURSING ACTIONS**

**Prevention/Treatment—*cont'd***

**RATIONALES**

Malnutrition also has a depressant effect on the immune system, which increases the client's risk of oral cavity infection.

16. Administer topical anesthetics, oral protective pastes or coating agents, topical and systemic analgesics, and antimicrobials if ordered.

16. Topical anesthetics, oral protective pastes or coating agents, and analgesics promote comfort if the oral mucous membrane is inflamed or if breakdown is present. This allows the client to increase oral intake of nutrients, which helps maintain health of the oral mucosa. Antimicrobials prevent or treat infection of the oral mucosa.

17. Consult physician if dryness, irritation, discomfort, and/or lesions of the oral cavity persist or worsen.

17. Notifying the physician allows for modification of the treatment plan.

## ❖ Nursing Diagnosis: *Pain*

### Definition

A state in which an individual experiences and reports the presence of severe discomfort or an uncomfortable sensation.

### Desired Outcome

The client will experience diminished pain as evidenced by:
a. verbalization of pain relief
b. relaxed facial expression and body positioning
c. increased participation in activities
d. stable vital signs.

### Documentation

a. Verbal description of pain
b. Numerical rating of pain intensity
c. Nonverbal signs of pain
d. Factors that aggravate and alleviate pain
e. Participation in activities
f. Therapeutic interventions
g. Client/family teaching

**NURSING ACTIONS**

**Assessments**

1. Determine how the client usually responds to pain.

**RATIONALES**

1. Sensitivity and reaction to pain are subjective and are influenced by previous experiences with pain, age, sex, emotional factors, and cultural background. An awareness of the client's usual response to painful stimuli enables the nurse to better evaluate the level of pain and facilitates the development of effective strategies to minimize the pain experience.

2. Assess for signs and symptoms of pain (e.g. verbal complaints of pain, wrinkled brow, clenched fists, reluctance to move, restlessness, diaphoresis, facial pallor, increased B/P, tachycardia).

2. Early recognition of signs and symptoms of pain allows for prompt intervention and improved pain control.

| NURSING ACTIONS | RATIONALES |
|---|---|
| **Assessments—*cont'd*** | |
| 3. Assess client's perception of pain including location, intensity, and type. Use a numerical scale to rate intensity. | 3. An awareness of the location, intensity, and type of pain being experienced helps determine the most appropriate intervention(s) for pain management. A numerical rating scale provides as objective a description as possible for a subjective experience and facilitates consistency when interpreting and communicating about the pain experience. This allows for a clearer understanding of the pain being experienced by the client. |
| 4. Assess for factors that seem to aggravate and alleviate pain. | 4. Knowledge of factors that aggravate and alleviate the client's pain helps the nurse formulate an effective individualized plan for pain management. |
| **Prevention/Treatment** | |
| 5. Implement measures to reduce fear and anxiety about the pain experience (e.g. assure client that his/her need for pain relief is understood and will be met, plan methods for achieving pain control with client, perform preoperative or preprocedure teaching). | 5. Fear and anxiety about pain decrease an individual's threshold and tolerance for pain, which reduces his/her ability to cope with the pain. The spiral effect that pain and anxiety have on each other needs to be interrupted in order to prevent escalation of the pain experience. |
| 6. Administer medication before any painful treatments or procedures and before pain becomes severe. | 6. Administering medication before a painful experience reduces the severity of the pain. Analgesics are also more effective if given before pain becomes severe because severe or prolonged pain takes longer to subside despite appropriate interventions. |
| 7. Provide or assist with nonpharmacological measures for pain relief (e.g. cutaneous stimulation techniques such as pressure, massage, hot and cold applications, transcutaneous electrical nerve stimulation [TENS], and vibration; relaxation techniques such as progressive relaxation exercises and meditation; distraction by quiet conversation, music, rhythmic massage, and diversional activities; guided imagery; position change). | 7. Nonpharmacological approaches for pain management are effective because:<br>a. they are thought to use the gate control mechanism of pain relief in which the gating mechanism in the dorsal horn of the spinal cord is inhibited and pain impulses are subsequently not transmitted<br>b. some techniques (i.e. TENS, acupuncture, placebos) may stimulate the production of endorphins, which reduce pain by inhibiting the conduction of pain impulses in the central nervous system |

| NURSING ACTIONS<br>Prevention/Treatment—*cont'd* | RATIONALES |
|---|---|
| | c. they reduce the client's anxiety about the pain experience, which interrupts the pain/anxiety spiral. |
| 8. Administer analgesics if ordered. | 8. Analgesics relieve or decrease pain by inhibiting the transmission of pain impulses, reducing the cortical response to painful stimuli, and/or altering the client's perception of the pain experience. |
| 9. Consult physician about an order for patient-controlled analgesia (PCA) if indicated. | 9. The use of PCA allows the client to self-administer analgesics within parameters established by the physician. This method facilitates pain management by minimizing waiting time, providing more continuous pain relief, and increasing the client's control over the pain. |
| 10. Consult physician if above measures fail to provide adequate pain relief. | 10. Notifying the physician allows for modification of the treatment plan. |

## ❖ Nursing Diagnosis: *Self-Concept Disturbance*

This diagnostic label includes the nursing diagnoses of body image disturbance, self-esteem disturbance, and altered role performance.

### Definitions

**Body Image Disturbance:** Disruption in the way one perceives one's body image.

**Self-Esteem Disturbance:** Negative self-evaluation/feelings about self or self-capabilities, which may be directly or indirectly expressed.

**Altered Role Performance:** Disruption in the way one perceives one's role performance.

### Desired Outcome

The client will demonstrate beginning adaptation to changes in appearance, level of independence, body functioning, life style, and roles as evidenced by:

a. verbalization of feelings of self-worth
b. maintenance of relationships with significant others
c. active participation in activities of daily living
d. active interest in personal appearance
e. willingness to resume usual roles and participate in social activities
f. verbalization of a beginning plan for adapting life style to meet restrictions imposed by injury or disease process and its treatment.

### Documentation

a. Verbal and nonverbal responses to changes that have occurred
b. Coping mechanisms used to deal with changes in body functioning and/or appearance
c. Reaction of significant others to changes in client's body functioning and/or appearance
d. Willingness to touch and talk about changes in body
e. Participation in activities of daily living
f. Client/family teaching
g. Referrals to community agencies

| NURSING ACTIONS | RATIONALES |
|---|---|
| **Assessments** | |
| 1. Assess for signs and symptoms of a self-concept disturbance (e.g. verbal or nonverbal cues denoting a negative response to change in body functioning or appearance such as denial of or preoccupation with changes that have occurred, refusal to look at or touch a body part, or withdrawal from significant others). | 1. Early recognition of signs and symptoms of self-concept disturbance allows for prompt intervention. |
| 2. Determine the meaning of the change in body image and/or functioning to the client by encouraging him/her to verbalize feelings and by noting nonverbal responses to changes experienced. | 2. An understanding of what the change means to the client provides a basis for planning care. |
| **Prevention/Treatment** | |
| 3. Implement measures to assist client through the beginning phases of grieving (e.g. shock, disbelief, denial, anger, sadness, depression). Do not reinforce maladaptive denial of situation. | 3. Loss of a body part or a change in body functioning typically initiates a grieving response. Successful resolution of grief is essential for acceptance of changes experienced and integration of these changes into self-concept. Denial is a protective defense mechanism initially used following a loss or change that allows the client to mobilize strengths and resources. If allowed to persist, denial becomes maladaptive and inhibits grief work. |
| 4. Discuss with client improvements in appearance and/or body functioning that can realistically be expected. | 4. Realistic expectations about appearance and/or body functioning facilitate goal setting and are essential for positive adaptation to the changes experienced and integration of these changes into self-concept. |
| 5. Implement measures to assist client to increase self-esteem (e.g. limit negative self-assessment, encourage positive comments about self, assist to identify strengths, give positive feedback about accomplishments and behaviors that are indicative of high self-esteem). | 5. Self-esteem is a major component of one's view of self. It is a product of self-evaluation, reflected appraisals, social expectations, and perceptions of personal competence. An increase in self-esteem has a positive effect on the client's self-concept. |
| 6. Assist client to identify and use coping techniques that have been helpful in the past. | 6. Coping techniques help the client to manage or reduce the anxiety and stress that result when changes in appearance and/or body functioning occur. This reduction in anxiety and stress facilitates adaptation to these changes and development of a positive self-concept. |

| NURSING ACTIONS | RATIONALES |
|---|---|
| **Prevention/Treatment—*cont'd*** | |
| 7. Implement measures to assist client to adjust to alteration(s) in sexual functioning if appropriate (e.g. encourage questions and discussion about changes experienced, facilitate communication between client and his/her partner, discuss ways to be creative in expressing sexuality). | 7. Sexual functioning is an important component of one's sense of self. Assistance may be necessary to help the client adjust to changes experienced and/or identify alternative ways of sexual expression congruent with the client's beliefs about self. |
| 8. Implement measures to assist client to adapt to changes in body functioning and/or appearance (e.g. instruct in use of assistive devices, assist with clothing selection that minimizes changes in body contour). | 8. Adaptive measures can help to minimize obvious changes in body appearance and/or functioning and subsequently reduce the impact of these changes on self-concept. |
| 9. Assist client with usual grooming and makeup habits if necessary. | 9. Appearance is an essential component of self-esteem and one's concept of self. Maintaining an appearance he/she is comfortable with has a positive effect on the client's self-concept. |
| 10. Promote activities that require client to confront the body changes that have occurred (e.g. exercise, grooming, bathing). Be aware that the integration of changes in body image do not usually occur until 2-6 months after the actual physical change has occurred. | 10. Activities that require the client to acknowledge and deal with the changes that have occurred in his/her body facilitate the incorporation of the changes into the brain's schemata of the body. |
| 11. Demonstrate acceptance of client with techniques such as touch and frequent visits. Encourage significant others to do the same. | 11. Acceptance by others facilitates the client's positive integration of a new body image. Frequent visits and the use of touch convey a feeling of acceptance to the client. This enhances his/her feelings of self-worth and assists in the development of a positive self-concept. |
| 12. Assess for and support behaviors suggesting positive adaptation to changes that have occurred (e.g. willingness to care for wounds, compliance with treatment plan, verbalization of feelings of self-worth, maintenance of relationships with significant others). | 12. Supporting behaviors indicative of positive adaptation to changes encourages the client to repeat these behaviors. Repetition of adaptive behaviors facilitates the development of a positive self-concept. |
| 13. Encourage significant others to allow client to do what he/she is able. | 13. Allowing the client to do as much as he/she is able facilitates the re-establishment of independence, which enhances feelings of self-esteem. |
| 14. Encourage client contact with | 14. Feedback from others is often a |

| NURSING ACTIONS | RATIONALES |
|---|---|
| **Prevention/Treatment—*cont'd*** | |
| others if a change in appearance and body functioning has occurred. | critical factor in the development of one's self-image. When a change in appearance and/or body functioning has occurred, contact with others provides the client with the opportunity to obtain feedback, test and establish a new self-image, and begin to adapt to the changes that have occurred. |
| 15. Assist client's and significant others' adjustment by listening, facilitating communication, and providing information. | 15. Listening, facilitating communication, and providing information assist the client and significant others to cope with the present situation. Effective coping facilitates their integration of the changes that have occurred. |
| 16. Assist client and significant others to have similar expectations and understanding of future life style and to identify ways that personal and family goals can be adjusted rather than abandoned. | 16. Congruent expectations of client and significant others facilitates their working together to meet common goals. Adjustment, rather than abandonment, of personal and family goals reduces the feeling of loss and increases the probability of positive adaptation to the changes that have occurred. |
| 17. Teach client the rationale for treatments, encourage maximum participation in treatment regimen, and allow choices whenever possible. | 17. An understanding of the reasons for treatments, active participation in treatment regimen, and the opportunity to make choices on one's behalf enable the client to maintain a sense of control, which enhances his/her self-esteem. |
| 18. Encourage client to pursue usual roles and interests and to continue involvement in social activities. If previous roles, interests, and hobbies cannot be pursued, encourage development of new ones. | 18. The ability to pursue usual roles and activities has a positive effect on the client's self-esteem. The same effect can be achieved if the client is successful in new roles and activities that he/she chooses. |
| 19. Provide information about and encourage use of community agencies and support groups (e.g. vocational rehabilitation; sexual, family, individual, and/or financial counseling). | 19. Community agencies and support groups provide the opportunity for the client to see that he/she is not experiencing a unique problem, to share feelings and concerns, to profit from the experience of others with similar difficulties, and to learn new skills necessary to rebuild self-esteem. All of these factors help the client to establish a positive self-concept. |
| 20. Consult physician about psychological counseling if | 20. Psychological counseling may be necessary to facilitate |

| NURSING ACTIONS | RATIONALES |
| --- | --- |
| **Prevention/Treatment—*cont'd*** | |
| client desires or if he/she seems unwilling or unable to adapt to changes resulting from the disease process and/or its treatment. | positive adaptation to the changes in body structure and/or functioning that have occurred. |

## ❖ Nursing Diagnosis: *Skin Integrity, Impaired, High Risk for*

### Definition

A state in which the individual's skin is at risk of being adversely altered.

### Desired Outcome

The client will maintain skin integrity as evidenced by:
a. absence of redness and irritation
b. no skin breakdown.

### Documentation

a. Skin condition
b. Therapeutic interventions
c. Client teaching

| NURSING ACTIONS | RATIONALES |
| --- | --- |
| **Assessments** | |
| 1. Inspect the skin (especially bony prominences, dependent areas, pruritic areas, perineum, and areas of decreased sensation and/or edema) for pallor, redness, and breakdown. | 1. Early recognition of signs of impaired skin integrity allows for prompt intervention. |
| **Prevention** | |
| 2. Implement measures to prevent prolonged and/or excessive pressure on any area of the skin:<br>a. assist client to turn at least every 2 hours; use all four sides (prone, lateral [left/right], dorsal) unless contraindicated<br>b. instruct or assist client to shift weight at least every 30 minutes<br>c. position client properly with pads and cushions as needed<br>d. keep bed linens wrinkle-free<br>e. ensure that braces, casts, and restraints are applied properly<br>f. obtain an air-filled or air-fluidized mattress for client while he/she is immobilized. | 2. Prolonged and/or excessive pressure on a skin area obstructs capillary blood flow to that area. The resultant hypoxia, impaired flow of nutrients, and accumulation of waste products in the area of obstructed blood flow make that tissue more susceptible to breakdown. Measures that prevent the excessive pressure or ensure that pressure is relieved often enough to avoid obstruction of capillary flow help maintain skin integrity. |
| 3. Gently massage around reddened areas at least every 2 hours. | 3. Massage stimulates circulation to the skin and underlying tissues. The improved blood flow helps maintain skin integrity by increasing the supply of oxygen and nutrients available to the cells and by removing waste products of |

| NURSING ACTIONS<br>**Prevention — *cont'd*** | RATIONALES |
|---|---|
| | metabolism. To avoid damaging the capillaries, massage should be gentle rather than deep and massage over reddened areas and bony prominences should be avoided. |
| 4. Implement measures to prevent shearing: | 4. When shearing (one tissue layer sliding past another in an opposite direction) occurs, the capillaries in the affected area are kinked, stretched, or severed. This compromises the area's blood supply and increases the risk of tissue breakdown. |
| a. perform actions to keep superficial skin from adhering to the bottom sheet when client moves (e.g. apply thin layer of powder or cornstarch to bottom sheet or skin, lift and move client carefully using turn sheet and adequate assistance) | a. Keeping the superficial skin from adhering to the sheet when the client changes position ensures that all skin layers move in the same direction as the client moves. |
| b. limit length of time client is in semi-Fowler's position to 30-minute intervals. | b. A client in a semi-Fowler's position often slides down in the bed. When this occurs, his/her superficial skin tends to remain stationary while the underlying tissues and skeletal structures shift position. Limiting the length of time the client is in a semi-Fowler's position reduces the risk of shearing. |
| 5. Implement measures to reduce friction between the skin and another surface (e.g. place sheepskin under client, apply thin layer of powder or cornstarch to bottom sheet or client's skin, lift and move client carefully using turn sheet and adequate assistance). | 5. The outermost layers of skin can be damaged or removed when dragged along a rough surface such as a sheet or chair cushion. Reducing friction helps prevent skin surface abrasion. |
| 6. Keep client's skin clean. | 6. Microorganisms are present in sebum and dead skin cells. Keeping the skin clean removes many of these microorganisms, which, if allowed to accumulate, increase the risk of infection and subsequent skin breakdown. |
| 7. Implement measures to keep skin free of excessive moisture:<br>a. apply a thin layer of cornstarch to bottom sheet or skin and to opposing skin surfaces<br>b. keep bed linens dry | 7. Excessive moisture on the skin softens the epidermal cells and makes them less resistant to damage. It also harbors microorganisms that can cause infection and increases the possibility of friction between |

| NURSING ACTIONS | RATIONALES |
|---|---|
| **Prevention—*cont'd*** | |
| c. protect skin from wound drainage (e.g. change dressing when damp, apply a drainage collection device if needed). | the skin and the surface it is against. Removing excessive moisture reduces the risk of skin irritation and subsequent breakdown. |
| 8. Increase activity as allowed and tolerated. | 8. Activity stimulates circulation, which helps maintain skin integrity by increasing the flow of oxygen and nutrients to the skin and underlying tissues. In addition, increasing activity reduces the possibility of prolonged pressure on any area as a result of decreased mobility. |
| 9. Maintain an optimal nutritional status. | 9. An inadequate nutritional status results in muscle atrophy, a decrease in the amount of subcutaneous tissue, and skin that is thin and less elastic. Subsequently, the skin and tissue are more vulnerable to injury because they are less able to withstand minor trauma. In addition, a malnourished client is more susceptible to the effects of pressure because there is less padding between the skin and underlying bone. Good nutrition helps maintain a positive nitrogen balance, which reduces the risk of muscle and tissue breakdown and helps maintain skin integrity. |
| 10. Implement measures to prevent drying of the skin: | 10. Dry skin is more prone to cracking and has decreased elasticity, which makes it susceptible to damage. |
| a. encourage a fluid intake of 2500 ml/day unless contraindicated | a. An adequate fluid intake helps ensure that the skin remains well hydrated. |
| b. provide a mild soap for bathing | b. Sebum has a lubricating effect on the skin. Using a mild rather than a harsh soap allows some sebum to remain on the skin, which helps prevent dryness. |
| c. apply a moisturizing lotion and/or emollient to skin at least once a day. | c. Moisturizing lotion and some emollients provide a source of moisture to the skin. Emollients also form a protective barrier on the epidermis, which reduces the evaporation of moisture. |
| 11. Protect skin from contact with urine and feces (e.g. perform actions to prevent incontinence and/or diarrhea, keep perineal area clean and dry, apply a protective ointment or cream to perineal area). | 11. The moisture in urine and feces softens epidermal cells and increases friction between skin surfaces and between the skin and bed linen. In addition, the normal acidity of urine and the digestive |

**NURSING ACTIONS**

**Prevention—*cont'd***

**RATIONALES**

enzymes present in feces irritate the skin. Measures to control incontinence and diarrhea, remove feces and urine from skin, and protect skin from these irritants help to maintain skin integrity.

12. If edema is present, handle edematous areas carefully and implement measures to reduce fluid accumulation in dependent areas (e.g. instruct client in and assist with range of motion exercises, elevate affected extremities whenever possible).

12. Since fluid-filled cells break down more easily, it is important to handle all edematous areas carefully. In addition, circulation in edematous tissue is compromised because there is an increase in the distance between the capillaries and the cells. By reducing the fluid in the tissue, oxygen and nutrients more readily reach the skin and underlying tissue.

13. If the client is experiencing pruritus, implement measures to reduce the itching sensation (e.g. apply cool compress to pruritic area, administer prescribed antihistamines) and keep his/her nails trimmed and/or apply mittens if necessary.

13. The client experiencing pruritus is likely to scratch the affected areas, which irritates the skin and can cause excoriation. Implementing measures to reduce the itching sensation helps prevent scratching. Trimming the client's nails and/or applying mittens reduces the risk of trauma to the skin if he/she does scratch the pruritic areas.

14. Notify physician if skin breakdown occurs.

14. Notifying the physician allows for modification of treatment plan.

## ❖ Nursing Diagnosis: *Sleep Pattern Disturbance*

### Definition

Disruption of sleep time causes discomfort or interferes with desired life-style.

### Desired Outcome

The client will attain optimal amounts of sleep within the parameters of the treatment regimen as evidenced by:

a. statements of feeling well rested
b. usual mental status
c. absence of frequent yawning, dark circles under eyes, and hand tremors.

### Documentation

a. Complaints of sleep pattern disturbance
b. Mental status
c. Physical appearance and behavior indicating sleep loss
d. Therapeutic interventions
e. Client teaching

**NURSING ACTIONS**

**Assessments**

1. Assess for signs and symptoms of a sleep pattern disturbance (e.g. verbal complaints of difficulty falling asleep, sleep interruptions, or not feeling well rested; irritability;

**RATIONALES**

1. Early recognition of signs and symptoms of a sleep pattern disturbance allows for prompt intervention.

| NURSING ACTIONS | RATIONALES |
|---|---|
| **Assessments—*cont'd*** | |
| lethargy; disorientation; frequent yawning; dark circles under eyes; slight hand tremors). | |
| 2. Determine client's usual sleep habits. | 2. Knowledge of the client's usual sleep-wake cycle and the routines that help to induce and maintain his/her sleep enables the nurse to plan interventions aimed at preventing a sleep pattern disturbance. |
| **Prevention/Treatment** | |
| 3. Discourage long periods of sleep during the day unless signs and symptoms of sleep deprivation exist or daytime sleep is usual for client. | 3. A change in the client's normal sleep-wake cycle causes desynchronization of his/her circadian rhythm and can result in a poorer quality of sleep. |
| 4. Implement measures to reduce fear and anxiety (e.g. maintain a calm, confident manner when working with client; assist client to identify specific stressors and ways to cope with them). | 4. Fear and anxiety stimulate the sympathetic nervous system, which results in the release of catecholamines into the bloodstream. The subsequent increase in mental activity makes it difficult for the client to fall asleep. The increased level of catecholamines also shortens the duration of non-rapid eye movement (NREM) and rapid eye movement (REM) sleep, which results in a poorer quality of sleep. |
| 5. Encourage participation in relaxing diversional activities during the evening. | 5. Involvement in relaxing activities in the evening promotes or shortens sleep induction. |
| 6. Discourage intake of fluids high in caffeine (e.g. coffee, tea, colas), especially in the evening. | 6. Caffeine acts as a central nervous system stimulant and can interfere with relaxation and sleep induction. Caffeine also acts as a diuretic and can cause an interruption in sleep if the client awakens in response to the urge to urinate. |
| 7. Offer client a high-protein evening snack (e.g. milk, cheese, nuts) unless contraindicated. | 7. When high-protein foods/fluids such as milk, cheese, and nuts are digested, they produce the amino acid, L-tryptophan, which is believed to help induce and maintain sleep. |
| 8. Allow client to continue usual sleep practices (e.g. position, time, bedtime rituals such as reading and meditating). | 8. Adherence to usual sleep practices promotes emotional and physical relaxation that assists the client to maintain his/her usual sleep-wake cycle. |
| 9. Satisfy basic needs such as comfort and warmth before sleep. | 9. When basic needs are met, the client is better able to relax because of the reduction in mental and/or physical stimulation. This facilitates |

| NURSING ACTIONS<br>**Prevention/Treatment—*cont'd*** | RATIONALES |
|---|---|
| | sleep induction and reduces the probability of frequent awakenings. |
| 10. Have client empty bladder just before bedtime. | 10. A full bladder stimulates an urge to urinate, which can interrupt the client's sleep. Emptying the bladder just before bedtime reduces the risk of the client awakening more frequently and/or earlier than desired. |
| 11. Maintain a quiet, restful atmosphere; have sleep mask and earplugs available for client if needed. | 11. Environmental activity, noise, and light can interfere with the client's ability to fall asleep and stay asleep. Reducing the stimuli helps prevent a sleep pattern disturbance. |
| 12. Ensure good room ventilation. | 12. A well-ventilated environment promotes comfort, making it easier for the client to fall asleep and stay asleep. |
| 13. If client has orthopnea, assist him/her to assume a position that facilitates breathing (e.g. head of bed elevated with arms supported on pillows, resting forward on overbed table with good pillow support, sitting in a chair) and maintain oxygen therapy during sleep. | 13. Hypoxemia stimulates the client's arousal system and can make it difficult for him/her to fall asleep and stay asleep. The additional drop in oxygen saturation that occurs during REM sleep because of muscle relaxation and subsequent decreased breathing efforts further increases the risk of awakening during this phase of the sleep cycle. Proper positioning and administration of supplemental oxygen help ease breathing efforts and reduce hypoxemia, which facilitates sleep and reduces the number of awakenings. |
| 14. Administer sedative-hypnotics if ordered. | 14. Sedative-hypnotics are central nervous system depressants that promote sleep by reducing anxiety, shortening sleep induction, and/or reducing arousal level (wakefulness). These medications should be used for only a short time because they interfere with the length of REM sleep and can actually create a disturbance in the client's sleep-wake cycle. |
| 15. Implement measures to reduce interruptions during sleep (e.g. restrict visitors, group care whenever possible) so that client is able to sleep undisturbed for 80- to 100-minute intervals. | 15. One sleep cycle takes 80-100 minutes to complete. Each time the cycle is interrupted, it begins again with NREM stage 1 sleep so the client loses portions of NREM and/or REM sleep. When the client is deprived of NREM sleep, lethargy and depression occur. Loss of REM sleep results in irritability and anxiety. |

**NURSING ACTIONS** / **RATIONALES**

**Prevention/Treatment—*cont'd***

Reducing the frequency of sleep interruptions helps ensure that the client progresses through all of the sleep stages and is able to maintain a near-normal sleep-wake cycle.

16. Consult physician if signs and symptoms of sleep deprivation persist or worsen.

16. Notifying the physician allows for modification of treatment plan.

## ❖ Nursing Diagnosis: *Swallowing, Impaired*

### Definition

The state in which an individual has decreased ability to voluntarily pass fluids and/or solids from the mouth to the stomach.

### Desired Outcome

The client will experience an improvement in swallowing as evidenced by:

a. verbalization of same
b. absence of food in oral cavity after swallowing
c. absence of coughing and choking when eating and drinking.

### Documentation

a. Verbalization of difficulty swallowing
b. Stasis of food in oral cavity
c. Coughing or choking when eating or drinking
d. Consistency of foods/fluids client is able to swallow without difficulty
e. Therapeutic interventions
f. Client/family teaching

**NURSING ACTIONS** / **RATIONALES**

**Assessments**

1. Assess for signs and symptoms of impaired swallowing (e.g. statements of difficulty swallowing, stasis of food in oral cavity, coughing or choking when eating or drinking).

1. Early recognition of signs and symptoms of impaired swallowing allows for prompt intervention.

2. Assist with tests to evaluate client's swallowing (e.g. videofluoroscopy, manometry) if ordered.

2. Swallowing is a complex act that consists of voluntary and involuntary neuromotor components. Studies that evaluate the client's ability to swallow help identify the specific physiological dysfunction, which aids in planning effective interventions.

**Prevention/Treatment**

3. Implement measures to reduce oral and pharyngeal discomfort if indicated (e.g. instruct client to gargle with a saline solution, administer topical and/or systemic analgesics as ordered).

3. Oral and pharyngeal discomfort can interfere with the client's ability to complete the oral phase of swallowing, which includes chewing and manipulating the food/fluid toward the back, upper portion of the mouth.

4. If client has viscous oral secretions, implement

4. Thick, ropy oral secretions interfere with movement of

| NURSING ACTIONS | RATIONALES |
|---|---|
| **Prevention/Treatment—*cont'd*** | |
| measures to liquefy these secretions (e.g. encourage a fluid intake of 2500 ml/day unless contraindicated, administer a papain product before meals as ordered). | food in the mouth. Liquefying these secretions makes it easier for a bolus of food to be formed and moved to the back of the mouth. Liquefying the secretions also helps ensure that the bolus that is formed is moist so that it stays intact and triggers an effective swallowing reflex. |
| 5. If client's mouth is dry, implement measures to stimulate salivation (e.g. provide oral care before meals, give client a piece of sour candy to suck on just before meals). | 5. Saliva lubricates food and makes it easier to chew, form into a bolus, and manipulate toward the back of the mouth. A formed, moist bolus more effectively triggers the swallowing reflex and moves more easily through the cricopharyngeal juncture and the esophagus. |
| 6. Consult speech pathologist or therapist about methods for dealing with client's specific swallowing impairment. | 6. Discussing the client's specific swallowing impairment with persons who are knowledgeable about ways to manage swallowing difficulties aids in the development of a plan of care that most effectively helps improve the client's swallowing. |
| 7. Instruct and assist client to select foods/fluids that are appropriate for his/her swallowing ability. Some general guidelines include: | 7. Impaired swallowing can be a result of structural or neurological disorders. The consistency of foods and fluids a client can swallow effectively varies depending on the actual impairment. |
| a. avoiding foods that tend to fall apart in mouth (e.g. applesauce, some pureed foods) if client has impaired tongue control | a. Clients with impaired tongue movement have difficulty keeping foods that tend to fall apart in the mouth in a bolus that can be transferred to the back of the mouth. Some food may flow to the back of the mouth, but because it is not in a bolus, it will not trigger a strong swallowing reflex. |
| b. avoiding foods that are sticky (e.g. peanut butter, soft bread, bananas) | b. Sticky foods are difficult to propel through the mouth because they tend to adhere to various structures, especially the hard palate. It is also difficult to form these foods into the distinct bolus needed to trigger the swallowing reflex. |
| c. moistening dry foods with gravy or sauces (e.g. catsup, sour cream, salad dressing) | c. Moist foods are more easily formed into a bolus. The formed, moist bolus more effectively triggers the swallowing reflex and moves with greater ease |

| NURSING ACTIONS<br>**Prevention/Treatment—*cont'd*** | RATIONALES |
|---|---|
| | through the mouth and esophagus. |
| d. selecting thick rather than thin fluids or thickening thin fluids with substances such as "Thick-it," gelatin, or baby cereal if client has a delayed swallowing reflex and/or poor tongue control | d. Thin fluids are difficult to keep in a bolus and tend to pass rapidly through the mouth. As a result, they can pour over the back of the tongue without triggering an effective swallow. Thick fluids remain more cohesive and are able to stimulate the swallowing reflex more effectively. |
| e. selecting foods that have a distinct texture if sensory and/or motor function of the mouth is diminished. | e. Foods with a distinct texture stimulate the tactile receptors in the mouth and subsequently the motor responses necessary for chewing and moving the bolus to the back of the mouth. |
| 8. Place client in a high Fowler's position for meals and snacks. | 8. A high Fowler's position uses gravity to aid in the flow of foods/fluids through the cricopharyngeal juncture and the esophagus. |
| 9. Instruct and assist client to position his/her head in a manner that promotes effective swallowing when eating and drinking. For example: | 9. Proper head positioning while eating and drinking helps the client to compensate for his/her particular swallowing impairment and achieve a more normal swallow. |
| a. if client has difficulty chewing and maneuvering a bolus of food in his/her mouth, instruct him/her to tilt head down when chewing and forming a bolus, then tilt head back when ready to swallow | a. Tilting the head down allows client more time to chew and form a bolus because the food is in the front of the mouth where it does not trigger the swallowing reflex. Once the bolus is formed, tilting the head back facilitates movement of the bolus to the back of the mouth so that the swallowing reflex can be triggered. NOTE: Tilting head back is safe only if the client has normal pharyngeal and laryngeal control and is therefore unlikely to aspirate. |
| b. if client is experiencing sensory and/or motor impairment of one side of the face or mouth, instruct him/her to tilt head toward the unaffected side when eating and drinking. | b. Tilting the head toward the unaffected side helps direct food/fluid toward that side. Advantages to this are that the unaffected side:<br>1. has more effective chewing ability and better tongue movement so that a bolus is more effectively formed, maintained, and mobilized |

| NURSING ACTIONS<br>Prevention/Treatment—*cont'd* | RATIONALES |
|---|---|
| | 2. has more tension in the buccal musculature so that food/fluid is less likely to collect in the sulcus between the cheek and the mandible<br>3. is more sensitive and will trigger a stronger swallowing reflex when the bolus reaches the back of the mouth. |
| 10. Serve foods/fluids that are hot or cold instead of room temperature. | 10. Foods/fluids that are hot or cold tend to trigger a more effective swallowing reflex because they have a greater stimulatory effect on the sensory receptors in the mouth. |
| 11. Instruct and assist client to use assistive devices (e.g. long-handled spoon) to place food that does not need to be chewed in the back of his/her mouth if tongue movement is impaired. | 11. The swallowing reflex is triggered when a bolus of food is pressed against the posterior wall of the pharynx. Placing food that can be swallowed safely without chewing in the back of the mouth facilitates swallowing if the client is unable to effectively move food posteriorly with his/her tongue. |
| 12. If client has motor and sensory dysfunction of one side of the mouth or face, instruct and assist him/her to place food in the unaffected side of the mouth. | 12. If the client has unilateral weakness of the tongue and cheek muscles, food is likely to get trapped in the sulcus between the cheek and the mandible. In addition, decreased tongue movement on the affected side makes it more difficult for the client to manipulate food and move it to the back of the mouth. Placing food in the unaffected side of the mouth helps promote a more effective swallow. |
| 13. Encourage client to concentrate on the act of swallowing. | 13. The first part of the swallowing process is voluntary. By focusing on chewing and moving food/fluid to the back of the mouth so that the swallowing reflex can be triggered, the client can achieve a more effective swallow. |
| 14. Instruct client to avoid putting too much food/fluid in mouth at one time. | 14. Overfilling the mouth makes it difficult for the client to form a distinct bolus and effectively move it along in the mouth so that it triggers the swallowing reflex. |
| 15. Encourage client to perform exercises to strengthen tongue and facial muscles if indicated (e.g. drinking through a straw unless contraindicated; opening | 15. Strong tongue and facial muscles increase the client's ability to chew food, form a bolus, and direct the bolus toward the back of the mouth, |

| NURSING ACTIONS | RATIONALES |
|---|---|
| **Prevention/Treatment—*cont'd*** | |
| mouth and moving tongue anteriorly, posteriorly, and laterally; pushing tongue upward against resistance using an object such as a tongue blade, popsicle, or sucker). | where it can trigger the swallowing reflex. |
| 16. Consult physician if swallowing difficulties persist or worsen. | 16. Notifying the physician allows for modification of treatment plan. |

## ❖ Nursing Diagnosis: *Tissue Perfusion, Altered*

This section focuses on altered systemic tissue perfusion rather than any one of the types specified by NANDA in order to provide the reader with more comprehensive information.

### Definition

The state in which an individual experiences a decrease in nutrition and oxygenation at the cellular level due to a deficit in capillary blood supply.

### Desired Outcome

The client will maintain adequate systemic tissue perfusion as evidenced by:

a. B/P within normal range
b. usual mental status
c. extremities warm with absence of pallor and cyanosis
d. palpable peripheral pulses
e. capillary refill time less than 3 seconds
f. absence of exercise-induced pain
g. balanced intake and output.

### Documentation

a. Blood pressure
b. Mental status
c. Skin color and temperature
d. Peripheral pulses
e. Capillary refill time
f. Exercise-induced pain
g. Intake and output
h. Therapeutic interventions
i. Client teaching

| NURSING ACTIONS | RATIONALES |
|---|---|
| **Assessments** | |
| 1. Assess for and report signs and symptoms of diminished tissue perfusion (e.g. hypotension, restlessness, confusion, cool extremities, pallor or cyanosis of extremities, diminished or absent peripheral pulses, slow capillary refill, claudication, angina, oliguria). | 1. Early recognition and reporting of signs and symptoms of diminished tissue perfusion allow for prompt intervention. |
| **Prevention/Treatment** | |
| 2. Administer intravenous fluids and/or blood if ordered. | 2. Intravenous fluids and/or blood help maintain vascular volume, which is essential for adequate tissue perfusion. |
| 3. Maintain a minimum fluid intake of 2500 ml/day unless contraindicated. | 3. Adequate hydration is essential for maintenance of a vascular volume sufficient to maintain adequate tissue perfusion. |
| 4. Instruct client to change from a horizontal to vertical position slowly if he/she has postural hypotension. | 4. Changing from a horizontal to vertical position slowly allows time for the baroreceptors to adjust to an upright position |

**NURSING ACTIONS**

**Prevention/Treatment—*cont'd***

**RATIONALES**

and thereby helps maintain adequate blood pressure and cerebral blood flow.

5. Discourage positions such as crossing legs, pillows under knees, use of knee gatch, and sitting for long periods.

5. These positions exert pressure on vessels in the lower extremities, which compromises blood flow.

6. If client is on bed rest, instruct and assist with range of motion exercises at least 3 times/day and active foot and leg exercises every 1-2 hours. Elevate foot of bed for 20-minute intervals several times/shift unless contraindicated.

6. When a client is on bed rest, blood pools in the extremities as a result of decreased muscle activity. Range of motion exercises help reduce venous stasis. The rhythmic muscle contractions that occur during active foot and leg exercises cause intermittent compression of the veins, which improves venous return. Elevation of the lower extremities promotes venous return by gravity flow.

7. If client's activity is limited and/or venous insufficiency is a problem, consult physician about an order for elastic stockings or bandages.

7. Elastic stockings or bandages prevent venous stasis and promote venous return by exerting constant, even pressure on the tissues and vessels in the lower extremities.

8. Encourage and assist client with ambulation as soon as allowed and tolerated.

8. Ambulation causes the skeletal muscles in the lower extremities to contract. The pumping effect that this has on the deep veins promotes venous return.

9. Implement measures to improve cardiac output (e.g. administer positive inotropic agents, vasodilators, and/or antiarrhythmics if ordered; promote rest; discourage smoking) if decreased cardiac output is contributing to inadequate tissue perfusion.

9. Improved cardiac output enhances tissue perfusion by increasing arterial and venous blood flow.

10. Implement measures to prevent vasoconstriction:

10. Vasoconstriction narrows vessel lumens, which results in diminished blood flow through the affected vessels. Vasoconstriction may also increase afterload with a resultant decrease in cardiac output and systemic tissue perfusion.

   a. perform actions to reduce stress

   a. Stress stimulates the sympathetic nervous system, which results in vasoconstriction.

   b. discourage smoking

   b. Nicotine increases catecholamine output, which subsequently causes vasoconstriction.

   c. perform actions to keep client from getting cold (e.g. maintain a comfortable room temperature, provide

   c. A compensatory mechanism for body coldness is peripheral vasoconstriction (occurs as a result of

| NURSING ACTIONS | RATIONALES |
|---|---|
| **Prevention/Treatment—*cont'd*** | |
| adequate clothing and blankets). | stimulation of the posterior hypothalamic sympathetic centers). |
| 11. Consult physician if signs and symptoms of diminished tissue perfusion persist or worsen. | 11. Notifying the physician allows for modification of treatment plan. |

## ❖ Nursing Diagnosis: *Urinary Elimination, Altered: Incontinence*

NANDA identifies five types of urinary incontinence. A client can experience a combination of types of incontinence and the actions for various types often are similar. The information presented here focuses on incontinence in general rather than a specific type.

### Definition

The state in which the individual experiences an involuntary loss or passage of urine.

### Desired Outcome

The client will experience urinary continence.

### Documentation

a. Episodes of incontinence
b. Statements of being unable to control urinary elimination
c. Therapeutic interventions
d. Client teaching

| NURSING ACTIONS | RATIONALES |
|---|---|
| **Assessments** | |
| 1. Assess for and report urinary incontinence. | 1. Early recognition and reporting of urinary incontinence allow for prompt intervention. |
| 2. Assist with urodynamic studies (e.g. cystometrogram) if ordered. | 2. Urodynamic studies may be done to determine the cause(s) of urinary incontinence. The studies provide information about bladder filling, capacity, and emptying. |
| **Prevention/Treatment** | |
| 3. Offer bedpan or urinal or assist client to commode or bathroom every 2-3 hours if indicated. | 3. A client who is unaware of or unable to respond to the urge to urinate experiences incontinence when the pressure within the bladder becomes greater than the pressure exerted by the urinary sphincters. Routinely emptying the bladder before the pressure becomes too great reduces the risk of incontinence. |
| 4. Allow client to assume a normal position for voiding (usually sitting for females and standing for males) unless contraindicated. | 4. A sitting or standing position uses gravity to facilitate bladder emptying. The more completely the bladder is emptied, the less risk there is of incontinence. |
| 5. Provide easy access to bathroom and assist client to | 5. If client is having difficulty controlling urination, any delay |

| NURSING ACTIONS | RATIONALES |
|---|---|
| **Prevention/Treatment—*cont'd*** | |
| select clothing that is easy to remove (e.g. pajamas with Velcro closures or elastic waistband). | in getting to the bathroom and removing clothing so he/she can urinate increases the risk of incontinence. |
| 6. Instruct client to perform perineal exercises (e.g. stopping and starting stream during voiding; squeezing buttocks together, then relaxing the muscles) unless contraindicated. | 6. Perineal exercises help strengthen the periurethral and pelvic muscles. As the strength of these muscles improves, the closing force of the external urinary sphincter increases and the risk of incontinence decreases. |
| 7. Instruct client to space fluids evenly throughout the day rather than drinking a large quantity at one time. | 7. Drinking a large amount of fluid at one time results in rapid filling of the bladder. This increases bladder pressure and the subsequent risk of incontinence. |
| 8. Limit oral fluid intake in the evening. | 8. As the client's bladder fills and bladder pressure increases during sleep, he/she is less likely to be aware of and/or able to respond to the urge to urinate. By limiting fluid intake in the evening, bladder filling during the night is decreased, which reduces the risk of incontinence. |
| 9. Instruct client to avoid drinking beverages containing caffeine such as colas, coffee, and tea. | 9. Caffeine increases urine formation because of its mild diuretic effect. As the amount of urine increases, pressure in the bladder rises and the risk of incontinence increases. |
| 10. Administer the following medications if ordered: | |
| a. cholinergics (e.g. bethanechol) | 10. a. If incontinence results from incomplete bladder emptying, cholinergic drugs may be prescribed to stimulate contraction of the detrusor muscle. This enhances bladder emptying and reduces the risk of incontinence. |
| b. muscle relaxants (e.g. oxybutynin chloride, flavoxate hydrochloride, baclofen) and/or sympathomimetic agents (e.g. ephedrine). | b. Hyperactivity of the bladder muscle can cause a sudden increase in pressure in the bladder and result in incontinence, especially if there is decreased bladder outlet resistance. Muscle relaxants may be prescribed to reduce detrusor muscle activity and thereby reduce the risk of incontinence. If decreased bladder outlet resistance is contributing to the incontinence, sympathomimetic agents may be given to increase the tone of the urinary sphincters. |

**NURSING ACTIONS** / **RATIONALES**

**Prevention/Treatment—*cont'd***

11. Consult physician if urinary incontinence persists.

11. Notifying the physician allows for modification of treatment plan.

## ❖ Nursing Diagnosis: *Urinary Retention*

### Definition

The state in which the individual experiences incomplete emptying of the bladder.

### Desired Outcome

The client will not experience urinary retention as evidenced by:
a. voiding at normal intervals
b. no complaints of bladder fullness and suprapubic discomfort
c. absence of bladder distention and dribbling of urine
d. balanced intake and output.

### Documentation

a. Frequency of urination and amount voided each time
b. Complaints of bladder fullness and/or suprapubic discomfort
c. Bladder distention
d. Evidence or statements of dribbling of urine
e. Intake and output
f. Therapeutic interventions
g. Patency of urinary catheter if present
h. Client teaching

**NURSING ACTIONS** / **RATIONALES**

**Assessments**

1. Assess for signs and symptoms of urinary retention:
   a. frequent voiding of small amounts (25-60 ml) of urine
   b. complaints of bladder fullness or suprapubic discomfort
   c. bladder distention
   d. dribbling of urine
   e. output less than intake.

1. Early recognition of signs and symptoms of urinary retention allows for prompt intervention.

2. Assist with urodynamic studies (e.g. cystometrogram) if ordered.

2. Urodynamic studies may be indicated when neurogenic dysfunction is the suspected cause of urinary retention. The studies provide information about bladder filling, capacity, and emptying.

**Prevention/Treatment**

3. Instruct client to urinate when the urge is first felt.

3. As the bladder fills, its stretch receptors periodically stimulate the micturition center in the sacral portion of the spinal cord. Parasympathetic impulses then cause the detrusor muscle (smooth muscle of the bladder) to contract, the internal sphincter relaxes, and urine enters the urethra. If the client allows the reflex to continue, the perineal muscles and the external urinary sphincter relax and voiding occurs. If he/she feels the urge to urinate and

| NURSING ACTIONS<br>**Prevention/Treatment—*cont'd*** | RATIONALES |
|---|---|
| | does not allow the reflex to continue, voiding will not occur and the urge to urinate disappears until the bladder fills more. If the bladder fills too much or is chronically distended, the stretch receptors become less sensitive and subsequently do not effectively stimulate micturition when the bladder fills. |
| 4. Implement measures to promote relaxation during voiding attempts (e.g. provide privacy, play soft music, encourage client to read). | 4. When the client is relaxed, he/she is better able to relax the perineal muscles and external urinary sphincter and allow voiding to occur. |
| 5. If client is having difficulty voiding, run water, place his/her hands in warm water, and/or pour warm water over his/her perineum unless contraindicated. | 5. These measures facilitate voiding by providing sensory stimulation, which helps trigger the micturition reflex. The measures also promote voluntary relaxation of the perineal muscles and external urinary sphincter. |
| 6. Allow client to assume a normal position for voiding (usually sitting for females and standing for males) unless contraindicated. | 6. A sitting or standing position uses gravity to facilitate bladder emptying. Allowing the client to assume a normal voiding position also promotes relaxation, which facilitates voiding. |
| 7. Instruct client to lean his/her upper body forward and/or gently press downward on the lower abdomen when attempting to void unless contraindicated. | 7. Leaning forward or gently pressing downward on the lower abdomen increases pressure on the bladder. This pressure helps create a sensation of bladder fullness, which stimulates the micturition reflex. |
| 8. Instruct client to perform the Valsalva maneuver during urination unless contraindicated. | 8. An increase in intra-abdominal pressure may increase the sensation of bladder fullness and subsequently stimulate the micturition reflex. This increase in pressure also promotes more complete bladder emptying provided urinary sphincters are relaxed. |
| 9. Administer cholinergic drugs (e.g. bethanechol) if ordered. | 9. Cholinergic drugs promote urination by stimulating contraction of the detrusor muscle. |
| 10. If an indwelling urinary catheter is present, implement measures to ensure its patency (e.g. keep tubing free of kinks, keep collection bag below bladder level, irrigate catheter if clots or sediment are present or urine output is declining). | 10. Maintaining patency of the indwelling catheter prevents urinary retention. |
| 11. Consult physician if signs and symptoms of urinary retention persist. | 11. Notifying the physician allows for modification of treatment plan. |

UNIT
# III

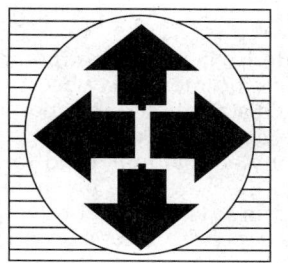

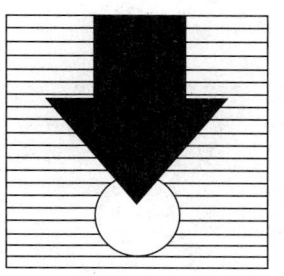

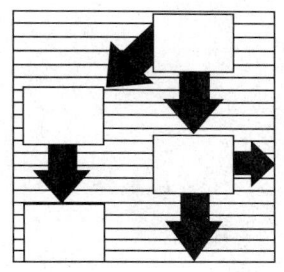

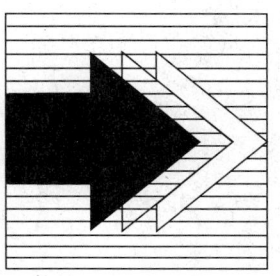

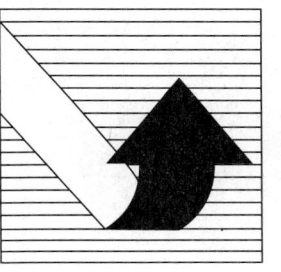

# *Nursing Care of the Elderly Client*

# The Elderly Client

The elderly client is a common recipient of health care in the United States today because of the marked shift in the age distribution of the population. Older persons are in the final stage of development, the stage during which many adaptations need to be made by the client because of the inevitable physiological changes that occur with aging. The extent or degree of the changes that take place depends on genetic and environmental factors as well as on the client's previous attention to health maintenance. As a client reaches old age, there may also be many changes in roles, relationships, and ability to maintain his/her usual life style. These factors create certain psychosocial concerns that need to be addressed.

**This care plan focuses on the elderly client hospitalized for management of a medical-surgical condition.** It includes the nursing diagnoses that reflect the biopsychosocial changes that commonly occur with old age and are intensified with the stressors of an acute illness and hospitalization. **This care plan should be used in conjunction with the appropriate medical and/or surgical care plans in this text.**

**NURSING/ COLLABORATIVE DIAGNOSES**

## 1. NURSING DIAGNOSIS: Altered tissue perfusion

related to:
a. decreased cardiac output associated with:
   1. age-related decrease in contractile strength and reduced compliance of the myocardium
   2. increased cardiac workload resulting from an increase in vascular resistance, thickened and rigid cardiac valves, and stress of current illness;
b. increased vascular resistance associated with loss of elasticity and narrowing of vessels resulting from degeneration of elastin, changes in collagen deposition, and accumulation of substances such as calcium and lipids;
c. decrease in baroreceptor sensitivity;
d. peripheral pooling of blood associated with venous dilation and loss of muscle tone in extremities.

| Desired Outcome | Nursing Actions and ***Selected Purposes/Rationales*** |
|---|---|
| 1. The client will maintain adequate tissue perfusion as evidenced by:<br>a. B/P within normal range for client<br>b. usual mental status<br>c. absence of vertigo and syncope<br>d. extremities warm with absence of pallor and cyanosis<br>e. palpable peripheral pulses<br>f. capillary refill time less than 3 seconds<br>g. BUN and serum creatinine within normal limits for an elderly client<br>h. balanced intake and output<br>i. absence of exercise-induced pain. | 1.a. Assess for and report signs and symptoms of:<br>1. decreased cardiac output (can lead to diminished tissue perfusion):<br>a. variations in B/P (may be increased because of compensatory vasoconstriction; may be decreased when compensatory mechanisms and pump fail)<br>b. irregular pulse (the incidence of arrhythmias increases with age and is of concern *because of the coexisting decrease in cardiac reserve*)<br>c. increase in loudness of existing systolic murmurs or presence of diastolic murmur (soft systolic murmurs are often present in elderly clients *because of sclerosed valves*)<br>d. development of or an increase in loudness of $S_3$ and/or $S_4$ gallop rhythm (an $S_4$ can be present in a healthy elderly client)<br>e. development of or increase in fatigue and weakness<br>f. development of or increase in dyspnea<br>g. increased crackles (crackles in the morning are a common finding in an elderly client)<br>h. peripheral edema<br>i. jugular vein distention (JVD)<br>j. abnormal ECG readings (expected age-related changes include left axis deviation, some prolongation of all conduction intervals, and lower voltage of waves)<br>k. chest x-ray results showing cardiomegaly, pleural effusion, or pulmonary edema<br>2. diminished tissue perfusion:<br>a. significant decrease in B/P (elevated systolic and diastolic pressures are often present in elderly clients *because of increased rigidity of the aorta and a generalized increase in peripheral vascular resistance*)<br>b. decline in systolic B/P of greater than 20 mm Hg when client changes from a lying to sitting or standing position (in an elderly client, there is often a decline in systolic B/P of 15-20 mm Hg with this position change *because of a decrease in baroreceptor sensitivity*)<br>c. restlessness, confusion<br>d. vertigo, syncope<br>e. cool, pale, or cyanotic skin<br>f. diminished or absent peripheral pulses<br>g. capillary refill time greater than 3 seconds<br>h. elevated BUN and serum creatinine (BUN and serum creatinine tend to be slightly elevated *because of the age-related decline in renal function*)<br>i. oliguria<br>j. claudication<br>k. angina. |

| Desired Outcome | Nursing Actions and ***Selected Purposes/Rationales*** |
|---|---|

b. Implement measures *to maintain adequate tissue perfusion:*
   1. perform actions *to reduce cardiac workload and help maintain an adequate cardiac output:*
      a. maintain client in a semi- to high Fowler's position unless contraindicated
      b. instruct client to avoid activities that create a Valsalva response (e.g. straining to have a bowel movement, holding breath while moving) *in order to prevent the marked increase in venous return and preload that occurs with exhalation*
      c. implement measures to promote rest and conserve energy (see Nursing Diagnosis 9, action b.1)
      d. implement measures to maintain an adequate respiratory status (see Nursing Diagnosis 2, action c) *in order to promote adequate tissue oxygenation*
      e. discourage smoking *(smoking has a cardiostimulatory effect, causes vasoconstriction, and reduces oxygen availability)*
      f. discourage excessive intake of beverages high in caffeine such as coffee, tea, and colas *(caffeine is a myocardial stimulant and increases myocardial oxygen consumption)*
      g. increase activity gradually
   2. maintain a fluid intake of 1500-2000 ml/day unless contraindicated; if oral intake is inadequate or contraindicated, maintain intravenous fluid therapy as ordered (be alert to the greater risk for fluid overload in the elderly client *because of the age-related decline in the kidney's ability to excrete large volumes of water in response to sudden volume excess)*
   3. perform actions *to reduce peripheral pooling of blood and increase venous return:*
      a. instruct client in and assist with active foot and leg exercises every 1-2 hours during periods of decreased activity
      b. consult physician about order for elastic stockings or bandages; if applied, make sure they are not applied too tightly and remove for 30-60 minutes at least twice daily
      c. if client is on bed rest, elevate foot of bed for 20-minute intervals several times a shift unless contraindicated
      d. encourage ambulation as allowed and tolerated
   4. instruct and assist client to change from a horizontal to vertical position slowly *in order to allow time for autoregulatory mechanisms to adjust to upright position*
   5. discourage positions that compromise blood flow in lower extremities (e.g. crossing legs, pillow under knees, use of knee gatch, sitting for long periods, prolonged standing)
   6. maintain a comfortable room temperature and provide client with adequate clothing and blankets *(exposure to cold causes generalized vasoconstriction).*

c. Consult physician if signs and symptoms of diminished tissue perfusion persist or worsen.

## 2. NURSING DIAGNOSIS: Impaired respiratory function:*

a. **ineffective breathing pattern** related to:
   1. loss of alveolar elasticity (results in reduced efficiency of air expulsion)
   2. decreased chest expansion associated with calcification of costal cartilage and weakened respiratory muscles

* This diagnostic label includes the following nursing diagnoses: ineffective breathing pattern, ineffective airway clearance, and impaired gas exchange.

3. decreased responsiveness of chemoreceptors to hypoxia and hypercapnea;

b. **ineffective airway clearance** related to stasis of secretions associated with decreased activity and an age-related decrease in ciliary activity and cough effectiveness;

c. **impaired gas exchange** related to:
   1. loss of effective lung surface associated with secretion accumulation and changes in alveolar walls and septal tissue
   2. reduced airflow associated with loss of alveolar elasticity, restricted chest expansion, and premature closure of small airways
   3. decreased pulmonary blood flow (especially in bases) associated with a generalized decrease in tissue perfusion.

| Desired Outcome | Nursing Actions and ***Selected Purposes/Rationales*** |
|---|---|
| 2. The client will experience adequate respiratory function as evidenced by:<br>a. normal rate, rhythm, and depth of respirations<br>b. absence of dyspnea<br>c. usual or improved breath sounds<br>d. usual mental status<br>e. usual skin color<br>f. blood gases within normal range for an elderly client. | 2.a. Assess for and report signs and symptoms of impaired respiratory function:<br>1. rapid, shallow, slow, or irregular respirations<br>2. dyspnea, orthopnea<br>3. use of accessory muscles when breathing<br>4. adventitious breath sounds (e.g. crackles [rales], rhonchi); crackles may be heard, especially on initial morning assessment, *as a result of some alveolar collapse associated with age and decreased activity*<br>5. diminished or absent breath sounds (diminished sounds are often present in the elderly client *because of reduced airflow)*<br>6. restlessness, irritability<br>7. confusion, somnolence<br>8. central cyanosis (a late sign).<br>b. Monitor for and report the following:<br>1. abnormal blood gases ($PaO_2$ is normally lower in the elderly client)<br>2. significant changes in oximetry results (oxygen saturation is normally lower in the elderly client)<br>3. abnormal chest x-ray results.<br>c. Implement measures *to maintain an adequate respiratory status:*<br>1. place client in a semi- to high Fowler's position unless contraindicated; position with pillows *to prevent slumping*<br>2. assist client to turn from side to side every 2 hours while in bed<br>3. instruct client to deep breathe or use incentive spirometer at least every 2 hours<br>4. instruct client in and assist with diaphragmatic (abdominal) and pursed-lip breathing techniques if indicated<br>5. perform actions *to facilitate removal of pulmonary secretions:*<br>a. instruct and assist client to cough or "huff" every 1-2 hours<br>b. implement measures *to liquefy secretions:*<br>1. maintain a fluid intake of 1500-2000 ml/day unless contraindicated<br>2. humidify inspired air as ordered<br>c. if client has difficulty mobilizing secretions:<br>1. assist with or perform postural drainage, percussion, and vibration if ordered<br>2. consult physician about use of a diluent or mucolytic agent via nebulizer or IPPB<br>3. suction as needed<br>6. assist with IPPB treatments if ordered<br>7. discourage smoking *(smoke causes bronchoconstriction, increases mucus production, further impairs ciliary function, and decreases oxygen availability)*<br>8. maintain oxygen therapy as ordered<br>9. instruct client to avoid intake of gas-forming foods (e.g. beans, cabbage, cauliflower, onions), carbonated beverages, and large meals *in order to prevent gastric distention and pressure on the diaphragm* |

| Desired Outcome | Nursing Actions and ***Selected Purposes/Rationales*** |
|---|---|
| | 10. maintain activity restrictions as ordered; increase activity gradually as allowed and tolerated<br>11. administer central nervous system depressants judiciously *because of their respiratory depressant effects* (the possibility of respiratory depression is increased in elderly clients *because of their altered metabolism, distribution, and excretion of drugs and decreased responsiveness of chemoreceptors to hypoxia and hypercapnea)*; hold medication and consult physician if respiratory rate is less than 12/minute.<br>d. Consult physician if signs and symptoms of impaired respiratory function persist or worsen. |

## 3. NURSING DIAGNOSIS: High risk for fluid volume deficit

related to:

a. age-related decrease in total body water;
b. decreased fluid intake associated with:
   1. restrictions imposed by current illness and/or treatment plan
   2. diminished thirst sensation
   3. desire to avoid nocturia and/or urinary incontinence;
c. age-related decline in kidney's ability to conserve water when a deficit is caused by disease or environmental factors.

| Desired Outcome | Nursing Actions and ***Selected Purposes/Rationales*** |
|---|---|
| 3. The client will not experience a fluid volume deficit as evidenced by:<br>a. normal skin and tongue turgor for client<br>b. moist mucous membranes<br>c. weight loss no greater than 0.5 kg/day<br>d. B/P and pulse within normal range for client with no further increase in postural hypotension<br>e. small vein filling time less than 3-5 seconds<br>f. BUN and Hct within normal range for age<br>g. usual mental status<br>h. balanced intake and output<br>i. urine specific gravity within normal range. | 3.a. Assess for and report signs and symptoms of fluid volume deficit:<br>1. decreased skin turgor (not always a reliable indicator *because decreased skin turgor is a normal age-related change;* turgor is best assessed over the forehead or sternum in an elderly client)<br>2. decreased tongue turgor (the tongue will be smaller than usual and have more than one longitudinal furrow)<br>3. dry mucous membranes, thirst (may not be reliable indicators *because saliva production and sensation of thirst are diminished in elderly clients)*<br>4. weight loss greater than 0.5 kg/day<br>5. low B/P and/or decline in systolic B/P of greater than 20 mm Hg when client sits up (not a reliable indicator of fluid volume unless compared with client's baseline B/P *because postural hypotension often occurs in elderly clients)*<br>6. weak, rapid pulse<br>7. delayed small vein filling time (longer than 3-5 seconds)<br>8. elevated BUN and Hct<br>9. confusion<br>10. decreased urine output with increased specific gravity (reflects an actual rather than potential fluid volume deficit).<br>b. Implement measures *to prevent fluid volume deficit:*<br>1. maintain a fluid intake of 1500-2000 ml/day and instruct client to adhere to this regimen following discharge unless contraindicated<br>2. maintain intravenous fluid therapy if ordered (administer intravenous fluids cautiously *because the elderly client is also at risk for fluid overload).* |

## 4. NURSING DIAGNOSIS: Altered nutrition: less than body requirements

related to:
a. decreased oral intake associated with:
   1. anorexia resulting from factors such as depression, loneliness, diminished sense of smell and/or taste, early satiety, and dyspepsia
   2. difficulty chewing and swallowing food resulting from poor dentition, a decreased amount of saliva, and weakened chewing and swallowing muscles
   3. decreased ability to purchase and/or prepare healthy foods;
b. decreased utilization of nutrients associated with impaired digestion resulting from:
   1. decreased ability to chew foods thoroughly
   2. reduced secretion of digestive enzymes (e.g. salivary ptyalin, hydrochloric acid, pepsin, lipase);
c. reduced absorption of nutrients associated with hypochlorhydria and atrophy of the absorptive surface of the intestine.

| Desired Outcome | Nursing Actions and ***Selected Purposes/Rationales*** |
|---|---|
| 4. The client will maintain an adequate nutritional status as evidenced by:<br>a. weight within normal range for client's age, height, and body frame<br>b. normal serum albumin, Hct, Hb, and lymphocyte levels for client's age<br>c. usual strength and activity tolerance<br>d. healthy oral mucous membrane. | 4.a. Assess for and report signs and symptoms of malnutrition:<br>1. weight below normal for client's age, height, and body frame; when using height and weight charts, be aware that weight is expected to decline gradually with age<br>2. low serum albumin, Hct, Hb, and lymphocyte levels<br>3. weakness and fatigue<br>4. stomatitis.<br>b. Monitor percentage of meals and snacks client consumes. Report a pattern of inadequate intake.<br>c. Implement measures *to maintain an adequate nutritional status:*<br>1. perform actions *to improve oral intake:*<br>a. implement measures to relieve dyspepsia, gastric fullness, and gas pain (see Nursing Diagnosis 5, action c)<br>b. increase activity as allowed and tolerated *(activity stimulates appetite and promotes gastric emptying, which reduces feeling of gastric fullness)*<br>c. obtain a dietary consult if necessary to assist client in selecting foods/fluids that meet nutritional needs as well as personal and cultural preferences whenever possible<br>d. maintain a clean environment and a relaxed, pleasant atmosphere<br>e. provide oral care before meals<br>f. serve small portions of nutritious foods/fluids that are appealing to client (visual appeal is especially important if sense of smell is diminished)<br>g. encourage significant others to bring in client's favorite foods unless contraindicated and eat with him/her *to make eating more of a familiar social experience*<br>h. if client has dentures, assist him/her to put them in before meals; if dentures do not fit properly, consult physician about referral to a dentist<br>i. provide a soft, ground, or pureed diet if client has difficulty chewing<br>j. implement measures *to compensate for taste alterations and/or dislike of prescribed diet:*<br>1. serve foods warm *to stimulate sense of smell*<br>2. encourage client to experiment with different flavorings and seasonings<br>3. instruct client to use salt substitutes and salt-free herbs and spices if he/she is on low-sodium diet |

| Desired Outcome | Nursing Actions and ***Selected Purposes/Rationales*** |
|---|---|
| | 4. encourage client to add extra sweeteners to foods unless contraindicated<br>k. limit fluid intake (unless it has a high nutritional value) with meals *to reduce early satiety and subsequent decreased food intake*<br>l. allow adequate time for meals; reheat food if necessary<br>2. ensure that meals are well balanced and high in essential nutrients; offer high-protein supplements between meals if client is having difficulty maintaining an adequate caloric intake<br>3. administer vitamins and minerals if ordered.<br>d. Perform a 72-hour calorie count if ordered. Report totals to dietitian and physician.<br>e. Consult physician regarding alternative methods of providing nutrition (e.g. parenteral nutrition, tube feedings) if client does not consume enough food or fluids to meet nutritional needs. |

## 5. NURSING DIAGNOSIS: Altered comfort: dyspepsia, gastric fullness, and/or gas pain

related to:
a. irritation of esophageal and gastric mucosa associated with thinning of esophageal and gastric linings;
b. impaired digestion of many foods associated with reduced secretion of digestive enzymes (e.g. hydrochloric acid, pepsin, lipase);
c. delayed esophageal and gastric emptying associated with altered lower esophageal sphincter pressure and decreased gastroesophageal motility;
d. accumulation of intestinal gas associated with decreased peristalsis.

| Desired Outcome | Nursing Actions and ***Selected Purposes/Rationales*** |
|---|---|
| 5. The client will experience diminished dyspepsia, gastric fullness, and gas pain as evidenced by:<br>a. verbalization of same<br>b. relaxed facial expression and body positioning<br>c. diminished eructation. | 5.a. Assess for verbal complaints of indigestion, fullness, or gas pain.<br>b. Assess for nonverbal signs of dyspepsia, gastric fullness, or gas pain (e.g. grimacing, clutching and guarding of abdomen, rubbing epigastric area, restlessness, reluctance to move, frequent eructation, reluctance to eat).<br>c. Implement measures *to reduce dyspepsia, gastric fullness, and gas pain:*<br>1. perform actions *to reduce gastroesophageal reflux:*<br>a. provide small, frequent meals rather than 3 large ones<br>b. instruct client to ingest foods and fluids slowly<br>c. maintain client in high Fowler's position during and for at least 30 minutes after meals and snacks<br>2. instruct client to avoid the following foods/fluids:<br>a. those that may irritate the gastroesophageal mucosa (e.g. spicy foods; citrus fruits and juices; caffeine-containing beverages such as coffee, tea, and colas)<br>b. those that are hard to digest (e.g. fried foods)<br>3. perform actions *to reduce accumulation of gas and fluid in gastrointestinal tract:*<br>a. encourage and assist client with frequent position changes and ambulation as allowed and tolerated *(activity stimulates peristalsis and expulsion of flatus)*<br>b. instruct client to avoid activities such as gum-chewing and smoking *in order to reduce air swallowing*<br>c. encourage client to drink warm liquids *in order to stimulate peristalsis* |

d. instruct client to avoid intake of carbonated beverages and gas-producing foods (e.g. cabbage, onions, beans)
e. encourage client to eructate and expel flatus whenever the urge is felt

4. administer the following medications if ordered:
   a. antacids and cytoprotective agents (e.g. sucralfate) *to protect the gastroesophageal mucosa*
   b. antiflatulents (e.g. simethicone) *to reduce gas accumulation*
   c. gastrointestinal stimulants (e.g. metoclopramide, biscodyl) *to increase gastrointestinal motility.*

d. Consult physician if signs and symptoms of dyspepsia, gastric fullness, or gas pain persist or worsen.

## 6. NURSING DIAGNOSIS: Sensory/perceptual alterations:

a. **visual** related to lens opacity and yellowing; loss of ability of lens to accommodate; change in the consistency of the vitreous humor; decreased pupil size; changes in the cornea, macula, and retina; and reduced ocular muscle function;
b. **auditory** related to degenerative changes in sensorineural and conduction pathways in the ear and cerumen accumulation;
c. **gustatory** related to a diminished sense of smell and possible atrophy of the taste buds (there is only a modest, quality-specific loss of taste in healthy elderly clients);
d. **olfactory** related to a decline in olfactory nerve function and a decreased number of sensory cells in the nasal lining;
e. **kinesthetic** related to a decreased central nervous system response to vestibular and kinesthetic stimuli;
f. **tactile** related to changes in the skin and a decreased number of nerve endings in the fingertips, palms, and lower extremities.

| Desired Outcome | Nursing Actions and ***Selected Purposes/Rationales*** |
|---|---|
| 6. The client will demonstrate adaptation to altered sensory/perceptual function as evidenced by:<br>a. appropriate verbal and nonverbal responses<br>b. expected level of participation in self-care activities and treatment plan<br>c. safe responses to environmental stimuli. | 6.a. Assess client for the following:<br>1. vision changes (e.g. statements of decreased visual acuity, altered depth perception, inability to adjust to changes in lighting, increased sensitivity to glare, or altered color perception; overreaching or underreaching for objects)<br>2. decreased auditory ability (e.g. verbal complaints of not being able to hear or understand what others are saying, inappropriate responses to auditory stimuli, irritability, increased volume of speech, staring at other person's lips during conversation, moving closer to others when they speak)<br>3. altered taste and smell (e.g. statements of same, decreased food intake, heavy use of sugar or seasonings)<br>4. diminished kinesthetic sense (e.g. unsteadiness on feet, swaying, uncoordinated movements)<br>5. diminished tactile sensation (e.g. statements of diminished feeling in extremities, holding or touching very hot objects, use of heating pad at higher than expected temperatures).<br>b. If client's vision is impaired:<br>1. provide adequate lighting in room at all times |

| Desired Outcome | Nursing Actions and ***Selected Purposes/Rationales*** |
|---|---|

2. avoid bright lighting and provide incandescent rather than fluorescent lighting *(opacities in the lens create an intense glare in bright light)*
3. avoid sudden changes in light intensity *(elderly clients often adjust more slowly to changes in lighting)*
4. reduce the glare from windows by partially closing blinds or curtains
5. use a red night light *to facilitate adaptation to a darkened environment and improve night vision*
6. provide large-print reading material if available
7. keep frequently used items within the visual field *(the visual field narrows with aging)*
8. encourage client to wear his/her glasses; make sure glasses are clean
9. provide auditory rather than visual diversionary activities if indicated
10. inform client of resources available if he/she desires additional information about visual aids (e.g. American Foundation for the Blind, publications such as Aids for the Blind)
11. assist with activities such as filling out menus and reading mail and legal documents as needed.

c. If client's hearing is impaired:
   1. assess auditory canal for excessive cerumen accumulation; if present, consult physician regarding removal of ear wax
   2. implement measures *to facilitate communication:*
      a. provide adequate lighting in room *so client can read lips and see facial expressions and gestures*
      b. reduce environmental noise
      c. get client's attention (e.g. touch his/her shoulder, stand within visual field) before beginning conversation
      d. remind client to use his/her hearing aid; ensure that it is functioning well, positioned correctly, and free of cerumen
      e. face client and stay within 3-6 feet of him/her while speaking
      f. avoid chewing gum, eating, and covering mouth while talking to client
      g. lower tone of voice, speak slightly louder than usual, and avoid talking rapidly
      h. avoid lowering voice at end of sentences
      i. use simple sentences
      j. articulate clearly but avoid overenunciation of words
      k. rephrase sentences if client does not understand what is being said
      l. employ related nonverbal cues such as facial expressions or gestures when appropriate
      m. use alternative forms of communication (e.g. word cards, paper and pencil, magic slate) if indicated
      n. respond to client's call signal in person rather than over intercommunication system
   3. encourage client to have an audiometric examination if indicated; provide client and significant others with information about available resources (e.g. audiologists, local chapter of hearing association).

d. Implement measures to compensate for taste alterations if present (see Nursing Diagnosis 4, action c.1.j).

e. Implement measures to prevent burns (see Nursing Diagnosis 16, action a.2) if client has diminished tactile sensation.

f. Implement measures to reduce the risk for falls (see Nursing Diagnosis 16, action a.1) if client's vision and/or sense of position or balance seems impaired.

g. Instruct client and significant others in above methods of adapting to sensory/perceptual alterations.

h. Consult physician if sensory/perceptual alterations worsen.

## 7. NURSING DIAGNOSIS: High risk for impaired skin integrity

related to:
a. increased fragility of the skin associated with decreased nutritional status and age-related dryness, loss of elasticity, and thinning of skin;
b. frequent contact with irritants if urinary incontinence is present;
c. ischemia of the skin and subcutaneous tissue associated with decreased tissue perfusion and prolonged pressure on tissues if mobility is decreased (ischemia resulting from pressure occurs more readily in elderly clients because they have a decreased amount of subcutaneous fat).

| Desired Outcome | Nursing Actions and ***Selected Purposes/Rationales*** |
|---|---|
| 7. The client will maintain skin integrity as evidenced by:<br>a. absence of redness and irritation<br>b. no skin breakdown. | 7.a. Inspect the skin (especially bony prominences, dependent areas, edematous areas, and perineum) for pallor, redness, and breakdown.<br>b. Implement measures *to prevent skin breakdown:*<br>1. assist client to turn at least every 2 hours (elderly clients may require more frequent position change *because of decreased tissue perfusion and reduced amounts of protective subcutaneous fat)*<br>2. gently massage around reddened areas at least every 2 hours<br>3. perform actions *to prevent shearing* (shearing occurs when one tissue layer slides past another) *and skin surface abrasion:*<br>a. apply a thin layer of powder or cornstarch to bottom sheet or skin *to absorb moisture (moist skin is more likely to adhere to sheet) and reduce friction*<br>b. lift and move client carefully using a turn sheet and adequate assistance<br>c. limit length of time client is in semi-Fowler's position to 30 minutes *(in this position, client tends to slide down in bed)*<br>4. instruct or assist client to shift weight every 30 minutes<br>5. if fade time (length of time it takes for reddened area to fade after pressure is removed) is greater than 15 minutes, increase frequency of position changes and provide more effective methods of cushioning, padding, and positioning<br>6. keep skin clean and dry<br>7. keep bed linens dry and wrinkle-free<br>8. apply a thin layer of powder or cornstarch to areas with opposing skin surfaces (e.g. axillae, perineum, beneath breasts) if indicated *to absorb moisture and/or reduce friction*<br>9. provide devices to reduce pressure on the skin, decrease shearing, and/or prevent moisture build-up (e.g. alternating pressure mattress or pad, sheepskin, elbow and heel protectors)<br>10. encourage client to wear socks while in bed *(helps reduce friction on heels)*<br>11. increase activity as allowed and tolerated<br>12. perform actions *to reduce dryness of the skin:*<br>a. avoid use of harsh soaps and hot water; use superfatted soap and tepid water for bathing<br>b. apply moisturizing lotion and/or emollient to skin at least once a day<br>c. assist client with total bath or shower every other day rather than daily<br>d. encourage a fluid intake of 1500-2000 ml/day unless contraindicated |

| Desired Outcome | Nursing Actions and ***Selected Purposes/Rationales*** |
|---|---|
| | 13. perform actions *to prevent skin irritation resulting from urinary incontinence:*<br>a. implement measures to reduce episodes of urinary incontinence (see Nursing Diagnosis 12, action e.2)<br>b. assist client to thoroughly cleanse and dry perineal area with soft tissue or cloth after each episode of incontinence; apply a protective ointment or cream (e.g. Desitin, A & D ointment, Vaseline)<br>c. provide incontinence pads if needed to absorb moisture; do not allow skin to come in contact with plastic portion of the pads<br>14. use caution with application of heat or cold to areas of decreased sensation or circulatory impairment<br>15. perform actions to maintain an adequate nutritional status (see Nursing Diagnosis 4, action c)<br>16. perform actions to maintain adequate tissue perfusion (see Nursing Diagnosis 1, action b).<br>c. If skin breakdown occurs:<br>1. notify physician<br>2. continue with above measures to prevent further irritation and breakdown<br>3. perform decubitus care as ordered or per standard hospital procedure<br>4. assess client closely and report signs and symptoms of infection (e.g. elevated temperature; redness, warmth, and edema around area of breakdown; unusual drainage from site). |

## 8. NURSING DIAGNOSIS: Altered oral mucous membrane: dryness, irritation, and breakdown

related to:
a. thinning of the oral mucosa associated with epithelial atrophy;
b. decreased saliva production associated with a gradual decline in salivary gland activity.

| Desired Outcome | Nursing Actions and ***Selected Purposes/Rationales*** |
|---|---|
| 8. The client will maintain a moist, intact oral mucous membrane. | 8.a. Assess client for dryness, irritation, and breakdown of the oral mucosa.<br>b. Implement measures *to decrease dryness and irritation of the oral mucous membrane:*<br>1. instruct and assist client to perform good oral hygiene as often as needed; avoid products such as lemon-glycerin swabs and mouthwashes containing alcohol *(these products have a drying or irritating effect on the oral mucous membrane)*<br>2. encourage client to rinse mouth frequently with water<br>3. lubricate client's lips with K-Y jelly, ChapStick, Blistex, or mineral oil frequently<br>4. encourage client to breathe through nose rather than mouth<br>5. encourage client not to smoke *(smoking irritates and dries the mucosa)*<br>6. encourage a fluid intake of 1500-2000 ml/day unless contraindicated<br>7. perform actions *to increase salivary flow:*<br>a. encourage client to chew sugarless gum or suck on sugarless, sour, hard candy<br>b. offer hot tea with lemon or warm lemonade at regular intervals unless contraindicated<br>8. encourage client to use artificial saliva *to lubricate the mucous membrane.* |

c. If oral mucosa is irritated or cracked, implement measures *to relieve discomfort and promote healing:*
   1. assist client to select soft, bland foods
   2. instruct client to avoid foods/fluids that are extremely hot
   3. use a soft bristle brush, sponge-tipped applicator, or low-pressure power spray for oral hygiene
   4. if client has dentures that fit poorly, remove and replace only for meals
   5. administer topical anesthetics, oral protective pastes or coating agents, and topical and systemic analgesics if ordered.

d. Consult physician if dryness, irritation, breakdown, or discomfort persists.

## 9. NURSING DIAGNOSIS: Activity intolerance

related to:
a. delayed oxygen diffusion to the tissues associated with decreased functional reserve capacity of the respiratory and cardiac systems during stress/illness;
b. decrease in strength and endurance associated with the muscle atrophy that occurs with aging;
c. inadequate nutritional status;
d. difficulty resting and sleeping.

| Desired Outcome | Nursing Actions and ***Selected Purposes/Rationales*** |
|---|---|
| 9. The client will demonstrate an increased tolerance for activity as evidenced by:<br>a. verbalization of feeling less fatigued and weak<br>b. ability to perform activities of daily living without exertional dyspnea, chest pain, diaphoresis, dizziness, and a significant change in vital signs. | 9.a. Assess for signs and symptoms of activity intolerance:<br>1. statements of fatigue and weakness<br>2. exertional dyspnea, chest pain, diaphoresis, or dizziness<br>3. abnormal heart rate response to activity (e.g. increase in rate of 20 beats/minute above resting rate, decrease in rate, rate not returning to preactivity level within 10 minutes after stopping activity, change from regular to irregular rate); be aware that the pulse rate increases only slightly with activity and returns to preactivity level slowly in an elderly client<br>4. decreased systolic B/P or a significant increase (10-15 mm Hg) in systolic or diastolic pressure with activity.<br>b. Implement measures *to improve activity tolerance:*<br>1. perform actions *to promote rest and/or conserve energy:*<br>a. maintain activity restrictions as ordered<br>b. minimize environmental activity and noise<br>c. organize nursing care to allow for periods of uninterrupted rest<br>d. limit the number of visitors and their length of stay<br>e. assist client with self-care activities as needed<br>f. keep supplies and personal articles within easy reach<br>g. instruct client in energy-saving techniques (e.g. using shower chair when showering, sitting to brush teeth or comb hair)<br>h. implement measures to reduce fear and anxiety (see Nursing Diagnosis 19, action b)<br>i. implement measures to promote sleep (see Nursing Diagnosis 14, action c)<br>2. perform actions to maintain adequate cardiac output and tissue perfusion (see Nursing Diagnosis 1, action b)<br>3. perform actions to maintain an adequate respiratory status (see Nursing Diagnosis 2, action c) |

| Desired Outcome | Nursing Actions and ***Selected Purposes/Rationales*** |
|---|---|
| | 4. perform actions to maintain an adequate nutritional status (see Nursing Diagnosis 4, action c)<br>5. increase client's activity gradually as allowed and tolerated; periods of activity should be short, frequent, and interspersed with rest periods.<br>c. Instruct client to:<br>1. report a decreased tolerance for activity; caution client that tolerance for vigorous activity may be diminished *because of age-related changes in thermoregulatory mechanisms and sympathetic responses*<br>2. stop any activity that causes chest pain, shortness of breath, dizziness, or extreme fatigue or weakness<br>3. continue with a regular exercise program following discharge to improve activity tolerance.<br>d. Consult physician if signs and symptoms of activity intolerance persist or worsen. |

## 10. NURSING DIAGNOSIS: Impaired physical mobility

related to:

a. decreased muscle strength associated with the loss of muscle mass that occurs with aging;
b. activity intolerance associated with decreased functional reserve capacity of the respiratory and cardiac systems during stress and illness, inadequate nutritional status, and difficulty resting and sleeping;
c. joint aching and stiffness that may be present as a result of degenerative changes in the joints;
d. fear of falling;
e. activity limitations imposed by current diagnosis and/or treatment plan.

| Desired Outcome | Nursing Actions and ***Selected Purposes/Rationales*** |
|---|---|
| 10. The client will maintain an optimal level of physical mobility within prescribed activity restrictions. | 10.a. Implement measures *to maintain an optimal level of physical mobility:*<br>1. perform actions to improve activity tolerance (see Nursing Diagnosis 9, action b)<br>2. perform actions to prevent falls (see Nursing Diagnosis 16, action a.1) *in order to reduce client's fear of injury*<br>3. perform actions to maintain an adequate nutritional status (see Nursing Diagnosis 4, action c) *in order to reduce the loss of lean muscle mass*<br>4. instruct client in and assist with use of mobility aids (e.g. cane, walker) if indicated<br>5. instruct client in and assist with range of motion exercises at least 3 times/day unless contraindicated<br>6. if client complains of joint aching or stiffness:<br>a. encourage him/her to perform mild exercise of affected joint(s) upon awakening in the morning *in order to reduce stiffness*<br>b. consult physician regarding application of heat to affected joint(s)<br>7. encourage activity and participation in self-care as allowed and tolerated<br>8. encourage client to continue a regular exercise program following discharge.<br>b. Provide praise and encouragement for all efforts to increase physical mobility.<br>c. Encourage the support of significant others. Allow them to assist with range of motion exercises, positioning, and activity if desired. |

d. Consult physician if client is unable to achieve expected level of mobility or if range of motion becomes more restricted.

## 11. NURSING DIAGNOSIS: Self-care deficit

related to:
a. impaired physical mobility;
b. decreased activity tolerance;
c. lack of motivation and/or presence of cognitive impairments that result in the elderly client attaching less importance to or forgetting usual grooming and hygiene practices.

| Desired Outcome | Nursing Actions and ***Selected Purposes/Rationales*** |
|---|---|
| 11. The client will perform self-care activities within physical limitations and activity restrictions imposed by the treatment plan. | 11.a. With client, develop a realistic plan for meeting daily physical needs.<br>b. Encourage maximum independence within physical limitations and prescribed activity restrictions.<br>c. Implement measures *to facilitate client's ability to perform self-care activities:*<br>1. schedule care at a time when client is most likely to be able to participate (e.g. after rest periods, not immediately after meals or treatments)<br>2. keep needed objects within easy reach<br>3. consult occupational therapist about assistive devices available (e.g. long-handled hairbrush and shoehorn) if indicated<br>4. allow adequate time for the accomplishment of self-care activities, remembering that elderly clients tend to be slower in reacting to stimuli and in moving<br>5. perform actions to maintain an optimal level of mobility (see Nursing Diagnosis 10, action a).<br>d. Provide positive feedback for all efforts and accomplishments of self-care.<br>e. Assist the client with activities he/she is unable to perform independently.<br>f. Inform significant others of client's abilities to perform own care. Explain the importance of encouraging and allowing client to maintain an optimal level of independence and allowing client to complete activities at his/her own pace. |

## 12. NURSING DIAGNOSIS: Altered urinary elimination:

a. **frequency** related to decrease in bladder capacity, decreased ability to concentrate urine associated with a decline in the number of functioning nephrons, and instability of detrusor muscle;
b. **urgency** related to decreased bladder capacity, decreased sensation of the urge to void until bladder is full, detrusor muscle instability, and/or irritation of bladder stretch receptors (may result from overdistention);
c. **retention** related to obstruction of bladder outlet by an enlarged prostate in men, pressure on the bladder outlet associated with fecal impaction if present, reduced bladder muscle tone, and/or decreased neural control over micturition;
d. **incontinence** related to:
   1. an incompetent bladder outlet associated with degenerative changes in sup-

port structures, external urinary sphincter, and urethra and/or atrophic vaginitis/urethritis
2. overdistention of the bladder associated with loss of bladder muscle tone, decreased neural control over micturition, and/or bladder outlet obstruction by an enlarged prostate in men or fecal impaction
3. age-related increase in detrusor muscle instability
4. inability to get to toilet in time to urinate associated with unfamiliar environment and impaired physical mobility and difficulty removing clothing associated with reduced manual dexterity.

| Desired Outcome | Nursing Actions and ***Selected Purposes/Rationales*** |
|---|---|
| 12. The client will maintain or regain optimal urinary elimination as evidenced by:<br>a. voiding at normal intervals<br>b. no complaints of urgency, frequency, bladder fullness, or suprapubic discomfort<br>c. absence of bladder distention<br>d. absence of incontinence<br>e. balanced intake and output. | 12.a. Determine client's usual urinary elimination pattern.<br>b. Assess for signs and symptoms of altered urinary elimination:<br>1. frequent voiding of small amounts (25-60 ml) of urine<br>2. nocturia<br>3. complaints of urgency, frequency, bladder fullness, or suprapubic discomfort<br>4. bladder distention<br>5. incontinence<br>6. output less than intake.<br>c. Catheterize client if ordered *to determine the amount of residual urine.*<br>d. Assist with urodynamic studies (e.g. uroflowmetry, cystometry, urethral pressure profilometry, electromyography, cystourethroscopy) if performed *to determine cause for altered urinary elimination.*<br>e. Implement measures *to promote optimal urinary elimination:*<br>1. perform actions *to prevent or treat urinary retention:*<br>a. offer bedpan or urinal or assist client to bedside commode or bathroom every 2-3 hours if indicated<br>b. instruct client to urinate when urge is first felt<br>c. perform actions *to promote relaxation during voiding attempts* (e.g. provide privacy, play soft music, encourage client to read)<br>d. perform actions *to provide sensory stimulation that may help trigger the micturition reflex and promote voluntary relaxation of the perineal muscles and external urinary sphincter* (e.g. run water, place client's hands in warm water, pour warm water over perineum)<br>e. allow client to assume a normal position for voiding unless contraindicated<br>f. instruct client to lean his/her upper body forward and/or gently press downward on lower abdomen during voiding attempts unless contraindicated *in order to put pressure on the bladder (pressure helps trigger the micturition reflex and promotes more complete bladder emptying)*<br>g. instruct client to perform the Valsalva maneuver during urination unless contraindicated<br>h. perform actions to prevent or treat constipation (see Nursing Diagnosis 13, actions d and e) *in order to reduce additional pressure on bladder outlet*<br>i. administer cholinergic drugs (e.g. bethanechol) if ordered *to stimulate bladder contraction*<br>j. consult physician about intermittent catheterization or insertion of an indwelling catheter if signs and symptoms of urinary retention persist<br>2. perform actions *to prevent or treat urinary incontinence:*<br>a. offer bedpan or urinal or assist client to bedside commode or bathroom every 2-3 hours or more frequently depending on the client's usual urinary elimination pattern |

b. allow client to assume a normal position for voiding unless contraindicated *in order to promote complete bladder emptying*
c. provide easy access to bathroom and assist client to select clothing that is easy to remove (e.g. pajamas with Velcro closures or elastic waistband) *in order to reduce delays in toileting*
d. instruct client to perform perineal exercises (e.g. stopping and starting stream during voiding; squeezing buttocks together, then relaxing the muscles) several times a day *in order to improve urinary sphincter tone and strengthen pelvic floor muscles;* instruct client to continue these exercises following discharge, emphasizing that it will take several weeks of exercise before improvement may be noted
e. instruct client to space fluids evenly throughout the day rather than drinking a large quantity at one time *(rapid filling of bladder can result in incontinence if client has decreased urinary sphincter control)*
f. limit oral fluid intake in the evening *to decrease the possibility of nighttime incontinence*
g. instruct client to avoid drinking beverages containing caffeine *(caffeine is a mild diuretic and may make urinary control more difficult)*
h. administer the following medications if ordered (medications selected to promote optimal urinary elimination will depend on anticipated side effects of the drug on other body systems):
    1. sympathomimetic agents (e.g. ephedrine) *to relax the detrusor muscle and increase contraction of urinary sphincter*
    2. anticholinergic agents (e.g. propantheline, oxybutynin) *to reduce or block detrusor contractions if detrusor instability is determined to be the cause of incontinence*
    3. cholinergic agents (e.g. bethanechol) *to stimulate bladder contractions and promote complete bladder emptying*
    4. low-dose estrogen preparations *to treat atrophic vaginitis/urethritis if present*
i. if urinary incontinence persists:
    1. utilize biofeedback techniques if appropriate *to assist client to regain control over the external urinary sphincter and pelvic floor musculature*
    2. instruct and assist client with bladder retraining program if appropriate
    3. consult physician regarding intermittent catheterization, insertion of an indwelling catheter, or use of an external catheter or penile clamp.

## 13. NURSING DIAGNOSIS: Constipation

related to:
a. decreased intake of fluids and foods high in fiber;
b. atony of intestines (may occur with chronic laxative/enema use);
c. decreased gastrointestinal motility associated with decreased activity and anxiety;
d. difficulty evacuating rectum associated with weakened abdominal and pelvic floor muscles;
e. failure to respond to the urge to defecate.

| Desired Outcome | Nursing Actions and ***Selected Purposes/Rationales*** |
|---|---|
| 13. The client will not experience constipation as evidenced by:<br>a. usual frequency of bowel movements<br>b. passage of soft, formed stool<br>c. absence of headache, anorexia, abdominal distention and pain, rectal pressure, and straining at stool. | 13.a. Ascertain client's usual bowel elimination habits.<br>b. Assess for signs and symptoms of constipation (e.g. decrease in frequency of stools; passage of hard, formed stools; headache; anorexia; abdominal distention and pain; feeling of fullness or pressure in rectum; straining at stool).<br>c. Assess bowel sounds. Report a pattern of decreasing bowel sounds.<br>d. Implement measures *to prevent constipation:*<br>1. encourage client to defecate whenever the urge is felt<br>2. assist client to toilet or bedside commode or place in high Fowler's position on bedpan for bowel movements unless contraindicated; provide privacy and adequate ventilation<br>3. encourage client to relax during attempts to defecate *in order to promote relaxation of the pelvic floor musculature and external anal sphincter*<br>4. instruct client to increase intake of foods high in fiber (e.g. bran, whole grains, raw fruits and vegetables, dried fruits) unless contraindicated<br>5. instruct client to maintain a minimum fluid intake of 1500-2000 ml/day unless contraindicated<br>6. encourage client to drink warm liquids upon arising in the morning *in order to initiate the gastrocolic and duodenocolic reflexes and stimulate peristalsis*<br>7. increase activity as tolerated<br>8. encourage client to perform isometric abdominal strengthening exercises unless contraindicated<br>9. perform actions to reduce fear and anxiety (see Nursing Diagnosis 19, action b)<br>10. administer laxatives, stool softeners, and/or enemas if ordered<br>11. instruct client to continue with actions to promote regular bowel function following discharge (e.g. maintain a fluid intake of at least 6-8 glasses/day; increase intake of foods high in fiber, particularly bran; participate in regular exercise program).<br>e. Check for impaction if client has not had a bowel movement in 3 days, if he/she is passing liquid stool, or if other signs and symptoms of constipation are present. Administer oil retention and/or cleansing enemas as ordered followed by digital removal of stool if necessary. |

## 14. NURSING DIAGNOSIS: Sleep pattern disturbance

related to:

a. fear, anxiety, decreased activity, unfamiliar environment, and discomfort associated with present illness;
b. age-related nocturia;
c. age-related changes in the stages of sleep resulting in frequent arousal periods and an increase in total awake time.

| Desired Outcome | Nursing Actions and ***Selected Purposes/Rationales*** |
|---|---|
| 14. The client will attain optimal amounts of sleep within the parameters of the | 14.a. Assess for signs and symptoms of a sleep pattern disturbance (e.g. verbal complaints of difficulty falling asleep, sleep interruptions, or not feeling well rested; irritability; lethargy; disorientation; frequent yawning; dark circles under eyes; slight hand tremors). |

treatment regimen as evidenced by:
a. statements of feeling well rested
b. usual mental status
c. absence of frequent yawning, dark circles under eyes, and hand tremors.

b. Determine the client's usual sleep habits.
c. Implement measures *to promote sleep:*
   1. assist client to determine the part of the night that he/she sleeps the best; arrange time of sleep to coincide with his/her particular body rhythms whenever possible
   2. discourage long periods of sleep during the day unless signs and symptoms of sleep deprivation exist; be aware that short naps may be necessary for the elderly client *in order to compensate for increased awake time at night and to obtain adequate amounts of restorative sleep*
   3. perform actions to reduce fear and anxiety (see Nursing Diagnosis 19, action b)
   4. perform actions to reduce dyspepsia, gastric fullness, and gas pain if present (see Nursing Diagnosis 5, action c) and discomfort associated with client's diagnosis and treatment
   5. inform client of normal changes in sleep pattern that occur with aging *in order to reduce concerns about quantity of sleep necessary to maintain health*
   6. encourage participation in relaxing diversional activities during the evening
   7. discourage intake of fluids high in caffeine (e.g. coffee, tea, colas), especially in the evening
   8. offer client a high-protein evening snack (e.g. milk, cheese) unless contraindicated
   9. allow client to continue usual sleep practices (e.g. position; bedtime rituals such as taking a warm bath, reading, and meditating) if possible
   10. satisfy basic needs such as comfort and warmth before sleep
   11. instruct client to limit intake of fluids in the evening and empty bladder just before bedtime *in order to reduce nocturia*
   12. maintain a quiet, restful atmosphere; have earplugs available for client if needed
   13. utilize relaxation techniques (e.g. progressive relaxation exercises, back massage, meditation, soft music) before sleep
   14. ensure good room ventilation
   15. administer sedative-hypnotics if ordered; administer these agents cautiously *because the metabolism, distribution, and excretion of drugs is often altered in the elderly client*
   16. perform actions *to reduce interruptions during sleep (80-100 minutes of uninterrupted sleep are usually needed to complete one sleep cycle):*
       a. restrict visitors
       b. group care (e.g. medications, treatments, physical care, assessments) whenever possible.
d. Consult physician if signs and symptoms of sleep deprivation persist or worsen.

## 15. NURSING DIAGNOSIS: High risk for infection

related to:
a. stasis of respiratory secretions associated with decreased activity and age-related decrease in ciliary activity and cough effectiveness;
b. decreased effectiveness of both the cellular and humoral components of the immune system;
c. inadequate nutritional status;

d. urinary stasis associated with incomplete bladder emptying and decreased activity;
e. favorable environment for growth of pathogens in vagina associated with an increase in the pH of vaginal secretions (results from age-related estrogen depletion).

| Desired Outcome | Nursing Actions and ***Selected Purposes/Rationales*** |
|---|---|
| 15. The client will remain free of infection as evidenced by:<br>a. absence of fever and chills<br>b. pulse within normal limits<br>c. normal breath sounds<br>d. voiding clear urine without complaints of burning and increased frequency and urgency<br>e. absence of heat, pain, redness, swelling, and unusual drainage in any area<br>f. usual mental status<br>g. WBC and differential counts within normal range for elderly client<br>h. negative results of cultured specimens. | 15.a. Assess for and report signs and symptoms of infection:<br>1. increase in temperature above client's usual level (be aware that normal temperature in the elderly client may be less than 37° C)<br>2. chills<br>3. increased pulse (the elderly client may not demonstrate the classic elevation in pulse rate that occurs with infection *because of his/her decreased sympathetic responses)*<br>4. abnormal breath sounds<br>5. cloudy, foul-smelling urine<br>6. complaints of burning when urinating<br>7. complaints of increased urinary frequency or urgency<br>8. presence of WBCs, bacteria, and/or nitrites in urine<br>9. heat, pain, redness, swelling, or unusual drainage in any area<br>10. confusion, decreased level of consciousness<br>11. elevated WBC count and/or significant change in differential.<br>b. Obtain specimens (e.g. urine, vaginal, mouth, sputum, blood) for culture as ordered. Report positive results.<br>c. Implement measures *to prevent infection:*<br>1. maintain a fluid intake of at least 1500-2000 ml/day unless contraindicated<br>2. use good handwashing technique and encourage client to do the same<br>3. maintain meticulous aseptic technique during all invasive procedures (e.g. catheterizations, venous and arterial punctures, injections)<br>4. change intravenous tubings and solutions and rotate insertion sites according to hospital policy<br>5. change equipment and solutions used for procedures such as irrigations, wound care, and tube feedings according to hospital policy<br>6. protect client from others with infections and instruct him/her to continue this after discharge<br>7. perform actions to maintain an adequate nutritional status (see Nursing Diagnosis 4, action c)<br>8. perform actions *to prevent irritation and breakdown of the oral mucous membrane:*<br>a. refer to Nursing Diagnosis 8, actions b and c for measures to decrease irritation and breakdown associated with dryness<br>b. if client has dentures, emphasize the importance of having them checked regularly *to ensure proper fit* and having cracks, chips, and rough surfaces repaired immediately<br>9. perform actions to maintain an adequate respiratory status (see Nursing Diagnosis 2, action c) *in order to reduce the risk of respiratory tract infection*<br>10. perform actions to prevent or treat urinary retention (see Nursing Diagnosis 12, action e.1) *in order to prevent urinary stasis*<br>11. perform actions *to prevent introduction of microorganisms into the urinary tract* (e.g. assist client with perineal care as needed, instruct and assist female client to wipe from front to back after urinating and defecating, maintain sterile technique during urinary catheterization) |

12. perform actions to prevent skin breakdown (see Nursing Diagnosis 7, action b)
13. instruct client to receive vaccinations for pneumococcal pneumonia, tetanus, diphtheria, and influenza at recommended intervals if appropriate.

## 16. NURSING DIAGNOSIS: High risk for trauma

related to:

a. falls associated with:
   1. dizziness, syncope, or drop attacks (sudden, unexplained fall without loss of consciousness) resulting from decreased cerebral tissue perfusion (can occur because of age-related decrease in cardiac output, vascular changes, and postural hypotension)
   2. impaired vision (e.g. decreased visual acuity, peripheral and night vision, and depth perception; glare intolerance)
   3. loss of balance and tripping resulting from gait abnormalities (e.g. decreased step height and length), increase in postural sway, delayed reaction time, inability to adjust center of gravity rapidly, reduced coordination, and impaired proprioception
   4. weakness resulting from decreased muscle strength and the general deconditioning that occurs with reduced physical activity;

b. burns associated with age-related decrease in tactile sensation.

| Desired Outcome | Nursing Actions and ***Selected Purposes/Rationales*** |
|---|---|
| 16. The client will not experience falls or burns. | 16.a. Implement measures *to reduce the risk for trauma:*<br>1. perform actions *to prevent falls:*<br>a. keep bed in low position with side rails up when client is in bed<br>b. keep needed items within easy reach and assist client to identify their location<br>c. encourage client to request assistance whenever needed; have call signal within easy reach<br>d. use lap belt when client is in chair if indicated<br>e. instruct client to wear well-fitting slippers/shoes with nonslip soles and low heels when ambulating<br>f. keep floor free of clutter and wipe up spills promptly<br>g. instruct and assist client to get out of bed slowly *in order to reduce dizziness associated with postural hypotension*<br>h. carefully position tubings and equipment so that they will not interfere with ambulation<br>i. accompany client during ambulation and use a transfer safety belt if he/she is weak or dizzy<br>j. provide ambulatory aids (e.g. walker, cane) if client is weak or unsteady on feet<br>k. reinforce instructions from physical therapist on correct ambulation and transfer techniques<br>l. if vision is impaired, orient client to surroundings, room, and arrangement of furniture and identify obstacles during ambulation<br>m. instruct client to move slowly, use wider stance when ambulating, and avoid rapidly turning head or body *in order to prevent loss of balance*<br>n. instruct client to ambulate in well-lit areas and to use handrails if needed |

| Desired Outcome | Nursing Actions and ***Selected Purposes/Rationales*** |
|---|---|
| | o. do not rush client; allow adequate time for ambulation to the bathroom and in hallway<br>p. make sure that bathtub and shower have nonslip bottom surfaces and that shower chair, secure bath mat, call light, hand grips, and adequate lighting are present<br>q. implement measures to increase strength and activity tolerance (see Nursing Diagnosis 9, action b) and maintain an optimal level of physical mobility (see Nursing Diagnosis 10, action a)<br>2. perform actions *to prevent burns:*<br>a. let hot foods and fluids cool slightly before serving<br>b. supervise client while smoking if indicated<br>c. assess temperature of bath water and heating pad before and during use<br>3. administer central nervous system depressants judiciously.<br>b. Include client and significant others in planning and implementing measures to prevent falls and burns. Discuss:<br>1. the need to evaluate home for environmental hazards (e.g. thick or loose carpets, inadequate or loose railings, insufficient lighting) and make necessary modifications<br>2. the importance of continuing appropriate safety precautions after discharge.<br>c. If injury does occur, initiate appropriate first aid and notify physician. |

## 17. COLLABORATIVE DIAGNOSES:

### Potential complications:

a. **pathologic fractures** related to osteoporosis associated with an imbalance between bone resorption and bone formation resulting from decreased estrogen levels in women, calcium deficiency (results from decreased dietary intake and decreased absorption due to vitamin D deficiency), and decreased activity;

b. **drug toxicity** related to:
1. increase in cell receptor sensitivity to many drugs (e.g. diazepam, metoclopramide, digoxin, aminophylline, warfarin, opiates)
2. changes in usual distribution of drugs associated with decreased serum protein, administration of multiple medications, decreased tissue perfusion, and changes in body composition particularly the proportion of fat to lean body mass
3. impaired metabolism and excretion of drugs associated with diminished liver and kidney function
4. synergistic effect that occurs with some combinations of medications (elderly clients are often taking a number of medications).

| Desired Outcomes | Nursing Actions and ***Selected Purposes/Rationales*** |
|---|---|
| 17.a. The client will not experience pathologic fractures as evidenced by:<br>1. usual mobility and range of motion<br>2. absence of unusual motion, abnormal joint position, and obvious deformity of any body part | 17.a. 1. Assess for and report signs and symptoms of pathologic fractures (e.g. decrease in mobility or range of motion, motion at site where motion does not usually occur, abnormal joint position or obvious deformity, pain or swelling over skeletal structures).<br>2. Monitor x-ray reports and notify physician of findings of pathologic fractures.<br>3. Implement measures *to prevent pathologic fractures:*<br>a. caution client to avoid coughing, sneezing, and straining at stool; consult physician regarding an order for an antitussive, antihistamine, and/or laxative if indicated<br>b. move client carefully; obtain adequate assistance as needed |

3. absence of pain and swelling over skeletal structures
4. x-ray reports showing absence of fractures.

c. when turning client, logroll and support all extremities
d. use smooth movements when moving client; avoid pulling or pushing on body parts
e. correctly apply brace or cervical collar as ordered
f. instruct client in the use of correct body mechanics and the need to avoid lifting heavy objects
g. perform actions to prevent falls (see Nursing Diagnosis 16, action a.1)
h. perform actions *to prevent or delay bone demineralization:*
   1. assist client to maintain maximum mobility *(weight-bearing reduces bone breakdown)*
   2. consult physician about use of a tilt table to facilitate weight-bearing if client is immobile
   3. administer calcium preparations, vitamin D, and medications *that inhibit bone resorption* (e.g. estrogen preparations) if ordered
   4. emphasize need for client to follow a regular exercise program after discharge.

4. If fractures occur:
   a. maintain activity restrictions if ordered
   b. apply external stabilization device (e.g. cervical collar, brace, splint, sling) if ordered
   c. prepare client for surgery (e.g. internal fixation) if planned
   d. administer analgesics, anti-inflammatory agents, and/or muscle relaxants if ordered *to control pain*
   e. provide emotional support to client and significant others.

17.b. The client will not develop drug toxicity as evidenced by absence of signs and symptoms commonly associated with drug toxicity such as:
1. ataxia, agitation, confusion, slurred speech, and seizure activity
2. anorexia, nausea, vomiting, and diarrhea
3. arrhythmias and postural hypotension
4. dyspnea and stridor
5. rash and/or urticaria
6. oliguria.

17.b.1. Assess client for signs and symptoms that might be indicative of drug toxicity (e.g. ataxia, agitation, confusion, slurred speech, seizure activity, anorexia, nausea, vomiting, diarrhea, arrhythmias, postural hypotension, dyspnea, stridor, rash, urticaria, oliguria). Be aware that the signs and symptoms will vary depending on drugs being taken.

2. Implement measures *to prevent drug toxicity:*
   a. be alert to possible drug interactions and nursing implications for the elderly; hold dose and consult physician if medication or dose appears contraindicated
   b. administer central nervous system depressants judiciously
   c. inform client of common adverse effects of drugs being taken and ways to avoid toxicity; encourage him/her to report adverse effects or any other unusual symptoms immediately
   d. obtain baseline vital signs and laboratory studies to facilitate assessment of renal and hepatic function and effects of medications on these systems
   e. monitor blood levels (e.g. peak, trough) of drugs as ordered and report results to physician; be aware that the elderly client may experience toxic effects when drug levels are within the "normal" therapeutic range
   f. prior to discharge:
      1. provide client and family members with clear, simple, written instructions for taking medications prescribed; include drug name, dose, schedule, route of administration, special precautions such as incompatible foods or drugs, and adverse reactions to observe for
      2. assist client to set up a system for remembering to take medication as prescribed (e.g. divided pill container, use of timer)
      3. emphasize the importance of taking only those medications that are prescribed, following the directions carefully, and keeping the physician informed of adverse effects experienced.

3. If signs and symptoms of drug toxicity occur, withhold dose and notify physician.

## 18. NURSING DIAGNOSIS: Sexual dysfunction

related to:

a. decreased libido associated with:
   1. fear of rejection resulting from feelings of loss of physical attractiveness
   2. inadequate opportunities for sexual expression and infrequent sexual activity resulting from lack of available partner
   3. misconceptions about sexual functioning in old age
   4. fear of urinary incontinence
   5. anxiety and depression
   6. inability to achieve orgasm each time;

b. dyspareunia associated with decreased vaginal lubrication, reduced elasticity and shortening of the vagina, and thinning of the vaginal walls (results in increased pressure on lower abdominal organs during thrusting) associated with decreased estrogen levels;

c. impotence associated with:
   1. performance anxiety, fatigue, and depression
   2. fear of rejection
   3. decreased penile responsiveness to vibration and light touch
   4. impaired circulation to the penis resulting from vascular disease (e.g. diabetes) if present
   5. side effects of medications such as thiazide diuretics and antihypertensive agents that are used to treat common chronic diseases of the elderly.

| Desired Outcome | Nursing Actions and ***Selected Purposes/Rationales*** |
|---|---|
| 18. The client will demonstrate beginning acceptance of changes in sexual functioning as evidenced by:<br>a. verbalization of a perception of self as sexually acceptable and adequate<br>b. statements reflecting beginning adjustment to effects of aging on sexual functioning<br>c. maintenance of relationship with significant other. | 18.a. Assess for symptoms of sexual dysfunction (e.g. verbalization of sexual concerns or inability to achieve sexual satisfaction, failure to maintain relationship with significant other).<br>b. Determine client's definition of healthy sexuality, usual pattern of sexual expression, recent changes in usual patterns, and knowledge of age-related changes in sexual functioning. Be aware that the client may be reluctant to express concerns *because of common stereotype that elderly are not sexually active.*<br>c. Implement measures *to promote optimal sexual functioning:*<br>1. inform client of age-related changes in sexual functioning (e.g. sexual responses are slower and less intense, erections take longer to achieve but can be maintained longer, seminal fluid volume is reduced, erection is rapidly lost after orgasm, refractory time between orgasms is longer); explain that continued sexual activity may delay some of these changes; encourage questions and clarify misconceptions<br>2. facilitate communication between client and his/her partner; focus on feelings shared by the couple and assist them to identify changes that may affect their sexual relationship<br>3. discuss ways to be creative in expressing sexuality (e.g. massage, fantasies, cuddling)<br>4. arrange for uninterrupted privacy during hospital stay if desired by couple<br>5. perform actions to improve client's self-concept (see Nursing Diagnosis 20, actions c-s)<br>6. if dyspareunia is a problem:<br>a. encourage female client to use a water-soluble lubricant before sexual intercourse *to reduce vaginal dryness*<br>b. suggest experimentation with different positions during intercourse *to reduce lower abdominal discomfort*<br>c. administer estrogen if ordered *to promote vaginal wall hypertrophy and reduce vaginal dryness* |

7. if impotence is a problem:
   a. encourage client to discuss it with physician *(impotence may be due to reversible factors such as medication therapy, alcohol, smoking, or poorly controlled chronic disease conditions)*
   b. assure client that occasional episodes of impotence are normal
   c. suggest alternative methods of sexual gratification if appropriate
   d. encourage client to discuss various treatment options (e.g. penile prosthesis, external vacuum device) with physician if appropriate
8. reinforce the importance of rest before sexual activity
9. if incontinence of urine is a problem, encourage client to void just before intercourse and other sexual activity.

d. Include partner in above discussions and encourage his/her continued support of the client.
e. Consult physician if counseling appears indicated.

## 19. NURSING DIAGNOSIS: Anxiety

related to unfamiliar environment; signs and symptoms of current diagnosis; lack of understanding of diagnostic tests, diagnosis, and treatment plan; financial concerns; and effects of diagnosis on health status, usual roles, and ability to live independently.

| Desired Outcome | Nursing Actions and ***Selected Purposes/Rationales*** |
|---|---|
| 19. The client will experience a reduction in anxiety as evidenced by:<br>a. verbalization of feeling less anxious and fearful<br>b. usual sleep pattern<br>c. relaxed facial expression and body movements<br>d. stable vital signs<br>e. usual perceptual ability and interactions with others. | 19.a. Assess client for signs and symptoms of anxiety (e.g. verbalization of fears and concerns, insomnia, tenseness, tremors, irritability, restlessness, tachypnea, tachycardia, increase in blood pressure, narrowed perceptual field, withdrawal, noncompliance with treatment plan). Validate perceptions carefully, remembering that sympathetic responses are often diminished in the elderly.<br>b. Implement measures *to reduce fear and anxiety:*<br>1. orient client to hospital environment, equipment, and routines<br>2. introduce staff who will be participating in his/her care; if possible, maintain consistency in staff assigned to his/her care *in order to provide feelings of stability and comfort with the environment*<br>3. assure client that staff members are nearby; respond to call signal as soon as possible<br>4. maintain a calm, supportive, confident manner when interacting with client<br>5. encourage verbalization of fear and anxiety; provide feedback<br>6. explain all diagnostic tests<br>7. reinforce physician's explanations and clarify misconceptions the client has about his/her diagnosis, treatment plan, and prognosis<br>8. allow client time to adjust psychologically to planned procedures<br>9. provide a calm, restful environment<br>10. instruct client in relaxation techniques and encourage participation in diversional activities<br>11. assist client to identify specific stressors and ways to cope with them<br>12. encourage significant others to project a caring, concerned attitude without obvious anxiousness<br>13. if surgical intervention is indicated, begin preoperative teaching<br>14. encourage client to discuss his/her concerns about the cost of health |

| Desired Outcome | Nursing Actions and ***Selected Purposes/Rationales*** |
|---|---|
| | care and about future living situation; obtain a social service consult to assist client with financial planning and finding an alternative living situation if indicated<br>15. administer antianxiety agents if ordered; give these agents cautiously because the metabolism, distribution, and excretion of drugs are often altered in the elderly.<br>c. Include significant others in orientation and teaching sessions and encourage their continued support of the client.<br>d. Provide information based on current needs of client and significant others at a level they can understand. Encourage questions and clarification of information provided.<br>e. Consult physician if above actions fail to control fear and anxiety. |

## 20. NURSING DIAGNOSIS: Self-concept disturbance*

related to:

a. changes in appearance and body functioning (e.g. graying and thinning of hair; increase in length and width of nose and ears; dry, wrinkled skin; reduced height; increase and change in distribution of body fat; reduction in lean body mass; impotence; decreased bladder control; diminished visual acuity, hearing, taste sensation, sense of smell, and tactile sensation);
b. increased dependence on others to meet basic needs;
c. feelings of powerlessness;
d. changes in usual life style and roles associated with decreased strength and endurance and sensory/perceptual alterations.

---

*This diagnostic label includes the nursing diagnoses of body image disturbance, self-esteem disturbance, and altered role performance.

| Desired Outcome | Nursing Actions and ***Selected Purposes/Rationales*** |
|---|---|
| 20. The client will demonstrate beginning adaptation to changes in appearance, body functioning, level of independence, life style, and roles as evidenced by:<br>a. verbalization of feelings of self-worth and sexual adequacy<br>b. maintenance of relationships with significant others<br>c. active participation in activities of daily living<br>d. active interest in personal appearance<br>e. willingness to pursue usual roles and participate in social activities | 20.a. Assess for signs and symptoms of a self-concept disturbance (e.g. verbal or nonverbal cues denoting a negative response to changes in body functioning or appearance such as denial of or preoccupation with the changes that have occurred or withdrawal from significant others).<br>b. Determine the meaning of changes in appearance, body functioning, life style, and roles to the client by encouraging him/her to verbalize feelings and by noting nonverbal responses to the changes experienced.<br>c. Be aware that the client may grieve the changes that have occurred. Assist him/her through the beginning phases of grieving (e.g. shock, disbelief, denial, anger, sadness, depression).<br>d. Implement measures *to assist client to increase self-esteem* (e.g. limit negative self-assessment, encourage positive comments about self, assist to identify strengths, give positive feedback about accomplishments and behaviors that are indicative of high self-esteem).<br>e. Assist client to identify and utilize coping techniques that have been helpful in the past.<br>f. Reinforce measures that may assist client to adjust to altered sexual functioning (see Nursing Diagnosis 18, action c).<br>g. Implement measures to assist client to adapt to sensory/perceptual alterations (see Nursing Diagnosis 6, actions b-f).<br>h. If client is incontinent, instruct in ways to minimize the problem *so that socialization is possible* (e.g. placing disposable liners in underwear, wearing absorbent undergarments such as Attends). |

f. verbalization of a beginning plan for adapting life style to meet restrictions imposed by the aging process and current diagnosis.

i. Assist client with usual grooming and makeup habits if necessary.
j. Implement measures *to assist the client to maintain his/her sexual identity* (e.g. do not expose client unnecessarily during assessments, procedures, and care; do not discuss incontinence episodes in front of client's visitors; assist client with bathing, makeup, hair-styling, and shaving before visitors arrive).
k. Implement measures to reduce client's feelings of powerlessness (see Nursing Diagnosis 21, actions c-n).
l. Demonstrate acceptance of client using techniques such as touch and frequent visits. Encourage significant others to do the same.
m. Assess for and support behaviors suggesting positive adaptation to changes that have occurred (e.g. interest in personal appearance, verbalization of feelings of self-worth, maintenance of relationships with significant others).
n. Assist client's and significant others' adjustment by listening, facilitating communication, and providing information.
o. Assist client and significant others to have similar expectations and understanding of future life style and to identify ways that personal and family goals can be adjusted rather than abandoned.
p. Encourage visits and support from significant others.
q. Encourage client to pursue usual roles and interests and continue involvement in social activities. If previous roles, interests, and hobbies cannot be pursued, encourage development of new ones.
r. Instruct client in ways to promote and maintain optimal body functioning after discharge (e.g. maintain good nutritional status, participate in an active exercise program).
s. Provide information about and encourage use of community agencies and support groups (e.g. senior centers; family, individual, and/or financial counseling; Help for Incontinent People [HIP]).
t. Consult physician about psychological counseling if client desires or if he/she seems unwilling or unable to adapt to changes resulting from the aging process.

## 21. NURSING DIAGNOSIS: Powerlessness

related to:
a. increased dependence on others to meet basic needs;
b. inability to pursue usual life activities and roles associated with age-related changes in body functioning, current diagnosis and its treatment, and inadequate financial resources;
c. inability to control many of the changes that occur with aging.

| Desired Outcome | Nursing Actions and ***Selected Purposes/Rationales*** |
|---|---|
| 21. The client will demonstrate increased feelings of control over his/her situation as evidenced by:<br>a. verbalization of same<br>b. active participation in the planning of care | 21.a. Assess for behaviors that may indicate feelings of powerlessness (e.g. verbalization of lack of control over self-care or current situation, anger, apathy, hostility, excessive dependency, lack of participation in care planning or self-care).<br>b. Obtain information from client and significant others regarding client's usual response to situations in which he/she has had limited control (e.g. loss of job, financial stress).<br>c. Evaluate with client his/her perceptions of current situation, strengths, weaknesses, expectations, and parts of current situation that are under his/her control. Correct misinformation and inaccurate perceptions and |

| Desired Outcome | Nursing Actions and ***Selected Purposes/Rationales*** |
|---|---|
| c. participation in self-care activities within physical limitations. | encourage discussion of feelings about areas in which he/she perceives a lack of control. |
| | d. Assist client to establish realistic short- and long-term goals. |
| | e. Discuss a living will and advanced directives for health care with client and significant others if appropriate; provide assistance if needed to complete necessary documents. |
| | f. Reinforce physician's explanations about the aging process, disease condition or injury, and treatment plan. Clarify misconceptions. |
| | g. Support realistic hope about the probability of future independence. |
| | h. Remind client of his/her right to ask questions about changes that are occurring, current condition, and plan of care. |
| | i. Support client's efforts to increase knowledge of and control over condition. Provide relevant pamphlets and audiovisual materials. |
| | j. Include client in the planning of care, encourage maximum participation in the treatment plan, and allow choices whenever possible *to promote a sense of control.* |
| | k. Provide information about scheduled procedures and tests *so that unpredictability is eliminated as much as possible and a feeling of control is promoted.* |
| | l. Consult physician about arranging for physical and occupational therapists to perform a physical functional assessment. Implement recommendations about assistive devices and environmental modifications that would allow client more independence in performing activities of daily living. |
| | m. Encourage significant others to allow client to do as much as he/she is able *so that a feeling of independence can be maintained.* |
| | n. Encourage client to be as active as possible in making decisions about his/her living situation. |
| | o. Encourage client's participation in self-help groups if indicated. |

## 22. NURSING DIAGNOSIS: Social isolation

related to:

a. decreased sensory and motor functioning;
b. reduced opportunities for socialization associated with inadequate financial resources, death or disability of friends and family members, negative attitude of others toward including the elderly in activities, reluctance to establish new relationships and try new activities, and/or placement in a long-term care facility;
c. decreased desire to communicate with others associated with an imbalance between the effort required to interact with others and the anticipated rewards of the interaction;
d. fear of injury such as falls in unfamiliar surroundings;
e. withdrawal from others associated with fear of embarrassment resulting from functional changes such as incontinence or hearing loss.

| Desired Outcome | Nursing Actions and ***Selected Purposes/Rationales*** |
|---|---|
| 22. The client will experience a decreased sense of isolation as evidenced by: | 22.a. Ascertain client's usual degree of social interaction. |
| a. maintenance of | b. Assess for indications of social isolation (e.g. absence of supportive significant others; uncommunicative and withdrawn; expression of feelings of rejection, being different from others, or aloneness imposed by others; hostility; sad, dull affect). |

relationships with significant others and casual acquaintances
b. verbalization of decreasing feelings of aloneness and rejection.

c. Implement measures *to decrease social isolation:*
   1. assist client to identify reasons for feeling isolated and alone; aid him/her in developing a plan of action to reduce these feelings
   2. use touch to demonstrate acceptance of client
   3. encourage significant others to visit
   4. encourage client to maintain telephone contact with others
   5. schedule time each day to sit and talk with client
   6. assist client to identify a few persons he/she feels comfortable with and encourage interactions with them
   7. make objects such as telephone, TV, radio, and newspapers accessible to client
   8. have significant others bring client's favorite objects from home and place in room
   9. change room assignments as feasible *to provide client with roommate with similar interests;* encourage their interaction
   10. discuss with family the possibility of using behavior modification techniques if indicated to assist client to develop more social types of behavior (e.g. initiation of social contact with others, participation in group activities)
   11. emphasize the importance of maintaining active friendships and seeking out new relationships; encourage participation in support groups if appropriate
   12. encourage client to participate in structured activity programs following discharge; provide information about community senior centers and the programs they offer.

## 23. NURSING DIAGNOSIS: Ineffective management of therapeutic regimen

related to:
a. lack of motivation, inadequate support and supervision, and insufficient financial resources;
b. confusion about appropriate health care practices and a decreased level of trust associated with conflicting advice from multiple health care providers;
c. conflicting values between client and health care providers;
d. knowledge deficit regarding current diagnosis, medications and treatments prescribed, and consequences of failure to comply with treatment plan.

| Desired Outcome | Nursing Actions and ***Selected Purposes/Rationales*** |
|---|---|
| 23. The client will demonstrate the probability of effective management of therapeutic regimen as evidenced by:<br>a. willingness to learn about and participate in treatments and care<br>b. statements reflecting ways to modify personal habits and | 23.a. Assess for indications that the client may be unable to effectively manage the therapeutic regimen:<br>1. statements reflecting that he/she was unable to manage care at home<br>2. failure to adhere to treatment plan while in hospital (e.g. not adhering to dietary modifications, refusing medications, refusing to ambulate)<br>3. statements reflecting a lack of understanding of the factors that will cause further progression of current illness and/or accelerate aging process<br>4. statements reflecting an unwillingness or inability to modify personal habits and integrate necessary treatments into life style<br>5. statements reflecting view that his/her situation is hopeless and that efforts to comply are useless. |

| Desired Outcome | Nursing Actions and ***Selected Purposes/Rationales*** |
|---|---|
| integrate treatments into life style<br>c. statements reflecting an understanding of the implications of not following the prescribed treatment plan. | b. Implement measures *to promote effective management of the therapeutic regimen:*<br>1. discuss with client the specific factors that may inhibit his/her management of care (e.g. inadequate financial resources, religious or cultural conflicts, lack of support systems)<br>2. explain the aging process and current diagnosis in terms the client can understand; stress the fact that adherence to the treatment plan is necessary in order to delay and/or prevent complications associated with the diagnosis and minimize some of the changes that occur with aging<br>3. assist client to clarify his/her values and to identify ways to incorporate the therapeutic goals and priorities into value system<br>4. encourage questions and clarify misconceptions the client has about aging and his/her diagnosis and effects of each<br>5. perform actions to promote trust in caregivers (e.g. validate conflicting advice, explain reasons for treatment plan)<br>6. encourage client to participate in treatment plan (e.g. take medications as prescribed, perform recommended exercises)<br>7. provide instruction regarding medications and treatments prescribed; allow time for return demonstration of procedures; determine areas of difficulty and misunderstanding and reinforce teaching as necessary<br>8. provide client with written instructions about medications and treatments<br>9. assist client to identify ways he/she can incorporate treatments into life style; focus on modifications of life style rather than complete change if possible<br>10. encourage client to discuss his/her financial concerns; obtain a social service consult to assist client with financial planning and to obtain financial aid if indicated<br>11. provide information about and encourage utilization of community resources that can assist client to make necessary life style changes if appropriate<br>12. encourage client to attend follow-up educational classes if appropriate<br>13. reinforce behaviors suggesting future compliance with the therapeutic regimen (e.g. statements reflecting plans for integrating treatments into life style, active participation in exercise program, changes in personal habits)<br>14. include significant others in explanations and teaching sessions and encourage their support; reinforce the need for client to assume responsibility for managing as much of care as possible.<br>c. Consult physician about referrals to community health agencies if continued instruction, support, or supervision is needed. |

## 24. NURSING DIAGNOSIS: Altered family processes

related to:

a. financial, physical, and psychological stresses associated with family member's illness and/or progressive disability;
b. inadequate knowledge about the normal aging process, client's current diagnosis, and necessary care;
c. inadequate support services;
d. decreased ability of client to fulfill usual family roles;
e. guilt associated with need to change client's living situation resulting from family's inability to provide necessary care.

| Desired Outcome | Nursing Actions and ***Selected Purposes/Rationales*** |
|---|---|
| 24. The family members* will demonstrate beginning adjustment to changes in functioning of family member and family roles and structure as evidenced by:<br>a. meeting client's needs<br>b. verbalization of ways to adapt to required role and life-style changes<br>c. active participation in decision making and client's rehabilitation<br>d. positive interactions with one another. | 24.a. Assess for signs and symptoms of altered family processes (e.g. inability to meet client's needs, statements of not being able to accept client's disabilities or make necessary role and life-style changes, inability to make decisions, inability or refusal to participate in client's care and/or rehabilitation, negative family interactions).<br>b. Identify components of the family and their patterns of communication and role expectations.<br>c. Implement measures *to facilitate family members' adjustment to age- or diagnosis-related changes in client and resultant changes in family roles and structure:*<br>1. encourage family members to verbalize feelings about changes in client and the effect of these on family structure; actively listen to each family member and maintain a nonjudgmental attitude about feelings shared<br>2. instruct client and family about normal aging processes (e.g. sensory deficits, decreased muscle strength, reduced coordination)<br>3. reinforce physician's explanation of the effects of the current diagnosis and planned treatment and rehabilitation<br>4. assist family members to gain a realistic perspective of client's situation, conveying as much hope as appropriate<br>5. provide privacy *so that family members can share their feelings with one another;* stress the importance of and facilitate the use of good communication techniques<br>6. assist family members to progress through their own grieving processes; explain that they may encounter times when they need to focus on meeting their own rather than the client's needs<br>7. emphasize the need for family members to obtain adequate rest and nutrition and to identify and utilize stress management techniques *so they are better able to emotionally and physically deal with changes experienced*<br>8. encourage and assist family members to identify coping strategies for dealing with client's age-related functional changes and changes in health status and their effect on the family<br>9. assist family members to identify realistic goals and ways of reaching these goals<br>10. include family members in decision making about client and his/her care; convey appreciation for their input and continued support of client<br>11. encourage and allow family members to participate in client's care and rehabilitation; instruct family in any special procedures and allow them to practice with supervision in the hospital prior to discharge of the client<br>12. assist family members to identify resources that could assist them in coping with their feelings and meeting their immediate and long-term needs (e.g. counseling and social services; pastoral care; service, church, and support groups); initiate a referral if indicated.<br>d. Consult physician if family members continue to demonstrate difficulty adapting to changes in client's functioning, roles, and family structure. |

*The term *family members* is being used here to include client's significant others.

UNIT

# IV

# *Nursing Care of the Client Having Surgery*

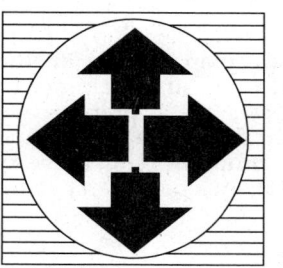

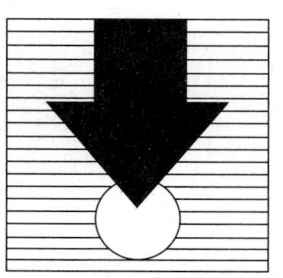

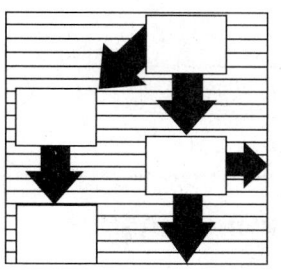

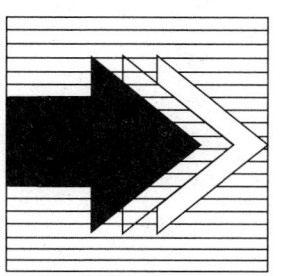

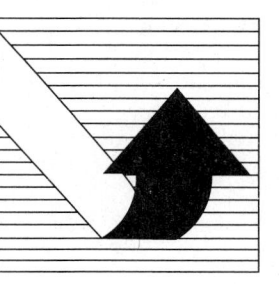

# Preoperative Care

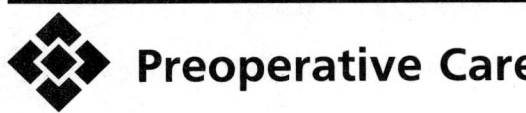

**This care plan focuses on the adult client who is scheduled for a surgical procedure.** The goals of preoperative care are to prepare the client physically and psychologically for the surgery and for the postoperative period. Thorough preoperative preparation greatly reduces the client's postoperative fear and anxiety and the risk of postoperative complications. Basic preoperative care is discussed here. In order to individualize this care plan, the client's emotional and physiological status, the type of anesthesia to be used, and the planned surgical procedure must be considered. **This care plan is to be used in conjunction with each surgical care plan.**

## PREOPERATIVE CRITERIA

Prior to surgery, the client will:

- share thoughts and feelings about the impending surgery and its anticipated effects
- verbalize an understanding of usual preoperative care and postoperative sensations and care
- demonstrate the ability to perform activities designed to prevent postoperative complications.

## NURSING DIAGNOSES



## 1. NURSING DIAGNOSIS: Anxiety

related to:
a. unfamiliar environment and separation from significant others;
b. anticipated loss of control, effects of anesthesia, and surgical findings;
c. lack of understanding of diagnostic tests and planned surgical procedure;
d. economic factors associated with hospitalization;
e. potential embarrassment or loss of dignity associated with body exposure;
f. risk of disease if blood transfusions are necessary;
g. anticipated discomfort, disfigurement, limitations, and changes in usual life style and roles;
h. possibility of death.

| Desired Outcome | Nursing Actions and ***Selected Purposes/Rationales*** |
|---|---|
| 1. The client will experience a reduction in anxiety as evidenced by:<br>a. verbalization of feeling less anxious and fearful<br>b. usual sleep pattern | 1.a. Gather the following data from the client during the preoperative period:<br>1. fears, misconceptions, and level of understanding of planned surgical procedure<br>2. perception of anticipated results of surgery<br>3. significance of the surgical procedure and hospitalization<br>4. previous surgical and hospital experiences<br>5. availability of adequate support systems. |

c. relaxed facial expression and body movements
d. stable vital signs
e. usual perceptual ability and interactions with others.

b. Assess client for signs and symptoms of anxiety (e.g. verbalization of fears and concerns, insomnia, tenseness, tremors, irritability, restlessness, diaphoresis, tachypnea, tachycardia, elevated blood pressure, facial pallor or flushing, narrowed perceptual field, withdrawal).
c. Implement measures *to reduce fear and anxiety:*
   1. orient client to hospital environment, equipment, and routines
   2. introduce staff who will be participating in his/her care; if possible maintain consistency in staff assigned to his/her care *to provide feelings of stability and comfort with the environment*
   3. assure client that staff members are nearby; respond to call signal as soon as possible
   4. maintain a calm, supportive, confident manner when interacting with client
   5. encourage verbalization of fear and anxiety; provide feedback
   6. reinforce physician's explanations and clarify misconceptions the client has about the surgical procedure (e.g. purpose, size and location of incision, outcome)
   7. explain all presurgical diagnostic tests
   8. instruct client regarding preoperative routines and postoperative care (see Nursing Diagnosis 4, actions a.1-4 and b.1)
   9. enable client *to maintain a sense of control by:*
      a. including him/her in planning of preoperative care and allowing choices whenever possible
      b. explaining purpose and importance of the written consent form (e.g. indicates voluntary and informed consent, protects against unsanctioned surgery)
   10. provide a calm, restful environment
   11. instruct client in relaxation techniques and encourage participation in diversional activities
   12. assist client to identify specific stressors and ways to cope with them
   13. assure client that pain relief needs will be met postoperatively
   14. assure client that blood is screened carefully and that his/her risk for blood-borne disease is minimal
   15. initiate financial and/or social services referrals if indicated
   16. encourage significant others to project a caring, concerned attitude without obvious anxiousness
   17. arrange for visit from clergy if client desires
   18. administer antianxiety agents if ordered.
d. Include significant others in orientation and teaching sessions and encourage their continued support of client.
e. Provide information based on current needs of client and significant others at a level they can understand. Encourage questions and clarification of information provided.
f. Consult physician if above actions fail to control fear and anxiety.

---

## 2. NURSING DIAGNOSIS: Sleep pattern disturbance

related to fear, anxiety, activities to prepare client for the surgical experience, and unfamiliar environment.

| Desired Outcome | Nursing Actions and ***Selected Purposes/Rationales*** |
|---|---|
| 2. The client will attain optimal amounts of sleep | 2.a. Assess for signs and symptoms of a sleep pattern disturbance (e.g. verbal complaints of difficulty falling asleep, sleep interruptions, or not feeling |

| Desired Outcome | Nursing Actions and ***Selected Purposes/Rationales*** |
|---|---|
| within the parameters of the treatment regimen as evidenced by:<br>a. statements of feeling well rested<br>b. usual mental status<br>c. absence of frequent yawning, dark circles under eyes, and hand tremors. | well rested; irritability; lethargy; disorientation; frequent yawning; dark circles under eyes; slight hand tremors).<br>b. Determine the client's usual sleep habits.<br>c. Implement measures *to promote sleep:*<br>1. perform actions to reduce fear and anxiety (see Nursing Diagnosis 1, action c)<br>2. encourage participation in relaxing diversional activities during the evening<br>3. discourage intake of fluids high in caffeine (e.g. coffee, tea, colas), especially in the evening<br>4. offer client a high-protein evening snack (e.g. milk, cheese) unless contraindicated<br>5. allow client to continue usual sleep practices (e.g. position, time, bedtime rituals such as reading and meditating) if possible<br>6. satisfy basic needs such as comfort and warmth before sleep<br>7. have client empty bladder just before bedtime<br>8. maintain a quiet, restful atmosphere; have earplugs available for client if needed<br>9. use relaxation techniques (e.g. progressive relaxation exercises, back massage, meditation, soft music) before sleep<br>10. ensure good room ventilation<br>11. administer sedative-hypnotics if ordered<br>12. perform actions *to reduce interruptions during sleep (80-100 minutes of uninterrupted sleep are usually needed to complete one sleep cycle):*<br>a. restrict visitors<br>b. group care (e.g. medications, treatments, physical care, assessments) whenever possible. |

## 3. NURSING DIAGNOSIS: Anticipatory grieving

related to potential loss of or change in a body part and/or usual body functioning.

| Desired Outcome | Nursing Actions and ***Selected Purposes/Rationales*** |
|---|---|
| 3. The client will demonstrate beginning progression through the grieving process as evidenced by:<br>a. verbalization of feelings about anticipated change in body image and usual body functioning<br>b. expression of grief<br>c. participation in preoperative care and self-care activities<br>d. use of available support systems. | 3.a. Assess for signs and symptoms of anticipatory grieving (e.g. change in eating habits, inability to concentrate, insomnia, anger, noncompliance, withdrawal from significant others). Be aware that client's response to the anticipated loss will be affected by factors such as previous experience with loss, age, developmental stage, available support systems, spiritual and cultural background, current health status, and significance of the anticipated loss.<br>b. Implement measures *to facilitate the grieving process:*<br>1. assist client to acknowledge the anticipated losses *so grief work can begin;* assess for factors that may hinder and facilitate acknowledgment<br>2. discuss the grieving process and assist client to accept the phases of grieving (phases vary among theorists but progress from shock and alarm to acceptance) as an expected response to anticipated losses<br>3. provide an atmosphere of care and concern (e.g. provide privacy, be available and nonjudgmental, display empathy and respect) *so client will feel free to verbalize feelings*<br>4. perform actions *to promote trust* (e.g. answer questions honestly, provide requested information) |

5. encourage the verbal expression of anger and sadness about the losses that may be experienced; recognize displacement of anger and assist client to see the actual cause of angry feelings and resentment
6. encourage client to express his/her feelings in whatever ways are comfortable (e.g. writing, drawing, conversation)
7. assist client to identify personal strengths that have helped him/her to cope in previous situations of loss
8. support realistic hope about changes that may result from surgery
9. support behaviors suggesting successful grief work (e.g. verbalizing feelings about anticipated losses, expressing sorrow, focusing on ways to adapt to losses that will occur)
10. explain the phases of the grieving process to significant others; encourage their support and understanding
11. assist significant others in their adjustment to losses that will be experienced by the client by encouraging them to voice their concerns and preparing them for anticipated changes in the client
12. provide information regarding counseling services and support groups that might assist client and significant others in working through grief
13. arrange for a visit from clergy if desired by client.

c. Consult physician regarding a referral for counseling if signs of dysfunctional grieving (e.g. persistent denial of the anticipated loss, excessive anger or sadness, hysteria, suicidal behaviors) occur.

## 4. NURSING DIAGNOSIS: Knowledge deficit

regarding hospital routines associated with surgery, physical preparation for the surgical procedure, sensations that normally occur following surgery and anesthesia, and postoperative care.

| Desired Outcomes | Nursing Actions and ***Selected Purposes/Rationales*** |
|---|---|
| 4.a. The client will verbalize an understanding of usual preoperative care and postoperative sensations and care. | 4.a.1. Provide information about usual preoperative routines for the surgery to be performed (e.g. blood work, ECG, urinalysis, chest x-ray, insertion of urinary catheter and/or nasogastric tube, bowel and skin preparation, removal of prosthetic devices).<br>2. Provide information related to:<br>a. scheduled time and estimated length of surgery<br>b. food and fluid restrictions before surgery<br>c. preoperative medications<br>d. body position during surgical procedure<br>e. induction and recovery rooms (e.g. purpose and estimated length of stay)<br>f. sensations that normally occur following surgery and anesthesia.<br>3. Reinforce teaching and information provided by the anesthesiologist and the surgeon.<br>4. Inform client of the anticipated postoperative care:<br>a. equipment (e.g. dressings, intravenous lines, drainage tubes, traction devices, elastic stockings or bandages, intermittent pneumatic compression stockings or boots)<br>b. activity limitations and expectations<br>c. dietary modifications<br>d. treatments (e.g. respiratory care, circulatory management, wound care) and expected frequency |

| Desired Outcomes | Nursing Actions and ***Selected Purposes/Rationales*** |
|---|---|
| | e. assessments (e.g. intake and output, lung sounds, vital signs, neurological checks, bowel sounds) and expected frequency<br>f. medications (e.g. antiemetics, analgesics, antimicrobials)<br>g. methods for controlling pain (e.g. positioning, medications, transcutaneous electrical nerve stimulation, progressive relaxation exercises, patient-controlled analgesia [PCA]).<br>5. Allow time for questions and clarification. Provide feedback. |
| 4.b. The client will demonstrate the ability to perform activities designed to prevent postoperative complications. | 4.b.1. Demonstrate activities that the client will be expected to perform postoperatively. These may include:<br>a. effective coughing and deep breathing<br>b. correct use of incentive spirometer<br>c. active foot and leg exercises<br>d. correct methods for changing position and increasing activity (e.g. moving slowly, keeping body in proper alignment, using good body mechanics, requesting assistance when needed).<br>2. Allow time for questions, clarification, and return demonstration. |

# Postoperative Care

The postoperative phase begins when the client is transferred from surgery to the recovery area and ends when he/she has recovered from the surgical intervention. **This care plan focuses on postoperative care of an adult client who has received a general anesthetic and has been transferred from the recovery area to the clinical care unit.** The goals of care are to prevent complications and to assist the client to attain an optimal health status postoperatively. **This care plan should be used in conjunction with all surgical care plans.**

## DISCHARGE CRITERIA

Prior to discharge, the client will:

- ❖ tolerate prescribed diet
- ❖ tolerate expected level of activity
- ❖ have surgical pain controlled
- ❖ have no signs and symptoms of complications
- ❖ identify ways to prevent postoperative infection
- ❖ demonstrate the ability to perform wound care
- ❖ state signs and symptoms to report to the health care provider
- ❖ share thoughts and feelings about the surgery, diagnosis, prognosis, and treatment plan
- ❖ verbalize an understanding of and a plan for adhering to recommended follow-up care including future appointments with health care provider, dietary modifications, activity level, treatments, and medications prescribed.

**NURSING/ COLLABORATIVE DIAGNOSES**



## 1. NURSING DIAGNOSIS: Altered tissue perfusion

related to:
a. hypovolemia associated with fluid loss and decreased fluid intake;
b. peripheral pooling of blood associated with decreased activity and diminished vasomotor response resulting from anesthesia and some medications (e.g. narcotic analgesics, central-acting muscle relaxants).

| Desired Outcome | Nursing Actions and ***Selected Purposes/Rationales*** |
|---|---|
| 1. The client will maintain adequate tissue perfusion as evidenced by:<br>a. B/P within normal | 1.a. Assess for and report signs and symptoms of diminished tissue perfusion (e.g. significant decrease in B/P, postural hypotension, syncope when changing to an upright position, restlessness, confusion, cool extremities, pallor or cyanosis of extremities, diminished or absent peripheral pulses, slow capillary refill, oliguria). |

| Desired Outcome | Nursing Actions and ***Selected Purposes/Rationales*** |
|---|---|
| range for client and stable with position change<br>b. usual mental status<br>c. extremities warm with absence of pallor and cyanosis<br>d. palpable peripheral pulses<br>e. capillary refill time less than 3 seconds<br>f. balanced intake and output within 48 hours after surgery. | b. Implement measures *to maintain adequate tissue perfusion:*<br>1. maintain a minimum fluid intake of 2500 ml/day unless contraindicated; if oral intake is inadequate or contraindicated, maintain intravenous fluid therapy as ordered<br>2. administer blood and blood products as ordered<br>3. instruct client to change from a horizontal to vertical position slowly *in order to allow time for autoregulatory mechanisms to adjust to upright position*<br>4. perform actions *to prevent peripheral pooling of blood and increase venous return:*<br>a. instruct and assist client to perform active foot and leg exercises every 1-2 hours while awake<br>b. encourage and assist with ambulation as soon as ordered (client should be instructed to pick up feet instead of shuffling *in order to maximize muscular contractions)*<br>c. discourage positions that compromise blood flow in lower extremities (e.g. crossing legs, pillows under knees, sitting for long periods)<br>d. consult physician regarding order for elastic stockings or bandages if prolonged activity restriction is expected; if applied, remove for 30-60 minutes at least twice daily<br>e. apply/maintain intermittent pneumatic compression stockings or boots if ordered<br>5. perform actions *to prevent vasoconstriction:*<br>a. implement measures to reduce stress<br>b. discourage smoking<br>c. implement measures *to keep client from getting cold* (e.g. maintain a comfortable room temperature, provide adequate clothing and blankets).<br>c. Consult physician if signs and symptoms of diminished tissue perfusion persist or worsen. |

## 2. NURSING DIAGNOSIS: Ineffective breathing pattern

related to fear, anxiety, pain, depressant effects of anesthesia and some medications (e.g. narcotic analgesics, central-acting muscle relaxants), abdominal distention, positioning, weakness, and fatigue.

| Desired Outcome | Nursing Actions and ***Selected Purposes/Rationales*** |
|---|---|
| 2. The client will maintain an effective breathing pattern as evidenced by:<br>a. normal rate and depth of respirations<br>b. absence of dyspnea<br>c. blood gases within normal range. | 2.a. Assess for signs and symptoms of an ineffective breathing pattern (e.g. shallow or slow respirations, tachypnea, dyspnea, use of accessory muscles when breathing).<br>b. Monitor for and report the following:<br>1. abnormal blood gases<br>2. significant changes in oximetry results.<br>c. Implement measures *to improve breathing pattern:*<br>1. perform actions to reduce fear and anxiety (see Nursing Diagnosis 20, action b)<br>2. perform actions to reduce pain (see Nursing Diagnosis 6, action e)<br>3. perform actions to reduce the accumulation of gastrointestinal gas and fluid (see Nursing Diagnosis 7.A, action 3) *in order to decrease pressure on the diaphragm* |

4. perform actions to increase strength and improve activity tolerance (see Nursing Diagnosis 10, action b)
5. instruct client to deep breathe or use incentive spirometer at least every 2 hours
6. assist with IPPB treatments as ordered
7. instruct client to breathe slowly if he/she is hyperventilating
8. place client in a semi- to high Fowler's position unless contraindicated; position with pillows *to prevent slumping*
9. assist client to turn from side to side at least every 2 hours while in bed
10. increase activity as allowed and tolerated
11. administer central nervous system depressants judiciously; hold medication and consult physician if respiratory rate is less than 12/minute.

d. Consult physician if:
  1. ineffective breathing pattern continues
  2. signs and symptoms of impaired gas exchange (e.g. restlessness, irritability, confusion, decreased $PaO_2$ and increased $PaCO_2$ levels) are present.

## 3. NURSING DIAGNOSIS: Ineffective airway clearance

related to:

a. blockage of pharynx by the base of the tongue associated with muscular flaccidity resulting from effects of anesthesia and some medications (e.g. narcotic analgesics, central-acting muscle relaxants);
b. stasis of secretions associated with:
  1. decreased activity
  2. poor cough effort resulting from the effects of anesthesia and some medications (e.g. narcotic analgesics, central-acting muscle relaxants), pain, weakness, and fatigue;
c. increased secretions associated with irritation of the respiratory tract (can result from inhalation anesthetics and endotracheal intubation);
d. tenacious secretions associated with fluid loss and decreased fluid intake.

| Desired Outcome | Nursing Actions and ***Selected Purposes/Rationales*** |
|---|---|
| 3. The client will maintain clear, open airways as evidenced by:<br>a. normal breath sounds<br>b. normal rate and depth of respirations<br>c. absence of dyspnea<br>d. absence of cyanosis. | 3.a. Assess for signs and symptoms of ineffective airway clearance (e.g. abnormal breath sounds; rapid, shallow respirations; dyspnea; cyanosis).<br>b. Implement measures *to promote effective airway clearance:*<br>1. position client on side and/or insert an artificial airway if necessary *to prevent obstruction of airway by tongue*<br>2. perform actions to reduce pain (see Nursing Diagnosis 6, action e)<br>3. instruct and assist client to turn, deep breathe, and cough or "huff" every 1-2 hours<br>4. increase activity as allowed and tolerated<br>5. perform actions *to facilitate removal of pulmonary secretions:*<br>a. implement measures *to liquefy tenacious secretions:*<br>1. maintain a fluid intake of at least 2500 ml/day unless contraindicated<br>2. humidify inspired air as ordered<br>b. assist with administration of diluent and mucolytic agents via nebulizer or IPPB treatment as ordered<br>c. perform tracheal suctioning if needed |

| Desired Outcome | Nursing Actions and ***Selected Purposes/Rationales*** |
|---|---|
| | 6. discourage smoking (*smoke causes bronchoconstriction, increases mucus production, and impairs ciliary function)*<br>7. protect client from exposure to irritants such as smoke, flowers, and perfume (*can cause bronchospasm and increased mucus production)*<br>8. reinforce correct use of incentive spirometer and assist with IPPB treatments if ordered *to promote bronchodilation and movement of secretions*<br>9. administer central nervous system depressants judiciously.<br>c. Consult physician if:<br>1. signs and symptoms of ineffective airway clearance persist<br>2. signs and symptoms of impaired gas exchange (e.g. restlessness, irritability, confusion, decreased $PaO_2$ and increased $PaCO_2$ levels) are present. |

## 4. NURSING/ COLLABORATIVE DIAGNOSIS:

**Altered fluid and electrolyte balance:**

a. **fluid volume deficit** related to blood loss; loss of fluid associated with vomiting, nasogastric tube drainage, and/or profuse wound drainage; and inadequate fluid replacement;

b. **hypokalemia, hypochloremia, and metabolic alkalosis** related to loss of electrolytes and hydrochloric acid associated with vomiting and nasogastric tube drainage;

c. **fluid volume excess or water intoxication** related to vigorous fluid therapy during and immediately following surgery and an increased secretion of antidiuretic hormone (output of ADH is stimulated by trauma, pain, anesthetic agents, and narcotic analgesics).

| Desired Outcomes | Nursing Actions and ***Selected Purposes/Rationales*** |
|---|---|
| 4.a. The client will maintain fluid and electrolyte balance as evidenced by:<br>1. normal skin turgor<br>2. moist mucous membranes<br>3. stable weight<br>4. B/P and pulse within normal range for client and stable with position change<br>5. small vein filling time less than 3-5 seconds<br>6. balanced intake and output within 48 hours after surgery<br>7. urine specific gravity within normal range<br>8. return of | 4.a.1. Assess for and report signs and symptoms of:<br>a. fluid volume deficit:<br>1. decreased skin turgor, dry mucous membranes, thirst<br>2. sudden weight loss of 2% or greater<br>3. low B/P and/or postural hypotension<br>4. weak, rapid pulse<br>5. delayed small vein filling time (longer than 3-5 seconds)<br>6. continued low urine output 48 hours after surgery with increased specific gravity (reflects an actual rather than potential fluid volume deficit)<br>7. elevated BUN<br>b. hypokalemia (e.g. cardiac arrhythmias, postural hypotension, muscle weakness, paresthesias, nausea and vomiting, continued abdominal distention and hypoactive or absent bowel sounds)<br>c. hypochloremia and metabolic alkalosis (e.g. dizziness, irritability, paresthesias, muscle twitching or spasms, hypoventilation).<br>2. Monitor serum electrolyte and blood gas results. Report abnormal values.<br>3. Implement measures *to prevent or treat fluid and electrolyte imbalances:*<br>a. perform actions to prevent nausea and vomiting (see Nursing Diagnosis 7.B, action 2)<br>b. if a nasogastric tube is present, irrigate it with normal saline rather than water<br>c. administer fluid and electrolyte replacements if ordered |

peristalsis within expected time
9. absence of cardiac arrhythmias, muscle weakness, paresthesias, twitching, spasms, and dizziness
10. BUN, serum electrolytes, and blood gases within normal range.

d. maintain a fluid intake of at least 2500 ml/day unless contraindicated
e. when oral intake is allowed and tolerated, assist client to select foods/fluids high in potassium (e.g. bananas, orange juice, potatoes, raisins, figs, apricots, dates, cantaloupe, tomato juice).

4. Consult physician if signs and symptoms of fluid and electrolyte imbalances persist or worsen.

4.b. The client will not experience fluid volume excess or water intoxication as evidenced by:
1. stable weight
2. stable B/P
3. absence of an $S_3$ heart sound
4. balanced intake and output within 48 hours following surgery
5. usual mental status
6. normal breath sounds
7. BUN, Hct, and serum sodium and osmolality levels within normal range
8. absence of dyspnea, orthopnea, edema, and distended neck veins
9. small vein emptying time less than 3-5 seconds
10. CVP within normal range.

4.b.1. Assess for and report signs and symptoms of fluid volume excess and water intoxication:
a. weight gain
b. elevated B/P (B/P may not be elevated if fluid has shifted out of vascular space)
c. presence of an $S_3$ heart sound
d. intake that continues to be greater than output 48 hours postoperatively (for the first 48 hours after surgery, output is expected to be less than intake *due to increased secretion of ADH)*
e. change in mental status
f. crackles (rales), diminished or absent breath sounds
g. low serum sodium and osmolality (indicates water intoxication)
h. decreased BUN and Hct (low Hct could also indicate blood loss)
i. decreased urine specific gravity
j. dyspnea, orthopnea
k. edema (peripheral edema reflects fluid volume excess; cellular edema reflects water intoxication)
l. distended neck veins
m. delayed small vein emptying time (longer than 3-5 seconds)
n. elevated CVP (use internal jugular vein pulsation method to estimate CVP if monitoring device not present).

2. Monitor chest x-ray results. Report findings of pulmonary vascular congestion, pleural effusion, or pulmonary edema.
3. Implement measures *to prevent or treat fluid volume excess and water intoxication:*
a. administer fluid replacement therapy judiciously, especially within first 48 hours after surgery
b. maintain fluid restrictions if ordered
c. administer diuretics if ordered.
4. Consult physician if signs and symptoms of fluid volume excess or water intoxication persist or worsen.

## 5. NURSING DIAGNOSIS: Altered nutrition: less than body requirements

related to:
a. decreased oral intake associated with prescribed dietary modifications, discomfort, fatigue, nausea, and dislike of prescribed diet;
b. inadequate nutritional replacement therapy;
c. loss of nutrients associated with vomiting;
d. increased nutritional needs associated with the increased metabolic rate that occurs during wound healing.

| Desired Outcome | Nursing Actions and ***Selected Purposes/Rationales*** |
|---|---|
| 5. The client will maintain an adequate nutritional status as evidenced by:<br>a. weight within normal range for client's age, height, and body frame<br>b. normal BUN and serum albumin, Hct, Hb, transferrin, and lymphocyte levels<br>c. triceps skinfold thickness within normal range<br>d. usual strength and activity tolerance<br>e. healthy oral mucous membrane. | 5.a. Assess for and report signs and symptoms of malnutrition:<br>1. weight below normal for client's age, height, and body frame<br>2. abnormal BUN and low serum albumin, Hct, Hb, transferrin, and lymphocyte levels (decreased Hct and Hb may also result from blood loss)<br>3. triceps skinfold thickness less than normal<br>4. weakness and fatigue<br>5. stomatitis.<br>b. Assess for return of bowel function every 2-4 hours. Notify physician when client has normal bowel sounds and is expelling flatus *so that oral intake can be resumed as soon as possible.*<br>c. When oral intake is allowed, monitor percentage of meals and snacks client consumes. Report pattern of inadequate intake.<br>d. Implement measures *to maintain an adequate nutritional status:*<br>1. when food or fluid is allowed, perform actions *to improve oral intake:*<br>a. implement measures to prevent nausea and vomiting (see Nursing Diagnosis 7.B, action 2)<br>b. implement measures to reduce discomfort (see Nursing Diagnoses 6, action e; 7.A, action 3; and 7.C)<br>c. increase activity as allowed and tolerated *(activity stimulates appetite)*<br>d. encourage a rest period before meals *to minimize fatigue*<br>e. obtain a dietary consult if necessary to assist client in selecting foods/fluids that meet nutritional needs and prescribed dietary modifications as well as personal and cultural preferences whenever possible<br>f. maintain a clean environment and a relaxed, pleasant atmosphere<br>g. provide oral care before meals<br>h. serve small portions of nutritious foods/fluids that are appealing to client<br>i. encourage significant others to bring in client's favorite foods unless contraindicated<br>j. allow adequate time for meals; reheat food if necessary<br>k. limit fluid intake (unless it has a high nutritional value) with meals *to reduce early satiety and subsequent decreased food intake*<br>2. ensure that meals are well balanced and high in essential nutrients; offer dietary supplements between meals if indicated<br>3. administer vitamins and minerals if ordered.<br>e. Perform a 72-hour calorie count if ordered. Report totals to dietitian and physician.<br>f. Consult physician regarding alternative methods of providing nutrition (e.g. parenteral nutrition, tube feedings) if client does not consume enough food or fluids to meet nutritional needs. |

## 6. NURSING DIAGNOSIS: Pain

related to tissue trauma and reflex muscle spasms associated with the surgery; irritation from drainage tubes; and stress on surgical area associated with deep breathing, coughing, and/or movement.

| Desired Outcome | Nursing Actions and ***Selected Purposes/Rationales*** |
|---|---|
| 6. The client will experience diminished pain as evidenced by:<br>a. verbalization of pain relief<br>b. relaxed facial expression and body positioning<br>c. increased participation in activities<br>d. stable vital signs. | 6.a. Determine how the client usually responds to pain.<br>b. Assess client's perception of pain including location, intensity, and type. Use a numerical scale to rate intensity.<br>c. Assess for nonverbal signs of pain (e.g. wrinkled brow, clenched fists, reluctance to move, restlessness, diaphoresis, facial pallor, increased B/P, tachycardia).<br>d. Assess for factors that seem to aggravate and alleviate pain.<br>e. Implement measures *to reduce pain:*<br>1. perform actions *to reduce fear and anxiety about the pain experience* (e.g. assure client that his/her need for pain relief will be met)<br>2. medicate prior to any painful treatments or procedures and before pain becomes severe<br>3. provide or assist with nonpharmacological measures for pain relief (e.g. back rub, position change, relaxation techniques, transcutaneous electrical nerve stimulation, guided imagery, quiet conversation, restful environment, diversional activities)<br>4. instruct and assist client to support abdominal or chest incision with a pillow or hands when turning, coughing, and deep breathing<br>5. if client has an abdominal incision, instruct him/her to bend knees while coughing and deep breathing *in order to reduce tension on abdominal muscles and incision*<br>6. securely anchor drainage tubes *to decrease tissue irritation resulting from movement of tubes*<br>7. encourage client to use patient-controlled analgesia (PCA) device as instructed<br>8. administer analgesics, anti-inflammatory agents, and muscle relaxants if ordered.<br>f. Consult physician if above measures fail to provide adequate pain relief. |

## 7.A. NURSING DIAGNOSIS: Altered comfort: abdominal distention and gas pain

related to accumulation of gas and fluid associated with:
1. decreased peristalsis resulting from manipulation of the bowel during abdominal surgery and depressant effects of anesthesia and some medications (e.g. narcotic analgesics, central-acting muscle relaxants);
2. decreased activity.

| Desired Outcome | Nursing Actions and ***Selected Purposes/Rationales*** |
|---|---|
| 7.A. The client will experience diminished abdominal distention and gas pain as evidenced by:<br>1. verbalization of decreased abdominal fullness and pain<br>2. relaxed facial expression and body positioning<br>3. decrease in abdominal girth. | 7.A.1. Assess for verbal complaints of abdominal fullness or gas pain.<br>2. Assess for nonverbal signs of abdominal distention or gas pain (e.g. clutching or guarding of abdomen, restlessness, reluctance to move, grimacing, increasing abdominal girth).<br>3. Implement measures *to reduce the accumulation of gastrointestinal gas and fluid:*<br>a. encourage and assist client with frequent position changes and ambulation as soon as allowed and tolerated *(activity stimulates peristalsis and expulsion of flatus)*<br>b. instruct the client to avoid activities such as chewing gum and smoking *in order to reduce air swallowing*<br>c. maintain patency of nasogastric, gastric, or intestinal tube if present<br>d. maintain food and fluid restrictions as ordered<br>e. when oral intake is allowed, instruct client to avoid intake of |

| Desired Outcome | Nursing Actions and ***Selected Purposes/Rationales*** |
|---|---|
| | carbonated beverages and gas-producing foods (e.g. cabbage, onions, beans)<br>f. encourage client to expel flatus whenever the urge is felt<br>g. consult physician regarding insertion of a rectal tube or administration of a return flow enema if indicated<br>h. encourage use of nonnarcotic analgesics once the period of severe pain has subsided *(narcotic analgesics depress gastrointestinal activity)*<br>i. administer gastrointestinal stimulants (e.g. metoclopramide, bisacodyl) if ordered *to increase gastrointestinal motility.*<br>4. Consult physician if signs and symptoms of abdominal distention and gas pain persist or worsen. |

## 7.B. NURSING DIAGNOSIS: Altered comfort: nausea and vomiting

related to stimulation of the vomiting center associated with:

1. stimulation of the afferent vagal and/or sympathetic pathways resulting from visceral irritation associated with abdominal distention;
2. cortical stimulation resulting from pain and stress.

| Desired Outcome | Nursing Actions and ***Selected Purposes/Rationales*** |
|---|---|
| 7.B. The client will experience relief of nausea and vomiting as evidenced by:<br>1. verbalization of relief of nausea<br>2. absence of vomiting. | 7.B.1. Assess client for nausea and vomiting.<br>2. Implement measures *to prevent nausea and vomiting:*<br>a. perform actions to reduce the accumulation of gastrointestinal gas and fluid (see Nursing Diagnosis 7.A, action 3)<br>b. perform actions to reduce pain (see Nursing Diagnosis 6, action e)<br>c. perform actions to reduce fear and anxiety (see Nursing Diagnosis 20, action b)<br>d. eliminate noxious sights and odors from the environment *(noxious stimuli cause cortical stimulation of the vomiting center)*<br>e. encourage client to take deep, slow breaths when nauseated<br>f. instruct client to change positions slowly *(rapid movement stimulates the afferent vestibulocerebellar pathway with resultant stimulation of the chemoreceptor trigger zone)*<br>g. provide oral hygiene every 2 hours or before meals if oral intake is allowed and after each emesis<br>h. when oral intake is allowed:<br>1. advance diet slowly (usually beginning with clear liquids and progressing to solid food)<br>2. avoid serving foods with an overpowering aroma; remove lids from hot foods before entering room<br>3. provide small, frequent meals rather than 3 large ones<br>4. instruct client to ingest foods and fluids slowly<br>5. instruct client to avoid foods/fluids that irritate the gastric mucosa (e.g. spicy foods; caffeine-containing beverages such as coffee, tea, and colas)<br>6. encourage client to eat dry foods (e.g. toast, crackers) and avoid drinking liquids with meals if nauseated<br>7. instruct client to avoid foods high in fat *(fat delays gastric emptying)*<br>8. instruct client to rest after eating with head of bed elevated<br>i. administer antiemetics and gastrointestinal stimulants (e.g. metoclopramide) if ordered.<br>3. Consult physician if above measures fail to control nausea and vomiting. |

## 7.C. NURSING DIAGNOSIS: Altered comfort: hiccoughs

related to irritation of the phrenic nerve associated with gastric distention, abdominal distention, and/or gastric or abdominal tube(s).

| Desired Outcome | Nursing Actions and ***Selected Purposes/Rationales*** |
|---|---|
| 7.C. The client will not experience persistent hiccoughs. | 7.C.1. Implement measures *to prevent irritation of the phrenic nerve:*<br>a. perform actions to reduce the accumulation of gastrointestinal gas and fluid (see Nursing Diagnosis 7.A, action 3)<br>b. instruct client to avoid drinking very hot or cold liquids *to prevent reflex irritation of the phrenic nerve*<br>c. securely anchor gastric and abdominal tubes if present *in order to minimize movement of the tubes and subsequent irritation of the phrenic nerve.*<br>2. Implement measures *to control hiccoughs if they occur:*<br>a. instruct client to perform techniques such as breathing deeply, rebreathing into a paper bag, holding breath, applying gentle pressure to closed eyelids for several minutes, allowing 1 teaspoon of granulated sugar to dissolve in mouth, or drinking water while holding breath unless contraindicated<br>b. administer phenothiazines if ordered *to reduce diaphragmatic spasms.*<br>3. Consult physician if hiccoughs persist. Be prepared to assist with the following treatments for intractable hiccoughs if ordered:<br>a. gastric suction *to decrease gastric distention*<br>b. removal of gastric or abdominal tubes *(these may be irritating the phrenic nerve)*<br>c. inhalation of carbon dioxide *(the depressant effect of $CO_2$ reduces spasm of the diaphragm)*<br>d. phrenic nerve block. |

## 8. NURSING DIAGNOSIS: Altered oral mucous membrane: dryness

related to:
a. fluid volume deficit associated with fluid loss and fluid restrictions;
b. decreased salivation associated with food and fluid restrictions and some medications (e.g. anesthetic agents, narcotic analgesics).

| Desired Outcome | Nursing Actions and ***Selected Purposes/Rationales*** |
|---|---|
| 8. The client will maintain a moist, intact oral mucous membrane. | 8.a. Assess client for dryness of the oral mucosa.<br>b. Implement measures *to relieve dryness of the oral mucous membrane:*<br>1. instruct and assist client to perform good oral hygiene as often as needed; avoid use of products such as lemon-glycerin swabs and commercial mouthwashes containing alcohol *(these products have a drying or irritating effect on the oral mucous membrane)*<br>2. encourage client to rinse mouth frequently with water or dilute mouthwash<br>3. lubricate client's lips frequently with K-Y jelly, ChapStick, Blistex, or mineral oil<br>4. encourage client to breathe through nose rather than mouth |

| Desired Outcome | Nursing Actions and ***Selected Purposes/Rationales*** |
|---|---|
| | 5. encourage client not to smoke *(smoking irritates and dries the mucosa)*<br>6. maintain intravenous fluid therapy as ordered *to improve hydration*<br>7. encourage client to suck on sour, hard candy unless contraindicated *in order to stimulate salivation*<br>8. increase oral fluid intake as soon as allowed and tolerated *to improve hydration and stimulate salivation.*<br>c. Consult physician if signs and symptoms of parotitis (e.g. swelling of the parotid glands, ear pain, difficulty swallowing, fever) occur. |

## 9. NURSING DIAGNOSIS: Actual/High risk for impaired skin integrity

related to:
a. disruption of skin associated with the surgical procedure;
b. delayed wound healing associated with decreased nutritional status and inadequate blood supply to wound area;
c. irritation of skin associated with contact with wound drainage, pressure from drainage tubes, and use of tape.

| Desired Outcomes | Nursing Actions and ***Selected Purposes/Rationales*** |
|---|---|
| 9.a. The client will experience normal healing of surgical wound(s) as evidenced by:<br>1. gradual reduction in redness and swelling at wound site<br>2. presence of granulation tissue if healing is by secondary or tertiary intention<br>3. intact, approximated wound edges if healing is by primary intention. | 9.a.1. Assess for and report signs and symptoms of impaired wound healing (e.g. increasing redness and swelling at wound site, pale or necrotic tissue in wounds healing by secondary or tertiary intention, separation of wound edges in wounds healing by primary intention).<br>2. Implement measures *to promote wound healing:*<br>a. perform actions to maintain an adequate nutritional status (see Nursing Diagnosis 5, action d)<br>b. perform actions *to maintain adequate circulation to wound area:*<br>1. implement measures to maintain adequate tissue perfusion (see Nursing Diagnosis 1, action b)<br>2. do not apply dressings tightly unless ordered *(excessive pressure impairs circulation to the area)*<br>c. perform actions *to protect the wound from mechanical injury:*<br>1. ensure that dressings are secure enough to keep them from rubbing and irritating wound<br>2. carefully remove tape and dressings when performing wound care<br>3. remind client to keep hands away from wound area<br>4. implement measures to prevent falls (see Nursing Diagnosis 17, action a)<br>d. perform actions *to decrease stress on wound area:*<br>1. instruct and assist client to support the involved area when moving<br>2. instruct and assist client to splint abdominal and chest wounds when coughing; consult physician regarding an order for an antitussive if persistent cough is present<br>3. apply an abdominal binder during periods of activity if ordered *for additional support following abdominal surgery*<br>4. implement measures to reduce the accumulation of gastrointestinal gas and fluid (see Nursing Diagnosis 7.A, action 3) in clients who have had abdominal surgery |

5. implement measures to prevent nausea and vomiting (see Nursing Diagnosis 7.B, action 2) in clients who have had chest, back, or abdominal surgery
e. perform actions to prevent wound infection (see Nursing Diagnosis 16, action b.4).
3. If signs and symptoms of impaired wound healing occur:
a. perform or assist with wound care (e.g. debridement, packing, irrigation) as ordered
b. prepare client for surgical revision of the wound if planned.

9.b. The client will maintain skin integrity as evidenced by:
1. absence of redness and irritation
2. no skin breakdown.

9.b.1. Inspect skin areas that are in contact with wound drainage, tape, and drainage tubings for signs of irritation and breakdown.
2. Implement measures *to prevent skin irritation and breakdown:*
a. perform actions *to prevent wound drainage from contacting or remaining on skin:*
1. inspect dressings, wounds, and areas around drains and puncture sites; cleanse skin and change dressings when appropriate
2. maintain patency of drainage tubes *to decrease risk of leakage around the tubes*
3. apply a collection pouch over drains and incisions that are draining continuously and/or copiously
4. apply a protective barrier (e.g. Stomahesive, ReliaSeal) to skin that is likely to be in frequent contact with drainage
b. when positioning client, ensure that he/she is not lying on drainage tubings *(pressure on the skin can compromise circulation to that area; in addition, if the tubing is occluded, there is an increased risk for leakage of drainage around the tube)*
c. secure all tubings *to prevent excessive movement and subsequent irritation of mucous membranes and skin*
d. apply a water-soluble lubricant to external nares every 2-4 hours *to decrease irritation from nasogastric tube and nasal airway or cannula*
e. perform actions *to decrease skin irritation resulting from the use of tape:*
1. use only necessary amount of tape
2. use hypoallergenic tape whenever possible
3. use Montgomery straps or tubular netting *to avoid repeated application and removal of tape if frequent dressing changes are anticipated*
4. when removing tape, pull it in the direction of hair growth; use adhesive solvents if necessary.
3. If skin breakdown occurs:
a. notify physician
b. continue with above measures to prevent further irritation and breakdown
c. perform wound care as ordered or per standard hospital procedure
d. assess client closely and report signs and symptoms of infection (e.g. elevated temperature; redness, warmth, and edema around incision or area of breakdown; unusual drainage from site).

## 10. NURSING DIAGNOSIS: Activity intolerance

related to:
a. tissue hypoxia associated with diminished tissue perfusion and anemia resulting from blood loss during surgery;
b. inadequate nutritional status;
c. difficulty resting and sleeping associated with discomfort, fear, and anxiety.

| Desired Outcome | Nursing Actions and ***Selected Purposes/Rationales*** |
|---|---|
| 10. The client will demonstrate an increased tolerance for activity as evidenced by:<br>a. verbalization of feeling less fatigued and weak<br>b. ability to perform activities of daily living without exertional dyspnea, chest pain, diaphoresis, dizziness, and a significant change in vital signs. | 10.a. Assess for signs and symptoms of activity intolerance:<br>1. statements of fatigue and weakness<br>2. exertional dyspnea, chest pain, diaphoresis, or dizziness<br>3. abnormal heart rate response to activity (e.g. increase in rate of 20 beats/minute above resting rate, decrease in rate, rate not returning to preactivity level within 3 minutes after stopping activity, change from regular to irregular rate)<br>4. decreased systolic B/P or a significant increase (10-15 mm Hg) in systolic or diastolic pressure with activity.<br>b. Implement measures *to improve activity tolerance:*<br>1. perform actions *to promote rest and/or conserve energy:*<br>a. maintain activity restrictions as ordered<br>b. minimize environmental activity and noise<br>c. organize nursing care to allow for periods of uninterrupted rest<br>d. limit number of visitors and their length of stay<br>e. assist client with self-care activities as needed<br>f. keep supplies and personal articles within easy reach<br>g. instruct client in energy-saving techniques (e.g. using shower chair when showering, sitting to brush teeth or comb hair)<br>h. implement measures to reduce fear and anxiety (see Nursing Diagnosis 20, action b)<br>i. implement measures to promote sleep (see Nursing Diagnosis 15, action c)<br>j. implement measures to reduce discomfort (see Nursing Diagnoses 6, action e; 7.A, action 3; 7.B, action 2; and 7.C)<br>2. perform actions to maintain adequate tissue perfusion (see Nursing Diagnosis 1, action b)<br>3. perform actions to improve breathing pattern and facilitate airway clearance (see Nursing Diagnoses 2, action c and 3, action b) *in order to promote maximum tissue oxygenation*<br>4. maintain oxygen therapy as ordered<br>5. perform actions to maintain an adequate nutritional status (see Nursing Diagnosis 5, action d)<br>6. administer whole blood or packed red cells if ordered<br>7. increase client's activity gradually as allowed and tolerated.<br>c. Instruct client to:<br>1. report a decreased tolerance for activity<br>2. stop any activity that causes chest pain, shortness of breath, dizziness, or extreme fatigue or weakness.<br>d. Consult physician if signs and symptoms of activity intolerance persist or worsen. |

## 11. NURSING DIAGNOSIS: Impaired physical mobility

related to:

a. decreased activity tolerance associated with tissue hypoxia, inadequate nutritional status, and difficulty resting and sleeping;
b. pain and nausea;
c. depressant effects of anesthesia and some medications (e.g. narcotic analgesics, central-acting muscle relaxants);
d. fear of falling, dislodging tubes, and compromising surgical wound;
e. activity restrictions imposed by the treatment plan.

| Desired Outcome | Nursing Actions and ***Selected Purposes/Rationales*** |
|---|---|
| 11. The client will achieve maximum physical mobility within the limitations imposed by the surgical procedure and postoperative treatment plan. | 11.a. Implement measures *to increase mobility:*<br>1. perform actions to improve activity tolerance (see Nursing Diagnosis 10, action b)<br>2. perform actions to reduce pain (see Nursing Diagnosis 6, action e)<br>3. perform actions to prevent nausea and vomiting (see Nursing Diagnosis 7.B, action 2)<br>4. schedule attempts to increase activity when analgesics and/or antiemetics are at peak effect<br>5. encourage use of nonnarcotic analgesics once severe pain has subsided<br>6. perform actions *to decrease client's fear of injury:*<br>a. implement measures to prevent falls (see Nursing Diagnosis 17, action a)<br>b. secure all dressings and tubings *to decrease risk of inadvertent removal during activity*<br>7. assure client that level of activity ordered will enhance rather than compromise healing process<br>8. encourage activity and participation in self-care as allowed and tolerated; put side rails up and provide overhead trapeze if appropriate *to promote independent movement.*<br>b. Provide praise and encouragement for all efforts to increase physical mobility.<br>c. Encourage the support of significant others. Allow them to assist client with activity if desired.<br>d. Consult physician if client is unable to achieve expected level of mobility. |

## 12. NURSING DIAGNOSIS: Self-care deficit

related to impaired physical mobility associated with activity intolerance, pain, nausea, depressant effects of some medications, fear of dislodging tubes and compromising surgical wound, and activity restrictions.

| Desired Outcome | Nursing Actions and ***Selected Purposes/Rationales*** |
|---|---|
| 12. The client will perform self-care activities within physical limitations and postoperative activity restrictions. | 12.a. With client, develop a realistic plan for meeting daily physical needs.<br>b. Encourage maximum independence within physical limitations and postoperative activity restrictions.<br>c. Implement measures *to facilitate the client's ability to perform self-care activities:*<br>1. schedule care at time when client is most likely to be able to participate (e.g. when analgesics are at peak effect, after rest periods, not immediately after meals or treatments)<br>2. keep needed objects within easy reach<br>3. allow adequate time for accomplishment of self-care activities<br>4. perform actions to increase physical mobility (see Nursing Diagnosis 11, action a).<br>d. Provide positive feedback for all efforts and accomplishments of self-care.<br>e. Assist the client with activities he/she is unable to perform independently.<br>f. Inform significant others of client's abilities to perform own care. Explain the importance of encouraging and allowing client to maintain an optimal level of independence within prescribed activity restrictions and his/her activity tolerance level. |

## 13. NURSING DIAGNOSIS: Urinary retention

related to:
a. inability to urinate associated with sympathetic nervous system stimulation of bladder and urinary sphincters resulting from pain, fear, and anxiety;
b. decreased bladder muscle tone and perception of bladder fullness associated with depressant effects of some medications (e.g. anesthetic agents, narcotic analgesics, central-acting muscle relaxants).

| Desired Outcome | Nursing Actions and ***Selected Purposes/Rationales*** |
|---|---|
| 13. The client will not experience urinary retention as evidenced by:<br>a. voiding at normal intervals<br>b. no complaints of bladder fullness and suprapubic discomfort<br>c. absence of bladder distention and dribbling of urine<br>d. balanced intake and output within 48 hours following surgery. | 13.a. Determine client's usual urinary elimination pattern.<br>b. Assess for signs and symptoms of urinary retention:<br>1. frequent voiding of small amounts (25-60 ml) of urine<br>2. complaints of bladder fullness or suprapubic discomfort<br>3. bladder distention<br>4. dribbling of urine.<br>c. Monitor intake and output. Consult physician if there is no urine output within 6-12 hours after surgery or if intake and output are not balanced within 48 hours after surgery (for first 48 hours postoperatively, urine output is expected to be less than intake *due to blood loss and increased secretion of ADH).*<br>d. Implement measures *to prevent urinary retention:*<br>1. instruct client to urinate when the urge is first felt<br>2. perform actions *to promote relaxation during voiding attempts* (e.g. provide privacy, play soft music, encourage client to read)<br>3. perform actions *to provide sensory stimulation that may help trigger the micturition reflex and promote voluntary relaxation of the perineal muscles and external urinary sphincter* (e.g. run water, place client's hands in warm water, pour warm water over perineum)<br>4. allow client to assume a normal position for voiding unless contraindicated<br>5. instruct client to lean his/her upper body forward and/or gently press downward on lower abdomen during voiding attempts unless contraindicated *in order to put pressure on the bladder (pressure helps trigger the micturition reflex and promotes more complete bladder emptying)*<br>6. perform actions to reduce postoperative pain (see Nursing Diagnosis 6, action e)<br>7. encourage use of nonnarcotic analgesics once period of severe pain has subsided<br>8. administer cholinergic drugs (e.g. bethanechol) if ordered *to stimulate bladder contraction.*<br>e. Consult physician regarding intermittent catheterization or insertion of an indwelling catheter if above actions fail to alleviate urinary retention.<br>f. If urinary catheter is present, prevent urinary retention by maintaining patency of the catheter (e.g. keep tubing free of kinks, irrigate as ordered). |

## 14. NURSING DIAGNOSIS: Constipation

related to:
a. decreased gastrointestinal motility associated with anesthesia, manipulation of bowel during abdominal surgery, narcotic analgesics, and decreased activity;
b. decreased fluid intake;
c. decreased intake of foods high in fiber.

**Desired Outcome** | **Nursing Actions and *Selected Purposes/Rationales***

14. The client will not experience constipation as evidenced by:
    a. usual frequency of bowel movements when usual oral intake is resumed
    b. passage of soft, formed stool
    c. absence of headache, anorexia, increasing abdominal distention and pain, rectal pressure, and straining at stool.

14.a. Ascertain client's usual bowel elimination habits.
   b. Assess for signs and symptoms of constipation (e.g. decrease in frequency of stools; passage of hard, formed stools; headache; anorexia; increasing abdominal distention and pain; feeling of fullness or pressure in rectum; straining at stool).
   c. Assess bowel sounds. Report diminishing sounds or sounds that do not return to normal when expected.
   d. Implement measures *to prevent constipation:*
      1. increase activity as allowed and tolerated
      2. encourage client to defecate whenever the urge is felt
      3. assist client to the bathroom or bedside commode or place in high Fowler's position on bedpan for bowel movements unless contraindicated; provide privacy and adequate ventilation
      4. encourage client to relax during attempts to defecate *in order to promote relaxation of the pelvic floor musculature and external anal sphincter*
      5. encourage use of nonnarcotic analgesics once period of severe pain has subsided
      6. when oral intake is allowed:
         a. instruct client to maintain a minimum fluid intake of 2500 ml/day unless contraindicated
         b. encourage client to drink warm liquids upon arising in the morning *in order to initiate the gastrocolic and duodenocolic reflexes and stimulate peristalsis*
         c. when diet advances, instruct client to increase intake of foods high in fiber (e.g. bran, whole-grain breads and cereals, raw fruits and vegetables) unless contraindicated
      7. administer laxatives, stool softeners, and/or enemas if ordered.
   e. Consult physician if signs and symptoms of constipation persist.

## 15. NURSING DIAGNOSIS: Sleep pattern disturbance

related to fear, anxiety, discomfort, inability to assume usual sleep position, and frequent assessments and treatments.

**Desired Outcome** | **Nursing Actions and *Selected Purposes/Rationales***

15. The client will attain optimal amounts of sleep within the parameters of the treatment regimen as evidenced by:
    a. statements of feeling well rested
    b. usual mental status
    c. absence of frequent yawning, dark circles under eyes, and hand tremors.

15.a. Assess for signs and symptoms of a sleep pattern disturbance (e.g. verbal complaints of difficulty falling asleep, sleep interruptions, or not feeling well rested; irritability; lethargy; disorientation; frequent yawning; dark circles under eyes; slight hand tremors).
   b. Determine the client's usual sleep habits.
   c. Implement measures *to promote sleep:*
      1. discourage long periods of sleep during the day unless signs and symptoms of sleep deprivation exist or daytime sleep is usual for client
      2. perform actions to reduce fear and anxiety (see Nursing Diagnosis 20, action b)
      3. perform actions to reduce discomfort (see Nursing Diagnoses 6, action e; 7.A, action 3; 7.B, action 2; and 7.C)
      4. encourage participation in relaxing diversional activities during the evening
      5. when oral intake is allowed:
         a. discourage intake of fluids high in caffeine (e.g. coffee, tea, colas), especially in the evening

| Desired Outcome | Nursing Actions and ***Selected Purposes/Rationales*** |
|---|---|

b. offer client a high-protein evening snack (e.g. milk, cheese) unless contraindicated
6. allow client to continue usual sleep practices (e.g. position, time, bedtime rituals such as reading and meditating) if possible
7. satisfy needs such as comfort and warmth whenever possible
8. have client empty bladder just before bedtime
9. maintain a quiet, restful atmosphere; have earplugs available for client if needed
10. use relaxation techniques (e.g. progressive relaxation exercises, back massage, meditation, soft music) before sleep
11. ensure good room ventilation
12. administer sedative-hypnotics if ordered
13. perform actions *to reduce interruptions during sleep (80-100 minutes of uninterrupted sleep are usually needed to complete one sleep cycle):*
    a. restrict visitors
    b. group care (e.g. medications, treatments, physical care, assessments) whenever possible.

d. Consult physician if signs and symptoms of sleep deprivation persist or worsen.

## 16. NURSING DIAGNOSIS: High risk for infection:

a. **pneumonia** related to stasis of pulmonary secretions and aspiration (if it occurs);
b. **wound infection** related to wound contamination and decreased resistance to infection associated with diminished tissue perfusion of wound area and inadequate nutritional status;
c. **urinary tract infection** related to:
    1. increased bacterial growth associated with urinary stasis
    2. introduction of pathogens associated with an indwelling catheter if present.

| Desired Outcomes | Nursing Actions and ***Selected Purposes/Rationales*** |
|---|---|
| 16.a. The client will not develop pneumonia as evidenced by:<br>1. normal breath sounds<br>2. resonant percussion note over lungs<br>3. absence of tachypnea<br>4. cough productive of clear mucus only<br>5. afebrile status<br>6. absence of pleuritic pain<br>7. WBC count returning toward normal | 16.a.1. Assess for and report signs and symptoms of pneumonia:<br>a. abnormal breath sounds (e.g. crackles [rales], pleural friction rub, bronchial breath sounds, diminished or absent breath sounds)<br>b. dull percussion note over affected lung area<br>c. increase in respiratory rate<br>d. cough productive of purulent, green, or rust-colored sputum<br>e. chills and fever<br>f. pleuritic pain<br>g. persistent elevation or increase in WBC count.<br>2. Monitor oximetry and blood gas results. Report abnormal findings.<br>3. Monitor chest x-ray results. Report findings indicative of pneumonia.<br>4. Obtain sputum specimen for culture if ordered. Report abnormal results.<br>5. Implement measures *to prevent pneumonia:*<br>a. perform actions to maintain an effective breathing pattern and airway clearance (see Nursing Diagnoses 2, action c and 3, action b)<br>b. perform actions to reduce risk for aspiration (see Nursing Diagnosis 18, action c)<br>c. encourage and assist client to perform good oral hygiene *in order to* |

8. blood gases within normal range for client
9. negative sputum culture.

*reduce the colonization of bacteria in the oropharynx and subsequent aspiration of these microorganisms*
d. protect client from persons with respiratory tract infections.
6. If signs and symptoms of pneumonia occur:
a. continue with above measures
b. administer oxygen as ordered
c. administer antimicrobials if ordered
d. perform or assist with respiratory physiotherapy (e.g. postural drainage, chest percussion and vibration)
e. refer to Care Plan on Pneumonia for additional care measures.

16.b. The client will remain free of wound infection as evidenced by:
1. absence of chills and fever
2. absence of redness, heat, and swelling around wounds
3. usual drainage from wounds
4. WBC and differential counts returning toward normal
5. negative cultures of wound drainage.

16.b.1. Assess for and report signs and symptoms of wound infection (e.g. chills; fever; redness, warmth, and swelling of wound area; unusual wound drainage; foul odor from wound area).
2. Monitor for and report persistent elevation of WBC count and significant change in differential.
3. Obtain cultures of wound drainage as ordered. Report positive results.
4. Implement measures *to prevent wound infection:*
a. perform actions to promote wound healing (see Nursing Diagnosis 9, action a.2)
b. use good handwashing technique and encourage client to do the same
c. instruct client to avoid touching incisions, dressings, drainage tubings, and open wounds
d. maintain meticulous aseptic technique during all dressing changes and wound care
e. protect client from others with infections
f. administer antimicrobials if ordered.
5. If signs and symptoms of infection are present, continue with above actions.

16.c. The client will remain free of urinary tract infection as evidenced by:
1. clear urine
2. no unusual odor to urine
3. absence of frequency, urgency, and burning on urination
4. absence of chills and fever
5. absence of nitrites, bacteria, and WBCs in urine
6. negative urine culture.

16.c.1. Assess for and report signs and symptoms of urinary tract infection (e.g. cloudy, foul-smelling urine; complaints of frequency, urgency, or burning on urination; chills; elevated temperature).
2. Monitor urinalysis and report presence of nitrites, bacteria, and/or WBCs.
3. Obtain a urine specimen for culture and sensitivity if ordered. Report abnormal results.
4. Implement measures *to prevent urinary tract infection:*
a. perform actions to prevent urinary retention (see Nursing Diagnosis 13, actions d and f)
b. instruct female client to wipe from front to back after urinating or defecating
c. assist client with perineal care every shift and after each bowel movement
d. maintain fluid intake of at least 2500 ml/day unless contraindicated
e. increase activity as allowed and tolerated *to decrease urinary stasis*
f. maintain sterile technique during urinary catheterizations and irrigations
g. if an indwelling urinary catheter is present:
1. secure the catheter tubing to lower abdomen or thigh on males or to thigh on females *to minimize risk of accidental traction and subsequent trauma to the bladder and urethra*
2. perform catheter care as often as needed *to prevent accumulation of mucus around the meatus*
3. keep urine collection container lower than level of the bladder at all times *to prevent reflux or stasis of urine*
4. remove catheter as soon as allowed *(risk for urinary tract infection increases the longer the catheter is in place).*
5. If signs and symptoms of urinary tract infection are present:
a. continue with the above actions
b. administer antimicrobials if ordered.

## 17. NURSING DIAGNOSIS: High risk for trauma

related to falls associated with:
a. weakness and fatigue;
b. postural hypotension resulting from peripheral pooling of blood and blood loss during surgery;
c. central nervous system depressant effects of some medications;
d. presence of drainage tubings or equipment.

| Desired Outcome | Nursing Actions and ***Selected Purposes/Rationales*** |
|---|---|
| 17. The client will not experience falls. | 17.a. Implement measures *to prevent falls:*<br>1. keep bed in low position with side rails up when client is in bed<br>2. keep needed items within easy reach<br>3. encourage client to request assistance whenever needed; have call signal within easy reach<br>4. use lap belt when client is in chair if indicated<br>5. instruct client to wear well-fitting slippers/shoes with nonslip soles and low heels when ambulating<br>6. keep floor free of clutter and wipe up spills promptly<br>7. instruct and assist client to get out of bed slowly *in order to reduce dizziness associated with postural hypotension*<br>8. carefully position tubings and equipment so that they will not interfere with ambulation<br>9. provide ambulatory aids (e.g. walker, cane) if client is weak or unsteady on feet<br>10. accompany client during ambulation and use a transfer safety belt if he/she is weak or dizzy<br>11. instruct client to ambulate in well-lit areas and to utilize handrails if needed<br>12. do not rush client; allow adequate time for ambulation to the bathroom and in hallway<br>13. make sure that shower area has a nonslip bottom surface and that shower chair, secure bath mat, call light, hand grips, and adequate lighting are present<br>14. perform actions to increase strength and improve activity tolerance (see Nursing Diagnosis 10, action b).<br>b. Include client and significant others in planning and implementing measures to prevent falls.<br>c. If client falls, initiate first aid measures if appropriate and notify physician. |

## 18. NURSING DIAGNOSIS: High risk for aspiration

related to:
a. decreased level of consciousness and absent or diminished gag reflex associated with depressant effects of anesthesia and narcotic analgesics;
b. flat, supine positioning.

| Desired Outcome | Nursing Actions and ***Selected Purposes/Rationales*** |
|---|---|
| 18. The client will not aspirate secretions or foods/fluids as evidenced by:<br>a. clear breath sounds<br>b. resonant percussion note over lungs<br>c. absence of cough, tachypnea, and dyspnea. | 18.a. Assess for signs and symptoms of aspiration of secretions or foods/fluids (e.g. rhonchi, dull percussion note over affected lung area, cough, tachypnea, dyspnea, tachycardia).<br>b. Monitor chest x-ray results. Report findings of pulmonary infiltrate.<br>c. Implement measures *to reduce the risk for aspiration:*<br>1. withhold oral foods/fluids and place client in a side-lying position unless contraindicated if gag reflex is absent or client is not alert<br>2. have suction equipment readily available for use<br>3. perform oropharyngeal suctioning and provide oral hygiene as often as needed *to remove secretions*<br>4. perform actions to prevent nausea and vomiting (see Nursing Diagnosis 7.B, action 2)<br>5. perform actions to reduce accumulation of gastrointestinal gas and fluid (see Nursing Diagnosis 7.A, action 3) *in order to prevent gastric distention and possible regurgitation*<br>6. place client in high Fowler's position during and for at least 30 minutes after eating or drinking unless contraindicated.<br>d. If signs and symptoms of aspiration occur:<br>1. perform tracheal suctioning<br>2. notify physician<br>3. prepare client for chest x-ray. |

## 19. COLLABORATIVE DIAGNOSES:

**Potential complications:**

a. **hypovolemic shock** related to hemorrhage and fluid volume deficit associated with excessive fluid loss and inadequate fluid replacement;

b. **atelectasis** related to shallow respirations, stasis of secretions in the alveoli and bronchioles, and decreased surfactant production (results from inadequate deep breathing and changes in regional blood flow in the lungs);

c. **thromboembolism** related to:
   1. venous stasis associated with decreased activity, positioning during and following surgery, fluid volume deficit, and abdominal distention (the distended intestine may put pressure on the abdominal vessels)
   2. hypercoagulability associated with increased release of tissue thromboplastin into the blood (occurs as a result of surgical trauma)
   3. decreased fibrinolytic activity (occurs in response to surgical trauma)
   4. trauma to vein walls during surgery;

d. **paralytic ileus** related to manipulation of intestines during abdominal surgery, effects of anesthesia and some medications (e.g. central nervous system depressants), hypokalemia, and hypovolemia (can cause decreased blood supply to the intestine);

e. **dehiscence** related to:
   1. inadequate wound closure
   2. stress on incision line associated with persistent coughing, distention, or vomiting
   3. poor wound healing associated with decreased tissue perfusion of wound area, inadequate nutritional status, and infection.

| Desired Outcomes | Nursing Actions and ***Selected Purposes/Rationales*** |
|---|---|
| 19.a. The client will not develop hypovolemic shock as evidenced by: | 19.a.1. Assess for and report excessive bleeding and gastrointestinal and wound drainage, persistent vomiting, and/or difficulty maintaining intravenous or oral fluid intake as ordered.<br>2. Monitor RBC, Hct, and Hb levels. Report declining values. |

| Desired Outcomes | Nursing Actions and ***Selected Purposes/Rationales*** |
|---|---|
| 1. usual mental status<br>2. stable vital signs<br>3. skin warm, dry, and usual color<br>4. palpable peripheral pulses<br>5. urine output at least 30 ml/hour. | 3. Assess for and report signs and symptoms of hypovolemic shock:<br>a. restlessness, agitation, confusion<br>b. significant decrease in B/P<br>c. postural hypotension<br>d. rapid, thready pulse<br>e. rapid respirations<br>f. cool, moist skin<br>g. pallor, cyanosis<br>h. diminished or absent peripheral pulses<br>i. urine output less than 30 ml/hour.<br>4. Implement measures *to prevent hypovolemic shock:*<br>a. if bleeding occurs, apply firm, prolonged pressure to area if possible<br>b. perform actions to prevent fluid volume deficit (see Nursing Diagnosis 4, actions a.3 a-d).<br>5. If signs and symptoms of hypovolemic shock occur:<br>a. continue with above measures to control bleeding and prevent fluid volume deficit<br>b. place client flat in bed with legs elevated unless contraindicated<br>c. monitor vital signs frequently<br>d. administer oxygen as ordered<br>e. administer blood products and/or volume expanders if ordered<br>f. prepare client for insertion of hemodynamic monitoring devices (e.g. central venous catheter, intra-arterial catheter) if indicated<br>g. provide emotional support to client and significant others. |
| 19.b. The client will not develop atelectasis as evidenced by:<br>1. normal breath sounds<br>2. resonant percussion note over lungs<br>3. unlabored respirations at 14-20/minute<br>4. pulse rate within normal range for client<br>5. afebrile status. | 19.b.1. Assess for and report signs and symptoms of atelectasis (e.g. diminished or absent breath sounds, dull percussion note over affected area, increased respiratory rate, dyspnea, tachycardia, elevated temperature).<br>2. Monitor chest x-ray results. Report findings of atelectasis.<br>3. Implement measures *to prevent atelectasis:*<br>a. perform actions to improve breathing pattern (see Nursing Diagnosis 2, action c)<br>b. perform actions to promote effective airway clearance (see Nursing Diagnosis 3, action b).<br>4. If signs and symptoms of atelectasis occur:<br>a. increase frequency of turning, coughing or "huffing," deep breathing, and use of incentive spirometer<br>b. consult physician if signs and symptoms of atelectasis persist or worsen. |
| 19.c.1. The client will not develop a deep vein thrombus as evidenced by:<br>a. absence of pain, tenderness, heaviness, swelling, and distended superficial vessels in extremities<br>b. usual temperature of extremities<br>c. negative Homan's sign. | 19.c.1.a. Assess for and report signs and symptoms of a deep vein thrombus:<br>1. pain, tenderness, or heavy feeling in extremity<br>2. increase in circumference of extremity<br>3. distention of superficial vessels in extremity<br>4. unusual warmth of extremity<br>5. positive Homan's sign (not always a reliable indicator).<br>b. Implement measures *to prevent thrombus formation:*<br>1. perform actions to prevent peripheral pooling of blood (see Nursing Diagnosis 1, action b.4)<br>2. maintain a minimum fluid intake of 2500 ml/day (unless contraindicated) *to prevent fluid volume deficit and increased blood viscosity, which leads to venous stasis*<br>3. administer anticoagulants (e.g. low-dose heparin, warfarin) or antiplatelet agents (e.g. low-dose aspirin) if ordered.<br>c. If signs and symptoms of a deep vein thrombus occur:<br>1. maintain client on bed rest until activity orders received<br>2. elevate foot of bed 15-20° above heart level if ordered (use knee gatch to maintain knees in a slightly flexed position) |

3. discourage positions that compromise blood flow (e.g. pillows under knees, crossing legs, sitting for long periods)
4. apply heating pad or warm moist packs to affected area if ordered
5. prepare client for diagnostic studies (e.g. venography, duplex ultrasound, impedance plethysmography) if indicated
6. administer anticoagulants (e.g. heparin, warfarin) if ordered
7. prepare client for the following if planned:
   a. vena caval interruption (e.g. insertion of an intracaval filtering device)
   b. thrombectomy
8. refer to Care Plan on Deep Vein Thrombosis for additional care measures.

19.c.2. The client will not experience a pulmonary embolism as evidenced by:
a. absence of sudden chest pain
b. unlabored respirations at 14-20/minute
c. pulse 60-100 beats/minute
d. usual mental status
e. blood gases within normal range.

19.c.2.a. Assess for and report signs and symptoms of a pulmonary embolism (e.g. sudden chest pain, dyspnea, tachypnea, tachycardia, restlessness, apprehension, low $PaO_2$).

b. Implement measures *to prevent a pulmonary embolism:*
1. perform actions to prevent and treat a deep vein thrombus (see actions c.1.b and c.1.c in this diagnosis)
2. do not exercise, check for Homan's sign in, or massage any extremity known to have a thrombus
3. caution client to avoid activities that create a Valsalva response (e.g. straining to have bowel movement, holding breath while moving) *in order to prevent dislodgment of existing thrombi.*

c. If signs and symptoms of a pulmonary embolism occur:
1. maintain client on strict bed rest in a semi- to high Fowler's position
2. maintain oxygen therapy as ordered
3. prepare client for diagnostic tests (e.g. blood gases, ventilation-perfusion lung scan, pulmonary angiography)
4. administer anticoagulants (e.g. continuous intravenous heparin, warfarin) if ordered
5. prepare client for the following if planned:
   a. vena caval interruption (e.g. insertion of an intracaval filtering device) *to prevent further pulmonary emboli*
   b. embolectomy
6. provide emotional support to client and significant others
7. refer to Care Plan on Pulmonary Embolism for additional care measures.

19.d. The client will not develop a paralytic ileus as evidenced by:
1. absence or resolution of abdominal pain and cramping
2. soft, nondistended abdomen
3. gradual return of bowel sounds
4. passage of flatus.

19.d.1. Assess for and report signs and symptoms of paralytic ileus (e.g. development of or persistent abdominal pain and cramping; firm, distended abdomen; absent bowel sounds; failure to pass flatus).

2. Implement measures *to prevent paralytic ileus:*
   a. increase activity as soon as allowed and tolerated
   b. perform actions to maintain fluid and electrolyte balance (see Nursing Diagnosis 4, action a.3) in order *to prevent hypokalemia and the resultant decrease in peristalsis*
   c. perform actions to maintain adequate tissue perfusion (see Nursing Diagnosis 1, action b) in order *to maintain adequate blood supply to the bowel*
   d. administer gastrointestinal stimulants (e.g. metoclopramide) if ordered.

3. If signs and symptoms of paralytic ileus occur:
   a. continue with above measures
   b. withhold all oral intake
   c. insert nasogastric tube and maintain suction as ordered
   d. assess for and report signs of bowel necrosis (e.g. fever, increased or persistent elevation of WBCs, significant decline in B/P and increase in pulse).

| Desired Outcomes | Nursing Actions and ***Selected Purposes/Rationales*** |
|---|---|
| 19.e. The client will not experience dehiscence as evidenced by intact, approximated wound edges. | 19.e.1. Assess for and report evidence of dehiscence (separation of edges of the wound).<br>2. Implement measures to promote wound healing (see Nursing Diagnosis 9, action a.2) *in order to decrease the risk of dehiscence.*<br>3. If dehiscence occurs:<br>a. apply skin closures (e.g. butterfly tape, Steri-Strips) to the incision line and/or assist with resuturing the wound if indicated<br>b. if client has an abdominal incision, assess for and immediately report signs and symptoms of evisceration (e.g. client statements that "something popped" or "gave way," sudden drainage of serosanguineous peritoneal fluid from wound, protrusion of intestinal contents). |

## 20. NURSING DIAGNOSIS: Anxiety

related to unfamiliar environment; pain; lack of understanding of surgical procedure performed, diagnosis, and postoperative treatment plan; changes in body image and roles; and financial concerns.

| Desired Outcome | Nursing Actions and ***Selected Purposes/Rationales*** |
|---|---|
| 20. The client will experience a reduction in anxiety as evidenced by:<br>a. verbalization of feeling less anxious and fearful<br>b. usual sleep pattern<br>c. relaxed facial expression and body movements<br>d. stable vital signs<br>e. usual perceptual ability and interactions with others. | 20.a. Assess client for signs and symptoms of anxiety (e.g. verbalization of fears and concerns, insomnia, tenseness, tremors, irritability, restlessness, diaphoresis, tachycardia, tachypnea, elevated blood pressure, facial pallor or flushing, narrowed perceptual field, withdrawal, noncompliance with treatment plan). Validate perceptions carefully, remembering that some behavior may result from factors such as pain, fluid and electrolyte imbalances, and infection.<br>b. Implement measures *to reduce fear and anxiety:*<br>1. orient client to hospital environment, equipment, and routines<br>2. introduce staff who will be participating in his/her care; if possible, maintain consistency in staff assigned to his/her care *to provide feelings of stability and comfort with the environment*<br>3. assure client that staff members are nearby; respond to call signal as soon as possible<br>4. maintain a calm, supportive, confident manner when interacting with client<br>5. encourage verbalization of fear and anxiety; provide feedback<br>6. reinforce the physician's explanations and clarify any misconceptions the client has about the diagnosis, surgical procedure performed, treatment plan, and prognosis<br>7. perform actions to reduce pain (see Nursing Diagnosis 6, action e)<br>8. provide a calm, restful environment<br>9. instruct client in relaxation techniques and encourage participation in diversional activities<br>10. assist client to identify specific stressors and ways to cope with them<br>11. arrange for visit from clergy if client desires<br>12. initiate financial and/or social service referrals if indicated<br>13. encourage significant others to project a caring, concerned attitude without obvious anxiousness<br>14. administer antianxiety agents if ordered. |

c. Include significant others in orientation and teaching sessions and encourage their continued support of the client.
d. Provide information based on current needs of client and significant others at a level they can understand. Encourage questions and clarification of information provided.
e. Consult physician if above actions fail to control fear and anxiety.

## 21. NURSING DIAGNOSIS: Knowledge deficit

regarding follow-up care.

| Desired Outcomes | Nursing Actions and ***Selected Purposes/Rationales*** |
|---|---|
| 21.a. The client will identify ways to prevent postoperative infection. | 21.a. Instruct client in ways to prevent postoperative infection:<br>1. continue with coughing (if allowed) and deep breathing every 2 hours while awake<br>2. reinforce continued use of incentive spirometer if indicated<br>3. increase activity as ordered<br>4. avoid contact with persons who have infections<br>5. avoid crowds during flu and cold seasons<br>6. decrease or stop smoking<br>7. drink at least 10 glasses of liquid/day<br>8. maintain a balanced nutritional intake<br>9. maintain proper balance of rest and activity<br>10. maintain good personal hygiene (especially oral care, handwashing, and perineal care)<br>11. avoid touching any wound unless it is completely healed<br>12. maintain sterile or clean technique as ordered during wound care. |
| 21.b. The client will demonstrate the ability to perform wound care. | 21.b.1. Discuss the rationale for, frequency of, and equipment necessary for the prescribed wound care.<br>2. Provide client with the necessary equipment (e.g. dressings, irrigating solution, tape) for wound care and with names and addresses of places where additional equipment can be obtained.<br>3. Demonstrate wound care and proper cleansing of any reusable equipment. Allow time for questions, clarification, and return demonstration. |
| 21.c. The client will state signs and symptoms to report to the health care provider. | 21.c. Instruct the client to report the following signs and symptoms:<br>1. persistent low-grade or significantly elevated (38.3° C [101° F]) temperature<br>2. difficulty breathing<br>3. chest pain<br>4. cough productive of purulent, green, or rust-colored sputum<br>5. increasing weakness or inability to tolerate prescribed activity level<br>6. increasing discomfort or discomfort not controlled by prescribed medications and treatments<br>7. continued nausea or vomiting<br>8. increasing abdominal distention and/or discomfort<br>9. separation of wound edges<br>10. increasing redness, warmth, pain, or swelling around wound<br>11. unusual or excessive drainage from any wound site<br>12. pain, redness, or swelling in calf of one or both legs<br>13. urine retention<br>14. frequency, urgency, or burning on urination<br>15. cloudy, foul-smelling urine. |

| Desired Outcomes | Nursing Actions and ***Selected Purposes/Rationales*** |
|---|---|
| 21.d. The client will verbalize an understanding of and a plan for adhering to recommended follow-up care including future appointments with health care provider, dietary modifications, activity level, treatments, and medications prescribed. | 21.d.1. Reinforce importance of keeping scheduled follow-up appointments with the health care provider.<br>2. Reinforce physician's instructions about dietary modifications. Obtain a dietary consult for client if needed.<br>3. Reinforce physician's instructions on suggested activity level and treatment plan.<br>4. Explain the rationale for, side effects of, and importance of taking medications prescribed.<br>5. Implement measures to improve client compliance:<br>a. include significant others in teaching sessions if possible<br>b. encourage questions and allow time for reinforcement and clarification of information provided<br>c. provide written instructions on scheduled appointments with health care provider, dietary modifications, activity level, treatment plan, medications prescribed, and signs and symptoms to report. |

UNIT
V

# *Nursing Care of the Immobile Client*

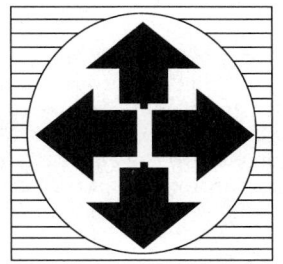

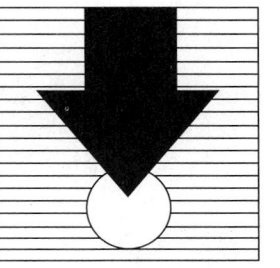

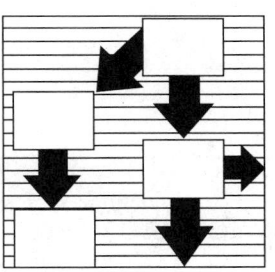

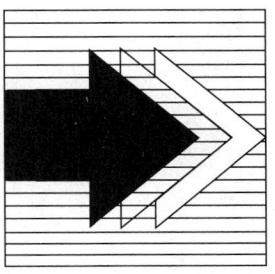

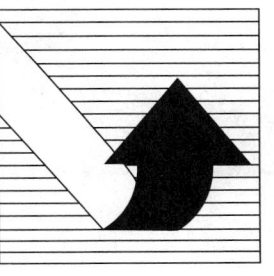

# Immobility

Immobility refers to a limitation of physical activity as a result of a disease process, trauma, or therapeutic intervention. Immobility for periods greater than 48 to 72 hours will result in changes in all body systems. **This care plan focuses on the adult client who is on complete bed rest for a prolonged period during hospitalization.** Goals of care are to maintain comfort, prevent complications, and educate the client regarding follow-up care. Many of the actions included in the care plan will help prevent disuse syndrome, which is a deterioration of body systems as a result of prescribed or unavoidable musculoskeletal inactivity.

## DISCHARGE CRITERIA

Prior to discharge, the client will:

- have no signs or symptoms of complications
- verbalize an understanding of ways to prevent complications associated with continued decreased mobility
- demonstrate techniques for meeting self-care needs
- state signs and symptoms to report to the health care provider
- identify community agencies that may provide assistance with home care and transportation
- verbalize an understanding of and a plan for adhering to recommended follow-up care including future appointments with health care provider and physical therapist, exercise regimen, and medications prescribed.

## NURSING/COLLABORATIVE DIAGNOSES

## 1. NURSING DIAGNOSIS: Ineffective breathing pattern

related to:
a. depressant effects of some medications (e.g. narcotic analgesics, sedatives, central-acting muscle relaxants) that may be given for treatment of current diagnosis;
b. impaired lung/chest wall expansion associated with:
   1. recumbent positioning (in this position, full expansion of the lungs is restricted by the bed surface and by the abdominal contents pushing up against the diaphragm)
   2. weakness
   3. eventual fixation of intercostal joints in an expiratory state (joints become fixed as a result of a prolonged lack of usual inspiratory movement).

| Desired Outcome | Nursing Actions and ***Selected Purposes/Rationales*** |
|---|---|
| 1. The client will maintain an effective breathing pattern as evidenced by:<br>a. normal rate and depth of respirations<br>b. blood gases within normal range. | 1.a. Assess for signs and symptoms of an ineffective breathing pattern (e.g. shallow or slow respirations).<br>b. Monitor for and report the following:<br>1. abnormal blood gases<br>2. significant change in oximetry results.<br>c. Implement measures *to improve breathing pattern:*<br>1. place client in a semi- to high Fowler's position unless contraindicated; position client with pillows *to prevent slumping*<br>2. turn client at least every 2 hours<br>3. instruct client to deep breathe or use incentive spirometer at least every 2 hours<br>4. assist with IPPB treatments as ordered<br>5. instruct client to avoid intake of gas-forming foods (e.g. beans, cauliflower, cabbage, onions), carbonated beverages, and large meals *in order to prevent gastric distention and pressure on the diaphragm*<br>6. increase activity as allowed<br>7. administer central nervous system depressants judiciously; hold medication and consult physician if respiratory rate is less than 12/minute.<br>d. Consult physician if:<br>1. ineffective breathing pattern continues<br>2. signs and symptoms of impaired gas exchange (e.g. restlessness, irritability, confusion, decreased $PaO_2$ and increased $PaCO_2$ levels) are present. |

## 2. NURSING DIAGNOSIS: Ineffective airway clearance

related to stasis of secretions associated with poor cough effort and decreased mobility.

| Desired Outcome | Nursing Actions and ***Selected Purposes/Rationales*** |
|---|---|
| 2. The client will maintain clear, open airways as evidenced by:<br>a. normal breath sounds | 2.a. Assess for signs and symptoms of ineffective airway clearance (e.g. abnormal breath sounds; rapid, shallow respirations; dyspnea; cyanosis).<br>b. Implement measures *to promote effective airway clearance:*<br>1. instruct and assist client to turn, deep breathe, and cough or "huff" every 1-2 hours |

| Desired Outcome | Nursing Actions and ***Selected Purposes/Rationales*** |
|---|---|
| b. normal rate and depth of respirations<br>c. absence of dyspnea<br>d. absence of cyanosis. | 2. perform actions *to facilitate removal of secretions:*<br>a. implement measures *to liquefy tenacious secretions:*<br>1. maintain a fluid intake of at least 2500 ml/day unless contraindicated<br>2. humidify inspired air as ordered<br>b. assist with administration of diluent and mucolytic agents via nebulizer or IPPB treatment as ordered<br>c. assist with or perform postural drainage, percussion, and vibration if ordered<br>d. perform nasal, oral, pharyngeal, or tracheal suctioning if needed<br>3. discourage smoking *(smoke causes bronchoconstriction, increases mucus production, and impairs ciliary function)*<br>4. protect client from exposure to irritants such as smoke, flowers, and perfume *(can cause bronchospasm and increased mucus production)*<br>5. reinforce correct use of incentive spirometer and assist with IPPB treatments if ordered *to promote bronchodilation and movement of secretions*<br>6. administer central nervous system depressants judiciously<br>7. increase activity as allowed.<br>c. Consult physician if:<br>1. signs and symptoms of ineffective airway clearance persist<br>2. signs and symptoms of impaired gas exchange (e.g. restlessness, irritability, confusion, decreased $PaO_2$ and increased $PaCO_2$ levels) are present. |

## 3. NURSING DIAGNOSIS: Altered nutrition: less than body requirements

related to:

a. decreased oral intake associated with:
   1. anorexia resulting from boredom, depression, a slowed metabolic rate, and early satiety that occurs with decreased gastrointestinal motility
   2. difficulty feeding self as a result of impaired or limited physical mobility;

b. imbalance in rate of catabolism and anabolism (in the immobilized person, catabolic processes occur at a faster rate than anabolic processes).

| Desired Outcome | Nursing Actions and ***Selected Purposes/Rationales*** |
|---|---|
| 3. The client will maintain an adequate nutritional status as evidenced by:<br>a. weight within normal range for client's age, height, and body frame<br>b. normal BUN and serum albumin, Hct, Hb, transferrin, and lymphocyte levels<br>c. triceps skinfold thickness within normal range<br>d. no further decline in strength and activity tolerance | 3.a. Assess for and report signs and symptoms of malnutrition:<br>1. weight below normal for client's age, height, and body frame<br>2. abnormal BUN and low serum albumin, Hct, Hb, transferrin, and lymphocyte levels<br>3. triceps skinfold thickness less than normal<br>4. weakness and fatigue<br>5. stomatitis.<br>b. Monitor percentage of meals and snacks client consumes. Report a pattern of inadequate intake.<br>c. Implement measures *to maintain an adequate nutritional status:*<br>1. perform actions *to improve oral intake:*<br>a. obtain a dietary consult if necessary to assist client in selecting foods/fluids that meet nutritional needs as well as personal and cultural preferences whenever possible<br>b. encourage a rest period before meals *to minimize fatigue*<br>c. maintain a clean environment and relaxed, pleasant atmosphere<br>d. provide oral care before meals |

e. healthy oral mucous membrane.

e. serve small portions of nutritious foods/fluids that are appealing to client
f. implement measures to prevent constipation (see Nursing Diagnosis 9, action d) *in order to reduce feeling of fullness*
g. encourage significant others to bring in client's favorite foods unless contraindicated and eat with him/her *to make eating more of a familiar social experience*
h. encourage significant others to be present to assist client with meals if needed
i. allow adequate time for meals; reheat food if necessary
j. limit fluid intake (unless it has a high nutritional value) with meals *to reduce early satiety and subsequent decreased food intake*
k. enable client to feed self if possible; if client needs to be fed, offer foods/fluids in the order he/she prefers
l. increase activity as allowed *(activity stimulates appetite)*

2. ensure that meals are well balanced and high in essential nutrients; offer high-protein, high-calorie dietary supplements between meals if indicated
3. administer vitamins (vitamin C in particular is essential for rebuilding depleted protein stores) and minerals if ordered.

d. Perform a 72-hour calorie count if ordered. Report totals to dietitian and physician.
e. Consult physician regarding alternative methods of providing nutrition (e.g. parenteral nutrition, tube feedings) if client does not consume enough food or fluids to meet nutritional needs.

## 4. NURSING DIAGNOSIS: High risk for impaired skin integrity

related to:
a. ischemia of the skin and subcutaneous tissue associated with prolonged pressure on tissues as a result of decreased mobility;
b. damage to the skin and/or subcutaneous tissue associated with friction or shearing;
c. increased fragility of the skin associated with dependent edema and inadequate nutritional status.

| Desired Outcome | Nursing Actions and ***Selected Purposes/Rationales*** |
|---|---|

4. The client will maintain skin integrity as evidenced by:
   a. absence of redness and irritation
   b. no skin breakdown.

4.a. Inspect the skin, especially bony prominences and dependent areas, for pallor, redness, and breakdown.

b. Implement measures *to prevent skin breakdown:*
   1. assist client to turn at least every 2 hours; use all 4 sides (prone, lateral [right/left], dorsal) unless contraindicated
   2. gently massage around reddened areas at least every 2 hours
   3. perform actions *to prevent shearing* (shearing occurs when one tissue layer slides past another) *and skin surface abrasion:*
      a. apply a thin layer of powder or cornstarch to bottom sheet or skin *to absorb moisture (moist skin is more likely to adhere to sheet) and reduce friction*
      b. lift and move client carefully using a turn sheet and adequate assistance
      c. limit length of time client is in semi-Fowler's position to 30 minutes *(in this position, client tends to slide down in bed)*
   4. instruct or assist client to shift weight every 30 minutes

| Desired Outcome | Nursing Actions and ***Selected Purposes/Rationales*** |
|---|---|

5. if fade time (length of time it takes for reddened area to fade after pressure is removed) is greater than 15 minutes, increase frequency of position changes and/or provide more effective methods of cushioning, padding, and positioning
6. keep skin clean and dry
7. keep bed linens dry and wrinkle-free
8. apply a thin layer of powder or cornstarch to areas with opposing skin surfaces (e.g. axillae, perineum, beneath breasts) if indicated *to absorb moisture and/or reduce friction*
9. provide devices to reduce pressure on the skin, decrease shearing, and/or prevent moisture build-up (e.g. Clinitron bed, alternating pressure mattress or pad, flotation pad, sheepskin)
10. perform actions *to prevent drying of the skin:*
    a. encourage a fluid intake of 2500 ml/day unless contraindicated
    b. provide a mild soap for bathing
    c. apply moisturizing lotion and/or emollient to skin at least once a day
11. perform actions to maintain an adequate nutritional status (see Nursing Diagnosis 3, action c)
12. if edema is present:
    a. perform actions *to reduce fluid accumulation in dependent areas:*
        1. instruct client in and assist with range of motion exercises
        2. elevate affected extremities whenever possible
    b. handle edematous areas carefully
13. increase activity as allowed.

c. If skin breakdown occurs:
    1. notify physician
    2. continue with above measures to prevent further irritation and breakdown
    3. perform decubitus care as ordered or per standard hospital procedure
    4. assess client closely and report signs and symptoms of infection (e.g. elevated temperature; redness, warmth, and edema around area of breakdown; unusual drainage from site).

## 5. NURSING DIAGNOSIS: Activity intolerance

related to:

a. decrease in available energy associated with slowed metabolic rate;
b. loss of muscle mass, tone, and strength associated with disuse and inadequate nutritional status;
c. eventual decrease in cardiac reserve associated with:
    1. a progressive increase in resting heart rate (increases approximately 0.5 beats/minute/day when a person is immobile)
    2. increased cardiac workload resulting from the increased venous return in a recumbent position
    3. weakening of the myocardium resulting from prolonged inactivity (not usually a factor until client has been immobilized for 3 weeks or longer);
d. difficulty resting and sleeping associated with inability to assume usual sleep position, frequent assessments and treatments, fear, anxiety, and unfamiliar environment.

| Desired Outcome | Nursing Actions and ***Selected Purposes/Rationales*** |
|---|---|

**Desired Outcome**

5. The client will demonstrate an increased tolerance for activity as evidenced by:
   a. verbalization of feeling less fatigued and weak
   b. ability to perform activities of daily living within physical limitations/restrictions without exertional dyspnea, chest pain, diaphoresis, dizziness, and a significant change in vital signs.

**Nursing Actions and *Selected Purposes/Rationales***

5.a. Assess for signs and symptoms of activity intolerance:
   1. statements of fatigue and weakness
   2. exertional dyspnea, chest pain, diaphoresis, or dizziness
   3. abnormal heart rate response to activity (e.g. increase in rate of 20 beats/minute above resting rate, decrease in rate, rate not returning to preactivity level within 3 minutes after stopping activity, change from regular to irregular rate)
   4. decreased systolic B/P or a significant increase (10-15 mm Hg) in systolic or diastolic pressure with activity.

b. Implement measures *to improve activity tolerance:*
   1. perform actions *to promote rest and/or conserve energy:*
      a. minimize environmental activity and noise
      b. organize nursing care to allow for periods of uninterrupted rest
      c. limit the number of visitors and their length of stay
      d. assist client with self-care activities as needed
      e. keep supplies and personal articles within easy reach
      f. implement measures to reduce fear and anxiety (see Nursing Diagnosis 13, action b)
      g. implement measures to promote sleep (see Nursing Diagnosis 10, action c)
   2. perform additional actions *to reduce cardiac workload and help maintain adequate cardiac reserve:*
      a. place client in a semi- to high Fowler's position periodically if allowed
      b. instruct client to avoid activities that create a Valsalva response (e.g. straining to have a bowel movement, holding breath while moving)
      c. implement measures to improve breathing pattern and airway clearance (see Nursing Diagnoses 1, action c and 2, action b) *in order to promote adequate tissue oxygenation*
      d. discourage smoking and excessive intake of beverages high in caffeine such as coffee, tea, and colas *(nicotine and caffeine increase cardiac workload and myocardial oxygen utilization, thereby decreasing oxygen availability)*
   3. perform actions to help maintain muscle strength (see Nursing Diagnosis 6, actions a.1-4)
   4. perform actions to maintain an adequate nutritional status (see Nursing Diagnosis 3, action c)
   5. when activity can be increased:
      a. increase activity gradually
      b. instruct client in energy-saving techniques (e.g. using shower chair when showering, sitting to brush teeth or comb hair).

c. Instruct client to:
   1. report a decreased tolerance for activity
   2. stop any activity that causes chest pain, shortness of breath, dizziness, or extreme fatigue or weakness.

d. Consult physician if signs and symptoms of activity intolerance persist or worsen.

## 6. NURSING DIAGNOSIS: Impaired physical mobility

related to:
a. activity limitations imposed by current diagnosis and/or treatment plan;
b. loss of muscle mass, tone, and strength associated with prolonged disuse and inadequate nutritional status.

| Desired Outcome | Nursing Actions and ***Selected Purposes/Rationales*** |
|---|---|
| 6. The client will maintain maximum physical mobility within limitations imposed by the disease or injury and treatment plan. | 6.a. Implement measures *to maintain optimal joint mobility and muscle function during period of immobility:*<br>1. instruct client in and assist with range of motion exercises at least 3 times/day unless contraindicated<br>2. reinforce instructions, activities, and exercise plan recommended by physical and occupational therapists<br>3. assist with use of electrical stimulation devices that promote muscle strengthening<br>4. encourage participation in self-care as allowed; put side rails up and provide overhead trapeze unless contraindicated *to promote independent movement*<br>5. perform actions to reduce the risk of contractures (see Collaborative Diagnosis 12, actions d.2-6)<br>6. perform actions to maintain an adequate nutritional status (see Nursing Diagnosis 3, action c) *in order to help maintain muscle mass, tone, and strength.*<br>b. Encourage the support of significant others. Allow them to assist with range of motion exercises and positioning if desired. |

## 7. NURSING DIAGNOSIS: Self-care deficit

related to:
a. activity limitations imposed by current diagnosis and/or treatment plan;
b. activity intolerance associated with decreased metabolic rate, cardiac deconditioning, loss of muscle strength, and difficulty resting and sleeping.

| Desired Outcome | Nursing Actions and ***Selected Purposes/Rationales*** |
|---|---|
| 7. The client will perform self-care activities within physical limitations and activity restrictions imposed by treatment plan. | 7.a. With client, develop a realistic plan for meeting daily physical needs.<br>b. Encourage client to perform as much of self-care as possible within physical limitations and activity restrictions imposed by the treatment plan.<br>c. Implement measures *to facilitate client's ability to perform self-care activities:*<br>1. schedule care at a time when client is most likely to be able to participate (e.g. when analgesics are at peak effect, after rest periods, not immediately after meals or treatments)<br>2. keep needed objects within easy reach<br>3. perform actions to increase activity tolerance (see Nursing Diagnosis 5, action b)<br>4. perform actions to maintain optimal joint mobility and muscle function (see Nursing Diagnosis 6, action a) |

5. consult occupational therapist about assistive devices available if indicated
6. allow adequate time for accomplishment of self-care activities.

d. Provide positive feedback for all efforts and accomplishments of self-care.
e. Assist the client with activities he/she is unable to perform independently.
f. Inform significant others of client's abilities to perform own care. Explain importance of encouraging and allowing client to maintain an optimal level of independence within prescribed activity restrictions and physical capabilities.

## 8. NURSING DIAGNOSIS: Urinary retention

related to:

a. pooling of urine in kidney and bladder associated with prolonged horizontal positioning;
b. difficulty urinating associated with anxiety regarding use of bedpan or urinal;
c. incomplete bladder emptying associated with:
   1. horizontal positioning (the gravity needed for complete bladder emptying is lost)
   2. decreased bladder muscle tone resulting from the generalized loss of muscle tone that occurs with prolonged immobility.

| Desired Outcome | Nursing Actions and ***Selected Purposes/Rationales*** |
|---|---|
| 8. The client will not experience urinary retention as evidenced by:<br>a. voiding at normal intervals<br>b. no complaints of bladder fullness or suprapubic discomfort<br>c. absence of bladder distention and dribbling of urine<br>d. balanced intake and output. | 8.a. Determine client's usual urinary elimination pattern.<br>b. Assess for signs and symptoms of urinary retention:<br>1. frequent voiding of small amounts (25-60 ml) of urine<br>2. complaints of bladder fullness or suprapubic discomfort<br>3. bladder distention<br>4. dribbling of urine<br>5. output less than intake.<br>c. Catheterize client if ordered *to determine the amount of residual urine.*<br>d. Implement measures *to prevent urinary retention:*<br>1. instruct client to urinate when the urge is first felt<br>2. perform actions *to promote relaxation during voiding attempts* (e.g. provide privacy, play soft music, encourage client to read)<br>3. perform actions *to provide sensory stimulation that may help trigger the micturition reflex and promote voluntary relaxation of the perineal muscles and external urinary sphincter* (e.g. run water, place client's hands in warm water, pour warm water over perineum)<br>4. allow client to assume a normal position for voiding unless contraindicated<br>5. instruct and/or assist client to lean his/her upper body forward and/or gently press downward on lower abdomen during voiding attempts unless contraindicated *in order to put pressure on the bladder area (pressure helps trigger the micturition reflex and promotes more complete bladder emptying)*<br>6. administer cholinergic drugs (e.g. bethanechol) if ordered *to stimulate bladder contraction.*<br>e. Consult physician about intermittent catheterization or insertion of an indwelling catheter if above actions fail to alleviate urinary retention. |

## 9. NURSING DIAGNOSIS: Constipation

related to:
a. diminished defecation reflex associated with:
   1. suppression of urge to defecate because of reluctance to use bedpan
   2. decreased gravity filling of lower rectum resulting from horizontal positioning;
b. weakened abdominal muscles associated with generalized loss of muscle tone resulting from prolonged immobility;
c. decreased gastrointestinal motility associated with decreased activity and the increased sympathetic nervous system activity that occurs with anxiety.

| Desired Outcome | Nursing Actions and ***Selected Purposes/Rationales*** |
|---|---|
| 9. The client will not experience constipation as evidenced by:<br>a. usual frequency of bowel movements<br>b. passage of soft, formed stool<br>c. absence of headache, anorexia, abdominal distention and pain, rectal pressure, and straining at stool. | 9.a. Ascertain client's usual bowel elimination habits.<br>b. Assess for signs and symptoms of constipation (e.g. decrease in frequency of stools; passage of hard, formed stools; headache; anorexia; abdominal distention and pain; feeling of fullness or pressure in rectum; straining at stool).<br>c. Assess bowel sounds. Report a pattern of decreasing bowel sounds.<br>d. Implement measures *to prevent constipation:*<br>1. encourage client to defecate whenever the urge is felt<br>2. place client in high Fowler's position for bowel movements unless contraindicated; provide privacy and adequate ventilation<br>3. encourage client to relax during attempts to defecate *in order to promote relaxation of the pelvic floor musculature and the external anal sphincter*<br>4. instruct client to increase intake of foods high in fiber (e.g. nuts, bran, whole-grain breads and cereals, raw fruits and vegetables, dried fruits) unless contraindicated<br>5. instruct client to maintain a minimum fluid intake of 2500 ml/day unless contraindicated<br>6. encourage client to drink warm liquids upon arising in the morning *in order to initiate the gastrocolic and duodenocolic reflexes and stimulate peristalsis*<br>7. encourage client to perform isometric abdominal strengthening exercises unless contraindicated<br>8. increase activity as allowed<br>9. administer laxatives, stool softeners, and/or enemas if ordered.<br>e. Check for impaction if client has not had a bowel movement in 3 days, if he/she is passing liquid stool, or if other signs and symptoms of constipation are present. Administer oil retention and/or cleansing enemas as ordered followed by digital removal of stool if necessary. |

## 10. NURSING DIAGNOSIS: Sleep pattern disturbance

related to current illness/injury, decreased physical activity, fear, anxiety, inability to assume usual sleep position, frequent assessments or treatments, and unfamiliar environment.

| Desired Outcome | Nursing Actions and ***Selected Purposes/Rationales*** |
|---|---|
| 10. The client will attain optimal amounts of sleep within the parameters of the treatment regimen as evidenced by:<br>a. statements of feeling well rested<br>b. usual mental status<br>c. absence of frequent yawning, dark circles under eyes, and hand tremors. | 10.a. Assess for signs and symptoms of a sleep pattern disturbance (e.g. verbal complaints of difficulty falling asleep, not feeling well rested, or sleep interruptions; irritability; disorientation; lethargy; frequent yawning; dark circles under eyes; slight hand tremors).<br>b. Determine the client's usual sleep habits.<br>c. Implement measures *to promote sleep:*<br>1. perform actions to reduce fear and anxiety (see Nursing Diagnosis 13, action b)<br>2. discourage long periods of sleep during the day unless signs and symptoms of sleep deprivation exist or daytime sleep is usual for client<br>3. encourage participation in relaxing diversional activities during the evening<br>4. discourage intake of fluids high in caffeine (e.g. coffee, tea, colas), especially in the evening<br>5. offer client a high-protein evening snack (e.g. milk, cheese, nuts) unless contraindicated<br>6. allow client to continue usual sleep practices (e.g. position, time, bedtime rituals such as reading and meditating) if possible<br>7. satisfy basic needs such as comfort and warmth before sleep<br>8. have client empty bladder just before bedtime<br>9. maintain a quiet, restful atmosphere; have earplugs available for client if needed<br>10. use relaxation techniques (e.g. progressive relaxation exercises, back massage, mediation, soft music) before sleep<br>11. ensure good room ventilation<br>12. administer sedative-hypnotics if ordered<br>13. perform actions *to reduce interruptions during sleep (80-100 minutes of uninterrupted sleep are usually needed to complete one sleep cycle)*<br>a. restrict visitors<br>b. group care (e.g. medications, treatments, physical care, assessments) whenever possible.<br>d. Consult physician if signs and symptoms of sleep deprivation persist or worsen. |

## 11. NURSING DIAGNOSIS: High risk for infection:

a. **pneumonia** related to stasis of secretions in the lungs (secretions provide a good medium for bacterial growth);
b. **urinary tract infection** related to:
   1. increased bacterial growth associated with urinary stasis and the increased urine alkalinity that results from hypercalciuria (with prolonged immobility, excess calcium is released from the bones and excreted in the urine)
   2. entry of pathogens associated with the presence of an indwelling catheter or tears in the bladder mucosa if the bladder becomes distended.

| Desired Outcomes | Nursing Actions and ***Selected Purposes/Rationales*** |
|---|---|
| 11.a. The client will not develop pneumonia as evidenced by:<br>1. normal breath sounds | 11.a.1. Assess for and report signs and symptoms of pneumonia:<br>a. abnormal breath sounds (e.g. crackles [rales], pleural friction rub, bronchial breath sounds, diminished or absent breath sounds)<br>b. dull percussion note over affected lung area<br>c. tachypnea |

| Desired Outcomes | Nursing Actions and ***Selected Purposes/Rationales*** |
|---|---|
| 2. resonant percussion note over lungs<br>3. absence of tachypnea<br>4. cough productive of clear mucus only<br>5. afebrile status<br>6. absence of pleuritic pain<br>7. blood gases and WBC count within normal range for client<br>8. negative sputum culture. | d. cough productive of purulent, green, or rust-colored sputum<br>e. chills and fever<br>f. pleuritic pain<br>g. elevated WBC count.<br>2. Monitor oximetry and blood gas results. Report abnormal findings.<br>3. Obtain sputum specimen for culture if ordered. Report abnormal results.<br>4. Monitor chest x-ray results. Report findings indicative of pneumonia.<br>5. Implement measures *to prevent pneumonia:*<br>a. perform actions to improve breathing pattern (see Nursing Diagnosis 1, action c) and promote effective airway clearance (see Nursing Diagnosis 2, action b)<br>b. protect client from persons with respiratory tract infections<br>c. encourage and assist client to perform good oral care *in order to reduce the colonization of bacteria in the oropharynx and subsequent aspiration of these microorganisms.*<br>6. If signs and symptoms of pneumonia occur:<br>a. continue with above measures<br>b. administer oxygen as ordered<br>c. administer antimicrobials if ordered<br>d. refer to Care Plan on Pneumonia for additional care measures. |
| 11.b. The client will remain free of urinary tract infection as evidenced by:<br>1. clear urine<br>2. no unusual odor to urine<br>3. absence of frequency, urgency, and burning on urination<br>4. absence of chills and fever<br>5. absence of nitrites, bacteria, and WBCs in urine<br>6. negative urine culture. | 11.b.1. Assess for and report signs and symptoms of urinary tract infection (e.g. cloudy, foul-smelling urine; complaints of frequency, urgency, or burning on urination; chills; elevated temperature).<br>2. Monitor urinalysis and report presence of nitrites, bacteria, and/or WBCs.<br>3. Obtain a urine specimen for culture and sensitivity if ordered. Report abnormal results.<br>4. Implement measures *to prevent urinary tract infection:*<br>a. perform actions to prevent urinary stasis (see Collaborative Diagnosis 12, action c.5.a)<br>b. perform actions to maintain urine acidity (see Collaborative Diagnosis 12, action c.5.d) *in order to inhibit bacterial growth*<br>c. maintain a fluid intake of at least 2500 ml/day unless contraindicated<br>d. instruct female client to wipe from front to back after urinating or defecating<br>e. assist client with perineal care every shift and after each bowel movement<br>f. maintain sterile technique during urinary catheterization and irrigations<br>g. if an indwelling urinary catheter is present:<br>1. secure the catheter tubing to lower abdomen or thigh on males or to thigh on females *to minimize risk of accidental traction and subsequent trauma to the bladder and urethra*<br>2. perform catheter care as often as needed *to prevent accumulation of mucus around the meatus*<br>3. keep urine collection container below bladder level at all times *to prevent reflux or stasis of urine*<br>4. change catheter according to hospital policy.<br>5. If signs and symptoms of urinary tract infection are present:<br>a. continue with above actions<br>b. administer antimicrobials if ordered. |

## 12. COLLABORATIVE DIAGNOSES:

**Potential complications:**

a. **thromboembolism** related to venous stasis associated with decreased mobility;
b. **atelectasis** related to shallow respirations, stasis of secretions in the alveoli and bronchioles, and decreased surfactant production (can result from inadequate deep breathing and changes in regional blood flow in the lungs) associated with prolonged recumbent positioning;
c. **renal calculi** related to:
   1. accumulation and deposition of calcium in the renal pelvis associated with urinary stasis and decreased urine formation (a result of decreased renal blood flow that can occur with prolonged immobility)
   2. change in the calcium/citric acid ratio associated with:
      a. increased renal excretion of calcium resulting from disuse osteoporosis
      b. reduction in the formation of acid end products of metabolism as a result of inactivity;
d. **contractures** related to an increase in fibrous connective tissue around joints and excessive calcium deposits in soft tissues around the joints associated with prolonged immobility of the joints;
e. **pathologic fractures** related to the osteoporosis that can develop with prolonged immobility.

| Desired Outcomes | Nursing Actions and ***Selected Purposes/Rationales*** |
|---|---|
| 12.a.1. The client will not develop a deep vein thrombus as evidenced by:<br>a. absence of pain, tenderness, heaviness, swelling, and distended superficial vessels in extremities<br>b. usual temperature of extremities<br>c. negative Homan's sign. | 12.a.1.a. Assess for and report signs and symptoms of a deep vein thrombus:<br>1. pain, tenderness, or heavy feeling in extremity<br>2. increase in circumference of extremity<br>3. distention of superficial vessels in extremity<br>4. unusual warmth of extremity<br>5. positive Homan's sign (not always a reliable indicator).<br>b. Implement measures *to prevent thrombus formation:*<br>1. encourage and assist client to perform active foot and leg exercises every 1-2 hours while awake<br>2. instruct client to avoid positions that compromise blood flow (e.g. pillows under knees, crossing legs, sitting for long periods)<br>3. elevate foot of bed for 20-minute intervals several times a shift unless contraindicated<br>4. consult physician about order for elastic stockings or bandages; if applied, remove for 30-60 minutes at least twice daily<br>5. apply/maintain intermittent pneumatic compression stockings or boots if ordered<br>6. maintain a minimum fluid intake of 2500 ml/day unless contraindicated *to prevent fluid volume deficit and increased blood viscosity, which leads to venous stasis*<br>7. administer anticoagulants (e.g. low-dose heparin, warfarin) or antiplatelet agents (e.g. low-dose aspirin) if ordered<br>8. progress activity as allowed.<br>c. If signs and symptoms of a deep vein thrombus occur:<br>1. maintain client on bed rest until activity orders are received<br>2. elevate foot of bed 15-20° above heart level if ordered (use knee gatch to maintain knees in a slightly flexed position)<br>3. discourage positions that compromise blood flow (e.g. pillows under knees, crossing legs, sitting for long periods)<br>4. apply heating pad or warm moist packs to affected area if ordered<br>5. prepare client for diagnostic studies (e.g. venography, duplex ultrasound, impedance plethysmography) if indicated<br>6. administer anticoagulants (e.g. heparin, warfarin) if ordered |

| Desired Outcomes | Nursing Actions and ***Selected Purposes/Rationales*** |
|---|---|
| | 7. prepare client for the following if planned:<br>a. injection of a thrombolytic agent (e.g. streptokinase)<br>b. vena caval interruption (e.g. insertion of an intracaval filtering device)<br>c. thrombectomy<br>8. refer to Care Plan on Deep Vein Thrombosis for additional care measures. |
| 12.a.2. The client will not experience a pulmonary embolism as evidenced by:<br>a. absence of sudden chest pain<br>b. unlabored respirations at 14-20/minute<br>c. pulse 60-100 beats/minute<br>d. usual mental status<br>e. blood gases within normal range. | 12.a.2.a. Assess for and report signs and symptoms of pulmonary embolism (e.g. sudden chest pain, dyspnea, tachypnea, tachycardia, restlessness, apprehension, low $PaO_2$).<br>b. Implement measures *to prevent a pulmonary embolism:*<br>1. perform actions to prevent and treat a deep vein thrombus (see actions a.1.b and c in this diagnosis)<br>2. do not exercise, check for Homan's sign in, or massage any extremity known to have a thrombus<br>3. caution client to avoid activities that create a Valsalva response (e.g. straining to have a bowel movement, holding breath while moving) *in order to prevent dislodgment of existing thrombi.*<br>c. If signs and symptoms of a pulmonary embolism occur:<br>1. maintain client on strict bed rest in a semi- to high Fowler's position<br>2. maintain oxygen therapy as ordered<br>3. prepare client for diagnostic tests (e.g. blood gases, ventilation-perfusion lung scan, pulmonary angiography)<br>4. administer anticoagulants (e.g. continuous intravenous heparin, warfarin) if ordered<br>5. prepare client for the following if planned:<br>a. injection of a thrombolytic agent (e.g. streptokinase, urokinase, tissue plasminogen activator [tPA])<br>b. vena caval interruption (e.g. insertion of an intracaval filtering device) *to prevent further pulmonary emboli*<br>c. embolectomy<br>6. provide emotional support to client and significant others<br>7. refer to Care Plan on Pulmonary Embolism for additional care measures. |
| 12.b. The client will not develop atelectasis as evidenced by:<br>1. normal breath sounds<br>2. resonant percussion note over lungs<br>3. unlabored respirations at 14-20/minute<br>4. pulse rate within normal range for client<br>5. afebrile status. | 12.b.1. Assess for and report signs and symptoms of atelectasis (e.g. diminished or absent breath sounds, dull percussion note over affected area, increased respiratory rate, dyspnea, tachycardia, elevated temperature).<br>2. Monitor chest x-ray results. Report findings of atelectasis.<br>3. Implement measures *to prevent atelectasis:*<br>a. perform actions to maintain an effective breathing pattern (see Nursing Diagnosis 1, action c)<br>b. perform actions to maintain effective airway clearance (see Nursing Diagnosis 2, action b).<br>4. If signs and symptoms of atelectasis occur:<br>a. increase frequency of turning, coughing or "huffing," deep breathing, and use of incentive spirometer<br>b. consult physician if signs and symptoms of atelectasis persist or worsen. |
| 12.c. The client will not develop renal calculi as evidenced by:<br>1. absence of flank pain, hematuria, urinary frequency | 12.c.1. Assess for and report signs and symptoms of renal calculi (e.g. dull, aching or severe, colicky flank pain; hematuria; urinary frequency or urgency; nausea; vomiting).<br>2. Monitor serum calcium levels and report elevations.<br>3. Obtain a urine specimen for analysis if ordered. Report the presence of crystals and/or high levels of calcium. |

and urgency, nausea, and vomiting
2. clear urine without calculi.

4. Monitor pH of urine. Report a pH above 6.5 *(calcium salts are more likely to precipitate in an alkaline urine).*
5. Implement measures *to prevent calcium stone formation:*
   a. perform actions *to prevent urinary stasis:*
      1. assist client to change positions at least every 2 hours; elevate head of bed periodically unless contraindicated
      2. progress activity as allowed
      3. implement measures to prevent urinary retention (see Nursing Diagnosis 8, action d)
      4. maintain patency of urinary catheter if present
   b. encourage a minimum fluid intake of 2500 ml/day unless contraindicated *to help prevent urinary stasis and promote adequate renal blood flow and urine formation*
   c. perform actions to prevent or delay bone demineralization (see action e.3.a in this diagnosis) *in order to reduce the amount of calcium present in the urine*
   d. perform actions *to maintain urine acidity:*
      1. assist the client with active-resistive exercises *(muscle activity produces an acid end product, which helps maintain a normal calcium/citric acid ratio)*
      2. encourage client to increase intake of foods/fluids that form an acid ash (e.g. cranberry juice, prune juice, meat, eggs, poultry, fish, plums, whole grains)
      3. instruct client to decrease intake of milk, most fruits and vegetables, and carbonated beverages *(these tend to alkalinize urine)*
      4. administer medications if ordered *to acidify the urine* (e.g. ascorbic acid)
      5. prevent urinary tract infections *(urea-splitting organisms tend to alkalinize urine)*
   e. instruct client to reduce intake of foods/fluids high in oxalate (e.g. cocoa, chocolate, fruit cocktail, tangerines, berries, peanuts, peanut butter, rhubarb, spinach, broccoli) *in order to help prevent precipitation of calcium stones.*
6. If signs and symptoms of renal calculi occur:
   a. strain all urine carefully and save any calculi for analysis; report finding to physician
   b. encourage maximum fluid intake allowed
   c. administer analgesics as ordered
   d. prepare client for removal of calculi (e.g. extracorporeal shock wave lithotripsy [ESWL], percutaneous ultrasonic or laser lithotripsy) if planned.

12.d. The client will regain or maintain normal range of motion.

12.d.1. Assess for complaints of joint stiffness and limitations in range of motion.
2. Implement general measures *to prevent contractures:*
   a. maintain proper body alignment at all times; mattress should be firm enough to provide adequate body support
   b. perform actions to maintain optimal joint mobility and muscle function during period of immobility (see Nursing Diagnosis 6, actions a.1-4).
3. Implement measures *to prevent hip and knee contractures:*
   a. place client in a flat, supine position at least every 4 hours
   b. limit length of time client is in high Fowler's position (usually no longer than 1 hour at a time)
   c. avoid use of knee gatch and pillows under knees
   d. instruct client to do quadriceps- and gluteal-setting exercises if able *in order to maintain muscle strength and tone and improve ability to perform range of motion exercises of hips and knees*
   e. when client is in a supine or Fowler's position, place trochanter roll

| Desired Outcomes | Nursing Actions and ***Selected Purposes/Rationales*** |
|---|---|
| | or sandbag along outer aspect of each thigh *to prevent external rotation of the hips.*<br>4. Implement measures *to prevent footdrop:*<br>a. instruct and assist client to perform active foot exercises every 1-2 hours while awake<br>b. use a footboard, sandbags, pillows, high-topped tennis shoes, foam boots, or foot positioners if necessary *to keep feet in neutral or slightly dorsiflexed position*<br>c. keep bed linen from exerting excessive pressure on toes and feet.<br>5. Implement measures *to prevent contractures in upper extremities:*<br>a. encourage client to use upper extremities to perform self-care and assist in moving unless contraindicated<br>b. reposition upper extremities at least every 2 hours<br>c. use handroll and wrist splints if indicated.<br>6. Use a small rather than large pillow to support client's head and shoulders *in order to prevent a neck flexion contracture.*<br>7. Consult physician if range of motion becomes restricted. |
| 12.e. The client will not experience pathologic fractures as evidenced by:<br>1. usual mobility and range of motion<br>2. absence of unusual motion, abnormal joint position, and obvious deformity of any body part<br>3. absence of pain and swelling over skeletal structures<br>4. x-ray reports showing absence of fractures. | 12.e.1. Assess for and report signs and symptoms of pathologic fractures (e.g. further decrease in mobility or range of motion, motion at site where motion does not usually occur, abnormal joint position or obvious deformity, pain or swelling over skeletal structures).<br>2. Monitor x-ray reports and notify physician of findings of pathologic fractures.<br>3. Implement measures *to prevent pathologic fractures:*<br>a. perform actions *to prevent or delay bone demineralization:*<br>1. consult physician about the use of a tilt table while client is immobile<br>2. assist client with weight-bearing activities as soon as allowed *(weight-bearing reduces bone breakdown)*<br>3. administer medications *that inhibit bone resorption* (e.g. calcitonin) if ordered<br>b. if evidence of osteoporosis exists:<br>1. caution client to avoid coughing, sneezing, and straining at stool; consult physician regarding an order for an antitussive, antihistamine, and/or laxative if indicated<br>2. move client carefully; obtain adequate assistance as needed<br>3. when turning client, logroll and support all extremities<br>4. use smooth movements when moving client; avoid pulling or pushing on body parts<br>5. correctly apply brace or cervical collar as ordered.<br>4. If fractures occur:<br>a. apply external stabilization device (e.g. cervical collar, brace, splint, sling) if ordered<br>b. administer analgesics, anti-inflammatory agents, and/or muscle relaxants if ordered *to control pain*<br>c. prepare client for surgery (e.g. internal fixation) if planned<br>d. provide emotional support to client and significant others. |

## 13. NURSING DIAGNOSIS: Anxiety

related to unfamiliar environment; lack of understanding of diagnosis, diagnostic tests, and treatments; financial concerns; and feelings of confinement.

| Desired Outcome | Nursing Actions and ***Selected Purposes/Rationales*** |
|---|---|
| 13. The client will experience a reduction in anxiety as evidenced by:<br>a. verbalization of feeling less anxious and fearful<br>b. usual sleep pattern<br>c. relaxed facial expression and body movements<br>d. stable vital signs<br>e. usual perceptual ability and interactions with others. | 13.a. Assess client for signs and symptoms of anxiety (e.g. verbalization of fears and concerns, insomnia, tenseness, tremors, irritability, restlessness, diaphoresis, tachypnea, tachycardia, elevated blood pressure, facial pallor or flushing, narrowed perceptual field, withdrawal, noncompliance with treatment plan).<br>b. Implement measures *to reduce fear and anxiety:*<br>1. orient client to hospital environment, equipment, and routines; explain the purpose for and operation of a kinetic bed if indicated<br>2. introduce staff who will be participating in his/her care; if possible, maintain consistency in staff assigned to his/her care *to provide feelings of stability and comfort with the environment*<br>3. assure client that staff members are nearby; respond to call signal as soon as possible<br>4. keep door and bed and window curtains open as much as possible *to reduce feeling of confinement*<br>5. maintain a calm, supportive, confident manner when interacting with client<br>6. encourage verbalization of fear and anxiety; provide feedback<br>7. reinforce physician's explanations and clarify misconceptions client has about his/her diagnosis, treatment plan, and prognosis<br>8. explain all diagnostic tests<br>9. provide a calm, restful environment<br>10. instruct client in relaxation techniques and encourage participation in diversional activities<br>11. assist client to identify specific stressors and ways to cope with them<br>12. initiate financial and/or social service referrals if indicated<br>13. encourage significant others to project a caring, concerned attitude without obvious anxiousness<br>14. administer antianxiety agents if ordered.<br>c. Include significant others in orientation and teaching sessions and encourage their continued support of the client.<br>d. Provide information based on current needs of client and significant others at a level they can understand. Encourage questions and clarification of information provided.<br>e. Consult physician if above actions fail to control fear and anxiety. |

## 14. NURSING DIAGNOSIS: Self-concept disturbance*

related to dependence on others to meet basic needs, feelings of powerlessness, and change in body functioning and usual roles and life style associated with physical limitations and/or prescribed activity restrictions.

*This diagnostic label includes the nursing diagnoses of body image disturbance, self-esteem disturbance, and altered role performance.

| Desired Outcome | Nursing Actions and ***Selected Purposes/Rationales*** |
|---|---|
| 14. The client will demonstrate beginning adaptation to changes in body functioning, life style, roles, and level of | 14.a. Assess for signs and symptoms of a self-concept disturbance (e.g. verbal or nonverbal cues denoting a negative response to changes in body functioning such as denial of or preoccupation with changes that have occurred or withdrawal from significant others).<br>b. Determine the meaning of feelings of dependency and changes in body |

| Desired Outcome | Nursing Actions and ***Selected Purposes/Rationales*** |
|---|---|
| independence as evidenced by:<br>a. verbalization of feelings of self-worth<br>b. maintenance of relationships with significant others<br>c. active participation in activities of daily living<br>d. active interest in personal appearance. | functioning, life style, and roles to the client by encouraging him/her to verbalize feelings and by noting nonverbal responses to the changes experienced.<br>c. Discuss with client improvements in body functioning and ability to resume usual roles and life style that can realistically be expected.<br>d. Implement measures *to assist client to increase self-esteem* (e.g. limit negative self-assessment, encourage positive comments about self, assist to identify strengths, give positive feedback about accomplishments).<br>e. Assist client to identify and use coping techniques that have been helpful in the past.<br>f. Assist client with usual grooming and makeup habits if necessary.<br>g. Implement measures to reduce client's feelings of powerlessness (see Nursing Diagnosis 15, actions c-m).<br>h. Assess for and support behaviors suggesting positive adaptation to changes that have occurred (e.g. verbalization of feelings of self-worth, maintenance of relationships with significant others).<br>i. Assist client's and significant others' adjustment by listening, facilitating communication, and providing information.<br>j. Encourage visits and support from significant others.<br>k. Encourage client to continue involvement in interests and hobbies if possible. If previous interests and hobbies cannot be pursued, encourage development of new ones during period of immobilization.<br>l. Provide information about and encourage use of community agencies and support groups (e.g. vocational rehabilitation; family, individual, and/or financial counseling).<br>m. Consult physician about psychological counseling if client desires or if he/she seems unwilling or unable to adapt to changes that have occurred as a result of the disease or injury and its treatment. |

## 15. NURSING DIAGNOSIS: Powerlessness

related to:
a. physical limitations and/or prescribed activity restrictions;
b. dependence on others to meet basic needs;
c. alterations in roles, relationships, and future plans.

| Desired Outcome | Nursing Actions and ***Selected Purposes/Rationales*** |
|---|---|
| 15. The client will demonstrate increased feelings of control over his/her situation as evidenced by:<br>a. verbalization of same<br>b. active participation in planning of care<br>c. participation in self- | 15.a. Assess for behaviors that may indicate feelings of powerlessness (e.g. verbalization of lack of control over self-care or current situation, anger, apathy, hostility, excessive dependency, lack of participation in self-care or care planning).<br>b. Obtain information from client and significant others regarding client's usual response to situations in which he/she has had limited control (e.g. loss of job, financial stress).<br>c. Evaluate with client his/her perceptions of current situation, strengths, weaknesses, expectations, and parts of current situation that are under his/her control. Correct misinformation and inaccurate perceptions and |

| | |
|---|---|
| care activities within physical limitations. | encourage discussion of feelings about areas in which he/she perceives a lack of control. |
| | d. Reinforce physician's explanations about the disease or injury and treatment plan. Clarify misconceptions. |
| | e. Support realistic hope about probability of future independence and ability to resume usual roles and life style. |
| | f. Remind client of his/her right to ask questions about condition and treatment regimen. |
| | g. Support client's efforts to increase knowledge of and control over condition. Provide relevant pamphlets and audiovisual materials. |
| | h. Include client in the planning of care, encourage maximum participation in the treatment plan, and allow choices whenever possible *to promote a sense of control.* |
| | i. Consult occupational therapist if indicated about assistive devices and environmental modifications that would allow client more independence in performing activities of daily living. |
| | j. Inform client of scheduled procedures and tests *so that unpredictability is eliminated as much as possible and a feeling of control is promoted.* |
| | k. Encourage significant others to allow client to do as much as he/she is able *so that a feeling of independence can be maintained.* |
| | l. Assist client to establish realistic short- and long-term goals. |
| | m. Encourage client's participation in self-help groups if indicated. |

## 16. NURSING DIAGNOSIS: Social isolation

related to inability to participate in usual activities, limited contact with peers, and decreased contact/awareness of events in the outside world associated with prolonged immobility.

| Desired Outcome | Nursing Actions and ***Selected Purposes/Rationales*** |
|---|---|
| 16. The client will experience a decreased sense of isolation as evidenced by:<br>a. maintenance of relationships with significant others<br>b. verbalization of decreasing feelings of aloneness and rejection. | 16.a. Ascertain client's usual degree of social interaction.<br>b. Assess for indications of social isolation (e.g. absence of supportive significant others; uncommunicative and withdrawn; expression of feelings of rejection, being different from others, or aloneness imposed by others; hostility; sad, dull affect).<br>c. Implement measures *to decrease social isolation:*<br>1. assist client to identify reasons for feeling isolated and alone; aid him/her in developing a plan of action to reduce these feelings<br>2. encourage significant others to visit<br>3. encourage client to maintain telephone contact with others<br>4. schedule time each day to sit and talk with client<br>5. make objects such as clock, TV, radio, newspapers, and greeting cards accessible to client<br>6. have significant others bring client's favorite objects from home and place in room<br>7. move client periodically to a more stimulating environment (e.g. hall, lounge, garden) when condition allows<br>8. change room assignments as feasible *to provide client with roommate with similar interests.* |

## 17. NURSING DIAGNOSIS: Knowledge deficit

regarding follow-up care.

| Desired Outcomes | Nursing Actions and ***Selected Purposes/Rationales*** |
|---|---|
| 17.a. The client will verbalize an understanding of ways to prevent complications associated with continued decreased mobility. | 17.a.1. Provide instructions regarding ways to prevent respiratory tract infection:<br>a. avoid contact with persons having respiratory tract infections<br>b. drink at least 10 glasses of liquid/day<br>c. continue with respiratory care (e.g. postural drainage, incentive spirometer, coughing and deep breathing) as long as mobility is impaired<br>d. avoid smoking.<br>2. Provide instructions regarding ways to prevent urinary tract infection:<br>a. drink at least 10 glasses of liquid/day<br>b. void whenever the urge is felt<br>c. maintain urine acidity by:<br>1. increasing intake of food/fluids that form an acid ash (e.g. cranberry juice, prune juice, meat, eggs, poultry, fish, plums, whole grains)<br>2. limiting intake of milk, carbonated beverages, and citrus fruits<br>3. taking acidifying agents (e.g. ascorbic acid) as prescribed.<br>3. Provide instructions regarding ways to prevent urinary calcium stone formation:<br>a. drink at least 10 glasses of liquid/day<br>b. void whenever the urge is felt<br>c. maintain urine acidity (see action a.2.c in this diagnosis)<br>d. avoid excessive intake of foods high in calcium and vitamin D (e.g. dairy products)<br>e. avoid excessive intake of foods/fluids high in oxalate (e.g. cocoa, chocolate, fruit cocktail, tangerines, berries, peanuts, peanut butter, rhubarb, spinach, broccoli).<br>4. Provide instructions regarding ways to prevent a thromboembolism:<br>a. drink at least 10 glasses of liquid/day<br>b. avoid placing pillows under knees, crossing legs, and prolonged sitting<br>c. perform active foot and leg exercises every 1-2 hours during periods of inactivity<br>d. wear elastic stockings as prescribed<br>e. do not massage extremities.<br>5. Provide instructions regarding ways to prevent fainting spells associated with position change:<br>a. wear elastic stockings as prescribed<br>b. change from a lying to sitting or standing position slowly.<br>6. Provide instructions regarding ways to prevent skin breakdown:<br>a. change positions at least every 2 hours<br>b. avoid pressure on any reddened or irritated area<br>c. keep skin lubricated, clean, and dry<br>d. place an alternating pressure pad, foam pad, or gel-filled flotation pad on bed and chair if prone to skin breakdown or if activity is severely limited.<br>7. Provide instructions regarding ways to prevent constipation:<br>a. drink at least 10 glasses of liquid/day<br>b. increase intake of foods high in fiber (e.g. nuts, bran, whole-grain breads and cereals, raw fruits and vegetables, dried fruits) |

c. defecate whenever the urge is felt
d. assume a natural position for defecation if possible.

| | |
|---|---|
| 17.b. The client will demonstrate techniques for meeting self-care needs. | 17.b.1. Assist the client to identify techniques that will allow him/her to perform as much self-care as possible.<br>2. Reinforce occupational therapist's instructions about use of assistive devices.<br>3. Allow time for return demonstration of self-care techniques and use of assistive devices. |
| 17.c. The client will state signs and symptoms to report to the health care provider. | 17.c. Instruct client to report the following signs and symptoms:<br>1. temperature elevation lasting longer than 3 days<br>2. skin breakdown<br>3. cough productive of purulent, green, or rust-colored sputum<br>4. pain or swelling in any extremity<br>5. chest pain<br>6. flank pain<br>7. frequency, urgency, or burning on urination<br>8. cloudy, foul-smelling urine<br>9. nausea and vomiting<br>10. increased restriction of any joint motion. |
| 17.d. The client will identify community agencies that may provide assistance with home care and transportation. | 17.d.1. Provide information about community agencies that may provide assistance to client with home care or transportation (e.g. home health agencies, Meals on Wheels, church groups, transportation agencies).<br>2. Initiate a referral if indicated. |
| 17.e. The client will verbalize an understanding of and a plan for adhering to recommended follow-up care including future appointments with health care provider and physical therapist, exercise regimen, and medications prescribed. | 17.e.1. Reinforce the importance of keeping follow-up appointments with health care provider and physical therapist.<br>2. Reinforce physician's instructions regarding exercises and activity limitations.<br>3. Explain the rationale for, side effects of, and importance of taking medications prescribed.<br>4. Implement measures to improve client compliance:<br>a. include significant others in teaching sessions if possible<br>b. encourage questions and allow time for reinforcement and clarification of information provided<br>c. provide written instructions regarding scheduled appointments with health care provider and physical therapist, medications prescribed, and signs and symptoms to report. |

UNIT
# VI

# *Nursing Care of the Client Who Is Dying*

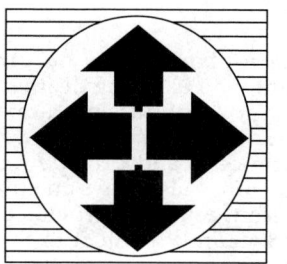

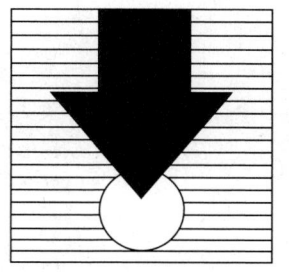

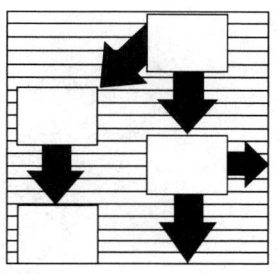

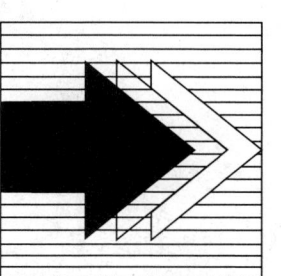

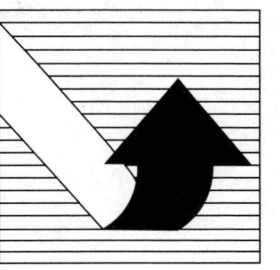

# Terminal Care

**This care plan focuses on care of the hospitalized adult client who is facing death in the very near future.** The major goals of nursing care are to maintain an optimal level of comfort; facilitate progression through the grieving process; and provide for a peaceful, dignified death. The nurse also plays an important role in assisting the significant others to provide effective support to the dying person and to adjust to their loss of that person.

This care plan does not deal with any particular medical diagnosis. The nursing diagnoses included are those that are relatively common to all persons facing death. Causal statements and actions for the nursing diagnoses will need to be individualized for each client and his/her underlying disease process and death trajectory. Care plans that pertain to the client's specific medical diagnosis will provide additional guidelines for nursing care during the terminal stages of that illness.

**Use in conjunction with the Care Plan on Immobility and care plans that pertain to the client's medical diagnosis.**

**NURSING DIAGNOSES**



**Refer to Care Plan on Immobility and care plans that pertain to the client's medical diagnosis for additional diagnoses.**

## 1. NURSING DIAGNOSIS: Impaired respiratory function:*

a. **ineffective breathing pattern** related to:
   1. fear, anxiety, and pain
   2. respiratory depressant and/or stimulant effects of hypoxia, hypercapnia, diminished cerebral blood flow, or neurological impairments that may be present as a result of the underlying disease process
   3. respiratory depressant effects of some medications (e.g. narcotic analgesics, central-acting muscle relaxants)
   4. impaired lung/chest wall expansion associated with recumbent positioning (in this position, full expansion of the lungs is restricted by the bed surface and by the abdominal contents pushing up against the diaphragm), weakness, abdominal distention, and/or pleural effusion (may occur as a result of the underlying disease process);

b. **ineffective airway clearance** related to:
   1. fluid accumulation in the alveoli and bronchioles associated with pulmonary edema if present as a result of the underlying disease process
   2. accumulation of tenacious secretions associated with fluid volume deficit, poor cough effort, and decreased mobility
   3. airway obstruction associated with underlying disease process and/or aspiration;

c. **impaired gas exchange** related to:
   1. loss of effective lung tissue associated with the underlying disease process
   2. a thickened alveolar-capillary membrane associated with pulmonary edema if present and stasis of pulmonary secretions.

*This diagnostic label includes the following nursing diagnoses: ineffective breathing pattern, ineffective airway clearance, and impaired gas exchange.

| Desired Outcome | Nursing Actions and ***Selected Purposes/Rationales*** |
|---|---|
| 1. The client will experience adequate respiratory function as evidenced by:<br>a. usual rate, rhythm, and depth of respirations<br>b. decreased dyspnea<br>c. usual or improved breath sounds<br>d. usual mental status<br>e. usual skin color<br>f. blood gases within normal range for client. | 1.a. Assess for signs and symptoms of impaired respiratory function:<br>1. rapid, shallow, slow, or irregular respirations<br>2. dyspnea, orthopnea<br>3. use of accessory muscles when breathing<br>4. adventitious breath sounds (e.g. crackles [rales], rhonchi)<br>5. diminished or absent breath sounds<br>6. restlessness, irritability<br>7. confusion, somnolence<br>8. central cyanosis (a late sign).<br>b. Monitor for and report the following:<br>1. abnormal blood gases<br>2. significant changes in oximetry results<br>3. abnormal chest x-ray results.<br>c. Implement measures *to improve respiratory status:*<br>1. perform actions to reduce pain (see Nursing Diagnosis 4, action e)<br>2. perform actions to decrease accumulation of gastrointestinal gas and fluid (see Nursing Diagnosis 5.C, action 3) *in order to decrease pressure on the diaphragm*<br>3. perform actions to decrease fear and anxiety (see Nursing Diagnosis 18)<br>4. place client in a semi- to high Fowler's position unless contraindicated; position client with pillows *to prevent slumping*<br>5. instruct client to breathe slowly if he/she is hyperventilating<br>6. assist client to turn from side to side at least every 2 hours<br>7. instruct client to deep breathe or use incentive spirometer at least every 2 hours<br>8. perform actions to reduce the risk for aspiration (see Nursing Diagnosis 17, action d) |

| Desired Outcome | Nursing Actions and ***Selected Purposes/Rationales*** |
|---|---|
| | 9. perform actions *to facilitate removal of secretions:*<br>a. instruct and assist client to cough or "huff" every 1-2 hours<br>b. implement measures *to liquefy tenacious secretions:*<br>1. encourage maximum fluid intake allowed and tolerated<br>2. humidify inspired air as ordered<br>c. assist with administration of diluent and mucolytic agents via nebulizer or IPPB treatment if ordered<br>d. perform oral, pharyngeal, and/or tracheal suctioning if necessary (deep suctioning should be avoided in final stage of dying process)<br>10. maintain oxygen therapy as ordered<br>11. discourage smoking *(smoke causes bronchoconstriction, increases mucus production, impairs ciliary function, and decreases oxygen availability)*<br>12. protect client from exposure to irritants such as smoke, flowers, and perfume *(can cause bronchospasm and increased mucus production)*<br>13. encourage activity as tolerated<br>14. administer the following medications if ordered:<br>a. diuretics *to decrease pulmonary fluid accumulation*<br>b. morphine sulfate *to reduce apprehension associated with dyspnea and decrease pulmonary vascular congestion (the vasodilatory action of morphine sulfate reduces cardiac workload and improves left ventricular emptying, which results in increased blood return from the pulmonary veins)*<br>c. bronchodilators (e.g. theophylline)<br>15. prepare client for thoracentesis or paracentesis if performed *to facilitate lung expansion.*<br>d. Consult physician about an order for an anticholinergic medication (e.g. atropine) *to reduce bronchial secretions if the final stage of dying process is prolonged, frequent suctioning is necessary, or the sound of excessive secretions is disturbing to significant others.*<br>e. Consult physician if dyspnea persists, worsens, or is causing client discomfort. |

## 2. NURSING DIAGNOSIS: Fluid volume deficit

related to:
a. decreased oral fluid intake associated with dysphagia, nausea, anorexia, fatigue, weakness, dyspnea, and/or decreased level of consciousness;
b. increased fluid loss associated with vomiting, diarrhea, and/or diaphoresis if client has a fever.

| Desired Outcome | Nursing Actions and ***Selected Purposes/Rationales*** |
|---|---|
| 2. The client will not experience a fluid volume deficit as evidenced by:<br>a. normal skin turgor<br>b. moist mucous membranes<br>c. stable weight<br>d. B/P and pulse within normal range for | 2.a. Assess for signs and symptoms of fluid volume deficit:<br>1. decreased skin turgor<br>2. dry mucous membranes, thirst<br>3. sudden weight loss of 2% or greater<br>4. low B/P and/or postural hypotension<br>5. weak, rapid pulse<br>6. delayed small vein filling time (longer than 3-5 seconds)<br>7. elevated BUN and Hct<br>8. decreased urine output (reflects an actual rather than potential fluid volume deficit). |

| Desired Outcome | Nursing Actions and ***Selected Purposes/Rationales*** |
|---|---|
| client and stable with position change<br>e. small vein filling time less than 3-5 seconds<br>f. BUN and Hct within normal range<br>g. balanced intake and output. | b. Implement measures *to prevent or treat fluid volume deficit:*<br>1. perform actions to prevent nausea and vomiting (see Nursing Diagnosis 5.A, action 2)<br>2. perform actions to control diarrhea if present (see Nursing Diagnosis 12, action d)<br>3. perform actions to reduce fever if present (e.g. administer tepid sponge bath and/or apply cool cloths to groin and axillae, administer antipyretics if ordered)<br>4. encourage the maximum fluid intake allowed and tolerated; if client is unable to drink from a glass and/or is too weak to drink through a straw:<br>a. give frequent sips of water or juice using a syringe<br>b. use a spoon to provide small amounts of ice chips.<br>c. Consult physician if signs and symptoms of fluid volume deficit persist or worsen or create discomfort for the client. Encourage significant others and client to discuss the positive and negative aspects of intravenous therapy and/or placement of a feeding tube with physician. |

## 3. NURSING DIAGNOSIS: Impaired swallowing

related to dry mouth and depressed swallowing reflex, and impaired tongue movement associated with weakness and fatigue and decreased level of consciousness.

| Desired Outcome | Nursing Actions and ***Selected Purposes/Rationales*** |
|---|---|
| 3. The client will experience an improvement in swallowing as evidenced by:<br>a. verbalization of same<br>b. absence of food in oral cavity after swallowing<br>c. absence of coughing and choking when eating and drinking. | 3.a. Assess for signs and symptoms of impaired swallowing (e.g. statements of difficulty swallowing, stasis of food in the oral cavity, coughing or choking when eating or drinking).<br>b. Implement measures *to improve ability to swallow:*<br>1. perform actions to reduce dryness of the oral mucous membrane (see Nursing Diagnosis 7, action b)<br>2. place client in high Fowler's position for meals and snacks; head and neck should be tilted forward slightly *to facilitate elevation of the larynx and posterior movement of the tongue*<br>3. assist client to select foods that require little or no chewing and are easily swallowed (e.g. custard, eggs, canned fruit, mashed potatoes)<br>4. avoid serving foods that are sticky (e.g. peanut butter, soft bread, bananas)<br>5. serve foods/fluids that are hot or cold instead of room temperature *(the more extreme temperatures stimulate the sensory receptors and swallowing reflex)*<br>6. moisten dry foods with gravy or sauces (e.g. catsup, sour cream, salad dressing)<br>7. perform actions *to stimulate salivation at mealtime in order to further reduce dry mouth:*<br>a. provide oral care before meals<br>b. provide sour, hard candy for client to suck on just before meals unless contraindicated<br>c. serve foods that are visually pleasing<br>d. place a piece of lemon or sour pickle on client's plate<br>8. instruct client to avoid putting too much food/fluid in mouth at one time<br>9. encourage client to concentrate on the act of swallowing |

| Desired Outcome | Nursing Actions and ***Selected Purposes/Rationales*** |
|---|---|
| | 10. consult speech pathologist or occupational therapist about methods for dealing with impaired swallowing if appropriate; reinforce recommended techniques.<br>c. Consult physician if swallowing difficulties persist or worsen. |

## 4. NURSING DIAGNOSIS: Pain

related to:
a. disease process;
b. unwillingness to take pain medication associated with fear of disappointing caregiver, loss of control, oversedation, and addiction; feeling that pain is a sign of weakness or has redemptive qualities; and/or need to be stoic.

| Desired Outcome | Nursing Actions and ***Selected Purposes/Rationales*** |
|---|---|
| 4. The client will experience diminished pain as evidenced by:<br>a. verbalization of pain relief<br>b. relaxed facial expression and body positioning<br>c. increased participation in activities<br>d. stable vital signs. | 4.a. Determine how client usually responds to pain.<br>b. Assess client's perception of pain including location, intensity, and type. Use a numerical scale to rate intensity.<br>c. Assess for nonverbal signs of pain (e.g. wrinkled brow, clenched fists, reluctance to move, guarding of affected body part, restlessness, agitation, diaphoresis, facial pallor, increased B/P, tachycardia).<br>d. Assess for factors that seem to aggravate and alleviate pain.<br>e. Implement measures *to reduce pain:*<br>1. perform actions *to reduce fear and anxiety about the pain experience* (e.g. assure client that his/her need for pain relief is understood and will be met)<br>2. plan methods for achieving pain relief (e.g. nonpharmacological measures, scheduled or "as necessary" administration of analgesics, methods of alternating or combining medications, medications at bedside [e.g. morphine elixir] to take as needed, patient-controlled analgesia [PCA]) with client *in order to assist him/her to maintain a sense of control over the pain experience*<br>3. medicate prior to any painful treatments or procedures and before pain becomes severe<br>4. provide or assist with nonpharmacological measures for pain relief (e.g. cutaneous stimulation techniques such as pressure, massage, heat and cold applications, transcutaneous electrical nerve stimulation, or vibration; relaxation techniques such as progressive relaxation exercises and meditation; distraction by quiet conversation, music, rhythmic massage, or diversional activities; guided imagery; position change)<br>5. administer analgesics as ordered; assist with titration of prescribed medications *in order to achieve adequate pain relief with minimal side effects;* assure client that drug addiction is not a concern.<br>f. Consult physician if above measures fail to provide adequate pain relief. |

## 5.A. NURSING DIAGNOSIS: Altered comfort: nausea and vomiting

related to stimulation of the vomiting center associated with:
1. stimulation of the afferent vagal and/or sympathetic pathways resulting from visceral irritation associated with abdominal distention if present;

2. cortical stimulation resulting from pain and stress;
3. stimulation of the chemoreceptor trigger zone by some medications (e.g. morphine sulfate, meperidine hydrochloride).

| Desired Outcome | Nursing Actions and ***Selected Purposes/Rationales*** |
|---|---|
| 5.A. The client will experience relief of nausea and vomiting as evidenced by:<br>1. verbalization of relief of nausea<br>2. absence of vomiting. | 5.A.1. Assess client for nausea and vomiting.<br>2. Implement measures *to prevent nausea and vomiting:*<br>a. perform actions to reduce accumulation of gastrointestinal gas and fluid (see Nursing Diagnosis 5.C, action 3)<br>b. perform actions to reduce pain (see Nursing Diagnosis 4, action e)<br>c. perform actions to reduce fear and anxiety (see Nursing Diagnosis 18)<br>d. eliminate noxious sights and odors from the environment *(noxious stimuli cause cortical stimulation of the vomiting center)*<br>e. encourage client to take deep, slow breaths when nauseated<br>f. instruct client to change positions slowly *(rapid movement stimulates the afferent vestibulocerebellar pathway with resultant stimulation of the chemoreceptor trigger zone)*<br>g. provide oral hygiene after each emesis and before meals<br>h. if oral intake is allowed:<br>1. avoid serving foods with an overpowering aroma; remove lids from hot foods before entering room<br>2. provide small, frequent meals; instruct client to ingest foods and fluids slowly<br>3. encourage client to eat dry foods (e.g. toast, crackers) and avoid drinking liquids with meals if nauseated<br>4. instruct client to avoid foods/fluids that irritate gastric mucosa (e.g. spicy foods; caffeine-containing beverages such as coffee, tea, and colas)<br>5. instruct client to avoid foods high in fat *(fat delays gastric emptying)*<br>6. instruct client to rest after eating with head of bed elevated<br>i. administer antiemetics and gastrointestinal stimulants (e.g. metoclopramide) if ordered.<br>3. If above measures fail to control nausea and vomiting:<br>a. consult physician<br>b. be prepared to insert a nasogastric tube and maintain suction as ordered. |

## 5.B. NURSING DIAGNOSIS: Altered comfort: pruritus

related to dry skin associated with underlying disease process and/or fluid volume deficit.

| Desired Outcome | Nursing Actions and ***Selected Purposes/Rationales*** |
|---|---|
| 5.B. The client will experience relief of pruritus as evidenced by:<br>1. verbalization of same<br>2. no scratching or rubbing of skin. | 5.B.1. Assess client's pruritus including onset, characteristics, location, and factors that aggravate and alleviate it.<br>2. Instruct client in and/or implement measures *to relieve pruritus:*<br>a. apply cool, moist compresses to pruritic areas<br>b. maintain a cool environment<br>c. perform actions *to reduce skin dryness:*<br>1. use tepid water and mild soaps for bathing |

| Desired Outcome | Nursing Actions and ***Selected Purposes/Rationales*** |
|---|---|
| | 2. apply oil-based agents to skin immediately after bathing when skin is hydrated<br>3. apply emollient creams or ointments frequently<br>4. limit bathing to every other day<br>5. use a room humidifier *to maintain moisture in the air and reduce fluid loss by evaporation*<br>d. add emollients, cornstarch, baking soda, or oatmeal preparations to bath water<br>e. pat skin dry, making sure to dry thoroughly<br>f. encourage participation in diversional activity<br>g. use relaxation techniques<br>h. encourage client to wear loose cotton garments; launder clothing in mild soap<br>i. use cutaneous stimulation techniques (e.g. pressure, massage, vibration, stroking with a soft brush) at site of itching or acupressure points<br>j. administer antihistamines and topical corticosteroids if ordered.<br>3. Consult physician if above measures fail to alleviate pruritus or if the skin becomes excoriated. |

## 5.C. NURSING DIAGNOSIS:

**Altered comfort: abdominal distention and gas pain**

related to an accumulation of gas and fluid associated with decreased gastrointestinal motility resulting from depressant effects of some medications (e.g. narcotic analgesics, central-acting muscle relaxants) and decreased activity.

| Desired Outcome | Nursing Actions and ***Selected Purposes/Rationales*** |
|---|---|
| 5.C. The client will experience diminished abdominal distention and gas pain as evidenced by:<br>1. verbalization of decreased abdominal fullness and pain<br>2. relaxed facial expression and body positioning<br>3. decrease in abdominal girth. | 5.C.1. Assess for verbal complaints of abdominal fullness or gas pain.<br>2. Assess for nonverbal signs of abdominal distention or gas pain (e.g. clutching or guarding of abdomen, restlessness, reluctance to move, grimacing, increasing abdominal girth).<br>3. Implement measures *to reduce the accumulation of gastrointestinal gas and fluid:*<br>a. encourage and assist client with frequent position changes and ambulation as tolerated *(activity stimulates peristalsis and expulsion of flatus)*<br>b. instruct client to avoid activities such as chewing gum and smoking *in order to reduce air swallowing*<br>c. maintain patency of nasogastric or intestinal tube if present<br>d. maintain food and fluid restrictions as ordered<br>e. encourage client to drink warm liquids *to stimulate peristalsis*<br>f. instruct client to avoid intake of carbonated beverages and gas-producing foods (e.g. cabbage, onions, beans)<br>g. encourage client to eructate and expel flatus whenever the urge is felt<br>h. consult physician about insertion of a rectal tube or administration of a return flow enema if indicated |

i. encourage use of nonnarcotic analgesics if possible *(narcotic analgesics depress gastrointestinal activity)*
j. administer the following medications if ordered:
   1. antiflatulents (e.g. simethicone) *to reduce gas accumulation*
   2. gastrointestinal stimulants (e.g. metoclopramide, bisacodyl) *to increase gastrointestinal motility.*

4. Consult physician if signs and symptoms of abdominal distention or gas pain persist or worsen.

## 5.D. NURSING DIAGNOSIS: Altered comfort: hiccoughs

related to irritation of the phrenic nerve associated with such things as gastric or abdominal distention, some abdominal or central nervous system tumors, and/or gastric or abdominal tubes.

| Desired Outcome | Nursing Actions and ***Selected Purposes/Rationales*** |
|---|---|
| 5.D. The client will not experience persistent hiccoughs. | 5.D.1. Implement measures *to prevent irritation of the phrenic nerve:*<br>a. perform actions to reduce accumulation of gastrointestinal gas and fluid (see Nursing Diagnosis 5.C, action 3)<br>b. instruct client to avoid drinking very hot or cold liquids *to avoid reflex irritation of the phrenic nerve*<br>c. if gastric or abdominal tubes are present, anchor them securely *in order to minimize movement of the tubes and subsequent phrenic nerve irritation.*<br>2. Implement measures *to control hiccoughs if they occur:*<br>a. instruct client to perform techniques such as breathing deeply, rebreathing into a paper bag, or holding breath if appropriate<br>b. administer phenothiazines if ordered *to reduce diaphragmatic spasms.*<br>3. Consult physician if hiccoughs persist. Be prepared to assist with the following treatments for intractable hiccoughs if ordered:<br>a. gastric suction *to decrease gastric distention*<br>b. removal of gastric or abdominal tubes *(these may be irritating the phrenic nerve)*<br>c. inhalation of carbon dioxide *(the depressant effect of $CO_2$ reduces spasm of the diaphragm)*<br>d. phrenic nerve block. |

## 6. NURSING DIAGNOSIS: High risk for impaired skin integrity

related to:
a. ischemia of the skin and subcutaneous tissue associated with prolonged pressure on tissues resulting from decreased mobility;
b. damage to the skin and/or subcutaneous tissue associated with friction or shearing;

c. frequent contact with irritants associated with persistent diarrhea or incontinence of urine or stool;
d. increased fragility of skin associated with inadequate nutritional status, dryness, and dependent edema;
e. excessive scratching associated with pruritus if present.

| Desired Outcome | Nursing Actions and ***Selected Purposes/Rationales*** |
|---|---|
| 6. The client will maintain skin integrity as evidenced by:<br>a. absence of redness and irritation<br>b. no skin breakdown. | 6.a. Inspect the skin (especially bony prominences; dependent, edematous, and pruritic areas; and perianal area) for pallor, redness, and breakdown.<br>b. Refer to Care Plan on Immobility, Nursing Diagnosis 4, action b (pp. 141-142), for measures to prevent skin breakdown.<br>c. Implement additional measures *to maintain skin integrity:*<br>1. perform actions *to prevent skin irritation resulting from diarrhea and incontinence of urine or stool:*<br>a. implement measures to reduce the episodes of urinary and bowel incontinence and to control diarrhea (see Nursing Diagnoses 10, actions b and c; 13, action b; and 12, action d)<br>b. assist client to thoroughly cleanse and dry perineal area with soft tissue or cloth after each episode of diarrhea and incontinence; apply a protective ointment or cream (e.g. Desitin, A & D ointment, Vaseline)<br>c. apply a drainable fecal collector if bowel incontinence is a persistent problem or diarrhea is severe<br>d. provide incontinence pads if needed to absorb moisture; do not allow skin to come in contact with plastic portion of the pads<br>2. perform actions *to prevent skin irritation resulting from scratching:*<br>a. implement measures to relieve pruritus (see Nursing Diagnosis 5.B, action 2)<br>b. keep nails trimmed and/or apply mittens if necessary<br>c. instruct client to apply firm pressure to pruritic areas rather than scratching<br>3. perform actions to prevent or treat fluid volume deficit (see Nursing Diagnosis 2, action b) *in order to reduce risk of skin breakdown associated with dryness.*<br>d. If skin breakdown occurs:<br>1. notify physician<br>2. continue with above measures to prevent further irritation and breakdown<br>3. perform decubitus care as ordered or per standard hospital procedure (extensiveness of treatment is usually limited to that necessary to maintain comfort in the final stages of life)<br>4. assess client closely and report signs and symptoms of infection (e.g. elevated temperature; redness, warmth, and edema around area of breakdown; unusual drainage from site). |

## 7. NURSING DIAGNOSIS: Altered oral mucous membrane: dryness

related to:
a. decreased salivation associated with fluid volume deficit, decreased oral intake, and some medications (e.g. tricyclic antidepressants, anticholinergics, narcotic analgesics, phenothiazines);
b. prolonged oxygen therapy administered by mask;
c. chronic mouth breathing.

| Desired Outcome | Nursing Actions and ***Selected Purposes/Rationales*** |
|---|---|
| 7. The client will maintain a moist, intact oral mucous membrane. | 7.a. Assess client frequently for dryness of the oral mucosa.<br>b. Implement measures *to relieve dryness of the oral mucous membrane:*<br>1. assist client to perform good oral hygiene as often as needed; avoid products such as lemon-glycerin swabs and commercial mouthwashes containing alcohol *(these have a drying or irritating effect on the oral mucous membrane)*<br>2. rinse mouth frequently with water or dilute mouthwash<br>3. lubricate client's lips frequently with K-Y jelly, ChapStick, Blistex, or mineral oil<br>4. encourage client to breathe through nose rather than his/her mouth<br>5. encourage client not to smoke *(smoking irritates and dries the mucosa)*<br>6. perform actions to prevent or treat fluid volume deficit (see Nursing Diagnosis 2, action b)<br>7. if salivary production is diminished:<br>a. perform actions *to increase salivary flow:*<br>1. encourage client to suck on sour, hard candy if allowed<br>2. offer hot tea with lemon or warm lemonade at regular intervals unless contraindicated<br>b. encourage client to use artificial saliva *to lubricate the mucous membrane.*<br>c. If oral mucosa is irritated or cracked, implement measures *to relieve discomfort and promote healing:*<br>1. if client is alert and able to take nourishment by mouth, assist him/her to select soft, bland foods<br>2. instruct client to avoid foods/fluids that are extremely hot<br>3. use a soft bristle brush, gauze-wrapped tongue blade, sponge-tipped applicator, or low-pressure power spray for oral hygiene<br>4. apply carbamide peroxide (e.g. Gly-Oxide, Proxigel) to irritated areas<br>5. administer topical anesthetics, oral protective pastes or coating agents, and topical and systemic analgesics if ordered.<br>d. Consult physician if dryness, irritation, and/or discomfort persist. |

## 8. NURSING DIAGNOSIS: Impaired physical mobility

related to weakness, fatigue, dyspnea, sensory and motor deficits associated with the disease process, reluctance to move because of pain and nausea, and/or decreased level of consciousness.

| Desired Outcome | Nursing Actions and ***Selected Purposes/Rationales*** |
|---|---|
| 8. The client will achieve maximum physical mobility within limitations imposed by terminal state. | 8.a. Implement measures *to increase mobility:*<br>1. perform actions to reduce pain and prevent nausea (see Nursing Diagnoses 4, action e and 5.A, action 2)<br>2. perform actions to improve respiratory status (see Nursing Diagnosis 1, action c) *in order to relieve dyspnea*<br>3. provide adequate rest periods before activity sessions<br>4. instruct client in and assist with active and/or passive range of motion exercises at least 3 times/day unless contraindicated<br>5. instruct client in and assist with use of mobility aids (e.g. cane, walker) if appropriate<br>6. provide assistive devices appropriate for client's specific sensory and motor deficits if indicated |

| Desired Outcome | Nursing Actions and ***Selected Purposes/Rationales*** |
|---|---|
| | 7. consult with occupational and/or physical therapists about ways to facilitate client's mobility if appropriate.<br>b. Provide praise and encouragement for all efforts to maintain or increase physical mobility.<br>c. Encourage the support of significant others. Allow them to assist with range of motion exercises, positioning, and activity if desired. |

## 9. NURSING DIAGNOSIS: Self-care deficit

related to altered thought processes and impaired physical mobility associated with sensory and motor deficits, pain, nausea, weakness, fatigue, dyspnea, and/or decreased level of consciousness.

| Desired Outcome | Nursing Actions and ***Selected Purposes/Rationales*** |
|---|---|
| 9. The client will perform self-care activities within physical limitations. | 9.a. Refer to Care Plan on Immobility, Nursing Diagnosis 7 (pp. 141-145), for measures related to planning for and meeting client's self-care needs.<br>b. Implement measures to increase mobility (see Nursing Diagnosis 8, action a) *in order to further facilitate client's ability to perform self-care.* |

## 10. NURSING DIAGNOSIS: Altered urinary elimination: incontinence

related to:

a. decreased ability to respond to the urge to urinate associated with decreased level of consciousness and impaired physical mobility;
b. poor urinary sphincter control associated with decreased level of consciousness.

| Desired Outcome | Nursing Actions and ***Selected Purposes/Rationales*** |
|---|---|
| 10. The client will experience urinary continence. | 10.a. Assess for urinary incontinence.<br>b. Implement measures *to maintain or regain urinary continence:*<br>1. offer bedpan or urinal or assist client to commode or bathroom every 2-3 hours<br>2. allow client to assume a normal position for voiding unless contraindicated *in order to promote complete bladder emptying*<br>3. have urinal, bedside commode, or bedpan readily available to client *in order to reduce delays in toileting*<br>4. instruct client to space fluids evenly throughout the day rather than drinking a large quantity at one time *(rapid filling of bladder can result in incontinence if client has decreased urinary sphincter control)* |

5. limit oral fluid intake in the evening *to decrease possibility of nighttime incontinence*
6. instruct client to avoid drinking beverages containing caffeine *(caffeine is a mild diuretic and may make urinary control more difficult).*

c. If urinary incontinence persists:
1. consult physician about intermittent catheterization, insertion of indwelling catheter, or use of external catheter
2. provide client with or apply disposable undergarments (e.g. Depends, Attends) if indicated.

## 11. NURSING DIAGNOSIS: Constipation

related to:
a. diminished defecation reflex associated with decreased neural responses in terminal state and decreased gravity filling of lower rectum resulting from prolonged horizontal positioning;
b. decreased ability to respond to the urge to defecate associated with weakened abdominal muscles, impaired physical mobility, and decreased level of consciousness;
c. decreased gastrointestinal motility associated with decreased activity, increased sympathetic nervous system activity that occurs with anxiety, and use of some medications (e.g. opiates, antacids containing aluminum or calcium);
d. decreased intake of fluid and foods high in fiber.

| Desired Outcome | Nursing Actions and ***Selected Purposes/Rationales*** |
|---|---|
| 11. The client will maintain a bowel routine that provides optimal comfort. | 11.a. Refer to Care Plan on Immobility, Nursing Diagnosis 9 (p. 146), for measures related to assessment, prevention, and management of constipation.<br>b. Implement additional measures *to prevent constipation:*<br>1. establish a routine time for defecation based on client's usual bowel elimination pattern<br>2. perform actions to reduce fear and anxiety (see Nursing Diagnosis 18)<br>3. assist client to toilet or place in high Fowler's position or on bedside commode for bowel movements unless contraindicated; provide privacy and adequate ventilation<br>4. assist with titration of laxative agents (e.g. combination of stool softener and bulk-forming agent or lubricant with a peristaltic stimulant)<br>5. if client is taking antacids containing aluminum or calcium, consult physician about alternating them with antacids containing magnesium. |

## 12. NURSING DIAGNOSIS: Diarrhea

related to:
a. increased intestinal motility associated with high levels of fear and anxiety and excessive use of laxatives and/or antacids containing magnesium;

b. reduction in usual bowel flora if client is receiving an antimicrobial agent;
c. increased water in the bowel associated with high-osmolality supplemental feedings or excessive use of stool softeners.

| Desired Outcome | Nursing Actions and ***Selected Purposes/Rationales*** |
|---|---|
| 12. The client will have fewer bowel movements and more formed stool. | 12.a. Ascertain client's usual bowel elimination habits.<br>b. Assess for and report signs and symptoms of diarrhea (e.g. frequent, loose stools; urgency; abdominal pain and cramping).<br>c. Assess bowel sounds regularly. Report an increase in frequency of bowel sounds.<br>d. Implement measures *to control diarrhea if it occurs:*<br>1. perform actions to reduce fear and anxiety (see Nursing Diagnosis 18)<br>2. discourage smoking *(nicotine has a stimulant effect on the gastrointestinal tract)*<br>3. if diarrhea is related to antimicrobial therapy, encourage intake of flora-containing foods (e.g. yogurt, buttermilk)<br>4. if client is receiving a commercial dietary supplement, dilute it and instruct him/her to drink it slowly; consult physician about use of a low-osmolality preparation (e.g. Osmolite, Jevity)<br>5. if client is taking antacids containing magnesium, consult physician about alternating them with antacids containing aluminum or calcium<br>6. administer the following antidiarrheal agents if ordered:<br>a. opiate or opiate-like substances (e.g. loperamide, diphenoxylate hydrochloride) *to decrease gastrointestinal motility*<br>b. bulk-forming agents (e.g. methylcellulose, psyllium hydrophilic mucilloid, calcium polycarbophil) *to absorb water in the bowel, which results in a more formed stool*<br>c. intestinal flora modifiers (e.g. *Lactobacillus acidophilus,* Lactinex, Bacid) *to promote recolonization of normal intestinal flora.*<br>e. Consult physician if diarrhea persists. |

## 13. NURSING DIAGNOSIS: Bowel incontinence

related to:
a. decreased ability to respond to the urge to defecate associated with decreased level of consciousness and impaired physical mobility;
b. poor anal sphincter control associated with decreased level of consciousness.

| Desired Outcome | Nursing Actions and ***Selected Purposes/Rationales*** |
|---|---|
| 13. The client will maintain optimal bowel control as evidenced by absence of or decreased episodes of incontinence. | 13.a. Monitor for episodes of bowel incontinence.<br>b. Implement measures *to reduce the risk of bowel incontinence:*<br>1. perform actions to control diarrhea if present (see Nursing Diagnosis 12, action d)<br>2. have commode or bedpan readily available to client.<br>c. If bowel incontinence persists:<br>1. consult physician about:<br>a. use of a rectal tube, drainable fecal collector, or insertion of a rectal Foley catheter if client is experiencing constant drainage of liquid stool<br>b. daily bowel care *to routinely evacuate contents of lower colon and reduce episodes of incontinence* |

2. provide client with disposable liners for underwear or disposable undergarments such as Attends
3. use room deodorants as necessary.

## 14. NURSING DIAGNOSIS: Altered thought processes

related to:
a. drug toxicity associated with organ failure;
b. fluid volume deficit and electrolyte imbalances associated with decreased oral intake, increased fluid loss, and specific imbalances that may result from underlying disease process;
c. cerebral hypoxia or cerebral tissue damage associated with the underlying disease process;
d. uncontrolled pain.

| Desired Outcome | Nursing Actions and ***Selected Purposes/Rationales*** |
|---|---|
| 14. The client will maintain optimal thought processes. | 14.a. Assess client for altered thought processes (e.g. impaired memory, shortened attention span, slowed verbal response time, confusion).<br>b. Ascertain from significant others client's usual level of intellectual functioning.<br>c. If client shows evidence of altered thought processes:<br>1. assess for possible causes (e.g. drug toxicity, pain, hypoxia, fluid and electrolyte imbalances) and treat accordingly<br>2. reorient client to person, place, time, and others as necessary<br>3. address client by name<br>4. encourage significant others to bring in client's favorite objects and place in room<br>5. approach client in a slow, calm manner; allow adequate time for communication<br>6. repeat instructions as necessary using clear, simple language and short sentences<br>7. keep environmental stimuli to a minimum<br>8. have client perform only one activity at a time and allow adequate time for performance of activities<br>9. encourage significant others to spend time with and to be supportive of client; instruct them in methods of dealing with client's altered thought processes<br>10. leave light on at night *to facilitate client's orientation to surroundings.* |

## 15. NURSING DIAGNOSIS: Sleep pattern disturbance

related to decreased physical activity, fear, anxiety, unfamiliar environment, discomfort, diarrhea, and inability to assume usual sleep position associated with orthopnea.

| Desired Outcome | Nursing Actions and ***Selected Purposes/Rationales*** |
|---|---|
| 15. The client will attain optimal amounts of | 15.a. Refer to Care Plan on Immobility Nursing Diagnosis 10 (p. 147), for measures related to assessment and promotion of sleep. |

| Desired Outcome | Nursing Actions and ***Selected Purposes/Rationales*** |
|---|---|
| sleep (see Care Plan on Immobility, Nursing Diagnosis 10 [p. 147], for outcome criteria). | b. Implement additional measures *to promote sleep:*<br>1. perform actions to reduce fear and anxiety (see Nursing Diagnosis 18)<br>2. perform actions to reduce discomfort (see Nursing Diagnoses 4, action e; 5.A, action 2; 5.B, action 2; 5.C, action 3; and 5.D)<br>3. perform actions to control diarrhea (see Nursing Diagnosis 12, action d) if present<br>4. if client has orthopnea, assist him/her to assume a position *that will facilitate breathing* (e.g. head of bed elevated with arms supported on pillows, resting forward on overbed table with good pillow support, sitting in a chair)<br>5. maintain oxygen therapy during sleep if indicated. |

## 16. NURSING DIAGNOSIS: High risk for trauma

related to falls, burns, and cuts associated with weakness, confusion, and decreased level of consciousness.

| Desired Outcome | Nursing Actions and ***Selected Purposes/Rationales*** |
|---|---|
| 16. The client will not experience falls, burns, or cuts. | 16.a. Implement measures *to prevent trauma:*<br>1. perform actions *to prevent falls:*<br>a. keep bed in low position with side rails up when client is in bed<br>b. keep needed items within easy reach<br>c. encourage client to request assistance whenever needed; have call signal within easy reach<br>d. use lap belt when client is in chair if indicated<br>e. instruct client to wear well-fitting slippers/shoes with nonslip soles and low heels when ambulating<br>f. keep floor free of clutter and wipe up spills promptly<br>g. instruct and assist client to get out of bed slowly *in order to reduce dizziness associated with postural hypotension*<br>h. carefully position tubing and equipment so that they will not interfere with ambulation<br>i. accompany client during ambulation and use transfer safety belt if he/she is weak or dizzy<br>j. provide ambulatory aids (e.g. walker, cane) if client is weak or unsteady on feet<br>k. reinforce instructions from physical therapist on correct transfer and ambulation techniques<br>l. instruct client to ambulate in well-lit areas and to use handrails if needed<br>m. do not rush client; allow adequate time for ambulation to the bathroom and in hallway<br>n. make sure that bathtub and shower have nonslip bottom surfaces and that shower chair, secure bath mat, call light, hand grips, and adequate lighting are present<br>2. perform actions *to prevent burns:*<br>a. let hot foods and fluids cool slightly before serving<br>b. supervise client while smoking if indicated<br>c. assess temperature of bath water and heating pad before and during use<br>3. assist client with tasks that require fine motor skills (e.g. shaving) *in order to prevent cuts* |

4. if client is confused:
   a. reorient frequently to surroundings and necessity of adhering to safety precautions
   b. provide constant supervision (e.g. staff member, significant other) if indicated
   c. consult physician about the temporary use of jacket or wrist restraints if necessary
   d. administer antianxiety and antipsychotic medications if ordered.

b. Include client and significant others in planning and implementing measures to prevent trauma.

c. If injury does occur, initiate appropriate first aid and notify physician.

## 17. NURSING DIAGNOSIS: High risk for aspiration

related to impaired swallowing and depressed cough and gag reflexes associated with a decreased level of consciousness.

### Desired Outcome

17. The client will not aspirate secretions or foods/fluids as evidenced by:
    a. clear or usual breath sounds
    b. resonant percussion note over lungs
    c. absence of cough and tachypnea
    d. absence of or no increase in dyspnea.

### Nursing Actions and ***Selected Purposes/Rationales***

17.a. Assess for signs and symptoms of aspiration of secretions or foods/fluids (e.g. rhonchi, dull percussion note over affected lung area, cough, tachypnea, tachycardia, increased dyspnea, presence of tube feeding in tracheal aspirate).

b. Monitor chest x-ray results. Report findings of pulmonary infiltrate.

c. If client is receiving tube feedings, add food coloring to the solution *so that it can be readily identified in tracheal aspirate.*

d. Implement measures *to reduce the risk for aspiration:*
   1. position client in side-lying or semi- to high Fowler's position at all times
   2. have suction equipment readily available for use
   3. perform oropharyngeal suctioning and oral hygiene as often as needed *to remove excess secretions*
   4. perform actions to prevent nausea and vomiting (see Nursing Diagnosis 5.A, action 2)
   5. perform actions to reduce the accumulation of gastrointestinal gas and fluid (see Nursing Diagnosis 5.C, action 3) *in order to reduce the risk of gastric distention and regurgitation*
   6. withhold oral food/fluids if gag reflex is depressed or absent, client is not alert, or he/she is experiencing dysphagia
   7. if client is receiving tube feedings:
      a. check tube placement before each feeding or on a routine basis if continuous feeding
      b. maintain continuous tube feeding infusion rate as ordered; administer intermittent tube feedings slowly
      c. maintain client in semi- to high Fowler's position during and for at least 30 minutes after feeding
      d. stop tube feeding and notify physician if residuals exceed established parameters
   8. if client is taking foods/fluids orally:
      a. perform actions to improve ability to swallow (see Nursing Diagnosis 3, action b)
      b. provide small, frequent meals rather than 3 large ones *to decrease the risk of gastric distention and regurgitation*
      c. allow ample time for meals

| Desired Outcome | Nursing Actions and ***Selected Purposes/Rationales*** |
|---|---|
| | d. maintain client in high Fowler's position for at least 30 minutes after meals and snacks<br>e. assist client with oral hygiene after eating *to ensure that food particles do not remain in mouth.*<br>e. If signs and symptoms of aspiration occur:<br>1. perform tracheal suctioning<br>2. notify physician<br>3. prepare client for chest x-ray if ordered. |

## 18. NURSING DIAGNOSIS: Anxiety

related to separation from significant others and familiar environment; feelings of abandonment, loneliness, and that life has been meaningless; the unknown; loss of control over life and body functioning; discomfort; dyspnea; changes in body image; concern about the welfare of significant others and loss of loved ones; unfinished business; unresolved conflicts; recognition of nonbeing; and religious conflicts.

| Desired Outcome | Nursing Actions and ***Selected Purposes/Rationales*** |
|---|---|
| 18. The client will experience a reduction in anxiety as evidenced by:<br>a. verbalization of feeling less anxious and fearful<br>b. usual sleep pattern<br>c. relaxed facial expression and body movements<br>d. stable vital signs<br>e. statements reflecting resolution of unfinished business, conflicts, and concerns. | 18.a. Refer to Care Plan on Immobility, Nursing Diagnosis 13 (p. 153), for measures related to assessment and reduction of fear and anxiety.<br>b. Implement additional measures *to reduce fear and anxiety:*<br>1. perform actions to reduce discomfort (see Nursing Diagnoses 4, action e; 5.A, action 2; 5.B, action 2; 5.C, action 3; and 5.D)<br>2. perform actions to improve respiratory status (see Nursing Diagnosis 1, action c) *in order to relieve dyspnea*<br>3. assist client to direct his/her own death trajectory (e.g. inform him/her of options available for care, encourage personal decision making, restrict visitors if he/she chooses)<br>4. spend time with client *to reduce feelings of loneliness and isolation*<br>5. encourage reminiscence about life experiences if he/she desires *to promote feelings of meaningfulness about the life he/she has lived*<br>6. encourage client to verbalize feelings about changes in body image<br>7. assist client to formulate plans for completing unfinished business and providing for care of significant others if appropriate<br>8. encourage client and significant others to share feelings of anxiety and loss with one another<br>9. encourage significant others to stay with client and participate in his/her care if their presence seems to relieve the client's fear and anxiety; offer support to significant others as necessary<br>10. arrange for a visit with clergy if desired by client or significant others. |

## 19. NURSING DIAGNOSIS: Grieving*

related to loss of control over his/her life and usual body processes, changes in body image, loss of significant others, and imminent death.

*This diagnostic label includes anticipatory grieving and grieving following the actual losses.

| Desired Outcome | Nursing Actions and ***Selected Purposes/Rationales*** |
|---|---|
| 19. The client will demonstrate progression through the grieving process as evidenced by:<br>a. verbalization of feelings about dying<br>b. expression of grief<br>c. use of available support systems. | 19.a. Assess for signs and symptoms of grieving (e.g. change in eating habits, inability to concentrate, insomnia, anger, noncompliance, withdrawal from significant others, denial). Be aware that client's response to his/her death will be affected by factors such as previous experience with a loss, age, developmental state, available support systems, spiritual and cultural background, current health status, significance of death, and the particular phase of grieving he/she is in (the phases of grieving vary among theorists but generally progress from shock and alarm to acceptance).<br>b. Observe for verbal and nonverbal cues indicative of the stages of grieving according to Kübler-Ross (1969):<br>1. denial (e.g. noncompliance with treatment plan, avoidance of the words "dying" or "death," making long-range plans, hyperactivity, relating symptoms experienced to a minor problem)<br>2. anger (e.g. abusive language; negative remarks about staff, family, and hospital; overcompliance; inappropriate responses to unpleasant procedures or current circumstances)<br>3. bargaining (e.g. magical thinking, making personal sacrifices, verbalizing renewed spiritual faith)<br>4. depression (e.g. expression of sadness, crying, withdrawal, change in sleep patterns and activity level)<br>5. acceptance (e.g. decreasing interest in the environment and visitors except for a significant few, decreased interest in talking or in treatment plan, increased desire to rest and sleep, verbalization of acceptance of death).<br>c. Implement measures *to facilitate the grieving process:*<br>1. assist client to acknowledge that death is imminent *so that grief work can progress;* assess for factors that hinder and facilitate acknowledgment<br>2. discuss the grieving process and assist client to accept the phases of grieving as an expected response to actual and/or anticipated losses<br>3. allow time for client to progress through the phases of grieving; be aware that not every phase is expressed by all individuals, that phases do not necessarily occur in sequential order, and that recurrence of phases is common during the course of an illness and the dying process<br>4. assist client to identify personal strengths that have helped him/her to cope in previous situations of loss<br>5. encourage client to express his/her feelings in whatever ways are comfortable (e.g. writing, drawing, conversation)<br>6. perform actions *to support the client and facilitate movement through the following stages of grieving:*<br>a. denial:<br>1. do not reinforce denial of terminal state, yet be aware that a period of denial is essential for client to mobilize inner strengths and resources<br>2. reinforce what client has been told about his/her current status<br>3. allow client to move toward the reality of the situation at his/her own pace<br>4. do not provide false reassurances but support expressions or feelings of hope<br>5. perform actions *to promote trust* (e.g. answer questions honestly, provide requested information)<br>b. anger:<br>1. recognize displacement of anger and assist client to see actual cause of angry feelings and resentment<br>2. encourage verbal expression of thoughts and anger but establish limits on abusive behavior if demonstrated |

| Desired Outcome | Nursing Actions and ***Selected Purposes/Rationales*** |
|---|---|

3. include client in planning of care, encourage maximum participation in treatment plan, and allow choices whenever possible *to enable client to maintain a sense of control*

c. bargaining:
1. assist client to look at available options realistically; discuss expectations and treatment options with him/her
2. observe for possible guilt feelings; encourage verbalization and provide feedback
3. encourage significant others to spend time with client
4. provide accurate information and reinforce teaching about the disease process and grieving *in order to help the client see the reality of the situation*

d. depression:
1. allow client to express feelings of sadness and to cry; acknowledge his/her expressions of grief
2. listen empathetically if client chooses to verbalize feelings; emphasize that his/her response to impending death is normal
3. sit quietly with client; use touch if appropriate
4. encourage those most significant to client to spend time with him/her; explain that depression facilitates the process of detachment that is essential to the client in adjusting to death

e. acceptance:
1. follow client cues in relation to desire for conversation, presence of others, and involvement in care
2. accept lack of interest in environment, world events, people, and treatments; recognize that client is detaching from life and avoid false cheer and hope
3. sit with the client when there are not tasks to perform; use touch as appropriate *to demonstrate caring*
4. recognize that the client may be experiencing feelings of isolation and loneliness if he/she has reached the stage of acceptance but the significant others have not
5. if desired by client, assist with after-death arrangements (e.g. funeral, religious service, who should be called); be careful not to interject your own beliefs

7. perform actions *to assist the client to maintain a positive self-concept and feel good about the life he/she has experienced:*
a. visit frequently and encourage verbalization about past events, life accomplishments, interests, and feelings
b. help client to focus on positive rather than negative aspects of his/her life experience
c. maintain a nonjudgmental attitude about the kind of life client has led and his/her beliefs
d. encourage participation in decisions about care
e. encourage and assist client with good physical hygiene and grooming; suggest use of personal rather than hospital clothing *to assist client to maintain his/her identity*

8. explain the phases of the grieving process to significant others; encourage their support and understanding
9. facilitate communication between the client and significant others; be aware that they may be in different phases of the grieving process
10. provide information about counseling services and support groups that might assist client and significant others in working through grief
11. arrange for visit from clergy if desired by client.

d. Consult physician regarding referral for counseling if signs of dysfunctional grieving (e.g. persistent denial of losses, excessive anger or sadness, hysteria, suicidal behaviors) occur.

## 20. NURSING DIAGNOSIS: Hopelessness

related to deteriorating physical condition, feelings of abandonment, and inability to reach self-fulfillment associated with terminal state.

| Desired Outcome | Nursing Actions and ***Selected Purposes/Rationales*** |
|---|---|
| 20. The client will maintain hope as evidenced by:<br>a. verbal expression of same<br>b. maintenance of satisfying relationships with others<br>c. participation in self-care and decision making as able<br>d. identification of realistic goals. | 20.a. Assess client for signs and symptoms of hopelessness (e.g. statements of feeling hopeless, decreased response to significant others, decreased participation in self-care and decision making, decreased verbalization, flat affect).<br>b. Implement measures *to assist client to reduce feelings of hopelessness:*<br>1. perform actions to facilitate the grieving process (see Nursing Diagnosis 19, action c)<br>2. if client has religious beliefs, encourage the use of them as a support system; support his/her renewal of spiritual being by creating an environment in which these beliefs can be openly acknowledged and practiced<br>3. allow client to retain as much control as possible over activities of daily living; involve him/her in as much self-care and decision making as feasible<br>4. assist client to identify goals that are achievable in the time that he/she has left, ways to continue working toward goals previously set even if not possible to achieve them totally, and the purpose remaining in his/her life such as role model or advisor to significant others.<br>c. Consult physician if client demonstrates increased feelings of hopelessness. |

## 21. NURSING DIAGNOSIS: Altered family processes

related to excessive anxiety, grief, disorganization and role changes within the family unit, inadequate support system, and exhaustion associated with long-term care of the dying family member.

| Desired Outcome | Nursing Actions and ***Selected Purposes/Rationales*** |
|---|---|
| 21. The family members* will demonstrate beginning adjustment to loss of client and changes in family roles and structure as evidenced by:<br>a. meeting client's needs<br>b. verbalization of ways to adapt to | 21.a. Assess for signs and symptoms of altered family processes (e.g. inability to meet client's needs, statements of not being able to accept client's imminent death or to make necessary role and life-style changes, inability to make decisions, infrequent visits, inappropriate response to client's situation, verbalization of guilt, preoccupation with other aspects of life, negative family interactions).<br>b. Identify components of the family and their patterns of communication and role expectations.<br>c. Implement measures *to facilitate family members' adjustment to imminent loss of client and altered family roles and structure:*<br>1. encourage and assist family members to verbalize feelings about the death of the client and the effect of it on their life style and family |

*The term "family members" is being used here to include client's significant others.

| Desired Outcome | Nursing Actions and ***Selected Purposes/Rationales*** |
|---|---|
| required role and life-style changes<br>c. active participation in decision making and client's care<br>d. positive interactions with one another. | structure; actively listen to each family member and maintain a nonjudgmental attitude about feelings shared<br>2. assist family members to confront the reality of the client's imminent death when they are ready; encourage them to imagine life after death of the client and to set some personal goals if appropriate<br>3. reinforce physician's explanation about the dying process and what to expect<br>4. provide privacy *so that family members can share their feelings and grief with one another;* stress the importance of and facilitate the use of good communication techniques<br>5. explain the process of grieving that everyone experiences in adjusting to a loss<br>6. assist family members to progress through their own grieving process; explain that they may encounter times when they need to focus on meeting their own rather than the client's needs<br>7. emphasize the need for family members to obtain adequate rest and nutrition and to identify and use stress management techniques *so that they are better able to emotionally and physically deal with the death of the client;* assure them that the client will be well cared for in their absence<br>8. encourage and assist family members to identify coping strategies for dealing with the client's death and its effect on those left behind<br>9. include family members in decision making about client and his/her care; convey appreciation of their input and continued support of the client<br>10. encourage and allow family members to participate in client's care if desired by both client and family members<br>11. assist family members to make necessary postmortem arrangements for client (e.g. funeral home, burial place, clergy visitation)<br>12. provide accurate information to family members about:<br>a. the current status of client<br>b. behaviors to expect as the client progresses through terminal stages of disease and his/her own grieving<br>c. ways they can best assist in meeting client's needs<br>13. instruct family members in signs of approaching death (e.g. reduced level of consciousness; reduced urine output; cool, mottled extremities; labored breathing or periods of no breathing)<br>14. prepare family members for the sound of changes in respiration associated with accumulation of secretions in major airways when death is imminent; describe the sound and explain that it is usually not disturbing or uncomfortable for the client<br>15. when appropriate, help and encourage family members to "let go" of client and say goodbye<br>16. assist family members to identify resources that can assist them in coping with their feelings and in meeting their immediate and long-term needs (e.g. counseling and social services; pastoral care; service, bereavement, and church groups; Hospice); initiate a referral if indicated<br>17. assist family members to contact appropriate persons (e.g. funeral home director, clergy) when death occurs.<br>d. Consult physician if family members continue to demonstrate difficulty adjusting to the loss of the client and changes in their roles and family structure. |

## Reference

Kübler-Ross, E. On death and dying. New York: Macmillan, 1969.

UNIT

# VII

# *Nursing Care of the Client Receiving Treatment for Neoplastic Disorders*

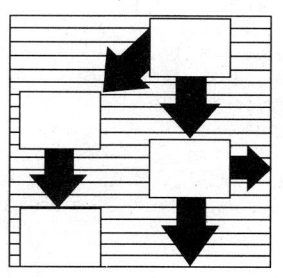

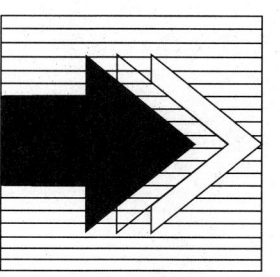

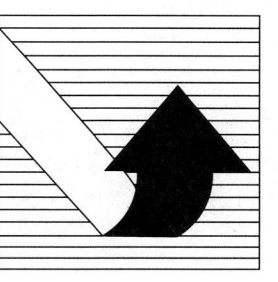

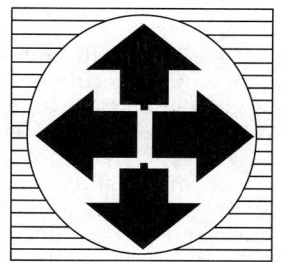

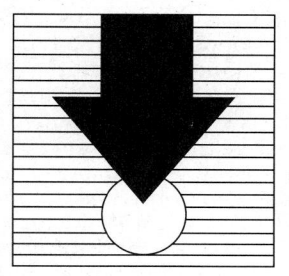

# Brachytherapy

Brachytherapy is the continuous delivery of radiation to a malignancy at a specific body site by placing the radioactive source close to or within the tumor. Brachytherapy can deliver a higher dose of radiation than is possible with external radiation therapy (teletherapy) and does so with minimal damage occurring to the surrounding healthy tissue because of the rapid fall in dose outside the implanted area. It can be used as a primary treatment or in combination with external radiation therapy and/or surgery to treat cancers of the head and neck, prostate, lung, brain, liver, colon, and bladder. Brachytherapy can be sealed or unsealed, temporary or permanent, and local or systemic. The method of application selected depends on the type, location, and size of the tumor; its radiocurability; the sensitivity of surrounding normal tissue; and the age and general physical condition of the client. The radioactive isotope used depends on the site to be treated, lesion size, availability and half-life of the isotope, and financial and safety concerns.

The most common types of brachytherapy are interstitial implants using iridium 192 ($^{192}Ir$) seeds or wire or iodine 125 ($^{125}I$) seeds and intracavitary implants using cesium 137 ($^{137}Cs$). Both types are sealed and temporary. Interstitial implants are used in the treatment of skin, brain, prostate, and oral cavity lesions, whereas intracavitary implants are used primarily in treating gynecological malignancies. With both interstitial and intracavitary implants, varying kinds of applicators (e.g. hollow needles, templates, plastic tubes, Fletcher-Suit) are surgically placed in the tissue or cavity to be treated, and the radioactive source is usually "after-loaded" when the client returns to his/her room. The implant is commonly left in place for 24-72 hours and delivers a dose of 40-60 cGy (centigrays)/hour. Remote after-loading systems, which eliminate personnel exposure to the radioactive source during the loading and unloading process, are also being used for low- and high-dose rate intracavity brachytherapy. These systems allow for retraction of the radioactive source by means of a transfer tube into a shielded bedside safe whenever personnel and/or family members enter the client's room.

Brachytherapy using unsealed isotopes is also commonly done. These isotopes can be ingested, injected, or implanted permanently in a body part. Unsealed interstitial implants using $^{125}I$ or gold 198 ($^{198}Au$) typically have been used in the treatment of pancreatic, prostate, and neck cancers. Iodine 131 ($^{131}I$) is commonly used to treat thyroid cancer and Graves' disease. It is ingested and metabolized by the body before being concentrated in the thyroid gland in 3-5 days. Although not in common use, colloidal forms of phosphorus 32 ($^{32}P$) and $^{198}Au$ can be injected into the pleural or peritoneal cavity to treat local disease or related effusions and/or ascites.

Another type of brachytherapy, surface brachytherapy, is accomplished by placing a radioactive source in a mold, which is then placed on or adjacent to an external body surface. It is used to treat sites such as small surface lesions that are difficult to access in other ways.

**This care plan focuses on the adult client hospitalized for brachytherapy.** The nursing care required will depend on the isotope used, its method of administration, and the general physiological condition of the client. Before the initiation of brachytherapy, the goals of care are to reduce fear and anxiety and educate the client regarding the therapy and expected side effects. During and following the treatment, the goals of care are to maintain comfort, prevent complications, and educate the client regarding follow-up care.

## DISCHARGE CRITERIA

Prior to discharge, the client will:

- verbalize appropriate safety precautions related to brachytherapy
- identify measures to increase comfort and prevent complications associated with vaginal irradiation
- share thoughts and feelings about the diagnosis of cancer and need for radiation therapy
- state signs and symptoms to report to the health care provider
- identify community resources that can assist with adjustment to the effects of the diagnosis and its treatment
- verbalize an understanding of and a plan for adhering to recommended follow-up care including future appointments with health care provider and radiologist and medications prescribed.

**NURSING DIAGNOSES**

**Preradiation**

**1.** Anxiety△ *183*
**2.** Knowledge deficit△ *183*

**See Standardized Preoperative Care Plan for additional diagnoses.**

**Radiation and Postradiation**

**1.** Pain:
  **a.** muscle aches
  **b.** pain at or around implant site△ *186*
**2.** Impaired physical mobility△ *187*
**3.** Self-care deficit△ *187*
**4.** Knowledge deficit△ *187*

## PRERADIATION

**Use in conjunction with the Standardized Preoperative Care Plan.**

### 1. NURSING DIAGNOSIS: Anxiety

related to:
a. lack of knowledge and preconceived ideas about treatment with radiation and its effect on physiological functioning;
b. anticipated loss of control, effects of anesthesia, and discomfort;
c. unfamiliar environment and financial concerns;
d. diagnosis of cancer.

| Desired Outcome | Nursing Actions and ***Selected Purposes/Rationales*** |
|---|---|
| 1. The client will experience a reduction in anxiety (see Standardized Preoperative Care Plan, Nursing Diagnosis 1 [pp. 108-109], for outcome criteria). | 1. Refer to Standardized Preoperative Care Plan, Nursing Diagnosis 1 (pp. 108-109), for measures related to assessment and reduction of fear and anxiety.<br>2. Implement additional measures *to reduce fear and anxiety;*<br>a. reinforce physician's explanations and clarify misconceptions client has about the diagnosis of cancer, treatment plan and its effects, and prognosis<br>b. provide information related to the specific type of brachytherapy the client will be receiving (see Preradiation Nursing Diagnosis 2, action b). |

### 2. NURSING DIAGNOSIS: Knowledge deficit

regarding:
a. hospital routines associated with brachytherapy;
b. placement of radioactive source;
c. precautions necessary to protect staff and significant others from exposure to radiation and prevent dislodgment of the radioactive source.

| Desired Outcome | Nursing Actions and ***Selected Purposes/Rationales*** |
|---|---|
| 2. The client will verbalize an understanding of usual preradiation and postradiation care. | 2.a. Refer to Standardized Preoperative Care Plan, Nursing Diagnosis 4, actions a.1-4 (pp. 111-112), for teaching related to routine preoperative and postoperative care.<br>b. Provide additional information regarding care associated with the type of brachytherapy the client will be receiving:<br>1. if the client is to receive a sealed, temporary interstitial or intracavitary implant:<br>a. reinforce preoperative teaching (a general anesthetic may be used)<br>b. explain that localization x-rays will be done following insertion of the applicator(s) in order to determine accuracy of placement and dosimetry<br>c. explain the manual loading procedure; reassure client that it is not painful<br>d. if a remote after-loading system will be used:<br>1. explain the process and indications for loading and unloading the radioactive source<br>2. explain that only essential care will be given (e.g. basic hygiene, change of soiled linen) by staff and visiting hours will be restricted so that radioactive source will not be unloaded for extended periods<br>e. if the radioactive source will be manually loaded and unloaded, explain the precautions that will be taken while the radioactive source is in place:<br>1. time and distance requirements should be followed by all who come in contact with the client<br>2. only essential care will be given (e.g. basic hygiene, change of soiled linen) in order to minimize staff exposure to radiation<br>3. each visitor will be limited to 30 minutes/day, children under 18 and women who may be or are pregnant will not be permitted to visit, and visitors must maintain a distance of 6 feet from the radioactive source<br>f. assure client that redness, edema, and drainage around applicator insertion sites are normal<br>g. explain that a minimum fluid intake of 2500 ml/day will be encouraged to promote elimination of the by-products of tumor breakdown<br>h. assure client that personal belongings will not be contaminated<br>i. explain that body fluids will not be contaminated<br>j. if a perineal or vaginal implant is planned:<br>1. inform client that sensations of rectal fullness, lower abdominal pressure, and low back pain may be experienced due to pressure of applicator and vaginal packing (vaginal packing is inserted to separate the bladder and rectum from the radioactive source and to maintain applicator position)<br>2. instruct client in isometric leg exercises that should be performed at regular intervals while on bed rest<br>3. explain purpose for thigh-high elastic hose the client will wear while on bed rest<br>4. inform client that applicator will be checked for correct position at least twice/shift to monitor for dislodgment<br>5. explain precautions that will be taken to prevent dislodgment of the implant:<br>a. complete bed rest will be required with head of bed slightly elevated<br>b. only minimal movement will be allowed (some physicians allow client to logroll from side to side 3-4 times/day)<br>c. a urinary catheter will be inserted to reduce the need for frequent use of bedpan (the catheter also maintains bladder |

decompression and inhibits close contact of bladder with radioactive source)

d. an enema will be given and a liquid or low-residue diet may be prescribed preoperatively to cleanse the bowel and decrease the chance that the client will have a bowel movement after implant insertion; a fracture pan will be used if bowel movement is necessary

e. no perineal care will be given unless absolutely necessary

k. if a brain implant is planned:

1. reinforce physician's explanation about the stereotactic equipment that will be used to implant radioactive source:
   a. describe the stereotactic frame using pictures or diagrams and explain how it will be applied
   b. discuss the use of the CT scanner in conjunction with the stereotactic frame (this is done to facilitate precise placement of the radioactive source)
   c. explain that local anesthesia will be used during the procedure
   d. explain that while the frame is being applied, pressure from the ear bars may cause temporary discomfort; emphasize that the bars will be removed once the frame is in place
2. clarify the physician's explanation about the amount of scalp hair that will be removed for the procedure
3. explain the safety precautions that will be followed while the radioactive source is in place (these will vary depending on the isotope used)
4. explain that self-care will be encouraged to minimize staff exposure to the radioactive source
5. arrange for a visit to the intensive care unit if client is expected to be there following implant insertion

2. if the client is to receive oral $^{131}I$:
   a. explain that the isotope will be mixed with water and that he/she should drink it through a straw (may also be given in capsule form)
   b. instruct client to notify staff if he/she is nauseous; emphasize the importance of not vomiting, particularly during first 4 hours after ingestion of the isotope in order to retain it and prevent contamination of others
   c. reinforce physician's explanation that stool, urine, sweat, saliva, and other body fluids will be highly contaminated for about 4 days
   d. emphasize the need to wear hospital clothing to prevent contamination of personal articles
   e. explain that articles in the room and on the floor will be covered with plastic to prevent contamination
   f. instruct client in good handwashing technique; stress the need to wash hands carefully, particularly after contact with urine, for 14 days after ingestion of the isotope
   g. instruct client to flush toilet at least 2 times after each voiding for 14 days after ingestion of the isotope to dilute the excreted isotope
   h. instruct male client to sit while urinating to prevent splashing of urine
   i. assure client that body fluids are no longer contaminated once the isotope is metabolized and excreted (usually 2 weeks after discharge)

3. if the client is to receive an intracavitary injection of colloidal $^{32}P$ or $^{198}Au$:
   a. explain that there are no isolation requirements (the isotope emits beta particles and is hazardous only if the colloidal substance leaks from body) but that staff will wear gloves when handling dressings or linens in case leakage has occurred

| Desired Outcome | Nursing Actions and ***Selected Purposes/Rationales*** |
|---|---|
| | b. explain that he/she will be assisted to turn frequently to ensure equal distribution of the colloidal substance within the body cavity<br>c. explain that the colloidal substance is dyed so that leakage is easily recognized by stains on dressings or linens<br>4. if the client is receiving a permanent implant of $^{125}I$ in a tumor or body part (e.g. prostate, neck, pancreas):<br>a. explain that neither client nor his/her body fluids are contaminated because the range of radiation for $^{125}I$ is only about 2 cm but that time and distance precautions will be followed during hospitalization<br>b. caution client to notify staff immediately if a seed is found in urine or wound dressing<br>5. if client is receiving a permanent implant of $^{198}Au$ seeds into the prostate:<br>a. explain that $^{198}Au$ seeds have a very short half-life (2.7 days) and safety precautions will be necessary during that time<br>b. inform client that his urine will need to be filtered before being disposed of in the toilet to monitor for seed dislodgment.<br>c. Allow adequate time for questions and clarification of information provided. |

## RADIATION AND POSTRADIATION

### 1. NURSING DIAGNOSIS: Pain:

a. **muscle aches** related to prescribed activity restrictions (required for some intracavitary and interstitial implants);
b. **pain at or around implant site** related to:
   1. contractions of hollow organ into which an intracavitary implant has been placed
   2. tissue trauma associated with placement of applicator(s) used to hold the radioactive source in place.

| Desired Outcome | Nursing Actions and ***Selected Purposes/Rationales*** |
|---|---|
| 1. The client will experience diminished pain as evidenced by:<br>a. verbalization of same<br>b. relaxed facial expression and body positioning<br>c. stable vital signs. | 1.a. Determine how client usually responds to pain.<br>b. Assess client's perception of pain including location, intensity, and type. Use a numerical scale to rate intensity.<br>c. Assess for nonverbal signs of pain (e.g. wrinkled brow; clenched fists; guarding of implant site; reluctance to move; restlessness; rubbing hips, shoulders, or lower back; diaphoresis; facial pallor; increased B/P; tachycardia).<br>d. Assess for factors that seem to aggravate and alleviate pain.<br>e. Implement measures *to reduce pain:*<br>1. support body parts with pillows if a particular body position needs to be maintained<br>2. provide or assist with nonpharmacological measures for relief of pain (e.g. back rub, position change as allowed, relaxation techniques, quiet conversation, restful environment, diversional activities), being careful to adhere to time and distance requirements |

3. place an alternating pressure mattress or pad on bed *to reduce discomfort associated with restricted body movement*
4. administer analgesics if ordered.

f. Consult physician if above measures fail to provide adequate relief of pain.

## 2. NURSING DIAGNOSIS: Impaired physical mobility

related to:
a. prescribed activity restrictions associated with the need to maintain accurate placement of the radioactive source;
b. reluctance to move associated with pain and/or fear of dislodging applicator(s).

| Desired Outcome | Nursing Actions and ***Selected Purposes/Rationales*** |
|---|---|
| 2. The client will achieve maximum physical mobility within prescribed activity restrictions. | 2.a. Implement measures *to increase mobility if allowed:*<br>1. perform actions to reduce pain (see Radiation and Postradiation Nursing Diagnosis 1, action e)<br>2. assure client that the device containing the radioactive source will not dislodge if activity restrictions are adhered to (mobility restrictions will depend on the type of applicator and/or location of the implant)<br>3. instruct client in exercises that can be performed in bed without affecting implant placement and encourage him/her to do them frequently<br>4. encourage activity and participation in self-care activities as allowed.<br>b. Provide praise and encouragement for all efforts to maintain level of mobility allowed. |

## 3. NURSING DIAGNOSIS: Self-care deficit

related to:
a. reluctance to move associated with pain and/or fear of dislodging applicator(s);
b. prescribed activity restrictions during the time the radioactive source is in place.

| Desired Outcome | Nursing Actions and ***Selected Purposes/Rationales*** |
|---|---|
| 3. The client will perform self-care activities within restrictions imposed by the treatment plan. | 3.a. With client, develop a realistic plan for meeting daily physical needs.<br>b. Encourage maximum independence within prescribed activity restrictions.<br>c. Implement measures *to facilitate client's ability to perform self-care activities:*<br>1. schedule care at a time when client is most likely to be able to participate (e.g. when analgesics are at peak effect, after rest periods)<br>2. keep needed objects within easy reach.<br>d. Provide positive feedback for all efforts toward and accomplishments of self-care.<br>e. Reinforce preradiation teaching that the nursing staff will assist only with necessary hygiene activities that the client is unable to perform independently. |

## 4. NURSING DIAGNOSIS: Knowledge deficit
regarding follow-up care.

| Desired Outcomes | Nursing Actions and ***Selected Purposes/Rationales*** |
|---|---|
| 4.a. The client will verbalize appropriate safety precautions related to brachytherapy. | 4.a.1. If client has received systemic $^{131}I$, provide the following instructions:<br>a. use separate toilet facilities if possible, flush toilet at least twice after urinating, and sit when urinating to prevent splashing of urine (urine contains the highest levels of radioactive iodine)<br>b. wash hands several times a day, particularly after toileting, to minimize contamination of any objects touched<br>c. take a bath or shower daily; rinse the bath tub or shower stall well after use<br>d. avoid shared use of items such as soap, comb, brush, toothbrush, makeup, clothing, linen, dishes, and eating utensils<br>e. launder clothing and wash dishes separately from those of others; rinse sink for at least 2-3 minutes after washing dishes<br>f. minimize physical contact with others, particularly pregnant women and children (perspiration and saliva contain small amounts of radioactive iodine)<br>g. adhere to radiologist's guidelines regarding distance requirements and limitations on time spent with others<br>h. if breastfeeding, stop until permission to resume is given by radiologist (radioactive iodine is excreted in breast milk)<br>i. sleep alone for the first week after hospital discharge<br>j. strictly adhere to contraceptive measures for 6 weeks following discharge<br>k. continue to adhere to precautions for the length of time specified by the radiologist.<br>2. Notify radiologist if a medical emergency occurs or if unexpected medical procedures need to be done in the 6 week period following discharge.<br>3. If client has had a temporary interstitial or intracavitary implant, reinforce the fact that no precautions are necessary after discharge.<br>4. If client has received a permanent implant of $^{125}I$ into the prostate, provide the following information:<br>a. distance requirements need to be adhered to for 2 months following insertion of the implant (i.e. 6 feet should be maintained from women who are or may be pregnant, children under 4 years should not sit on client's lap)<br>b. seed loss can occur during urination, particularly for 1 month postimplant; if this occurs, the seed should be retrieved if possible using tweezers or pliers, wrapped in foil, and returned to the Radiation Oncology Unit for disposal (the seeds are the size of a grain of rice and are considered inert after 1 year)<br>c. a condom needs to be used during intercourse for 2 months following the implant insertion. |
| 4.b. The client will identify measures to increase comfort and prevent complications associated with vaginal irradiation. | 4.b.1. If client has received vaginal irradiation:<br>a. instruct in correct douche technique if appropriate (povidine-iodine [betadine] or vinegar douche may be ordered to cleanse the vagina and decrease inflammation)<br>b. explain that a pink to tan vaginal discharge is normal for 7-10 days after removal of the implant<br>c. instruct client to abstain from using tampons and to change sanitary napkins every 4 hours |

d. reinforce physician's explanation about the possibility of vaginal stenosis occurring and ways to prevent permanent sealing of vaginal walls (e.g. intercourse 3 times/week as soon as allowed, use of vaginal dilator [obturator] for 5-10 minutes 3 times/week)
e. if client is sexually active:
   1. explain that intercourse can be resumed in 2-3 weeks
   2. encourage her to try various positions for intercourse to compensate for shortening and narrowing of vagina (some clients may lose the upper 2/3 of the vaginal vault)
   3. explain that having male partner use a condom will prevent the burning sensation that may result when semen comes in contact with the fragile vaginal tissue
   4. explain that a water-soluble lubricant can be used to reduce discomfort if dryness associated with decreased vaginal secretions is problematic.

2. Allow time for questions, clarification, and demonstration of techniques.

| | |
|---|---|
| 4.c. The client will state signs and symptoms to report to the health care provider. | 4.c. Instruct client to report the following:<br>1. unusual discharge, odor, or excessive bleeding from irradiated area<br>2. signs and symptoms of radiation cystitis (e.g. blood in urine, pain on urination, urinary frequency or urgency)<br>3. signs and symptoms of tissue fibrosis within the treatment area (e.g. BOWEL: inability to move bowels, distended abdomen, loss of appetite, alternating diarrhea and constipation; SKIN: uneven texture, changes in appearance of surface blood vessels; VAGINA: pain or difficulty with sexual intercourse)<br>4. increasing pain in irradiated area<br>5. significant, unexplained weight loss<br>6. excessive depression or difficulty coping<br>7. persistent urgency, frequency, or burning on urination and/or increased temperature after removal of a gynecological implant (these symptoms are an expected response to the inflammation that occurs 8-10 days after removal of the radioactive source but the health care provider should be notified if symptoms do not diminish by day 15). |
| 4.d. The client will identify community resources that can assist with adjustment to the effects of the diagnosis and its treatment. | 4.d.1. Provide information about and encourage use of community resources that can assist the client and significant others with adjustment to effects of the diagnosis and radiation therapy (e.g. local support groups, American Cancer Society, counselors, social service agencies, Make Today Count, Hospice).<br>2. Initiate a referral if indicated. |
| 4.e. The client will verbalize an understanding of and a plan for adhering to recommended follow-up care including future appointments with health care provider and radiologist and medications prescribed. | 4.e.1. Reinforce the importance of keeping follow-up appointments with the health care provider and radiologist.<br>2. Teach the client the rationale for, side effects of, and importance of taking prescribed medications (e.g. antimicrobials).<br>3. Implement measures to improve client compliance:<br>a. include significant others in teaching sessions if possible<br>b. encourage questions and allow time for reinforcement and clarification of information provided<br>c. provide written instructions on future appointments with health care provider and radiologist, medications prescribed, and signs and symptoms to report. |

# Chemotherapy

This care plan focuses on the use of cytotoxic drugs (chemotherapeutic agents) in the treatment of cancer. The drugs are used alone or with surgery and/or radiation therapy to achieve a cure or to control or relieve symptoms associated with advanced disease.

The goal of curative chemotherapy is to eliminate all malignant cells without causing permanent damage to normal ones. Success of the therapy depends on the size, type, and location of the tumor in addition to the client's physiological condition, prior treatment with radiation and/or chemotherapy, and the status of his/her immune system.

Cytotoxic drugs are classified according to their chemical structure or their effect on the cell life cycle. Some are cell cycle–nonspecific (e.g. alkylating agents, nitrosoureas, antibiotics) and will destroy a cell regardless of its phase of replication. Others are cell cycle–specific (e.g. antimetabolites, plant alkaloids) and are most effective against the cells that are actively replicating.

Cytotoxic drugs are thought to kill a fixed percentage of the tumor cells with each dose because only a fraction of the tumor cell mass is in the process of dividing and therefore is sensitive to the drugs. Cell kill is hypothesized to be the greatest when the growth fraction of the tumor is the highest. Cells in the resting phase are less responsive to chemotherapeutic agents and are better able to repair themselves if damaged during treatment.

Clients with cancer are usually treated with a combination of drugs given simultaneously or in a particular sequence or protocol. The additive and sometimes synergistic effects that occur when drugs are used together allow an increased percentage of tumor cell kill without a concomitant increase in drug-induced toxicities. Drugs are selected for combination based on their effectiveness, action on the cell cycle, toxic effects, and nadir.

Cytotoxic drugs do not discriminate between the normal and the cancerous cell and, as a result, the client may experience certain side effects and/or toxic effects following their administration. The drugs have the greatest effect on rapidly dividing cancerous and normal cells (e.g. bone marrow, skin, hair follicles, lining of the gastrointestinal tract). Because of this lack of selectivity between the cancerous and the normal cell, nursing care of the recipient of the drugs is indeed a challenge.

**This care plan focuses on the adult client hospitalized for an initial or subsequent cycle of chemotherapy and/or management of side effects of treatment with cytotoxic agents.** The major goals of care are to maintain comfort; prevent complications; and educate the client about chemotherapy, expected side effects, and toxic effects to be reported. The nurse also plays a major role in assisting the client and significant others to cope with actual and anticipated changes in body image, life style, and roles as a result of cancer and chemotherapy.

## DISCHARGE CRITERIA

Prior to discharge, the client will:

- have no signs and symptoms of toxic effects of cytotoxic agents
- have side effects of cytotoxic agents under control
- identify ways to prevent infection during periods of lowered immunity
- demonstrate the ability to take an oral and an axillary temperature correctly
- demonstrate appropriate oral hygiene techniques
- identify techniques to control nausea and vomiting
- verbalize ways to improve appetite and nutritional status
- verbalize ways to manage and cope with persistent fatigue
- verbalize ways to prevent bleeding when platelet counts are low
- verbalize ways to adjust to alterations in reproductive and sexual functioning
- demonstrate the ability to care for a central venous catheter, a peritoneal catheter, or an implanted infusion device if in place
- verbalize an understanding of the care and precautions necessary if an Ommaya reservoir is in place
- verbalize an understanding of an implanted infusion pump and precautions necessary if one is in place
- state signs and symptoms of complications to report to the health care provider
- share thoughts and feelings about changes in body image resulting from chemotherapy
- identify community resources that can assist with home management and adjustment to the diagnosis of cancer and chemotherapy and its effects

❖ verbalize an understanding of and a plan for adhering to recommended follow-up care including medications prescribed and schedule for chemotherapy, laboratory studies, and future appointments with health care provider.

**NURSING/ COLLABORATIVE DIAGNOSES**



## 1. NURSING DIAGNOSIS: Anxiety

related to lack of knowledge about chemotherapy including administration procedure, expected side effects, and impact on usual life style and roles; unfamiliar environment; financial concerns; and diagnosis of cancer with potential for premature death.

| Desired Outcome | Nursing Actions and ***Selected Purposes/Rationales*** |
|---|---|
| 1. The client will experience a reduction in anxiety as evidenced by:<br>a. verbalization of feeling less anxious and fearful | 1.a. Assess client on admission for:<br>1. fears, misconceptions, and level of understanding of chemotherapy and its effects on body functioning, life style, and roles<br>2. perception of anticipated results of planned chemotherapeutic regimen<br>3. feelings about past experiences with chemotherapy or other treatments for cancer |

| Desired Outcome | Nursing Actions and ***Selected Purposes/Rationales*** |
|---|---|
| b. usual sleep pattern<br>c. relaxed facial expression and body movements<br>d. stable vital signs<br>e. usual perceptual ability and interactions with others. | 4. availability of an adequate support system<br>5. signs and symptoms of anxiety (e.g. verbalization of fears and concerns, insomnia, tenseness, tremors, irritability, restlessness, diaphoresis, tachypnea, tachycardia, elevated blood pressure, facial pallor or flushing, narrowed perceptual field, withdrawal, noncompliance with treatment plan); validate perceptions carefully, remembering that some behavior may be a result of physiological changes associated with the disease process.<br>b. Implement measures *to reduce fear and anxiety:*<br>1. orient client to hospital environment, equipment, and routines<br>2. introduce staff who will be participating in his/her care; if possible, maintain consistency in staff assigned to his/her care *to provide feelings of stability and comfort with the environment*<br>3. assure client that staff members are nearby; respond to call signal as soon as possible<br>4. maintain a calm, supportive, confident manner when interacting with client<br>5. encourage verbalization of fear and anxiety; provide feedback<br>6. explain all tests that may be done before the initiation of chemotherapy (e.g. blood and urine studies, ECG, radionuclide angiography, pulmonary function studies)<br>7. reinforce physician's explanations and clarify misconceptions the client has about how prescribed drugs work, expected side effects, and potential drug toxicities<br>8. provide a calm, restful environment<br>9. instruct client in relaxation techniques and encourage participation in diversional activities<br>10. perform actions to assist the client to cope with the diagnosis of cancer and chemotherapy and its effects (see Nursing Diagnosis 15, action c)<br>11. initiate financial and/or social service referrals if indicated<br>12. encourage significant others to project a caring, concerned attitude without obvious anxiousness<br>13. initiate preoperative teaching if placement of a peritoneal or central venous catheter, Ommaya reservoir, or implanted infusion device is planned<br>14. administer antianxiety agents if ordered.<br>c. Include significant others in orientation and teaching sessions and encourage their continued support of the client.<br>d. Provide information based on current needs of client and significant others at a level they can understand. Encourage questions and clarification of information provided.<br>e. Consult physician if above actions fail to control fear and anxiety. |

## 2. NURSING DIAGNOSIS: Altered nutrition: less than body requirements

related to:

a. decreased oral intake associated with:
   1. oral, pharyngeal, and esophageal pain resulting from mucositis if it has developed
   2. anorexia resulting from factors such as depression, fear, anxiety, fatigue, discomfort, early satiety, and an altered sense of taste;

b. loss of nutrients associated with vomiting and diarrhea if present;

c. impaired utilization of nutrients associated with:
   1. accelerated and inefficient metabolism of proteins, carbohydrates, and fats resulting from the disease process
   2. decreased absorption of nutrients resulting from loss of intestinal absorptive surface if mucositis has developed
   3. utilization of available nutrients by the malignant cells rather than the host.

| Desired Outcome | Nursing Actions and ***Selected Purposes/Rationales*** |
|---|---|
| 2. The client will maintain an adequate nutritional status as evidenced by:<br>a. weight within normal range for client's age, height, and body frame<br>b. normal BUN and serum albumin, Hct, Hb, and transferrin levels<br>c. triceps skinfold thickness within normal range<br>d. usual strength and activity tolerance<br>e. healthy oral mucous membrane. | 2.a. Assess for and report signs and symptoms of malnutrition:<br>1. weight below normal for client's age, height, and body frame<br>2. abnormal BUN and low serum albumin, Hct, Hb, and transferrin levels<br>3. triceps skinfold thickness less than normal<br>4. weakness and fatigue<br>5. stomatitis.<br>b. Monitor percentage of meals and snacks client consumes. Report a pattern of inadequate intake.<br>c. Implement measures *to maintain an adequate nutritional status:*<br>1. perform actions *to improve oral intake:*<br>a. implement measures to reduce nausea and vomiting (see Nursing Diagnosis 5, action b)<br>b. implement measures to reduce oral, pharyngeal, esophageal, and abdominal pain (see Nursing Diagnosis 4, action c)<br>c. implement measures to assist client to adjust psychologically to the diagnosis of cancer and treatment with chemotherapy (see Nursing Diagnoses 14, actions d-n; 15, action c; and 16, action b)<br>d. implement measures *to compensate for taste alteration:*<br>1. encourage the client to select fish, cold chicken, eggs, and cheese as protein sources if beef or pork tastes bitter or rancid<br>2. provide meat for breakfast if aversion to meat tends to increase as day progresses<br>3. add extra sweeteners to foods if acceptable to client<br>4. experiment with different flavorings, seasonings, and textures<br>5. serve food warm *to stimulate sense of smell*<br>e. implement measures to improve client's ability to swallow (see Nursing Diagnosis 3, action b)<br>f. increase activity as tolerated *(activity stimulates appetite)*<br>g. obtain a dietary consult if necessary to assist client in selecting foods/fluids that meet nutritional needs as well as personal and cultural preferences whenever possible<br>h. encourage a rest period before meals *to minimize fatigue*<br>i. maintain a clean environment and a relaxed, pleasant atmosphere<br>j. provide oral hygiene before meals<br>k. provide largest amount of calories and protein when appetite is the best (usually at breakfast)<br>l. serve small portions of nutritious foods/fluids that are appealing to client<br>m. encourage significant others to bring in client's favorite foods and eat with him/her *to make eating more of a familiar social experience*<br>n. limit fluid intake (unless it has a high nutritional value) with meals *to reduce early satiety and subsequent decreased food intake*<br>o. allow adequate time for meals; reheat food if necessary<br>2. ensure that meals are well balanced and high in essential nutrients; offer sweetened, high-calorie, high-protein dietary supplements (e.g. milk shakes, puddings, or eggnog made with cream or powdered milk reconstituted with whole milk) between meals if indicated<br>3. perform actions to control diarrhea (see Nursing Diagnosis 10, action d)<br>4. administer vitamins and minerals if ordered. |

| Desired Outcome | Nursing Actions and ***Selected Purposes/Rationales*** |
|---|---|
| | d. Perform a 72-hour calorie count if ordered. Report totals to dietitian and physician.<br>e. Consult physician regarding alternative methods of providing nutrition (e.g. parenteral nutrition, tube feedings) if client does not consume enough food or fluids to meet nutritional needs. |

## 3. NURSING DIAGNOSIS: Impaired swallowing

related to:
a. oral, pharyngeal, and esophageal pain associated with mucositis resulting from the effects of cytotoxic drugs;
b. dry mouth and viscous oral secretions associated with changes in the quantity and quality of saliva resulting from stomatitis and decreased oral intake.

| Desired Outcome | Nursing Actions and ***Selected Purposes/Rationales*** |
|---|---|
| 3. The client will experience an improvement in swallowing as evidenced by:<br>a. verbalization of same<br>b. absence of food in oral cavity after swallowing<br>c. absence of coughing and choking when eating and drinking. | 3.a. Assess for signs and symptoms of impaired swallowing (e.g. statements of difficulty swallowing, stasis of food in oral cavity, coughing or choking when eating or drinking).<br>b. Implement measures *to improve ability to swallow:*<br>1. perform actions to reduce oral, pharyngeal, and esophageal pain (see Nursing Diagnosis 4, action c)<br>2. perform actions to prevent or reduce the severity of stomatitis and reduce dryness of the oral mucous membrane (see Nursing Diagnosis 7, action d)<br>3. assist client to select foods that require little or no chewing and are easily swallowed (e.g. custard, eggs, canned fruit, mashed potatoes)<br>4. avoid serving foods that are sticky (e.g. peanut butter, soft bread, bananas)<br>5. moisten dry foods with gravy or sauces (e.g. sour cream, salad dressing)<br>6. perform actions *to stimulate salivation:*<br>a. provide oral care before meals<br>b. provide a piece of sour candy for client to suck on just before meals unless contraindicated<br>c. serve foods that are visually pleasing<br>d. place a piece of lemon or sour pickle on client's plate<br>7. encourage client to avoid milk and milk products (unless boiled) and chocolate *(when combined with saliva, they produce very thick secretions).*<br>c. Consult physician if swallowing difficulties persist or worsen. |

## 4. NURSING DIAGNOSIS: Pain: oral, pharyngeal, esophageal, and/or abdominal

related to mucositis associated with effects of cytotoxic drugs on the rapidly dividing cells of gastrointestinal mucosa.

| Desired Outcome | Nursing Actions and ***Selected Purposes/Rationales*** |
|---|---|
| 4. The client will experience diminished oral, pharyngeal, esophageal, and/or abdominal pain as evidenced by:<br>a. verbalization of pain relief<br>b. ability to swallow without difficulty<br>c. relaxed facial expression and body positioning. | 4.a. Assess client for:<br>1. complaints of oral, pharyngeal, esophageal, and/or abdominal pain<br>2. statements of inability to tolerate spicy, acidic, or hot foods/fluids<br>3. difficulty swallowing<br>4. wrinkled brow, restlessness, clutching abdomen.<br>b. Assess client's perception of pain including location, intensity, and type. Use a numerical scale to rate intensity.<br>c. Implement measures *to reduce oral, pharyngeal, esophageal, and/or abdominal pain:*<br>1. perform actions to prevent or reduce the severity of stomatitis (see Nursing Diagnosis 7, actions d and e)<br>2. instruct client to avoid substances that might further irritate the gastrointestinal mucosa (e.g. extremely hot, spicy, or acidic foods/fluids; dry or hard foods; raw fruits and vegetables)<br>3. offer cool, soothing liquids such as nonacidic juices, ices, and ice cream<br>4. instruct client to gargle with a saline solution every 2 hours *to soothe the oral mucous membrane*<br>5. administer topical anesthetics, oral protective pastes or coating agents, topical or systemic analgesics, and antacids if ordered.<br>d. Consult physician if pain persists or worsens. |

## 5. NURSING DIAGNOSIS: Altered comfort: nausea and vomiting

related to:
1. direct stimulation of the vomiting center by cytotoxic drugs and by-products of cellular destruction;
2. indirect stimulation of the vomiting center associated with:
   a. stimulation of the chemoreceptor trigger zone by cytotoxic drugs
   b. stimulation of the afferent vagal and/or sympathetic pathways resulting from inflammation of the gastrointestinal mucosa if present
   c. cortical stimulation resulting from pain, stress, and a learned conditioned response to previous experience with nausea and vomiting after the administration of cytotoxic drugs.

| Desired Outcome | Nursing Actions and ***Selected Purposes/Rationales*** |
|---|---|
| 5. The client will experience a reduction in nausea and vomiting as evidenced by:<br>a. verbalization of decreased nausea<br>b. reduction in the number of episodes of vomiting. | 5.a. Assess client for nausea and vomiting.<br>b. Implement measures *to reduce nausea and vomiting:*<br>1. perform actions to reduce fear and anxiety (see Nursing Diagnosis 1, action b)<br>2. perform actions to reduce pain (see Nursing Diagnosis 4, action c)<br>3. convey an attitude that nausea and vomiting might not occur *(not every client experiences nausea and vomiting every time)*<br>4. administer the following medications as ordered 1-24 hours before initiating chemotherapy and routinely for the expected period of nausea and vomiting for the specific chemotherapeutic agents being administered:<br>a. phenothiazines (e.g. perphenazine, prochlorperazine)<br>b. butyrophenones (e.g. droperidol, haloperidol)<br>c. gastrointestinal stimulants (e.g. metoclopramide)<br>d. benzodiazepines (e.g. lorazepam, diazepam) *to decrease anxiety and/or induce amnesia in order to lessen the possibility of client's developing a conditioned response to chemotherapy* |

| Desired Outcomes | Nursing Actions and ***Selected Purposes/Rationales*** |
|---|---|
| | e. corticosteroids (e.g. dexamethasone)<br>f. serotonin inhibitors (e.g. ondansetron)<br>5. administer intravenous cytotoxic drugs slowly unless contraindicated *to decrease stimulation of the vomiting center*<br>6. if feasible, administer the cytotoxic drugs at night *so client will sleep and experience less nausea*<br>7. provide sour, hard candy for client to suck on if he/she can taste the drug<br>8. eliminate noxious sights and odors from the environment *(noxious stimuli cause cortical stimulation of the vomiting center)*<br>9. encourage client to take deep, slow breaths when nauseated<br>10. encourage client to change positions slowly *(rapid movement stimulates the afferent vestibulocerebellar pathway with resultant stimulation of the chemoreceptor trigger zone)*<br>11. provide oral hygiene every two hours and after each emesis<br>12. provide carbonated beverages for client to sip if nauseated<br>13. avoid serving foods with an overpowering aroma; remove lids from hot foods before entering room<br>14. provide small, frequent meals; instruct client to ingest foods and fluids slowly<br>15. encourage client to eat dry foods (e.g. toast, crackers) and avoid drinking liquids with meals if nauseated<br>16. instruct client to avoid foods/fluids that irritate the gastric mucosa (e.g. spicy foods; caffeine-containing beverages such as coffee, tea, and colas)<br>17. instruct client to avoid foods high in fat *(fat delays gastric emptying)*<br>18. instruct client to rest after eating.<br>c. Consult physician if above measures fail to control nausea and vomiting. |

## 6. NURSING DIAGNOSIS: High risk for impaired skin integrity

related to:

a. frequent contact of the skin with irritants associated with diarrhea if present;
b. damage to the skin and/or subcutaneous tissue associated with prolonged pressure on tissues, friction, or shearing if mobility is decreased;
c. increased skin fragility associated with malnutrition and dryness (a result of the effects of cytotoxic drugs on sebaceous and sweat glands).

| Desired Outcome | Nursing Actions and ***Selected Purposes/Rationales*** |
|---|---|
| 6. The client will maintain skin integrity as evidenced by:<br>a. absence of redness and irritation<br>b. no skin breakdown. | 6.a. Inspect the skin, especially bony prominences and dependent areas, for pallor, redness, and breakdown.<br>b. Implement measures *to prevent skin breakdown:*<br>1. assist client to turn at least every 2 hours; use all 4 sides (prone, lateral [left/right], dorsal) unless contraindicated<br>2. gently massage around reddened areas at least every 2 hours<br>3. perform actions *to prevent shearing* (shearing occurs when one tissue layer slides past another) *and skin surface abrasion:*<br>a. apply a thin layer of powder or cornstarch to bottom sheet or skin |

*to absorb moisture (moist skin is more likely to adhere to sheet) and reduce friction*
   b. lift and move client carefully using a turn sheet and adequate assistance
   c. limit length of time client is in semi-Fowler's position to 30 minutes *(in this position, client tends to slide down in bed)*
4. instruct or assist client to shift weight every 30 minutes
5. if fade time (length of time it takes for reddened area to fade after pressure is removed) is greater than 15 minutes, increase frequency of position changes
6. keep skin clean and dry
7. keep bed linens dry and wrinkle-free
8. apply a thin layer of powder or cornstarch to areas with opposing skin surfaces (e.g. axillae, perineum, beneath breasts) if indicated *to absorb moisture and/or reduce friction*
9. increase activity as tolerated
10. provide devices to reduce pressure on the skin, decrease shearing, and/or prevent moisture build-up (e.g. alternating pressure mattress or pad, flotation pad, sheepskin)
11. perform actions *to prevent drying of the skin:*
    a. encourage a fluid intake of 2500 ml/day unless contraindicated
    b. provide a mild soap for bathing
    c. apply moisturizing lotion and/or emollient to skin at least once a day
12. perform actions *to prevent skin irritation resulting from diarrhea:*
    a. implement measures to control diarrhea (see Nursing Diagnosis 10, action d)
    b. assist client to cleanse and dry perineal area thoroughly with soft tissue or cloth after each bowel movement; apply a protective ointment or cream (e.g. Desitin, A & D ointment, Vaseline)
    c. apply a drainable fecal collector if diarrhea is a persistent problem
    d. provide incontinence pads if needed to absorb moisture; do not allow skin to come in contact with plastic portion of pads
13. perform actions to maintain an adequate nutritional status (see Nursing Diagnosis 2, action c).

c. If skin breakdown occurs:
   1. notify physician
   2. continue with above measures to prevent further irritation and breakdown
   3. perform decubitus care as ordered or per standard hospital procedure
   4. assess client closely and report signs and symptoms of infection (e.g. elevated temperature; redness, warmth, and edema around area of breakdown; unusual drainage from site).

## 7. NURSING DIAGNOSIS: Altered oral mucous membrane:

a. **dryness** related to reduced oral intake;
b. **stomatitis** related to:
   1. malnutrition and inadequate oral hygiene
   2. disruption in the renewal process of mucosal epithelial cells associated with toxic effects of cytotoxic drugs (particularly antimetabolities, antibiotics, and plant alkaloids)
   3. infection, particularly gingival, during the period of myelosuppression.

**Desired Outcome**

7. The client will maintain a healthy oral cavity as evidenced by:
   a. absence of inflammation
   b. pink, moist, intact mucosa
   c. no complaints of oral dryness and burning
   d. ability to swallow without discomfort.

**Nursing Actions and *Selected Purposes/Rationales***

7.a. Assess client for dryness of the oral mucosa.

b. Assess for and report signs and symptoms of stomatitis (e.g. inflamed and/or ulcerated oral mucosa, complaints of oral dryness and burning, dysphagia, leukoplakia, viscous saliva).

c. Culture suspicious oral lesions as ordered. Report positive results.

d. Implement measures *to prevent or reduce the severity of stomatitis and/or relieve dryness of the oral mucous membrane:*
   1. reinforce importance of and assist client with oral hygiene after meals and snacks; avoid products such as lemon-glycerin swabs and commercial mouthwashes containing alcohol *(these products have a drying or irritating effect on the oral mucous membrane)*
   2. have client rinse mouth frequently with warm saline; baking soda and water; or a solution of salt, baking soda, and water (frequency and consistency of performing oral hygiene is more important than product used)
   3. use a soft-bristle brush, sponge-tipped applicator, or low-pressure power spray for oral hygiene
   4. lubricate client's lips with Vaseline, K-Y jelly, ChapStick, Blistex, or mineral oil frequently
   5. encourage client to breathe through nose rather than mouth *in order to reduce mouth dryness*
   6. encourage a fluid intake of at least 2500 ml/day unless contraindicated
   7. encourage client not to smoke *(smoking irritates and dries the mucosa)*
   8. if stomatitis is not severe, encourage client to use artificial saliva *to lubricate the oral mucous membrane*
   9. instruct client to avoid substances that might further irritate the oral mucosa (e.g. extremely hot, spicy, or acidic foods/fluids)
   10. perform actions to maintain an adequate nutritional status (see Nursing Diagnosis 2, action c)
   11. consult physician regarding an order for a prophylactic antimicrobial agent.

e. If stomatitis is not controlled:
   1. increase frequency of oral hygiene
   2. if client has dentures, remove and replace only for meals.

f. Administer topical anesthetics, oral protective pastes or coating agents, and topical and systemic analgesics if ordered.

g. Consult physician if signs and symptoms of dryness and stomatitis persist or worsen.

## 8. NURSING DIAGNOSIS: Fatigue

related to:*
a. accumulation of cellular waste products associated with rapid lysis of cancerous and normal cells exposed to cytotoxic drugs;
b. difficulty resting and sleeping;
c. fear, anxiety, and depression;
d. increased energy expenditure associated with an increase in the metabolic rate resulting from continuous, active tumor growth;
e. malnutrition.

*Some of the etiological factors presented here are under investigation.

| Desired Outcome | Nursing Actions and ***Selected Purposes/Rationales*** |
|---|---|
| 8. The client will experience a reduction in fatigue as evidenced by:<br>a. verbalization of feelings of increased energy<br>b. ability to perform usual activities of daily living<br>c. increased interest in surroundings and ability to concentrate<br>d. decreased emotional lability. | 8.a. Assess for signs and symptoms of fatigue (e.g. verbalization of unremitting, overwhelming lack of energy and inability to maintain usual routines; lack of interest in surroundings; decreased ability to concentrate; increased emotional lability).<br>b. Inform client that a feeling of persistent fatigue is expected as a result of the disease itself and as a side effect of chemotherapy.<br>c. Assist client to identify personal patterns of fatigue (e.g. time of day, after certain activities) and to plan activities so that times of greatest fatigue are avoided.<br>d. Implement measures *to reduce fatigue:*<br>1. perform actions *to promote rest and/or conserve energy:*<br>a. schedule several short rest periods during the day<br>b. minimize environmental activity and noise<br>c. limit the number of visitors and their length of stay<br>d. assist client with self-care activities as needed<br>e. keep supplies and personal articles within easy reach<br>f. implement measures to reduce fear and anxiety (see Nursing Diagnosis 1, action b)<br>g. implement measures to promote sleep (see Nursing Diagnosis 11, action c)<br>h. implement measures to reduce discomfort (see Nursing Diagnoses 4, action c and 5, action b)<br>i. instruct client in energy-saving techniques (e.g. using shower chair when showering, sitting to brush teeth or comb hair)<br>2. perform actions to maintain an adequate nutritional status (see Nursing Diagnosis 2, action c)<br>3. encourage client to maintain a fluid intake of at least 2500 ml/day *to promote elimination of the by-products of cellular breakdown*<br>4. perform actions to facilitate client's psychological adjustment to the diagnosis of cancer and the treatment regimen and its effects (see Nursing Diagnoses 14, actions d-n; 15, action c; and 16, action b).<br>e. Consult physician if signs and symptoms of fatigue worsen. |

## 9. NURSING DIAGNOSIS: Self-care deficit

related to:

a. fatigue, weakness, and discomfort;

b. sedation associated with effects of some medications administered to control nausea and vomiting.

| Desired Outcome | Nursing Actions and ***Selected Purposes/Rationales*** |
|---|---|
| 9. The client will perform self-care activities within physical limitations. | 9.a. With client, develop a realistic plan for meeting daily physical needs.<br>b. Encourage maximum independence within limitations imposed by fatigue, discomfort, and weakness.<br>c. Implement measures *to facilitate client's ability to perform self-care activities:*<br>1. perform actions to reduce fatigue (see Nursing Diagnosis 8, action d)<br>2. schedule care at a time when client is most likely to be able to participate (e.g. following rest periods, before chemotherapy administration)<br>3. allow adequate time for accomplishment of self-care activities. |

| Desired Outcome | Nursing Actions and ***Selected Purposes/Rationales*** |
|---|---|
| | d. Assist the client with those activities he/she is unable to perform independently. |

## 10. NURSING DIAGNOSIS: Diarrhea

related to increased intestinal motility associated with extreme fear and anxiety and inflammation and ulceration of the gastrointestinal mucosa resulting from effects of cytotoxic drugs (particularly fluorouracil and methotrexate) on rapidly dividing epithelial cells.

| Desired Outcome | Nursing Actions and ***Selected Purposes/Rationales*** |
|---|---|
| 10. The client will maintain usual bowel elimination pattern. | 10.a. Ascertain client's usual bowel elimination habits.<br>b. Assess for signs and symptoms of diarrhea (e.g. frequent, loose stools; urgency; abdominal pain and cramping).<br>c. Assess bowel sounds regularly. Report an increase in frequency of bowel sounds.<br>d. Implement measures *to control diarrhea:*<br>1. perform actions *to rest the bowel:*<br>a. restrict oral intake if ordered<br>b. when oral intake is allowed:<br>1. gradually progress from fluids to small meals<br>2. instruct client to avoid foods/fluids that may stimulate or irritate the inflamed bowel:<br>a. those high in fiber (e.g. whole-grain cereals, raw fruits and vegetables)<br>b. gas producers (e.g. cabbage, beans, onions, cauliflower)<br>c. those that are spicy or extremely hot or cold<br>d. those high in lactose (e.g. milk, milk products)<br>e. those high in fat (e.g. butter, cream, fried foods)<br>c. implement measures to reduce fear and anxiety (see Nursing Diagnosis 1, action b)<br>d. encourage client to rest<br>e. discourage smoking *(nicotine has a stimulant effect on the gastrointestinal tract)*<br>2. administer the following antidiarrheal agents if ordered:<br>a. opiate or opiate-like substances (e.g. loperamide, diphenoxylate hydrochloride) *to decrease gastrointestinal motility*<br>b. bulk-forming agents (e.g. methylcellulose, psyllium hydrophilic mucilloid, calcium polycarbophil) *to absorb water in the bowel, which results in a more formed stool.*<br>e. Consult physician if diarrhea persists or worsens. |

## 11. NURSING DIAGNOSIS: Sleep pattern disturbance

related to:
a. nausea, vomiting, and pain;
b. anxiety, fear, and depression;
c. frequent need to defecate associated with diarrhea if present.

| Desired Outcome | Nursing Actions and ***Selected Purposes/Rationales*** |
|---|---|
| 11. The client will attain optimal amounts of sleep within the parameters of the treatment regimen as evidenced by:<br>a. statements of feeling well rested<br>b. usual mental status<br>c. absence of frequent yawning, dark circles under eyes, and hand tremors. | 11.a. Assess for signs and symptoms of a sleep pattern disturbance (e.g. verbal complaints of difficulty falling asleep, not feeling well rested, or sleep interruptions; irritability; lethargy; disorientation; frequent yawning; dark circles under eyes; slight hand tremors).<br>b. Determine the client's usual sleep habits.<br>c. Implement measures *to promote sleep:*<br>1. discourage long periods of sleep during the day unless signs and symptoms of sleep deprivation exist or daytime sleep is usual for client<br>2. perform actions to reduce discomfort (see Nursing Diagnoses 4, action c and 5, action b)<br>3. perform actions to control diarrhea (see Nursing Diagnosis 10, action d)<br>4. perform actions to reduce fear and anxiety (see Nursing Diagnosis 1, action b)<br>5. encourage participation in relaxing diversional activities during the evening<br>6. discourage intake of fluids high in caffeine (e.g. coffee, tea, colas), especially in the evening<br>7. offer client a high-protein evening snack unless contraindicated<br>8. allow client to continue usual sleep practices (e.g. position, time, bedtime rituals such as reading and meditating) if possible<br>9. satisfy basic needs such as comfort and warmth before sleep<br>10. have client empty bladder just before bedtime<br>11. use relaxation techniques (e.g. progressive relaxation exercises, back massage, meditation, soft music) before sleep<br>12. maintain a quiet, restful atmosphere; have earplugs available for client if needed<br>13. ensure good room ventilation<br>14. administer sedative-hypnotics if ordered<br>15. perform actions *to reduce interruptions during sleep (80-100 minutes of uninterrupted sleep are usually needed to complete one sleep cycle):*<br>a. restrict visitors<br>b. group care (e.g. medications, treatments, physical care, assessments) whenever possible.<br>d. Consult physician if signs and symptoms of sleep deprivation persist or worsen. |

## 12. NURSING DIAGNOSIS: High risk for infection

related to:

a. lowered natural resistance associated with:
   1. malnutrition and general debilitation
   2. chemotherapy-induced bone marrow suppression and long-term treatment with corticosteroids
   3. disruption in normal, endogenous microbial flora resulting from antimicrobial therapy
   4. impaired immune system functioning resulting from certain malignancies (e.g. Hodgkin's disease, lymphoma, multiple myeloma, leukemia);

b. break in mucosal surfaces associated with delayed cellular renewal resulting from effects of cytotoxic agents;

c. break in integrity of the skin associated with placement of a central venous catheter (e.g. Groshong), implanted infusion device (e.g. Port-a-Cath), or peritoneal catheter (e.g. Tenckhoff);

d. stasis of secretions in lungs and urinary stasis if mobility is decreased.

**Desired Outcome**

12. The client will remain free of infection as evidenced by:
    a. absence of fever and chills
    b. pulse within normal limits
    c. normal breath sounds
    d. voiding clear urine without complaints of frequency, urgency, and burning
    e. absence of heat, pain, redness, swelling, and unusual drainage in any area
    f. no complaints of increased weakness and fatigue
    g. WBC and differential counts within normal range for client
    h. negative results of cultured specimens.

**Nursing Actions and *Selected Purposes/Rationales***

12.a. Assess for and report signs and symptoms of infection (be aware of subtle changes in client since signs of infection may be very minimal as a result of immunosuppression):
   1. increase in client's usual temperature
   2. chills
   3. increased pulse
   4. abnormal breath sounds
   5. cloudy, foul-smelling urine
   6. complaints of frequency, urgency, or burning when urinating
   7. presence of WBCs, bacteria, and/or nitrites in urine
   8. heat, pain, redness, swelling, or unusual drainage in any area
   9. complaints of increased weakness or fatigue
   10. increase in WBC count and/or significant change in differential.

b. Monitor absolute neutrophil count (WBC count multiplied by the percentage of neutrophils). Report values below 1000/mm$^3$.

c. Obtain specimens (e.g. urine, vaginal, mouth, sputum, blood) for culture as ordered. Report positive results.

d. Implement measures *to reduce the risk for infection:*
   1. protect client from others with infections and those who have recently been vaccinated *(a person may have a subclinical infection after a vaccination)*
   2. use good handwashing technique and encourage client to do the same
   3. maintain a fluid intake of at least 2500 ml/day unless contraindicated
   4. perform actions to maintain an adequate nutritional status (see Nursing Diagnosis 2, action c)
   5. encourage a low-bacteria diet (e.g. cooked foods, no fresh fruit) if the client is immunosuppressed
   6. perform actions to prevent or reduce severity of stomatitis and relieve dryness of the oral mucous membrane (see Nursing Diagnosis 7, actions d and e)
   7. perform actions to prevent skin breakdown (see Nursing Diagnosis 6, action b)
   8. avoid invasive procedures (e.g. urinary catheterizations, arterial and venous punctures, injections) whenever possible; if such procedures are necessary, perform them using meticulous aseptic technique
   9. give meticulous attention to any break in the skin; cleanse area carefully with antiseptic solution at least twice daily or as ordered
   10. change intravenous tubings and solutions and rotate insertion sites according to hospital policy
   11. change equipment and solutions used for procedures such as irrigations, wound care, and tube feedings according to hospital policy
   12. initiate measures to prevent constipation (e.g. encourage client to defecate whenever the urge is felt, encourage a minimum fluid intake of 2500 ml/day, encourage increased intake of foods high in fiber, administer laxatives and stool softeners as ordered) *in order to prevent damage to the rectal mucosa from hard stool*
   13. avoid unnecessary rectal invasion (e.g. temperature taking, enemas, suppositories, rectal tube) *to prevent trauma to rectal mucosa and possible abscess formation*
   14. perform actions to reduce stress and discomfort (see Nursing Diagnoses 1, action b; 4, action c; and 5, action b) *in order to prevent excessive secretion of cortisol (cortisol inhibits the immune response)*
   15. perform actions *to prevent stasis of respiratory secretions* (e.g. assist client to turn, cough, and deep breathe; increase activity as tolerated)
   16. perform actions to prevent urinary retention (e.g. instruct client to

void when the urge is first felt, promote relaxation during voiding attempts) *in order to prevent urinary stasis*

17. perform actions *to prevent the introduction of microorganisms into the urinary tract* (e.g. assist client with perineal care as needed, instruct and assist female client to wipe from front to back after urinating and defecating, maintain sterile technique during urinary catheterization)
18. instruct and assist client in proper care of the exit site of a central venous catheter or insertion site of an implanted infusion device and/or peritoneal catheter (see Nursing Diagnosis 17, actions i.1-3)
19. administer the following as ordered:
    a. antimicrobial agents (usually initiated when the neutropenic client becomes febrile or may be administered prophylactically if the neutrophil count is less than 500/mm$^3$)
    b. colony-stimulating factors (e.g. Filgrastim) *to stimulate granulocyte production.*

## 13. COLLABORATIVE DIAGNOSES:

**Potential complications:**

a. **bleeding** related to thrombocytopenia associated with chemotherapy-induced bone marrow suppression;
b. **impaired renal function** related to:
    1. direct toxic effects of some cytotoxic agents (e.g. cisplatin, high-dose methotrexate and mithramycin, streptozocin) on renal cells
    2. nephropathy associated with:
        a. excessive uric acid accumulation resulting from the rapid lysis of large numbers of tumor cells
        b. precipitation of certain drugs (e.g. high doses of methotrexate) in the renal tubules and collecting ducts as a result of low urinary pH and inadequate hydration before, during, and after drug administration;
c. **hemorrhagic cystitis** related to irritation of the bladder mucosa by toxic metabolites of cyclophosphamide and ifosfamide;
d. **local tissue irritation and sloughing** related to extravasation of vesicant drugs (e.g. doxorubicin, daunorubicin, vinblastine, vincristine);
e. **cardiac arrhythmias** related to cardiotoxic effects of certain cytotoxic drugs (primarily doxorubicin and daunorubicin);
f. **inflammation and fibrosis of lung tissue** related particularly to the administration of bleomycin and carmustine;
g. **neurotoxicity** related to demyelination of nerve fibers (occurs primarily with the vinca alkaloids and cisplatin);
h. **anaphylactic reaction** related to a hypersensitivity response to a cytotoxic drug (occurs primarily with cisplatin and L-asparaginase).

| Desired Outcomes | Nursing Actions and ***Selected Purposes/Rationales*** |
|---|---|
| 13.a. The client will not experience unusual bleeding as evidenced by:<br>1. skin and mucous membranes free of petechiae, purpura, ecchymoses, and active bleeding<br>2. absence of unusual joint pain | 13.a.1. Assess client for and report signs and symptoms of unusual bleeding:<br>a. petechiae, purpura, or ecchymoses<br>b. gingival bleeding<br>c. prolonged bleeding from puncture sites<br>d. epistaxis, hemoptysis<br>e. unusual joint pain<br>f. frank or occult blood in stool, urine, or vomitus<br>g. increase in abdominal girth<br>h. menorrhagia<br>i. restlessness, confusion<br>j. declining B/P and increased pulse rate<br>k. decline in Hct and Hb levels. |

**Desired Outcomes** | **Nursing Actions and *Selected Purposes/Rationales***

3. absence of frank and occult blood in stool, urine, and vomitus
4. no increase in abdominal girth
5. usual menstrual flow
6. usual mental status
7. vital signs within normal range for client
8. stable or improved Hct and Hb.

2. Monitor platelet count and coagulation test results (e.g. bleeding time). Report abnormal values.
3. If platelet count is low, coagulation test results are abnormal, or Hct and Hb levels decline, test all stools, urine, and vomitus for occult blood. Report positive results.
4. Implement measures *to prevent bleeding:*
   a. use the smallest gauge needle possible when giving injections and performing venous and arterial punctures
   b. apply gentle, prolonged pressure to puncture sites after injections, venous and arterial punctures, and diagnostic tests such as bone marrow aspiration
   c. take B/P only when necessary and avoid overinflating the cuff
   d. caution client to avoid activities that increase the risk for trauma (e.g. shaving with a straight-edge razor, using stiff-bristle toothbrush or dental floss)
   e. avoid procedures that can cause injury to rectal mucosa (e.g. taking temperatures rectally, inserting a rectal suppository or tube, administering an enema)
   f. pad side rails if client is confused or restless
   g. perform actions *to reduce the risk for falls* (e.g. keep bed in low position with side rails up when client is in bed, avoid unnecessary clutter in room, instruct client to wear slippers/shoes with nonslip soles when ambulating)
   h. instruct client to avoid blowing nose forcefully or straining to have a bowel movement; consult physician about order for decongestants, stool softeners, and/or laxatives if indicated
   i. administer the following if ordered:
      1. estrogen-progestin preparations *to suppress menses*
      2. platelets
      3. whole blood.
5. If bleeding occurs and does not subside spontaneously:
   a. apply firm, prolonged pressure to bleeding area(s) if possible
   b. if epistaxis occurs, place client in high Fowler's position and apply pressure and ice pack to nasal area
   c. maintain oxygen therapy as ordered
   d. perform gastric lavage as ordered *to control gastric bleeding*
   e. administer blood products (e.g. platelets) as ordered
   f. assess for and report signs and symptoms of hypovolemic shock (e.g. restlessness; confusion; significant decrease in B/P; rapid, thready pulse; rapid respirations; cool, pale skin; urine output less than 30 ml/hour).

13.b. The client will maintain adequate renal function as evidenced by:
1. urine output at least 30 ml/hour
2. urine specific gravity, BUN, serum creatinine, and creatinine clearance within normal range.

13.b.1. Assess for and report a urine output below 100 ml/hour during and for 24 hours after administration of nephrotoxic drugs (consult physician about insertion of a urinary catheter if output cannot be monitored accurately).
2. Assess for and report signs and symptoms of impaired renal function (e.g. urine output less than 30 ml/hour, urine specific gravity fixed at or less than 1.010, elevated BUN and serum creatinine levels).
3. Collect a 24-hour urine specimen if ordered. Report decreased creatinine clearance.
4. Implement measures *to maintain adequate renal function:*
   a. hydrate client with at least 150 ml fluid/hour unless contraindicated for 6-24 hours before administration of drugs known to be nephrotoxic (e.g. cisplatin, high-dose methotrexate and mithramycin, streptozocin)
   b. administer intravenous fluids as ordered during administration of nephrotoxic drugs and for 24 hours after therapy *to maintain a high rate of glomerular blood flow*

c. administer the following medications as ordered:
   1. diuretics (e.g. furosemide, mannitol) *to promote more rapid plasma clearance of the cytotoxic agent*
   2. xanthine oxidase inhibitor (e.g. allopurinol) *to decrease the formation of uric acid*
   3. sodium bicarbonate *to alkalinize the urine and subsequently increase the solubility of uric acid in the urine and prevent the precipitation of methotrexate in renal tubules and collecting ducts*
   4. leucovorin calcium (folinic acid) *to diminish the toxic effects of methotrexate on the renal cells.*

5. If signs and symptoms of impaired renal function occur:
   a. continue with above actions
   b. assess for and report signs of acute renal failure (e.g. oliguria or anuria; weight gain; edema; elevated B/P; lethargy and confusion; increasing BUN and serum creatinine, phosphorus, and potassium levels)
   c. prepare client for dialysis if indicated
   d. refer to Care Plan on Renal Failure for additional care measures.

13.c. The client will not develop hemorrhagic cystitis as evidenced by absence of dysuria, urinary frequency and urgency, and hematuria.

13.c.1. Assess for and report signs and symptoms of hemorrhagic cystitis (e.g. dysuria, urinary frequency and/or urgency, frank or occult blood in urine).

2. Implement measures *to prevent hemorrhagic cystitis:*
   a. encourage a minimum fluid intake of 2500 ml/day; if client is unable to tolerate oral fluids, consult physician about an order for intravenous fluids *to ensure adequate hydration and reduce concentration of toxic drug metabolites in the bladder*
   b. administer cyclophosphamide early in the day and encourage client to void every 2 hours and before going to bed *in order to prevent stasis of toxic drug metabolites in the bladder*
   c. administer mesna (Mesnex) as ordered *to interact with and inactivate the toxic drug metabolites of ifosfamide and cyclophosphamide.*

3. If signs and symptoms of hemorrhagic cystitis occur:
   a. discontinue cytotoxic drug administration and notify physician
   b. continue with fluid administration as ordered
   c. administer diuretics as ordered *to increase urine output and thereby decrease the concentration of toxic drug metabolites in the urine*
   d. insert a urinary catheter if ordered *to decrease the risk for urinary stasis and thereby minimize contact of toxic drug metabolites with the bladder mucosa*
   e. assist with or perform bladder irrigations as ordered *to facilitate removal of drug metabolites and flush clots from the bladder*
   f. maintain continuous bladder irrigation with silver nitrate or alum solution if ordered *to stop bleeding*
   g. prepare client for the following if planned:
      1. cystoscopy to cauterize bleeding vessels
      2. intravesical instillation of formalin *to control persistent, severe bleeding*
   h. provide emotional support to client and significant others.

13.d. The client will not experience drug extravasation as evidenced by:
   1. absence of swelling and erythema at drug infusion site
   2. no complaints of stinging or burning pain at infusion site.

13.d.1. Assess for signs and symptoms of drug extravasation (e.g. swelling around drug infusion site, erythema at infusion site several hours after drug administration, client complaints of stinging or burning pain at infusion site).

2. Differentiate between a flare reaction and extravasation if giving doxorubicin. (With a flare reaction, swelling and erythema occur within minutes, usually extend along vein line, and disappear in 60-90 minutes. A good blood return is also present and the client experiences itching rather than pain at the infusion site.)

3. Ensure that the infusion site and surrounding tissue are visible at all times.

Desired Outcomes | Nursing Actions and ***Selected Purposes/Rationales***

4. Implement measures *to prevent drug extravasation:*
   a. select the best vein possible for vesicant drug administration:
      1. do not use a vein that has been previously used for vesicant agents
      2. use a site in forearm if possible; avoid the antecubital fossa and small veins in the hand
      3. do not use an existing intravenous site unless no other site is available and blood return is excellent
      4. avoid extremities with compromised circulation
   b. do not perform multiple punctures in the same vein *in order to prevent leakage from the vessel after infusion has begun*
   c. tape needle securely
   d. perform actions *to ensure that the drug is infusing into the vein:*
      1. test patency of vein with a minimum of 5 ml of normal saline before administration of cytotoxic drug
      2. check blood return after every 3-4 ml if giving the drug by direct push
      3. stay with client while a vesicant drug is infusing; check site every 2-3 minutes
   e. perform actions *to prevent increased irritation of the vein:*
      1. dilute drug according to manufacturer's recommendations
      2. administer drug at recommended rate of infusion
   f. stop infusion if there is any indication that the drug is not infusing properly (e.g. poor or absent blood return, client complaints of pain at infusion site)
   g. when the drug infusion is complete, flush needle with a minimum of 30 ml of normal saline; apply pressure to site for at least 4 minutes after needle removal *to minimize oozing.*
5. If signs and symptoms of drug extravasation occur:
   a. stop infusion immediately
   b. treat area of extravasation as ordered (treatment varies depending on drug used) or per standard hospital procedure
   c. assess the site closely every shift for signs of inflammation and necrosis
   d. provide emotional support to client and significant others.

13.e. The client will experience resolution of cardiac arrhythmias if they occur as evidenced by:
1. regular apical pulse at 60-100 beats/minute
2. equal apical and radial pulses
3. absence of syncope and palpitations
4. ECG reading showing normal sinus rhythm.

13.e.1. Assess for and report signs and symptoms of cardiac arrhythmias (e.g. irregular apical pulse; pulse rate below 60 or above 100 beats/minute; apical-radial pulse deficit; syncope; palpitations; abnormal rate, rhythm, or configurations on ECG).

2. Monitor liver and kidney function studies and report abnormal results *(cardiotoxicity can result from delayed metabolism or excretion of cytotoxic drugs by the liver or kidneys).*
3. If cardiac arrhythmias occur:
   a. initiate cardiac monitoring if ordered
   b. prepare client for ECG if ordered
   c. administer antiarrhythmic agents (e.g. lidocaine, quinidine, procainamide, propanolol, amiodarone) if ordered
   d. restrict client's activity based on his/her tolerance and severity of the arrhythmia
   e. maintain oxygen therapy as ordered
   f. assess cardiovascular status frequently and report signs and symptoms of inadequate tissue perfusion (e.g. decline in B/P; cool, clammy, mottled skin; cyanosis; diminished peripheral pulses; declining urine output; restlessness and agitation; shortness of breath)
   g. have emergency cart readily available for defibrillation, cardioversion, or cardiopulmonary resuscitation.

| | |
|---|---|
| 13.f. The client will experience decreased signs and symptoms of pulmonary inflammation and fibrosis if they occur as evidenced by:<br>1. decreased coughing<br>2. afebrile status<br>3. decreased dyspnea<br>4. improved breath sounds<br>5. improved chest x-ray and pulmonary function studies. | 13.f.1. Assess for signs and symptoms of pulmonary inflammation and fibrosis (e.g. dry, hacking, persistent cough; fever; tachypnea; dyspnea on exertion; crackles) particularly if client is reaching total allowable cumulative dose of cytotoxic agent(s) known to cause pulmonary toxicity.<br>2. Monitor for and report significant changes in oximetry results.<br>3. Monitor for and report changes in chest x-ray reports and pulmonary function studies.<br>4. If signs and symptoms of pulmonary inflammation and fibrosis occur:<br>a. discontinue infusion of cytotoxic agent as ordered<br>b. prepare client for lung biopsy if planned<br>c. administer the following medications if ordered:<br>1. corticosteroids *to reduce inflammatory response*<br>2. bronchodilators<br>d. implement measures *to improve gas exchange:*<br>1. place client in a semi- to high Fowler's position unless contraindicated<br>2. instruct and assist client to turn, cough, and deep breathe at least every 2 hours<br>3. reinforce correct use of incentive spirometer at least every 2 hours<br>4. assist with IPPB treatments if ordered<br>5. maintain oxygen therapy as ordered<br>e. provide emotional support to client and significant others<br>f. consult physician if signs and symptoms of pulmonary inflammation and fibrosis worsen. |
| 13.g. The client will experience resolution of signs and symptoms of neurotoxicity if they occur as evidenced by usual motor and sensory function. | 13.g.1. Assess for and report signs and symptoms of neurotoxicity (e.g. constipation, ataxia, numbness and tingling of extremities, unusual muscle weakness, gait disturbances, difficulty with fine motor movements, footdrop or wristdrop, hearing loss, blurred vision, impaired color perception or discrimination).<br>2. Assure client that most changes in neurological function may be reversible if reported immediately and the neurotoxic drug is discontinued.<br>3. If signs and symptoms of neurotoxicity occur:<br>a. administer laxatives and stool softeners as ordered *to prevent constipation*<br>b. implement measures *to prevent falls* (e.g. keep bed in low position with side rails up when client is in bed, avoid unnecessary clutter in room, instruct client to wear slippers/shoes with nonslip soles when ambulating)<br>c. implement measures *to prevent footdrop* (e.g. instruct client to perform active foot exercises every 1-2 hours while awake; use footboard, high-topped tennis shoes, or foot positioners to keep feet in a neutral or slightly dorsiflexed position)<br>d. implement measures *to prevent wristdrop* (e.g. instruct client to perform active wrist exercises every 1-2 hours while awake, provide a wrist splint if necessary)<br>e. implement measures *to prevent burns* (e.g. let hot foods/fluids cool slightly before serving, assess temperature of bath water before and during bathing)<br>f. avoid use of cold applications on areas of decreased sensation<br>g. implement measures *to facilitate communication if hearing is impaired* (e.g. face client when speaking, use related nonverbal cues such as facial expressions and gestures, respond to client's call signal in person rather than over the intercommunication system)<br>h. implement measures *to help client adapt to impaired vision* (e.g. identify yourself when entering room and before any physical contact, describe activities and reasons for various noises in room, |

| Desired Outcomes | Nursing Actions and ***Selected Purposes/Rationales*** |
|---|---|
| | assist client with personal hygiene he/she is unable to perform independently)<br>i. assist client with tasks that require fine motor skills (e.g. shaving) *in order to prevent cuts*<br>j. consult physician if signs and symptoms of neurotoxicity persist or worsen. |
| 13.h. The client will not develop an anaphylactic reaction as evidenced by:<br>1. usual mental status<br>2. usual skin color<br>3. absence of urticaria and pruritus<br>4. no complaints of abdominal cramps<br>5. absence of dyspnea, wheezing, and stridor<br>6. stable vital signs<br>7. absence of facial and peripheral edema<br>8. usual speaking ability. | 13.h.1. Assess for and report signs and symptoms of an anaphylactic reaction (usually some or all of the signs and symptoms will occur within minutes of drug administration):<br>a. anxiety, agitation<br>b. flushing of skin<br>c. generalized urticaria and pruritus<br>d. abdominal cramps<br>e. dyspnea, wheezing, stridor<br>f. irregular and/or increased pulse rate, decline in B/P<br>g. edema of face, hands, and feet<br>h. inability to speak.<br>2. Implement measures *to prevent an anaphylactic reaction:*<br>a. consult physician before giving any drug that is the same as or similar to one the client has reacted to previously<br>b. administer a test dose before giving drug if appropriate.<br>3. If signs and symptoms of an anaphylactic reaction occur:<br>a. discontinue the cytotoxic drug but keep intravenous line open with a normal saline solution<br>b. administer oxygen as ordered<br>c. administer the following medications if ordered:<br>1. sympathomimetics (e.g. epinephrine) *to relieve bronchospasm and stimulate peripheral vasoconstriction*<br>2. antihistamines (e.g. diphenhydramine) *to reduce the sensitivity reaction and control pruritus and urticaria*<br>3. bronchodilators (e.g. theophylline) *to relieve bronchospasm*<br>4. corticosteroids *to reduce the allergic response and maintain usual vascular wall permeability*<br>d. assess for and report signs and symptoms of anaphylactic shock (e.g. increased restlessness; significant decrease in B/P; rapid, thready pulse; increased dyspnea; cool, pale skin)<br>e. provide emotional support to client and significant others. |

## 14. NURSING DIAGNOSIS: Self-concept disturbance*

related to:

a. changes in appearance associated with the side effects of chemotherapy (e.g. alopecia, excessive weight loss, skin and nail changes) and external drug infusion catheter if present;
b. possible alteration in usual sexual activities associated with weakness, fatigue, reduced levels of testosterone (can occur with chemotherapy for prostate or testicular cancer or lymphoma), psychological factors, and vaginal discomfort (may result from mucositis);
c. possible temporary or permanent infertility associated with gonadal dysfunction resulting from extensive therapy with cytotoxic drugs (particularly alkylating agents and nitrosoureas);
d. increased dependence on others to meet self-care needs;
e. changes in life style and roles associated with effects of the disease process and its treatment.

*This diagnostic label includes the nursing diagnoses of body image disturbance, self-esteem disturbance, and altered role performance.

| Desired Outcome | Nursing Actions and ***Selected Purposes/Rationales*** |
|---|---|
| 14. The client will demonstrate beginning adaptation to changes in appearance, body functioning, life style, and roles as evidenced by:<br>a. verbalization of feelings of self-worth and sexual adequacy<br>b. maintenance of relationships with significant others<br>c. active participation in activities of daily living<br>d. active interest in personal appearance<br>e. willingness to pursue usual roles and participate in social activities<br>f. verbalization of a beginning plan for adapting life style to meet restrictions imposed by the disease process and residual effects of chemotherapy. | 14.a. Assess for signs and symptoms of a self-concept disturbance (e.g. verbal or nonverbal cues denoting a negative response to changes in body functioning or appearance such as denial of or preoccupation with changes that have occurred or withdrawal from significant others).<br>b. Determine the meaning of the changes in appearance, body functioning, life style, and roles to the client by encouraging him/her to verbalize feelings and by noting nonverbal responses to changes experienced.<br>c. Implement measures to facilitate the grieving process (see Nursing Diagnosis 16, action b).<br>d. Discuss with client improvements in appearance and functioning that can realistically be expected.<br>e. Implement measures *to assist client to increase self-esteem* (e.g. limit negative self-assessment, encourage positive comments about self, assist to identify strengths, give positive feedback about accomplishments and behaviors that are indicative of high self-esteem).<br>f. Reinforce actions to assist client to cope with effects of chemotherapy (see Nursing Diagnosis 15, action c).<br>g. Implement measures *to assist client to adapt to the following changes in body functioning and appearance if appropriate:*<br>1. alopecia:<br>a. inform client that hair loss can be expected approximately 2 weeks after initiation of chemotherapy; may be sudden, gradual, partial, or complete; and can include scalp hair, pubic hair, beard, eyebrows, and eyelashes<br>b. reassure client that hair loss is temporary (regrowth sometimes occurs before cessation of treatment but usually occurs 2-3 months after it)<br>c. inform client that hair regrowth may be a different color, texture, and consistency<br>d. encourage client to cut long hair *to decrease the anxiety related to seeing large quantities of hair fall out*<br>e. inform client that he/she can reduce rate of scalp hair loss by:<br>1. brushing hair gently using a soft-bristle brush<br>2. avoiding use of harsh shampoos<br>3. wearing an ice cap and/or scalp tourniquet if offered during drug administration to reduce blood supply and therefore contact of the cytotoxic agent with hair follicles<br>f. encourage client to wear a wig, scarf, false eyelashes, or makeup if desired *to camouflage hair loss;* contact the American Cancer Society for a wig if client desires one but is unable to obtain it<br>g. encourage use of the wig before hair loss *to facilitate adjustment to wig and its integration into self-image*<br>2. skin and vein hyperpigmentation:<br>a. inform client that skin and vein hyperpigmentation may occur if he/she is receiving cytotoxic drugs such as bleomycin, busulfan, methotrexate, and fluorouracil<br>b. inform client that skin and vein discoloration is usually temporary<br>c. instruct client to avoid exposure to sunlight and to use sun screen to prevent an increase in hyperpigmentation and photosensitivity reactions<br>d. assist client to identify types of clothing that can be worn to camouflage hyperpigmented areas<br>3. nail changes:<br>a. inform client that his/her nails may thicken and stop growing, develop ridges, darken, and detach from nail bed during treatment with certain cytotoxic drugs (e.g. cyclophosphamide, doxorubicin, bleomycin, fluorouracil) |

| Desired Outcome | Nursing Actions and ***Selected Purposes/Rationales*** |
|---|---|
| | b. reassure client that normal nail growth will resume when chemotherapy is completed<br>4. infertility:<br>a. clarify physician's explanation that infertility is a possible permanent effect of chemotherapy<br>b. discuss alternative methods of becoming a parent (e.g. artificial insemination, adoption) if of concern to client<br>5. impotence:<br>a. encourage client to discuss issue with physician (impotence usually resolves after cessation of therapy)<br>b. suggest alternative methods of sexual gratification if appropriate<br>c. discuss ways to be creative in expressing sexuality (e.g. massage, fantasies, cuddling).<br>h. Assist client with usual grooming and makeup habits if necessary.<br>i. Assess for and support behaviors suggesting positive adaptation to changes that have occurred (e.g. interest in personal appearance, maintenance of relationships with significant others).<br>j. Assist client's and significant others' adjustment to changes by listening, facilitating communication, and providing information.<br>k. Encourage significant others to allow client to do what he/she is able *so that independence can be re-established and/or self-esteem redeveloped.*<br>l. Encourage client contact with others *so that he/she can test and establish a new self-image.*<br>m. Encourage visits and support from significant others.<br>n. Encourage client to pursue usual roles and interests and continue involvement in social activities. If previous roles, interests, and hobbies cannot be pursued, encourage development of new ones.<br>o. Consult physician about psychological counseling if client desires or if he/she seems unwilling or unable to adapt to changes that have occurred as a result of cancer and its treatment. |

## 15. NURSING DIAGNOSIS: Ineffective individual coping

related to an inadequate support system, persistent discomfort associated with the side effects of chemotherapy, fear, anxiety, chronic fatigue, and uncertainty of the effectiveness of chemotherapy.

| Desired Outcome | Nursing Actions and ***Selected Purposes/Rationales*** |
|---|---|
| 15. The client will demonstrate the use of effective coping skills as evidenced by:<br>a. verbalization of ability to cope with diagnosis of cancer and chemotherapy and its effects<br>b. use of appropriate problem-solving techniques<br>c. willingness to | 15.a. Assess for and report signs and symptoms of ineffective individual coping (e.g. verbalization of inability to cope; inability to ask for help, problem solve, or meet basic needs; reluctance to participate in treatment plan; destructive behavior toward self or others; inappropriate use of defense mechanisms; inability to meet role expectations).<br>b. Assess client's perception of current situation including precipitating factors and effectiveness of coping mechanisms.<br>c. Implement measures *to promote effective coping:*<br>1. allow time for client to adjust psychologically to diagnosis, need for chemotherapy, side effects of drugs administered, and anticipated changes in life style and roles<br>2. assist client to recognize and manage inappropriate denial if it is present |

participate in treatment plan and meet basic needs
d. absence of destructive behavior toward self and others
e. appropriate use of defense mechanisms
f. recognition and use of available support systems.

3. perform actions to reduce fear and anxiety (see Nursing Diagnosis 1, action b)
4. perform actions to reduce discomfort (see Nursing Diagnoses 4, action c and 5, action b)
5. perform actions to reduce fatigue (see Nursing Diagnosis 8, action d)
6. encourage verbalization about current situation and ways comparable situations have been handled in the past
7. assist client to identify personal strengths and resources that can be used to facilitate coping with the current situation
8. demonstrate acceptance of client but set limits on inappropriate behavior
9. create an atmosphere of trust and support
10. arrange for a visit with another individual who has been successfully treated for cancer with cytotoxic drugs
11. include client in planning of care, encourage maximum participation in treatment plan, and allow choices when possible *to enable him/her to maintain a sense of control*
12. instruct client in effective problem-solving techniques (e.g. accurate identification of stressors, determination of various options to solve problem)
13. assist client to maintain usual daily routines whenever possible
14. assist client as he/she starts to plan for necessary life-style and role changes after discharge; help client to identify priorities and attainable goals
15. assist client and significant others to identify ways that personal and family goals can be adjusted rather than abandoned
16. administer antianxiety and/or antidepressant agents if ordered
17. assist client to identify and use available support systems; provide information regarding available community resources that can assist client and significant others in coping with effects of chemotherapy and diagnosis of cancer (e.g. American Cancer Society; support groups; individual, family, and financial counselors)
18. encourage continued emotional support from significant others
19. encourage client to share with significant others the kind of support that would be most beneficial (e.g. listening, inspiring hope, providing reassurance and accurate information)
20. support behaviors suggesting positive adaptation to changes experienced (e.g. willingness to care for central venous catheter, compliance with treatment plan, verbalization of the ability to cope, use of effective problem-solving strategies).

d. Consult physician about psychological counseling if appropriate. Initiate a referral if necessary.

---

## 16. NURSING DIAGNOSIS: Grieving*

related to:
a. changes in body image and usual roles and life style;
b. diagnosis of cancer with potential for premature death.

*This diagnostic label includes anticipatory grieving and grieving following the actual losses.

| Desired Outcome | Nursing Actions and ***Selected Purposes/Rationales*** |
|---|---|
| 16. The client will demonstrate beginning | 16.a. Assess for signs and symptoms of grieving (e.g. change in eating habits, inability to concentrate, insomnia, anger, noncompliance, withdrawal |

| Desired Outcome | Nursing Actions and ***Selected Purposes/Rationales*** |
|---|---|
| progression through the grieving process as evidenced by:<br>a. verbalization of feelings about the diagnosis of cancer and chemotherapy<br>b. expression of grief<br>c. participation in the treatment plan and self-care activities<br>d. use of available support systems<br>e. verbalization of a plan for integrating prescribed follow-up care into life style. | from significant others, denial of losses). Be aware that client's response to the diagnosis of cancer and losses experienced will be affected by factors such as previous experience with loss, age, developmental stage, available support systems, spiritual and cultural background, current health status, and significance of the diagnosis and losses experienced.<br>b. Implement measures *to facilitate the grieving process:*<br>1. assist client to acknowledge the losses experienced *so grief work can begin;* assess for factors that may hinder and facilitate acknowledgment<br>2. discuss the grieving process and assist client to accept the phases of grieving as an expected response to actual and/or anticipated losses<br>3. allow time for client to progress through the phases of grieving (phases vary among theorists but progress from shock and alarm to acceptance); be aware that not every phase is expressed by all individuals, that recurrence of phases is common, and that the grieving process may take months to years<br>4. provide an atmosphere of care and concern (e.g. provide privacy, be available and nonjudgmental, display empathy and respect) *so client will feel free to verbalize feelings*<br>5. perform actions *to promote trust* (e.g. answer questions honestly, provide requested information)<br>6. encourage the verbal expression of anger and sadness about the diagnosis and losses experienced; recognize displacement of anger and assist client to see the actual cause of angry feelings and resentment<br>7. encourage client to express his/her feelings in whatever ways are comfortable (e.g. writing, drawing, conversation)<br>8. perform actions to promote effective coping (see Nursing Diagnosis 15, action c)<br>9. support realistic hope about the prognosis and the temporary nature of most of the physical changes<br>10. support behaviors suggesting successful grief work (e.g. verbalizing feelings about the diagnosis and losses, focusing on ways to adapt to losses)<br>11. explain the phases of the grieving process to significant others; encourage their support and understanding<br>12. facilitate communication between the client and significant others; be aware that they may be in different phases of the grieving process<br>13. provide information regarding counseling services and support groups that might assist client in working through grief<br>14. arrange for visit from clergy if desired by client.<br>c. Consult physician regarding referral for counseling if signs of dysfunctional grieving (e.g. persistent denial of diagnosis or losses, excessive anger or sadness, hysteria, suicidal behaviors) occur. |

## 17. NURSING DIAGNOSIS: Knowledge deficit

regarding follow-up care.

| Desired Outcomes | Nursing Actions and ***Selected Purposes/Rationales*** |
|---|---|
| 17.a. The client will identify ways to prevent infection | 17.a.1. Explain to client that his/her resistance to infection is reduced when WBC counts are low. Emphasize need to adhere closely to recommended techniques to prevent infection. |

during periods of lowered immunity.

2. Instruct the client in ways to prevent infection:
   a. avoid crowds, persons with any sign of infection, and persons recently vaccinated
   b. avoid any trauma to skin or mucous membranes
   c. take axillary rather than oral temperature if stomatitis is present
   d. lubricate skin frequently to prevent dryness and subsequent cracking
   e. cleanse any breaks in the skin with a recommended antiseptic solution as directed
   f. use excellent handwashing technique
   g. maintain sterile technique when caring for a central venous or peritoneal catheter, Ommaya reservoir, or implanted infusion device (e.g. MediPort) if in place
   h. avoid any unnecessary rectal invasion (e.g. temperature taking, enemas, suppositories, sexual activity) to prevent rectal trauma
   i. if hemorrhoids are present, avoid situations that could aggravate them (e.g. constipation, sitting for prolonged periods)
   j. avoid constipation to prevent damage to the rectal mucosa from hard or impacted stool
   k. wash perianal area thoroughly with soap and water after each bowel movement and after sexual activity; instruct female client to always wipe from front to back after urination and defecation
   l. drink at least 10 glasses of liquid/day
   m. cough and deep breathe or use incentive spirometer every 2 hours until usual activity is resumed
   n. stop smoking
   o. perform meticulous oral hygiene after meals and at bedtime
   p. avoid douching unless ordered (douching disturbs normal vaginal flora and may cause trauma to the vaginal mucosa)
   q. maintain an optimal nutritional status (e.g. diet high in protein, calories, vitamins, and minerals)
   r. avoid intake of foods with a high bacteria content (e.g. fresh fruit, uncooked foods)
   s. avoid sharing eating utensils
   t. maintain an adequate balance between activity and rest.

17.b. The client will demonstrate the ability to take an oral and axillary temperature correctly.

17.b.1. Demonstrate the correct way to take an oral and axillary temperature.
2. Allow time for questions, clarification, and return demonstration.

17.c. The client will demonstrate appropriate oral hygiene techniques.

17.c.1. Explain the rationale for and importance of frequent oral hygiene.
2. Provide instructions regarding oral hygiene techniques:
   a. cleanse mouth after eating and at bedtime; increase frequency to every 2 hours if stomatitis is present
   b. use a soft-bristle toothbrush to prevent trauma to fragile mucous membranes
   c. rinse mouth with the following solutions as prescribed:
      1. salt and water (1 tsp: 1 quart)
      2. hydrogen peroxide and normal saline or water (1:4) or baking soda and water (1 T: 1 quart) if crusting, debris, and/or tenacious mucus are present (solutions containing hydrogen peroxide should be mixed just before using and mouth should be rinsed thoroughly with a saline solution after use to avoid further damage to the oral mucous membrane)
   d. avoid commercial mouthwashes that have an alcohol base (these are drying to oral mucosa).

17.d. The client will identify techniques

17.d. Instruct client in methods to control nausea and vomiting:
1. eat foods that are cool or room temperature (hot foods frequently have an overpowering aroma that stimulates nausea)

| Desired Outcomes | Nursing Actions and ***Selected Purposes/Rationales*** |
|---|---|
| to control nausea and vomiting. | 2. eat dry foods (e.g. toast, crackers) or sour foods (e.g. lemon drops, pickles, lemon ice) or sip cold carbonated beverages if nausea is present<br>3. eat several small meals instead of 3 large ones<br>4. avoid drinking liquids with meals<br>5. select bland foods (e.g. mashed potatoes, applesauce, cottage cheese) rather than fatty, spicy foods (e.g. fried potatoes, chili)<br>6. rest after eating<br>7. if feasible, have someone else prepare the food<br>8. avoid offensive odors and sights<br>9. cleanse mouth frequently<br>10. take deep, slow breaths when nauseated<br>11. take antiemetics on a regular basis for prescribed length of time and if nausea is persistent. |
| 17.e. The client will verbalize ways to improve appetite and nutritional status. | 17.e. Instruct client in ways to improve appetite and maintain an adequate nutritional status:<br>1. try fish, cheese, and eggs as protein sources instead of beef and pork if taste distortion is a problem<br>2. increase amount of sugar or sweeteners and seasonings usually used in foods and beverages<br>3. eat in a pleasant environment with company if possible<br>4. perform frequent meticulous oral hygiene to eliminate disagreeable tastes in mouth<br>5. try recommended methods of controlling nausea (see action d in this diagnosis)<br>6. eat several high-calorie, high-protein, nutritious small meals/day rather than 3 large ones<br>7. take vitamins and minerals as prescribed. |
| 17.f. The client will verbalize ways to manage and cope with persistent fatigue. | 17.f. Instruct client in ways to manage and cope with persistent fatigue:<br>1. view fatigue as a protective mechanism rather than a problematic limitation<br>2. determine ways in which daily patterns of activity can be modified to conserve energy and prevent excessive fatigue (e.g. spread light and heavy tasks throughout the day, take short rests during an activity whenever possible, sit during an activity whenever possible, take several short rest periods during the day instead of one long one)<br>3. determine if life demands are realistic in light of physical state and adjust short- and long-term goals accordingly<br>4. avoid situations that are particularly fatiguing such as those that are boring, frustrating, or require prolonged or strenuous physical activity<br>5. participate in a regular aerobic exercise program to improve cardiovascular and respiratory fitness, reduce anxiety and stress, and build up tolerance for activity. |
| 17.g. The client will verbalize ways to prevent bleeding when platelet counts are low. | 17.g.1. Instruct client in ways to minimize risk of bleeding:<br>a. avoid taking aspirin, aspirin-containing compounds, and ibuprofen<br>b. use an electric rather than a straight-edge razor<br>c. floss and brush teeth gently<br>d. cut nails and cuticles carefully<br>e. use caution when ambulating to prevent falls or bumps<br>f. avoid situations that could result in injury (e.g. contact sports)<br>g. avoid straining to have a bowel movement<br>h. avoid blowing nose forcefully<br>i. avoid constrictive clothing<br>j. use an ample amount of water-soluble lubricant prior to sexual intercourse and avoid anal sexual activity, douching, use of rectal suppositories, and enemas in order to prevent trauma to the mucous membranes |

k. avoid heavy lifting.
2. Instruct client to control any bleeding by applying firm, prolonged pressure to the area if possible.

17.h. The client will verbalize ways to adjust to alterations in reproductive and sexual functioning.

17.h.1. Assure client that many of the side effects of chemotherapy (e.g. decreased libido, impotence) are temporary or can be treated.
2. Explain to the female client that ovarian failure during chemotherapy may result in irritability, hot flashes, and other symptoms of premature menopause.
3. Instruct client in the childbearing years to use contraception (many cytotoxic drugs cause genetic abnormalities in the developing fetus).
4. Encourage client to rest before sexual activity if fatigue is a problem.
5. Instruct client in measures to decrease discomfort associated with decreased vaginal secretions and mucositis:
   a. use an ample amount of water-soluble lubricant prior to intercourse
   b. use vaginal steroid cream if prescribed to ease dryness and inflammation if present
   c. take a sitz bath 2-3 times a day
   d. avoid intercourse until mucositis of the vaginal canal resolves.
6. Instruct client to take hormone replacements (e.g. estrogen, testosterone) as prescribed.

17.i. The client will demonstrate the ability to care for a central venous catheter, a peritoneal catheter, or an implanted infusion device if in place.

17.i.1. Provide instructions related to care of a central venous catheter (e.g. Groshong) if appropriate:
   a. change dressing if present according to protocol using aseptic technique
   b. observe exit site for changes in appearance, redness, swelling, and unusual drainage
   c. flush catheter according to protocol to maintain patency
   d. replace injection cap as directed
   e. tape catheter securely to the chest wall to prevent accidental dislodgment
   f. notify physician if unable to flush catheter, if signs and symptoms of infection occur at exit site, or if catheter appears to be leaking.
2. Provide instructions related to care of a peritoneal catheter if in place:
   a. change dressing daily according to protocol utilizing aseptic technique
   b. keep catheter capped between treatments
   c. keep water below the level of the catheter when taking a tub bath (a tub bath may be taken 7-10 days after catheter insertion)
   d. observe for and notify physician if any of the following occur:
      1. redness, swelling, or change in appearance of exit site
      2. unusual drainage from exit site
      3. increasing abdominal pain
      4. chills or fever
      5. increased abdominal distention between treatments
      6. persistent nausea or vomiting
      7. dyspnea.
3. Provide instructions related to care of an implanted infusion device (e.g. MediPort, Port-a-Cath) if in place:
   a. keep appointment to have device flushed or flush as instructed
   b. avoid trauma to insertion site
   c. notify physician if area around infusion device becomes reddened or painful.
4. Allow time for questions, clarification, and return demonstration of procedures.

17.j. The client will verbalize an understanding of the care and precautions necessary if an

17.j. Provide instructions related to care and precautions necessary if an Ommaya reservoir is in place:
1. wash site daily with soap and water
2. observe for and report redness, drainage, or discomfort at insertion site; stiff neck; or persistent headache

| Desired Outcomes | Nursing Actions and ***Selected Purposes/Rationales*** |
|---|---|
| Ommaya reservoir is in place. | 3. avoid activities that could result in trauma to the head and damage to the reservoir (e.g. contact sports). |
| 17.k. The client will verbalize an understanding of an implanted infusion pump and precautions necessary if one is in place. | 17.k.1. Reinforce physician's explanation about the purpose of the pump and how it works.<br>2. Instruct client to avoid activities that could result in abdominal trauma and dislodgment of pump.<br>3. Caution client to notify physician if:<br>a. air travel is planned (client should carry an explanatory letter since pump may trigger airport weapon security devices; flow rate of pump may also need to be adjusted if the flight time is lengthy)<br>b. body temperature is elevated more than 2° F for more than 24 hours (an increase in vapor pressure in the pump can increase flow rate)<br>c. he/she plans to move to an area of greater or lesser altitude (alterations in the pump's flow rate may need to be made)<br>d. redness, swelling, or drainage occurs at incisional or refilling site.<br>4. Emphasize importance of keeping appointments to have pump refilled (permanent blockage of the catheter can occur if pump is allowed to empty completely). |
| 17.l. The client will state signs and symptoms of complications to report to the health care provider. | 17.l. Instruct client to observe for and report the following:<br>1. signs and symptoms of infection (stress that usual signs of infection are diminished in people with altered bone marrow function and/or a suppressed immune system and that it is necessary to monitor closely for the following signs and symptoms):<br>a. temperature above 38° C (100.4° F)<br>b. changes in odor, color, or consistency of urine or pain on urination<br>c. white patches in mouth or vagina<br>d. crusted ulcerations around or in oral cavity<br>e. swollen, reddened, coated tongue<br>f. painful rectal or vaginal area<br>g. redness, increased pain, or bleeding of hemorrhoids<br>h. changes in the appearance or temperature of skin, particularly around puncture sites<br>i. persistent productive or nonproductive cough<br>2. signs and symptoms of bleeding (e.g. excessive bruising, black stools, persistent nosebleeds or bleeding from gums, sudden swelling in joints, red or smoke-colored urine, blood in vomitus)<br>3. signs and symptoms of hemorrhagic cystitis (e.g. blood in urine, pain on urination, urinary frequency or urgency)<br>4. signs and symptoms of extravasation (e.g. redness, pain, swelling, and/or skin changes at infusion site)<br>5. signs and symptoms of pulmonary dysfunction (e.g. shortness of breath; persistent, dry, hacking cough; fever)<br>6. signs and symptoms of dehydration (e.g. dry mouth, significant weight loss, concentrated urine, lightheadedness)<br>7. signs and symptoms of cardiotoxicity (e.g. irregular or rapid heart rate, increased weakness and fatigue, shortness of breath, unexplained weight gain, swelling of extremities); emphasize that cardiotoxicity can occur several days to months after administration of drugs known to cause it<br>8. signs and symptoms of neurotoxicity (e.g. numbness and tingling of extremities, change in hearing acuity, blurred vision or change in ability to perceive and discriminate color, constipation, change in motor function and coordination)<br>9. persistent diarrhea, nausea, vomiting, and/or decreased oral intake<br>10. significant weight loss<br>11. inability to cope with the effects of the diagnosis and treatment. |

| | |
|---|---|
| 17.m. The client will identify community resources that can assist with home management and adjustment to the diagnosis of cancer and chemotherapy and its effects. | 17.m.1. Provide information about and encourage use of community resources that can assist client and significant others with home management and adjustment to diagnosis of cancer and chemotherapy and its effects (e.g. American Cancer Society, counselors, social service agencies, Meals on Wheels, Make Today Count, Hospice, local community support groups).<br>2. Initiate a referral if indicated. |
| 17.n. The client will verbalize an understanding of and a plan for adhering to recommended follow-up care including medications prescribed and schedule for chemotherapy, laboratory studies, and future appointments with health care provider. | 17.n.1. Thoroughly explain rationale for, side effects of, and importance of taking medications prescribed.<br>2. Reinforce physician's explanation of planned chemotherapy schedule.<br>3. Discuss with client any difficulties he/she might have adhering to the schedule and assist in planning ways to overcome these.<br>4. Reinforce importance of keeping appointments for chemotherapy and laboratory studies.<br>5. Reinforce importance of keeping follow-up appointments with health care provider.<br>6. Implement measures to improve client compliance:<br>a. include significant others in teaching sessions<br>b. encourage questions and allow time for reinforcement and clarification of information provided<br>c. provide written instructions regarding ways to maintain nutritional status, future appointments with health care provider and laboratory, medications prescribed, and signs and symptoms to report. |

# External Radiation Therapy (Teletherapy)

Radiation therapy is one of the four major modes of treatment for cancer. It is used alone or in combination with surgery, chemotherapy, or biotherapy to achieve palliative or curative results. Radiation therapy, which can be either external (teletherapy) or internal (brachytherapy), is a local treatment in which cellular destruction occurs only at the treatment site. It is most effective on well-oxygenated tumors with a high growth fraction. Unfortunately, radiation therapy is not a selective process and changes in cellular structure and function occur in both the cancerous and the normal cell within the treatment field. The normal cell, however, has a greater capacity for self-repair.

Radiation therapy is a complex process that produces an effect on the cell that begins immediately and continues for an unlimited period. The time of cellular death and the side effects experienced by the client depend on the number of grays (Gy) or centigrays (cGy) received, whether or not both strands of DNA are broken, the condition of the cellular membrane, the mitotic rate of the cell, and the damage to the cell's reproductive abilities. The side effects that all clients receiving external radiation may experience are a skin reaction at the radiation treatment site(s), fatigue, malaise, and anorexia. Other side effects experienced depend on the anatomical site being radiated, mitotic rate of the cells within the treatment field, fractionation of the dose, total dose delivered, and general condition of the client.

**This care plan focuses on the adult client hospitalized for initiation of external radiation therapy or the adult client who is currently undergoing treatment on an outpatient basis and is admitted because of difficulty tolerating certain side effects.** The major goals of care are to maintain comfort; prevent complications; and educate the client about radiation therapy, expected side effects, and toxic effects to be reported. The nurse also plays a major role in assisting the client and significant others to cope with actual and anticipated changes in body image, life style, and roles as a result of cancer and radiation therapy.

## DISCHARGE CRITERIA

Prior to discharge, the client will:

- ❖ have no complications of radiation therapy
- ❖ demonstrate the ability to perform appropriate skin care at sites of irradiation
- ❖ identify techniques to control nausea and vomiting
- ❖ verbalize ways to improve appetite and nutritional status
- ❖ identify ways to reduce the risk of dental caries and periodontal disease and demonstrate appropriate oral hygiene techniques
- ❖ identify ways to prevent bleeding if platelet counts are low
- ❖ identify ways to prevent infection if WBC counts are low
- ❖ verbalize an understanding of and ways to manage the effects of radiation therapy on sexual and reproductive functioning
- ❖ verbalize ways to manage and cope with persistent fatigue
- ❖ state signs and symptoms to report to the health care provider
- ❖ share feelings and thoughts about the diagnosis of cancer and the effects of radiation therapy on body image
- ❖ identify community resources that can assist with home management and adjustment to the diagnosis of cancer and radiation therapy and its effects
- ❖ verbalize an understanding of and a plan for adhering to recommended follow-up care including medications prescribed and future appointments with health care provider, radiation department, and laboratory.

## NURSING/ COLLABORATIVE DIAGNOSES



## 1. NURSING DIAGNOSIS: Anxiety

related to:

a. lack of knowledge and preconceived ideas about radiation therapy and its potential effects on physiological functioning and usual life style and roles;
b. unfamiliar environment and financial concerns;
c. diagnosis of cancer with potential for premature death.

| Desired Outcome | Nursing Actions and ***Selected Purposes/Rationales*** |
|---|---|

1. The client will experience a reduction in anxiety as evidenced by:
   a. verbalization of feeling less anxious and fearful
   b. usual sleep pattern
   c. relaxed facial expression and body movements
   d. stable vital signs
   e. usual perceptual ability and interactions with others.

1.a. Assess client on admission for:
   1. fears, misconceptions, and level of understanding of radiation therapy and its therapeutic and nontherapeutic effects
   2. concerns about particular side effects of radiation and their effect on his/her life style
   3. significance to client of the site to be irradiated
   4. perception of the impact of daily radiation therapy for several weeks on usual life style, roles, and personal relationships
   5. availability of an adequate support system
   6. past experience with radiation therapy or other treatments for cancer
   7. signs and symptoms of anxiety (e.g. verbalization of fears and concerns, insomnia, tenseness, tremors, irritability, restlessness, diaphoresis, tachypnea, tachycardia, elevated blood pressure, facial pallor or flushing, narrowed perceptual field, withdrawal, noncompliance with treatment plan); validate perceptions carefully, remembering that some behavior may be a result of the disease process.

b. Implement measures *to reduce fear and anxiety:*
   1. orient client to hospital environment, equipment, and routines
   2. introduce staff who will be participating in his/her care; if possible, maintain consistency in staff assigned to his/her care *to provide feelings of stability and comfort with the environment*
   3. assure client that staff members are nearby; respond to call signal as soon as possible
   4. maintain a calm, supportive, confident manner when interacting with client
   5. encourage verbalization of fear and anxiety; provide feedback
   6. provide information about radiation therapy:
      a. explain how radiation therapy works and why the total radiation dose prescribed is fractionated
      b. inform client that he/she will be alone in the room during the few minutes of therapy but will be observed continuously via a television monitor; explain that he/she will be able to communicate by means of an intercommunication system
      c. inform client that the machine may click or make a whirring noise but that no discomfort will be felt during treatment
      d. assure client that his/her body, body fluids, and clothing will not be radioactive
      e. instruct client about the expected general side effects of radiation therapy (e.g. fatigue; anorexia; itchy, dry, reddened skin; dry or moist desquamation and increase in skin pigmentation at radiation site) and anticipated side effects for the particular site being irradiated; explain when they can be expected to occur and resolve
      f. explain the treatment simulation process the client will experience before initiation of therapy (the simulation process is done to determine accurately the treatment field[s] and design of devices such as molds, plaster casts, or lead blocks that are necessary to immobilize or position client and/or shield vital body organs within the treatment field[s])
      g. inform client that vital organs within the radiation treatment field(s) are shielded during treatment to prevent unnecessary exposure to radiation; assure client that the treatment field(s) will include the smallest amount of normal tissue possible and that field(s) may be changed or reduced as the tumor shrinks in size
      h. explain how treatment field(s) will be outlined (e.g. skin markings with an indelible dye, ink, or felt tip marker); inform client that the markings will be replaced by pinpoint tattoos once the reproducibility of the field is ensured

| Desired Outcome | Nursing Actions and ***Selected Purposes/Rationales*** |
|---|---|
| | 7. arrange for client and significant others to visit the radiation department and meet those individuals responsible for his/her care<br>8. prepare client for his/her waiting room experiences with others receiving therapy; emphasize that each individual has a different treatment plan, response, and prognosis and that comparison should be avoided<br>9. reinforce physician's explanations and clarify misconceptions client has about the diagnosis of cancer, treatment plan and its effects, and prognosis<br>10. provide a calm, restful environment<br>11. instruct client in relaxation techniques and encourage participation in diversional activities<br>12. perform actions to assist client to cope with radiation therapy and its effects (see Nursing Diagnosis 14, action c)<br>13. initiate financial and/or social service referrals if indicated<br>14. encourage significant others to project a caring, concerned attitude without obvious anxiousness<br>15. administer antianxiety agents if ordered.<br>c. Include significant others in orientation and teaching sessions and encourage their continued support of client.<br>d. Provide information based on current needs of client and significant others at a level they can understand. Encourage questions and clarification of information provided.<br>e. Consult physician if above actions fail to control fear and anxiety. |

## 2. NURSING DIAGNOSIS: Altered nutrition: less than body requirements

related to:
a. decreased oral intake associated with:
   1. anorexia resulting from factors such as depression, fear, anxiety, fatigue, discomfort, early satiety, and altered sense of taste (can result from damage to the taste buds and salivary glands following administration of 1000-2000 cGy to the head and neck area)
   2. impaired swallowing resulting from pharyngitis, esophagitis, dry mouth, and/or viscous oral secretions if present as a result of treatment to the head, neck, or mediastinum;
b. loss of nutrients associated with vomiting and diarrhea if present;
c. impaired utilization of nutrients associated with:
   1. accelerated and inefficient metabolism of proteins, carbohydrates, and fats resulting from the disease process
   2. decreased absorption of nutrients resulting from loss of intestinal absorptive surface if mucositis has developed (can occur with treatment to the abdomen or lower back)
   3. utilization of available nutrients by the malignant cells rather than the host.

| Desired Outcome | Nursing Actions and ***Selected Purposes/Rationales*** |
|---|---|
| 2. The client will maintain an adequate nutritional status as evidenced by:<br>a. weight within normal range for client's age, height, and body frame<br>b. normal BUN and | 2.a. Assess for and report signs and symptoms of malnutrition:<br>1. weight below normal for client's age, height, and body frame<br>2. abnormal BUN and low serum albumin, Hct, Hb, and transferrin levels<br>3. triceps skinfold thickness less than normal<br>4. weakness and fatigue<br>5. stomatitis.<br>b. Monitor percentage of meals and snacks client consumes. Report a pattern of inadequate intake. |

serum albumin, Hct, Hb, and transferrin levels
c. triceps skinfold thickness within normal range
d. usual strength and activity tolerance
e. healthy oral mucous membrane.

c. Implement measures *to maintain an adequate nutritional status:*
  1. perform actions *to improve oral intake:*
     a. implement measures to control nausea and vomiting (see Nursing Diagnosis 5.A, action 2)
     b. implement measures to reduce pain (see Nursing Diagnosis 4, action e)
     c. implement measures to assist client to adjust psychologically to the diagnosis of cancer and treatment with radiation therapy (see Nursing Diagnoses 13, actions d-n; 14, action c; and 15, action b)
     d. implement measures to improve client's ability to swallow (see Nursing Diagnosis 3, action b)
     e. implement measures *to compensate for taste alteration* (loss of sense of taste occurs within 2 weeks of initiation of radiation treatment to head and neck, persists for 4-6 weeks after completion of therapy, and usually is not permanent):
        1. encourage client to select fish, cold cooked chicken, eggs, and cheese as protein sources if beef or pork tastes bitter or rancid
        2. provide meat for breakfast if aversion to meat tends to increase during day
        3. add extra sweeteners to foods if acceptable to client
        4. experiment with different flavorings, seasonings, and textures
        5. serve food warm *to stimulate the sense of smell*
     f. increase activity as tolerated *(activity stimulates appetite)*
     g. obtain a dietary consult if necessary to assist client in selecting foods/fluids that meet nutritional needs as well as personal and cultural preferences whenever possible
     h. encourage a rest period before meals *to minimize fatigue*
     i. maintain a clean environment and a relaxed, pleasant atmosphere
     j. provide oral hygiene before meals
     k. provide largest amount of calories and protein when appetite is best (usually at breakfast)
     l. serve small portions of nutritious foods/fluids that are appealing to client
     m. encourage significant others to bring in client's favorite foods and eat with him/her *to make eating more of a familiar social experience*
     n. limit fluid intake (unless it has a high nutritional value) with meals *to reduce early satiety and subsequent decreased food intake*
     o. allow adequate time for meals; reheat food if necessary
  2. ensure that meals are well balanced and high in essential nutrients; offer high-protein, high-calorie dietary supplements between meals if indicated
  3. perform activities to control diarrhea (see Nursing Diagnosis 9, action d)
  4. administer vitamins and minerals if ordered.

d. Perform a 72-hour calorie count if ordered. Report totals to dietitian and physician.
e. Consult physician about alternative methods of providing nutrition (e.g. parenteral nutrition, tube feedings) if client does not consume enough food or fluids to meet nutritional needs.

## 3. NURSING DIAGNOSIS: Impaired swallowing

related to:
a. oral, pharyngeal, or esophageal pain associated with inflammation and/or ulceration of the mucosa if the treatment field includes the head, neck, or mediastinum;

b. dry mouth and viscous oral secretions associated with:
   1. destruction of the salivary glands (particularly the parotids) if the treatment field includes the head and neck area
   2. decreased oral intake.

| Desired Outcome | Nursing Actions and ***Selected Purposes/Rationales*** |
|---|---|
| 3. The client will experience an improvement in swallowing as evidenced by:<br>a. verbalization of same<br>b. absence of food in oral cavity after swallowing<br>c. absence of coughing and choking when eating and drinking. | 3.a. Assess for signs and symptoms of impaired swallowing (e.g. statements of difficulty swallowing, stasis of food in oral cavity, coughing or choking when eating or drinking).<br>b. Implement measures *to improve ability to swallow:*<br>1. perform actions to reduce oral, pharyngeal, and esophageal pain (see Nursing Diagnosis 4, action e.5)<br>2. perform actions to decrease dryness of the oral mucous membrane (see Nursing Diagnosis 7, action a.2)<br>3. assist client to select foods that require little or no chewing and are easily swallowed (e.g. custard, eggs, canned fruit, mashed potatoes)<br>4. avoid serving foods that are sticky (e.g. peanut butter, soft bread, bananas)<br>5. moisten dry foods with gravy or sauces (e.g. sour cream, salad dressing)<br>6. perform actions *to stimulate salivation:*<br>a. provide oral care before meals<br>b. provide a piece of sour, sugarless candy for client to suck on just before meals unless contraindicated<br>c. serve foods that are visually pleasing<br>d. place a piece of lemon or sour pickle on client's plate<br>7. perform actions *to reduce and/or liquefy viscous oral secretions:*<br>a. encourage a fluid intake of 2500 ml/day unless contraindicated<br>b. encourage client to avoid milk and milk products (unless boiled) and chocolate *(when combined with saliva, they produce very thick secretions).*<br>c. Consult physician if swallowing difficulties persist or worsen. |

## 4. NURSING DIAGNOSIS: Pain

related to inflammation and/or moist desquamation (if it occurs) in irradiated area(s).

| Desired Outcome | Nursing Actions and ***Selected Purposes/Rationales*** |
|---|---|
| 4. The client will experience diminished pain as evidenced by:<br>a. verbalization of decreased pain<br>b. relaxed facial expression and body positioning<br>c. increased participation in activities<br>d. stable vital signs. | 4.a. Determine how client usually responds to pain.<br>b. Assess client's perception of pain including location, intensity, and type. Use a numerical scale to rate intensity.<br>c. Assess for nonverbal signs of pain (e.g. wrinkled brow, guarding of irradiated area, clenched fists, reluctance to move, restlessness, diaphoresis, facial pallor, increased B/P, tachycardia).<br>d. Assess for factors that seem to aggravate and alleviate pain.<br>e. Implement measures *to reduce pain:*<br>1. perform actions *to reduce fear and anxiety about the pain experience* (e.g. assure client that his/her need for pain relief will be met)<br>2. medicate prior to any painful treatments or procedures and before pain becomes severe<br>3. perform actions *to reduce pain associated with moist desquamation:*<br>a. keep irradiated site clean and dry<br>b. apply hydrogel dressings (e.g. Vigilon, Geliperm) if ordered or |

position a covered bed cradle over affected area *to reduce airflow over exposed nerve endings*

4. perform actions *to reduce perianal pain* (can occur if the perineum is in the treatment field or if diarrhea is present):
   a. provide a foam pad for client to sit on
   b. consult physician about an order for sitz bath unless contraindicated
   c. implement measures to decrease skin irritation and prevent breakdown associated with diarrhea (see Nursing Diagnosis 6, action b.4)
   d. avoid taking temperature rectally or administering rectal suppositories
5. perform actions *to reduce oral, pharyngeal, and esophageal pain* (can occur with radiation exposure of approximately 3000 cGy to the head, neck, and mediastinum):
   a. implement measures to reduce severity of stomatitis (see Nursing Diagnosis 7, actions b.3-5)
   b. offer cool, soothing liquids such as nonacidic juices, ices, and ice cream
   c. instruct client to gargle with a saline solution every 2 hours *to soothe the oral mucous membrane*
6. provide or assist with nonpharmacological measures for pain relief (e.g. back rub, position change, relaxation techniques, guided imagery, quiet conversation, restful environment, diversional activities)
7. plan methods for achieving pain control with client *in order to assist him/her to maintain a sense of control over the pain experience*
8. administer analgesics if ordered.

f. Consult physician if above measures fail to provide adequate pain relief.

---

**5.A. NURSING DIAGNOSIS:**

**Altered comfort: nausea and vomiting**

related to:
1. direct stimulation of the vomiting center associated with:
   a. cerebral inflammation (occurs with irradiation of the whole brain)
   b. absorption of waste products of cellular destruction if client is receiving a large daily fraction of radiation or daily treatments over a period of several weeks;
2. indirect stimulation of the vomiting center associated with:
   a. stimulation of the afferent vagal and/or sympathetic pathways resulting from visceral irritation associated with inflammation of the gastrointestinal mucosa (occurs when areas of chest, back, abdomen, and pelvis are irradiated)
   b. cortical stimulation resulting from stress and pain.

| Desired Outcome | Nursing Actions and ***Selected Purposes/Rationales*** |
|---|---|
| 5.A. The client will experience relief of nausea and vomiting as evidenced by:<br>1. verbalization of relief of nausea<br>2. absence of vomiting. | 5.A.1. Assess client for nausea and vomiting (tends to occur within 1-3 hours after treatment).<br>2. Implement measures *to control nausea and vomiting:*<br>a. perform actions to reduce fear and anxiety (see Nursing Diagnosis 1, action b)<br>b. perform actions to reduce pain (see Nursing Diagnosis 4, action e)<br>c. eliminate noxious sights and odors from the environment *(noxious stimuli cause cortical stimulation of the vomiting center)*<br>d. encourage client to take deep, slow breaths when nauseated |

| Desired Outcome | Nursing Actions and ***Selected Purposes/Rationales*** |
|---|---|
| | e. encourage client to change positions slowly *(rapid movement stimulates the afferent vestibulocerebellar pathway with resultant stimulation of the chemoreceptor trigger zone)*<br>f. provide oral hygiene after each emesis and before meals<br>g. maintain food and fluid restrictions if ordered (client may be placed on a clear liquid or bland diet for short periods if nausea is severe)<br>h. instruct client to avoid foods/fluids for 3 hours before and after treatments<br>i. provide carbonated beverages for client to sip if nauseated<br>j. avoid serving foods with an overpowering aroma; remove lids from hot foods before entering room<br>k. provide small, frequent meals; instruct client to ingest foods and fluids slowly<br>l. if nausea tends to peak after each treatment, instruct client to eat his/her major meal of the day at least 3 hours before treatment and to eat lightly for the rest of the day<br>m. encourage client to eat dry foods (e.g. toast, crackers) and avoid drinking liquids with meals if nauseated<br>n. instruct client to avoid foods/fluids that irritate the gastric mucosa (e.g. spicy foods; caffeine-containing beverages such as coffee, tea, and colas)<br>o. instruct client to avoid foods high in fat *(fat delays gastric emptying)*<br>p. instruct client to rest after eating<br>q. administer antiemetics if ordered (these are often given 1-2 hours before radiation therapy and every 4-6 hours for 12 hours after treatment).<br>3. Consult physician if above measures fail to control nausea and vomiting. |

## 5.B. NURSING DIAGNOSIS: Altered comfort: pruritus

related to dry skin associated with decreased function of sebaceous and sweat glands within the treatment field (gland function may cease if dose exceeds 4500-6000 cGy).

| Desired Outcome | Nursing Actions and ***Selected Purposes/Rationales*** |
|---|---|
| 5.B. The client will experience relief of pruritus as evidenced by:<br>1. verbalization of same<br>2. no scratching or rubbing of skin. | 5.B.1. Assess skin within the treatment field, particularly body folds and thin epidermal areas (e.g. face, axilla, perineum), for dryness and itching.<br>2. Instruct client in and/or implement measures *to relieve pruritus in the treatment area:*<br>a. perform actions *to promote capillary constriction:*<br>1. apply cool, moist compresses to pruritic areas<br>2. maintain a cool environment<br>b. perform actions *to reduce skin dryness:*<br>1. use tepid water and mild soaps for bathing being careful not to remove skin markings<br>2. apply water-based lubricant lotions (e.g. Lubriderm, Eucerin) frequently (lanolin lotions can also be used but must be removed before treatments)<br>3. limit bathing to every other day<br>4. encourage a fluid intake of 2500 ml/day unless contraindicated |

c. add emollients, cornstarch, baking soda, or oatmeal preparations to bath water
d. apply cornstarch to areas of dry desquamation (cornstarch should not be used if moist desquamation is present)
e. pat skin dry, making sure to dry thoroughly
f. encourage participation in diversional activities
g. use relaxation techniques
h. use cutaneous stimulation techniques (e.g. stroking with a soft brush) at sites of itching or acupressure points (skin within the treatment field should never be rubbed or massaged)
i. encourage client to wear loose cotton garments; launder clothing in mild soap
j. administer antihistamines and apply a mild corticosteroid cream if ordered (topical corticosteroids are used with caution *because they can cause diffuse thinning of the skin).*

3. Consult physician if above measures fail to relieve pruritus or if the skin becomes excoriated.

## 6. NURSING DIAGNOSIS: Actual/High risk for impaired skin integrity

related to:
a. dry desquamation of irradiated site(s) associated with increased sensitivity of skin in certain areas (e.g. opposing skin surfaces, face, perineum) and destruction of rapidly dividing epithelial cells of the skin (occurs with a cumulative dose of 3000-4000 cGy);
b. moist desquamation of irradiated area(s), particularly if client is receiving electron beam therapy, associated with inability of basal cells to provide sufficient differentiated, cornified cells (occurs with doses above 4500 cGy or lower cumulative doses if client is receiving concurrent chemotherapy);
c. increased skin fragility associated with:
   1. tissue edema resulting from vascular changes in irradiated area(s)
   2. malnutrition;
d. excessive scratching associated with pruritus;
e. damage to the skin and/or subcutaneous tissue associated with prolonged pressure on the tissues, friction, or shearing if mobility is decreased;
f. frequent contact of the skin with irritants associated with diarrhea if present.

| Desired Outcome | Nursing Actions and ***Selected Purposes/Rationales*** |
|---|---|
| 6. The client will maintain or regain skin integrity as evidenced by:<br>a. minimal redness and irritation within the treatment field<br>b. absence of redness and irritation in other body areas<br>c. no skin breakdown. | 6.a. Inspect the following areas for pallor, redness, and breakdown:<br>1. treatment field(s)<br>2. opposing skin surfaces such as buttocks, groin, axillae, and breasts<br>3. bony prominences<br>4. dependent, pruritic, and edematous areas<br>5. perineum.<br>b. Implement measures *to maintain or regain skin integrity:*<br>1. perform actions *to prevent or treat skin irritation or breakdown within the treatment field(s):*<br>a. cleanse irradiated area(s) gently each shift with tepid water and mild soap (may be contraindicated initially when skin markings rather than tattoos are used)<br>b. pat skin dry using soft materials, paying particular attention to opposing skin surfaces within the treatment field(s)<br>c. expose irradiated area(s) to the air as much as possible, avoiding extremes in temperature |

| Desired Outcome | Nursing Actions and ***Selected Purposes/Rationales*** |
|---|---|

d. avoid use of tape within irradiated area(s)
e. instruct client to:
   1. wear loose cotton clothing
   2. avoid use of perfumed lotions or soaps, cosmetics, and deodorants *to prevent chemical irritation (many of these products contain heavy metals that will augment effects of radiation on the skin)*
   3. apply cornstarch to areas of dry desquamation *to reduce friction*
   4. use water-based (hydrophilic), mild, lubricant lotions (e.g. Lubriderm, Eucerin, Aquaphor) *to reduce skin dryness and subsequent cracking*
   5. avoid use of hydrophobic products (e.g. petroleum jelly) *because they are difficult to remove*
   6. use an electric rather than a straight-edge razor if it is absolutely necessary to shave in irradiated area(s)
   7. avoid applications of heat and cold to irradiated area(s)
f. implement measures to relieve pruritus (see Nursing Diagnosis 5.B, action 2) *in order to minimize the risk of scratching*
g. implement measures *to treat a moist desquamation reaction if it has occurred:*
   1. if open method of treatment is prescribed:
      a. cleanse area well with warm saline, water, or a dilute solution of chlorhexidine gluconate 3 times/day; apply an astringent soak if ordered
      b. keep involved area exposed to the air as much as possible
   2. if semi-open method of treatment is prescribed:
      a. apply a weak astringent soak (e.g. dilute Domboro solution) for 15 minutes 3 times/day
      b. apply a hydrogel primary wound dressing (e.g. Vigilon, Geliperm) or a nonadherent dressing (e.g. Adaptic) as ordered
   3. if closed method of treatment is prescribed, apply occlusive dressings *to maintain a moist environment*
   4. apply a topical antimicrobial agent as ordered if signs and symptoms of a localized infection occur

2. perform actions *to prevent skin breakdown resulting from decreased mobility:*
   a. assist client to turn at least every 2 hours; use all 4 sides (prone, lateral [left/right], dorsal) unless contraindicated
   b. gently massage around reddened areas at least every 2 hours
   c. implement measures *to prevent shearing* (shearing occurs when one tissue layer slides past another) *and skin surface abrasion:*
      1. apply a thin layer of powder or cornstarch to bottom sheet or skin *to absorb moisture (moist skin is more likely to adhere to sheet) and reduce friction*
      2. lift and move client carefully using a turn sheet and adequate assistance
      3. limit length of time client is in semi-Fowler's position to 30 minutes *(in this position, client tends to slide down in bed)*
   d. instruct or assist client to shift weight every 30 minutes
   e. if fade time (length of time it takes for reddened area to fade after pressure is removed) is greater than 15 minutes, increase frequency of position changes
   f. keep skin clean and dry
   g. keep bed linens dry and wrinkle-free
   h. provide devices to reduce pressure on the skin, decrease shearing, and/or prevent moisture build-up (e.g. alternating pressure mattress or pad, flotation pad, sheepskin)
   i. increase activity as tolerated
3. apply a thin layer of powder or cornstarch to areas with opposing skin

surfaces (e.g. axillae, perineum, beneath breasts) unless contraindicated *to absorb moisture and/or reduce friction*

4. perform actions *to decrease skin irritation and prevent breakdown associated with diarrhea:*
    a. implement measures to control diarrhea (see Nursing Diagnosis 9, action d)
    b. assist client to cleanse and dry perineal area thoroughly with soft tissue or cloth after each bowel movement; apply a protective ointment or cream (e.g. Desitin, A & D ointment) being sure to remove it before treatments if rectal area is within treatment field(s)
    c. apply a drainable fecal collector unless contraindicated if diarrhea is severe
    d. provide incontinence pads if needed to absorb moisture; do not allow skin to come in contact with plastic portion of pads
5. if edema is present:
    a. perform actions *to reduce fluid accumulation in dependent areas:*
        1. instruct client in and assist with range of motion exercises
        2. elevate affected extremities whenever possible
    b. handle edematous areas carefully
6. perform actions *to prevent skin breakdown associated with scratching:*
    a. implement measures to relieve pruritus (see Nursing Diagnosis 5.B, action 2)
    b. keep nails trimmed and/or apply mittens if necessary
7. perform actions to maintain an adequate nutritional status (see Nursing Diagnosis 2, action c).

c. If unexpected skin irritation or breakdown occurs:
    1. notify physician
    2. continue with above measures to prevent further irritation and breakdown
    3. perform decubitus ulcer and other wound care as ordered or per standard hospital procedure
    4. assess client closely and report signs and symptoms of infection (e.g. elevated temperature; redness, warmth, and edema around area of breakdown; unusual drainage from site).

---

## 7. NURSING DIAGNOSIS: Altered oral mucous membrane:

a. **dryness** related to decreased oral intake and destruction of salivary glands if the treatment field includes the head and neck;
b. **stomatitis** related to malnutrition, inadequate oral hygiene, and disruption in the normal renewal process of mucosal epithelial cells if the oral cavity is irradiated.

| Desired Outcomes | Nursing Actions and ***Selected Purposes/Rationales*** |
|---|---|
| 7.a. The client will maintain a moist, intact oral mucous membrane. | 7.a.1. Assess client every shift for dryness of the oral mucosa (reduction in salivary flow may occur after a cumulative dose of as little as 1000 cGy to the head and neck area and may persist for many months after treatment; dryness will be permanent after a radiation exposure of over 6000 cGy).<br>2. Implement measures *to decrease dryness of oral mucous membrane:*<br>a. instruct and assist client to perform good oral hygiene after eating and as often as needed<br>b. encourage client to rinse or spray mouth frequently with water<br>c. instruct client to avoid products such as lemon-glycerin swabs and |

| Desired Outcomes | Nursing Actions and ***Selected Purposes/Rationales*** |
|---|---|
| | commercial mouthwashes containing alcohol *(these products have a drying or irritating effect on the oral mucous membrane)*<br>d. lubricate client's lips with Vaseline, K-Y jelly, ChapStick, Blistex, or mineral oil frequently<br>e. encourage client to breathe through nose rather than mouth<br>f. encourage client not to smoke *(smoking irritates and dries the mucosa)*<br>g. encourage a fluid intake of at least 2500 ml/day unless contraindicated<br>h. if stomatitis is not severe, encourage client to use artificial saliva *to lubricate the mucous membrane*<br>i. if some salivary production is occurring, encourage the client to suck on sour, hard, sugarless candy or chew sugarless gum *to stimulate salivation.* |
| 7.b. The client will maintain a healthy oral cavity as evidenced by:<br>1. absence of inflammation<br>2. pink, intact mucosa<br>3. no complaints of oral dryness and burning<br>4. ability to swallow without discomfort<br>5. usual consistency of saliva. | 7.b.1. Assess client for and report signs and symptoms of stomatitis such as inflamed and/or ulcerated oral mucosa, complaints of oral dryness or burning, dysphagia, leukoplakia, and viscous saliva. (Stomatitis usually begins by the end of the second week of therapy and persists for up to 4 weeks following the cessation of treatment. Signs and symptoms initially appear on the buccal surfaces and/or palate.)<br>2. Culture suspicious oral lesions as ordered. Report positive results.<br>3. Implement measures *to prevent or reduce the severity of stomatitis:*<br>a. perform actions to reduce dryness of the oral mucous membrane (see action a.2 in this diagnosis)<br>b. have client rinse mouth every 1-2 hours with warm saline; baking soda and water; or a solution of salt, baking soda, and water<br>c. use a soft-bristle brush, sponge-tipped applicator, or low-pressure power spray for oral hygiene<br>d. instruct client to avoid substances that might further irritate the oral mucosa (e.g. extremely hot, spicy, or acidic foods/fluids)<br>e. perform actions to maintain an adequate nutritional status (see Nursing Diagnosis 2, action c)<br>f. consult physician regarding an order for a prophylactic antimicrobial agent.<br>4. If stomatitis is not controlled:<br>a. increase frequency of oral hygiene<br>b. if client has dentures, remove and replace only for meals.<br>5. Administer topical anesthetics, oral protective pastes or coating agents, and topical and systemic analgesics if ordered.<br>6. Consult physician if signs and symptoms of stomatitis persist or worsen. |

## 8. NURSING DIAGNOSIS: Fatigue

related to*:

a. accumulation of cellular waste products associated with rapid lysis of cancerous and normal cells exposed to radiation;
b. difficulty resting and sleeping;
c. fear, anxiety, and depression;
d. increased energy expenditure associated with an increase in the metabolic rate resulting from continuous active tumor growth;
e. malnutrition.

*Some of the etiological factors presented here are under investigation.

| Desired Outcome | Nursing Actions and ***Selected Purposes/Rationales*** |
|---|---|
| 8. The client will experience a reduction in fatigue as evidenced by:<br>a. verbalization of feelings of increased energy<br>b. ability to perform usual activities of daily living<br>c. increased interest in surroundings and ability to concentrate<br>d. decreased emotional lability. | 8.a. Assess for signs and symptoms of fatigue (e.g. verbalization of unremitting, overwhelming lack of energy and inability to maintain usual routines; lack of interest in surroundings; decreased ability to concentrate; increased emotional lability).<br>b. Inform client that a feeling of persistent fatigue is expected as a result of the disease itself and is a side effect of radiation therapy.<br>c. Assist client to identify personal patterns of fatigue (e.g. time of day, after treatments or certain activities) and to plan activities so that times of greatest fatigue are avoided.<br>d. Implement measures *to reduce fatigue:*<br>1. perform actions *to promote rest and/or conserve energy:*<br>a. schedule several short rest periods during the day<br>b. minimize environmental activity and noise<br>c. limit the number of visitors and their length of stay<br>d. assist client with self-care activities as needed<br>e. keep supplies and personal articles within easy reach<br>f. implement measures to reduce fear and anxiety (see Nursing Diagnosis 1, action b)<br>g. implement measures to promote sleep (see Nursing Diagnosis 10, action c)<br>h. implement measures to reduce discomfort (see Nursing Diagnoses 4, action e; 5.A, action 2; and 5.B, action 2)<br>i. instruct client in energy-saving techniques (e.g. using shower chair when showering, sitting to brush teeth or comb hair)<br>2. perform actions to maintain an adequate nutritional status (see Nursing Diagnosis 2, action c)<br>3. encourage client to maintain a fluid intake of at least 2500 ml/day *to promote elimination of the by-products of cellular breakdown*<br>4. perform actions to facilitate client's psychological adjustment to the diagnosis of cancer and the treatment regimen and its effects (see Nursing Diagnoses 1, action b; 13, actions d-n; 14, action c; and 15, action b).<br>e. Consult physician if signs and symptoms of fatigue worsen. |

## 9. NURSING DIAGNOSIS: Diarrhea

related to:

a. decreased absorption of water from the intestines associated with destruction of the villi and microvilli if the treatment field includes the pelvis, abdomen, or lower back;
b. increased intestinal motility associated with extreme fear and anxiety and inflammation, denuding, and ulceration of the gastrointestinal mucosa if the treatment field includes the pelvis, abdomen, or lower back.

| Desired Outcome | Nursing Actions and ***Selected Purposes/Rationales*** |
|---|---|
| 9. The client will have fewer bowel movements and more formed stool. | 9.a. Ascertain client's usual bowel elimination habits.<br>b. Assess for signs and symptoms of diarrhea (e.g. frequent, loose stools; urgency; abdominal pain and cramping). Diarrhea will usually begin after 1500-3000 cGy have been received and end 2-3 weeks after cessation of treatment. |

| Desired Outcome | Nursing Actions and ***Selected Purposes/Rationales*** |
|---|---|
| | c. Assess bowel sounds regularly. Report an increase in frequency of bowel sounds.<br>d. Implement measures *to control diarrhea:*<br>1. perform actions *to rest the bowel:*<br>a. restrict oral intake if ordered<br>b. when oral intake is allowed:<br>1. gradually progress from fluids to small meals<br>2. instruct client to avoid foods/fluids that may stimulate or irritate the inflamed bowel:<br>a. those high in fiber (e.g. whole-grain cereals, raw fruits and vegetables)<br>b. gas producers (e.g. cabbage, beans, onions, cauliflower)<br>c. those that are spicy or extremely hot or cold<br>d. those high in lactose (e.g. milk, milk products)<br>e. those high in fat (e.g. butter, cream, fried foods)<br>c. implement measures to reduce fear and anxiety (see Nursing Diagnosis 1, action b)<br>d. encourage client to rest<br>e. discourage smoking *(nicotine has a stimulant effect on the gastrointestinal tract)*<br>2. administer the following antidiarrheal agents if ordered:<br>a. opiate or opiate-like substances (e.g. loperamide, diphenoxylate hydrochloride) *to decrease gastrointestinal motility*<br>b. bulk-forming agents (e.g. methylcellulose, psyllium hydrophilic mucilloid, calcium polycarbophil) *to absorb water in the bowel, which results in a more formed stool.*<br>e. Consult physician if diarrhea persists. |

## 10. NURSING DIAGNOSIS: Sleep pattern disturbance

related to:
a. pain, nausea, vomiting, pruritus, and severe xerostomia;
b. anxiety, fear, and depression;
c. frequent need to defecate associated with diarrhea if present.

| Desired Outcome | Nursing Actions and ***Selected Purposes/Rationales*** |
|---|---|
| 10. The client will attain optimal amounts of sleep within the parameters of the treatment regimen as evidenced by:<br>a. statements of feeling well rested<br>b. usual mental status<br>c. absence of frequent yawning, dark circles under eyes, and hand tremors. | 10.a. Assess for signs and symptoms of a sleep pattern disturbance (e.g. verbal complaints of difficulty falling asleep, not feeling well rested, or sleep interruptions; irritability; lethargy; disorientation; frequent yawning; dark circles under eyes; slight hand tremors).<br>b. Determine the client's usual sleep habits.<br>c. Implement measures *to promote sleep:*<br>1. discourage long periods of sleep during the day unless signs and symptoms of sleep deprivation exist or daytime sleep is usual for client<br>2. perform actions to reduce fear and anxiety (see Nursing Diagnosis 1, action b)<br>3. perform actions to reduce discomfort (see Nursing Diagnoses 4, action e; 5.A, action 2; and 5.B, action 2)<br>4. perform actions to control diarrhea (see Nursing Diagnosis 9, action d) |

5. if client has xerostomia, instruct him/her to use artificial saliva before sleep *to prevent the dry, choking sensation that often occurs during sleep*
6. encourage participation in relaxing diversional activities during the evening
7. discourage intake of fluids high in caffeine (e.g. coffee, tea, colas), especially in the evening
8. offer client a high-protein evening snack unless contraindicated
9. allow client to continue usual sleep practices (e.g. position, time, bedtime rituals such as reading and meditating) if possible
10. satisfy basic needs such as comfort and warmth before sleep
11. have client empty bladder just before bedtime
12. use relaxation techniques (e.g. progressive relaxation exercises, back massage, meditation, soft music) before sleep
13. maintain a quiet, restful atmosphere; have earplugs available for client if needed
14. ensure good room ventilation
15. administer sedative-hypnotics if ordered
16. perform actions *to reduce interruptions during sleep (80-100 minutes of uninterrupted sleep are usually needed to complete one sleep cycle):*
    a. restrict visitors
    b. group care (e.g. medications, treatments, physical care, assessments) whenever possible.

d. Consult physician if signs and symptoms of sleep deprivation persist or worsen.

## 11. NURSING DIAGNOSIS: High risk for infection

related to:

a. break in the integrity of the skin associated with dry or moist desquamation;
b. lowered natural resistance associated with:
   1. malnutrition
   2. neutropenia resulting from bone marrow suppression if large amounts of active bone marrow are included in the treatment field(s);
c. stasis of respiratory secretions and urinary stasis if mobility is decreased.

| Desired Outcome | Nursing Actions and ***Selected Purposes/Rationales*** |
|---|---|
| 11. The client will remain free of infection as evidenced by:<br>a. absence of fever and chills<br>b. pulse within normal limits<br>c. normal breath sounds<br>d. voiding clear urine without complaints of frequency, urgency, and burning<br>e. absence of redness, heat, pain, swelling, | 11.a. Assess for and report signs and symptoms of infection:<br>1. elevated temperature<br>2. chills<br>3. increased pulse<br>4. abnormal breath sounds<br>5. cloudy, foul-smelling urine<br>6. complaints of frequency, urgency, or burning when urinating<br>7. presence of WBCs, bacteria, and/or nitrites in urine<br>8. redness, heat, pain, swelling, or unusual drainage in any area<br>9. complaints of increased weakness or fatigue<br>10. elevated WBC count and/or significant change in differential.<br>b. Obtain specimens (e.g. urine, vaginal, mouth, sputum, blood, moist desquamation sites) for culture as ordered. Report positive results.<br>c. Implement measures *to reduce the risk for infection:*<br>1. protect client from others with infections and those who have recently been vaccinated *(a person may have a subclinical infection after a vaccination)* |

| Desired Outcome | Nursing Actions and ***Selected Purposes/Rationales*** |
|---|---|
| and unusual drainage in any area<br>f. no complaints of increased weakness and fatigue<br>g. WBC and differential counts within normal range for client<br>h. negative results of cultured specimens. | 2. use good handwashing technique and encourage client to do the same<br>3. maintain a fluid intake of at least 2500 ml/day unless contraindicated<br>4. perform actions to maintain an adequate nutritional status (see Nursing Diagnosis 2, action c)<br>5. encourage a low-bacteria diet (e.g. cooked foods, no fresh fruit) if client is immunosuppressed<br>6. perform actions to decrease dryness of the oral mucous membrane and/or reduce severity of stomatitis (see Nursing Diagnosis 7, actions a.2, b.3, and b.4)<br>7. perform actions to maintain or regain skin integrity (see Nursing Diagnosis 6, action b)<br>8. give meticulous attention to any break in skin integrity; provide wound care as ordered<br>9. avoid invasive procedures (e.g. urinary catheterizations, arterial and venous punctures, injections) whenever possible; if such procedures are necessary, perform them using meticulous aseptic technique<br>10. change intravenous tubings and solutions and rotate insertion sites according to hospital policy<br>11. change equipment and solutions used for procedures such as irrigations, wound care, and tube feedings according to hospital policy<br>12. initiate measures to prevent constipation (e.g. encourage client to defecate whenever the urge is felt, encourage a minimum fluid intake of 2500 ml/day, administer laxatives and stool softeners as ordered) *in order to prevent damage to the rectal mucosa from hard stool*<br>13. avoid unnecessary rectal invasion (e.g. temperature taking, enemas, suppositories, rectal tube) *to prevent trauma to rectal mucosa and possible abscess formation*<br>14. perform actions to reduce stress and discomfort (see Nursing Diagnoses 1, action b; 4, action e; 5.A, action 2; and 5.B, action 2) *in order to prevent excessive secretion of cortisol (cortisol inhibits the immune response)*<br>15. perform actions *to prevent stasis of respiratory secretions* (e.g. assist client to turn, cough, and deep breathe; increase activity as tolerated)<br>16. perform actions to prevent urinary retention (e.g. instruct client to urinate when the urge is first felt, promote relaxation during voiding attempts) *in order to prevent urinary stasis*<br>17. perform actions *to prevent the introduction of microorganisms into the urinary tract* (e.g. assist client with perineal care as needed, instruct and assist female client to wipe from front to back after urinating and defecating, maintain sterile technique during urinary catheterization)<br>18. administer the following if ordered:<br>a. antimicrobial agents (usually initiated when the neutropenic client becomes febrile or may be administered prophylactically if the neutrophil count is less than 500/mm$^3$)<br>b. colony-stimulating factors (e.g. Filgrastim) *to stimulate granulocyte production.* |

## 12. COLLABORATIVE DIAGNOSES:

**Potential complications:**

a. **bleeding** related to thrombocytopenia associated with bone marrow suppression if large amounts of active bone marrow are included in the treatment field(s);
b. **radiation cystitis** related to irritation of the bladder mucosa (occurs after radiation exposure of the bladder to 3000-4000 cGy).

| Desired Outcomes | Nursing Actions and ***Selected Purposes/Rationales*** |
|---|---|

12.a. The client will not experience unusual bleeding as evidenced by:
1. skin and mucous membranes free of petechiae, purpura, ecchymoses, and active bleeding
2. absence of unusual joint pain
3. no increase in abdominal girth
4. absence of frank and occult blood in stool, urine, and vomitus
5. usual menstrual flow
6. usual mental status
7. vital signs within normal range for client
8. stable or improved Hct and Hb.

12.a.1. Assess client for and report signs and symptoms of unusual bleeding:
- a. petechiae, purpura, or ecchymoses
- b. gingival bleeding
- c. prolonged bleeding from puncture sites
- d. epistaxis, hemoptysis
- e. unusual joint pain
- f. increase in abdominal girth
- g. frank or occult blood in stool, urine, or vomitus
- h. menorrhagia
- i. restlessness, confusion
- j. declining B/P and increased pulse rate
- k. decline in Hct and Hb levels.

2. Monitor platelet count and coagulation test results (e.g. bleeding time). Report abnormal values.
3. If platelet count is low, coagulation test results are abnormal, or Hct and Hb levels decline, test all stools, urine, and vomitus for occult blood. Report positive results.
4. Implement measures *to prevent bleeding:*
   - a. use the smallest gauge needle possible when giving injections and performing venous and arterial punctures
   - b. apply gentle, prolonged pressure to puncture sites after injections and venous and arterial punctures
   - c. take B/P only when necessary and avoid overinflating the cuff
   - d. caution client to avoid activities that increase the risk for trauma (e.g. shaving with a straight-edge razor, using stiff-bristle toothbrush or dental floss)
   - e. avoid procedures that can cause injury to rectal mucosa (e.g. taking temperature rectally, inserting a rectal suppository, administering an enema)
   - f. pad side rails if client is confused or restless
   - g. perform actions *to reduce the risk for falls* (e.g. keep bed in low position with side rails up when client is in bed, avoid unnecessary clutter in room, instruct client to wear slippers/shoes with nonslip soles when ambulating)
   - h. instruct client to avoid blowing nose forcefully or straining to have a bowel movement; consult physician regarding an order for decongestants, stool softeners, and/or laxatives if indicated
   - i. administer the following if ordered:
     1. estrogen-progestin preparations *to suppress menses*
     2. platelets
     3. whole blood.
5. If bleeding occurs and does not subside spontaneously:
   - a. apply firm, prolonged pressure to bleeding area(s) if possible
   - b. if epistaxis occurs, place client in a high Fowler's position and apply pressure and ice pack to nasal area
   - c. maintain oxygen therapy as ordered
   - d. perform gastric lavage as ordered *to control gastric bleeding*
   - e. administer blood products as ordered
   - f. assess for and report signs and symptoms of hypovolemic shock (e.g. restlessness; confusion; significant decrease in B/P; rapid, thready pulse; rapid respirations; cool, pale skin; urine output less than 30 ml/hour)
   - g. provide emotional support to client and significant others.

12.b. The client will experience resolution of radiation cystitis if it occurs as evidenced by:

12.b.1. Assess for and report signs and symptoms of radiation cystitis (e.g. dysuria, urinary frequency and/or urgency, frank or occult blood in the urine). Acute symptoms may appear 3-4 weeks after radiation therapy is initiated and persist for 1 month following the completion of treatment.

| Desired Outcomes | Nursing Actions and ***Selected Purposes/Rationales*** |
|---|---|
| 1. decreasing complaints of dysuria and urinary frequency and urgency<br>2. absence of hematuria. | 2. If signs and symptoms of radiation cystitis occur:<br>a. implement measures *to reduce discomfort associated with cystitis:*<br>1. encourage a minimum fluid intake of 2500 ml/day *to keep urine dilute and thereby reduce further irritation of the bladder lining*<br>2. administer urinary tract analgesics, antispasmodics, and antimicrobials if ordered<br>b. assist with or perform bladder irrigations *to remove clots and maintain urinary flow*<br>c. maintain continuous bladder irrigation with silver nitrate or alum solution if ordered *to stop bleeding*<br>d. prepare client for the following if planned:<br>1. cystoscopy to cauterize bleeding vessels<br>2. intravesical instillation of formalin *to control persistent, severe bleeding*<br>e. provide emotional support to client and significant others. |

## 13. NURSING DIAGNOSIS: Self-concept disturbance*

related to:

a. changes in appearance (e.g. temporary or permanent hair loss within the treatment field; skin changes such as erythema, telangiectasia, uneven skin texture, or hyperpigmentation within the treatment field[s]; excessive weight loss);
b. possible alteration in usual sexual activities associated with:
   1. fatigue, decreased levels of testosterone (if testes are in the treatment field), psychological factors, and vaginal and/or urethral discomfort (if the lower abdomen, pelvis, or perineal area is irradiated)
   2. temporary or permanent impotence resulting from psychological factors, decreased levels of testosterone (if testes are in the treatment field), and/or pelvic nerve injury if included within the treatment field;
c. altered reproductive function:
   1. permanent sterility associated with exposure of testes or ovaries to radiation (600 cGy or more to testes or 500-600 cGy to ovaries will cause permanent sterility)
   2. potential for genetic mutations associated with sperm or ova chromosomal damage resulting from irradiation of the gonads (oophoropexy is frequently done in a woman of childbearing age to prevent ovarian exposure);
d. increased dependence on others to meet self-care needs;
e. changes in life style and roles associated with the effects of the disease process and its treatment.

*This diagnostic label includes the nursing diagnoses of body image disturbance, self-esteem disturbance, and altered role performance.

| Desired Outcome | Nursing Actions and ***Selected Purposes/Rationales*** |
|---|---|
| 13. The client will demonstrate beginning adaptation to changes in appearance, body functioning, life style, and roles as evidenced by:<br>a. verbalization of | 13.a. Assess for signs and symptoms of a self-concept disturbance (e.g. verbal or nonverbal cues denoting a negative response to changes in body functioning or appearance such as denial of or preoccupation with changes that have occurred or withdrawal from significant others).<br>b. Determine the meaning of the changes in appearance, body functioning, life style, and roles to the client by encouraging him/her to verbalize feelings and by noting nonverbal responses to changes experienced.<br>c. Implement measures to facilitate the grieving process (see Nursing Diagnosis 15, action b). |

feelings of self-worth and sexual adequacy
b. maintenance of relationships with significant others
c. active participation in activities of daily living
d. active interest in personal appearance
e. willingness to pursue usual roles and participate in social activities
f. verbalization of a beginning plan for adapting life style to meet restrictions imposed by the disease process and the residual effects of radiation therapy.

d. Discuss with client improvements in appearance and functioning that can realistically be expected.
e. Implement measures *to assist client to increase self-esteem* (e.g. limit negative self-assessment, encourage positive comments about self, assist to identify strengths, give positive feedback about accomplishments and behaviors that are indicative of high self-esteem).
f. Reinforce actions to assist client to cope with effects of radiation therapy (see Nursing Diagnosis 14, action c).
g. Implement measures *to assist client to adapt to the following changes in appearance and body functioning if appropriate:*
   1. alopecia:
      a. inform client that hair loss usually begins 2-3 weeks after initiation of therapy
      b. reassure client that regrowth of hair within the treatment field will occur within 2-3 months after cessation of therapy if the loss is temporary (temporary or patchy loss will usually occur with a radiation dose of 1500-3000 cGy; delayed hair growth or complete, permanent hair loss within the treatment field may result from a radiation exposure above 5000 cGy; explain that regrowth may be a different color, texture, and thickness)
      c. instruct the client in ways *to minimize scalp hair loss if thinning or partial hair loss is anticipated:*
         1. brush and comb hair gently
         2. wash hair only when necessary and avoid harsh shampoo, cream rinse, and other hair care products
         3. do not use hair dryers, curling irons, curlers, or constrictive decorations (e.g. clips, rubber bands) on hair
      d. encourage the client to wear a wig, scarf, or turban if desired to conceal hair loss; contact the American Cancer Society for a wig if client is unable to obtain one but desires to do so
      e. encourage use of the wig before hair loss *to facilitate adjustment to wig and its integration into body image;* caution client to remove wig several times/day to allow for exposure of treatment area to the air
   2. skin changes within the treatment field:
      a. reinforce physician's explanation about skin changes that will occur and when they can be expected
      b. suggest possible clothing styles that will make changes in skin texture and pigmentation less obvious
   3. sterility or chromosomal damage:
      a. clarify physician's explanation about probable effects of radiation therapy on the gonads if they are in the treatment field
      b. discuss alternative methods of becoming a parent (e.g. artificial insemination, adoption) if of concern to client
   4. impotence:
      a. reinforce physician's explanation about the temporary or permanent nature of impotence; if it will be permanent, encourage client to discuss various treatment options (e.g. penile prosthesis) with physician
      b. suggest alternative methods of sexual gratification if appropriate
      c. discuss ways to be creative in expressing sexuality (e.g. massage, fantasies, cuddling).
h. Assist client with usual grooming and makeup habits if necessary.
i. Assess for and support behaviors suggesting positive adaptation to changes that have occurred (e.g. interest in personal appearance, maintenance of relationships with significant others).
j. Encourage significant others to allow client to do what he/she is able *so that independence can be re-established and/or self-esteem redeveloped.*
k. Assist client's and significant others' adjustment by listening, facilitating communication, and providing information.

| Desired Outcome | Nursing Actions and ***Selected Purposes/Rationales*** |
|---|---|
| | l. Encourage visits and support from significant others.<br>m. Encourage client to pursue usual roles and interests and to continue involvement in social activities. If previous roles, interests, and hobbies cannot be pursued, encourage development of new ones.<br>n. Provide information about and encourage use of community agencies and support groups (e.g. vocational rehabilitation; sexual, family, individual, and/or financial counseling).<br>o. Consult physician about psychological counseling if client desires or if he/she seems unwilling or unable to adapt to changes resulting from cancer and radiation therapy. |

## 14. NURSING DIAGNOSIS: Ineffective individual coping

related to persistent discomfort associated with side effects of radiation therapy, chronic fatigue, fear, anxiety, uncertainty of the effectiveness of radiation therapy, and an inadequate support system.

| Desired Outcome | Nursing Actions and ***Selected Purposes/Rationales*** |
|---|---|
| 14. The client will demonstrate the use of effective coping skills as evidenced by:<br>a. verbalization of ability to cope with the diagnosis of cancer and radiation therapy and its effects<br>b. use of appropriate problem-solving techniques<br>c. willingness to participate in treatment plan and meet basic needs<br>d. absence of destructive behavior toward self and others<br>e. appropriate use of defense mechanisms<br>f. recognition and use of available support systems. | 14.a. Assess for and report signs and symptoms of ineffective individual coping (e.g. verbalization of inability to cope; inability to ask for help, problem solve, or meet basic needs; reluctance to participate in treatment plan; destructive behavior toward self or others; inappropriate use of defense mechanisms; inability to meet role expectations).<br>b. Assess client's perception of current situation including precipitating factors and effectiveness of coping mechanisms.<br>c. Implement measures *to promote effective coping:*<br>1. allow time for client to adjust psychologically to the diagnosis, radiation therapy and possible side effects, and anticipated changes in life style and roles<br>2. assist client to recognize and manage inappropriate denial if it is present<br>3. perform actions to reduce discomfort (see Nursing Diagnoses 4, action e; 5.A, action 2; and 5.B, action 2)<br>4. perform actions to reduce fear and anxiety (see Nursing Diagnosis 1, action b)<br>5. perform actions to reduce fatigue (see Nursing Diagnosis 8, action d)<br>6. encourage verbalization about current situation and ways comparable situations have been handled in the past<br>7. assist client to identify personal strengths and resources that can be used to facilitate coping with the current situation<br>8. demonstrate acceptance of client but set limits on inappropriate behavior<br>9. create an atmosphere of trust and support<br>10. arrange for a visit with another individual who has been successfully treated for cancer with radiation therapy<br>11. include client in planning of care, encourage maximum participation in treatment plan, and allow choices when possible *to enable him/her to maintain a sense of control*<br>12. instruct client in effective problem-solving techniques (e.g. accurate identification of stressors, determination of various options to solve problem) |

13. assist client to maintain usual daily routines whenever possible
14. assist client as he/she starts to plan for necessary life-style and role changes after discharge; help client to identify priorities and attainable goals
15. assist the client and significant others to identify ways that personal and family goals can be adjusted rather than abandoned
16. administer antianxiety and/or antidepressant agents if ordered
17. assist client to identify and use available support systems; provide information regarding available community resources that can assist client and significant others in coping with effects of radiation therapy and the diagnosis of cancer (e.g. American Cancer Society; support groups; individual, family and/or financial counseling)
18. discuss any difficulties client may have in meeting the schedule for radiation treatments (usually 5 days/week for 3-8 weeks depending on site, dose, and desired therapeutic effect); refer to community agencies and/or support groups if transportation is a problem
19. encourage continued emotional support from significant others
20. encourage the client to share with significant others the kind of support that would be most beneficial (e.g. listening, inspiring hope, providing reassurance and accurate information)
21. support behaviors suggesting positive adaptation to changes experienced (e.g. compliance with treatment plan, maintenance of personal appearance, verbalization of the ability to cope, use of effective problem-solving strategies).

d. Consult physician about psychological counseling if appropriate. Initiate a referral if necessary.

## 15. NURSING DIAGNOSIS: Grieving*

related to:
a. changes in body image and usual life style and roles;
b. diagnosis of cancer with potential for premature death.

*This diagnostic label includes anticipatory grieving and grieving following the actual losses.

| Desired Outcome | Nursing Actions and ***Selected Purposes/Rationales*** |
|---|---|
| 15. The client will demonstrate beginning progression through the grieving process as evidenced by:<br>a. verbalization of feelings about the diagnosis of cancer and radiation therapy and its effects<br>b. expression of grief<br>c. participation in treatment plan and self-care activities<br>d. use of available support systems<br>e. verbalization of a | 15.a. Assess for signs and symptoms of grieving (e.g. change in eating habits, inability to concentrate, insomnia, anger, noncompliance, withdrawal from significant others, denial of losses). Be aware that client's response to the diagnosis of cancer and losses experienced will be affected by factors such as previous experience with loss, age, developmental stage, available support systems, spiritual and cultural background, current health status, and significance of the diagnosis and losses to him/her.<br>b. Implement measures *to facilitate the grieving process:*<br>1. assist client to acknowledge the losses experienced *so grief work can begin;* assess for factors that may hinder and facilitate acknowledgment<br>2. discuss the grieving process and assist client to accept the phases of grieving as an expected response to actual and/or anticipated losses<br>3. allow time for client to progress through the phases of grieving (phases vary among theorists but progress from shock and alarm to acceptance); be aware that not every phase is expressed by all individuals, that recurrence of phases is common, and that the grieving process may take months to years |

| Desired Outcome | Nursing Actions and ***Selected Purposes/Rationales*** |
|---|---|
| plan for integrating prescribed follow-up care into life style. | 4. provide an atmosphere of care and concern (e.g. provide privacy, be available and nonjudgmental, display empathy and respect) *so client will feel free to verbalize feelings*<br>5. perform actions *to promote trust* (e.g. answer questions honestly, provide requested information)<br>6. encourage the verbal expression of anger and sadness about the diagnosis and losses experienced; recognize displacement of anger and assist client to see the actual cause of angry feelings and resentment<br>7. encourage client to express his/her feelings in whatever ways are comfortable (e.g. writing, drawing, conversation)<br>8. perform actions to promote effective coping (see Nursing Diagnosis 14, action c)<br>9. support realistic hope about the prognosis and the temporary nature of most of the changes in appearance<br>10. support behaviors suggesting successful grief work (e.g. verbalizing feelings about the diagnosis, expressing sorrow, focusing on ways to adapt to losses)<br>11. explain the phases of the grieving process to significant others; encourage their support and understanding<br>12. facilitate communication between the client and significant others; be aware that they may be in different phases of the grieving process<br>13. provide information regarding counseling services and support groups that might assist client in working through grief<br>14. arrange for visit from clergy if desired by client.<br>c. Consult physician about referral for counseling if signs of dysfunctional grieving (e.g. persistent denial of losses, excessive anger or sadness, hysteria, suicidal behaviors) occur. |

## 16. NURSING DIAGNOSIS: Knowledge deficit

regarding follow-up care.

| Desired Outcomes | Nursing Actions and ***Selected Purposes/Rationales*** |
|---|---|
| 16.a. The client will demonstrate the ability to perform appropriate skin care at sites of irradiation. | 16.a.1. Reinforce teaching about the expected skin reaction at the sites of irradiation (e.g. redness, tanned appearance, peeling, itching, loss of hair, decreased perspiration).<br>2. Instruct the client to:<br>a. cleanse irradiated areas gently using a mild soap and tepid water, being careful not to wash off skin markings<br>b. pat skin dry with a soft cotton towel<br>c. avoid rubbing, scratching, and massaging irradiated skin<br>d. relieve itching by:<br>1. applying cornstarch to areas of dry desquamation<br>2. adding emollients, cornstarch, baking soda, or oatmeal preparations to bath water<br>e. relieve dryness by applying A & D ointment or lanolin cream as prescribed<br>f. avoid use of deodorant if treatment field includes axilla<br>g. check with physician before using cosmetics or perfumed lotions or creams in treatment area |

h. protect irradiated skin from exposure to temperature extremes and wind
i. avoid exposure of treated skin areas to direct sunlight during treatment period and for at least 1 month after therapy is complete (burns can occur easily because melanin production in new epidermal cells is slowed)
j. wear soft cotton garments next to treatment area; use mild soap to launder clothing
k. avoid wearing tight or constrictive clothing over irradiated area in order to reduce mechanical irritation
l. avoid shaving and using tape within treatment field; use an electric razor if shaving is absolutely necessary
m. care for a moist desquamation reaction by:
   1. performing wound care and applying sterile dressings as prescribed (stretchable netting should be used instead of tape to hold dressings in place)
   2. exposing area to the air as much as possible.

3. Demonstrate care of treatment sites.
4. Allow time for questions, clarification, and return demonstration of skin and wound care.

16.b. The client will identify techniques to control nausea and vomiting.

16.b. Instruct client in the following techniques to control nausea and vomiting:
1. cleanse mouth frequently
2. avoid offensive odors and sights
3. avoid eating and food aromas 3 hours before and after treatments
4. eat several small meals/day instead of 3 large ones
5. eat the largest meal 3-4 hours before treatments and eat lightly for the rest of the day if nausea peaks after treatments
6. eat foods that are cool or at room temperature (hot foods frequently have an overpowering aroma that stimulates nausea)
7. eat dry foods (e.g. toast, crackers) or sour foods (e.g. lemon drops, pickles, lemon ice) or sip cold carbonated beverages if nausea is present
8. select bland foods (e.g. mashed potatoes, applesauce, cottage cheese) rather than fatty, spicy foods (e.g. fried potatoes, chili)
9. if feasible, have someone else prepare the food
10. avoid drinking liquids with meals
11. rest after eating
12. take deep, slow breaths when nauseated
13. follow prescribed antiemetic regimen if nausea is continuous.

16.c. The client will verbalize ways to improve appetite and nutritional status.

16.c. Instruct client in ways to improve appetite and maintain an adequate nutritional status:
1. try chicken, fish, cheese, and eggs as protein sources instead of beef and pork if taste distortion is a problem
2. increase the amount of sweeteners and seasonings usually used in foods or beverages
3. moisten dry foods with sauces, salad dressing, or sour cream
4. eat in a pleasant environment with company if possible
5. perform frequent oral hygiene to eliminate disagreeable tastes in mouth
6. try recommended methods of controlling nausea (see action b in this diagnosis)
7. increase intake of high-protein, high-calorie foods
8. eat several high-calorie, nutritious small meals rather than 3 large ones
9. take vitamins and minerals as prescribed.

16.d. The client will identify ways to reduce the risk of

16.d.1. Inform client that dental caries and periodontal disease can occur months to years after irradiation of the jaw, neck, or oral cavity.

| Desired Outcomes | Nursing Actions and ***Selected Purposes/Rationales*** |
|---|---|
| dental caries and periodontal disease and demonstrate appropriate oral hygiene techniques. | Emphasize that a meticulous daily oral hygiene program is essential, particularly if salivary flow is permanently reduced.<br>2. Instruct client in ways to reduce the risk of dental caries and periodontal disease:<br>a. use appropriate technique for cleansing teeth<br>b. brush teeth with a fluoridated toothpaste or fluoride gel (e.g. stannous fluoride 0.4%) several times a day for 3-4 minutes, particularly after eating<br>c. use a small, soft, flexible toothbrush<br>d. rinse with a topical fluoride solution (e.g. Fluorigard, Karigel) after brushing<br>e. use a dental and fluoride gel daily as ordered until salivary gland function has returned to normal.<br>3. If stomatitis is present, instruct client to:<br>a. irrigate mouth and cleanse teeth frequently with a gentle power spray using saline solution or water instead of brushing<br>b. rinse mouth every 4 hours with a baking soda and water solution followed by a thorough rinsing with saline if tenacious mucus, crusting, and/or debris are present.<br>4. Allow time for questions, clarification, and practice of oral hygiene techniques.<br>5. Instruct client to discuss any planned dental care with the radiologist and to inform the dentist that he/she is receiving or has had radiation to the oral cavity. |
| 16.e. The client will identify ways to prevent bleeding if platelet counts are low. | 16.e.1. Instruct client in ways to minimize the risk of bleeding:<br>a. avoid taking aspirin, aspirin-containing compounds, and ibuprofen<br>b. use an electric rather than a straight-edge razor<br>c. floss and brush teeth gently<br>d. cut nails carefully<br>e. use caution when ambulating to prevent falls or bumps<br>f. avoid blowing nose forcefully<br>g. avoid situations that could result in injury (e.g. contact sports)<br>h. avoid straining to have a bowel movement<br>i. avoid wearing constrictive clothing<br>j. use an ample amount of water-soluble lubricant prior to sexual intercourse and avoid anal sexual activity, douching, use of rectal suppositories, and enemas in order to prevent trauma to the mucous membranes<br>k. avoid heavy lifting.<br>2. Instruct client to control any bleeding by applying firm, prolonged pressure to the area(s) if possible. |
| 16.f. The client will identify ways to prevent infection if WBC counts are low. | 16.f.1. Explain to client that his/her resistance to infection is reduced when WBC counts are low. Emphasize the need to adhere closely to recommended techniques to prevent infection.<br>2. Instruct client in ways to prevent infection:<br>a. avoid crowds, persons with any sign of infection, and persons who have recently been vaccinated<br>b. avoid trauma to the skin and mucous membranes<br>c. take an axillary rather than an oral temperature if stomatitis is present<br>d. lubricate the skin outside irradiated area frequently to prevent dryness and subsequent cracking<br>e. cleanse and care for skin within treatment field as recommended (see action a.2 in this diagnosis)<br>f. use excellent handwashing technique<br>g. avoid unnecessary rectal invasion (e.g. temperature taking, enemas, suppositories, sexual activity) to prevent rectal trauma |

h. if hemorrhoids are present, avoid situations that could aggravate them (e.g. constipation, sitting for prolonged periods)
i. avoid constipation to prevent trauma to the rectal mucosa from hard or impacted stool
j. wash perianal area thoroughly with soap and water after each bowel movement and after sexual activity; inform female client to always wipe from front to back after defecating and urinating
k. avoid douching unless ordered (douching disturbs the normal vaginal flora and may cause trauma to the vaginal mucosa)
l. drink at least 10 glasses of liquid/day
m. cough and deep breathe or use incentive spirometer every 2 hours until usual activity level is resumed
n. stop smoking
o. perform meticulous oral hygiene as directed
p. maintain an optimal nutritional status (e.g. diet high in protein, calories, vitamins, and minerals)
q. avoid intake of foods with a high bacteria content (e.g. fresh fruit, uncooked foods)
r. avoid sharing eating utensils
s. maintain an adequate balance between activity and rest.

16.g. The client will verbalize an understanding of and ways to manage the effects of radiation therapy on sexual and reproductive functioning.

16.g.1. Clarify physician's explanation about the possible effects of irradiation on the gonads if included in the treatment field(s).
2. Assure client that many of the effects of radiation therapy on sexual and reproductive functioning are temporary or can be treated.
3. Explain that a temporary decrease in libido may occur as a result of radiation treatment.
4. Encourage client to rest before sexual activity if fatigue is a problem.
5. Instruct client in measures to decrease discomfort associated with decreased vaginal secretions and mucositis:
   a. use an ample amount of water-soluble lubricant to prevent trauma to the vaginal mucosa and increase lubrication during intercourse
   b. use a vaginal steroid cream if prescribed to ease dryness and inflammation
   c. take a sitz bath 2-3 times a day (this is contraindicated during the treatment period if the perineal area is in the treatment field)
   d. avoid intercourse until mucositis of the vaginal canal and/or urethra resolves
   e. have partner use a condom during intercourse to prevent contact of vaginal area with semen (semen can cause a burning sensation in the early months after vaginal irradiation).
6. Emphasize the need for frequent intercourse or vaginal dilatation once mucositis has resolved to prevent stenosis of the vaginal canal (may occur several weeks or months after cessation of treatment that includes the vaginal area).
7. Explain to the female client that ovarian failure during therapy may result in decreased libido, irritability, hot flashes, and other symptoms of premature menopause.
8. Inform the female client that her usual menstrual cycle will resume within 6 months to 1 year after treatment if sterility is temporary.
9. Emphasize the need for both male and female clients to practice birth control during treatment and for at least 2 years after it. Encourage both male and female clients to seek genetic counseling before attempting conception to ascertain the risk of chromosomal anomalies.
10. Instruct client to take hormone replacements as prescribed.

16.h. The client will verbalize ways to manage and cope with persistent fatigue.

16.h. Instruct client in ways to manage and cope with persistent fatigue:
1. view fatigue as a protective mechanism rather than a problematic limitation
2. determine ways that daily patterns of activity can be modified to conserve energy and prevent excessive fatigue (e.g. spread light and

| Desired Outcomes | Nursing Actions and ***Selected Purposes/Rationales*** |
|---|---|
| | heavy tasks throughout the day, take short rests during an activity whenever possible, take several short rest periods during the day instead of one long one)<br>3. determine if life demands are realistic in light of physical state and adjust short- and long-term goals accordingly<br>4. avoid situations that are particularly fatiguing such as those that are boring, frustrating, or require prolonged or strenuous physical activity<br>5. participate in a regular aerobic exercise program to improve cardiovascular and respiratory fitness, reduce anxiety and stress, and build up tolerance for activity. |
| 16.i. The client will state signs and symptoms to report to the health care provider. | 16.i. Instruct the client to observe for and report the following:<br>1. signs and symptoms of infection (stress that the usual signs of infection are diminished in people with a suppressed immune system and that it is necessary to monitor closely for the following signs and symptoms):<br>a. temperature above 38° C (100.4° F)<br>b. changes in odor, color, or consistency of urine or pain on urination<br>c. white patches in mouth or vagina<br>d. crusted ulcerations around or in oral cavity<br>e. swollen, reddened, coated tongue<br>f. painful rectal or vaginal area<br>g. redness, increased pain, or bleeding of hemorrhoids<br>h. changes in appearance or temperature of the skin, particularly around puncture sites<br>i. persistent or productive cough<br>j. unusual odor or drainage from treatment area<br>2. signs and symptoms of bleeding (e.g. excessive bruising, black stools, persistent nosebleeds or bleeding from gums, sudden swelling in joints, red or smoke-colored urine, blood in vomitus)<br>3. signs and symptoms of radiation cystitis (e.g. blood in the urine, pain on urination, urinary frequency or urgency)<br>4. signs and symptoms of radiation pneumonitis (e.g. shortness of breath; persistent, dry, hacking cough; fever); radiation pneumonitis can occur 2-3 months after cessation of treatment depending on total dose of radiation received, fractionation of dose, and volume of lung tissue within the treatment field<br>5. signs and symptoms of tissue fibrosis within treatment field (e.g. **LUNG**: increasing shortness of breath, cough, hemoptysis; **BOWEL**: inability to move bowels, distended abdomen, loss of appetite, alternating diarrhea and constipation; **ESOPHAGUS**: difficulty swallowing; **SKIN**: uneven texture; **VAGINA**: pain during intercourse)<br>6. excessive tooth decay<br>7. signs and symptoms of dehydration (e.g. dry mouth, weight loss, concentrated urine)<br>8. persistent nausea, vomiting, or decreased oral intake<br>9. significant weight loss<br>10. persistent diarrhea<br>11. increased pain in irradiated area<br>12. excessive depression or difficulty coping with the effects of the diagnosis and treatment. |
| 16.j. The client will identify community resources that can assist with home management and adjustment to the diagnosis of cancer | 16.j.1. Provide information about and encourage use of community resources that can assist the client and significant others with home management and adjustment to cancer and the effects of radiation therapy (e.g. local support groups, American Cancer Society, home health agencies, counselors, social service agencies, Meals on Wheels, Make Today Count, Hospice).<br>2. Initiate a referral if indicated. |

| Desired Outcomes | Nursing Actions and ***Selected Purposes/Rationales*** |
|---|---|
| and radiation therapy and its effects. | |
| 16.k. The client will verbalize an understanding of and a plan for adhering to recommended follow-up care including medications prescribed and future appointments with health care provider, radiation department, and laboratory. | 16.k.1. Explain the rationale for, side effects of, and importance of taking medications prescribed.<br>2. Reinforce physician's explanation of planned radiation therapy schedule.<br>3. Discuss with client any difficulties he/she might have adhering to the schedule and assist in planning ways to overcome these.<br>4. Reinforce the importance of keeping appointments for radiation treatments and follow-up laboratory studies.<br>5. Reinforce the importance of keeping follow-up appointments with health care provider.<br>6. Implement measures to improve client compliance:<br>a. include significant others in teaching sessions<br>b. encourage questions and allow time for reinforcement and clarification of information provided<br>c. provide written instructions regarding future appointments with health care provider, radiation department, and laboratory; medications prescribed; and signs and symptoms to report. |

UNIT
# VIII

# *Nursing Care of the Client with Disturbances of Neurological Function*

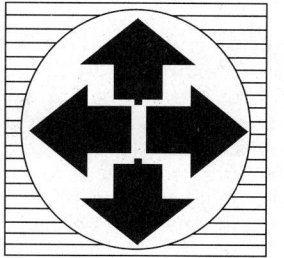

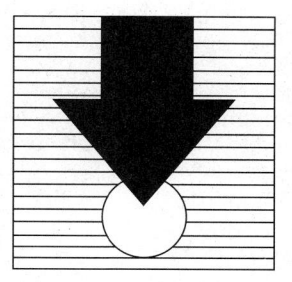

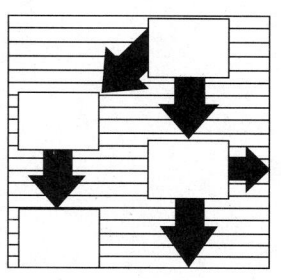

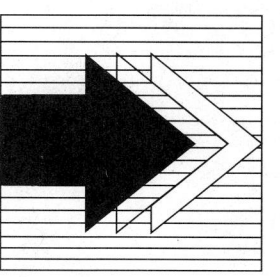

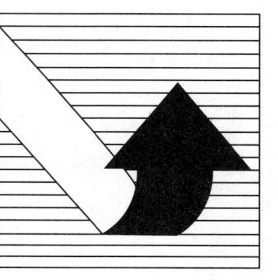

# Cerebrovascular Accident

A cerebrovascular accident (CVA), or stroke, is the result of an interruption in the blood supply to certain parts of the brain and is characterized by the sudden development of focal neurological deficits that last for at least 24 hours. These deficits range from mild symptoms such as tingling, weakness, and slight speech impairment to severe symptoms such as hemiplegia, aphasia, and visual field cuts. The type and extensiveness of neurological deficits that a client experiences depend on the particular area(s) of the brain affected by the ischemia and by the subsequent development of cerebral edema or cerebral necrosis.

Cerebrovascular accidents are classified according to etiology. The most common cause is a thrombosis that is most frequently associated with atherosclerosis. Thrombotic strokes are classified according to their stage of development (i.e. stroke in evolution [neurological deficits that continue to worsen over a period of a few days], completed stroke [neurological deficits that remain unchanged after 2 to 3 days]). Other causes of a CVA include an embolus; cerebral hemorrhage; generalized hypoxia (can occur with severe hypotension or severely decreased cardiac output resulting from conditions such as arrhythmias); and cerebral vessel spasm, constriction, or compression. Treatment following a CVA is determined by the etiology and the neurological deficits that are present.

**This care plan focuses on the adult client hospitalized with signs and symptoms of a CVA.** During the acute phase, the goals of care are to improve cerebral tissue perfusion, prevent life-threatening complications, and perform or assist the client with those activities he/she is unable to accomplish independently. The goals of care during the rehabilitation phase are to prevent complications and assist the client to attain an optimal level of functioning. This care plan focuses on the most common deficits that occur as a result of a CVA. The reader should refer to neurological texts for further information about the various speech, motor, and sensory deficits than can occur.

## DIAGNOSTIC TESTS

Carotid ultrasound
Computed tomography (CT)
Magnetic resonance imaging (MRI)
Electroencephalogram (EEG)
Cerebral angiography
Visual field examination
Positron emission tomography (PET)

## DISCHARGE CRITERIA

Prior to discharge, the client will:

- have improved cerebral tissue perfusion
- have improved or stable neurological function
- communicate an awareness of ways to decrease the risk of a recurrent CVA
- identify ways to manage sensory and verbal communication impairments and altered thought processes
- identify ways to manage urinary and bowel incontinence
- demonstrate measures to facilitate the performance of activities of daily living and increase physical mobility
- communicate an awareness of signs and symptoms to report to the health care provider
- share thoughts and feelings about the effects of the CVA on life style, roles, and self-concept
- communicate knowledge of community agencies that can assist with home management and adjustment to changes resulting from the CVA
- communicate an understanding of and a plan for adhering to recommended follow-up care including future appointments with health care provider and therapists and medications prescribed.

**Use in conjunction with the Care Plan on Immobility.**

**NURSING/ COLLABORATIVE DIAGNOSES**



**See Care Plan on Immobility for additional diagnoses.**

## 1. NURSING DIAGNOSIS: Altered cerebral tissue perfusion

related to decreased cerebral blood flow associated with thrombus, embolus, cerebral hemorrhage, and/or spasm or compression of cerebral vessel(s).

| Desired Outcome | Nursing Actions and ***Selected Purposes/Rationales*** |
|---|---|
| 1. The client will experience improved cerebral tissue perfusion as evidenced by:<br>a. absence of or reduction in dizziness, visual disturbances, and/or speech impairments<br>b. improved mental status<br>c. improved sensory and motor function. | 1.a. Assess the client for signs and symptoms of decreased cerebral tissue perfusion:<br>1. dizziness<br>2. visual disturbances (e.g. blurred or dimmed vision, diplopia, change in visual field)<br>3. aphasia<br>4. irritability and restlessness<br>5. decreased level of consciousness<br>6. paresthesias, paresis, paralysis.<br>b. Implement measures *to improve cerebral tissue perfusion:*<br>1. if a thrombus or embolus is present, administer the following medications if ordered:<br>a. anticoagulants (e.g. heparin, warfarin)<br>b. antiplatelet agents (e.g. aspirin) |

| Desired Outcome | Nursing Actions and ***Selected Purposes/Rationales*** |
|---|---|
| | 2. if intracerebral hemorrhage occurred as a result of cerebral aneurysm rupture, administer a hemostatic agent (e.g. aminocaproic acid) if ordered *to prevent the lysis of formed clots and subsequent rebleeding*<br>3. administer calcium-channel blockers (e.g. nimodipine) if ordered *to reduce cerebral vasospasm (the calcium that is released by the injured neural cells can cause vasospasm)*<br>4. perform actions to prevent and treat increased intracranial pressure (see Collaborative Diagnosis 17, actions a.2 and 3)<br>5. prepare client for surgery (e.g. evacuation of hematoma, repair of ruptured aneurysm) if planned.<br>c. Consult physician if signs and symptoms of decreased cerebral tissue perfusion worsen. |

## 2. NURSING DIAGNOSIS: Altered nutrition: less than body requirements

related to decreased oral intake associated with:

a. anorexia resulting from fear, anxiety, depression, and early satiety that occurs with decreased gastrointestinal motility (can result from decreased activity and anxiety);
b. difficulty feeding self as a result of impaired motor function of the affected arm, visual impairments, and/or spatial-perceptual difficulties;
c. difficulty chewing resulting from paresis or paralysis of the muscles of mastication on the affected side;
d. dysphagia.

| Desired Outcome | Nursing Actions and ***Selected Purposes/Rationales*** |
|---|---|
| 2. The client will maintain an adequate nutritional status (see Care Plan on Immobility, Nursing Diagnosis 3 [pp. 140-141], for outcome criteria). | 2.a. Refer to Care Plan on Immobility, Nursing Diagnosis 3 (pp. 140-141), for measures related to assessment and maintenance of an adequate nutritional status.<br>b. Implement additional measures *to improve oral intake and maintain an adequate nutritional status:*<br>1. perform actions to reduce fear and anxiety (see Nursing Diagnosis 19, actions b and c)<br>2. perform actions to facilitate client's psychological adjustment to the effects of the CVA (see Nursing Diagnoses 20, actions d-v; 21, action c; and 22, action b)<br>3. perform actions to prevent constipation (see Nursing Diagnosis 11) *in order to reduce feeling of fullness*<br>4. perform actions to improve ability to swallow (see Nursing Diagnosis 3, action c)<br>5. perform actions to enable client to feed self (see Nursing Diagnosis 9, action b.3). |

## 3. NURSING DIAGNOSIS: Impaired swallowing

related to paresis or paralysis of the muscles of deglutition on the affected side and diminished or absent swallowing reflex.

| Desired Outcome | Nursing Actions and ***Selected Purposes/Rationales*** |
|---|---|
| 3. The client will experience an improvement in swallowing as evidenced by:<br>a. communication of same<br>b. absence of food in oral cavity after swallowing<br>c. absence of coughing and choking when eating and drinking. | 3.a. Assess for signs and symptoms of impaired swallowing (e.g. communication of difficulty swallowing, stasis of food in oral cavity, coughing or choking when eating or drinking).<br>b. Assist with studies that evaluate client's ability to swallow (e.g. videofluoroscopy, manometry) if indicated.<br>c. Implement measures *to improve ability to swallow:*<br>1. place client in high Fowler's position for meals and snacks; head and neck should be tilted forward slightly *to facilitate elevation of the larynx and posterior movement of the tongue*<br>2. assist client to select foods that require little or no chewing and are easily swallowed (e.g. custard, eggs, canned fruit, mashed potatoes)<br>3. instruct client to avoid mixing foods of different texture in his/her mouth at the same time<br>4. avoid serving foods that are sticky (e.g. peanut butter, soft bread, bananas)<br>5. serve foods/fluids that are hot or cold instead of room temperature *(the more extreme temperatures stimulate the sensory receptors and swallowing reflex)*<br>6. serve thick fluids or thicken thin fluids with substances such as "Thick-it," gelatin, or baby cereal<br>7. moisten dry foods with gravy or sauces (e.g. catsup, salad dressing, sour cream)<br>8. utilize assistive devices (e.g. long-handled spoon) to place food in back of mouth on unaffected side if tongue movement is impaired<br>9. instruct client to avoid putting too much food/fluid in mouth at one time<br>10. encourage client to concentrate on the act of swallowing<br>11. if client has decreased lip control, instruct him/her to close lips with hand before swallowing<br>12. gently stroke client's throat when he/she is swallowing if indicated<br>13. consult speech pathologist or therapist about methods for dealing with impaired swallowing; reinforce recommended exercises and techniques.<br>d. Consult physician if swallowing difficulties persist or worsen. |

## 4. NURSING DIAGNOSIS: Sensory/perceptual alterations:

a. **visual** related to ischemia of visual pathways;
b. **kinesthetic** related to spatial-perceptual impairments associated with visual deficits and ischemia of portions of the nondominant cerebral hemisphere.

| Desired Outcome | Nursing Actions and ***Selected Purposes/Rationales*** |
|---|---|
| 4. The client will experience a reduction in and/or demonstrate beginning adaptation to sensory/perceptual alterations as evidenced by:<br>a. communication of same | 4.a. Assess for signs and symptoms of:<br>1. visual impairments such as homonymous hemianopsia and/or diplopia (e.g. lack of response to visual stimuli on side of hemiplegia, complaints of double vision, decreased participation in activities)<br>2. kinesthetic impairment (e.g. difficulty buttoning clothing, placing self in an upright position, or locating mouth when trying to feed self; decreased participation in activities).<br>b. Implement measures to improve cerebral tissue perfusion (see Nursing Diagnosis 1, action b) *in order to reduce cerebral ischemia.* |

| Desired Outcome | Nursing Actions and ***Selected Purposes/Rationales*** |
|---|---|
| b. increased participation in activities. | c. Implement measures *to assist client to adapt to changes in visual and/or kinesthetic functioning:*<br>1. provide an eyepatch or frosted lens for client to wear if diplopia is present<br>2. if client is experiencing homonymous hemianopsia:<br>a. position bed so that client receives the greatest amount of visual stimuli (e.g. when client is in bed, the door rather than a wall should be within his/her visual field)<br>b. after condition has stabilized, place items (e.g. television, clock, calendar, pictures) on affected side *to promote environmental scanning*<br>3. if client is experiencing kinesthetic impairments, place him/her in front of a full-length mirror during activities when possible after condition has stabilized *(viewing his/her reflection helps the client to identify vertical and horizontal planes)*<br>4. perform actions to facilitate performance of self-care activities (see Nursing Diagnosis 9, actions b.3 and 4).<br>d. Consult physician if sensory/perceptual alterations worsen or client is unable to adapt to the ones he/she is experiencing. |

## 5. NURSING DIAGNOSIS: Unilateral neglect

related to ischemia of portions of the nondominant cerebral hemisphere (usually the right hemisphere).

| Desired Outcome | Nursing Actions and ***Selected Purposes/Rationales*** |
|---|---|
| 5. The client will experience a gradual reduction in and/or demonstrate beginning adaptation to unilateral neglect as evidenced by:<br>a. awareness of stimuli on affected side<br>b. awareness of the affected side of body. | 5.a. Assess client for presence of unilateral neglect (e.g. not looking toward affected side, no response to stimuli on affected side, lack of awareness of affected extremities).<br>b. Implement measures to improve cerebral tissue perfusion (see Nursing Diagnosis 1, action b) *in order to reduce cerebral ischemia.*<br>c. If unilateral neglect is present:<br>1. ensure that affected extremities are positioned properly at all times<br>2. protect affected extremities from injury<br>3. after client's condition stabilizes, implement measures *to increase client's awareness of affected side:*<br>a. encourage client to handle affected extremities when bathing, dressing, and repositioning self<br>b. place some items (e.g. television, clock, calendar, pictures) on affected side *to increase the likelihood of the client viewing his/her affected extremities*<br>c. place familiar items (e.g. his/her favorite bracelet or watch, frequently worn shoe or slipper) on affected extremities *to assist client to recognize that the extremities are a part of his/her body*<br>4. consult physical and occupational therapists about additional ways to facilitate client's adaptation to unilateral neglect<br>5. inform significant others and health care personnel of approaches being used to increase client's awareness of affected side; encourage their use of these techniques<br>6. consult physician if client is unable to begin to adapt to unilateral neglect. |

## 6. NURSING DIAGNOSIS: Impaired verbal communication

related to:

a. loss of function of the muscles used to produce speech;
b. ischemia in the dominant cerebral hemisphere (ischemia of Wernicke's area in the temporoparietal lobe will result in receptive aphasia; ischemia of Broca's area in the frontal lobe will result in expressive aphasia).

| Desired Outcome | Nursing Actions and ***Selected Purposes/Rationales*** |
|---|---|
| 6. The client will communicate needs and desires effectively. | 6.a. Assess client for impaired verbal communication (e.g. inability to speak, difficulty forming words or sentences, difficulty expressing thoughts verbally, inappropriate verbalization). Validate verbal responses with an assessment of nonverbal behavior *in order to determine if client is experiencing receptive aphasia.*<br>b. Implement measures *to facilitate communication:*<br>1. answer call signal in person rather than using the intercommunication system<br>2. maintain a patient, calm approach; listen attentively and allow ample time for communication<br>3. maintain a calm, quiet environment *so that client can concentrate on communication efforts, does not have to speak loudly, and is able to hear others clearly*<br>4. ask questions that require short answers, eyeblinks, or nod of head if client is having difficulty speaking and/or is frustrated or fatigued<br>5. schedule rest periods before visiting hours and speech therapy sessions *to maximize communication ability during those times*<br>6. when speaking to client, face him/her; speak slowly; use direct, short statements; repeat key words; and avoid using unrelated gestures<br>7. provide materials such as magic slate, pad and pencil, word cards, and/or picture board if appropriate; try to ensure that placement of intravenous line does not interfere with use of these communication aids<br>8. consult speech pathologist regarding methods for dealing with speech impairments; reinforce exercises and techniques recommended.<br>c. Inform significant others and health care personnel of techniques being used to facilitate client's ability to communicate. Stress the importance of consistent use of these techniques.<br>d. Encourage significant others and staff to talk to client even if he/she is unresponsive or unable to communicate.<br>e. Consult physician if client experiences increasing impairment of verbal communication. |

## 7. NURSING DIAGNOSIS: High risk for impaired skin integrity

related to:

a. ischemia of the skin and subcutaneous tissue associated with prolonged pressure on tissues as a result of decreased mobility;
b. damage to the skin and/or subcutaneous tissue associated with friction or shearing;
c. increased fragility of the skin associated with dependent edema and inadequate nutritional status;
d. frequent contact of the skin with irritants associated with urinary and/or bowel incontinence.

| Desired Outcome | Nursing Actions and ***Selected Purposes/Rationales*** |
|---|---|
| 7. The client will maintain skin integrity as evidenced by:<br>a. absence of redness and irritation<br>b. no skin breakdown. | 7.a. Refer to Care Plan on Immobility, Nursing Diagnosis 4 (pp. 141-142), for measures related to assessment, prevention, and treatment of skin breakdown.<br>b. Implement additional measures *to prevent skin breakdown:*<br>1. perform actions *to prevent skin irritation resulting from incontinence:*<br>a. implement measures to reduce the risk of urinary and bowel incontinence (see Nursing Diagnoses 10, action b and 12, action b)<br>b. assist client to thoroughly cleanse and dry perineal area with soft tissue or cloth after each episode of incontinence; apply a protective ointment or cream (e.g. Desitin, A & D ointment, Vaseline)<br>c. apply a drainable fecal collector if bowel incontinence is a persistent problem<br>d. provide incontinence pads if needed to absorb moisture; do not allow skin to come in contact with plastic portion of the pads<br>2. perform actions to maintain an adequate nutritional status (see Nursing Diagnosis 2). |

## 8. NURSING DIAGNOSIS: Impaired physical mobility

related to:

a. activity limitations associated with decreased motor function and spatial-perceptual impairments;
b. loss of muscle tone during period of flaccidity of affected extremities (flaccid paralysis may be present during the first few days following a CVA);
c. hypertonia of affected extremities (as muscle tone returns after period of flaccidity, it often progresses to spasticity);
d. reluctance to move associated with fear of injuring self (occurs mainly with ischemia of the dominant hemisphere);
e. loss of muscle mass, tone, and strength associated with prolonged disuse and inadequate nutritional status.

| Desired Outcome | Nursing Actions and ***Selected Purposes/Rationales*** |
|---|---|
| 8. The client will achieve maximum physical mobility within limitations imposed by the CVA. | 8.a. Refer to Care Plan on Immobility, Nursing Diagnosis 6 (p. 144), for measures related to ways to increase mobility.<br>b. Implement additional measures *to increase mobility:*<br>1. provide adequate rest periods before activity sessions<br>2. administer muscle relaxants (e.g. baclofen, dantrolene) if ordered *to relieve spasticity in affected extremities*<br>3. perform actions to prevent falls (see Nursing Diagnosis 15, action a.1) *in order to decrease client's fear of injury*<br>4. instruct client in and assist with use of mobility aids (e.g. cane, walker) if appropriate<br>5. after client's condition has stabilized, assist with and reinforce the following if appropriate:<br>a. neurophysiologic and neurodevelopmental concept application (e.g. Bobath approach) *to promote more normal movement of the affected extremities*<br>b. neuromuscular re-education techniques (e.g. electromyographic biofeedback) *to improve muscle strength and reduce spasticity of the affected extremities* |

6. perform actions to maintain an adequate nutritional status (see Nursing Diagnosis 2) *in order to maintain muscle mass, tone, and strength.*

c. Provide praise and encouragement for all efforts to increase physical mobility.

d. Encourage the support of significant others. Allow them to assist with range of motion exercises, positioning, and activity if desired.

e. Consult physician if client is unable to achieve expected level of mobility or if range of motion becomes restricted.

## 9. NURSING DIAGNOSIS: Self-care deficit

related to impaired physical mobility, visual and spatial-perceptual impairments, apraxia, unilateral neglect, and altered thought processes.

| Desired Outcome | Nursing Actions and ***Selected Purposes/Rationales*** |
|---|---|
| 9. The client will perform self-care activities within physical limitations. | 9.a. Refer to Care Plan on Immobility, Nursing Diagnosis 7 (pp. 141-145), for measures to facilitate client's ability to perform self-care activities.<br>b. Implement additional measures *to facilitate client's ability to perform self-care activities:*<br>1. if apraxia is present, explain and demonstrate use of items such as toothbrush, comb, and washcloth as often as necessary<br>2. encourage client to wear eyepatch or frosted lens if diplopia is present<br>3. perform actions *to enable client to feed self:*<br>a. place foods/fluids within client's visual field until he/she learns to effectively utilize scanning techniques<br>b. place only a few items on the tray at one time if spatial-perceptual deficits are present<br>c. identify where items are placed on the plate and tray and open containers, cut meat, and butter bread as indicated<br>d. consult with occupational therapist about assistive devices available (e.g. broad-handled utensils, rocker knives, plate guards); reinforce use of these devices<br>4. perform actions *to enable client to dress self when condition is stabilized:*<br>a. encourage use of assistive devices such as button hooks, long-handled shoehorns, and pull loops for pants<br>b. encourage client to select clothing that is easy to put on and remove (e.g. clothing with zippers rather than buttons, loose-fitting clothing, shoes with Velcro fasteners rather than laces)<br>c. if client has difficulty distinguishing right from left, mark outer aspect of shoes with tape or label with R or L<br>5. perform actions to increase mobility (see Nursing Diagnosis 8) *in order to further facilitate the client's ability to perform self-care activities*<br>6. reinforce exercises and activities recommended by the occupational therapist to improve fine motor skills.<br>c. Provide positive feedback for all efforts and accomplishments of self-care.<br>d. Assist the client with activities he/she is unable to perform independently.<br>e. Inform significant others of client's abilities to perform own care. Explain importance of encouraging and allowing client to maintain an optimal level of independence. |

## 10. NURSING DIAGNOSIS: Altered urinary elimination: incontinence

related to:

a. increased reflex activity of the bladder and loss of voluntary control of urinary elimination associated with upper motor neuron involvement if it has occurred;
b. decreased ability to control urination associated with decreased level of consciousness or inability to recognize sensation of bladder fullness;
c. inability to get to bedside commode or bathroom in a timely manner associated with:
   1. delay in obtaining assistance resulting from inability to communicate the urge to urinate
   2. impaired physical mobility.

| Desired Outcome | Nursing Actions and ***Selected Purposes/Rationales*** |
|---|---|
| 10. The client will experience urinary continence. | 10.a. Assess for and report urinary incontinence.<br>b. Implement measures *to reduce the risk of urinary incontinence:*<br>1. offer bedpan or urinal or assist client to bedside commode or bathroom every 2-3 hours<br>2. allow client to assume a normal position for voiding unless contraindicated *in order to promote complete bladder emptying*<br>3. provide easy access to bathroom and assist client to select clothing that is easy to remove (e.g. pajamas with Velcro closures or elastic waistband) *in order to reduce delays in toileting*<br>4. if client is aphasic, establish an effective method for him/her to communicate the urge to urinate<br>5. instruct client to space fluids evenly throughout the day rather than drinking a large quantity at one time *(rapid filling of bladder can result in incontinence if client has decreased urinary sphincter control)*<br>6. limit oral fluid intake in the evening *to decrease possibility of nighttime incontinence*<br>7. instruct client to avoid drinking beverages containing caffeine *(caffeine is a mild diuretic and may make urinary control more difficult)*<br>8. if client is experiencing severe bladder spasticity, administer sympathomimetics (e.g. ephedrine) if ordered *to relax the detrusor muscle and increase the tone of the urinary sphincter.*<br>c. If urinary incontinence persists, consult physician about intermittent catheterization, insertion of indwelling catheter, or use of external catheter. |

## 11. NURSING DIAGNOSIS: Constipation

related to:

a. decreased gastrointestinal motility associated with decreased activity and the increased sympathetic nervous system activity that occurs with anxiety;
b. decreased intake of fluids and foods high in fiber associated with difficulty feeding self, chewing, and swallowing;
c. failure to respond to the urge to defecate associated with decreased level of consciousness or inability to recognize sensation of rectal fullness;
d. weakened abdominal muscles associated with generalized loss of muscle tone resulting from prolonged immobility.

| Desired Outcome | Nursing Actions and ***Selected Purposes/Rationales*** |
| --- | --- |
| 11. The client will not experience constipation (see Care Plan on Immobility, Nursing Diagnosis 9 [p. 146], for outcome criteria). | 11.a. Refer to Care Plan on Immobility, Nursing Diagnosis 9 (p. 146), for measures related to assessment, prevention, and management of constipation.<br>b. Implement additional measures *to prevent constipation:*<br>1. establish a routine time for defecation based on client's usual bowel elimination pattern<br>2. perform or, as the rehabilitation program progresses, assist client with digital stimulation of the rectum if indicated<br>3. perform actions to improve oral intake (see Nursing Diagnosis 2) *in order to increase intake of fluids and foods high in fiber.* |

## 12. NURSING DIAGNOSIS: Bowel incontinence

related to:

a. increased reflex activity of the bowel and loss of voluntary control of bowel elimination associated with upper motor neuron involvement if it has occurred;
b. decreased ability to control defecation associated with decreased level of consciousness or inability to recognize sensation of rectal fullness;
c. inability to get to bedside commode or bathroom in a timely manner associated with:
   1. delay in obtaining assistance resulting from inability to communicate need to defecate
   2. impaired physical mobility.

| Desired Outcome | Nursing Actions and ***Selected Purposes/Rationales*** |
| --- | --- |
| 12. The client will not experience bowel incontinence. | 12.a. Monitor for episodes of bowel incontinence.<br>b. Implement measures *to reduce the risk of bowel incontinence:*<br>1. initiate a bowel training program *so that the client will evacuate the lower colon at regularly scheduled intervals*<br>2. have commode or bedpan readily available to client<br>3. if client is aphasic, establish an effective method for him/her to communicate the urge to defecate<br>4. remove fecal impaction if present *(continuous stimulation of the defecation reflex by the fecal mass inhibits the internal anal sphincter and results in loss of ability to retain the mucus and fluid that collects proximal to and leaks around the fecal mass).*<br>c. If bowel incontinence persists, consult physician about revision of bowel training program. |

## 13. NURSING DIAGNOSIS: Altered thought processes

related to impaired cerebral functioning associated with cerebral ischemia.

| Desired Outcome | Nursing Actions and ***Selected Purposes/Rationales*** |
|---|---|
| 13. The client will experience improvement in thought processes as evidenced by:<br>a. improved attention span, memory, and problem-solving abilities<br>b. improved level of orientation<br>c. reduction in instances of inappropriate responses. | 13.a. Assess client for altered thought processes (e.g. shortened attention span, impaired memory, decreased ability to problem solve, confusion, inappropriate responses).<br>b. Ascertain from significant others client's usual level of intellectual and emotional functioning.<br>c. Implement measures to improve cerebral tissue perfusion (see Nursing Diagnosis 1, action b) *in order to reduce cerebral ischemia and subsequently improve thought processes.*<br>d. If client shows evidence of altered thought processes:<br>1. reorient to person, place, and time as necessary<br>2. address client by name<br>3. place familiar objects, clock, and calendar within client's view<br>4. face client when conversing with him/her<br>5. approach client in a slow, calm manner; allow adequate time for communication<br>6. repeat instructions as necessary using clear, simple language and short sentences<br>7. keep environmental stimuli to a minimum but avoid sensory deprivation<br>8. maintain a consistent and fairly structured routine<br>9. provide written or taped information whenever possible for client to review as often as necessary<br>10. have client perform only one activity at a time and allow adequate time for performance of activities<br>11. encourage client to make lists of planned activities, questions, and concerns<br>12. assist client to problem solve if necessary<br>13. implement measures *to stop emotional outbursts and inappropriate responses if they occur* (e.g. provide distraction by clapping hands, handing client an object to hold, or turning on the radio or television)<br>14. maintain realistic expectations of client's ability to learn, comprehend, and remember information provided<br>15. encourage significant others to be supportive of client; instruct them in methods of dealing with client's altered thought processes<br>16. discuss physiological basis for altered thought processes with client and significant others; inform them that intellectual and emotional functioning may improve gradually during the next 6-12 months<br>17. consult physician if altered thought processes worsen. |

## 14. NURSING DIAGNOSIS: High risk for infection: pneumonia

related to:
a. aspiration associated with difficulty swallowing, depressed cough and gag reflexes, and decreased level of consciousness;
b. stasis of secretions in the lungs associated with poor cough effort and decreased mobility (secretions provide a good medium for bacterial growth).

| Desired Outcome | Nursing Actions and ***Selected Purposes/Rationales*** |
|---|---|
| 14. The client will not develop pneumonia (see Care Plan on | 14.a. Refer to Care Plan on Immobility, Nursing Diagnosis 11, action a (pp. 147-148), for measures related to assessment, prevention, and treatment of pneumonia. |

| | |
|---|---|
| Immobility, Nursing Diagnosis 11, outcome a [pp. 147-148], for outcome criteria). | b. Implement measures to reduce the risk for aspiration (see Nursing Diagnosis 16, action d) *in order to further reduce the risk for pneumonia.* |

## 15. NURSING DIAGNOSIS: High risk for trauma

related to:

a. falls associated with motor, visual, and spatial-perceptual impairments; weakness; spasticity; quick, impulsive behavior (occurs primarily with involvement of the nondominant cerebral hemisphere); altered thought processes; and decreased level of consciousness;

b. burns and cuts associated with motor, sensory, and spatial-perceptual impairments; spasticity; and quick, impulsive behavior.

| Desired Outcome | Nursing Actions and *Selected Purposes/Rationales* |
|---|---|
| 15. The client will not experience falls, burns, or cuts. | 15.a. Implement measures *to reduce the risk for trauma:*<br>1. perform actions *to prevent falls:*<br>a. keep bed in low position with side rails up when client is in bed<br>b. keep needed items within easy reach and within client's visual field<br>c. encourage client to request assistance whenever needed; have call signal within easy reach<br>d. if vision is impaired:<br>1. orient client to surroundings, room, and arrangement of furniture and identify obstacles during ambulation<br>2. provide an eyepatch or frosted lens for client to wear if diplopia is present<br>3. encourage visual scanning if homonymous hemianopsia is present<br>e. use lap belt when client is in chair if indicated<br>f. instruct client to wear well-fitting slippers/shoes with nonslip soles and low heels when ambulating<br>g. keep floor free of clutter and wipe up spills promptly<br>h. accompany client during ambulation utilizing a transfer safety belt<br>i. provide ambulatory aids (e.g. walker, cane) if client is weak or unsteady on feet<br>j. reinforce instructions from physical therapist on correct transfer and ambulation techniques<br>k. instruct client to ambulate in well-lit areas and to utilize handrails if needed<br>l. do not rush client; allow adequate time for ambulation to the bathroom and in hallway<br>m. make sure that bathtub and shower have nonslip bottom surfaces and that shower chair, secure bath mat, call light, hand grips, and adequate lighting are present<br>n. implement measures *to reduce weakness:*<br>1. maintain an adequate nutritional status (see Nursing Diagnosis 2)<br>2. perform actions to improve activity tolerance (see Care Plan on Immobility, Nursing Diagnosis 5, action b [p. 143])<br>o. stabilize client's affected arm with a sling when he/she is out of bed *in order to improve balance* |

| Desired Outcome | Nursing Actions and ***Selected Purposes/Rationales*** |
|---|---|
| | 2. perform actions *to prevent burns:*<br>a. let hot foods/fluids cool slightly before serving<br>b. supervise client while smoking if indicated<br>c. assess temperature of bath water before and during use<br>3. assist client with tasks that require fine motor skills (e.g. shaving) *in order to prevent cuts*<br>4. if client is confused or irrational:<br>a. reorient frequently to surroundings and necessity of adhering to safety precautions<br>b. provide constant supervision (e.g. staff member, significant other) if indicated<br>c. consult physician about the temporary use of a jacket or wrist restraints if necessary<br>d. administer antianxiety and antipsychotic medications if ordered<br>5. administer muscle relaxants if ordered *to reduce spasticity of affected muscles.*<br>b. Include client and significant others in planning and implementing measures to prevent trauma.<br>c. If injury does occur, initiate appropriate first aid and notify physician. |

## 16. NURSING DIAGNOSIS: High risk for aspiration

related to impaired swallowing, depressed cough and gag reflexes, and decreased level of consciousness.

| Desired Outcome | Nursing Actions and ***Selected Purposes/Rationales*** |
|---|---|
| 16. The client will not aspirate secretions or foods/fluids as evidenced by:<br>a. clear breath sounds<br>b. resonant percussion note over lungs<br>c. absence of cough, tachypnea, and dyspnea. | 16.a. Assess for signs and symptoms of aspiration of secretions or foods/fluids (e.g. rhonchi, dull percussion note over affected lung area, cough, tachypnea, tachycardia, dyspnea, presence of tube feeding in tracheal aspirate).<br>b. Monitor chest x-ray results. Report findings of pulmonary infiltrate.<br>c. If client is receiving tube feedings, add food coloring to the solution *so that it can readily be identified in tracheal aspirate.*<br>d. Implement measures *to reduce the risk for aspiration:*<br>1. withhold oral foods/fluids and place client in side-lying position if he/she has a depressed or absent gag reflex, severe dysphagia, and/or is not alert<br>2. have suction equipment readily available for use<br>3. perform oropharyngeal suctioning, encourage client to use tonsil-tip suction, and provide oral hygiene as often as needed *to remove excess secretions*<br>4. if client is receiving tube feedings:<br>a. check tube placement before each feeding or on a routine basis if feeding is continuous<br>b. maintain continuous tube feeding infusion rate as ordered; administer intermittent tube feedings slowly<br>c. maintain client in a semi- to high Fowler's position during and for at least 30 minutes after feeding<br>d. stop tube feeding and notify physician if residuals exceed established parameters |

5. if oral intake is allowed:
   a. perform actions to improve ability to swallow (see Nursing Diagnosis 3, action c)
   b. allow ample time for meals
   c. instruct client to avoid laughing and talking while eating and drinking
   d. maintain client in high Fowler's position during and for at least 30 minutes after meals and snacks
   e. assist client with oral hygiene after eating *to ensure that food particles do not remain in mouth.*

e. If signs and symptoms of aspiration occur:
   1. perform tracheal suctioning
   2. notify physician
   3. prepare client for chest x-ray
   4. prepare client for bronchoscopy if ordered *to remove aspirated food particles.*

## 17. COLLABORATIVE DIAGNOSES:

**Potential complications:**

a. **increased intracranial pressure (IICP)** related to:
   1. cerebral hemorrhage or hematoma (can occur if CVA is caused by cerebral bleeding resulting from conditions such as ruptured cerebral aneurysm)
   2. cerebral edema associated with increased capillary permeability of the cerebral vessels and malfunction of the sodium pump resulting from cerebral ischemia;

b. **corneal irritation and abrasion** related to inability to close eye on affected side if facial nerve paresis or paralysis has occurred;

c. **subluxation of shoulder** related to muscle weakness and gravity pull on affected arm.

| Desired Outcomes | Nursing Actions and ***Selected Purposes/Rationales*** |
|---|---|
| 17.a. The client will not develop IICP as evidenced by:<br>1. usual or improved level of consciousness<br>2. no complaints of headache<br>3. stable or improved motor and sensory function<br>4. absence of vomiting, papilledema, and seizure activity<br>5. usual pupillary size and reactivity<br>6. stable vital signs. | 17.a.1. Assess for and report signs and symptoms of IICP:<br>a. restlessness, agitation, confusion, lethargy<br>b. complaints of headache<br>c. decreasing motor and sensory function<br>d. abnormal posturing (e.g. extension [decerebrate], flexion [decorticate])<br>e. vomiting (usually without nausea)<br>f. papilledema<br>g. seizures<br>h. change in pupil size or reactivity<br>i. altered respiratory pattern (e.g. Cheyne-Stokes, central neurogenic hyperventilation)<br>j. full, bounding, slow pulse<br>k. rise in systolic B/P with widening pulse pressure.<br>2. Implement measures *to prevent IICP:*<br>a. maintain fluid restrictions as ordered<br>b. administer osmotic diuretics (e.g. mannitol) and/or loop diuretics (e.g. furosemide) if ordered *to reduce cerebral edema*<br>c. perform actions *to promote adequate cerebral venous drainage:*<br>1. elevate head of bed 30-45° unless contraindicated<br>2. keep client's head and neck in midline position; avoid flexion, extension, and rotation of head and neck |

Desired Outcomes | Nursing Actions and ***Selected Purposes/Rationales***

3. administer stool softeners, antitussives, and antiemetics if ordered *to prevent straining to have a bowel movement, coughing, and vomiting (these conditions cause an increase in intrathoracic pressure that subsequently impedes venous return from the brain)*

d. perform actions *to prevent cerebral hypoxia and subsequent cerebral edema and vasodilation:*
   1. implement measures to improve cerebral tissue perfusion (see Nursing Diagnosis 1, action b)
   2. implement measures *to maintain a patent airway* (e.g. position client on side, suction if necessary)
   3. administer oxygen as ordered and before and after tracheal suctioning

e. perform additional actions *to prevent vasodilation of the cerebral vessels:*
   1. implement measures *to prevent an increase in blood pressure:*
      a. observe for and control conditions that can cause agitation (e.g. fear, anxiety, distended bladder)
      b. instruct client to avoid activities that result in isometric muscle contractions (e.g. pushing feet against footboard, tightly gripping side rails)
   2. assist with mechanical hyperventilation *(may be done to decrease arterial $CO_2$ and prevent subsequent vasodilation)*

f. schedule care so activities that could raise intracranial pressure (e.g. suctioning, bathing, repositioning) are not grouped together.

3. If signs and symptoms of IICP are present:
   a. continue with above actions
   b. initiate seizure precautions
   c. prepare client for the following if planned:
      1. insertion of an intracranial pressure monitoring device (e.g. intraventricular catheter, subarachnoid screw or bolt, epidural fiberoptic catheter or transducer, intraparenchymal catheter)
      2. surgical intervention (e.g. ligation of bleeding vessel, evacuation of expanding hematoma)
   d. provide emotional support to client and significant others.

17.b. The client will not experience corneal irritation or abrasion as evidenced by:
1. absence of excessive tearing and eye redness
2. no complaints of eye discomfort
3. usual visual acuity.

17.b.1. Assess for and report signs and symptoms of corneal irritation and abrasion (e.g. excessive tearing; reddened, itchy eye; sensation of foreign body in eye; eye pain; blurred vision).

2. Implement measures *to prevent corneal irritation and abrasion of eye on affected side:*
   a. reduce client's exposure to irritants such as powder, dust, and smoke
   b. have client wear his/her glasses *to protect eye*
   c. lubricate conjunctiva with isotonic eyedrops frequently
   d. tape eyelid shut if client is unable to close eye completely
   e. instruct client to avoid rubbing eye.

3. If signs and symptoms of irritation or abrasion occur:
   a. continue with above measures
   b. assist with removal of any foreign body in the eye
   c. administer antimicrobial and anti-inflammatory ophthalmic ointments or solutions if ordered
   d. consult physician if signs and symptoms of corneal irritation or abrasion persist or worsen.

17.c. The client will not experience subluxation of shoulder as evidenced by:
1. absence of shoulder pain,

17.c.1. Assess for and report signs and symptoms of subluxation of the shoulder (e.g. shoulder pain, tenderness, or swelling; decreased range of motion of shoulder).

2. Implement measures *to prevent subluxation of the shoulder on the affected side:*
   a. instruct client in and assist with active or passive range of motion to affected upper extremity *in order to improve muscle tone*

tenderness, and swelling
2. maintenance of full range of motion of shoulder.

b. when client is in bed or chair, position arm in correct alignment using pillows or lap board for support if necessary
c. assist client with application of an arm support before sitting up in bed or getting out of bed
d. use turn sheet or transfer belt when assisting client to move; never pull on his/her shoulder or arm.
3. If signs and symptoms of shoulder subluxation occur:
a. continue with above actions
b. apply heat or cold to area as ordered
c. administer anti-inflammatory medications and analgesics if ordered.

## 18. NURSING DIAGNOSIS: Sexual dysfunction

related to:
a. alteration in usual sexual activities associated with impaired motor function and lengthy hospitalization;
b. decreased libido and/or impotence associated with depression, impaired motor and sensory function, fear of urinary and bowel incontinence, self-concept disturbance, and fear of rejection by partner.

| Desired Outcome | Nursing Actions and ***Selected Purposes/Rationales*** |
|---|---|
| 18. The client will perceive self as sexually adequate and acceptable as evidenced by:<br>a. communication of same<br>b. maintenance of relationship with significant other. | 18.a. Assess for signs and symptoms of sexual dysfunction (e.g. communication of sexual concerns or inability to achieve sexual satisfaction, alteration in relationship with significant other, physical limitations imposed by CVA).<br>b. Provide accurate information about the effects of the CVA on sexual functioning. Encourage questions and clarify misconceptions.<br>c. Implement measures *to promote optimal sexual functioning:*<br>1. facilitate communication between client and his/her partner; focus on the feelings the couple share and assist them to identify changes that may affect their sexual relationship<br>2. discuss ways to be creative in expressing sexuality (e.g. massage, fantasies, cuddling)<br>3. arrange for uninterrupted privacy during hospital stay if desired by the couple<br>4. perform actions to improve client's self-concept (see Nursing Diagnosis 20, actions c-v)<br>5. if impotence is a problem:<br>a. encourage client to discuss it and various treatment options (e.g. penile prosthesis) with physician<br>b. suggest alternative methods of sexual gratification if appropriate<br>c. discuss alternative methods of parenting (e.g. adoption) if of concern to client<br>6. if appropriate, involve partner in care of client *to facilitate partner's adjustment to the changes in client's appearance and/or body functioning and subsequently decrease the possibility of partner's rejection of client*<br>7. if incontinence of urine or stool is a problem, encourage client to void and/or defecate just before intercourse and other sexual activity<br>8. encourage client to rest before sexual activity<br>9. discuss positions that may facilitate sexual activity (e.g. lying on affected side, client in supine position).<br>d. Include partner in above discussions and encourage his/her continued support of the client.<br>e. Consult physician if counseling appears indicated. |

## 19. NURSING DIAGNOSIS: Anxiety

related to impaired verbal communication and/or motor and sensory function; unfamiliar environment; lack of understanding of diagnosis, diagnostic tests, and treatments; uncertain prognosis; altered thought processes; financial concerns; and anticipated effect of the CVA on future life style and roles.

| Desired Outcome | Nursing Actions and ***Selected Purposes/Rationales*** |
|---|---|
| 19. The client will experience a reduction in anxiety (see Care Plan on Immobility, Nursing Diagnosis 13 [p. 153], for outcome criteria). | 19.a. Assess client for signs and symptoms of anxiety (e.g. communication of fears and concerns, insomnia, tenseness, tremors, irritability, restlessness, diaphoresis, tachypnea, elevated blood pressure, tachycardia, facial pallor or flushing, narrowed perceptual field, withdrawal, noncompliance with treatment plan). Validate perceptions carefully, remembering that some behaviors may result from neurological changes.<br>b. Refer to Care Plan on Immobility, Nursing Diagnosis 13, action b (p. 153), for measures to reduce fear and anxiety.<br>c. Implement additional measures *to reduce fear and anxiety:*<br>1. if speech or comprehension is impaired, establish an effective communication system (e.g. paper and pencil, word or picture board, magic slate, gestures) as soon as possible<br>2. if client is experiencing homonymous hemianopsia, approach on unaffected side within his/her visual field<br>3. simplify the client's environment as much as possible<br>4. explain that motor, sensory, and speech impairments and altered thought processes are often more extensive initially and may gradually improve<br>5. perform actions to assist client to cope with the diagnosis and its effects (see Nursing Diagnosis 21, action c). |

## 20. NURSING DIAGNOSIS: Self-concept disturbance*

related to:

a. change in appearance (e.g. hemiplegia, facial droop, ptosis) and sexual functioning;
b. life-style and role changes associated with motor and spatial-perceptual impairments and altered thought processes;
c. impaired verbal communication;
d. loss of self-control (e.g. automatic speech, emotional lability, inappropriate behavior);
e. urinary and bowel incontinence;
f. dependence on others to meet basic needs.

*This diagnostic label includes the nursing diagnoses of body image disturbance, self-esteem disturbance, and altered role performance.

| Desired Outcome | Nursing Actions and ***Selected Purposes/Rationales*** |
|---|---|
| 20. The client will demonstrate beginning adaptation to changes in appearance, physical and mental functioning, | 20.a. Assess for signs and symptoms of a self-concept disturbance (e.g. verbal or nonverbal cues denoting a negative response to changes in body functioning or appearance such as denial of or preoccupation with changes that have occurred, refusal to look at or touch a body part, or withdrawal from significant others). |

life style, and roles as evidenced by:
a. communication of feelings of self-worth and sexual adequacy
b. maintenance of relationships with significant others
c. active participation in activities of daily living
d. active interest in personal appearance
e. willingness to participate in social activities
f. communication of a beginning plan for adapting life style to meet changes in physical and mental functioning.

b. Determine the meaning of changes in appearance, physical and mental functioning, life style, and roles to the client by encouraging him/her to communicate feelings and by noting nonverbal responses to the changes experienced.
c. Implement measures to facilitate the grieving process (see Nursing Diagnosis 22, action b).
d. Discuss with client improvements in neurological functioning that can realistically be expected.
e. Implement measures *to assist client to increase self-esteem* (e.g. limit negative self-assessment, encourage positive comments about self, assist to identify strengths, give positive feedback about accomplishments and behaviors that are indicative of high self-esteem).
f. Reinforce measures to assist client to cope with effects of CVA (see Nursing Diagnosis 21, action c).
g. Reinforce measures to promote optimal sexual functioning (see Nursing Diagnosis 18, action c).
h. Discuss techniques the client can utilize *to adapt to altered thought processes:*
   1. encourage client to make lists and jot down messages and refer to these notes rather than relying on his/her memory
   2. instruct client to place self in a calm environment when making decisions
   3. encourage client to validate decisions, clarify information, and seek assistance problem-solving if indicated.
i. Instruct significant others in ways to manage client's emotional lability and inappropriate laughing, crying, or swearing (e.g. provide privacy; distract client by clapping hands, turning on television, or handing him/her an object).
j. Implement measures to reduce the risk of urinary and bowel incontinence (see Nursing Diagnoses 10, action b and 12, action b).
k. Implement measures *to assist client to adapt to changes in appearance:*
   1. instruct and assist client to position self with affected extremities well supported and in proper alignment *(if extremities are positioned awkwardly, the impairment is more obvious)*
   2. assist client with usual grooming and makeup habits.
l. Demonstrate acceptance of client using techniques such as touch and frequent visits. Encourage significant others to do the same.
m. Implement measures to facilitate communication (see Nursing Diagnosis 6, action b).
n. Reinforce use of assistive devices (e.g. plate guards, broad-handled utensils, universal cuff, button hook, long-handled shoehorn) and mobility aids (e.g. walker, cane) *to increase client's independence.*
o. Encourage significant others to allow client to do what he/she is able *so that independence can be re-established and/or self-esteem redeveloped.*
p. Use adjectives such as weak, affected, or right- or left-sided rather than "bad" when referring to side of hemiplegia.
q. Assess for and support behaviors suggesting positive adaptation to changes that have occurred (e.g. maintenance of relationships with significant others, increased participation in care, compliance with treatment plan).
r. Assist client's and significant others' adjustment by listening, facilitating communication, and providing information.
s. Assist client and significant others to have similar expectations and understanding of future life style.
t. Encourage visits and support from significant others.
u. Encourage client to continue involvement in social activities and to pursue usual roles and interests. If previous roles, interests, and hobbies cannot be pursued, encourage development of new ones.
v. Provide information about and encourage utilization of community

| Desired Outcome | Nursing Actions and ***Selected Purposes/Rationales*** |
|---|---|
| | agencies and support groups (e.g. stroke support groups; vocational rehabilitation; sexual, family, individual, and/or financial counseling).<br>w. Consult physician about psychological counseling if client desires or if he/she seems unwilling or unable to adapt to changes resulting from the CVA. |

## 21. NURSING DIAGNOSIS: Ineffective individual coping

related to fear; anxiety; decreased ability to communicate verbally; changes in motor and sensory function, thought processes, and future life style and roles; and need for lengthy rehabilitation.

| Desired Outcome | Nursing Actions and ***Selected Purposes/Rationales*** |
|---|---|
| 21. The client will demonstrate the use of effective coping skills as evidenced by:<br>a. communication of ability to cope with the effects of the CVA<br>b. utilization of appropriate problem-solving techniques<br>c. willingness to participate in treatment plan and meet basic needs<br>d. appropriate use of defense mechanisms<br>e. recognition and utilization of available support systems. | 21.a. Assess for and report signs and symptoms of ineffective individual coping (e.g. communication of inability to cope; inability to ask for help, problem-solve, or meet basic needs; reluctance to participate in treatment plan; inappropriate use of defense mechanisms; inability to meet role expectations). Validate perceptions carefully, remembering that some behaviors may be a result of neurological changes.<br>b. Assess client's perception of current situation including precipitating factors and effectiveness of coping mechanisms.<br>c. Implement measures *to promote effective coping:*<br>1. allow time for client to adjust psychologically to diagnosis and planned treatment, residual effects of CVA, and anticipated life-style and role changes<br>2. perform actions to facilitate communication (see Nursing Diagnosis 6, action b)<br>3. perform actions to reduce fear and anxiety (see Nursing Diagnosis 19, actions b and c)<br>4. assist client to recognize and manage inappropriate denial if it is present<br>5. encourage communication about current situation<br>6. assist client to identify personal strengths and resources that can be utilized to facilitate coping with the current situation<br>7. create an atmosphere of trust and support<br>8. arrange for a visit with another individual who has successfully adjusted to the effects of a CVA<br>9. include client in the planning of care, encourage maximum participation in treatment plan, and allow choices when possible *to enable him/her to maintain a sense of control*<br>10. instruct client in effective problem-solving techniques (e.g. accurate identification of stressors, determination of various options to solve problem)<br>11. assist client to maintain usual daily routines whenever possible<br>12. assist client as he/she starts to plan for necessary life-style and role changes after discharge; help client to identify priorities and attainable goals<br>13. assist client through methods such as role playing to prepare for negative reactions of others to his/her altered appearance and other neurological impairments<br>14. if client is incontinent, instruct in ways to minimize the problem *so* |

*that socialization with others is possible* (e.g. placing disposable liners in underwear, wearing absorbent undergarments such as Attends)

15. set up a home evaluation appointment with occupational and physical therapists before client's discharge *so that changes in home environment (e.g. installation of ramps and handrails, widening doorways, altering kitchen facilities) can be completed by discharge*
16. assist client and significant others to identify ways that personal and family goals can be adjusted rather than abandoned
17. inform client that he/she will have times when impairments worsen; assure client that this is usually temporary and the result of physical and/or emotional stress or fatigue rather than an indication of deteriorating neurological status
18. administer antianxiety and/or antidepressant agents if ordered
19. assist client to identify and utilize available support systems; provide information regarding available community resources that can assist client and significant others in coping with effects of the CVA (e.g. stroke support groups, local chapter of the American Heart Association)
20. encourage continued emotional support from significant others
21. encourage the client to share with significant others the kind of support that would be most beneficial (e.g. listening, inspiring hope, providing reassurance and accurate information)
22. support behaviors suggesting positive adaptation to changes experienced (e.g. participation in treatment plan and self-care activities, communication of ability to cope, utilization of effective problem-solving strategies).

d. Consult physician about psychological and vocational rehabilitation counseling if appropriate. Initiate a referral if necessary.

## 22. NURSING DIAGNOSIS: Grieving*

related to changes in motor and sensory function and thought processes and the effect of these changes on future life style and roles.

*This diagnostic label includes anticipatory grieving and grieving following the actual losses.

| Desired Outcome | Nursing Actions and ***Selected Purposes/Rationales*** |
|---|---|
| 22. The client will demonstrate beginning progression through the grieving process as evidenced by:<br>a. communication of feelings about the CVA and its effects<br>b. expression of grief<br>c. participation in treatment plan and self-care activities<br>d. utilization of available support systems<br>e. communication of a plan for integrating | 22.a. Assess for signs and symptoms of grieving (e.g. change in eating habits, inability to concentrate, insomnia, anger, noncompliance, withdrawal from significant others, denial of loss). Be aware that client's response to a loss will be affected by factors such as previous experience with loss, age, developmental stage, available support systems, spiritual and cultural background, current health status, and significance of the loss.<br>b. Implement measures *to facilitate the grieving process:*<br>1. assist client to acknowledge the losses experienced *so grief work can begin;* assess for factors that may hinder and facilitate acknowledgment<br>2. discuss the grieving process and assist client to accept the phases of grieving as an expected response to changes that have occurred<br>3. allow time for client to progress through the phases of grieving (phases vary among theorists but progress from shock and alarm to acceptance); be aware that not every phase is expressed by all individuals, that recurrence of phases is common, and that the grieving process may take months to years |

| Desired Outcome | Nursing Actions and ***Selected Purposes/Rationales*** |
|---|---|
| prescribed follow-up care into life style. | 4. provide an atmosphere of care and concern (e.g. provide privacy, be available and nonjudgmental, display empathy and respect) *so client will feel free to communicate feelings*<br>5. perform actions *to promote trust* (e.g. answer questions honestly, provide requested information)<br>6. encourage the communication of anger and sadness about the losses experienced; recognize displacement of anger and assist client to see the actual cause of angry feelings and resentment if demonstrated<br>7. encourage client to express his/her feelings in whatever ways are comfortable (e.g. writing, drawing, conversation)<br>8. perform actions to promote effective coping (see Nursing Diagnosis 21, action c)<br>9. perform actions *to support realistic hope about the effects of treatment on the residual impairments:*<br>a. focus on what the client is able to accomplish independently and with the use of assistive devices<br>b. reinforce knowledge that impairments may improve with time<br>c. reinforce positive effects of speech, physical, and occupational therapies and control of underlying cause of CVA (e.g. hypertension, diabetes)<br>10. support behaviors suggesting successful grief work (e.g. communicating feelings about losses, focusing on ways to adapt to losses, developing or renewing relationships)<br>11. explain the phases of the grieving process to significant others; encourage their support and understanding<br>12. facilitate communication between client and significant others; be aware that they may be in different phases of the grieving process<br>13. provide information regarding counseling services and support groups that might assist client in working through grief<br>14. arrange for visit from clergy if desired by client.<br>c. Consult physician regarding referral for counseling if signs of dysfunctional grieving (e.g. persistent denial of losses, excessive anger or sadness, hysteria, suicidal behaviors) occur. |

## 23. NURSING DIAGNOSIS: Altered family processes

related to change in family roles and structure associated with a family member's verbal, motor, and sensory impairments; altered thought processes; and need for lengthy rehabilitation.

| Desired Outcome | Nursing Actions and ***Selected Purposes/Rationales*** |
|---|---|
| 23. The family members* will demonstrate beginning adjustment to changes in functioning of family member and family roles and structure as evidenced by: | 23.a. Assess for signs and symptoms of altered family processes (e.g. inability to meet client's needs, statements of not being able to accept client's diagnosis of CVA and its effects or make necessary role and life-style changes, inability to make decisions, inability or refusal to participate in client's rehabilitation, negative family interactions).<br>b. Identify components of the family and their patterns of communication and role expectations.<br>c. Implement measures *to facilitate family members' adjustment to client's* |

*The term "family members" is being used here to include client's significant others.

a. meeting client's needs
b. verbalization of ways to adapt to required role and life-style changes
c. active participation in decision making and client's rehabilitation
d. positive interactions with one another.

*diagnosis, changes in his/her functioning within the family system, and altered family roles and structure:*

1. encourage verbalization of feelings about the CVA and its effects on family structure; actively listen to each family member and maintain a nonjudgmental attitude about feelings shared
2. reinforce physician's explanation about the CVA and planned treatment and rehabilitation
3. assist family members to gain a realistic perspective of client's situation, conveying as much hope as appropriate
4. provide privacy *so that family members and client can share their feelings with one another;* stress the importance of and facilitate the use of good communication techniques
5. assist family members to progress through their own grieving process; explain that they may encounter times when they need to focus on meeting their own rather than the client's needs
6. emphasize the need for family members to obtain adequate rest and nutrition and to identify and utilize stress management techniques *so that they are better able to emotionally and physically deal with the changes and losses experienced and the physical care of the client*
7. encourage and assist family members to identify coping strategies for dealing with the client's impairments and their effects on the family
8. assist family members to identify realistic goals and ways of reaching these goals
9. include family members in decision making about client and his/her care; convey appreciation for their input and continued support of client
10. encourage and allow family members to participate in client's care and rehabilitation as appropriate
11. assist family members to identify resources that could assist them in coping with their feelings and meeting their immediate and long-term needs (e.g. counseling and social services; pastoral care; service, church, and stroke support groups); initiate a referral if indicated.

d. Consult physician if family members continue to demonstrate difficulty adapting to changes in client's functioning, roles, and family structure.

## 24. NURSING DIAGNOSIS: Knowledge deficit

regarding follow-up care.

| Desired Outcomes | Nursing Actions and ***Selected Purposes/Rationales*** |
|---|---|
| 24.a. The client will communicate an awareness of ways to decrease the risk of a recurrent CVA. | 24.a.1. Assist client to recognize factors that may have contributed to the CVA (e.g. hypertension, hyperlipidemia, diabetes, obesity, atrial fibrillation, use of oral contraceptives).<br>2. Identify appropriate actions client can take to decrease risk of a recurrent CVA (e.g. take medications as prescribed, decrease stress, lose weight, stop smoking, modify diet, adhere to medical treatment plan to control hypertension and/or diabetes, use another form of birth control if taking oral contraceptives).<br>3. Provide information about resources that can help client to control risk factors (e.g. National Stroke Association; American Heart Association; smoking cessation, weight reduction, and stress management programs). Initiate a referral if indicated. |

| Desired Outcomes | Nursing Actions and ***Selected Purposes/Rationales*** |
|---|---|
| 24.b. The client will identify ways to manage sensory and verbal communication impairments and altered thought processes. | 24.b.1. Reinforce instructions regarding ways to adapt to visual impairments if present:<br>a. utilize scanning techniques if visual field cut is present<br>b. arrange home setting so that when in favorite chair or in bed, stimuli other than wall or furniture are within visual field<br>c. wear eyepatch or frosted lens if double vision persists.<br>2. Reinforce use of established communication techniques and continuation with speech therapy if indicated.<br>3. If spatial-perceptual deficits and/or unilateral neglect are present, stress need for assistance with usual daily activities and strict adherence to safety measures to prevent injury.<br>4. Reinforce methods of adapting to impaired memory and shortened attention span (e.g. make lists of planned activities, review taped or written instructions frequently).<br>5. Instruct client to request assistance when problem-solving and setting priorities and to seek validation of decisions if reasoning ability is impaired. |
| 24.c. The client will identify ways to manage urinary and bowel incontinence. | 24.c.1. Reinforce instructions regarding client's bladder and bowel training programs. Stress the importance of adhering to the programs in order to reduce the risk of incontinence.<br>2. Demonstrate procedures that are included in client's bladder training program (e.g. intermittent catheterization, application of an external catheter) and bowel training program (e.g. digital stimulation, insertion of a rectal suppository, administration of an enema). Allow time for questions, clarification, and return demonstration. |
| 24.d. The client will demonstrate measures to facilitate the performance of activities of daily living and increase physical mobility. | 24.d.1. Reinforce measures that the client is using to improve his/her ability to perform activities of daily living and increase physical mobility (e.g. participation in exercise program; use of assistive devices and mobility aids; continued concentration on body positioning, balance, and movement).<br>2. Allow time for questions, clarification, and return demonstration. |
| 24.e. The client will communicate an awareness of signs and symptoms to report to the health care provider. | 24.e.1. Refer to Care Plan on Immobility, Nursing Diagnosis 17, action c (p. 157), for signs and symptoms to report to health care provider.<br>2. Instruct client to report these additional signs and symptoms:<br>a. increased weakness or loss of sensation in extremities<br>b. increase in or development of visual disturbances such as tunnel vision, blurred vision, or transient blindness<br>c. increased lethargy, irritability, or confusion<br>d. increased difficulty chewing or swallowing<br>e. increased difficulty speaking or understanding verbal and nonverbal communication<br>f. increased difficulty maintaining balance<br>g. seizures (can develop months after the CVA as scar tissue forms in the ischemic area). |
| 24.f. The client will communicate knowledge of community agencies that can assist with home management and adjustment to changes resulting from the CVA. | 24.f.1. Provide information about community resources that can assist client and significant others with home management and adjustment to impairments in motor and sensory function and altered thought processes resulting from the CVA (e.g. home health agencies, stroke support groups, Meals on Wheels, social and financial services, local chapter of the American Heart Association, local service groups that can help obtain assistive devices, individual and family counselors).<br>2. Initiate a referral if indicated. |
| 24.g. The client will communicate an understanding of and a plan for adhering to | 24.g.1. Reinforce the importance of keeping follow-up appointments with health care provider and physical, occupational, and speech therapists.<br>2. Teach client the rationale for, side effects of, and importance of taking prescribed medications (e.g. anticoagulants, antihypertensives). |

recommended follow-up care including future appointments with health care provider and therapists and medications prescribed.

3. Implement measures to improve client compliance:
   a. include significant others in teaching sessions if possible
   b. encourage questions and allow time for reinforcement and clarification of information provided
   c. provide written instructions on scheduled appointments with health care provider and occupational, physical, and speech therapists; medications prescribed; signs and symptoms to report; and exercise program.

# Craniocerebral Trauma

The leading causes of craniocerebral trauma (head injury, traumatic brain injury [TBI]) are motor vehicle accidents, falls, sports injuries, and assaults. Examples of skull and brain injury that can occur include skull fracture; dural tear; cerebral contusion, concussion, and laceration; brain stem damage; and intracranial hemorrhage. Brain damage can occur during the initial injury and as a result of subsequent cerebral ischemia, hemorrhage, hematoma, and edema; seizure activity; and/or obstruction in the flow of cerebrospinal fluid. Following craniocerebral trauma, clients usually experience headache, some degree of irritability, and altered thought processes. Additional signs and symptoms vary depending on the area of the brain that has been affected. For example, tissue damage in the frontal lobe could result in loss of voluntary motor control, personality changes, and/or expressive aphasia; damage to the occipital lobe could cause visual disturbances; and damage to the temporal lobe could result in receptive aphasia and/or hearing impairment.

Craniocerebral trauma is classified according to location (e.g. skull, epidural area, brain stem), effect (e.g. concussion, diffuse axonal injury, subdural hematoma), and severity. The severity of trauma ranges from mild (usually a concussion) to severe, in which extensive contusion and/or laceration of brain tissue and possible brain stem injury occurs. Severe craniocerebral trauma usually involves a period of prolonged unconsciousness and results in permanent neurological impairments that require extensive rehabilitation and long-term care.

**This care plan focuses on the adult client hospitalized following craniocerebral trauma.** It deals mainly with nursing and collaborative diagnoses appropriate for a client who has regained consciousness after sustaining a moderate brain injury. Goals of care during the acute phase are to prevent life-threatening complications and perform or assist the client with those activities he/she is unable to do independently. After the client's condition has stabilized, care is focused on assisting him/her to adapt to residual neurological impairments. Nursing care and discharge teaching need to be individualized according to the areas of the brain affected and the extensiveness of the tissue damage. If the client has sustained more severe craniocerebral trauma, refer also to the Care Plans on Immobility and Cerebrovascular Accident.

## DIAGNOSTIC TESTS

Computed tomography (CT)
Magnetic resonance imaging (MRI)
Skull x-rays
Cerebral angiography
Brain scan
Positron emission tomography (PET)
Electroencephalogram (EEG)
Visual field examination
Evoked potentials (auditory, visual, and/or somatosensory)

## DISCHARGE CRITERIA

Prior to discharge, the client will:

- have improved cerebral tissue perfusion
- have improved or stable neurological function
- identify ways to adapt to neurological deficits that may persist following craniocerebral trauma
- identify ways to reduce headache

- state signs and symptoms to report to the health care provider
- share thoughts and feelings about residual neurological impairments
- identify community agencies that can assist with home management and adjustment to changes resulting from the injury
- verbalize an understanding of and a plan for adhering to recommended follow-up care including future appointments with health care provider and therapists and medications prescribed.

**NURSING/ COLLABORATIVE DIAGNOSES**



## 1. NURSING DIAGNOSIS: Altered cerebral tissue perfusion

related to decreased cerebral blood flow associated with:
a. cerebral hemorrhage resulting from tearing of blood vessels at the time of injury;
b. pressure on cerebral vessels resulting from hematoma formation and/or edema;
c. vascular spasm (can occur when vessels are damaged and stretched at time of injury).

| Desired Outcome | Nursing Actions and ***Selected Purposes/Rationales*** |
|---|---|
| 1. The client will experience improved cerebral tissue perfusion as evidenced by:<br>a. decrease in or absence of dizziness, visual disturbances, | 1.a. Assess client for signs and symptoms of decreased cerebral tissue perfusion:<br>1. dizziness<br>2. visual disturbances (e.g. blurred or dimmed vision, diplopia, change in visual field)<br>3. aphasia<br>4. irritability and restlessness |

| | |
|---|---|
| and/or speech impairments<br>b. improved mental status<br>c. improved or usual sensory and motor function. | 5. decreased level of consciousness<br>6. paresthesias, paresis, paralysis.<br>b. Implement measures *to improve cerebral tissue perfusion:*<br>1. perform actions to prevent and treat increased intracranial pressure (see Collaborative Diagnosis 9, actions a.2 and 3)<br>2. administer calcium-channel blockers (e.g. nimodipine) if ordered *to reduce cerebral vasospasm (the calcium that is released by the injured neural cells can cause vasospasm)*<br>3. prepare client for surgery (e.g. evacuation of hematoma, ligation of bleeding vessels) if planned.<br>c. Consult physician if signs and symptoms of decreased cerebral tissue perfusion worsen. |

## 2. NURSING DIAGNOSIS: Altered nutrition: less than body requirements

related to:

a. decreased oral intake associated with:
   1. anorexia resulting from fear, anxiety, pain, and anosmia (loss of sense of smell occurs frequently following craniocerebral trauma because the olfactory nerves are very sensitive to pressure)
   2. dysphagia (can occur with damage to cranial nerves IX and X)
   3. difficulty feeding self if visual disturbances are present (can occur as a result of damage to cranial nerves II, III, IV, or VI) or motor function is impaired
   4. prescribed dietary restrictions (may be necessary if client has a decreased level of consciousness or if damage to cranial nerves has resulted in a depressed or absent gag reflex or severe dysphagia);
b. increased nutritional needs associated with the increased metabolic rate that occurs following craniocerebral trauma.

| Desired Outcome | Nursing Actions and ***Selected Purposes/Rationales*** |
|---|---|
| 2. The client will maintain an adequate nutritional status as evidenced by:<br>a. weight within normal range for client's age, height, and body frame<br>b. normal BUN and serum albumin, Hct, Hb, transferrin, and lymphocyte levels<br>c. triceps skinfold thickness within normal range<br>d. usual strength and activity tolerance<br>e. healthy oral mucous membrane. | 2.a. Assess the client for signs and symptoms of malnutrition:<br>1. weight below normal for client's age, height, and body frame<br>2. abnormal BUN and low serum albumin, Hct, Hb, transferrin, and lymphocyte levels<br>3. triceps skinfold thickness less than normal<br>4. weakness and fatigue<br>5. stomatitis.<br>b. Monitor percentage of meals and snacks client consumes. Report a pattern of inadequate intake.<br>c. Implement measures *to maintain an adequate nutritional status:*<br>1. when food or fluid is allowed, perform actions *to improve oral intake:*<br>a. implement measures to reduce headache (see Nursing Diagnosis 3, action e)<br>b. implement measures to reduce fear and anxiety (see Nursing Diagnosis 10, action b)<br>c. implement measures to assist client to adapt to loss of or diminished sense of smell, visual impairments, impaired swallowing ability, and/or altered sense of taste if present (see Collaborative Diagnosis 9, actions d.2.a and b; d.2.d.2.b; and d.2.e)<br>d. increase activity as allowed and tolerated *(activity stimulates appetite)*<br>e. obtain a dietary consult if necessary to assist client in selecting foods/fluids that meet nutritional needs as well as personal and cultural preferences whenever possible<br>f. maintain a clean environment and a relaxed, pleasant atmosphere |

| Desired Outcome | Nursing Actions and ***Selected Purposes/Rationales*** |
|---|---|
| | g. provide oral care before meals<br>h. serve small portions of nutritious foods/fluids that are appealing to the client<br>i. encourage significant others to bring in client's favorite foods unless contraindicated and eat with him/her *to make eating more of a familiar social experience*<br>j. allow adequate time for meals; reheat food if necessary<br>k. implement measures to enable client to feed self (see Nursing Diagnosis 5, action c.6); if client needs to be fed, offer foods/fluids in the order he/she prefers<br>2. ensure that meals are well balanced and high in essential nutrients; offer dietary supplements between meals if indicated<br>3. administer vitamins and minerals if ordered.<br>d. Perform a 72-hour calorie count if ordered. Report totals to dietitian and physician.<br>e. Consult physician regarding alternative methods of providing nutrition (e.g. parenteral nutrition, tube feedings) if client does not consume enough food or fluids to meet nutritional needs. |

## 3. NURSING DIAGNOSIS: Pain: headache

related to:

a. trauma to the scalp, dura, and cerebral vessels and tissue;
b. stretching or compression of cerebral vessels and tissue associated with increased intracranial pressure if it occurs;
c. irritation of the meninges (occurs primarily if blood is present in the cerebrospinal fluid or meningitis develops).

| Desired Outcome | Nursing Actions and ***Selected Purposes/Rationales*** |
|---|---|
| 3. The client will obtain relief from headache as evidenced by:<br>a. verbalization of headache relief<br>b. relaxed facial expression and body positioning<br>c. increased participation in activities. | 3.a. Determine how the client usually responds to pain.<br>b. Assess client's perception of pain including location, intensity, and type. Utilize a numerical scale to rate intensity.<br>c. Assess for nonverbal signs of headache (e.g. grimacing, rubbing head, avoidance of bright lights and noises, reluctance to move).<br>d. Assess for factors that seem to aggravate and alleviate headache.<br>e. Implement measures *to relieve headache:*<br>1. perform actions *to minimize environmental stimuli* (e.g. provide a quiet environment, restrict visitors, dim lights)<br>2. avoid jarring bed or startling client *to minimize risk of sudden movements*<br>3. perform actions to prevent and treat increased intracranial pressure and meningitis (see Collaborative Diagnosis 9, actions a.2 and 3 and b.5 and 6)<br>4. provide nonpharmacological measures for headache relief (e.g. cool cloth to forehead, relaxation techniques)<br>5. administer nonnarcotic analgesics or codeine (other narcotic analgesics are usually contraindicated *because they have a greater depressant effect on the central nervous system)* if ordered.<br>f. Consult physician if above actions fail to relieve headache. |

## 4. NURSING DIAGNOSIS: Impaired physical mobility

related to:
a. motor and spatial-perceptual impairments if present;
b. activity restrictions imposed by the treatment plan;
c. reluctance to move associated with pain.

| Desired Outcome | Nursing Actions and ***Selected Purposes/Rationales*** |
|---|---|
| 4. The client will achieve maximum physical mobility within limitations imposed by the treatment plan and the effects of the injury. | 4.a. Implement measures *to increase mobility when allowed:*<br>1. instruct client in and assist with range of motion exercises at least 3 times/day unless contraindicated<br>2. instruct client in and assist with correct use of mobility aids (e.g. cane, walker) if appropriate<br>3. reinforce instructions, activities, and exercise plan recommended by physical and occupational therapists<br>4. perform actions to relieve headache (see Nursing Diagnosis 3, action e)<br>5. increase activity and participation in self-care as allowed and tolerated.<br>b. Provide praise and encouragement for all efforts to increase physical mobility.<br>c. Encourage the support of significant others. Allow them to assist with range of motion exercises, positioning, and activity if desired.<br>d. Consult physician if client is unable to achieve expected level of mobility or range of motion becomes restricted. |

## 5. NURSING DIAGNOSIS: Self-care deficit

related to impaired physical mobility, altered thought processes, and/or visual impairments (e.g. diplopia, visual field cut) if present.

| Desired Outcome | Nursing Actions and ***Selected Purposes/Rationales*** |
|---|---|
| 5. The client will perform self-care activities within physical limitations and prescribed activity restrictions. | 5.a. With client, develop a realistic plan for meeting daily physical needs.<br>b. Encourage client to perform as much of self-care as possible within physical limitations and activity restrictions imposed by the treatment plan.<br>c. Implement measures *to facilitate client's ability to perform self-care activities:*<br>1. perform actions to increase mobility when allowed (see Nursing Diagnosis 4, action a)<br>2. schedule care at a time when client is most likely to be able to participate (e.g. when analgesics are at peak effect, after rest periods, not immediately after meals or treatments)<br>3. keep needed objects within easy reach<br>4. allow adequate time for accomplishment of self-care activities<br>5. if vision is impaired:<br>a. inform client where items are placed on his/her plate and tray<br>b. instruct client to visually scan his/her environment to locate needed items<br>c. encourage client to wear an eyepatch or frosted lens if diplopia is present |

| Desired Outcome | Nursing Actions and ***Selected Purposes/Rationales*** |
|---|---|
| | 6. perform actions *to enable client to feed self:*<br>a. place only a few items on the tray at one time if spatial-perceptual deficits are present<br>b. consult with occupational therapist about assistive devices available (e.g. broad-handled utensils, rocker knives, plate guards); reinforce use of these devices<br>7. perform actions *to enable client to dress self when condition stabilizes:*<br>a. encourage use of assistive devices such as button hooks, long-handled shoehorns, and pull loops for pants<br>b. encourage client to select clothing that is easy to put on and remove (e.g. clothing with zippers rather than buttons, loose-fitting clothing, shoes with Velcro fasteners rather than laces)<br>c. if client has difficulty distinguishing right from left, mark outer aspect of shoes with tape or label with R or L<br>8. reinforce exercises and activities recommended by the occupational therapist to improve fine motor skills.<br>d. Provide positive feedback for all efforts and accomplishments of self-care.<br>e. Assist the client with activities he/she is unable to perform independently.<br>f. Inform significant others of client's abilities to perform own care. Explain importance of encouraging and allowing client to maintain an optimal level of independence within prescribed activity restrictions and physical limitations. |

## 6. NURSING DIAGNOSIS: Altered thought processes

related to impaired cerebral functioning associated with cerebral irritation and ischemia resulting from craniocerebral trauma.

| Desired Outcome | Nursing Actions and ***Selected Purposes/Rationales*** |
|---|---|
| 6. The client will experience improvement in thought processes as evidenced by:<br>a. improved attention span, memory, reasoning ability, and judgment<br>b. decreased irritability and aggressiveness<br>c. improved level of orientation. | 6.a. Assess client for altered thought processes (e.g. shortened attention span, impaired memory, decreased ability to concentrate, slowness in thinking and perceiving, poor reasoning ability or judgment, irritability, aggressiveness, inappropriate responses, confusion).<br>b. Ascertain from significant others client's usual level of intellectual and emotional functioning.<br>c. Implement measures to improve cerebral tissue perfusion (see Nursing Diagnosis 1, action b) *in order to reduce cerebral ischemia and subsequently improve thought processes.*<br>d. If client shows evidence of altered thought processes:<br>1. reorient client to person, place, and time as necessary<br>2. address client by name<br>3. place familiar objects, clock, and calendar within client's view<br>4. face client when conversing with him/her<br>5. approach client in a slow, calm manner; allow adequate time for communication<br>6. repeat instructions as necessary using clear, simple language and short sentences<br>7. keep environmental stimuli to a minimum but avoid sensory deprivation<br>8. maintain a consistent and fairly structured routine<br>9. provide written or taped information whenever possible for client to review as often as necessary |

10. have client perform only one activity at a time and allow adequate time for performance of activities
11. encourage client to make lists of planned activities, questions, and concerns
12. assist client to problem solve if necessary
13. implement measures *to stop emotional outbursts, aggressive behavior, and inappropriate responses if they occur* (e.g. provide distraction by clapping hands, decrease environmental stimuli by turning off television or radio and/or requesting that visitors leave for short while)
14. maintain realistic expectations of client's ability to learn, comprehend, and remember information provided
15. encourage significant others to be supportive of client; instruct them in methods of dealing with client's altered thought processes
16. discuss physiological basis for altered thought processes with client and significant others; inform them that intellectual and emotional functioning usually improve gradually but caution them that posttraumatic syndrome (a postconcussion syndrome manifested by persistent headache and altered thought processes) may persist for a few months to a year or more depending on the severity of the head injury
17. assist with neuropsychological testing if indicated
18. consult physician if altered thought processes worsen.

## 7. NURSING DIAGNOSIS: High risk for trauma

related to:

a. falls associated with motor, visual, and/or spatial-perceptual impairments if present; quick, impulsive behavior (can occur with injury involving the non-dominant cerebral hemisphere); ataxia (can occur with cerebellar injury); and altered thought processes;
b. burns and cuts associated with motor and spatial-perceptual impairments; quick, impulsive behavior; and altered thought processes.

| Desired Outcome | Nursing Actions and ***Selected Purposes/Rationales*** |
|---|---|
| 7. The client will not experience falls, burns, or cuts. | 7.a. Implement measures *to reduce the risk for trauma:*<br>1. perform actions *to prevent falls:*<br>a. keep bed in low position with side rails up when client is in bed<br>b. keep needed items within easy reach<br>c. encourage client to request assistance whenever needed; have call signal within easy reach<br>d. use lap belt when client is in chair if indicated<br>e. instruct client to wear well-fitting slippers/shoes with nonslip soles and low heels when ambulating<br>f. keep floor free of clutter and wipe up spills promptly<br>g. accompany client during ambulation utilizing a transfer safety belt<br>h. provide ambulatory aids (e.g. walker, cane) if client is weak or unsteady on feet<br>i. reinforce instructions from physical therapist on correct transfer and ambulation techniques<br>j. instruct client to ambulate in well-lit areas and to utilize handrails if needed<br>k. do not rush client; allow adequate time for ambulation to the bathroom and in hallway |

| Desired Outcome | Nursing Actions and ***Selected Purposes/Rationales*** |
|---|---|
| | l. if vision is impaired:<br>1. orient client to surroundings, room, and arrangement of furniture and identify obstacles during ambulation<br>2. instruct client to wear an eyepatch or frosted lens if diplopia is present<br>3. encourage visual scanning if a visual field cut is present<br>m. make sure that bathtub and shower have nonslip bottom surfaces and that shower chair, secure bath mat, call light, hand grips, and adequate lighting are present<br>2. perform actions *to prevent burns:*<br>a. let hot foods and fluids cool slightly before serving<br>b. supervise client while smoking if indicated<br>c. assess temperature of bath water before and during use<br>3. assist client with tasks that require fine motor skills (e.g. shaving) *in order to prevent cuts*<br>4. administer central nervous system depressants judiciously<br>5. if client is confused or irrational:<br>a. reorient frequently to surroundings and necessity of adhering to safety precautions<br>b. provide constant supervision (e.g. staff member, significant other) if indicated<br>c. consult physician about the temporary use of a jacket or wrist restraints if necessary or use of a floor bed (large mattress on floor with surrounding "wall" of mattresses or padding) if indicated<br>d. administer antianxiety and antipsychotic medications if ordered.<br>b. Include client and significant others in planning and implementing measures to prevent trauma.<br>c. If injury does occur, initiate appropriate first aid and notify physician. |

## 8. NURSING DIAGNOSIS: High risk for altered body temperature: increased

related to direct trauma to the hypothalamus and/or pressure on the hypothalamus associated with edema of the surrounding tissue.

| Desired Outcome | Nursing Actions and ***Selected Purposes/Rationales*** |
|---|---|
| 8. The client will maintain a normal body temperature. | 8.a. Assess for and report signs and symptoms of increased body temperature resulting from trauma to the hypothalamus (e.g. elevated temperature; pale, hot, dry skin).<br>b. Administer osmotic diuretics (e.g. mannitol) and/or loop diuretics if ordered *to decrease edema of the hypothalamus and surrounding tissue.*<br>c. If increased body temperature occurs:<br>1. implement external cooling measures (e.g. apply a hypothermia blanket if ordered, reduce room temperature, bathe client with tepid water)<br>2. administer antipyretics if ordered (antipyretics are often not ordered *because they have little, if any, effect on temperature elevation resulting from failure of central regulatory structures).* |

**9. COLLABORATIVE DIAGNOSES:**

**Potential complications:**

a. **increased intracranial pressure (IICP)** related to:
   1. cerebral bleeding and/or hematoma formation
   2. cerebral edema associated with increased capillary permeability of cerebral vessels and malfunction of the sodium pump resulting from cerebral tissue trauma and subsequent cerebral ischemia
   3. hydrocephalus associated with obstruction of normal cerebrospinal fluid (CSF) flow resulting from edema, hematoma, and/or presence of blood in the subarachnoid space
   4. cerebral vasodilation associated with cerebral hypoxia and/or an increased metabolic rate resulting from hyperthermia (can occur following trauma to the hypothalamus), seizure activity, or meningitis;

b. **meningitis** related to:
   1. irritation of the meninges associated with trauma to the meningeal vessels or presence of blood in the CSF
   2. introduction of microorganisms into the meninges or CSF associated with a tear in the dura (especially if frontal or temporal bone fracture has occurred);

c. **seizures** related to altered activity of the cerebral neurons associated with irritation of the brain tissue resulting from the injury and IICP and meningitis if they occur;

d. **cranial nerve damage** related to trauma to the nerves during the initial injury and/or compression of the nerves associated with the development of intracerebral hematoma or edema;

e. **diabetes insipidus** related to decreased production and/or impaired release of antidiuretic hormone (ADH) associated with trauma to the hypothalamus and/or pituitary gland;

f. **syndrome of inappropriate antidiuretic hormone (SIADH)** related to:
   1. increased production and/or release of ADH associated with trauma to the hypothalamus and/or pituitary gland
   2. stimulation of ADH output associated with pain, trauma, and stress;

g. **gastrointestinal (GI) bleeding** related to the development of a stress ulcer (stress-induced ulcer, stress-erosive gastritis, Cushing's ulcer) associated with:
   1. gastric ischemia resulting from vasoconstriction (occurs with sympathetic nervous system stimulation due to cerebral injury)
   2. hypersecretion of hydrochloric acid resulting from parasympathetic nervous system stimulation due to cerebral injury and stress.

| Desired Outcomes | Nursing Actions and ***Selected Purposes/Rationales*** |
|---|---|
| 9.a. The client will not develop IICP as evidenced by:<br>1. usual or improved level of consciousness<br>2. no complaints of increased headache<br>3. stable or improved motor and sensory function<br>4. absence of vomiting, papilledema, and seizure activity<br>5. usual pupillary size and reactivity<br>6. stable vital signs. | 9.a.1. Assess for and report signs and symptoms of IICP:<br>a. increased restlessness, agitation, confusion, or lethargy<br>b. complaints of increased headache<br>c. decreasing motor and sensory function<br>d. abnormal posturing (e.g. extension [decerebrate], flexion [decorticate])<br>e. vomiting (usually without nausea)<br>f. papilledema<br>g. seizures<br>h. change in pupil size or reactivity<br>i. altered respiratory pattern (e.g. Cheyne-Stokes, central neurogenic hyperventilation)<br>j. full, bounding, slow pulse<br>k. rise in systolic B/P with widening pulse pressure.<br>2. Implement measures *to prevent IICP:*<br>a. maintain fluid restrictions as ordered<br>b. administer osmotic diuretics (e.g. mannitol) and/or loop diuretics (e.g. furosemide) *to reduce cerebral edema* |

| Desired Outcomes | Nursing Actions and ***Selected Purposes/Rationales*** |
|---|---|
| | c. perform actions *to promote adequate cerebral venous drainage:*<br>1. elevate head of bed 30-45° unless contraindicated<br>2. keep head and neck in midline position; avoid flexion, extension, and rotation of head and neck<br>3. administer stool softeners, antitussives, and antiemetics if ordered *to prevent straining to have a bowel movement, coughing, and vomiting (these conditions cause an increase in intrathoracic pressure, which subsequently impedes venous return from the brain)*<br>d. perform actions *to prevent cerebral hypoxia and subsequent cerebral edema and vasodilation:*<br>1. implement measures to improve cerebral tissue perfusion (see Nursing Diagnosis 1, action b)<br>2. implement measures *to maintain a patent airway* (e.g. position client on side, suction if necessary)<br>3. administer central nervous system depressants judiciously; hold medication and consult physician if respiratory rate is less than 12/minute<br>4. administer oxygen as ordered and before and after tracheal suctioning<br>e. perform additional actions *to prevent vasodilation of cerebral vessels:*<br>1. implement measures *to prevent an increase in blood pressure:*<br>a. observe for and control conditions that can cause agitation (e.g. fear, anxiety, distended bladder)<br>b. instruct client to avoid activities that result in isometric muscle contractions (e.g. pushing feet against footboard, tightly gripping side rails)<br>2. implement measures *to prevent an increase in metabolic rate:*<br>a. administer anticonvulsants (eg. phenytoin, carbamazepine) if ordered *to prevent seizure activity*<br>b. perform actions to prevent and treat increased body temperature (see Nursing Diagnosis 8, actions b and c)<br>c. perform actions to prevent and treat meningitis (see actions b.5 and 6 in this diagnosis)<br>3. assist with mechanical hyperventilation (may be done *to decrease arterial $CO_2$ and prevent subsequent vasodilation)*<br>f. schedule care so activities that could raise intracranial pressure (e.g. suctioning, bathing, repositioning) are not grouped together.<br>3. If signs and symptoms of IICP are present:<br>a. continue with above actions<br>b. initiate seizure precautions<br>c. prepare client for the following if planned:<br>1. insertion of an intracranial pressure monitoring device (e.g. intraventricular catheter, subarachnoid screw or bolt, epidural fiberoptic catheter or transducer, intraparenchymal catheter)<br>2. lumbar or ventricular puncture *to remove excess CSF*<br>3. surgical intervention (e.g. ligation of bleeding vessel, aspiration of hematoma, elevation of depressed bone, removal of bone fragments)<br>4. barbiturate coma therapy (may be indicated if other measures fail to control IICP)<br>d. provide emotional support to client and significant others. |
| 9.b. The client will not develop meningitis as evidenced by:<br>1. absence of fever and chills<br>2. gradual resolution of headache | 9.b.1. Assess for and report signs and symptoms of a CSF leak *(indicates a tear in the dura):*<br>a. presence of glucose in nasal, ear, or wound drainage as shown by positive glucose reagent strip (e.g. Tes-Tape, Dextrostix) results; be aware that any drainage containing blood will also test positive for glucose |

3. absence of nuchal rigidity and photophobia
4. negative Kernig's and Brudzinski's signs
5. normal CSF analysis.

b. clear halo or watery, yellowish ring around bloody or serosanguineous drainage on dressing or pillowcase
c. complaints of postnasal drip
d. constant swallowing.

2. Assess for and report signs and symptoms of meningitis:
   a. fever, chills
   b. increasing or persistent headache
   c. nuchal rigidity
   d. photophobia
   e. positive Kernig's sign (inability to straighten knee when hip is flexed)
   f. positive Brudzinski's sign (flexion of hip and knee in response to forward flexion of the neck).
3. Assist with lumbar puncture if indicated. Document appearance of CSF (a milky appearance can indicate elevated WBC levels) and CSF pressure (pressure is often elevated with meningitis).
4. Monitor results of the CSF analysis and report increased WBC and protein levels.
5. Implement measures *to prevent meningitis:*
   a. assist with thorough cleansing and debridement of head wound if indicated
   b. use sterile technique when changing dressings and working with intracranial pressure monitoring device
   c. instruct client to keep hands away from head wound and dressing; use restraints or mittens if necessary
   d. if a CSF leak is present:
      1. instruct client to avoid excessive movement and activity (bed rest is usually ordered *to prevent further stress on the torn dura)*
      2. instruct client to avoid coughing, sneezing, blowing nose, or straining to have a bowel movement *(these activities raise intracranial pressure and can cause extension of the dural tear);* consult physician regarding an order for an antitussive, decongestant, stool softener, and laxative if indicated
      3. if CSF is leaking from nose:
         a. position client with head of bed elevated at least 20° unless contraindicated *to allow the fluid to drain*
         b. instruct client to avoid putting finger in nose
         c. do not perform nasal suctioning or insert a nasogastric tube
         d. do not attempt to clean nose unless ordered by physician
      4. if CSF is leaking from ear:
         a. position client on side of CSF leakage unless contraindicated *to allow the fluid to drain*
         b. instruct client to avoid putting finger in ear
         c. do not attempt to clean ear unless ordered by physician
      5. do not pack dressing into area of CSF leakage (nose, ear, or wound) *because it will interfere with the drainage of fluid;* place a sterile pad over area of CSF leakage to absorb drainage and change pad as soon as it becomes damp
      6. prepare client for surgical repair of the torn dura if the leak does not heal spontaneously
   e. administer antimicrobials if ordered prophylactically.
6. If signs and symptoms of meningitis occur:
   a. continue with above measures
   b. initiate seizure precautions *(cerebral irritation can cause seizures)*
   c. provide a quiet environment with dim lighting *to reduce discomfort associated with headache and photophobia*
   d. administer antimicrobials if ordered
   e. provide emotional support to client and significant others.

9.c. The client will not experience seizure

9.c.1. Assess for and report signs and symptoms of seizure activity (e.g. twitching [usually of face or hands], clonic-tonic movements).

| Desired Outcomes | Nursing Actions and ***Selected Purposes/Rationales*** |
|---|---|
| activity or injury if seizure occurs. | 2. Implement measures *to prevent seizures:*<br>a. perform actions to prevent and treat IICP (see actions a.2 and 3 in this diagnosis)<br>b. perform actions to prevent and treat meningitis (see actions b.5 and 6 in this diagnosis)<br>c. administer anticonvulsants (e.g. phenytoin, carbamazepine) if ordered.<br>3. Initiate and maintain seizure precautions:<br>a. have oral airway and suction equipment readily available<br>b. pad side rails with blankets or soft pads<br>c. keep bed in low position with side rails up when client is in bed.<br>4. If seizures do occur:<br>a. implement measures *to decrease risk of injury:*<br>1. ease client to the floor if he/she is sitting in chair or ambulating at onset of seizure<br>2. remain with but do not restrain client during seizure activity<br>3. do not force any object between clenched teeth or try to pry mouth open<br>4. remove from area items that may cause injury<br>5. place towel under client's head if he/she is on floor<br>6. as seizure activity subsides, perform actions *to maintain a patent airway* (e.g. turn client on his/her side, insert an oral airway, suction as needed)<br>b. observe for and report characteristics of seizures (e.g. progression, time elapsed)<br>c. administer intravenous anticonvulsants (e.g. phenytoin, phenobarbital) if ordered<br>d. provide emotional support to client and significant others. |
| 9.d. The client will experience adaptation to cranial nerve damage if it occurs. | 9.d.1. Assess for signs and symptoms of damage to the following cranial nerves:<br>a. olfactory (e.g. decreased or absent sense of smell)<br>b. optic, oculomotor, trochlear, or abducens (e.g. diplopia, visual field cut, decreased visual acuity, abnormal extraocular movements)<br>c. trigeminal (e.g. decreased or absent corneal reflex, difficulty chewing, pain when chewing)<br>d. vagus or glossopharyngeal (e.g. loss of gag reflex, difficulty swallowing, hoarseness, inability to speak clearly)<br>e. hypoglossal (e.g. difficulty chewing, swallowing, or speaking)<br>f. facial (e.g. facial ptosis, impaired sense of taste).<br>2. Implement measures *to help the client compensate for cranial nerve damage if is has occurred:*<br>a. if the olfactory nerve is affected, provide meals that are visually appealing *to help stimulate appetite*<br>b. if vision is impaired, provide an eyepatch or frosted lens *(helps reduce double vision),* instruct client in visual scanning techniques (if experiencing visual field cut), and assist client with self-care and ambulation if indicated<br>c. if the corneal reflex is absent or the client is unable to close his/her eye, perform actions *to protect the cornea from irritation and abrasion* (e.g. instruct client to avoid rubbing eye; reduce his/her exposure to dust, powder, and smoke; instill isotonic eyedrops frequently)<br>d. if the trigeminal, hypoglossal, vagus, and/or glossopharyngeal nerves are affected:<br>1. withhold oral foods/fluids until gag reflex returns and client is better able to chew and swallow *in order to reduce the risk for aspiration;* provide parenteral nutrition or tube feedings if indicated<br>2. when oral intake is allowed:<br>a. perform actions *to prevent aspiration* (e.g. place client in high |

Fowler's position during and for at least 30 minutes after meals and snacks, assist client with oral hygiene after eating *to ensure that food particles do not remain in mouth,* instruct client to avoid laughing and talking while eating and drinking)

b. perform actions *to improve client's ability to swallow* (e.g. avoid serving sticky foods such as peanut butter and bananas, assist client to select foods that require little or no chewing and are easily swallowed, serve thick fluids or thicken thin fluids with substances such as "Thick-it" or gelatin)

3. perform actions *to facilitate communication* (e.g. maintain quiet environment; provide pad and pencil, magic slate, or word cards; listen carefully when client speaks)
4. consult speech pathologist about additional ways to facilitate swallowing and communication

e. if the sensory component of the facial nerve is affected, instruct client to add extra sweeteners or seasonings to food/fluids if desired *in order to compensate for impaired sense of taste*

f. provide emotional support to client and significant others.

9.e. The client will not experience diabetes insipidus as evidenced by:
1. absence of polyuria and polydipsia
2. urine specific gravity within normal range.

9.e.1. Assess for and report signs and symptoms of diabetes insipidus:
a. polyuria (urine output can range from 4-10 or more liters/day)
b. polydipsia (if the client is able to tolerate oral liquids, he/she may drink 4-10 or more liters of fluid/day)
c. urine specific gravity less than 1.005.

2. Administer osmotic diuretics (e.g. mannitol) and/or loop diuretics (e.g. furosemide) if ordered *to decrease edema of the hypothalamus, pituitary gland, and surrounding tissue and subsequently reduce the risk for the development of diabetes insipidus.*

3. If signs and symptoms of diabetes insipidus occur:
a. maintain fluid intake equal to output *in order to prevent water deficit*
b. administer an ADH replacement (e.g. vasopressin, lypressin, desmopressin acetate [DDAVP]) if ordered
c. assess for and report signs and symptoms of water deficit (e.g. decreased skin turgor; dry mucous membranes; sudden weight loss of 2% or greater; low B/P and/or postural hypotension; weak, rapid pulse; elevated serum sodium and osmolality).

9.f. The client will not develop SIADH as evidenced by:
1. stable weight
2. balanced intake and output
3. stable or improved mental status
4. stable or improved muscle strength
5. decreased complaints of headache
6. absence of cellular edema, abdominal cramping, nausea, and seizure activity
7. urine specific gravity within normal limits
8. urine and serum sodium and osmolality levels within normal limits.

9.f.1. Assess for and report signs and symptoms of SIADH:
a. sudden weight gain
b. intake greater than output
c. increased irritability or confusion
d. increasing muscle weakness
e. complaints of persistent or increased headache
f. fingerprint edema over sternum (reflects cellular edema)
g. abdominal cramping, nausea
h. seizures
i. urine specific gravity greater than 1.012
j. elevated urine sodium and osmolality levels
k. low serum sodium and osmolality levels.

2. Implement measures *to reduce the risk for the development of SIADH:*
a. perform actions to reduce pain (see Nursing Diagnosis 3, action e)
b. perform actions to reduce fear and anxiety (see Nursing Diagnosis 10, action b)
c. administer osmotic diuretics (e.g. mannitol) and/or loop diuretics (e.g. furosemide) if ordered *to decrease edema of the hypothalamus, pituitary gland, and surrounding tissue.*

3. If signs and symptoms of SIADH occur:
a. maintain fluid restrictions if ordered (usually 500-700 ml/day) *to prevent further fluid retention*
b. encourage intake of foods/fluids high in sodium (e.g. tomato juice, cured meats, processed cheese, canned soups, catsup, canned vegetables, dill pickles, bouillon)

Desired Outcomes | Nursing Actions and ***Selected Purposes/Rationales***

c. initiate seizure precautions
d. administer the following if ordered:
  1. diuretics (usually furosemide) *to promote water excretion*
  2. intravenous infusion of isotonic or hypertonic saline solution *to treat hyponatremia*
  3. demeclocycline *to promote water excretion (inhibits the effect of ADH on the renal tubules)*
e. provide emotional support to client and significant others.

9.g. The client will not experience GI bleeding as evidenced by:
  1. no complaints of epigastric discomfort and fullness
  2. absence of frank and occult blood in stool and gastric contents
  3. B/P and pulse within normal range for client
  4. RBC, Hct, and Hb levels within normal range.

9.g.1. Assess for and report signs and symptoms of GI bleeding (e.g. complaints of epigastric discomfort or fullness, frank or occult blood in stool or gastric contents, decreased B/P, increased pulse).
2. Monitor RBC, Hct, and Hb levels. Report declining values.
3. Implement measures *to prevent ulceration of the gastric and duodenal mucosa:*
  a. perform actions to decrease fear and anxiety (see Nursing Diagnosis 10, action b)
  b. instruct client to avoid foods/fluids that stimulate hydrochloric acid secretion or irritate the gastric mucosa:
    1. coffee, caffeine-containing tea and colas
    2. spices such as black pepper, chili powder, and nutmeg
  c. administer histamine$_2$-receptor antagonists (e.g. cimetidine, ranitidine, famotidine), antacids, and cytoprotective agents (e.g. sucralfate) if ordered.
4. If signs and symptoms of GI bleeding occur:
  a. insert nasogastric tube and maintain suction as ordered
  b. assist with measures to control bleeding (e.g. gastric lavage, endoscopic electrocoagulation, selective arterial embolization, intravenous or intra-arterial administration of vasopressin) if ordered
  c. administer blood products and/or volume expanders if ordered
  d. prepare client for surgery (e.g. ligation of bleeding vessels, partial gastrectomy) if indicated
  e. provide emotional support to client and significant others
  f. refer to Care Plan on Peptic Ulcer for additional care measures.

## 10. NURSING DIAGNOSIS: Anxiety

related to impaired motor and/or sensory function; altered thought processes; uncertainty as to permanence of neurological deficits; unfamiliar environment; and lack of understanding of diagnostic tests, diagnosis, and treatments.

Desired Outcome | Nursing Actions and ***Selected Purposes/Rationales***

10. The client will experience a reduction in anxiety as evidenced by:
  a. verbalization of feeling less anxious and fearful
  b. usual sleep pattern
  c. relaxed facial expression and body movements

10.a. Assess client for signs and symptoms of anxiety (e.g. verbalization of fears and concerns, insomnia, tenseness, tremors, restlessness, diaphoresis, tachypnea, elevated blood pressure, tachycardia, facial pallor or flushing, narrowed perceptual field, withdrawal, noncompliance with treatment plan). Validate perceptions carefully, remembering that some behaviors may result from neurological changes.
b. Implement measures *to reduce fear and anxiety:*
  1. orient client to hospital environment, equipment, and routines
  2. introduce staff who will be participating in his/her care; if possible, maintain consistency in staff assigned to his/her care *to provide feelings of stability and comfort with the environment*

d. stable vital signs
e. usual perceptual ability and interactions with others.

3. assure client that staff members are nearby; respond to call signal as soon as possible
4. maintain a calm, supportive, confident manner when interacting with client
5. encourage verbalization of fear and anxiety; provide feedback
6. reinforce physician's explanations and clarify misconceptions client has about the injury, treatment plan, and prognosis
7. explain all diagnostic tests
8. provide a calm, restful environment
9. instruct client in relaxation techniques and encourage participation in diversional activities
10. perform actions to assist the client to cope with the effects of the injury (see Nursing Diagnosis 12, action c)
11. encourage significant others to project a caring, concerned attitude without obvious anxiousness
12. if surgical intervention is indicated, begin preoperative teaching
13. administer antianxiety agents if ordered.

c. Include significant others in orientation and teaching sessions and encourage their continued support of the client.
d. Provide information based on current needs of client and significant others at a level they can understand. Encourage questions and clarification of information provided.
e. Consult physician if above actions fail to control fear and anxiety.

## 11. NURSING DIAGNOSIS: Self-concept disturbance*

related to:
a. change in appearance (e.g. periocular edema and ecchymosis, loss of hair on head if an area was shaved to repair lacerations or perform cranial surgery);
b. changes in motor and sensory function;
c. dependence on others to meet basic needs;
d. anticipated changes in life style and roles associated with sensory and motor impairments and altered thought processes.

*This diagnostic label includes the nursing diagnoses of body image disturbance, self-esteem disturbance, and altered role performance.

| Desired Outcome | Nursing Actions and ***Selected Purposes/Rationales*** |
|---|---|
| 11. The client will demonstrate beginning adaptation to changes in appearance, physical and mental functioning, life style, and roles as evidenced by:<br>a. verbalization of feelings of self-worth<br>b. maintenance of relationships with significant others<br>c. active participation | 11.a. Assess for signs and symptoms of a self-concept disturbance (e.g. verbal or nonverbal cues denoting a negative response to changes in body functioning and appearance such as denial of or preoccupation with changes that have occurred, refusal to look at or touch affected body part, or withdrawal from significant others).<br>b. Determine the meaning of changes in appearance, physical and mental functioning, life style, and roles to the client by encouraging him/her to verbalize feelings and by noting nonverbal responses to the changes experienced.<br>c. Implement measures to facilitate the grieving process (see Nursing Diagnosis 13, action b).<br>d. Discuss with client improvements in appearance and neurological function that can realistically be expected. |

| Desired Outcome | Nursing Actions and ***Selected Purposes/Rationales*** |
|---|---|
| in activities of daily living<br>d. active interest in personal appearance<br>e. willingness to participate in social activities<br>f. verbalization of a beginning plan for adapting life style to meet changes in physical and mental functioning. | e. Implement measures *to assist client to increase self-esteem* (e.g. limit negative self-assessment, encourage positive comments about self, give positive feedback about accomplishments and behaviors that are indicative of high self-esteem, assist to identify strengths).<br>f. Implement measures to assist the client to cope with the effects of craniocerebral trauma (see Nursing Diagnosis 12, action c).<br>g. If periocular edema and ecchymosis are present:<br>1. reinforce that they are temporary (edema usually begins to subside 48-72 hours after the injury and ecchymosis usually disappears in 10-14 days)<br>2. instruct and assist client with measures *to reduce swelling* (e.g. cold compresses to affected area, lying on unaffected side, keeping head of bed elevated 30° unless contraindicated).<br>h. Implement measures *to reduce client's embarrassment about loss of hair* (e.g. assist with hair styling that makes shaved area less obvious, provide a scarf or surgical cap if desired). Reinforce the fact that the hair will grow back.<br>i. Assist client with usual grooming and makeup habits if necessary.<br>j. Discuss techniques the client can utilize *to adapt to altered thought processes:*<br>1. encourage client to make lists and jot down messages and to refer to these rather than relying on his/her memory<br>2. instruct the client to place self in a calm environment when making decisions<br>3. encourage client to validate decisions, clarify information, and seek assistance to problem-solve if indicated<br>4. encourage client to schedule adequate rest periods and reduce stressors *in order to decrease irritability.*<br>k. Instruct significant others in ways to manage client's emotional lability and inappropriate behavior (e.g. provide privacy, reduce environmental stimuli, distract client by clapping hands).<br>l. Reinforce use of assistive devices (e.g. plate guards, broad-handled utensils, universal cuff, button hook, long-handled shoehorn) and mobility aids (e.g. walker, cane) *to increase client's independence.*<br>m. Encourage significant others to allow client to do what he/she is able *so that independence can be re-established and/or self-esteem redeveloped.*<br>n. Demonstrate acceptance of client using techniques such as touch and frequent visits. Encourage significant others to do the same.<br>o. Assist client's and significant others' adjustment by listening, facilitating communication, and providing information.<br>p. Assess for and support behaviors suggesting positive adaptation to changes that have occurred (e.g. use of assistive devices to perform self-care, verbalization of feelings of self-worth, maintenance of relationships with significant others).<br>q. Assist client and significant others to have similar expectations and understanding of future life style.<br>r. Encourage visits and support from significant others.<br>s. Encourage client to continue involvement in social activities and to pursue usual roles and interests. If previous roles, interests, and hobbies cannot be pursued, encourage development of new ones.<br>t. Provide information about and encourage utilization of community agencies and support groups (e.g. head injury support groups, vocational rehabilitation, family and individual counseling) if appropriate.<br>u. Consult physician about psychological counseling if client desires or if he/she seems unwilling or unable to adapt to changes resulting from craniocerebral trauma. |

## 12. NURSING DIAGNOSIS: Ineffective individual coping

related to fear, anxiety, persistent headache, changes in motor and sensory function and thought processes, and possibility of lengthy rehabilitation and changes in future life style and roles.

| Desired Outcome | Nursing Actions and ***Selected Purposes/Rationales*** |
|---|---|
| 12. The client will demonstrate the use of effective coping skills as evidenced by:<br>a. verbalization of ability to cope with the effects of craniocerebral trauma<br>b. utilization of appropriate problem-solving techniques<br>c. willingness to participate in treatment plan and meet basic needs<br>d. absence of destructive behavior toward self and others<br>e. appropriate use of defense mechanisms<br>f. recognition and utilization of available support systems. | 12.a. Assess for and report signs and symptoms of ineffective individual coping (e.g. verbalization of inability to cope; inability to ask for help, problem solve, or meet basic needs; reluctance to participate in treatment plan; destructive behavior toward self or others; inappropriate use of defense mechanisms; inability to meet role expectations). Validate perceptions carefully, remembering that some behaviors may be the result of neurological changes.<br>b. Assess client's perception of current situation including precipitating factors and effectiveness of coping mechanisms.<br>c. Implement measures *to promote effective coping:*<br>1. allow time for client to adjust psychologically to planned treatment, residual effects of craniocerebral trauma, and anticipated life-style and role changes<br>2. perform actions to reduce fear and anxiety (see Nursing Diagnosis 10, action b)<br>3. perform actions to reduce headache (see Nursing Diagnosis 3, action e)<br>4. assist client to recognize and manage inappropriate denial if it is present<br>5. encourage verbalization about current situation<br>6. assist client to identify personal strengths and resources that can be utilized to facilitate coping with the current situation<br>7. demonstrate acceptance of client but set limits on inappropriate behavior<br>8. create an atmosphere of trust and support<br>9. arrange for a visit with another individual who has successfully recovered from craniocerebral trauma<br>10. include client in the planning of care, encourage maximum participation in treatment plan, and allow choices when possible *to enable him/her to maintain a sense of control*<br>11. instruct client in effective problem-solving techniques (e.g. accurate identification of stressors, determination of various options to solve problem)<br>12. assist client to maintain usual daily routines whenever possible<br>13. assist client as he/she starts to plan for necessary life-style and role changes after discharge; help client to identify priorities and attainable goals<br>14. set up a home evaluation appointment with occupational and physical therapists before client's discharge if indicated *so that changes in the home environment (e.g. installation of ramps and handrails, widening doorways, altering kitchen facilities) can be completed by discharge*<br>15. assist client and significant others to identify ways that personal and family goals can be adjusted rather than abandoned<br>16. inform client that he/she will have days when impairments worsen; assure client that this is usually temporary and the result of physical and/or emotional stress or fatigue rather than an indication of deteriorating neurological status |

| Desired Outcome | Nursing Actions and ***Selected Purposes/Rationales*** |
|---|---|
| | 17. administer antianxiety and/or antidepressant agents if ordered<br>18. assist client to identify and utilize available support systems; provide information regarding available community resources that can assist client and significant others in coping with effects of craniocerebral trauma (e.g. head injury support groups; individual, family, and financial counseling services)<br>19. encourage continued emotional support from significant others<br>20. encourage client to share with significant others the kind of support that would be most beneficial (e.g. listening, inspiring hope, providing reassurance and accurate information)<br>21. support behaviors suggesting positive adaptation to changes experienced (e.g. participation in treatment plan and self-care activities, communication of ability to cope, utilization of effective problem-solving strategies).<br>d. Consult physician about psychological and vocational rehabilitation counseling if appropriate. Initiate a referral if necessary. |

## 13. NURSING DIAGNOSIS: Grieving*

related to impaired motor and sensory function and altered thought processes and the effect of these changes on future life style and roles.

*This diagnostic label includes anticipatory grieving and grieving following the actual losses.

| Desired Outcome | Nursing Actions and ***Selected Purposes/Rationales*** |
|---|---|
| 13. The client will demonstrate beginning progression through the grieving process as evidenced by:<br>a. verbalization of feelings about the craniocerebral trauma and its effects<br>b. expression of grief<br>c. participation in treatment plan and self-care activities<br>d. utilization of available support systems<br>e. verbalization of a plan for integrating prescribed follow-up care into life style. | 13.a. Assess for signs and symptoms of grieving (e.g. change in eating habits, inability to concentrate, insomnia, anger, noncompliance, withdrawal from significant others, denial of loss). Be aware that client's response to a loss will be affected by factors such as previous experience with loss, age, developmental stage, available support systems, spiritual and cultural background, current health status, and significance of the loss.<br>b. Implement measures *to facilitate the grieving process:*<br>1. assist client to acknowledge the losses experienced *so grief work can begin;* assess for factors that may hinder and facilitate acknowledgment<br>2. discuss the grieving process and assist client to accept the phases of grieving as an expected response to actual and/or anticipated losses<br>3. allow time for client to progress through the phases of grieving (phases vary among theorists but progress from shock and alarm to acceptance); be aware that not every phase is expressed by all individuals, that recurrence of phases is common, and that the grieving process may take months to years<br>4. provide an atmosphere of care and concern (e.g. provide privacy, be available and nonjudgmental, display empathy and respect) *so client will feel free to verbalize feelings*<br>5. perform actions *to promote trust* (e.g. answer questions honestly, provide requested information)<br>6. encourage the verbal expression of anger and sadness about the losses experienced; recognize displacement of anger and assist client to see the actual cause of angry feelings and resentment; establish limits on abusive behavior if demonstrated |

7. encourage client to express his/her feelings in whatever ways are comfortable (e.g. writing, drawing, conversation)
8. perform actions to promote effective coping (see Nursing Diagnosis 12, action c)
9. perform actions *to support realistic hope about the effects of rehabilitation on the neurological impairments:*
    a. focus on what the client is able to accomplish independently and with the use of assistive devices
    b. reinforce knowledge that impairments may improve with time
    c. reinforce positive effects of physical and occupational therapies
10. support behaviors suggesting successful grief work (e.g. verbalizing feelings about losses in mental and physical functioning, focusing on ways to adapt to losses, learning needed skills, developing or renewing relationships)
11. explain the phases of the grieving process to significant others; encourage their support and understanding
12. facilitate communication between client and significant others; be aware that they may be in different phases of the grieving process
13. provide information about counseling services and support groups that might assist client in working through grief
14. arrange for a visit from clergy if desired by client.

c. Consult physician about referral for counseling if signs of dysfunctional grieving (e.g. persistent denial of losses, excessive anger or sadness, hysteria, suicidal behaviors) occur.

## 14. NURSING DIAGNOSIS: Altered family processes

related to change in family roles and structure associated with a family member's motor and sensory impairments, altered thought processes, and possible need for lengthy rehabilitation.

| Desired Outcome | Nursing Actions and ***Selected Purposes/Rationales*** |
|---|---|
| 14. The family members* will demonstrate beginning adjustment to changes in functioning of family member and family roles and structure as evidenced by:<br>a. meeting client's needs<br>b. verbalization of ways to adapt to required roles and life-style changes<br>c. active participation in decision making and client's rehabilitation<br>d. positive interactions with one another. | 14.a. Assess for signs and symptoms of altered family processes (e.g. inability to meet client's needs, statements of not being able to accept client's physical impairments and changes in thought processes or make necessary role and life-style changes, inability to make decisions, inability or refusal to participate in client's rehabilitation, negative family interactions).<br>b. Identify components of the family and their patterns of communication and role expectations.<br>c. Implement measures *to facilitate family members' adjustment to client's diagnosis, changes in his/her functioning within the family system, and altered family roles and structure:*<br>1. encourage verbalization of feelings about client's disabilities and the effect of these on their family structure; actively listen to each member and maintain a nonjudgmental attitude about feelings shared<br>2. reinforce physician's explanation about the effects of craniocerebral trauma and planned treatment and rehabilitation<br>3. assist family members to gain a realistic perspective of client's situation, conveying as much hope as appropriate<br>4. provide privacy *so that family members and client can share their feelings* |

*The term "family members" is being used here to include client's significant others.

| Desired Outcome | Nursing Actions and ***Selected Purposes/Rationales*** |
|---|---|
| | *with one another;* stress the importance of and facilitate the use of good communication techniques<br>5. assist family members to progress through their own grieving process; explain that they may encounter times when they need to focus on meeting their own rather than the client's needs<br>6. emphasize the need for family members to obtain adequate rest and nutrition and to identify and utilize stress management techniques *so that they are better able to emotionally and physically deal with the changes and losses experienced*<br>7. encourage and assist family members to identify coping strategies for dealing with the client's disabilities and the effects on the family<br>8. assist family members to identify realistic goals and ways of reaching these goals<br>9. include family members in decision making about client and his/her care; convey appreciation for their input and continued support of client<br>10. encourage and allow family members to participate in client's care and rehabilitation<br>11. assist family members to identify resources that could assist them in coping with their feelings and meeting their immediate and long-term needs (e.g. counseling and social services; pastoral care; service, church, and head injury support groups); initiate a referral if indicated.<br>d. Consult physician if family members continue to demonstrate difficulty adapting to changes in client's functioning, roles, and family structure. |

## 15. NURSING DIAGNOSIS: Knowledge deficit

regarding follow-up care.

| Desired Outcomes | Nursing Actions and ***Selected Purposes/Rationales*** |
|---|---|
| 15.a. The client will identify ways to adapt to neurological deficits that may persist following craniocerebral trauma. | 15.a.1. Instruct client in ways to adapt to neurological deficits* resulting from the craniocerebral trauma:<br>a. wear an eyepatch or frosted lens if double vision is a problem<br>b. utilize scanning techniques if visual field cut is present<br>c. utilize paper and pencil, magic slate, computer, pictures, and gestures to express self if verbal communication is impaired<br>d. write down messages and reminders and refer to written instructions repeatedly if experiencing difficulty concentrating or remembering<br>e. request assistance when problem-solving and setting priorities and seek validation of decisions if reasoning ability is impaired<br>f. continue with techniques and exercises to improve swallowing if indicated |

*Neurological deficits can range from a temporary increase in irritability or a slight facial droop to hemiplegia, aphasia, or severely altered thought processes depending on the areas of the brain that have been affected. Ways of adapting to a few of the more common deficits are included here. For more specific rehabilitative measures and a more extensive discussion of deficits, refer to textbooks on neurological nursing and the Care Plan on Cerebrovascular Accident.

| | |
|---|---|
| | g. prepare meals that are visually appealing to help stimulate appetite if senses of smell and/or taste are impaired<br>h. utilize devices (e.g. wheelchair, cane, walker, broad-handled eating utensils, plate guard) if motor function is impaired<br>i. plan daily activities to allow for adequate rest periods in order to reduce irritability that often occurs after craniocerebral trauma.<br>2. Allow time for questions, clarification, and return demonstration of techniques. |
| 15.b. The client will identify ways to reduce headache. | 15.b. Instruct client in ways to reduce headache (headache may persist for months following injury):<br>1. dim environmental lighting if possible or wear sunglasses when light is bright<br>2. reduce environmental noise whenever possible (e.g. lower volume on TV and radio)<br>3. avoid situations that increase stress<br>4. take analgesics as prescribed. |
| 15.c. The client will state signs and symptoms to report to the health care provider. | 15.c. Instruct client to report the following signs and symptoms:<br>1. increasing drowsiness<br>2. increased irritability or restlessness<br>3. changes in behavior, increased difficulty remembering or concentrating<br>4. new or increased weakness of extremities<br>5. decreased sensation in extremities<br>6. severe headache<br>7. new or increased difficulty speaking or understanding what others are saying<br>8. new or increased difficulty chewing or swallowing<br>9. increase in or development of changes in vision (e.g. double vision, blurred vision, visual field cuts)<br>10. dizziness, difficulty maintaining balance<br>11. bloody, yellowish, or clear drainage from nose or ears<br>12. stiff neck<br>13. sudden weight gain or loss<br>14. excessive thirst<br>15. unusual increase or decrease in amount of urination<br>16. unexplained fever<br>17. seizures. |
| 15.d. The client will identify community agencies that can assist with home management and adjustment to changes resulting from the injury. | 15.d.1. Inform client and significant others of community resources that can assist with home management and the adjustment to changes resulting from craniocerebral trauma (e.g. home health agencies, Meals on Wheels, social and financial services, head injury support groups, local service groups that can help obtain assistive devices, individual and family counseling services).<br>2. Initiate a referral if indicated. |
| 15.e. The client will verbalize an understanding of and a plan for adhering to recommended follow-up care including future appointments with health care provider and therapists and medications prescribed. | 15.e.1. Reinforce the importance of keeping follow-up appointments with health care provider and physical, occupational, and speech therapists.<br>2. Teach client the rationale for, side effects of, schedule for taking, and importance of taking medications prescribed (e.g. phenytoin, antimicrobials).<br>3. Implement measures to improve client compliance:<br>a. include significant others in teaching sessions if possible<br>b. encourage questions and allow time for reinforcement and clarification of information provided<br>c. provide written instructions on scheduled appointments with health care provider and occupational, physical, and speech therapists; medications prescribed; and signs and symptoms to report. |

# Craniotomy

A craniotomy involves an opening through the skull in order to gain access to intracranial structures. The surgery may be performed to remove space-occupying lesions (e.g. tumor, hematoma) or objects such as a bullet or bone fragments, repair a vascular abnormality (e.g. aneurysm, arteriovenous malformation), or improve ventricular drainage.

A craniotomy is described in relation to the tentorium (i.e. supratentorial, infratentorial) and by the operative approach (e.g. temporal, occipital, parietal). The neurological deficits that can occur following the surgical procedure depend primarily on the areas of the brain that are disrupted to gain access to the surgical area (e.g. speech may be impaired following a temporal approach, ataxia is expected after a cerebellar approach) and the amount and location of the brain tissue that is excised or traumatized at the surgical site.

**This care plan focuses on the adult client hospitalized for a craniotomy.** Preoperative goals of care are to decrease fear and anxiety and educate the client about postoperative expectations and management. Postoperatively, goals of care are to reduce pain, prevent complications, assist the client to adjust to any neurological impairments, and educate the client regarding follow-up care. Client care and discharge teaching need to be individualized based on the diagnosis and the neurological deficits he/she is experiencing. For more detailed coverage of nursing care measures for various neurological deficits, refer to the Care Plan on Cerebrovascular Accident.

## DIAGNOSTIC TESTS

Computed tomography (CT)
Magnetic resonance imaging (MRI)
Skull x-rays
Cerebral angiography
Brain scan
Positron emission tomography (PET)

## DISCHARGE CRITERIA

Prior to discharge, the client will:

- have adequate cerebral tissue perfusion
- have improved or stable neurological function
- have no signs and symptoms of complications
- identify ways to adapt to neurological deficits resulting from the underlying disease condition and/or the surgical procedure
- state signs and symptoms to report to the health care provider
- share thoughts and feelings about the diagnosis and neurological deficits that may be the result of the underlying disease process and/or the surgery
- identify community resources that can assist with home management and adjustment to changes resulting from the diagnosis and/or the surgery
- verbalize an understanding of and a plan for adhering to recommended follow-up care including future appointments with health care provider, activity level, pain management, medications prescribed, and wound care.

## NURSING/ COLLABORATIVE DIAGNOSES

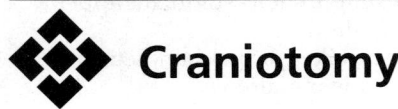

**See Standardized Preoperative and Postoperative Care Plans for additional diagnoses.**

## PREOPERATIVE

**Use in conjunction with the Standardized Preoperative Care Plan.**

### 1. NURSING DIAGNOSIS: Anxiety

related to:
a. unfamiliar environment and separation from significant others;
b. lack of understanding of diagnostic tests and planned surgical procedure;
c. anticipated loss of control, effects of anesthesia, and surgical findings;
d. financial concerns associated with hospitalization;
e. possibility of continued and/or new neurological impairments;
f. anticipated discomfort and changes in appearance (e.g. shaved head, scalp indentation) and usual life style and roles;
g. possibility of death.

| Desired Outcome | Nursing Actions and ***Selected Purposes/Rationales*** |
|---|---|
| 1. The client will experience a reduction in anxiety (see Standardized Preoperative Care Plan, Nursing Diagnosis 1 [pp. 108-109], for outcome criteria). | 1.a. Refer to Standardized Preoperative Care Plan, Nursing Diagnosis 1 (pp. 108-109), for measures related to assessment and reduction of fear and anxiety.<br>b. Implement additional measures *to reduce fear and anxiety:*<br>1. explain the necessity for intensive care monitoring after most craniotomies; orient to the intensive care unit and equipment that may be used (e.g. intracranial pressure monitoring device, ventricular drain, wound catheter, ventilator) if appropriate<br>2. identify and practice alternative forms of communication (e.g. magic slate, word cards and/or picture board, hand signals) if client is expected to be intubated or speech impairment is anticipated following surgery<br>3. perform actions *to reduce fear and anxiety about anticipated changes in physical appearance:*<br>a. assure client that when head dressing is removed, he/she can wear a surgical cap or scarf if desired (most physicians advise clients to avoid wearing a wig or hairpiece until sutures are removed)<br>b. inform client that incision lines are usually behind normal hairline and should not be apparent when hair grows back<br>c. discuss alternative hair styles that might make incision lines, cranial indentation, and/or shaved portion of scalp less apparent<br>d. assure client that the periocular edema and ecchymosis that may occur after surgery are temporary<br>e. if a craniectomy is planned, discuss the possibility of having a cranioplasty in a few months if appropriate<br>4. reinforce physician's explanations about anticipated effects of the surgery on neurological function; discuss resources available to assist client to adapt to anticipated impairments (e.g. speech, occupational, and physical therapists). |

## POSTOPERATIVE

**Use in conjunction with the Standardized Postoperative Care Plan.**

### 1. NURSING DIAGNOSIS: Pain: headache

related to:
a. trauma to the cerebral tissue associated with the surgical procedure;
b. stretching or compression of cerebral vessels and tissue associated with increased intracranial pressure if it occurs;
c. irritation of the meninges associated with bleeding from meningeal vessels, leakage of blood into the cerebrospinal fluid (CSF), and/or inflammation of the meninges.

| Desired Outcome | Nursing Actions and ***Selected Purposes/Rationales*** |
|---|---|
| 1. The client will obtain relief from headache as evidenced by:<br>a. verbalization of headache relief<br>b. relaxed facial expression and body positioning. | 1.a. Determine how the client usually responds to pain.<br>b. Assess client's perception of pain including location, intensity, and type. Utilize a numerical scale to rate intensity.<br>c. Assess for nonverbal signs of headache (e.g. grimacing, rubbing head, avoidance of bright lights and noises, reluctance to move).<br>d. Assess for factors that seem to aggravate and alleviate headache.<br>e. Implement measures *to relieve headache:*<br>1. perform actions *to minimize environmental stimuli* (e.g. provide a quiet environment, restrict visitors, dim lights)<br>2. avoid jarring bed or startling client *to minimize risk of sudden movements*<br>3. perform actions to prevent and treat increased intracranial pressure and meningitis (see Postoperative Collaborative Diagnosis 2, actions a.2 and 3 and b.5 and 6)<br>4. provide nonpharmacological measures for headache relief (e.g. cool cloth to forehead, back rub, relaxation techniques)<br>5. administer nonnarcotic analgesics or codeine (other narcotic analgesics are usually contraindicated *because they have a greater depressant effect on the central nervous system*) if ordered.<br>f. Consult physician if above actions fail to relieve headache. |

### 2. COLLABORATIVE DIAGNOSES: Potential complications:

a. **increased intracranial pressure (IICP)** related to:
   1. cerebral bleeding and/or hematoma formation following surgery
   2. cerebral edema associated with increased capillary permeability of cerebral vessels and malfunction of the sodium pump resulting from cerebral tissue trauma and subsequent cerebral ischemia
   3. hydrocephalus associated with obstruction of normal CSF flow resulting from edema, hematoma, presence of blood in the subarachnoid space, and/or occlusion of ventricular shunt if present
   4. cerebral vasodilation associated with cerebral hypoxia and/or an increased metabolic rate resulting from hyperthermia (can occur following surgical trauma to the hypothalamus), seizure activity, or meningitis;

b. **meningitis** related to:
   1. irritation of the meninges associated with trauma to the meningeal vessels or presence of blood in the CSF
   2. introduction of microorganisms into the meninges or CSF associated with an interruption in the dura, which is incised to gain access to the brain tissue;

c. **seizures** related to altered activity of the cerebral neurons associated with irritation of the brain tissue during surgery (especially if a supratentorial craniotomy was performed) or IICP and meningitis if they occur;
d. **diabetes insipidus** related to decreased production and/or impaired release of antidiuretic hormone (ADH) associated with altered function of the hypothalamus or pituitary gland (can occur because of surgical trauma or postoperative edema in that area);
e. **cranial nerve damage** related to trauma to the nerves prior to or during surgery and/or compression of the nerves associated with postoperative intracerebral hematoma or edema.

| Desired Outcomes | Nursing Actions and ***Selected Purposes/Rationales*** |
|---|---|
| 2.a. The client will not develop IICP as evidenced by:<br>1. usual or improved level of consciousness<br>2. no complaints of increased headache<br>3. stable or improved motor and sensory function<br>4. absence of vomiting, papilledema, and seizure activity<br>5. usual pupillary size and reactivity<br>6. stable vital signs. | 2.a.1. Assess for and report signs and symptoms of IICP:<br>a. restlessness, agitation, confusion, lethargy<br>b. complaints of increased headache<br>c. decreasing motor and sensory function<br>d. abnormal posturing (e.g. extension [decerebrate], flexion [decorticate])<br>e. vomiting (usually without nausea)<br>f. papilledema<br>g. seizures<br>h. change in pupil size or reactivity<br>i. altered respiratory pattern (e.g. Cheyne-Stokes, central neurogenic hyperventilation)<br>j. full, bounding, slow pulse<br>k. rise in systolic B/P with widening pulse pressure.<br>2. Implement measures *to prevent IICP:*<br>a. maintain fluid restrictions as ordered<br>b. administer osmotic diuretics (e.g. mannitol) and/or loop diuretics (e.g. furosemide) if ordered *to reduce cerebral edema*<br>c. perform actions *to promote adequate cerebral venous drainage:*<br>1. elevate head of bed 30-45° unless contraindicated<br>2. keep head and neck in midline position; avoid flexion, extension, and rotation of head and neck<br>3. administer stool softeners, antitussives, and antiemetics if ordered *to prevent straining to have a bowel movement, coughing, and vomiting (these conditions cause an increase in intrathoracic pressure, which subsequently impedes venous return from the brain)*<br>d. perform actions *to prevent cerebral hypoxia and subsequent cerebral edema and vasodilation:*<br>1. implement measures *to maintain a patent airway* (e.g. position client on side, suction if necessary)<br>2. administer central nervous system depressants judiciously; hold medication and consult physician if respiratory rate is less than 12/minute<br>3. administer oxygen as ordered and before and after tracheal suctioning<br>e. perform additional actions *to prevent vasodilation of cerebral vessels:*<br>1. implement measures *to prevent an increase in blood pressure:*<br>a. observe for and control conditions that can cause agitation (e.g. fear, anxiety, distended bladder)<br>b. instruct client to avoid activities that result in isometric muscle contractions (e.g. pushing feet against footboard, tightly gripping side rails)<br>2. implement measures *to prevent an increase in metabolic rate:*<br>a. administer anticonvulsants (e.g. phenytoin, carbamazepine) if ordered *to prevent seizure activity* |

| Desired Outcomes | Nursing Actions and ***Selected Purposes/Rationales*** |
|---|---|

b. perform actions to prevent and treat meningitis (see actions b.5 and 6 in this diagnosis)

c. if client is experiencing hyperthermia (may occur following trauma to the hypothalamus during surgery), perform actions *to reduce body temperature* (e.g. sponge his/her body with tepid water, obtain a hypothermia blanket as ordered)

3. assist with mechanical hyperventilation (may be done *to decrease arterial $CO_2$ and prevent subsequent vasodilation*)

f. schedule care so activities that could raise intracranial pressure (e.g. suctioning, bathing, repositioning) are not grouped together

g. position client on unoperative side if bone flap and/or large mass was removed *(helps prevent increased pressure and venous congestion in the operative area)*

h. if client has an internal shunt, perform actions *to maintain its patency* (e.g. avoid pressure on the shunt, tubing, and reservoir site; pump shunt as ordered)

i. if client has an external shunt, perform actions *to maintain its patency* (e.g. avoid kinks in tubing, keep client's head and drainage receptacle at the prescribed levels).

3. If signs and symptoms of IICP are present:
   a. continue with above actions
   b. initiate seizure precautions
   c. prepare client for the following if planned:
      1. insertion of an intracranial pressure monitoring device (e.g. intraventricular catheter, subarachnoid screw or bolt, epidural fiberoptic catheter or transducer, intraparenchymal catheter)
      2. lumbar or ventricular puncture *to remove excess CSF*
      3. surgical intervention (e.g. ligation of bleeding vessel, repair of blocked shunt, removal of bone flap or hematoma)
   d. provide emotional support to client and significant others.

**Desired Outcome**

2.b. The client will not develop meningitis as evidenced by:
1. absence of fever and chills
2. absence of nuchal rigidity and photophobia
3. gradual resolution of headache
4. negative Kernig's and Brudzinski's signs
5. normal CSF analysis.

**Nursing Actions**

2.b.1. Assess for and report signs and symptoms of a CSF leak *(indicates an opening in the dura):*
   a. presence of glucose in nasal, ear, or wound drainage as shown by positive glucose reagent strip (e.g. Tes-Tape, Dextrostix) results; be aware that any drainage containing blood will also test positive for glucose
   b. clear halo or a watery, yellowish ring around bloody or serosanguineous drainage on dressing or pillowcase
   c. complaints of postnasal drip
   d. constant swallowing.

2. Assess for and report signs and symptoms of meningitis:
   a. fever, chills
   b. nuchal rigidity
   c. photophobia
   d. increasing or persistent headache
   e. positive Kernig's sign (inability to straighten knee when hip is flexed)
   f. positive Brudzinski's sign (flexion of hip and knee in response to forward flexion of the neck).

3. Assist with lumbar puncture if indicated. Document appearance of CSF (a milky appearance can indicate elevated WBC levels) and CSF pressure (pressure is often elevated with meningitis).

4. Monitor results of CSF analysis and report increased WBC and protein levels.

5. Implement measures *to prevent meningitis:*
   a. use sterile technique when changing dressings and when working with an external ventricular shunt, wound drain, and intracranial pressure monitoring device

b. instruct client to keep hands away from drains and dressings; use restraints or mittens if necessary
c. if a CSF leak is present:
  1. instruct client to avoid excessive movement and activity (bed rest is usually ordered *to prevent further stress on the incised dura*)
  2. instruct client to avoid coughing, sneezing, blowing nose, and straining to have a bowel movement *(these activities raise intracranial pressure and can cause extension of the dural tear);* consult physician about an order for an antitussive, decongestant, laxative, and stool softener if indicated
  3. if CSF is leaking from nose:
     a. position client with head of bed elevated at least 20° unless contraindicated *to allow the fluid to drain*
     b. instruct client to avoid putting finger in nose
     c. do not perform nasal suctioning or insert a nasogastric tube
     d. do not attempt to clean nose unless ordered by physician
  4. if CSF is leaking from ear:
     a. position client on side of CSF leakage unless contraindicated *to allow the fluid to drain*
     b. instruct client to avoid putting finger in ear
     c. do not attempt to clean ear unless ordered by physician
  5. do not pack dressing into area of CSF leakage (nose, ear, or wound) *because it will interfere with the drainage of fluid;* place a sterile pad over area of CSF leakage to absorb drainage and change pad as soon as it becomes damp
  6. prepare client for surgical repair of the dura if leak does not heal spontaneously (the area usually heals without surgical intervention within 7-10 days)
d. administer antimicrobials if ordered prophylactically.

6. If signs and symptoms of meningitis occur:
   a. continue with above measures
   b. initiate seizure precautions *(cerebral irritation can cause seizures)*
   c. provide a quiet environment with dim lighting *to reduce discomfort associated with headache and photophobia*
   d. administer antimicrobials if ordered
   e. provide emotional support to client and significant others.

2.c. The client will not experience seizure activity or injury if seizure occurs.

2.c. 1. Assess for and report signs and symptoms of seizure activity (e.g. twitching [usually of face or hands], clonic-tonic movements).
2. Implement measures *to prevent seizures:*
   a. perform actions to prevent and treat IICP (see actions a.2 and 3 in this diagnosis)
   b. perform actions to prevent and treat meningitis (see actions b.5 and 6 in this diagnosis)
   c. administer anticonvulsants (e.g. phenytoin, carbamazepine) if ordered.
3. Initiate and maintain seizure precautions:
   a. have an oral airway and suction equipment readily available
   b. pad side rails with blankets or soft pads
   c. keep bed in low position with side rails up when client is in bed.
4. If seizures do occur:
   a. implement measures *to decrease risk of injury:*
      1. ease client to the floor if he/she is sitting in chair or ambulating at onset of seizure
      2. remain with but do not restrain client during seizure activity
      3. do not force any object between clenched teeth or try to pry mouth open
      4. remove from area items that may cause injury
      5. place towel under client's head if he/she is on the floor
      6. as seizure activity subsides, perform actions *to maintain a patent*

| Desired Outcomes | Nursing Actions and ***Selected Purposes/Rationales*** |
|---|---|
| | *airway* (e.g. turn client on his/her side, insert an oral airway, suction as needed)<br>b. observe for and report characteristics of seizures (e.g. progression, time elapsed)<br>c. administer intravenous anticonvulsants (e.g. phenytoin, phenobarbital) if ordered<br>d. provide emotional support to client and significant others. |
| 2.d. The client will not experience diabetes insipidus as evidenced by:<br>1. absence of polyuria and polydipsia<br>2. urine specific gravity within normal range. | 2.d.1. Assess for and report signs and symptoms of diabetes insipidus:<br>a. polyuria (urine output can range from 4-10 or more liters/day)<br>b. polydipsia (if the client is able to tolerate oral liquids, he/she may drink 4-10 or more liters of fluid/day)<br>c. urine specific gravity less than 1.005.<br>2. Administer osmotic diuretics (e.g. mannitol) and/or loop diuretics (e.g. furosemide) if ordered *to reduce edema of the hypothalamus, pituitary gland, and surrounding tissue and subsequently reduce the risk for the development of diabetes insipidus.*<br>3. If signs and symptoms of diabetes insipidus occur:<br>a. maintain fluid intake equal to output *in order to prevent water deficit*<br>b. administer an ADH replacement (e.g. vasopressin, lypressin, desmopressin acetate [DDAVP]) as ordered<br>c. assess for and report signs and symptoms of water deficit (e.g. decreased skin turgor; dry mucous membranes; sudden weight loss of 2% or greater; low B/P and/or postural hypotension; weak, rapid pulse; elevated serum sodium and osmolality). |
| 2.e. The client will experience beginning adaptation to cranial nerve damage if it occurs. | 2.e.1. Assess for signs and symptoms of damage to the following cranial nerves:<br>a. olfactory (e.g. decreased or absent sense of smell)<br>b. optic, oculomotor, trochlear, or abducens (e.g. diplopia, visual field cut, decreased visual acuity, abnormal extraocular movements)<br>c. trigeminal (e.g. decreased or absent corneal reflex, difficulty chewing, pain when chewing)<br>d. vagus or glossopharyngeal (e.g. loss of gag reflex, difficulty swallowing, hoarseness, inability to speak clearly)<br>e. hypoglossal (e.g. difficulty chewing, swallowing, or speaking)<br>f. facial (e.g. facial ptosis, impaired sense of taste).<br>2. Implement measures *to assist the client to adapt to cranial nerve damage if it has occurred:*<br>a. if the olfactory nerve is affected, provide meals that are visually appealing *to help stimulate appetite*<br>b. if vision is affected, provide an eyepatch or frosted lens *(helps reduce double vision),* instruct client in visual scanning techniques (if experiencing visual field cut), and assist client with self-care and ambulation if indicated<br>c. if the corneal reflex is absent or the client is unable to close his/her eye, perform actions *to protect the cornea from irritation and abrasion* (e.g. instruct client to avoid rubbing eye; reduce his/her exposure to dust, powder, and smoke; instill isotonic eyedrops frequently)<br>d. if the trigeminal, hypoglossal, vagus, and/or glossopharyngeal nerves are affected:<br>1. withhold oral foods/fluids until gag reflex returns and client is better able to chew and swallow *in order to reduce the risk for aspiration;* provide parenteral nutrition or tube feedings if indicated<br>2. when oral intake is allowed:<br>a. perform actions *to prevent aspiration* (e.g. place client in high Fowler's position during and for at least 30 minutes after meals and snacks, assist client with oral hygiene after eating *to ensure that food particles do not remain in mouth,* instruct client to avoid laughing and talking while eating and drinking) |

b. perform actions *to improve client's ability to swallow* (e.g. avoid serving sticky foods such as peanut butter and bananas, assist client to select foods that require little or no chewing and are easily swallowed, serve thick fluids or thicken thin fluids with substances such as "Thick-it" or gelatin)
3. perform actions *to facilitate communication* (e.g. maintain quiet environment; provide pad and pencil, magic slate, or word cards; listen carefully when client speaks)
4. consult speech pathologist about additional ways to facilitate swallowing and communication

e. if the sensory component of the facial nerve is affected, instruct client to add extra sweeteners or seasonings to foods/fluids if desired *in order to compensate for impaired sense of taste*

f. provide emotional support to client and significant others.

## 3. NURSING DIAGNOSIS: Self-concept disturbance*

related to:
a. changes in appearance (e.g. periocular edema and ecchymosis, skull indentation, loss of scalp hair);
b. dependence on others to meet basic needs;
c. anticipated changes in life style and roles associated with altered motor and sensory function (e.g. hemiplegia, visual disturbances, speech impairment) and usual thought processes (changes may occur as a result of cerebral tissue injury).

*This diagnostic label includes the nursing diagnoses of body image disturbance, self-esteem disturbance, and altered role performance.

| Desired Outcome | Nursing Actions and ***Selected Purposes/Rationales*** |
|---|---|
| 3. The client will demonstrate beginning adaptation to changes in appearance, physical and mental functioning, life style, and roles as evidenced by:<br>a. verbalization of feelings of self-worth<br>b. maintenance of relationships with significant others<br>c. active participation in activities of daily living<br>d. active interest in personal appearance<br>e. willingness to participate in social activities<br>f. verbalization of a beginning plan for adapting life style to meet changes resulting from the | 3.a. Assess for signs and symptoms of a self-concept disturbance (e.g. verbal or nonverbal cues denoting a negative response to changes in body functioning and appearance such as denial of or preoccupation with changes that have occurred, refusal to look in the mirror, or withdrawal from significant others).<br>b. Determine the meaning of the changes in appearance, physical and mental functioning, life style, and roles to the client by encouraging him/her to verbalize feelings and by noting nonverbal responses to the changes experienced.<br>c. Be aware that client may recognize and grieve the losses experienced. Assist him/her through the beginning phases of grieving (e.g. shock, disbelief, denial, anger, sadness, depression). Do not reinforce maladaptive denial of situation.<br>d. Discuss with client improvements in appearance and neurological function that can realistically be expected.<br>e. Implement measures *to assist client to increase self-esteem* (e.g. limit negative self-assessment, encourage positive comments about self, give positive feedback about accomplishments and behaviors that are indicative of high self-esteem, assist to identify strengths).<br>f. Assist the client to identify and utilize coping techniques that have been helpful in the past.<br>g. If periocular edema and ecchymosis are present:<br>1. reinforce that they are temporary (edema usually begins to subside 48-72 hours after surgery and ecchymosis usually disappears in 10-14 days) |

| Desired Outcome | Nursing Actions and ***Selected Purposes/Rationales*** |
|---|---|
| underlying disease process and/or residual effects of the surgery. | 2. instruct client in and assist with measures *to reduce swelling* (e.g. cold compresses to affected area, lying on unoperative side, keeping head of bed elevated 30° unless contraindicated).<br>h. Implement measures *to reduce client's embarrassment about partial or total loss of hair and misshapen skull if bone flap was removed* (e.g. provide client with a surgical cap or scarf if desired, assist client to obtain a wig or hairpiece when allowed). Reinforce the fact that the hair will grow back and, if indicated, a cranioplasty can be performed in a few months to restore original shape of the skull.<br>i. Assist client with usual grooming and makeup habits if necessary.<br>j. Discuss techniques the client can utilize *to adapt to altered thought processes if present:*<br>1. encourage client to make lists and jot down messages and to refer to these rather than relying on his/her memory<br>2. instruct the client to place self in a calm environment when making decisions<br>3. encourage client to validate decisions, clarify information, and seek assistance to problem-solve if indicated<br>4. encourage client to schedule adequate rest periods and reduce stressors *in order to decrease irritability.*<br>k. Demonstrate acceptance of client using techniques such as touch and frequent visits. Encourage significant others to do the same.<br>l. Assess for and support behaviors suggesting positive adaptation to changes that have occurred (e.g. scanning environment or wearing eyepatch if visual disturbances are present, utilizing alternative methods of communicating if speech is impaired, utilizing assistive devices to perform self-care activities).<br>m. Encourage significant others to allow client to do what he/she is able *so that independence can be re-established and/or self-esteem redeveloped.*<br>n. Encourage client contact with others *so that he/she can test and establish a new self-image.*<br>o. Assist client's and significant others' adjustment by listening, facilitating communication, and providing information.<br>p. Assist client and significant others to have similar expectations and understanding of future life style and to identify ways that personal and family goals can be adjusted rather than abandoned.<br>q. Teach client the rationale for treatments, encourage maximum participation in treatment regimen, and allow choices whenever possible *to enable him/her to maintain a sense of control over life.*<br>r. Encourage visits and support from significant others.<br>s. Encourage client to continue involvement in social activities and to pursue usual roles and interests. If previous roles, interests, and hobbies cannot be pursued, encourage development of new ones.<br>t. Provide information about and encourage utilization of community agencies and support groups (e.g. head injury support groups; vocational rehabilitation; American Cancer Society; family, individual, and/or financial counseling) if appropriate.<br>u. Consult physician about psychological counseling if client desires or if he/she seems unwilling or unable to adapt to changes resulting from the disease and/or the surgery. |

## 4. NURSING DIAGNOSIS: Knowledge deficit

regarding follow-up care.

| Desired Outcomes | Nursing Actions and ***Selected Purposes/Rationales*** |
| --- | --- |
| 4.a. The client will identify ways to adapt to neurological deficits resulting from the underlying disease condition and/or the surgical procedure. | 4.a.1. Instruct client in ways to adapt to neurological deficits* resulting from the underlying disease condition and/or the surgical procedure:<br>a. wear an eyepatch or frosted lens if double vision is a problem<br>b. utilize scanning techniques if visual field cut is present<br>c. utilize pencil and paper, magic slate, computer, pictures, and gestures to express self if verbal communication is impaired<br>d. write down messages and reminders and refer to written instructions repeatedly if experiencing difficulty concentrating or memory is impaired<br>e. request assistance when problem-solving and setting priorities and seek validation of decisions if reasoning ability is impaired<br>f. prepare meals that are visually appealing to help stimulate appetite if sense of smell and/or taste are diminished<br>g. utilize assistive devices (e.g. wheelchair, cane, walker, broad-handled eating utensils, plate guard) if motor function is impaired<br>h. plan daily activities to allow for adequate rest periods in order to reduce the irritability that often occurs after cerebral tissue trauma.<br>2. Allow time for questions, clarification, and return demonstration of techniques. |
| 4.b. The client will state signs and symptoms to report to the health care provider. | 4.b.1. Refer to Standardized Postoperative Care Plan, Nursing Diagnosis 21, action c (p. 135), for signs and symptoms to report to the health care provider.<br>2. Instruct client to report these additional signs and symptoms:<br>a. increasing drowsiness<br>b. increased irritability or restlessness<br>c. changes in behavior, decreased ability to concentrate<br>d. decreased sensation in extremities<br>e. new or increased weakness of extremities<br>f. difficulty speaking or understanding what others are saying<br>g. change in vision (e.g. double vision, blurred vision, visual field cuts)<br>h. increased difficulty chewing or swallowing<br>i. dizziness, difficulty maintaining balance<br>j. increased swelling at wound site<br>k. bloody, yellowish, or clear drainage from ears, nose, or incision<br>l. stiff neck<br>m. excessive thirst<br>n. excessive urination<br>o. severe or persistent headache<br>p. seizures. |
| 4.c. The client will identify community resources that can assist with home management and adjustment to changes resulting from the diagnosis and/or the surgery. | 4.c. 1. Inform client and significant others of community resources that can assist with home management and adjustment to neurological changes resulting from the diagnosis and/or surgery (e.g. physical, occupational, and speech therapists; Meals on Wheels; social services; home health agencies; American Cancer Society; head injury support groups).<br>2. Initiate a referral if indicated. |
| 4.d. The client will verbalize an understanding of and a plan for adhering to | 4.d.1. Refer to Standardized Postoperative Care Plan, Nursing Diagnosis 21 (pp. 135-136), for routine postoperative instructions and measures to improve client compliance.<br>2. Instruct client in ways to reduce headache if present (e.g. reduce |

*Neurological deficits can range from a temporary increase in irritability or a slight facial droop to hemiplegia, aphasia, or severely altered thought processes depending on the area(s) of the brain that have been affected. Ways of adapting to a few of the more common deficits are included here. For more specific rehabilitative measures and a more extensive discussion of deficits, refer to textbooks on neurological and neurosurgical nursing and the Care Plan on Cerebrovascular Accident.

| Desired Outcomes | Nursing Actions and ***Selected Purposes/Rationales*** |
|---|---|
| recommended follow-up care including future appointments with health care provider, activity level, pain management, medications prescribed, and wound care. | environmental lighting and noise whenever possible, avoid situations that increase stress, take analgesics as prescribed).<br>3. Explain the rationale for, side effects of, schedule for taking, and importance of taking the prescribed medications (e.g. phenytoin, antimicrobials). |

# Spinal Cord Injury

Spinal cord injury (spinal cord trauma) can result from a motor vehicle accident, fall, sports injury, or act of violence. It can be classified by the cause of cord injury (e.g. contusion, compression, transection, ischemia), direction of movement of the vertebrae or mechanism of injury (e.g. flexion, hyperextension, axial loading, flexion with rotation), level of injury (e.g. cervical, sacral), stability of the vertebral column (i.e. stable, unstable), and degree of cord involvement (i.e. complete, incomplete).

Immediately following spinal cord injury, spinal shock (complete loss of motor, sensory, autonomic, and reflex activity below the level of the injury) usually occurs. Spinal shock can last hours to months, with the usual duration being between 1 and 6 weeks. The neurological impairments that remain following the period of spinal shock depend upon the level of the cord injury (the higher the level, the greater the loss of body function) and the degree of cord involvement (if complete, there is total loss of sensory function and voluntary muscle control below the level of the injury; if incomplete, some of the motor and/or sensory fibers below the level of injury are able to function).

**This care plan focuses on the adult client hospitalized with a complete injury of the spinal cord at the level of the fifth cervical vertebra (C5).** After the period of spinal shock, a client with a complete cord injury at the C5 level experiences loss of motor function below the clavicles; however, full neck, upper shoulder, and some biceps control and elbow flexion are retained. Sensory function is intact above the clavicles and in certain areas of the deltoids and forearms. With rehabilitation, the client should be able to do things such as operate an electric wheelchair, feed self using assistive devices, utilize reflex activity to achieve an erection and stimulate bowel and bladder elimination, turn in bed, and operate some equipment (e.g. typewriter, computer, telephone) using assistive devices.

Initially, goals of care are to sustain life and prevent further cord damage by stabilizing the vertebral column and reducing spinal cord ischemia. Subsequently, goals of care are to mobilize the client, prevent complications, assist him/her to regain as much independence as possible, and facilitate psychological adjustment to the effects of the injury.

## DIAGNOSTIC TESTS

Cervical spine x-rays
Computed tomography (CT)
Magnetic resonance imaging (MRI)
Somatosensory-evoked potentials

## DISCHARGE CRITERIA

Prior to discharge, the client will:

- have no signs and symptoms of complications resulting from the spinal cord injury and decreased mobility
- identify ways to prevent complications associated with spinal cord injury and decreased mobility
- demonstrate the ability to correctly use and maintain assistive devices

- identify ways to manage altered bowel and bladder function
- state signs and symptoms to report to the health care provider
- identify community resources that can assist with home management and adjustment to changes resulting from spinal cord injury
- share thoughts and feelings about the effects of spinal cord injury on self-concept, life style, and roles
- verbalize an understanding of and a plan for adhering to recommended follow-up care including future appointments with health care provider and occupational and physical therapists and medications prescribed.

---

**NURSING/COLLABORATIVE DIAGNOSES**



**See Care Plan on Immobility for additional diagnoses.**

## 1. NURSING DIAGNOSIS: Anxiety

related to extensive loss of motor and sensory function; application of immobilization device to stabilize the cervical spine; lack of understanding of diagnostic tests, diagnosis, and treatment; unfamiliar environment; financial concerns; and anticipated effect of the spinal cord injury on life style and roles.

| Desired Outcome | Nursing Actions and ***Selected Purposes/Rationales*** |
|---|---|
| 1. The client will experience a reduction in anxiety as evidenced by:<br>a. verbalization of feeling less anxious and fearful<br>b. usual sleep pattern<br>c. relaxed facial expression<br>d. usual perceptual ability and interactions with others. | 1.a. Assess client for signs and symptoms of anxiety (e.g. verbalization of fears and concerns, insomnia, tenseness, irritability, facial pallor or flushing, narrowed perceptual field, withdrawal, noncompliance with treatment plan).<br>b. Implement measures *to reduce fear and anxiety:*<br>1. remain with client while immobilization device is being applied<br>2. explain necessity of frequent neurological checks<br>3. provide information about the insertion of skull pins:<br>a. assure client that the pins penetrate only the outer table of the skull, not the brain<br>b. assure client that very little pain is associated with the insertion but that the procedure will be quite loud since bone is such a good sound conductor<br>c. assure client that only a small amount of hair is clipped at each insertion site<br>d. explain that tongs and traction or a halo ring and traction or body jacket will be attached to the pins so that the cervical spine is immobilized and kept in correct alignment<br>4. explain the purpose and safety features of the turning frame or kinetic bed if appropriate<br>5. assure client that measures have been taken to keep him/her from falling off bed/frame (e.g. side rails up if in bed, safety straps on turning frame)<br>6. explain the sensations the client may experience when frame is turned (e.g. closed-in feeling, momentary dizziness); assure him/her that these sensations disappear when the turn is completed<br>7. once cervical spine immobilization is accomplished:<br>a. orient client to hospital environment, equipment, and routines<br>b. assure client that staff members are nearby; provide client with a call signal that has been adapted to meet his/her needs (e.g. voice-activated call light) and respond to call signal as soon as possible<br>c. introduce staff who will be participating in his/her care; if possible, maintain consistency in staff assigned to his/her care *to provide feelings of stability and comfort with the environment*<br>d. maintain a calm, supportive, confident manner when interacting with client<br>e. avoid startling client (e.g. speak client's name and identify yourself when entering room and before physical contact, place self in client's visual field whenever possible during care and conversation)<br>f. encourage verbalization of fear and anxiety; provide feedback<br>g. reinforce physician's explanations and clarify misconceptions client has about spinal cord injury, treatment plan, and prognosis<br>h. explain all diagnostic tests<br>i. explain that the flaccid paralysis and lack of reflex activity below the level of the cord injury that occurs immediately following the |

injury is a result of spinal shock; emphasize that some reflex activity will return after spinal shock subsides
- j. provide a calm, restful environment
- k. instruct client in relaxation techniques and encourage participation in diversional activities
- l. initiate financial and/or social service referrals if indicated
- m. perform actions to assist client to cope with effects of the injury (see Nursing Diagnosis 22, action c)
- n. encourage significant others to project a caring, concerned attitude without obvious anxiousness
- o. if comfortable for nurse and client, reinforce verbal messages of caring by touching areas where client has sensation (e.g. shoulders, head, neck); encourage significant others to do the same
- p. arrange for a visit from clergy if client desires.

c. Include significant others in orientation and teaching sessions and encourage their continued support of the client.
d. Provide information based on current needs of client and significant others at a level they can understand. Encourage questions and clarification of information provided.
e. Consult physician if above actions fail to control fear and anxiety.

## 2. NURSING DIAGNOSIS: Altered tissue perfusion

related to:
a. decreased cardiac output associated with:
1. suppression of the cardiac accelerator reflex resulting from loss of sympathetic nervous system control below the level of the injury (especially during period of spinal shock)
2. decreased venous return resulting from massive vasodilation below the level of the injury (occurs as a result of loss of sympathetic nervous system vasopressor activity [especially during period of spinal shock] and the subsequent unopposed parasympathetic nervous system activity);

b. peripheral pooling of blood associated with loss of sympathetic nervous system control over peripheral vessels below the level of the injury (especially during period of spinal shock) and loss of muscle tone in extremities resulting from paralysis of extremities and decreased mobility.

| Desired Outcome | Nursing Actions and ***Selected Purposes/Rationales*** |
|---|---|
| 2. The client will maintain adequate tissue perfusion as evidenced by:<br>a. B/P within normal range for client<br>b. usual mental status<br>c. extremities warm with absence of pallor and cyanosis<br>d. palpable peripheral pulses<br>e. capillary refill time less than 3 seconds<br>f. balanced intake and output. | 2.a. Assess for and report signs and symptoms of diminished tissue perfusion (e.g. hypotension, restlessness, confusion, cool extremities, pallor or cyanosis of extremities, diminished or absent peripheral pulses, slow capillary refill, oliguria).<br>b. Implement measures *to maintain adequate tissue perfusion:*<br>1. avoid activities that cause vagal stimulation (e.g. suctioning) unless absolutely necessary *in order to prevent a further reduction in pulse rate*<br>2. administer the following medications if ordered *to increase cardiac output:*<br>a. anticholinergics (e.g. atropine) *to increase heart rate*<br>b. sympathomimetics (e.g. dopamine) *to treat intractable hypotension and promote venous return*<br>3. perform actions *to prevent peripheral pooling of blood and/or increase venous return:*<br>a. perform passive range of motion exercises at least 3 times/day<br>b. avoid positions that compromise blood flow in the lower extremities (e.g. crossing legs, pillows under knees, sitting for long periods) |

| Desired Outcome | Nursing Actions and ***Selected Purposes/Rationales*** |
|---|---|
| | c. apply thigh-high elastic stockings as ordered; remove for 30-60 minutes at least twice daily<br>d. apply/maintain intermittent pneumatic compression stockings or boots if ordered<br>e. elevate lower extremities for 20-minute intervals several times a shift unless contraindicated<br>f. apply an abdominal binder if ordered before placing client in a sitting or upright position *(the binder increases pressure on the aorta, which reduces the amount of blood that flows to and pools in extremities)*<br>4. perform actions *to allow time for remaining autoregulatory mechanisms to adjust to position changes:*<br>a. change client's position slowly<br>b. gradually progress client to a sitting or upright position using a recliner wheelchair or tilt table when allowed and tolerated.<br>c. Consult physician if signs and symptoms of decreased tissue perfusion persist or worsen. |

## 3. NURSING DIAGNOSIS: Ineffective breathing pattern

related to:

a. impaired lung/chest wall expansion associated with:
   1. loss of abdominal and intercostal muscle function (innervation of these muscles occurs at the thoracic level)
   2. upward pressure on the diaphragm resulting from gastric distention (can occur if paralytic ileus develops during period of spinal shock)
   3. decreased activity and recumbent positioning (in this position, full expansion of the lungs is restricted by the bed or turning frame surface and by the abdominal contents pushing up against the diaphragm)
   4. pressure on the chest wall associated with improper fit or application of halo device body jacket or abdominal binder;

b. depressant effects of some medications (e.g. narcotic analgesics, central-acting muscle relaxants).

| Desired Outcome | Nursing Actions and ***Selected Purposes/Rationales*** |
|---|---|
| 3. The client will maintain an effective breathing pattern (see Care Plan on Immobility, Nursing Diagnosis 1 [p. 139], for outcome criteria). | 3.a. Refer to Care Plan on Immobility, Nursing Diagnosis 1 (p. 139), for measures related to assessment and improvement of breathing pattern.<br>b. Monitor for and report a significant decline in vital capacity measurements.<br>c. Implement additional measures *to improve breathing pattern:*<br>1. perform actions to treat paralytic ileus if it develops (see Collaborative Diagnosis 19, action b.2) *in order to reduce gastric distention and upward pressure on diaphragm*<br>2. if client needs an abdominal binder, make sure that it is positioned below the rib cage<br>3. if client is wearing a halo device body jacket, consult physician and orthotist about having it readjusted if it is restricting full expansion of client's chest wall<br>4. encourage and assist client to perform exercises that strengthen the accessory muscles used in breathing (e.g. shoulder shrugs *to strengthen the trapezius muscles*) when allowed and tolerated. |

## 4. NURSING DIAGNOSIS: Ineffective airway clearance

related to stasis of secretions associated with decreased mobility and poor cough effort (results from paralysis of abdominal and intercostal muscles and weakened diaphragm).

| Desired Outcome | Nursing Actions and ***Selected Purposes/Rationales*** |
|---|---|
| 4. The client will maintain clear, open airways (see Care Plan on Immobility, Nursing Diagnosis 2 [pp. 139-140], for outcome criteria). | 4.a. Refer to Care Plan on Immobility, Nursing Diagnosis 2 (pp. 139-140), for measures related to assessment and promotion of effective airway clearance.<br>b. Implement measures *to facilitate the client's cough efforts in order to further promote effective airway clearance:*<br>1. place client in a horizontal position during cough efforts unless contraindicated *(this position promotes a more effective forced expiration by decreasing the effects of gravity on the diaphragm)*<br>2. use an assisted coughing technique (e.g. place palm of hand below diaphragm and push upward as client exhales). |

## 5. NURSING DIAGNOSIS: Altered nutrition: less than body requirements

related to decreased oral intake associated with:

a. dietary restrictions during period of spinal shock if paralytic ileus develops;
b. anorexia resulting from boredom, fatigue, depression, a slowed metabolic rate (occurs with decreased activity), and early satiety that occurs with decreased gastrointestinal activity;
c. difficulty swallowing resulting from neck hyperextension and/or horizontal body position during the time that the cervical spine is immobilized;
d. difficulty feeding self resulting from loss of most of upper extremity motor function.

| Desired Outcome | Nursing Actions and ***Selected Purposes/Rationales*** |
|---|---|
| 5. The client will maintain an adequate nutritional status (see Care Plan on Immobility, Nursing Diagnosis 3 [pp. 140-141], for outcome criteria). | 5.a. Refer to Care Plan on Immobility, Nursing Diagnosis 3 (pp. 140-141), for measures related to assessment and maintenance of an adequate nutritional status.<br>b. Implement additional measures *to improve oral intake and maintain an adequate nutritional status:*<br>1. facilitate client's psychological adjustment to effects of spinal cord injury (see Nursing Diagnoses 21; 22, action c; 23; and 24, action b)<br>2. perform actions *to facilitate swallowing if client is on a turning frame* (e.g. place in prone position during meals, use a straw for all liquids)<br>3. perform actions *to facilitate swallowing if client's neck is in a hyperextended position while the cervical spine is being immobilized* (e.g. place in side-lying position during meals unless contraindicated, use a straw for all liquids)<br>4. feed client until he/she is able to feed self using assistive devices. |

## 6. NURSING DIAGNOSIS: Pain:

a. **headache** related to contractions of the neck muscles (can occur in response to stress);
b. **neck pain** related to nerve root irritation at the site of spinal cord injury, muscle stiffness while immobilization device is in place, and muscle strain associated with increased use of neck muscles following removal of immobilization device;
c. **upper arm and shoulder pain** related to muscle strain associated with increased use of biceps and shoulders as activity progresses.

| Desired Outcome | Nursing Actions and ***Selected Purposes/Rationales*** |
|---|---|
| 6. The client will experience diminished pain as evidenced by:<br>a. verbalization of same<br>b. relaxed facial expression<br>c. increased participation in activities when allowed. | 6.a. Determine how the client usually responds to pain.<br>b. Assess client's perception of pain including location, intensity, and type. Utilize a numerical scale to rate intensity.<br>c. Assess for nonverbal signs of pain (e.g. grimacing or tense facial expression, reluctance to turn head or move shoulders when increased activity is allowed, restlessness, facial pallor).<br>d. Assess for factors that seem to aggravate and alleviate pain.<br>e. Implement measures *to reduce pain:*<br>1. perform actions *to prevent or relieve headache:*<br>a. minimize environmental stimuli (e.g. provide a calm environment, restrict visitors, dim lights)<br>b. implement measures to reduce psychological stress (see Nursing Diagnoses 1, action b; 21; 22, action c; 23; and 24, action b)<br>c. avoid letting any object hit the skull pins, tongs, traction weights, and/or halo frame *(sound transmitted through these objects is intensified by their contact with the skull and loud noise is a noxious stimulus that can cause or intensify headache)*<br>d. apply cool cloth to forehead if client desires<br>2. perform actions *to prevent or relieve neck, upper arm, and/or shoulder pain:*<br>a. maintain immobilization of the cervical spine as ordered *to prevent nerve root irritation*<br>b. when moving client, provide support to neck and utilize turn sheet rather than pushing or pulling on shoulders and arms<br>c. apply neck support (e.g. soft cervical collar) if ordered following removal of immobilization device<br>d. massage client's upper arms and shoulders, being careful to avoid area around or over cervical spine until the injury has stabilized<br>e. consult physician about application of heat and/or cold to upper arms, shoulders, and neck<br>3. provide or assist with additional nonpharmacological measures for pain relief (e.g. position change if allowed, relaxation techniques, guided imagery, quiet conversation, diversional activities)<br>4. administer analgesics if ordered (narcotic analgesics are usually contraindicated *because of their respiratory depressant effect*).<br>f. Consult physician if above measures fail to provide adequate relief of pain. |

## 7. NURSING DIAGNOSIS: Ineffective thermoregulation

related to loss of nervous system feedback between the area below the level of cord injury and the hypothalamus (interruption of this feedback system results in the loss of compensatory responses to temperature changes [i.e. vasodilation, sweating, vasoconstriction, shivering] below the level of cord injury).

| Desired Outcome | Nursing Actions and ***Selected Purposes/Rationales*** |
|---|---|
| 7. The client will experience effective thermoregulation as evidenced by:<br>a. verbalization of comfortable body temperature above the level of the injury<br>b. absence of excessively warm or cool skin<br>c. temperature between 36-38° C. | 7.a. Assess for signs and symptoms of ineffective thermoregulation (e.g. complaints of feeling too warm or too cold, excessively warm or cool skin below the level of the injury).<br>b. Monitor client's temperature. Report if less than 36° C or greater than 38° C.<br>c. Implement measures *to maintain effective thermoregulation:*<br>1. perform actions *to prevent hypothermia:*<br>a. maintain room temperature at 70° F<br>b. provide extra clothing and bedding as necessary<br>c. protect client from drafts<br>d. apply warming blanket as ordered<br>e. provide warm liquids for client to drink<br>f. avoid taking client outdoors when it is very cold<br>2. perform actions *to prevent hyperthermia:*<br>a. maintain room temperature at 70° F<br>b. avoid use of excessive clothing and bedding<br>c. apply cooling blanket as ordered<br>d. remove extra clothing during physical and occupational therapy sessions<br>e. avoid taking client outdoors when it is very hot (especially if the humidity is high).<br>d. Consult physician if above measures fail to maintain effective thermoregulation. |

## 8. NURSING DIAGNOSIS: Sensory/perceptual alterations:

a. **visual** related to decreased ability to move head associated with immobilization device used to stabilize the cervical spine;
b. **tactile** related to loss of integrity of ascending spinal pathways at the level of the cord injury.

| Desired Outcomes | Nursing Actions and ***Selected Purposes/Rationales*** |
|---|---|
| 8.a. The client will experience adequate visual stimulation as evidenced by verbalization of same. | 8.a. Implement measures *to provide visual stimulation if the client's head movement or visual field is limited by the immobilization device:*<br>1. provide prism glasses for client's use<br>2. position mirrors in strategic places *to provide increased visualization of surroundings*<br>3. place self within client's visual field when talking with him/her; instruct others to do the same<br>4. put posters, pictures, and cards on the ceiling and suspend objects such as mobiles from ceiling (these will be within client's visual field when he/she is supine)<br>5. if client is on a turning frame, place objects of interest (e.g. posters, clock, flowers, cards, small TV, pictures) on the floor within client's visual field when he/she is in prone position. |

| Desired Outcomes | Nursing Actions and ***Selected Purposes/Rationales*** |
|---|---|
| 8.b. The client will experience adequate tactile stimulation as evidenced by verbalization of same. | 8.b.1. Ascertain areas of body where client can perceive tactile sensation (mainly head, neck, and shoulders).<br>2. Implement measures *to provide tactile stimulation:*<br>a. touch client on shoulders, head, and neck when appropriate; encourage significant others to do the same<br>b. obtain materials of various textures (e.g. cotton, leather) to rub gently on areas of sensation<br>c. consult occupational therapist for additional ways to provide tactile stimulation. |

## 9. NURSING DIAGNOSIS: High risk for impaired skin integrity

related to:

a. ischemia of the skin and subcutaneous tissue associated with prolonged pressure on tissues as a result of decreased mobility, halo device body jacket, and/or some assistive devices;
b. damage to the skin or subcutaneous tissue associated with friction or shearing;
c. increased fragility of the skin associated with dependent edema, decreased tissue perfusion, and inadequate nutritional status;
d. frequent contact with irritants associated with urinary incontinence if it occurs.

| Desired Outcome | Nursing Actions and ***Selected Purposes/Rationales*** |
|---|---|
| 9. The client will maintain skin integrity as evidenced by:<br>a. absence of redness and irritation<br>b. no skin breakdown. | 9.a. Inspect the skin (especially bony prominences, dependent and/or edematous areas, pin sites, perineum, area underneath halo device body jacket, and areas of sensory loss) for pallor, redness, and breakdown.<br>b. Refer to Care Plan on Immobility, Nursing Diagnosis 4, action b (pp. 141-142), for measures to prevent skin breakdown associated with decreased mobility.<br>c. Implement additional measures *to prevent skin breakdown:*<br>1. perform actions to maintain adequate tissue perfusion (see Nursing Diagnosis 2, action b)<br>2. perform actions to maintain an adequate nutritional status (see Nursing Diagnosis 5)<br>3. if client is wearing a halo device body jacket:<br>a. ensure that jacket lining and skin beneath it are kept clean and dry<br>b. make sure that clothing worn under the jacket is clean, dry, wrinkle-free, and made of cotton (some physicians allow client to wear a T-shirt under the jacket; others do not because they feel the shirt promotes slippage of the jacket)<br>c. cover all rough jacket edges with foam tape<br>d. consult physician and orthotist about having the jacket readjusted if it is placing excessive pressure on any skin area<br>4. perform actions to prevent urinary incontinence (see Nursing Diagnosis 12, actions d.2-4 and e)<br>5. if client is incontinent:<br>a. thoroughly cleanse and dry perineal area with soft tissue or cloth after each episode of incontinence; apply a protective ointment or cream (e.g. Desitin, A & D ointment, Vaseline)<br>b. provide incontinence pads to absorb moisture; do not allow skin to come in contact with plastic portion of the pads<br>6. perform actions to decrease spasticity (see Nursing Diagnosis 10, action |

a.9) *because spasms can cause movement and subsequent friction and make it difficult to keep client positioned properly*
7. ensure that wheelchair is not too small for client and that it is adequately cushioned
8. ensure that clothing and straps that secure assistive devices are not too tight.

d. If skin breakdown occurs:
1. notify physician
2. continue with above measures to prevent further irritation and breakdown
3. perform decubitus care as ordered or per standard hospital procedure
4. assess client closely and report signs and symptoms of infection (e.g. elevated temperature; redness, warmth, and edema around area of breakdown; unusual drainage from site).

## 10. NURSING DIAGNOSIS: Impaired physical mobility

related to:
a. activity limitations associated with quadriplegia and immobilization of the spine;
b. spasticity following the period of spinal shock associated with stimulation of the reflex arcs below the level of the injury;
c. decreased motivation associated with fatigue and the psychological response to the extensive motor and sensory losses that have occurred;
d. pain.

| Desired Outcome | Nursing Actions and ***Selected Purposes/Rationales*** |
|---|---|
| 10. The client will achieve maximum physical mobility within limitations imposed by the injury and the treatment plan. | 10.a. Implement measures *to increase mobility:*<br>1. facilitate client's psychological adjustment to the effects of the spinal cord injury (see Nursing Diagnoses 21; 22, action c; 23; and 24, action b)<br>2. perform actions to reduce pain (see Nursing Diagnosis 6, action e)<br>3. instruct client in and assist with active and active-resistive exercises of neck, shoulders, and biceps when allowed by physician<br>4. perform passive range of motion at least 3 times/day to areas below the level of the cord injury<br>5. reposition client at least every 2 hours and maintain proper alignment *in order to decrease the risk of contractures and further impaired mobility*<br>6. when activity is allowed, instruct client in ways to move his/her body (e.g. hook arm over side rail to assist in turning self, trigger flexor spasm of knees to help swing legs over side of bed during transfer to and from wheelchair)<br>7. instruct client in and assist with use of mobility aids (e.g. sliding board, electric wheelchair) as activity progresses<br>8. reinforce instructions, activities, and exercise plan recommended by physical and occupational therapists<br>9. perform actions *to reduce spasticity (spasms can interfere with attempts to increase mobility):*<br>a. avoid stimulating extremities or muscle groups (e.g. do not jar bed, do not touch easily stimulated areas unnecessarily)<br>b. implement measures to prevent conditions such as urinary tract |

| Desired Outcome | Nursing Actions and ***Selected Purposes/Rationales*** |
|---|---|
| | infection, muscle tightening from staying in one position too long, fatigue, and chills *(these conditions can result in the stimulation of various muscle groups)*<br>c. provide or assist with nonpharmacological measures for reducing spasticity (e.g. biofeedback, stretching exercises, position changes, local application of cold)<br>d. administer muscle relaxants (e.g. baclofen, dantrolene, diazepam) if ordered<br>10. provide adequate rest periods before activity sessions.<br>b. Provide praise and encouragement for all efforts to increase physical mobility.<br>c. Encourage the support of significant others. Allow them to assist with range of motion exercises, positioning, and activity if desired.<br>d. Consult physician if client is unable to achieve expected level of mobility or if range of motion becomes restricted. |

## 11. NURSING DIAGNOSIS: Self-care deficit

related to impaired physical mobility associated with quadriplegia, spasticity, decreased motivation, pain, and activity restrictions imposed by treatment plan.

| Desired Outcome | Nursing Actions and ***Selected Purposes/Rationales*** |
|---|---|
| 11. The client will demonstrate increased participation in self-care activities within the limitations imposed by the treatment plan and effects of the spinal cord injury. | 11.a. With client, develop a realistic plan for meeting daily physical needs. Inform client that with rehabilitation and use of assistive devices, he/she should be able to:<br>1. feed self once meal has been set up<br>2. wash face and chest<br>3. comb front and sides of hair, brush teeth, shave self with an electric razor<br>4. participate in dressing upper body.<br>b. When condition stabilizes and physician allows, implement measures *to facilitate client's ability to perform self-care activities:*<br>1. perform actions to increase mobility (see Nursing Diagnosis 10, action a)<br>2. consult occupational therapist regarding assistive devices available; reinforce use of these devices, which may include:<br>a. rocker feeder, overhead sling, plate guard, sandwich holder, and broad-handled and/or swivel utensils for feeding self<br>b. flexor-hinge splint or universal cuff to aid in brushing teeth, combing hair, and shaving self with electric razor<br>c. bath mitt for bathing face and chest<br>d. Velcro fasteners *to facilitate dressing upper body*<br>3. schedule care at a time when client is most likely to be able to participate (e.g. when analgesics are at peak effect, after rest periods, not immediately after physical therapy sessions or meals)<br>4. keep objects client can use independently within easy reach<br>5. allow adequate time for accomplishment of self-care activities.<br>c. Provide positive feedback for all efforts and accomplishments of self-care.<br>d. Perform for client the self-care activities that he/she is unable to accomplish. |

e. Inform significant others of client's abilities to participate in own care. Explain the importance of encouraging and allowing client to achieve an optimal level of independence.

## 12. NURSING DIAGNOSIS: Altered urinary elimination:

a. **retention** related to:
   1. atony of bladder wall and contraction of external urinary sphincter during period of spinal shock
   2. spasticity of the external urinary sphincter and/or loss of ability to coordinate bladder contraction and relaxation of the external urinary sphincter following period of spinal shock
   3. incomplete bladder emptying associated with horizontal positioning (in this position, the gravity needed for complete bladder emptying is lost);

b. **incontinence** related to:
   1. spasticity of the bladder following period of spinal shock (incontinence can occur if the bladder contracts strongly)
   2. inadvertent stimulation of the voiding reflex.

| Desired Outcome | Nursing Actions and ***Selected Purposes/Rationales*** |
|---|---|
| 12. The client will experience an optimal pattern of urinary elimination as evidenced by:<br>a. absence of bladder distention<br>b. balanced intake and output<br>c. absence of urinary incontinence. | 12.a. Assess for and report signs and symptoms of altered urinary elimination:<br>1. urinary retention (e.g. bladder distention, intake greater than output)<br>2. urinary incontinence.<br>b. Catheterize client if ordered *to determine amount of residual urine.*<br>c. Assist with urodynamic studies (e.g. cystometrogram) if ordered.<br>d. Implement measures *to promote optimal urinary elimination:*<br>1. perform actions *to prevent urinary retention during period of spinal shock:*<br>a. perform intermittent catheterizations or insert indwelling urinary catheter as ordered<br>b. implement measures *to maintain patency of urinary catheter if present* (e.g. keep tubing free of kinks)<br>2. following the period of spinal shock, perform actions *to promote complete bladder emptying and/or prevent bladder distention (a distended bladder can cause bladder spasms and subsequent incontinence):*<br>a. attempt to periodically initiate voiding by stimulating the trigger zones of the reflex sacral arc (e.g. tap suprapubic area, stroke or massage abdomen, stroke inner thigh, perform anal sphincter stretching, pull pubic hair); if voiding occurs, repeat stimulus as necessary *to empty the bladder*<br>b. if possible, place client on bedside commode or toilet when triggering voiding reflex or performing intermittent catheterization *(gravity facilitates complete bladder emptying)*<br>c. encourage client to space fluid intake evenly throughout the day rather than drinking a large quantity at one time *(if the bladder fills rapidly and frequency of emptying is not increased, bladder distention occurs)*<br>d. instruct client to limit intake of beverages containing caffeine such as colas, coffee, and tea *(caffeine is a mild diuretic; the increased urine production can result in bladder distention if the frequency of bladder emptying is not also increased)*<br>e. limit oral fluid intake in the evening *so that the bladder does not become overdistended during the night* (as rehabilitation progresses, most clients do not perform intermittent catheterization or attempt to trigger voiding during the night) |

| Desired Outcome | Nursing Actions and ***Selected Purposes/Rationales*** |
|---|---|
| | 3. instruct client and others to avoid stimulating the voiding reflex trigger zones at times other than during bladder care *in order to reduce the risk of incontinence*<br>4. administer central-acting muscle relaxants (e.g. baclofen) *to decrease spastic contraction of the bladder and subsequent risk of incontinence and to decrease tone of the external urinary sphincter (decreased sphincter tone allows for more complete bladder emptying during reflex voiding attempts).*<br>e. If urinary retention or incontinence persists:<br>1. carefully review bladder training program<br>2. prepare client for insertion of an indwelling catheter (urethral or suprapubic) if indicated<br>3. provide emotional support to client and significant others. |

## 13. NURSING DIAGNOSIS: Constipation

related to:

a. decreased gastrointestinal motility associated with:
   1. loss of autonomic nervous system function below the level of the injury during period of spinal shock
   2. decreased activity;

b. lack of awareness of stool in rectum associated with sensory loss below the level of the injury;

c. loss of central nervous system control over defecation reflex;

d. decreased gravity filling of lower rectum associated with horizontal positioning;

e. decreased intake of fluids and foods high in fiber.

| Desired Outcome | Nursing Actions and ***Selected Purposes/Rationales*** |
|---|---|
| 13. The client will not experience constipation as evidenced by:<br>a. usual frequency of bowel movements<br>b. passage of soft, formed stool<br>c. absence of abdominal distention<br>d. absence of or decrease in headache and anorexia. | 13.a. Ascertain client's usual bowel elimination habits.<br>b. Assess for signs and symptoms of constipation (e.g. decrease in frequency of stools; passage of hard, formed stools; abdominal distention; development of or increase in headache or anorexia).<br>c. Assess bowel sounds. Report a pattern of decreasing bowel sounds.<br>d. Implement measures *to prevent constipation* (the following are usually included in a bowel training program):<br>1. instruct client to increase intake of foods high in fiber (e.g. nuts, bran, whole-grain breads and cereals, raw fruits and vegetables, dried fruits) unless contraindicated<br>2. assist client to maintain a minimum fluid intake of 2500 ml/day unless contraindicated<br>3. encourage client to drink warm liquids *in order to initiate the gastrocolic and duodenocolic reflexes and stimulate peristalsis*<br>4. assist client to eat at scheduled times and adhere to a routine time for defecation; follow client's preinjury pattern if possible<br>5. increase activity as allowed and tolerated<br>6. perform digital stimulation and/or insert rectal suppository *to stimulate reflex peristalsis and emptying of rectum*<br>7. place client on toilet or bedside commode or place in high Fowler's position on bedpan for bowel movements unless contraindicated; provide privacy and adequate ventilation<br>8. allow ample time for bowel evacuation (may take up to an hour after rectal stimulation) |

9. if an analgesic is needed, encourage use of nonnarcotics rather than narcotics *to prevent further decrease in bowel activity*
10. administer laxatives, stool softeners, and/or enemas if ordered.

e. Check for impaction if client has not had a bowel movement in 3 days, if he/she is passing liquid stool, or if other signs and symptoms of constipation are present. Administer oil retention and/or cleansing enemas as ordered followed by digital removal of stool if necessary.
f. If constipation occurs, review bowel training program and revise it as needed.

## 14. NURSING DIAGNOSIS: Sleep pattern disturbance

related to:
a. inability to assume usual sleep position associated with loss of motor function and use of devices to immobilize the spine (e.g. halo device, turning frame);
b. frequent assessments and treatments;
c. fear and anxiety;
d. unfamiliar environment;
e. sudden, uncontrolled movement associated with spasticity following period of spinal shock.

| Desired Outcome | Nursing Actions and ***Selected Purposes/Rationales*** |
|---|---|
| 14. The client will attain optimal amounts of sleep within the parameters of the treatment regimen (see Care Plan on Immobility, Nursing Diagnosis 10 [p. 147], for outcome criteria). | 14.a. Refer to Care Plan on Immobility, Nursing Diagnosis 10 (p. 147), for measures related to assessment and promotion of sleep.<br>b. Implement additional measures *to promote sleep:*<br>1. assist client to assume a comfortable sleep position within limits of treatment plan (e.g. if client is more comfortable prone than supine, it may be possible to alter turning schedule to allow prone position for 3 rather than 2 hours during the night)<br>2. perform actions to decrease fear and anxiety (see Nursing Diagnosis 1, action b)<br>3. perform actions to reduce spasticity (see Nursing Diagnosis 10, action a.9). |

## 15. NURSING DIAGNOSIS: High risk for infection:

a. **pneumonia** related to stasis of secretions in the lungs (secretions provide a good medium for bacterial growth) and aspiration if it occurs;
b. **urinary tract infection** related to:
   1. increased bacterial growth associated with urinary stasis and the increased urine alkalinity that results from hypercalciuria (with prolonged immobility, excess calcium is released from the bones and excreted in the urine)
   2. entry of pathogens associated with presence of an indwelling catheter, performance of intermittent catheterizations, or tears in the bladder mucosa if the bladder becomes distended.

| Desired Outcomes | Nursing Actions and ***Selected Purposes/Rationales*** |
|---|---|
| 15.a. The client will not develop pneumonia (see Care Plan on | 15.a.1. Refer to Care Plan on Immobility, Nursing Diagnosis 11, action a (pp. 147-148), for measures related to assessment, prevention, and treatment of pneumonia. |

| Desired Outcomes | Nursing Actions and ***Selected Purposes/Rationales*** |
|---|---|
| Immobility, Nursing Diagnosis 11, outcome a [pp. 147-148], for outcome criteria). | 2. Implement additional measures *to prevent pneumonia:*<br>a. perform actions to improve breathing pattern and promote effective airway clearance (see Nursing Diagnoses 3 and 4)<br>b. perform actions to reduce the risk for aspiration (see Nursing Diagnosis 17, action c). |
| 15.b. The client will remain free of urinary tract infection as evidenced by:<br>1. clear urine<br>2. no unusual odor to urine<br>3. afebrile status<br>4. no increase in spasticity<br>5. absence of WBCs, bacteria, and nitrites in urine<br>6. negative urine culture. | 15.b.1. Assess for and report signs and symptoms of urinary tract infection (e.g. cloudy, foul-smelling urine; elevated temperature; increase in spasticity [bladder mucosal irritation triggers muscle spasms]).<br>2. Monitor urinalysis and report presence of WBCs, bacteria, and/or nitrites.<br>3. Obtain a urine specimen for culture and sensitivity if ordered. Report abnormal results.<br>4. Refer to Care Plan on Immobility, Nursing Diagnosis 11, actions b.4 and 5 (pp. 148), for measures related to prevention and treatment of urinary tract infection.<br>5. Implement measures to prevent urinary retention (see Nursing Diagnosis 12, actions d.1, 2, and 4 and e) *in order to further reduce the risk of urinary tract infection.* |

## 16. NURSING DIAGNOSIS: High risk for trauma

related to:
a. falls associated with loss of motor function, use of turning frame, and spasticity;
b. burns associated with loss of motor and sensory function.

| Desired Outcome | Nursing Actions and ***Selected Purposes/Rationales*** |
|---|---|
| 16. The client will not experience falls or burns. | 16.a. Implement measures *to reduce the risk for trauma:*<br>1. perform actions *to prevent falls:*<br>a. if client is in a standard hospital bed, keep bed in low position with side rails up<br>b. keep safety belts securely fastened when client is on a turning frame or stretcher or in a wheelchair<br>c. obtain adequate assistance when moving client; utilize instructions from physical therapist on correct transfer techniques<br>d. implement measures *to increase client's stability when in a wheelchair* (e.g. use wheelchair equipped with an anti-tipping device, fasten safety belt around upper body and chair to stabilize trunk, use H-straps to keep legs positioned properly)<br>e. do not rush client; allow adequate time for him/her to assist with transfers and position changes<br>2. perform actions *to prevent burns:*<br>a. let hot foods and fluids cool slightly before serving<br>b. supervise client while smoking<br>c. assess temperature of bath water before and during use<br>d. when client is in a wheelchair, instruct him/her to avoid placing self next to sources of heat (e.g. heater, stove)<br>3. encourage client to request assistance whenever needed; have a specially adapted call signal available to client at all times<br>4. perform actions to decrease spasticity (see Nursing Diagnosis 10, action a.9) *in order to reduce the risk of unexpected body movements.* |

b. Include client and significant others in planning and implementing measures to prevent trauma.
c. If injury does occur, initiate appropriate first aid and notify physician.

## 17. NURSING DIAGNOSIS: High risk for aspiration

related to:
a. decreased ability to clear tracheobronchial passages associated with inability to cough forcefully resulting from weakness of the diaphragm and paralysis of the abdominal and intercostal muscles;
b. reflux of gastric contents associated with accumulation of gas and fluid in the stomach as a result of decreased or absent gastrointestinal motility (especially during period of spinal shock);
c. difficulty swallowing associated with neck hyperextension and/or horizontal body positioning during the time that the cervical spine is immobilized.

| Desired Outcome | Nursing Actions and ***Selected Purposes/Rationales*** |
|---|---|
| 17. The client will not aspirate secretions or foods/fluids as evidenced by:<br>a. clear breath sounds<br>b. resonant percussion note over lungs<br>c. absence of cough, tachypnea, and dyspnea. | 17.a. Assess for signs and symptoms of aspiration of secretions or foods/fluids (e.g. rhonchi, dull percussion note over affected lung area, cough, tachypnea, dyspnea).<br>b. Monitor chest x-ray results. Report findings of pulmonary infiltrate.<br>c. Implement measures *to reduce the risk for aspiration:*<br>1. if client has absent bowel sounds, withhold oral foods/fluids and consult physician about insertion of a nasogastric tube for gastric decompression *to reduce the possibility of gastric reflux or vomiting and subsequent aspiration*<br>2. place client in a side-lying or prone position (if on turning frame) as often as possible during period of spinal shock when client's ability to clear upper airways is most severely compromised<br>3. have suction equipment readily available for use<br>4. perform oropharyngeal suctioning and provide oral hygiene as often as needed *to remove excess secretions*<br>5. when oral intake is allowed:<br>a. maintain client in the following position during and for at least 30 minutes after meals and snacks:<br>1. prone position if on turning frame<br>2. high Fowler's or side-lying position if in halo device<br>b. decrease environmental stimuli during meals and snacks *so client can concentrate on chewing and swallowing*<br>c. encourage client to use a straw for all liquids and to take small sips and sip slowly when drinking<br>d. provide small, frequent meals rather than 3 large ones *to decrease risk of gastric distention and regurgitation*<br>e. cut food in bite-size pieces and remind client to chew food thoroughly<br>f. allow ample time for meals<br>g. instruct client to avoid laughing and talking while eating and drinking<br>h. assist client with oral hygiene after eating *to ensure that food particles do not remain in mouth*<br>i. administer upper gastrointestinal stimulants (e.g. metoclopramide) if ordered *to decrease risk of gastric distention and regurgitation.* |

| Desired Outcome | Nursing Actions and ***Selected Purposes/Rationales*** |
|---|---|
| | d. If signs and symptoms of aspiration occur:<br>1. perform the assisted coughing maneuver if client begins to choke on food particles<br>2. notify physician<br>3. prepare client for chest x-ray<br>4. prepare client for bronchoscopy if ordered *to remove aspirated food particles.* |

## 18. NURSING DIAGNOSIS: Dysreflexia

related to loss of autonomic nervous system control below the level of the cord injury (can occur when reflex activity returns following period of spinal shock).

| Desired Outcome | Nursing Actions and ***Selected Purposes/Rationales*** |
|---|---|
| 18. The client will not experience dysreflexia as evidenced by:<br>a. vital signs within normal range for client<br>b. skin dry and usual color above the level of the injury<br>c. no complaints of headache, nasal congestion, and blurred vision. | 18.a. Assess for signs and symptoms of dysreflexia:<br>1. sudden rise in B/P (may go as high as 300/140 mm Hg)<br>2. bradycardia<br>3. flushing and profuse diaphoresis above level of injury<br>4. pounding headache<br>5. nasal congestion<br>6. blurred vision.<br>b. Implement measures *to prevent stimulation of the sympathetic nervous system below the level of the cord injury in order to prevent dysreflexia:*<br>1. perform actions to prevent distention of the bladder and bowel (see Nursing Diagnoses 12, actions d and e and 13, action d)<br>2. perform actions *to prevent pressure on any area of the client's body below the level of the cord injury:*<br>a. change his/her position frequently<br>b. ensure that overbed tray is not resting on client<br>c. ensure that clothing is not constrictive and shoes are not too tight<br>3. perform good nail care *(ingrown nails can cause sympathetic stimulation)*<br>4. perform actions to prevent and treat urinary tract infection (see Nursing Diagnosis 15, actions b.4 and 5)<br>5. apply a topical anesthetic agent to any existing pressure sore<br>6. apply a local anesthetic (e.g. Nupercainal ointment) or administer a ganglionic blocking agent (e.g trimethaphan, mecamylamine) if ordered before performing actions that may result in an exaggerated sympathetic response (e.g. urinary catheterization, removal of a fecal impaction, administration of an enema, bladder irrigation, care of any wound below the level of the injury).<br>c. If signs and symptoms of dysreflexia occur:<br>1. immediately raise head of bed and lower client's legs unless contraindicated *(this will usually decrease B/P significantly)*<br>2. monitor B/P and pulse frequently<br>3. assess for and, if possible, alleviate the condition causing sympathetic stimulation<br>4. notify physician immediately if signs and symptoms persist or if complications resulting from severe hypertension (e.g. seizures, intraocular hemorrhage, cerebrovascular accident, myocardial infarction) occur<br>5. administer intravenous antihypertensives (e.g. diazoxide, hydralazine, nitroprusside) if ordered |

6. notify all persons participating in client's care of his/her episode of dysreflexia *since such episodes can recur*
7. prepare client for pelvic or pudendal nerve block or posterior rhizotomy if indicated (these procedures may be necessary if dysreflexia recurs frequently)
8. provide emotional support to client and significant others.

---

## 19. COLLABORATIVE DIAGNOSES:

**Potential complications:**

a. **ascending spinal cord injury** related to further damage to and/or ischemia of the cord above the C5 level associated with vasospasm of damaged vessels, progressive edema, bleeding, compression of cord by hematoma or bone fragments, and/or ineffective immobilization of an unstable cord injury;
b. **paralytic ileus** related to absence of neural stimulation of the intestine associated with absence of autonomic nervous system and reflex activity below the level of the spinal cord injury during period of spinal shock;
c. **thromboembolism** related to venous stasis associated with decreased mobility and decreased vasomotor tone below the level of the injury;
d. **gastrointestinal (GI) bleeding** related to:
   1. development of a stress ulcer (continued stress causes vagal stimulation that results in gastric hyperacidity and multiple diffuse erosions of the gastric and duodenal mucosa)
   2. irritation of the gastric mucosa associated with side effects of certain medications (e.g. corticosteriods, some muscle relaxants);
e. **contractures** related to:
   1. increase in fibrous connective tissue around the joints and excessive calcium deposits in soft tissues around the joints (occurs with prolonged immobility of the joints)
   2. prolonged periods of hip flexion associated with use of wheelchair
   3. difficulty putting joints through full range of motion associated with severe spasticity if it occurs.

| Desired Outcomes | Nursing Actions and ***Selected Purposes/Rationales*** |
|---|---|
| 19.a. The client will not experience spinal cord injury above the level of C5 as evidenced by:<br>1. stable respiratory status<br>2. stable B/P and pulse<br>3. no further loss of motor and sensory function. | 19.a. 1. Assess for and report signs and symptoms of ascending spinal cord injury:<br>a. respiratory failure (e.g. rapid, shallow respirations; dusky or cyanotic skin color; drowsiness; confusion)<br>b. significant decrease in B/P and pulse<br>c. further loss of motor and sensory function.<br>2. Implement measures *to prevent spinal cord injury above the level of C5:*<br>a. perform actions *to maintain immobilization of the spine until stabilization has been accomplished:*<br>1. do not release or adjust skeletal traction or halo device unless ordered<br>2. if skeletal traction is present, keep traction rope and weights hanging freely<br>3. always use turn sheet and adequate assistance when repositioning client; never use the bars of the halo device as handles<br>4. check pin sites of halo or traction device every shift; notify physician if pins are loose<br>5. if immobilization device fails (e.g. pins fall out, traction weights drop, rods on halo device disconnect):<br>a. stabilize client's head, neck, and shoulders with hands and/or sandbags |

| Desired Outcomes | Nursing Actions and ***Selected Purposes/Rationales*** |
|---|---|
| | b. notify physician immediately<br>b. remind staff to utilize the jaw thrust method rather than hyperextending client's neck if respiratory distress occurs<br>c. perform actions *to prevent ascending spinal cord ischemia:*<br>1. implement measures to maintain adequate tissue perfusion (see Nursing Diagnosis 2, action b)<br>2. administer oxygen as ordered<br>3. implement measures to maintain an adequate respiratory status (see Nursing Diagnoses 3 and 4)<br>4. administer the following medications if ordered:<br>a. corticosteroids (e.g. methylprednisolone) *to decrease inflammation of and around the level of injury*<br>b. calcium-channel blockers (e.g. nimodipine) *to decrease vasospasm*<br>d. prepare client for decompression of the spinal cord (e.g. removal of hematoma or bone fragments) or surgical stabilization (e.g. fusion) if planned.<br>3. If signs and symptoms of ascending spinal cord injury occur:<br>a. continue with above actions<br>b. assist with intubation or tracheostomy and mechanical ventilation<br>c. provide emotional support to client and significant others. |
| 19.b. The client will have resolution of paralytic ileus if it occurs as evidenced by:<br>1. soft, nondistended abdomen<br>2. gradual return of bowel sounds<br>3. passage of flatus. | 19.b.1. Assess for and report signs and symptoms of paralytic ileus (e.g. firm, distended abdomen; absent bowel sounds; failure to pass flatus).<br>2. If signs and symptoms of paralytic ileus occur:<br>a. withhold all oral intake<br>b. insert nasogastric tube and maintain suction as ordered<br>c. assess for and report signs of bowel necrosis (e.g. fever, increased WBCs, decline in B/P). |
| 19.c.1. The client will not develop a deep vein thrombus as evidenced by:<br>a. absence of swelling and distended superficial vessels in extremities<br>b. usual temperature of extremities. | 19.c.1. a. Assess for and report signs and symptoms of a deep vein thrombus (e.g. increase in circumference of extremity, distention of superficial vessels in extremity, unusual warmth of extremity).<br>b. Refer to Care Plan on Immobility, Nursing Diagnosis 12, actions a.1.b and c (pp. 149-150), for measures related to prevention and treatment of a deep vein thrombus.<br>c. Implement additional measures *to prevent thrombus formation:*<br>1. position firm pillow between client's legs if spasms tend to cause legs to cross<br>2. instruct client to notify staff if legs cross *so that they can be repositioned properly.* |
| 19.c.2. The client will not experience a pulmonary embolism as evidenced by:<br>a. absence of sudden shoulder pain<br>b. unlabored respirations at 14-20/minute<br>c. usual mental status | 19.c.2. a. Assess for and report signs and symptoms of pulmonary embolism (e.g. sudden shoulder pain [this is a referred pain], dyspnea, tachypnea, restlessness, apprehension, low $PaO_2$).<br>b. Refer to Care Plan on Immobility, Nursing Diagnosis 12, actions a.2.b and c (p. 150), for measures related to prevention and treatment of a pulmonary embolism.<br>c. Implement additional measures *to prevent a pulmonary embolism:*<br>1. perform actions to prevent and treat a deep vein thrombus (see actions c.1.b and c in this diagnosis)<br>2. perform actions to prevent dysreflexia (see Nursing Diagnosis 18, action b) *in order to prevent a sudden increase in blood pressure and subsequent dislodgment of a thrombus if present.* |

| | |
|---|---|
| d. blood gases within normal range. | |
| 19.d. The client will not experience GI bleeding as evidenced by:<br>1. no complaints of shoulder pain<br>2. absence of frank and occult blood in stool and gastric contents<br>3. B/P within normal range for client<br>4. RBC, Hct, and Hb levels within normal range. | 19.d.1. Assess for and report signs and symptoms of GI bleeding (e.g. complaints of shoulder pain [this is a referred pain], frank or occult blood in stool or gastric contents, decreased B/P).<br>2. Monitor RBC, Hct, and Hb levels. Report declining values.<br>3. Implement measures *to prevent ulceration of the gastric and duodenal mucosa:*<br>a. perform actions to decrease fear and anxiety (see Nursing Diagnosis 1, action b)<br>b. instruct client to reduce intake of foods/fluids that stimulate hydrochloric acid secretion or irritate the gastric mucosa:<br>1. coffee, caffeine-containing teas and colas<br>2. spices such as black pepper, chili powder, and nutmeg<br>c. administer ulcerogenic medications (e.g. corticosteroids, some muscle relaxants) with meals or snacks *to decrease gastric irritation*<br>d. administer histamine$_2$ receptor antagonists (e.g. cimetidine, ranitidine, famotidine), antacids, and cytoprotective agents (e.g. sucralfate) if ordered.<br>4. If signs and symptoms of GI bleeding occur:<br>a. insert nasogastric tube and maintain suction as ordered<br>b. assist with measures to control bleeding (e.g. gastric lavage, endoscopic electrocoagulation, selective arterial embolization) if ordered<br>c. administer blood products and/or volume expanders if ordered<br>d. prepare client for surgery (e.g. ligation of bleeding vessels, partial gastrectomy) if indicated<br>e. provide emotional support to client and significant others<br>f. refer to Care Plan on Peptic Ulcer for additional care measures. |
| 19.e. The client will maintain normal range of motion. | 19.e.1. Refer to Care Plan on Immobility, Collaborative Diagnosis 12, action d (pp. 151-152), for measures related to assessment and prevention of contractures.<br>2. Implement additional measures *to reduce the risk of contractures:*<br>a. perform actions to reduce spasticity (see Nursing Diagnosis 10, action a.9)<br>b. position client in prone or supine position routinely unless contraindicated *to counteract prolonged periods of hip flexion resulting from wheelchair use.* |

## 20. NURSING DIAGNOSIS: Sexual dysfunction

related to:

a. decreased libido associated with:
   1. loss of sensory and voluntary motor function below the level of spinal cord injury
   2. presence of a urinary catheter and/or fear of urinary and bowel incontinence
   3. depression, altered self-concept
   4. fear of rejection by partner
   5. fear of dysreflexia (genital stimulation may cause dysreflexia);

b. decreased ability to control and maintain an erection associated with loss of ability to have a psychogenic erection (only reflexogenic erection is possible);

c. altered ejaculatory flow associated with impaired nerve function in the bladder neck (can result in retrograde rather than antegrade ejaculation).

| Desired Outcome | Nursing Actions and ***Selected Purposes/Rationales*** |
|---|---|
| 20. The client will demonstrate beginning acceptance of changes in sexual functioning as evidenced by:<br>a. verbalization of a perception of self as sexually acceptable and adequate<br>b. statements reflecting beginning adjustment to the effects of the spinal cord injury on sexual functioning<br>c. maintenance of relationship with significant other. | 20.a. Assess for signs and symptoms of sexual dysfunction (e.g. verbalization of sexual concerns or inability to achieve sexual satisfaction, alteration in relationship with significant other, limitations imposed by quadriplegia).<br>b. Provide accurate information about the effects of the spinal cord injury on sexual functioning. Encourage questions and clarify misconceptions.<br>c. Implement measures *to promote optimal sexual functioning:*<br>1. facilitate communication between client and his/her partner; focus on the feelings the couple share and assist them to identify changes that affect their sexual relationship<br>2. discuss ways to be creative in expressing sexuality (e.g. massage, fantasies, cuddling)<br>3. arrange for uninterrupted privacy during hospital stay if desired by the couple<br>4. perform actions to improve client's self-concept (see Nursing Diagnosis 21)<br>5. suggest alternative methods of sexual gratification and use of assistive devices if appropriate; encourage partner to explore erogenous areas on the client's lips, neck, and ears<br>6. inform male client and his partner of techniques for eliciting and maintaining reflexogenic erection (e.g. stimulate genitalia, stroke inner thigh, stimulate the rectum, manipulate the urinary catheter)<br>7. if client has difficulty maintaining an erection, encourage him to discuss the possibility of a penile prosthesis with physician if desired<br>8. if client experiences episodes of dysreflexia, instruct him/her to consult physician about ways to prevent it during sexual activity (e.g. take a ganglionic blocking agent before sexual activity, have partner apply a local anesthetic to client's genitals)<br>9. discuss alternative methods of parenting (e.g. adoption, sperm recovery, artificial insemination) if of concern to client<br>10. inform female client that vaginal lubrication can occur by local stimulation or can be enhanced by using a water-soluble lubricant<br>11. if client has an indwelling urethral catheter, instruct him/her on ways to fold and secure the catheter tubing prior to sexual intercourse<br>12. if incontinence of urine is a problem, instruct client to:<br>a. limit fluid intake 2 hours before sexual activity<br>b. have bladder emptied immediately before sexual activity<br>13. instruct client to perform bowel care several hours before sexual activity *in order to reduce the risk of stool evacuation if anal or rectal stimulation occurs during sexual activity*<br>14. if appropriate, involve partner in care of client *to facilitate partner's adjustment to the changes in client's appearance and body functioning and subsequently decrease the possibility of partner's rejection of client*<br>15. encourage client to rest before sexual activity<br>16. instruct client and partner to establish a relaxed, unhurried atmosphere for sexual activity<br>17. discuss positions that may facilitate sexual activity (e.g. lying on side, client in supine position)<br>18. provide explicit films and literature if desired by client and/or partner.<br>d. Include partner in above discussions and encourage his/her continued support of the client.<br>e. Consult physician when client is ready for sexual counseling and/or sexual counseling appears indicated. |

## 21. NURSING DIAGNOSIS: Self-concept disturbance*

related to:

a. dependence on others to meet self-care needs;
b. feelings of powerlessness;
c. change in appearance associated with temporary presence of devices to immobilize the spine, necessity of wheelchair use, and spasticity following period of spinal shock;
d. infertility (in males) associated with:
   1. possibility of retrograde ejaculation (can result from impaired nerve function in the bladder neck)
   2. decreased sperm formation and viability resulting from testicular atrophy and impaired temperature regulation in the testes;
e. changes in body functioning, life style, and roles.

*This diagnostic label includes the nursing diagnoses of body image disturbance, self-esteem disturbance, and altered role performance.

| Desired Outcome | Nursing Actions and ***Selected Purposes/Rationales*** |
|---|---|
| 21. The client will demonstrate beginning adaptation to changes in body functioning, appearance, life style, roles, and level of independence (see Care Plan on Immobility, Nursing Diagnosis 14 [pp. 153-154], for outcome criteria). | 21.a. Refer to Care Plan on Immobility, Nursing Diagnosis 14 (pp. 153-154), for measures related to assessment and promotion of a positive self-concept.<br>b. Implement additional measures *to promote a positive self-concept:*<br>1. reinforce actions to assist client to cope with effects of the spinal cord injury (see Nursing Diagnosis 22, action c)<br>2. perform actions to prevent urinary incontinence (see Nursing Diagnosis 12, actions d.2-4 and e)<br>3. perform actions to reduce client's feelings of powerlessness (see Nursing Diagnosis 23)<br>4. perform actions to facilitate the grieving process (see Nursing Diagnosis 24, action b)<br>5. avoid unnecessary exposure of client during care<br>6. assure client that immobilization device is temporary and will be removed as soon as internal stabilization of the spine occurs; if brace or collar is needed after removal of the skull pins, assist client to select clothing that makes the spinal support less obvious (e.g. high-collared shirts, loose-fitting shirts)<br>7. demonstrate acceptance of client using techniques such as touch and frequent visits; encourage significant others to do the same<br>8. promote activities that require client to confront the body changes that have occurred (e.g. exercise, grooming, eating); be aware that the integration of changes in body image does not usually occur until 2-6 months after the actual physical change has occurred<br>9. encourage client contact with others *so that he/she can test and establish a new self-image*<br>10. reinforce actions to assist client to adjust to alterations in sexual functioning (see Nursing Diagnosis 20, action c)<br>11. perform actions to increase the client's ability to perform self-care (see Nursing Diagnosis 11, action b) *in order to increase client's sense of independence*<br>12. provide privacy during client's attempts at self-care *in order to minimize embarrassment that he/she may feel because of neurological impairments*<br>13. encourage significant others to allow client to do what he/she is able *so that independence can be re-established and/or self-esteem redeveloped*<br>14. use the term "disabled" rather than "handicapped," "cripple," or "invalid"; avoid use of slang (e.g. quad, gimp). |

## 22. NURSING DIAGNOSIS: Ineffective individual coping

related to fear and anxiety; changes in body functioning, life style, and roles; feelings of powerlessness; need for lengthy rehabilitation; and inadequate support system.

| Desired Outcome | Nursing Actions and ***Selected Purposes/Rationales*** |
|---|---|
| 22. The client will demonstrate the use of effective coping skills as evidenced by:<br>a. verbalization of ability to cope with the effects of the spinal cord injury<br>b. utilization of appropriate problem-solving techniques<br>c. willingness to participate in treatment plan and rehabilitation program<br>d. absence of destructive behavior toward self<br>e. appropriate use of defense mechanisms<br>f. recognition and utilization of available support systems. | 22.a. Assess for and report signs and symptoms of ineffective individual coping (e.g. verbalization of inability to cope; inability to ask for help, problem solve, or meet basic needs; reluctance to participate in treatment plan; destructive behavior toward self; inappropriate use of defense mechanisms; inability to meet role expectations).<br>b. Assess client's perception of current situation including precipitating factors and effectiveness of coping mechanisms.<br>c. Implement measures *to promote effective coping:*<br>1. allow time for client to adjust psychologically to the diagnosis and planned treatment, residual effects of the spinal cord injury, and anticipated changes in life style and roles<br>2. perform actions to decrease fear and anxiety (see Nursing Diagnosis 1, action b)<br>3. assist client to recognize and manage inappropriate denial if it is present<br>4. encourage verbalization about current situation<br>5. assist client to identify personal strengths and resources that can be utilized to facilitate coping with the current situation<br>6. demonstrate acceptance of client but set limits on inappropriate behavior<br>7. create an atmosphere of trust and support<br>8. arrange for a visit with another individual who has successfully adjusted to a similar injury<br>9. perform actions to reduce client's feelings of powerlessness (see Nursing Diagnosis 23)<br>10. assist client to maintain usual daily routines whenever possible<br>11. instruct client in effective problem-solving techniques (e.g. accurate identification of stressors, determination of various options to solve problem)<br>12. if client is experiencing severe spasticity:<br>a. reinforce measures to reduce severity of the spasms (see Nursing Diagnosis 10, action a.9)<br>b. reinforce ways that spasms can be beneficial (e.g. help swing legs from bed to wheelchair, initiate arm movements, maintain an erection, evacuate bowels)<br>c. inform client that spasticity usually stabilizes in 1-2 years<br>13. inform client that there will be times when spasticity is worse, bowel and bladder programs are less effective, and efforts at self-care are less successful; assure him/her that these are temporary results of physical and/or emotional stress or fatigue rather than an indication of deteriorating neurological status<br>14. assist client as he/she starts to plan for necessary life-style and role changes; help client to identify priorities and attainable goals<br>15. assist client and significant others to identify ways that personal and family goals can be adjusted rather than abandoned<br>16. assist client through methods such as role playing to prepare for negative reactions of others to his/her quadriplegia<br>17. administer antianxiety and/or antidepressant agents if ordered |

18. assist client to find, hire, and train an attendant before discharge from the rehabilitative care unit
19. set up a home evaluation appointment with occupational and physical therapists before client's discharge *so that changes in the home environment (e.g. installation of ramps, widening doorways, altering bathroom facilities) can be completed by discharge*
20. assist client to identify and utilize available support systems; provide information regarding available community resources that can assist client and significant others in coping with effects of the spinal cord injury (e.g. spinal cord injury groups)
21. encourage continued emotional support from significant others
22. encourage the client to share with significant others the kind of support that would be most beneficial (e.g. listening, inspiring hope, providing reassurance and accurate information)
23. support behaviors suggesting positive adaptation to changes experienced (e.g. verbalization of ability to cope, utilization of available support systems, participation in rehabilitation program).

d. Consult physician about psychological and vocational rehabilitation counseling if appropriate. Initiate a referral if necessary.

## 23. NURSING DIAGNOSIS: Powerlessness

related to:
a. quadriplegia;
b. dependence on others to meet basic needs;
c. alterations in usual roles, relationships, and future plans associated with effects of the injury and need for extensive and lengthy rehabilitation.

| Desired Outcome | Nursing Actions and ***Selected Purposes/Rationales*** |
|---|---|
| 23. The client will demonstrate increasing feelings of control over his/her situation (see Care Plan on Immobility, Nursing Diagnosis 15 [pp. 154-155], for outcome criteria). | 23.a. Refer to Care Plan on Immobility, Nursing Diagnosis 15 (pp. 154-155), for measures related to assessment of feelings of powerlessness and measures to promote client's feeling of control over his/her situation.<br>b. Implement additional measures *to reduce client's feelings of powerlessness:*<br>1. perform actions to promote effective coping (see Nursing Diagnosis 22, action c) *in order to promote an increased sense of control over his/her situation*<br>2. support realistic hope about the effects of rehabilitation on future independence (within 3-6 months and with the aid of assistive devices, the client should be able to perform many activities including operating an electric wheelchair, feeding self once meal has been set up, washing face and chest, brushing teeth, and using a computer)<br>3. stress to persons coming in contact with client that an individual has an enormous potential for adjusting to a disability and that they need to avoid being overly sympathetic *(an overly sympathetic attitude can communicate a feeling of hopelessness)*<br>4. assist client to select wheelchairs (usually one manual and one electric one) that best meet mobility needs and can assist him/her to pursue a more active life style<br>5. encourage client to be as active as possible in making decisions about his/her living situation<br>6. provide client with information about technical advances (e.g. the Environmental Control System [ECS]) that can make independent operation of electronic devices such as lights, radio, television, and specially installed door openers and window shades possible |

| Desired Outcome | Nursing Actions and ***Selected Purposes/Rationales*** |
|---|---|
| | 7. discuss with significant others client's need to maintain as much control over his/her life as possible; stress the necessity of their encouraging and allowing the client to actively participate in the rehabilitation program and discharge planning. |

## 24. NURSING DIAGNOSIS: Grieving*

related to extensive loss of motor and sensory function and the effects of this loss on future life style and roles.

*This diagnostic label includes anticipatory grieving and grieving following the actual losses.

| Desired Outcome | Nursing Actions and ***Selected Purposes/Rationales*** |
|---|---|
| 24. The client will demonstrate beginning progression through the grieving process as evidenced by:<br>a. verbalization of feelings about the loss of motor and sensory function and its effects on his/her life<br>b. expression of grief<br>c. participation in treatment plan and self-care activities<br>d. utilization of available support systems<br>e. verbalization of a plan for integrating prescribed follow-up care into life style. | 24.a. Assess for signs and symptoms of grieving (e.g. change in eating habits, inability to concentrate, insomnia, anger, noncompliance, withdrawal from significant others, denial of loss). Be aware that client's response to a loss will be affected by factors such as previous experience with loss, age, developmental stage, available support systems, spiritual and cultural background, current health status, and significance of the loss.<br>b. Implement measures *to facilitate the grieving process:*<br>1. assist client to acknowledge the losses experienced *so grief work can begin;* assess for factors that may hinder and facilitate acknowledgment<br>2. discuss the grieving process and assist client to accept the phases of grieving as an expected response to the actual and anticipated losses<br>3. allow time for client to progress through the phases of grieving (phases vary among theorists but progress from shock and alarm to acceptance); be aware that not every phase is expressed by all individuals, that recurrence of phases is common, and that the grieving process may take months to years<br>4. provide an atmosphere of care and concern (e.g. provide privacy, be available and nonjudgmental, display empathy and respect) *so client will feel free to verbalize feelings*<br>5. perform actions *to promote trust* (e.g. answer questions honestly, provide requested information)<br>6. encourage the verbal expression of anger and sadness about the losses experienced; recognize displacement of anger and assist client to see actual cause of angry feelings and resentment; establish limits on abusive behavior if demonstrated<br>7. encourage client to express his/her feelings in whatever ways are comfortable (e.g. conversation); provide client with an acceptable outlet for frustration and anger (e.g. punching bag he/she can swing arms against, wheeling outside when able, privacy)<br>8. perform actions to promote effective coping (see Nursing Diagnosis 22, action c)<br>9. support realistic hope about effects of rehabilitation on future independence<br>10. support behaviors suggesting successful grief work (e.g. verbalizing feelings about losses, focusing on ways to adapt to losses, learning needed skills, developing or renewing relationships)<br>11. explain the phases of the grieving process to significant others; encourage their support and understanding |

12. facilitate communication between client and significant others; be aware that they may be in different phases of the grieving process
13. provide information about counseling services and support groups that might assist client in working through grief
14. arrange for visit from clergy if desired by client.

c. Consult physician about referral for counseling if signs of dysfunctional grieving (e.g. persistent denial of losses, excessive anger or sadness, hysteria, suicidal behaviors) occur.

## 25. NURSING DIAGNOSIS: Social isolation

related to inability to participate in usual activities, depression, limited contact with peers, and decreased contact/awareness of events in the outside world associated with quadriplegia and prolonged hospitalization.

| Desired Outcome | Nursing Actions and ***Selected Purposes/Rationales*** |
|---|---|
| 25. The client will experience a decreased sense of isolation (see Care Plan on Immobility, Nursing Diagnosis 16 [p. 155], for outcome criteria). | 25.a. Refer to Care Plan on Immobility, Nursing Diagnosis 16 (p. 155), for measures related to assessment of and ways to decrease social isolation.<br>b. Implement additional measures *to decrease social isolation:*<br>1. provide client with an effective method of contacting nurses' station (e.g. whistle, pressure-sensitive pad under shoulder or upper arm)<br>2. perform actions to reduce depression by implementing measures to facilitate client's psychological adjustment to effects of spinal cord injury (see Nursing Diagnoses 21; 22, action c; 23; and 24, action b)<br>3. set up a schedule of visiting times so that client will not go for long periods of time without visitors<br>4. assist client to identify a few persons with whom he/she feels comfortable and encourage interactions with them<br>5. encourage and assist client to maintain telephone contact with others; if possible, provide client with a speaker phone that has a dialing mechanism he/she can activate independently<br>6. encourage participation in support groups. |

## 26. NURSING DIAGNOSIS: Altered family processes

related to change in family roles and structure associated with a family member's sudden, catastrophic injury; permanent disability; and need for extensive rehabilitation.

| Desired Outcome | Nursing Actions and ***Selected Purposes/Rationales*** |
|---|---|
| 26. The family members* will demonstrate beginning adjustment | 26.a. Assess for signs and symptoms of altered family processes (e.g. inability to meet client's needs, statements of not being able to accept client's quadriplegia or make necessary role and life-style changes, inability to |

*The term "family members" is being used here to include client's significant others.

| Desired Outcome | Nursing Actions and ***Selected Purposes/Rationales*** |
|---|---|
| to changes in functioning of a family member and family roles and structure as evidenced by:<br>a. meeting client's needs<br>b. verbalization of ways to adapt to required role and life-style changes<br>c. active participation in decision making and client's rehabilitation<br>d. positive interactions with one another. | make decisions, inability or refusal to participate in client's rehabilitation, negative family interactions).<br>b. Identify components of the family and their patterns of communication and role expectations.<br>c. Implement measures *to facilitate family members' adjustment to client's diagnosis, changes in his/her functioning within the family system, and altered family roles and structure:*<br>1. encourage verbalization of feelings about client's quadriplegia and the effect of this on family structure; actively listen to each family member and maintain a nonjudgmental attitude about feelings shared<br>2. reinforce physician's explanations of the effects of the injury and planned treatment and rehabilitation<br>3. assist family members to gain a realistic perspective of client's situation, conveying as much hope as appropriate<br>4. provide privacy *so that family members and client can share their feelings with one another;* stress the importance of and facilitate the use of good communication techniques<br>5. assist family members to progress through their own grieving process; explain that they may encounter times when they need to focus on meeting their own rather than the client's needs<br>6. emphasize the need for family members to obtain adequate rest and nutrition and to identify and utilize stress management techniques *so that they are better able to emotionally and physically deal with the changes and losses experienced*<br>7. encourage and assist family members to identify coping strategies for dealing with the client's quadriplegia and its effects on the family<br>8. assist family members to identify realistic goals and ways of reaching these goals<br>9. include family members in decision making about client and his/her care; convey appreciation for their input and continued support of client<br>10. encourage and allow family members to participate in client's care and rehabilitation<br>11. assist family members to identify resources that could assist them in coping with their feelings and meeting their immediate and long-term needs (e.g. counseling and social services; pastoral care; service, church, and spinal cord injury groups); initiate a referral if indicated.<br>d. Consult physician if family members continue to demonstrate difficulty adapting to changes in client's functioning, roles, and family structure. |

## 27. NURSING DIAGNOSIS: Knowledge deficit

regarding follow-up care.*

*Although the client will not be able to independently perform many of the actions included in this diagnosis, he/she must be knowledgeable about them in order to provide proper instruction to significant others and attendant and maintain an active role in the rehabilitation process.

| Desired Outcomes | Nursing Actions and ***Selected Purposes/Rationales*** |
|---|---|
| 27.a. The client will identify ways to prevent complications | 27.a.1. Refer to Care Plan on Immobility, Nursing Diagnosis 17, action a (pp. 156-157), for instructions related to ways to prevent complications associated with decreased mobility. |

associated with spinal cord injury and decreased mobility.

2. Instruct client in ways to prevent complications associated with spinal cord injury:
   a. position firm pillow between legs if spasms tend to cause legs to cross (helps to prevent thrombus formation and adduction contractures)
   b. wear an abdominal binder when changing from a reclining to a sitting position and take vasoconstrictor drugs if prescribed to prevent dizziness and fainting
   c. elevate legs periodically during the day to promote venous return
   d. implement measures to reduce severe spasticity (e.g. avoid fatigue and chills, change position at least every 2 hours, take muscle relaxants as prescribed) in order to increase mobility and prevent contractures
   e. use full-length and long-handled mirrors to examine all skin surfaces in the morning and the evening
   f. obtain a kinetic bed for home use if possible
   g. implement measures to prevent hyperthermia (e.g. avoid direct sunlight in hot weather, avoid excessive clothing and bedding)
   h. implement measures to prevent hypothermia (e.g. wear adequate amounts of clothing, wear a hat when in a cold environment, drink warm liquids)
   i. implement measures to prevent falls (e.g. always use safety belt during transfers and when in chair, be certain to have adequate assistance for transfer activity)
   j. implement measures to prevent burns:
      1. always check temperature of shower or bath water before use (can use bath water thermometer or have attendant check water temperature)
      2. never smoke when alone
      3. let hot foods/fluids cool slightly before attempting to feed self
      4. never position self next to a stove, heater, or other major source of heat
      5. never use an electric heating pad or electric blanket
   k. implement measures to prevent dysreflexia:
      1. do not allow bladder or bowel to become distended
      2. change position frequently
      3. seek medical attention at first sign of infection, persistent pressure area, or ingrown toenail
      4. apply a topical anesthetic to any area being stimulated or take a ganglionic blocking agent as prescribed (may need to be taken routinely or before activities known to precipitate dysreflexia).
3. Demonstrate the following procedures to client, significant others, and attendant:
   a. assisted coughing technique
   b. skin care
   c. proper positioning and padding
   d. transfer techniques
   e. active and passive range of motion exercises
   f. application of elastic stockings, abdominal binder, and heel and elbow protectors
   g. emergency treatment of dysreflexia (e.g. elevate head of bed and lower client's legs, alleviate causative factor, administer ganglionic blocking agent).
4. Allow time for questions, clarification, and return demonstration.

27.b. The client will demonstrate the ability to correctly use and maintain assistive devices.

27.b.1. Reinforce instructions of physical and occupational therapists regarding use of assistive devices. Allow time for questions, clarification, and return demonstration.
2. Instruct client in proper maintenance of assistive devices (e.g. replace worn parts, clean wheel hubs and crossbars of wheelchairs per manufacturer's instruction, keep wheelchair tires properly inflated).

| Desired Outcomes | Nursing Actions and ***Selected Purposes/Rationales*** |
|---|---|
| 27.c. The client will identify ways to manage altered bowel and bladder function. | 27.c. 1. Reinforce bladder and bowel training programs. (Guidelines are included in Nursing Diagnoses 12, action d and 13, action d, but the specific program will vary for each client.)<br>2. Demonstrate bowel care (e.g. digital stimulation, insertion of suppositories, administration of enemas) and bladder care (e.g. stimulation techniques, intermittent catheterization, emptying of urinary collection bag). Allow time for questions, clarification, and return demonstration. |
| 27.d. The client will state signs and symptoms to report to the health care provider. | 27.d. Instruct the client to report the following:<br>1. cloudy, foul-smelling urine<br>2. nausea and vomiting<br>3. cough productive of purulent, green, or rust-colored sputum<br>4. difficulty breathing or increased shortness of breath with activity<br>5. sudden or persistent shoulder pain (this can be a referred pain)<br>6. fever<br>7. chills or profuse sweating (can occur above the level of the injury)<br>8. increase in spasticity (could indicate an infection below the level of the injury)<br>9. unsuccessful bowel and/or bladder programs<br>10. redness in any extremity<br>11. swelling that appears suddenly, occurs only in one extremity, or does not subside overnight<br>12. increased restriction of any joint motion<br>13. signs and symptoms of dysreflexia (e.g. pounding headache, ringing in ears, slow pulse, flushing and diaphoresis above level of injury, nasal congestion) that do not subside once the stimulus is removed<br>14. any area of persistent skin irritation or breakdown<br>15. indications of pregnancy (stress that appropriate prenatal care should be initiated as soon as possible). |
| 27.e. The client will identify community resources that can assist with home management and adjustment to changes resulting from spinal cord injury. | 27.e. 1. Inform client and significant others of community resources that can assist with home management and adjustment to changes resulting from spinal cord injury (e.g. spinal cord injury support and social groups; home health agencies; community health agencies; local service groups; financial, individual, family, and vocational rehabilitation counselors).<br>2. Initiate a referral if indicated. |
| 27.f. The client will verbalize an understanding of and a plan for adhering to recommended follow-up care including future appointments with health care provider and occupational and physical therapists and medications prescribed. | 27.f. 1. Reinforce the importance of keeping scheduled follow-up visits with health care provider and occupational and physical therapists.<br>2. Explain the rationale for, side effects of, and importance of taking prescribed medications.<br>3. Implement measures designed to improve client compliance:<br>a. include significant others and caregivers in teaching sessions<br>b. encourage questions and allow time for reinforcement and clarification of information provided<br>c. provide written instructions on scheduled appointments with health care provider and occupational and physical therapists, medications prescribed, and signs and symptoms to report. |

UNIT

# IX

# *Nursing Care of the Client with Disturbances of Cardiovascular Function*

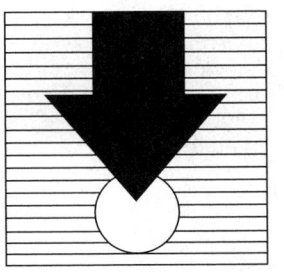

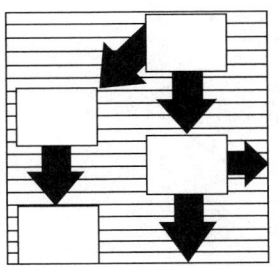

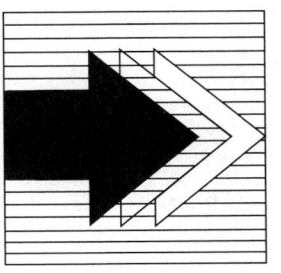

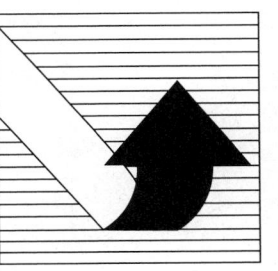

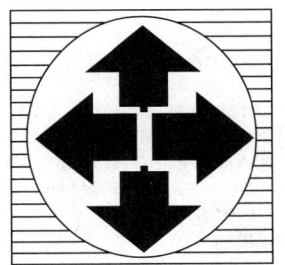

# Angina Pectoris

Angina pectoris is a syndrome characterized by transient episodes of retrosternal chest pain that are caused by an imbalance between myocardial oxygen supply and demand. The most common cause of angina pectoris is decreased coronary blood supply due to atherosclerosis of a major coronary artery. The atherosclerotic vessel is unable to dilate and therefore cannot supply sufficient blood to the myocardium at times when myocardial oxygen needs are increased. Other conditions that can compromise coronary blood flow are spasm and/or thrombosis of a coronary artery, hypotension, and aortic stenosis. Conditions that reduce oxygen availability and/or increase myocardial workload and oxygen demands (e.g. anemia, smoking, chronic lung disease, exercise, heavy meals, exposure to cold, stress, thyrotoxicosis, hypertension) may precipitate or increase the frequency of angina attacks by widening the gap between oxygen needs and availability.

The three major types of angina pectoris are stable (classic) angina, unstable (crescendo, preinfarction, progressive) angina, and variant (Prinzmetal's) angina. These types differ with regard to severity and frequency of attacks, refractoriness of the pain, and typical precipitants of the pain. Stable angina, the most common type, is usually precipitated by physical exertion or emotional stress, lasts 3 to 5 minutes, and is relieved by rest and nitroglycerin. In all types of angina, the pain usually occurs in the retrosternal area; may or may not radiate; and is described as heaviness or a pressing, squeezing, burning, or choking sensation.

**This care plan focuses on the adult client hospitalized during an episode of chest pain suspected to be angina.** The goals of care are to improve myocardial oxygen supply, relieve pain, prevent complications, and educate the client regarding follow-up care.

## DIAGNOSTIC TESTS

Electrocardiogram (ECG)
Cardiac enzymes/isoenzymes
Serum cholesterol and triglyceride levels and lipoprotein profile
Radionuclide imaging
Exercise electrocardiography (stress test)
Coronary angiography

## DISCHARGE CRITERIA

Prior to discharge, the client will:

- perform activities of daily living and ambulate without angina
- have angina controlled by oral medication
- verbalize a basic understanding of angina pectoris
- identify factors that may precipitate angina attacks and ways to control these factors
- identify modifiable cardiovascular risk factors and ways to reduce these factors
- verbalize an understanding of the rationale for and components of a diet low in saturated fat and cholesterol
- demonstrate accuracy in counting pulse
- verbalize an understanding of medications ordered including rationale, side effects, schedule for taking, and importance of taking as prescribed
- state signs and symptoms to report to the health care provider
- identify community resources that can assist in making necessary life-style changes and adjusting to the effects of angina pectoris
- verbalize an understanding of and a plan for adhering to recommended follow-up care including future appointments with health care provider.

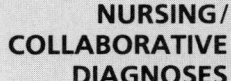

**NURSING/ COLLABORATIVE DIAGNOSES**



## 1. NURSING DIAGNOSIS: Altered tissue perfusion: myocardial

related to narrowing of the coronary artery(ies) associated with atherosclerosis, spasm, and/or thrombosis.

| Desired Outcome | Nursing Actions and ***Selected Purposes/Rationales*** |
|---|---|
| 1. The client will experience adequate myocardial tissue perfusion and oxygenation as evidenced by:<br>a. absence of chest pain<br>b. apical pulse regular and between 60-100 beats/minute. | 1.a. Assess for signs and symptoms of decreased myocardial tissue perfusion (e.g. chest pain, breathlessness, arrhythmias).<br>b. Implement measures *to improve myocardial tissue perfusion and/or oxygenation:*<br>1. maintain oxygen therapy as ordered<br>2. administer the following medications if ordered:<br>a. nitrates (e.g. nitroglycerin, isosorbide) *to dilate the coronary and peripheral (primarily venous) blood vessels, thereby improving myocardial blood flow and reducing cardiac workload and myocardial oxygen consumption*<br>b. beta-adrenergic blocking agents (e.g. atenolol, nadolol, metoprolol, propranolol) *to decrease myocardial contractility and heart rate, thereby reducing myocardial oxygen consumption*<br>c. calcium-channel blockers (e.g. verapamil, diltiazem, nifedipine, nicardipine) *to increase coronary blood flow and reduce cardiac workload by decreasing afterload and the force of myocardial contractility*<br>d. anticoagulants (e.g. intravenous heparin) and antiplatelet agents (e.g. low-dose aspirin) *to prevent obstruction of the coronary artery(ies) by thrombosis*<br>3. perform actions *to reduce cardiac workload and myocardial oxygen requirements:*<br>a. maintain activity restrictions as ordered<br>b. instruct client to avoid activities that create a Valsalva response (e.g. straining to have a bowel movement, holding breath while moving) *in order to prevent the marked increase in venous return and preload that occurs with exhalation*<br>c. implement measures *to promote emotional rest* (e.g. reduce fear and anxiety)<br>d. discourage excessive intake of beverages high in caffeine such as coffee, tea, and colas *(caffeine is a myocardial stimulant and increases myocardial oxygen consumption)*<br>e. discourage smoking *(smoke has a cardiostimulatory effect, causes vasoconstriction, and reduces oxygen availability).*<br>c. Consult physician if signs and symptoms of decreased myocardial tissue perfusion persist or worsen. |

## 2. NURSING DIAGNOSIS: Pain: radiating or nonradiating chest pain

related to decreased myocardial oxygenation (an insufficient oxygen supply forces the myocardium to convert to anaerobic metabolism; the end products of anaerobic metabolism act as irritants to myocardial neural receptors).

**Desired Outcome**

2. The client will experience diminished pain as evidenced by:
   a. verbalization of pain relief
   b. relaxed facial expression and body positioning
   c. increased participation in activities
   d. stable vital signs.

**Nursing Actions and *Selected Purposes/Rationales***

2.a. Determine how the client usually responds to pain.
- b. Assess client's perception of pain including location, intensity, and type. Utilize a numerical scale to rate intensity.
- c. Assess for nonverbal signs of pain (e.g. facial grimacing; clenched fists; rubbing of neck, jaw, or arm; reluctance to move; restlessness; diaphoresis; facial pallor; shallow, guarded respirations; increased B/P; tachycardia).
- d. Assess for factors that seem to aggravate and alleviate pain.
- e. Implement measures *to relieve pain:*
  1. administer nitroglycerin if ordered
  2. maintain client on bed rest in a semi- to high Fowler's position
  3. administer a narcotic analgesic if ordered if pain is unrelieved by rest and nitroglycerin within 15-20 minutes (narcotic analgesics are usually administered intravenously *because intramuscular injections are poorly absorbed if tissue perfusion is decreased; intramuscular injections also elevate serum enzyme levels, which makes assessment of myocardial damage more difficult)*
  4. provide or assist with nonpharmacological measures for pain relief (e.g. position change, relaxation techniques, restful environment).
- f. Consult physician if pain persists or worsens.
- g. Implement measures to improve myocardial tissue perfusion and oxygenation (see Nursing Diagnosis 1, action b) *in order to prevent recurrent episodes of angina.*

## 3. COLLABORATIVE DIAGNOSES: Potential complications:

a. **cardiac arrhythmias** related to myocardial irritability associated with myocardial hypoxia;
b. **myocardial infarction** related to prolonged myocardial ischemia.

**Desired Outcomes**

3.a. The client will not experience cardiac arrhythmias as evidenced by:
   1. regular apical pulse at 60-100 beats/minute
   2. equal apical and radial pulses
   3. absence of syncope and palpitations
   4. ECG reading

**Nursing Actions and *Selected Purposes/Rationales***

3.a.1. Assess for and report signs and symptoms of cardiac arrhythmias (e.g. irregular apical pulse; pulse rate below 60 or above 100 beats/minute; apical-radial pulse deficit; syncope; palpitations; abnormal rate, rhythm, or configurations on ECG).
- 2. Implement measures to improve myocardial tissue perfusion and oxygenation (see Nursing Diagnosis 1, action b) *in order to prevent cardiac arrhythmias.*
- 3. If cardiac arrhythmias occur:
  - a. initiate cardiac monitoring if not already being done
  - b. administer the following medications if ordered:
    1. Class I antiarrhythmics (e.g. quinidine, procainamide, lidocaine, tocainide, moricizine) *to delay the rate of depolarization*

showing normal sinus rhythm.

2. Class II antiarrhythmics (e.g. esmolol, propranolol) *to block effects of beta-adrenergic stimulation on the heart*
3. Class III antiarrhythmics (e.g. bretylium, amiodarone) *to prolong repolorization and the duration of the action potential*
4. Class IV antiarrhythmics (e.g. verapamil) *to block the slow calcium channels, which then prolongs conduction and refractory period in AV node and depresses automaticity in SA and AV nodes*

c. restrict client's activity based on his/her tolerance and severity of the arrhythmia
d. maintain oxygen therapy as ordered
e. assess cardiovascular status frequently and report signs and symptoms of inadequate tissue perfusion (e.g. decline in B/P; cool, clammy, mottled skin; cyanosis; diminished peripheral pulses; declining urine output; increased restlessness and agitation; shortness of breath)
f. have emergency cart readily available for cardioversion, defibrillation, or cardiopulmonary resuscitation.

3.b. The client will not experience a myocardial infarction as evidenced by:
1. resolution of chest pain within 15-20 minutes
2. stable vital signs
3. cardiac enzymes within normal range
4. absence of ST segment elevation, T wave inversion, and pathological Q wave on ECG reading.

3.b.1. Assess for and report signs and symptoms of a myocardial infarction (e.g. chest pain that lasts longer than 20 minutes; increase in pulse rate; significant change in B/P; labored respirations; elevation of cardiac enzymes [CK-MB is the first to increase]; ST segment elevation, T wave inversion, and/or pathological Q wave on ECG [ST segment elevation can also occur in Prinzmetal's angina]).

2. Implement measures to improve myocardial tissue perfusion and oxygenation (see Nursing Diagnosis 1, action b) *in order to prevent a myocardial infarction.*
3. If signs and symptoms of a myocardial infarction occur:
   a. initiate cardiac monitoring if not already being done
   b. maintain client on strict bed rest in a semi- to high Fowler's position
   c. maintain oxygen therapy as ordered
   d. prepare client for the following procedures that may be performed *to improve myocardial blood flow:*
      1. injection of a thrombolytic agent (e.g. streptokinase, tissue plasminogen activator [tPA], anistreplase [APSAC, Eminase])
      2. percutaneous transluminal coronary angioplasty (PTCA) and/or atherectomy
      3. insertion of an intra-aortic balloon pump (IABP)
   e. administer the following medications if ordered:
      1. morphine sulfate *to reduce pain and anxiety and decrease cardiac workload*
      2. nitrates *to improve coronary blood flow and reduce myocardial oxygen requirements*
      3. beta-adrenergic blocking agents *to reduce myocardial oxygen requirements by decreasing the heart rate and force of myocardial contractility*
   f. provide emotional support to client and significant others
   g. refer to Care Plan on Myocardial Infarction for additional care measures.

## 4. NURSING DIAGNOSIS: Anxiety

related to pain or threat of recurrent pain; lack of understanding of diagnostic tests, diagnosis, and treatment plan; unfamiliar environment; and effect of angina pectoris on future life style and roles.

| Desired Outcome | Nursing Actions and ***Selected Purposes/Rationales*** |
|---|---|
| 4. The client will experience a reduction in anxiety as evidenced by:<br>a. verbalization of feeling less anxious and fearful<br>b. usual sleep pattern<br>c. relaxed facial expression and body movements<br>d. stable vital signs<br>e. usual perceptual ability and interactions with others. | 4.a. Assess client for signs and symptoms of anxiety (e.g. verbalization of fears and concerns, insomnia, tenseness, tremors, irritability, restlessness, diaphoresis, tachypnea, tachycardia, elevated blood pressure, facial pallor or flushing, narrowed perceptual field, withdrawal, noncompliance with treatment plan).<br>b. Implement measures *to reduce fear and anxiety:*<br>1. provide care in a calm, supportive, confident manner<br>2. if client is having severe pain:<br>a. do not leave him/her alone during period of acute distress<br>b. perform actions to relieve pain (see Nursing Diagnosis 2, action e)<br>3. once period of acute distress has subsided:<br>a. orient client to hospital environment, equipment, and routines; include an explanation of cardiac monitoring equipment<br>b. keep cardiac monitor out of client's view and the sound turned as low as possible<br>c. introduce staff who will be participating in client's care; if possible, maintain consistency in staff assigned to his/her care *to provide feelings of stability and comfort with the environment*<br>d. assure client that staff members are nearby; respond to call signal as soon as possible<br>e. encourage verbalization of fear and anxiety; provide feedback<br>f. explain all diagnostic tests<br>g. reinforce physician's explanations and clarify misconceptions the client has about angina pectoris, the treatment plan, and prognosis; stress to client that he/she has not had a "heart attack"<br>h. reinforce physician's explanation of percutaneous transluminal coronary angioplasty (PTCA) and/or atherectomy if planned<br>i. initiate preoperative teaching if heart surgery is planned<br>j. provide a calm, restful environment<br>k. instruct client in relaxation techniques and encourage participation in diversional activities<br>l. assist client to identify specific stressors and ways to cope with them<br>m. allow client to discuss concerns about future life style and roles; focus on the need for alteration in rather than elimination of activities<br>n. encourage significant others to project a caring, concerned attitude without obvious anxiousness<br>o. administer antianxiety agents if ordered.<br>c. Include significant others in orientation and teaching sessions and encourage their continued support of the client.<br>d. Provide information based on current needs of client and significant others at a level they can understand. Encourage questions and clarification of information provided.<br>e. Consult physician if above actions fail to control fear and anxiety. |

## 5. NURSING DIAGNOSIS: Knowledge deficit

regarding follow-up care.

| Desired Outcomes | Nursing Actions and ***Selected Purposes/Rationales*** |
|---|---|
| 5.a. The client will verbalize a basic understanding of angina pectoris. | 5.a. Explain angina pectoris in terms that client can understand. Utilize teaching aids (e.g. pamphlets, diagrams) whenever possible. |
| 5.b. The client will identify factors that may precipitate angina attacks and ways to control these factors. | 5.b.1. Ask client if there is a pattern to angina attacks and precipitating factors.<br>2. Inform the client of factors that may precipitate angina pectoris (e.g. strenuous or isometric exercises, change in usual sexual habits and/or partner, consumption of a large meal, exposure to extreme cold, strong emotions, smoking).<br>3. Provide the following instructions regarding ways to reduce risk of precipitating an angina attack:<br>a. take sublingual nitroglycerin 5-10 minutes before strenuous activity or sexual intercourse and during times of high emotional stress<br>b. adhere to a regular isotonic exercise program (e.g. walking, biking, swimming)<br>c. avoid isometric exercises/activities (e.g. weight lifting, pushing, straining)<br>d. rest between activities<br>e. stop any activity that causes shortness of breath, palpitations, dizziness, or extreme fatigue and weakness<br>f. begin a cardiovascular fitness program when approved by physician<br>g. adhere to the following precautions regarding sexual activity:<br>1. avoid intercourse for 1-2 hours after a heavy meal or alcohol consumption and when fatigued or stressed<br>2. engage in sexual activity with usual partner, in a familiar environment, and in a position that minimizes exertion (e.g. side-lying, partner on top)<br>3. avoid hot or cold showers just before and after intercourse. |
| 5.c. The client will identify modifiable cardiovascular risk factors and ways to reduce these factors. | 5.c.1. Inform client that the following modifiable factors have been shown to contribute to cardiovascular disease:<br>a. obesity<br>b. hyperlipidemia<br>c. sedentary life style<br>d. smoking<br>e. hypertension<br>f. stressful life style.<br>2. Inform client that alcohol intake should not exceed 1 oz of ethanol (i.e. 2 oz of 100-proof whiskey, 8 oz of wine, 24 oz of beer) a day on a regular basis because there is evidence that excessive alcohol intake contributes to the development of hypertension and some forms of heart disease.<br>3. Assist client to identify ways he/she can make appropriate changes in life style to reduce above factors. Provide information about weight reduction plans; stress management classes; and cardiovascular fitness, smoking cessation, and alcohol rehabilitation programs if appropriate. Initiate a referral if indicated. |
| 5.d. The client will verbalize an understanding of the rationale for and components of a diet low in saturated fat and cholesterol. | 5.d.1. Explain the rationale for a diet low in saturated fat and cholesterol.<br>2. Provide the following instructions on ways to reduce intake of saturated fat and cholesterol:<br>a. reduce intake of red meat<br>b. trim visible fat off meat and remove all skin from poultry<br>c. eat no more than 2 whole eggs/week<br>d. avoid commercial baked goods<br>e. avoid dairy products containing more than 1% fat. |
| 5.e. The client will demonstrate accuracy in counting pulse. | 5.e.1. Teach client to count his/her pulse, being alert to the regularity of the rhythm.<br>2. Allow time for return demonstration and accuracy check. |
| 5.f. The client will verbalize an | 5.f. 1. Explain the rationale for, side effects of, and importance of taking the medications prescribed. |

| Desired Outcomes | Nursing Actions and ***Selected Purposes/Rationales*** |
|---|---|
| understanding of medications ordered including rationale, side effects, schedule for taking, and importance of taking as prescribed. | 2. If client is discharged on nitroglycerin, instruct to:<br>a. avoid drinking alcoholic beverages<br>b. have tablets readily available at all times<br>c. take a tablet before strenuous activity and in emotionally stressful situations<br>d. take one tablet when chest pain occurs and another every 5 minutes up to a total of 3 times if necessary; notify physician if pain persists<br>e. place tablet under tongue and allow it to dissolve thoroughly before swallowing<br>f. store tablets in a cool place in a light-resistant, airtight container; when opening bottle for initial use, remove cotton plug and do not replace it<br>g. replace tablets every 5 months or sooner if they do not relieve discomfort or do not cause a slight tingling/stinging sensation at sublingual site<br>h. avoid rising to a standing position quickly after taking nitroglycerin in order to reduce dizziness associated with its vasodilatory effect<br>i. recognize that dizziness, flushing, and mild headache may occur after taking nitroglycerin; instruct client to notify physician if fainting occurs or headache persists for more than a few days.<br>3. If nitroglycerin skin patches are prescribed:<br>a. provide instructions about correct application, skin care, need to rotate sites, and frequency of change<br>b. caution client that activities that increase blood flow to the skin (e.g. hot bath or shower, sauna) can cause a sudden reduction in blood pressure.<br>4. If client is discharged on a beta-adrenergic blocking agent (e.g. propranolol, metoprolol, atenolol, nadolol), instruct to:<br>a. take the medication at the same time every day<br>b. check pulse before taking medication; consult physician if pulse rate is unusually slow (it is expected that pulse will be lower than normal)<br>c. avoid skipping doses, trying to make up for missed doses, altering the prescribed dose, and discontinuing medication without physician's permission<br>d. change from a lying to a sitting or standing position slowly if dizziness is a problem<br>e. limit intake of alcoholic beverages<br>f. take medication 1 hour after meals if gastrointestinal distress occurs and report continued problems<br>g. monitor blood glucose on a regular basis if a diabetic (beta blockers may affect blood sugar).<br>5. If client is discharged on a calcium-channel blocker (e.g. nifedipine, nicardipine, verapamil, diltiazem), instruct to:<br>a. avoid skipping doses, altering the prescribed dose, and discontinuing medication without physician's permission<br>b. change from a lying to a sitting or standing position slowly in order to prevent dizziness<br>c. report any increase in frequency, duration, or severity of angina<br>d. avoid drinking alcoholic beverages<br>e. keep medication in a cool place in an airtight, light-resistant container.<br>6. Instruct client to take antilipemic agents (e.g. lovastatin, gemfibrozil, pravastatin, simvastatin) and antiplatelet agents (e.g. aspirin) as prescribed.<br>7. Instruct client to consult physician before taking other prescription and nonprescription medications.<br>8. Instruct client to inform all health care providers of medications being taken. |

| | |
|---|---|
| 5.g. The client will state signs and symptoms to report to the health care provider. | 5.g. Stress the importance of reporting the following signs and symptoms:<br>1. chest, arm, neck, or jaw pain unrelieved by rest and/or nitroglycerin taken every 5 minutes for 15 minutes<br>2. shortness of breath<br>3. irregular pulse or a resting pulse less than 56 or greater than 100 beats/minute<br>4. fainting spells<br>5. diminished activity tolerance<br>6. swelling of feet or ankles<br>7. increase in severity or frequency of angina attacks. |
| 5.h. The client will identify community resources that can assist in making necessary life-style changes and adjusting to the effects of angina pectoris. | 5.h.1. Provide information about community resources that can assist client in making life-style changes and adjusting to effects of angina pectoris (e.g. weight loss, smoking cessation, and stress management programs; American Heart Association; counseling services).<br>2. Initiate a referral if indicated. |
| 5.i. The client will verbalize an understanding of and a plan for adhering to recommended follow-up care including future appointments with health care provider. | 5.i. 1. Reinforce the importance of keeping follow-up appointments with health care provider.<br>2. Implement measures to improve client compliance:<br>a. include significant others in teaching sessions if possible<br>b. encourage questions and allow time for reinforcement and clarification of information provided<br>c. provide written instructions regarding future appointments with health care provider, dietary modifications, activity level, medications prescribed, and signs and symptoms to report. |

# Heart Failure

Heart failure is a syndrome in which the heart is unable to pump an adequate supply of blood to meet the body's metabolic needs. Inadequate emptying of the ventricles results in increased pressure in the cardiac chambers, which leads to decreased pulmonary and systemic venous return and subsequent vascular congestion. To compensate for decreased cardiac output, there is an increase in sympathetic nervous system activity, ventricular dilation to accommodate the increased volume (Frank-Starling response), stimulation of renin-angiotensin-aldosterone output and ADH release, and eventual ventricular hypertrophy. These compensatory mechanisms aid in maintaining an adequate cardiac output but eventually have a deleterious effect on the heart because they increase myocardial oxygen consumption.

Heart failure can result from conditions that cause myocardial dysfunction (e.g. myocardial infarction, coronary artery disease, cardiomyopathy, myocarditis, arrhythmias), abnormal volume overload (e.g. hypervolemia, valve incompetence), abnormal pressure overload (e.g. aortic stenosis, hypertension), filling disorders (e.g. restrictive pericarditis, valve stenosis), and increased metabolic demand (e.g. thyrotoxicosis, anemia). Heart failure is often classified as left-sided or right-sided, backward or forward, low-output or high-output, acute or chronic, and/or systolic (classic) or diastolic heart failure. The types of medications used for treatment are primarily dependent on whether failure is systolic (an impaired inotropic state characterized by ventricular dilation and inadequate ventricle emptying) or diastolic (impaired relaxation of the ventricles with decreased ventricular filling). Positive inotropic agents, as well as diuretics and vasodilators, are the mainstay of treatment in systolic or classic heart failure. Medications that decrease the force of myocardial contractility are indicated for treatment of diastolic failure.

Signs and symptoms of heart failure are dependent on which side of the heart is failing as well as whether there is forward or backward failure. Symptoms of forward failure are caused by low cardiac output. Symptoms of backward failure are associated with the ventricle failing to empty completely, which results in blood flow backup. In left-sided failure, there is reduced emptying of the left ventricle, which results in decreased systemic tissue perfusion as well as blood flow backup in the left atrium and pulmonary vasculature. Pulmonary vascular congestion leads to pulmonary edema with symptoms such as tachypnea, dyspnea, cough, and abnormal breath sounds. In right-sided failure, the effect of reduced function and emptying of the right ventricle is decreased pulmonary blood flow and backup of blood in the right atrium. This results in systemic venous congestion, which is manifested by peripheral edema and signs of major organ enlargement and dysfunction. Initially only one side of the heart may fail (more commonly the left side), but as failure progresses, both sides are usually affected.

As long as the body's compensatory mechanisms are able to maintain adequate tissue perfusion, a state of compensated heart failure exists. If the myocardium is severely damaged and intrinsic compensatory mechanisms fail to maintain adequate cardiac output and tissue perfusion, a state of decompensated heart failure exists. When this state persists and is no longer responsive to medical treatment, it is termed intractable or refractory heart failure.

**This care plan focuses on the adult client with signs and symptoms of acute classic biventricular heart failure hospitalized for diagnosis and treatment.** The goals of care are to reduce cardiac workload, improve cardiac output, prevent complications, promote an optimal level of functioning, and educate the client regarding follow-up care.

## DIAGNOSTIC TESTS

Chest x-ray
Echocardiography
Radionuclide imaging
Electrocardiogram (ECG)
Cardiac catheterization
Blood studies (e.g. blood gases, electrolytes, BUN, creatinine)
Oximetry

## DISCHARGE CRITERIA

Prior to discharge, the client will:

- ❖ have adequate cardiac output
- ❖ tolerate expected level of activity
- ❖ have resolution of fluid imbalance
- ❖ identify modifiable cardiovascular risk factors and ways to reduce these factors
- ❖ verbalize an understanding of the rationale for and components of a diet low in sodium
- ❖ demonstrate accuracy in counting pulse
- ❖ verbalize an understanding of medications ordered including rationale, side effects, schedule for taking, and importance of taking as prescribed
- ❖ state signs and symptoms to report to the health care provider
- ❖ identify community resources that can assist with home management and adjustment to changes resulting from heart failure
- ❖ share feelings and concerns about changes in body functioning and usual roles and life style
- ❖ verbalize an understanding of and a plan for adhering to recommended follow-up care including future appointments with health care provider and activity limitations.

---

**Use in conjunction with the Care Plan on Immobility.**

## NURSING/ COLLABORATIVE DIAGNOSES

**See Immobility Care Plan for additional diagnoses.**

## 1. NURSING DIAGNOSIS: Decreased cardiac output

related to impaired contractility or relaxation of the ventricles associated with ventricular dilation or hypertrophy.

| Desired Outcome | Nursing Actions and ***Selected Purposes/Rationales*** |
|---|---|
| 1. The client will have improved cardiac output as evidenced by:<br>a. B/P within normal range for client<br>b. apical pulse between 60-100 beats/minute and regular<br>c. resolution of gallop rhythms<br>d. verbalization of feeling less fatigued and weak<br>e. unlabored respirations at 14-20/minute<br>f. improved breath sounds<br>g. usual mental status<br>h. absence of vertigo and syncope<br>i. palpable peripheral pulses<br>j. improved skin temperature and color | 1.a. Assess for signs and symptoms of heart failure and decreased cardiac output:<br>1. variations in B/P (may be increased because of compensatory vasoconstriction; may be decreased when compensatory mechanisms and pump fail)<br>2. tachycardia, irregular pulse<br>3. pulsus alternans<br>4. presence of an $S_3$ heart sound or summation gallop<br>5. fatigue and weakness<br>6. dyspnea, tachypnea<br>7. cough (usually dry, hacking)<br>8. abnormal breath sounds (e.g. crackles [rales], wheezes, diminished sounds)<br>9. restlessness, change in mental status<br>10. vertigo, syncope<br>11. diminished or absent peripheral pulses<br>12. cool, clammy skin<br>13. pallor, mottling, or cyanosis of skin<br>14. capillary refill time greater than 3 seconds<br>15. oliguria<br>16. peripheral edema<br>17. jugular vein distention (JVD)<br>18. hemodynamic changes such as decreased CO and increased PAP, PCWP, and CVP (use internal jugular vein pulsation method to estimate CVP if monitoring device not present).<br>b. Monitor ECG readings and report arrhythmias. |

| Desired Outcome | Nursing Actions and ***Selected Purposes/Rationales*** |
|---|---|
| k. capillary refill time less than 3 seconds<br>l. balanced intake and output<br>m. decrease in peripheral edema and jugular vein distention<br>n. hemodynamic measurements such as cardiac output (CO), pulmonary artery pressure (PAP), pulmonary capillary wedge pressure (PCWP), and central venous pressure (CVP) returning toward normal range. | c. Monitor chest x-ray results. Report findings of cardiomegaly, pleural effusion, or pulmonary edema.<br>d. Implement measures *to improve cardiac output:*<br>1. perform actions *to reduce cardiac workload:*<br>a. place client in a semi- to high Fowler's position<br>b. instruct client to avoid activities that create a Valsalva response (e.g. straining to have a bowel movement, holding breath while moving) *in order to prevent the marked increase in venous return and preload that occurs with exhalation*<br>c. maintain activity restrictions as ordered<br>d. implement measures *to promote emotional rest* (e.g. reduce fear and anxiety)<br>e. implement measures to improve respiratory status (see Nursing Diagnosis 2, action c) *in order to improve alveolar gas exchange and promote adequate tissue oxygenation*<br>f. discourage smoking *(smoke has a cardiostimulatory effect, causes vasoconstriction, and reduces oxygen availability)*<br>g. provide small meals rather than large ones *(large meals require an increase in blood supply to gastrointestinal tract for digestion)*<br>h. discourage excessive intake of fluids high in caffeine such as coffee, tea, and colas *(caffeine is a myocardial stimulant and increases myocardial oxygen consumption)*<br>i. increase activity gradually as allowed and tolerated<br>j. implement measures to reduce fluid volume excess (see Nursing Diagnosis 3, action d.1)<br>2. administer the following medications if ordered:<br>a. positive inotropic agents (e.g. digitalis preparations, dobutamine, dopamine, milrinone, amrinone) *to improve myocardial contractility*<br>b. arterial dilators (e.g. hydralazine) *to decrease afterload*<br>c. nitrates (e.g. nitroglycerin, isosorbide) and balanced vasodilators (e.g. prazosin, nitroprusside) *to decrease preload and afterload*<br>d. angiotensin-converting enzyme inhibitors (e.g. captopril, lisinopril, enalapril) *to decrease peripheral vascular resistance and suppress aldosterone output.*<br>e. If signs and symptoms of decreased cardiac output persist or worsen:<br>1. consult physician<br>2. prepare client for insertion of intra-aortic balloon pump (IABP) or surgery (e.g. artificial heart or ventricular assist device implant) if indicated. |

## 2. NURSING DIAGNOSIS: Impaired respiratory function:*

a. **ineffective breathing pattern** related to:
   1. fear and anxiety
   2. decreased lung compliance (distensibility) associated with pleural effusion and accumulation of fluid in interstitial spaces and alveoli
   3. impaired lung/chest wall expansion associated with weakness, decreased mobility, and pressure on the diaphragm as a result of peritoneal fluid accumulation (if present)
   4. respiratory depressant and/or stimulant effects of hypoxia, hypercapnia, and diminished cerebral blood flow;

b. **ineffective airway clearance** related to:
   1. fluid accumulation in the airways associated with alveolar pulmonary edema
   2. stasis of secretions associated with decreased mobility and poor cough effort;

*This diagnostic label includes the following nursing diagnoses: ineffective breathing pattern, ineffective airway clearance, and impaired gas exchange.

c. **impaired gas exchange** related to:
   1. impaired diffusion of gases associated with accumulation of fluid in the pulmonary interstitium and alveoli
   2. decreased pulmonary tissue perfusion associated with decreased cardiac output.

| Desired Outcome | Nursing Actions and ***Selected Purposes/Rationales*** |
|---|---|
| 2. The client will experience adequate respiratory function as evidenced by:<br>a. normal rate, rhythm, and depth of respirations<br>b. decreased dyspnea<br>c. usual or improved breath sounds<br>d. usual mental status<br>e. usual skin color<br>f. blood gases within normal range. | 2.a. Assess for signs and symptoms of impaired respiratory function:<br>1. rapid, shallow, slow, or irregular respirations<br>2. dyspnea, orthopnea<br>3. use of accessory muscles when breathing<br>4. adventitious breath sounds (e.g. crackles [rales], wheezes)<br>5. diminished or absent breath sounds<br>6. dry, hacking cough or cough productive of frothy or blood-tinged sputum<br>7. restlessness, irritability<br>8. confusion, somnolence<br>9. central cyanosis (a late sign).<br>b. Monitor for and report the following:<br>1. abnormal blood gases<br>2. significant changes in oximetry results<br>3. abnormal chest x-ray results.<br>c. Implement measures *to improve respiratory status:*<br>1. perform actions to improve cardiac output (see Nursing Diagnosis 1, action d) *in order to improve pulmonary tissue perfusion and reduce fluid accumulation in the lungs*<br>2. perform actions to reduce fear and anxiety (see Nursing Diagnosis 13, action b)<br>3. instruct client to breathe slowly if he/she is hyperventilating<br>4. place client in a semi- to high Fowler's position; position overbed table so client can lean forward on it if desired<br>5. assist client to turn at least every 2 hours<br>6. instruct client to deep breathe or use incentive spirometer at least every 2 hours<br>7. perform actions to increase strength and activity tolerance (see Nursing Diagnosis 7)<br>8. perform actions *to facilitate removal of pulmonary secretions:*<br>a. instruct and assist client to cough or "huff" every 1-2 hours<br>b. implement measures *to liquefy tenacious secretions:*<br>1. humidify inspired air as ordered<br>2. maintain the maximum fluid intake allowed<br>c. assist with administration of diluent and mucolytic agents via nebulizer or IPPB treatment as ordered<br>d. assist with or perform postural drainage, percussion, and vibration if ordered<br>e. perform tracheal suctioning if needed<br>9. maintain oxygen therapy as ordered (initially, high concentrations under positive pressure may be given *to overcome the pressure barrier caused by alveolar fluid accumulation and to reduce the transudation of fluid from the capillaries*)<br>10. instruct client to avoid intake of gas-forming foods (e.g. beans, cauliflower, cabbage, onions), carbonated beverages, and large meals *in order to prevent gastric distention and a further increase in pressure on the diaphragm* |

| Desired Outcome | Nursing Actions and ***Selected Purposes/Rationales*** |
|---|---|
| | 11. discourage smoking *(smoke causes bronchoconstriction, increases mucus production, impairs ciliary function, and decreases oxygen availability)*<br>12. protect client from exposure to irritants such as smoke, flowers, and perfume *(can cause bronchospasm and increased mucus production)*<br>13. maintain activity restrictions; increase activity gradually as allowed and tolerated<br>14. administer central nervous system depressants judiciously; hold medication and consult physician if respiratory rate is less than 12/minute<br>15. administer the following medications if ordered:<br>a. diuretics *to decrease pulmonary fluid accumulation*<br>b. morphine sulfate *to decrease pulmonary vascular congestion (the vasodilatory action of morphine sulfate reduces cardiac workload and eventually improves left ventricular emptying, which results in increased blood return from the pulmonary veins); morphine also reduces the apprehension associated with dyspnea*<br>c. theophylline *to dilate the bronchioles (its mild diuretic effect also helps reduce pulmonary vascular congestion)*<br>16. assist with thoracentesis and/or paracentesis if performed *to allow increased lung expansion.*<br>d. Consult physician if signs and symptoms of impaired respiratory function persist or worsen. |

**3. NURSING/ COLLABORATIVE DIAGNOSIS:**

**Altered fluid balance:**

a. **fluid volume excess** related to:
   1. reduced glomerular filtration rate (GFR) associated with decreased renal blood flow
   2. activation of the renin-angiotensin-aldosterone mechanism (results in retention of sodium and water) associated with decreased renal blood flow
   3. increased ADH output associated with:
      a. stimulation of the baroreceptors if the systemic pressure is low
      b. stimulation of the osmoreceptors if osmotic pressure is increased as a result of aldosterone-induced sodium retention;

b. **third-spacing of fluid** related to:
   1. increased intravascular pressure associated with fluid volume excess
   2. low plasma colloid osmotic pressure if serum albumin is decreased as a result of malnutrition or impaired liver function (occurs with hepatic venous congestion).

| Desired Outcome | Nursing Actions and ***Selected Purposes/Rationales*** |
|---|---|
| 3. The client will experience resolution of fluid imbalance as evidenced by:<br>a. decline in weight toward client's normal<br>b. B/P and pulse within normal range for client and stable with position change | 3.a. Assess for signs and symptoms of the following:<br>1. fluid volume excess:<br>a. weight gain<br>b. elevated B/P (B/P may not be elevated if cardiac output is poor or fluid has shifted out of the vascular space)<br>c. presence of an $S_3$ heart sound or summation gallop<br>d. intake greater than output<br>e. change in mental status<br>f. crackles (rales)<br>g. low Hct (may be normal or even increased if fluid has shifted out of the vascular space) |

c. resolution of gallop rhythms
d. balanced intake and output
e. usual mental status
f. improved breath sounds
g. Hct returning toward normal range
h. decreased dyspnea and orthopnea
i. resolution of peripheral edema, ascites, and neck vein distention
j. small vein emptying time less than 3-5 seconds
k. CVP within normal range.

h. dyspnea, orthopnea
i. peripheral edema
j. distended neck veins
k. delayed small vein emptying time (longer than 3-5 seconds)
l. elevated CVP (use internal jugular vein pulsation method to estimate CVP if monitoring device not present)

2. third-spacing:
   a. ascites
   b. increased dyspnea and diminished or absent breath sounds
   c. evidence of vascular depletion (e.g. postural hypotension; weak, rapid pulse; decreased urine output).

b. Monitor chest x-ray results. Report findings of pulmonary vascular congestion, pleural effusion, or pulmonary edema.
c. Monitor serum albumin levels. Report below-normal levels *(albumin maintains plasma colloid osmotic pressure).*
d. Implement measures *to restore fluid balance:*
   1. perform actions *to reduce fluid volume excess:*
      a. restrict sodium intake as ordered
      b. maintain fluid restrictions if ordered
      c. encourage client to rest periodically in a recumbent position if tolerated *(lying flat promotes venous return, which results in lower venous hydrostatic pressure with subsequent reshifting of fluid back into vascular space; the increased fluid in the vascular space and improved renal blood flow that occur in a recumbent position result in increased excretion of sodium and water)*
      d. administer the following medications if ordered:
         1. diuretics (e.g. furosemide, bumetanide) *to increase excretion of water*
         2. positive inotropic agents and arterial vasodilators *to increase cardiac output and subsequently improve renal blood flow*
   2. perform actions *to prevent further third-spacing and promote mobilization of fluid back into the vascular space:*
      a. implement measures to reduce fluid volume excess (see action d.1 in this diagnosis)
      b. administer salt-poor albumin if ordered *to increase colloid osmotic pressure.*
e. Consult physician if signs and symptoms of fluid imbalance persist or worsen.

## 4. NURSING DIAGNOSIS: Altered nutrition: less than body requirements

related to:
a. decreased oral intake associated with nausea, weakness, fatigue, dyspnea, and dislike of the prescribed diet;
b. impaired absorption and transport of nutrients associated with poor tissue perfusion.

| Desired Outcome | Nursing Actions and ***Selected Purposes/Rationales*** |
|---|---|
| 4. The client will maintain an adequate nutritional status as evidenced by: a. dry weight within normal range for | 4.a. Assess for and report signs and symptoms of malnutrition: 1. dry weight below normal for client's age, height, and body frame 2. abnormal BUN and low serum albumin, Hct, Hb, transferrin, and lymphocyte levels 3. triceps skinfold thickness less than normal |

| Desired Outcome | Nursing Actions and ***Selected Purposes/Rationales*** |
|---|---|
| client's age, height, and body frame (dry weight is achieved after fluid volume excess has been resolved)<br>b. normal BUN and serum albumin, Hct, Hb, transferrin, and lymphocyte levels<br>c. triceps skinfold thickness within normal range<br>d. improved strength and activity tolerance<br>e. healthy oral mucous membrane. | 4. weakness and fatigue<br>5. stomatitis.<br>b. Monitor percentage of meals and snacks client consumes. Report a pattern of inadequate intake.<br>c. Implement measures *to maintain an adequate nutritional status:*<br>1. perform actions *to improve oral intake:*<br>a. implement measures to prevent nausea and vomiting (see Nursing Diagnosis 5, action b)<br>b. increase activity as allowed and tolerated *(activity stimulates appetite)*<br>c. obtain a dietary consult if necessary to assist client in selecting foods/fluids that meet nutritional needs, dietary restrictions, and personal and cultural preferences whenever possible<br>d. encourage a rest period before meals *to minimize fatigue*<br>e. maintain a clean environment and a relaxed, pleasant atmosphere<br>f. provide oral care before meals<br>g. serve small portions of nutritious foods/fluids that are appealing to the client<br>h. place client in a high Fowler's position for meals and provide supplemental oxygen therapy during meals if indicated *to help relieve dyspnea*<br>i. instruct client to use herbs, spices, and salt substitutes if approved by physician or dietitian *in order to make low-sodium diet more palatable*<br>j. allow adequate time for meals; reheat food if necessary<br>k. limit fluid intake (unless it has a high nutritional value) with meals *to reduce early satiety and subsequent decreased food intake*<br>2. perform actions to improve cardiac output (see Nursing Diagnosis 1, action d) *in order to increase tissue perfusion and the absorption and transport of nutrients*<br>3. ensure that meals are well balanced and high in essential nutrients; offer dietary supplements between meals if indicated<br>4. administer vitamins and minerals if ordered.<br>d. Perform a 72-hour calorie count if ordered. Report totals to dietitian and physician.<br>e. Consult physician regarding alternative methods of providing nutrition (e.g. parenteral nutrition, tube feedings) if client does not consume enough food or fluids to meet nutritional needs. |

## 5. NURSING DIAGNOSIS: Altered comfort: nausea and vomiting

related to stimulation of the vomiting center associated with:
a. stimulation of the afferent vagal and/or sympathetic pathways resulting from vascular congestion in the heart and gastrointestinal tract;
b. cortical stimulation resulting from stress;
c. chemoreceptor trigger zone stimulation by certain medications (e.g. digitalis preparations, morphine sulfate).

| Desired Outcome | Nursing Actions and ***Selected Purposes/Rationales*** |
|---|---|
| 5. The client will experience relief of nausea and vomiting as evidenced by:<br>a. verbalization of relief of nausea | 5.a. Assess client for nausea and vomiting.<br>b. Implement measures *to prevent nausea and vomiting:*<br>1. perform actions to improve cardiac output (see Nursing Diagnosis 1, action d) *in order to reduce vascular congestion in the heart and gastrointestinal tract* |

b. absence of vomiting.

2. monitor serum digoxin levels and report elevated values (be alert to a low serum potassium level *because it may precipitate digitalis toxicity)*
3. perform actions to reduce fear and anxiety (see Nursing Diagnosis 13, action b)
4. eliminate noxious sights and odors from the environment *(noxious stimuli cause cortical stimulation of the vomiting center)*
5. encourage client to take deep, slow breaths when nauseated
6. encourage client to change positions slowly *(rapid movement stimulates the afferent vestibulocerebellar pathway with resultant stimulation of the chemoreceptor trigger zone)*
7. provide oral hygiene after each emesis and before meals
8. provide small, frequent meals; instruct client to ingest foods and fluids slowly
9. avoid serving foods with an overpowering aroma; remove lids from hot foods before entering room
10. instruct client to avoid foods high in fat *(fat delays gastric emptying)*
11. instruct client to avoid foods/fluids that irritate gastric mucosa (e.g. spicy foods; caffeine-containing beverages such as coffee, tea, and colas)
12. instruct client to eat dry foods (e.g. toast, crackers) and avoid drinking liquids with meals if nauseated
13. instruct client to rest after eating with head of bed elevated
14. administer antiemetics if ordered.

c. Consult physician if above measures fail to control nausea and vomiting.

## 6. NURSING DIAGNOSIS: High risk for impaired skin integrity

related to:
a. ischemia of the skin and subcutaneous tissue associated with prolonged pressure on tissues as a result of decreased mobility;
b. damage to the skin and/or subcutaneous tissue associated with friction or shearing;
c. increased fragility of the skin associated with edema, poor tissue perfusion, and inadequate nutritional status.

| Desired Outcome | Nursing Actions and ***Selected Purposes/Rationales*** |
|---|---|
| 6. The client will maintain skin integrity as evidenced by:<br>a. absence of redness and irritation<br>b. no skin breakdown. | 6.a. Inspect the skin, especially bony prominences and dependent and edematous areas, for pallor, redness, and breakdown.<br>b. Refer to Care Plan on Immobility, Nursing Diagnosis 4, action b (pp. 141-142), for measures to prevent skin breakdown associated with decreased mobility.<br>c. Implement additional measures *to prevent skin breakdown:*<br>1. perform actions *to improve tissue perfusion and reduce edema:*<br>a. implement measures to increase cardiac output (see Nursing Diagnosis 1, action d)<br>b. implement measures to restore fluid balance (see Nursing Diagnosis 3, action d)<br>2. perform actions to maintain an adequate nutritional status (see Nursing Diagnosis 4, action c).<br>d. If skin breakdown occurs:<br>1. notify physician<br>2. continue with above measures to prevent further irritation and breakdown |

| Desired Outcome | Nursing Actions and ***Selected Purposes/Rationales*** |
|---|---|
| | 3. perform decubitus care as ordered or per standard hospital procedure<br>4. assess client closely and report signs and symptoms of infection (e.g. elevated temperature; redness, warmth, and edema around area of breakdown; unusual drainage from site). |

## 7. NURSING DIAGNOSIS: Activity intolerance

related to:

a. tissue hypoxia associated with impaired alveolar gas exchange and decreased cardiac output;
b. inadequate nutritional status;
c. difficulty resting and sleeping associated with dyspnea, frequent assessments and treatments, fear, and anxiety.

| Desired Outcome | Nursing Actions and ***Selected Purposes/Rationales*** |
|---|---|
| 7. The client will demonstrate an increased tolerance for activity (see Care Pan on Immobility, Nursing Diagnosis 5 [p. 143], for outcome criteria). | 7.a. Refer to Care Plan on Immobility, Nursing Diagnosis 5 (p. 143), for measures related to assessment and improvement of activity tolerance.<br>b. Implement additional measures *to promote rest and/or improve activity tolerance:*<br>1. maintain activity restrictions as ordered<br>2. perform actions to reduce fear and anxiety (see Nursing Diagnosis 13, action b)<br>3. perform actions to promote sleep (see Nursing Diagnosis 10)<br>4. perform actions to improve respiratory status (see Nursing Diagnosis 2, action c) *in order to relieve dyspnea and improve tissue oxygenation*<br>5. perform actions to increase cardiac output (see Nursing Diagnosis 1, action d)<br>6. perform actions to maintain an adequate nutritional status (see Nursing Diagnosis 4, action c)<br>7. increase client's activity gradually as allowed and tolerated; explain that activity is increased gradually *to prevent a sudden increase in cardiac workload.* |

## 8. NURSING DIAGNOSIS: Self-care deficit

related to weakness, fatigue, dyspnea, altered thought processes, and activity restrictions imposed by the treatment plan.

| Desired Outcome | Nursing Actions and ***Selected Purposes/Rationales*** |
|---|---|
| 8. The client will perform self-care activities within physical limitations and activity restrictions imposed by the treatment plan. | 8.a. Refer to Care Plan on Immobility, Nursing Diagnosis 7 (pp. 144-145) for measures related to planning for and meeting client's self-care needs.<br>b. Implement additional measures *to facilitate client's ability to perform self-care activities:*<br>1. perform actions to increase strength and activity tolerance (see Nursing Diagnosis 7)<br>2. perform actions to improve respiratory status and relieve dyspnea (see Nursing Diagnosis 2, action c) |

3. perform actions to improve cardiac output (see Nursing Diagnosis 1, action d) *in order to improve activity tolerance and increase cerebral blood flow and subsequently improve thought processes.*

## 9. NURSING DIAGNOSIS: Altered thought processes

related to:
a. cerebral hypoxia associated with impaired alveolar gas exchange and inadequate cerebral tissue perfusion (a result of decreased cardiac output);
b. altered fluid balance.

| Desired Outcome | Nursing Actions and ***Selected Purposes/Rationales*** |
|---|---|
| 9. The client will regain usual thought processes as evidenced by:<br>a. improved verbal response time<br>b. longer attention span<br>c. improved memory<br>d. improved level of orientation. | 9.a. Assess client for altered thought processes (e.g. slowed verbal responses, shortened attention span, impaired memory, confusion).<br>b. Ascertain from significant others client's usual level of intellectual functioning.<br>c. Implement measures *to improve thought processes:*<br>1. perform actions *to increase cerebral tissue oxygenation:*<br>a. implement measures to improve cardiac output (see Nursing Diagnosis 1, action d)<br>b. implement measures to improve respiratory status (see Nursing Diagnosis 2, action c)<br>2. perform actions to restore fluid balance (see Nursing Diagnosis 3, action d).<br>d. If client shows evidence of altered thought processes:<br>1. reorient client to person, place, and time as necessary<br>2. address client by name<br>3. place familiar objects, clock, and calendar within client's view<br>4. approach client in a slow, calm manner; allow adequate time for communication<br>5. repeat instructions as necessary using clear, simple language and short sentences<br>6. maintain a consistent and fairly structured routine and write out a schedule of activities for client to refer to if desired<br>7. have client perform only one activity at a time and allow adequate time for performance of activities<br>8. maintain realistic expectations of client's ability to learn, comprehend, and remember information provided; provide client with a written copy of instructions<br>9. encourage significant others to be supportive of client; instruct them in methods of dealing with client's altered thought processes<br>10. discuss physiological basis for altered thought processes with client and significant others; inform them that intellectual functioning is expected to improve as a result of treatment<br>11. consult physician if altered thought processes persist or worsen. |

## 10. NURSING DIAGNOSIS: Sleep pattern disturbance

related to unfamiliar environment, frequent assessments and treatments, decreased physical activity, fear, anxiety, and inability to assume usual sleep position associated with orthopnea.

| Desired Outcome | Nursing Actions and ***Selected Purposes/Rationales*** |
|---|---|
| 10. The client will attain optimal amounts of sleep within the parameters of the treatment regimen (see Care Plan on Immobility, Nursing Diagnosis 10 [p. 147], for outcome criteria). | 10.a. Refer to Care Plan on Immobility, Nursing Diagnosis 10 (p. 147), for measures related to assessment and promotion of sleep.<br>b. Implement additional measures *to promote sleep:*<br>1. perform actions to improve respiratory status (see Nursing Diagnosis 2, action c) *in order to relieve dyspnea*<br>2. if client has orthopnea, assist him/her to assume a position *that facilitates breathing* (e.g. head of bed elevated with arms supported on pillows, resting forward on overbed table with good pillow support, sitting in chair)<br>3. maintain oxygen therapy during sleep if indicated<br>4. perform actions to reduce fear and anxiety (see Nursing Diagnosis 13, action b). |

## 11. NURSING DIAGNOSIS: High risk for trauma

related to falls associated with:

a. weakness;
b. dizziness and syncope resulting from inadequate cerebral tissue oxygenation and hypotensive effects of vasodilators;
c. getting up without assistance as a result of restlessness, agitation, forgetfulness, and confusion.

| Desired Outcome | Nursing Actions and ***Selected Purposes/Rationales*** |
|---|---|
| 11. The client will not experience falls. | 11.a. Implement measures *to prevent falls:*<br>1. keep bed in low position with side rails up when client is in bed<br>2. keep needed items within easy reach<br>3. encourage client to request assistance whenever needed; have call signal within easy reach<br>4. use lap belt when client is in chair if indicated<br>5. instruct client to wear well-fitting slippers/shoes with nonslip soles and low heels when ambulating<br>6. keep floor free of clutter and wipe up spills promptly<br>7. accompany client during ambulation utilizing a transfer safety belt if he/she is weak or dizzy<br>8. provide ambulatory aids (e.g. walker, cane) if client is weak or unsteady on feet<br>9. instruct client to ambulate in well-lit areas and to utilize handrails if needed<br>10. do not rush client; allow adequate time for ambulation to the bathroom and in hallway<br>11. instruct and assist client to get out of bed slowly *in order to reduce dizziness associated with postural hypotension*<br>12. perform actions to improve cardiac output (see Nursing Diagnosis 1, action d) *in order to improve cerebral blood flow and reduce dizziness, syncope, and altered thought processes*<br>13. perform actions to increase strength and activity tolerance (see Nursing Diagnosis 7)<br>14. make sure that bathtub and shower have nonslip bottom surfaces and that shower chair, secure bath mat, call light, hand grips, and adequate lighting are present<br>15. administer central nervous system depressants judiciously |

16. if client is confused or irrational:
    a. reorient frequently to surroundings and necessity of adhering to safety precautions
    b. provide constant supervision (e.g. staff member, significant other) if indicated
    c. consult physician about the temporary use of jacket or wrist restraints if necessary
    d. administer antianxiety and antipsychotic medications if ordered.

b. Include client and significant others in planning and implementing measures to prevent falls.

c. If client falls, initiate first aid measures if appropriate and notify physician.

## 12. COLLABORATIVE DIAGNOSES:

**Potential complications:**

a. **renal failure** related to a prolonged or severe decrease in renal blood flow associated with low cardiac output, volume depletion (a result of third-spacing and/or excessive diuretic use), venous congestion, and vasodilator-induced hypotension;

b. **cardiac arrhythmias** related to myocardial irritability associated with myocardial hypoxia and increased catecholamine levels (catecholamines increase as a compensatory response to low cardiac output);

c. **thromboembolism** related to:
   1. venous stasis in the periphery associated with decreased cardiac output and decreased mobility
   2. stasis of blood in the heart associated with decreased ventricular emptying (risk increases if arrhythmias are present);

d. **cardiogenic shock** related to inability of heart, intrinsic compensatory mechanisms, and treatments to maintain adequate tissue perfusion to vital organs.

| Desired Outcomes | Nursing Actions and ***Selected Purposes/Rationales*** |
|---|---|
| 12.a. The client will maintain adequate renal function as evidenced by:<br>1. urine output at least 30 ml/hour<br>2. urine specific gravity, BUN, serum creatinine, and creatinine clearance within normal range. | 12.a.1. Assess for and report signs and symptoms of impaired renal function (e.g. urine output less than 30 ml/hour, urine specific gravity fixed at or less than 1.010, elevated BUN and serum creatinine levels).<br>2. Collect a 24-hour urine specimen if ordered. Report decreased creatinine clearance.<br>3. Implement measures *to maintain adequate renal blood flow:*<br>a. perform actions to improve cardiac output (see Nursing Diagnosis 1, action d)<br>b. perform actions to restore fluid balance (see Nursing Diagnosis 3, action d) *in order to reduce venous congestion and prevent hypovolemia resulting from third-spacing*<br>c. provide the maximum fluid intake allowed *to ensure adequate renal perfusion*<br>d. consult physician before giving vasodilators and diuretics if client is hypotensive.<br>4. If signs and symptoms of impaired renal function occur:<br>a. continue with above actions<br>b. administer diuretics if ordered *to increase urine output*<br>c. consult physician about possible need to reduce the digitalis dosage *(digitalis is excreted by the kidney and will quickly reach toxic levels when renal function is impaired)*<br>d. assess for and report signs of acute renal failure (e.g. oliguria or anuria; further weight gain; increasing edema; increased B/P; |

Desired Outcomes | Nursing Actions and ***Selected Purposes/Rationales***

lethargy and confusion; increasing BUN and serum creatinine, phosphorus, and potassium levels)
e. prepare client for dialysis if indicated
f. refer to Care Plan on Renal Failure for additional care measures if indicated.

12.b. The client will not experience cardiac arrhythmias as evidenced by:
1. regular apical pulse at 60-100 beats/minute
2. equal apical and radial pulses
3. absence of syncope and palpitations
4. ECG reading showing normal sinus rhythm.

12.b.1. Assess for and report signs and symptoms of cardiac arrhythmias (e.g. irregular apical pulse; pulse rate below 60 or above 100 beats/minute; apical-radial pulse deficit; syncope; palpitations; abnormal rate, rhythm, or configurations on ECG).
2. Implement measures *to prevent cardiac arrhythmias:*
   a. perform actions to improve cardiac output (see Nursing Diagnosis 1, action d) *in order to promote adequate myocardial tissue perfusion and oxygenation*
   b. perform actions to improve respiratory status (see Nursing Diagnosis 2, action c) *in order to improve tissue oxygenation.*
3. If cardiac arrhythmias occur:
   a. initiate cardiac monitoring if not already being done
   b. administer the following medications if ordered:
      1. Class I antiarrhythmics (e.g. quinidine, procainamide, lidocaine, tocainide, moricizine) *to delay the rate of depolarization*
      2. Class III antiarrhythmics (e.g. amiodarone) *to prolong repolarization and the duration of the action potential*
      3. cardiac glycosides (e.g. digitalis) *to decrease the heart rate*
   c. restrict client's activity based on his/her tolerance and severity of the arrhythmia
   d. maintain oxygen therapy as ordered
   e. assess cardiovascular status frequently and report signs and symptoms of a further decline in cardiac output and tissue perfusion
   f. have emergency cart readily available for cardioversion, defibrillation, or cardiopulmonary resuscitation.

12.c. The client will not develop a thromboembolism as evidenced by:
1. absence of pain, tenderness, heaviness, numbness, and swelling in extremities
2. usual temperature and color of extremities
3. palpable peripheral pulses
4. usual mental status
5. usual sensory and motor function
6. absence of sudden chest pain and increased dyspnea.

12.c.1. Assess for and report signs and symptoms of:
   a. deep vein thrombus (e.g. pain, tenderness, heaviness, swelling, unusual warmth, and/or positive Homan's sign in extremity)
   b. arterial embolus (e.g. diminished or absent peripheral pulses; pallor, coolness, numbness, and/or pain in extremity)
   c. cerebral ischemia (e.g. decreased level of consciousness, alteration in usual sensory and motor function)
   d. pulmonary embolism (e.g. sudden chest pain, increased dyspnea, increased restlessness and apprehension).
2. Implement measures to prevent and treat a deep vein thrombus and pulmonary embolism (see Care Plan on Immobility, Collaborative Diagnosis 12, actions a.1.b and c and a.2.b and c [pp. 149-150]).
3. Implement additional measures *to prevent the development of thromboemboli:*
   a. perform actions to improve cardiac output (see Nursing Diagnosis 1, action d)
   b. perform actions to treat cardiac arrhythmias if present (see action b.3 in this diagnosis)
   c. administer anticoagulants (e.g. warfarin, low-dose heparin) or antiplatelet agents (e.g. low-dose aspirin) if ordered.
4. If signs and symptoms of an arterial embolus occur:
   a. maintain client on strict bed rest with affected extremity in a level or slightly dependent position *to improve arterial blood flow*
   b. prepare client for the following if planned:
      1. diagnostic studies (e.g. Doppler ultrasound, arteriography)
      2. injection of a thrombolytic agent (e.g. streptokinase)
      3. embolectomy

c. administer anticoagulants (e.g. continuous intravenous heparin, warfarin) if ordered
d. provide emotional support to client and significant others.
5. If signs and symptoms of cerebral ischemia occur:
a. maintain client on bed rest with head of bed flat unless contraindicated
b. provide emotional support to client and significant others
c. refer to Care Plan on Cerebrovascular Accident for additional care measures if signs and symptoms persist.

12.d. The client will not develop cardiogenic shock as evidenced by:
1. stable or improved mental status
2. stable vital signs
3. palpable peripheral pulses
4. stable or improved skin temperature and color
5. urine output at least 30 ml/hour
6. PCWP within normal range.

12.d.1. Assess for and immediately report signs and symptoms of cardiogenic shock:
a. increased restlessness, lethargy, or confusion
b. systolic B/P below 90 mm Hg
c. rapid, thready pulse
d. diminished or absent peripheral pulses
e. increased coolness and duskiness or cyanosis of skin
f. urine output less than 30 ml/hour
g. elevated PCWP.
2. Implement measures *to prevent cardiogenic shock:*
a. perform actions to improve cardiac output (see Nursing Diagnosis 1, action d)
b. perform actions to treat cardiac arrhythmias if present (see action b.3 in this diagnosis).
3. If signs and symptoms of cardiogenic shock occur:
a. continue with above actions
b. maintain client on strict bed rest
c. maintain oxygen therapy as ordered
d. prepare client for diagnostic studies (e.g. two-dimensional echocardiogram, cardiac catheterization) if planned
e. administer the following medications if ordered:
1. sympathomimetics (e.g. dopamine, dobutamine, norepinephrine) *to increase cardiac output and maintain arterial pressure*
2. bipyridines (e.g. milrinone, amrinone) *to increase myocardial contractility and decrease systemic vascular resistance*
3. vasodilators (e.g. nitroprusside, nitroglycerin) *to decrease cardiac workload* (sympathomimetics are given in conjunction with vasodilators *to maintain mean arterial pressure)*
4. intravenous sodium bicarbonate *to correct acidosis* (reserved for treatment of severe acidosis when pH is less than 7.1)
f. assist with intubation and insertion of hemodynamic monitoring device (e.g. Swan-Ganz catheter) and intra-aortic balloon pump (IABP) if indicated
g. provide emotional support to client and significant others.

## 13. NURSING DIAGNOSIS: Anxiety

related to unfamiliar environment; difficulty breathing; and lack of understanding of diagnostic tests, the diagnosis, treatments, and prognosis.

| Desired Outcome | Nursing Actions and ***Selected Purposes/Rationales*** |
|---|---|
| 13. The client will experience a reduction | 13.a. Assess client for signs and symptoms of anxiety (e.g. verbalization of fears and concerns, insomnia, tenseness, tremors, irritability, |

| Desired Outcome | Nursing Actions and ***Selected Purposes/Rationales*** |
|---|---|
| in anxiety as evidenced by:<br>a. verbalization of feeling less anxious and fearful<br>b. usual sleep pattern<br>c. relaxed facial expression and body movements<br>d. stable vital signs<br>e. usual perceptual ability and interactions with others. | restlessness, increased dyspnea, diaphoresis, tachycardia, elevated blood pressure, facial pallor or flushing, narrowed perceptual field, withdrawal, noncompliance with treatment plan). Validate perceptions carefully, remembering that some behavior may result from tissue hypoxia or fluid imbalance.<br>b. Implement measures *to reduce fear and anxiety:*<br>1. maintain a calm, supportive, confident manner when interacting with client<br>2. if client is in acute respiratory distress:<br>a. do not leave him/her alone during this period<br>b. perform actions to improve respiratory status (see Nursing Diagnosis 2, action c)<br>c. perform actions *to reduce feeling of suffocation:*<br>1. open curtains and doors<br>2. limit the number of visitors in room at any one time<br>3. remove unnecessary equipment from room<br>4. administer oxygen via nasal cannula rather than mask if possible<br>3. encourage significant others to project a caring, concerned attitude without obvious anxiousness<br>4. once the period of acute respiratory distress has subsided:<br>a. orient client to hospital environment, equipment, and routines<br>b. introduce staff who will be participating in client's care; if possible, maintain consistency in staff assigned to his/her care *to provide feelings of stability and comfort with the environment*<br>c. assure client that staff members are nearby; respond to call signal as soon as possible<br>d. provide a calm, restful environment<br>e. keep cardiac monitor out of client's view and the sound turned as low as possible<br>f. encourage verbalization of fear and anxiety; provide feedback<br>g. explain all diagnostic tests<br>h. reinforce physician's explanations and clarify misconceptions the client has about heart failure, the treatment plan, and prognosis<br>i. instruct client in relaxation techniques and encourage participation in diversional activities<br>j. assist client to identify specific stressors and ways to cope with them (see Nursing Diagnosis 14, action c)<br>k. administer antianxiety agents if ordered.<br>c. Include significant others in orientation and teaching sessions and encourage their continued support of the client.<br>d. Provide information based on current needs of client and significant others at a level they can understand. Encourage questions and clarification of information provided.<br>e. Consult physician if above actions fail to control fear and anxiety. |

## 14. NURSING DIAGNOSIS: Ineffective individual coping

related to fear, anxiety, possible need to alter life style, knowledge that condition is chronic and will require lifelong medical supervision and medication therapy, and inadequate support system.

| Desired Outcome | Nursing Actions and ***Selected Purposes/Rationales*** |
|---|---|

14. The client will demonstrate the use of effective coping skills as evidenced by:
    a. verbalization of ability to cope
    b. utilization of appropriate problem-solving techniques
    c. willingness to participate in treatment plan and meet basic needs
    d. absence of destructive behavior toward self and others
    e. appropriate use of defense mechanisms
    f. recognition and utilization of available support systems.

14.a. Assess for and report signs and symptoms of ineffective individual coping (e.g. verbalization of inability to cope; inability to ask for help, problem solve, or meet basic needs; destructive behavior toward self or others; inappropriate use of defense mechanisms; inability to meet role expectations).

b. Assess client's perception of current situation including precipitating factors and effectiveness of coping mechanisms.

c. Implement measures *to promote effective coping:*
   1. allow time for client to adjust psychologically to diagnosis and planned treatment and anticipated changes in life style and roles
   2. assist client to recognize and manage inappropriate denial if it is present
   3. perform actions to reduce fear and anxiety (see Nursing Diagnosis 13, action b)
   4. encourage verbalization about current situation and ways comparable situations have been handled in the past
   5. assist client to identify personal strengths and resources that can be utilized to facilitate coping with the current situation
   6. create an atmosphere of trust and support
   7. include client in planning of care, encourage maximum participation in treatment plan, and allow choices when possible *to enable him/her to maintain a sense of control*
   8. instruct client in effective problem-solving techniques (e.g. accurate identification of stressors, determination of various options to solve problem)
   9. assist client to maintain usual daily routines whenever possible
   10. instruct client in relaxation and stress reduction techniques
   11. assist client as he/she starts to plan for necessary life-style and role changes after discharge; help client to identify priorities and attainable goals
   12. assist client and significant others to identify ways that personal and family goals can be adjusted rather than abandoned
   13. administer antianxiety and/or antidepressant agents if ordered
   14. assist client to identify and utilize available support systems; provide information about available community resources that can assist client and significant others in coping with the effects of heart failure
   15. encourage continued emotional support from significant others
   16. encourage client to share with significant others the kind of support that would be most beneficial (e.g. listening, inspiring hope, providing reassurance and accurate information)
   17. support behaviors suggesting positive adaptation to changes experienced (e.g. participation in treatment plan and self-care activities, communication of the ability to cope, utilization of effective problem-solving strategies).

d. Consult physician about psychological and vocational rehabilitation counseling if appropriate. Initiate a referral if necessary.

## 15. NURSING DIAGNOSIS: Ineffective management of therapeutic regimen

related to:

a. lack of understanding of the implications of not following the prescribed treatment plan;
b. difficulty modifying personal habits (e.g. smoking, alcohol intake, diet);
c. insufficient financial resources;

d. unpleasant side effects experienced with some medications used to manage heart failure (e.g. vasodilators, diuretics).

| Desired Outcome | Nursing Actions and ***Selected Purposes/Rationales*** |
|---|---|
| 15. The client will demonstrate the probability of effective management of the therapeutic regimen as evidenced by:<br>a. willingness to learn about and participate in treatments and care<br>b. statements reflecting ways to modify personal habits and integrate treatments into life style<br>c. statements reflecting an understanding of the implications of not following the prescribed treatment plan. | 15.a. Assess for indications that the client may be unable to effectively manage the therapeutic regimen:<br>1. statements reflecting that he/she was unable to manage care at home<br>2. failure to adhere to treatment plan while in hospital (e.g. not adhering to dietary modifications and fluid restrictions, refusing medications)<br>3. statements reflecting a lack of understanding of factors that may cause further progression of heart failure<br>4. statements reflecting an unwillingness or inability to modify personal habits and integrate necessary treatments into life style<br>5. statements reflecting the view that heart failure resolves completely or is hopeless and that efforts to comply with the treatment plan are useless<br>6. statements reflecting that medications are too expensive or that their side effects are too unpleasant.<br>b. Implement measures *to promote effective management of the therapeutic regimen:*<br>1. explain heart failure in terms the client can understand; stress the fact that heart failure is a chronic disease and that adherence to the treatment program is necessary in order to delay and/or prevent complications<br>2. encourage questions and clarify misconceptions the client has regarding heart failure and its effects<br>3. encourage client to participate in treatment plan<br>4. provide instructions on measuring intake and output, weighing self, counting pulse, and calculating dietary sodium content; allow time for return demonstration; determine areas of difficulty and misunderstanding and reinforce teaching as necessary<br>5. provide client with written instructions about medications, signs and symptoms to report, measuring intake and output, weighing self, counting pulse, and prescribed diet<br>6. assist client to identify ways he/she can incorporate treatments into life style; focus on modifications of life style rather than complete change<br>7. encourage the client to discuss his/her concerns regarding the cost of hospitalization, medications, and lifelong follow-up care; obtain a social service consult to assist the client with financial planning and to obtain financial aid if indicated<br>8. perform actions to promote effective coping (see Nursing Diagnosis 14, action c)<br>9. initiate and reinforce discharge teaching outlined in Nursing Diagnosis 16 *in order to promote a sense of control and self-reliance*<br>10. provide information about and encourage utilization of community resources that can assist client to make necessary life-style changes (e.g. cardiovascular fitness, weight loss, and smoking cessation programs)<br>11. reinforce behaviors suggesting future compliance with the therapeutic regimen (e.g. statements reflecting ways to modify personal habits, active interest and participation in treatment plan)<br>12. include significant others in explanations and teaching sessions and encourage their support; reinforce need for client to assume responsibility for managing as much of care as possible. |

c. Consult physician regarding referrals to community health agencies if continued instruction, support, or supervision is needed.

## 16. NURSING DIAGNOSIS: Knowledge deficit
regarding follow-up care.

| Desired Outcomes | Nursing Actions and ***Selected Purposes/Rationales*** |
|---|---|
| 16.a. The client will identify modifiable cardiovascular risk factors and ways to reduce these factors. | 16.a.1. Inform client that the following modifiable factors have been shown to contribute to cardiovascular disease:<br>a. obesity<br>b. hyperlipidemia<br>c. sedentary life style<br>d. smoking<br>e. hypertension<br>f. stressful life style.<br>2. Inform client that alcohol intake should not exceed 1 oz of ethanol (i.e. 2 oz of 100-proof whiskey, 8 oz of wine, 24 oz of beer) a day on a regular basis because there is evidence that excessive alcohol intake contributes to the development of hypertension and some forms of heart disease.<br>3. Assist client to identify ways he/she can make appropriate changes in life style to reduce the above factors. Provide information about weight reduction plans; stress management classes; and cardiovascular fitness, smoking cessation, and alcohol rehabilitation programs if appropriate. Initiate a referral if indicated. |
| 16.b. The client will verbalize an understanding of the rationale for and components of a diet low in sodium. | 16.b.1. Explain the rationale for a diet low in sodium.<br>2. Provide the following information about decreasing sodium intake:<br>a. be aware that the terms salt and sodium are often used interchangeably but are not synonymous; there is 40% sodium in table salt<br>b. read food labels and calculate sodium content of items (often expressed in milligrams [2 gm is 2000 mg])<br>c. do not add salt when cooking foods or to prepared foods; use low-sodium herbs and spices if desired<br>d. avoid canned soups and vegetables<br>e. avoid processed convenience foods and commercial sauces<br>f. avoid cured and smoked foods<br>g. avoid salty snack foods.<br>3. Obtain a dietary consult to assist client in planning meals that will meet prescribed dietary modifications. |
| 16.c. The client will demonstrate accuracy in counting pulse. | 16.c.1. Teach the client how to count his/her pulse, being alert to the regularity of the rhythm.<br>2. Allow time for return demonstration and accuracy check. |
| 16.d. The client will verbalize an understanding of medications ordered including rationale, side effects, schedule for taking, and importance of taking as prescribed. | 16.d.1. Explain the rationale for, side effects of, and importance of taking the medications prescribed.<br>2. If client is discharged on a digitalis preparation, instruct to:<br>a. take pulse before taking digitalis (should be a resting pulse rate taken at least 5 minutes after any activity); consult physician before taking medication if pulse rate is more irregular than usual or below 60 or above 120 beats/minute<br>b. promptly report a loss of usual appetite, nausea, vomiting, diarrhea, or visual disturbances. |

| Desired Outcomes | Nursing Actions and ***Selected Purposes/Rationales*** |
|---|---|
| | 3. If client is discharged on a diuretic, instruct to:<br>a. take once-daily doses or the larger dose in the morning to minimize nighttime urination<br>b. weigh self daily and keep a record of daily weights<br>c. change from a lying to standing position slowly if experiencing dizziness or lightheadedness with position change<br>d. increase intake of foods/fluids high in potassium (e.g. orange juice, bananas, figs, dates, potatoes, raisins, apricots, cantaloupe) if taking a potassium-depleting diuretic<br>e. notify physician if unable to tolerate food or fluids (*dehydration can develop rapidly if intake is poor and client continues to take diuretic*)<br>f. avoid salt substitutes with a high potassium content if discharged on a potassium-sparing diuretic (e.g. triamterene, spironolactone)<br>g. report the following signs and symptoms:<br>1. weight loss of more than 5 pounds a week<br>2. excessive thirst<br>3. severe dizziness or episodes of fainting<br>4. muscle weakness or cramping, nausea, vomiting, irregular pulse, or increased pulse rate.<br>4. If client is discharged on a vasodilator or angiotensin-converting enzyme inhibitor, instruct to:<br>a. change from a lying to standing position slowly if experiencing dizziness or lightheadedness with position change<br>b. avoid strenuous exercise, especially in hot weather, and hot baths and showers, steam room, and sauna<br>c. limit alcohol intake<br>d. report continued dizziness, lightheadedness, or fainting.<br>5. Instruct client to take medications on a regular basis and avoid skipping doses, altering prescribed dose, making up for missed doses, and discontinuing medication without permission of health care provider.<br>6. Instruct client to consult physician before taking other prescription and nonprescription medications.<br>7. Instruct client to inform all health care providers of medications being taken. |
| 16.e. The client will state signs and symptoms to report to the health care provider. | 16.e. Instruct client to report:<br>1. weight gain of more than 2 pounds in a day<br>2. increased swelling of ankles, feet, or abdomen<br>3. persistent cough<br>4. increasing shortness of breath<br>5. chest pain<br>6. increased weakness and fatigue<br>7. frequent nighttime urination<br>8. signs and symptoms of digitalis toxicity (see action d.2.b in this diagnosis)<br>9. side effects of diuretic therapy (see action d.3.g in this diagnosis). |
| 16.f. The client will identify community resources that can assist with home management and adjustment to changes resulting from heart failure. | 16.f. 1. Provide information regarding community resources that can assist with home management and adjustment to changes resulting from heart failure (e.g. Meals on Wheels, home health agencies, transportation services, American Heart Association, counseling services).<br>2. Initiate a referral if indicated. |
| 16.g. The client will verbalize an | 16.g.1. Reinforce the importance of keeping follow-up appointments with health care provider. |

understanding of and a plan for adhering to recommended follow-up care including future appointments with health care provider and activity limitations.

2. Provide the following instructions regarding activity:
   a. progress activity gradually and only as tolerated
   b. stop any activity that causes shortness of breath, chest pain, dizziness, or significant fatigue
   c. plan and adhere to rest periods during the day
   d. adhere to physician's recommendations about activities that should be avoided
   e. notify physician if activity tolerance declines
   f. reduce dyspnea and fatigue during sexual activity by:
      1. avoiding sexual activity when unusually fatigued
      2. waiting 1-2 hours after a heavy meal or alcohol intake before engaging in sexual activity
      3. identifying and using positions that minimize energy expenditure (e.g. side-lying, partner on top)
      4. using portable oxygen during sexual activities.
3. Refer to Nursing Diagnosis 15, action b, for measures to promote the client's ability to effectively manage the therapeutic regimen.

# Heart Surgery: Coronary Artery Bypass Grafting (CABG) or Valve Replacement

Heart surgery is performed for a variety of reasons including myocardial revascularization; valve repair or replacement; repositioning of vessels; heart transplant; and repair of septal defects, aneurysms, and coarctation of the aorta. Two common heart surgeries are coronary artery bypass grafting (CABG), which is done to treat severe coronary artery disease, and heart valve replacement. CABG involves removing a segment of the saphenous vein and grafting it to the aorta and to a point on the coronary artery distal to the obstruction. The internal mammary artery(ies) can also be used to bypass the occluded coronary artery(ies). Heart valve replacement involves replacing the stenotic or regurgitant valve with a mechanical prosthesis (e.g. Starr-Edwards valve, St. Jude valve) or a biological (tissue) valve (e.g. Carpentier-Edwards valve, Hancock valve).

Both CABG and valve replacement surgeries are performed through a median sternotomy. Cardiopulmonary bypass (extracorporeal circulation) is maintained during surgery by a heart-lung machine that performs vital gas exchange functions; maintains the desired body temperature; filters the blood for thrombi, emboli, and impurities; and recirculates the blood into the arterial system. Cardioplegia (paralysis of the heart) is induced by infusion of a cold solution containing potassium into the aortic root and pericardium. Prior to closing the chest, epicardial pacer wires are often placed on the atria and/or ventricles and connected to an external demand pacemaker. A chest tube is inserted to drain blood from the mediastinum; another may also be inserted to promote lung re-expansion if the pleura was opened.

**This care plan focuses on the adult client hospitalized for either coronary artery bypass grafting (CABG) or valve replacement surgery.** Preoperatively, a major goal of care is to reduce fear and anxiety. Goals of postoperative care are to maintain comfort, prevent complications, and educate the client regarding follow-up care.

## DIAGNOSTIC TESTS

Coronary angiography
Echocardiography
Cardiac catheterization
Electrocardiogram (ECG)
Blood studies (e.g. chemistry screen, type and cross match, coagulation screen, complete blood count)
Chest x-ray
Radionuclide imaging

## DISCHARGE CRITERIA

Prior to discharge, the client will:

- ❖ have adequate cardiac output
- ❖ tolerate expected level of activity
- ❖ have surgical pain controlled
- ❖ have no signs and symptoms of complications
- ❖ identify modifiable cardiovascular risk factors and ways to reduce these factors
- ❖ verbalize an understanding of the rationale for and components of a diet restricted in sodium, saturated fat, and cholesterol
- ❖ verbalize an understanding of activity restrictions and the rate of activity progression
- ❖ verbalize an understanding of medications ordered including rationale, side effects, schedule for taking, and importance of taking as prescribed
- ❖ state signs and symptoms to report to the health care provider
- ❖ identify community resources that can assist with cardiac rehabilitation and adjustment to having had heart surgery
- ❖ verbalize an understanding of and a plan for adhering to recommended follow-up care, including future appointments with health care provider, wound care, and pain management.

## NURSING/COLLABORATIVE DIAGNOSES



**See Standardized Preoperative and Postoperative Care Plans for additional diagnoses.**

## PREOPERATIVE

**Use in conjunction with the Standardized Preoperative Care Plan.**

## 1. NURSING DIAGNOSIS: Anxiety

related to:
a. unfamiliar environment;
b. lack of understanding of diagnostic tests, preoperative procedures/preparation, planned surgery, and postoperative course;
c. anticipated loss of control, effects of anesthesia, and postoperative discomfort;
d. financial concerns associated with surgery and hospitalization;
e. possible alterations in life style and roles;
f. risk of disease if blood transfusions are necessary;
g. possibility of death.

| Desired Outcome | Nursing Actions and ***Selected Purposes/Rationales*** |
|---|---|
| 1. The client will experience a reduction in anxiety (see Standardized Preoperative Care Plan, Nursing Diagnosis 1 [pp. 108-109], for outcome criteria). | 1.a. Refer to Standardized Preoperative Care Plan, Nursing Diagnosis 1 (pp. 108-109), for measures related to assessment and reduction of fear and anxiety.<br>b. Implement additional measures *to reduce fear and anxiety:*<br>1. explain procedures/special preparation (e.g. platelet apheresis, showering with bacteriostatic soap, antimicrobial therapy) that may be done preoperatively<br>2. assure client that blood is screened carefully and that risk for blood-borne disease is minimal if transfusions are necessary<br>3. arrange for a visit from an intensive care nurse or a visit to the intensive care unit; assure client and significant others that transfer to intensive care after heart surgery is routine<br>4. describe and explain the rationale for equipment and tubes that may be present postoperatively (e.g. cardiac monitoring equipment, ventilator, chest tube, arterial and venous lines, nasogastric tube, urinary catheter)<br>5. if bypass grafting is planned, inform client that he/she may have leg incisions as well as a chest incision<br>6. with client, establish an alternative method of communicating (e.g. magic slate, word board, flash cards, signals) to be used while he/she is on the ventilator<br>7. focus on postoperative care *(this promotes a feeling in client that he/she will survive surgery).* |

# POSTOPERATIVE

**Use in conjunction with the Standardized Postoperative Care Plan.**

## 1. NURSING DIAGNOSIS: Decreased cardiac output

related to mechanical and/or electrical dysfunction of the heart associated with:
a. pre-existing compromise in cardiac function;
b. trauma to the heart during surgery;
c. increased cardiac workload resulting from increased systemic vascular resistance (can occur because of an initial increase in catecholamine output and plasma renin levels and/or fluid overload);
d. decreased preload resulting from hypovolemia (can occur because of blood loss, loss of fluid from nasogastric tube, decreased fluid intake, and excessive diuresis) and hypotension (can occur if body is warmed rapidly following surgery and from effects of anesthetic and certain medications [e.g. narcotic analgesics, vasodilators]);
e. effects of hypothermia, hypoxemia, and acid-base and/or electrolyte imbalances on contractility and conductivity of the heart.

**Desired Outcome**

1. The client will maintain adequate cardiac output as evidenced by:
   a. B/P within range of 130-100/80-60
   b. apical pulse regular and between 60-100 beats/minute
   c. absence of or no increase in intensity of gallop rhythms
   d. increased strength and activity tolerance
   e. unlabored respirations at 14-20/minute
   f. absence of adventitious breath sounds
   g. usual mental status
   h. absence of vertigo and syncope
   i. palpable peripheral pulses
   j. skin warm, dry, and usual color
   k. capillary refill time less than 3 seconds
   l. urine output at least 30 ml/hour
   m. absence of peripheral edema and jugular vein distention
   n. hemodynamic measurements such as cardiac output (CO), pulmonary artery pressure (PAP), pulmonary capillary wedge pressure (PCWP), and central venous pressure (CVP) within normal limits.

**Nursing Actions and *Selected Purposes/Rationales***

1.a. Assess for and report signs and symptoms of:
   1. hypovolemia (e.g. low B/P; resting pulse rate greater than 100 beats/minute; postural hypotension; cool, pale, or cyanotic skin; diminished or absent peripheral pulses; urine output less than 30 ml/hour; low central venous, left atrial, and pulmonary pressures)
   2. hypotension (systolic B/P persistently below 100 mm Hg)
   3. decreased cardiac output:
      a. variations in B/P (may be increased because of compensatory vasoconstriction; may be decreased when compensatory mechanisms and pump fail)
      b. irregular pulse, tachycardia
      c. presence of gallop rhythm
      d. fatigue and weakness
      e. dyspnea, tachypnea
      f. crackles (rales)
      g. restlessness, change in mental status
      h. vertigo, syncope
      i. diminished or absent peripheral pulses
      j. cool, clammy skin
      k. pallor, mottling, or cyanosis of skin
      l. capillary refill time greater than 3 seconds
      m. oliguria
      n. peripheral edema
      o. jugular vein distention (JVD)
      p. hemodynamic changes such as decreased CO and increased PAP, PCWP, and CVP (use internal jugular vein pulsation method to estimate CVP if monitoring device not present).

b. Monitor for and report the following:
   1. arrhythmias on ECG reading
   2. chest x-ray results showing pulmonary vascular congestion, pulmonary edema, or pleural effusion
   3. abnormal blood gases
   4. significant change in oximetry results.

c. Implement measures *to maintain an adequate cardiac output:*
   1. perform actions *to prevent or treat hypovolemia:*
      a. administer blood and/or crystalloid or colloid solutions as ordered
      b. maintain a minimum fluid intake of 1000 ml/day unless ordered otherwise
      c. implement measures to prevent and control bleeding (see Postoperative Collaborative Diagnosis 6.B, actions 1.d and e)
   2. perform actions *to prevent or treat hypotension:*
      a. consult physician before giving negative inotropic agents, diuretics, and vasodilating agents if systolic B/P is below 100 mm Hg
      b. administer narcotic analgesics judiciously, being alert to the synergistic effect of the narcotic ordered and the anesthetic that was used during surgery
      c. gradually bring client's body temperature to normal if he/she is hypothermic
      d. administer sympathomimetics (e.g. norepinephrine, dopamine) if ordered
   3. administer the following medications if ordered:
      a. positive inotropic agents (e.g. dopamine, dobutamine, digitalis preparations) *to increase myocardial contractility*
      b. vasodilators (e.g. nitroprusside, nitroglycerin) *to reduce cardiac workload*
   4. perform actions *to reduce cardiac workload:*
      a. place client in a semi- to high Fowler's position

b. instruct client to avoid activities that create a Valsalva response (e.g. straining to have a bowel movement, holding breath while moving) *in order to prevent the marked increase in venous return and preload that occurs with exhalation*
c. implement measures *to promote rest* (e.g. maintain activity restrictions, administer prescribed pain medications, limit the number of visitors, reduce anxiety)
d. maintain oxygen therapy as ordered
e. discourage smoking *(smoke has a cardiostimulatory effect, causes vasoconstriction, and reduces oxygen availability)*
f. discourage excessive intake of beverages high in caffeine such as coffee, tea, and colas *(caffeine is a myocardial stimulant and increases myocardial oxygen consumption)*
g. implement measures to prevent or treat fluid volume excess (see Postoperative Nursing Diagnosis 3, action a)
h. increase activity gradually as allowed and tolerated.

d. Consult physician if signs and symptoms of decreased cardiac output persist or worsen.

---

**2. NURSING DIAGNOSIS: Ineffective breathing pattern**

related to:
a. respiratory depressant effects of anesthesia and some medications (e.g. narcotic analgesics);
b. decreased lung expansion associated with weakness and reluctance to breathe deeply because of chest incision pain and fear of dislodging chest tube.

| Desired Outcome | Nursing Actions and ***Selected Purposes/Rationales*** |
|---|---|
| 2. The client will maintain an effective breathing pattern (see Standardized Postoperative Care Plan, Nursing Diagnosis 2 [p. 114], for outcome criteria). | 2.a. Refer to Standardized Postoperative Care Plan, Nursing Diagnosis 2 (pp. 114-115), for measures related to assessment and management of ineffective breathing pattern.<br>b. Implement additional measures *to improve breathing pattern:*<br>1. monitor mechanical ventilation carefully *to ensure that ventilatory rate and pressures are correct*<br>2. assure client that the chest tube is sutured in place and that deep breathing will not dislodge the tube. |

---

**3. NURSING/ COLLABORATIVE DIAGNOSIS: Altered fluid and electrolyte balance:**

a. **fluid volume excess or water intoxication** related to:
  1. the hemodilution technique used to prime the heart-lung machine
  2. vigorous fluid replacement therapy during and immediately after surgery
  3. increased production of antidiuretic hormone (output of ADH is stimulated by trauma, pain, anesthetic agents, and narcotic analgesics)
  4. reabsorption of third-space fluid approximately 3 days after surgery
  5. renal or cardiac insufficiency;

b. **fluid volume deficit** related to blood loss, inadequate fluid replacement, and loss of fluid associated with nasogastric tube drainage and excessive diuresis;

c. **hypokalemia, hypochloremia, and/or metabolic alkalosis** related to loss of electrolytes and hydrochloric acid associated with nasogastric tube drainage (the hemodilution created by priming the heart-lung machine with large amounts of fluid also contributes to the electrolyte imbalances).

| Desired Outcomes | Nursing Actions and ***Selected Purposes/Rationales*** |
|---|---|
| 3.a. The client will not experience fluid volume excess or water intoxication (see Standardized Postoperative Care Plan, Nursing Diagnosis 4, outcome b [p. 117], for outcome criteria). | 3.a.1. Refer to Standardized Postoperative Care Plan, Nursing Diagnosis 4, action b (p. 117), for measures related to assessment, prevention, and management of fluid volume excess and water intoxication.<br>2. Implement additional measures *to prevent or treat fluid volume excess and water intoxication:*<br>a. perform actions to maintain adequate renal blood flow (see Postoperative Collaborative Diagnosis 6.B, action 4.c)<br>b. perform actions to maintain an adequate cardiac output (see Postoperative Nursing Diagnosis 1, action c)<br>c. maintain fluid and sodium restrictions as ordered (2500 ml fluid and 3-4 gm sodium restrictions are common). |
| 3.b. The client will not experience fluid volume deficit, hypokalemia, hypochloremia, and metabolic alkalosis (see Standardized Postoperative Care Plan, Nursing Diagnosis 4, outcome a [pp. 116-117], for outcome criteria). | 3.b. Refer to Standardized Postoperative Care Plan, Nursing Diagnosis 4, action a (pp. 116-117), for measures related to assessment, prevention, and treatment of fluid volume deficit, hypokalemia, hypochloremia, and metabolic alkalosis. |

## 4. NURSING DIAGNOSIS: Activity intolerance

related to:

a. tissue hypoxia associated with decreased cardiac output and anemia (results from hemodilution, blood loss, and red cell hemolysis [red cells are traumatized by the heart-lung machine]);

b. difficulty resting and sleeping associated with frequent assessments and treatments, discomfort, fear, and anxiety.

| Desired Outcome | Nursing Actions and ***Selected Purposes/Rationales*** |
|---|---|
| 4. The client will demonstrate an increased tolerance for activity (see Standardized Postoperative Care Plan, Nursing Diagnosis 10 [p. 124], for outcome criteria). | 4.a. Refer to Standardized Postoperative Care Plan, Nursing Diagnosis 10 (p. 124), for measures related to assessment and improvement of activity tolerance.<br>b. Implement additional measures *to improve activity tolerance:*<br>1. perform actions to maintain an adequate cardiac output (see Postoperative Nursing Diagnosis 1, action c)<br>2. perform actions to improve breathing pattern (see Postoperative Nursing Diagnosis 2) and promote effective airway clearance (see Standardized Postoperative Care Plan, Nursing Diagnosis 3, action b [pp. 115-116]), *in order to maintain adequate alveolar gas exchange*<br>3. encourage client to increase intake of foods high in iron (e.g. organ meats, dried fruit, dark green leafy vegetables, whole-grain or iron- |

enriched breads and cereals) and vitamin C (e.g. citrus fruits) *in order to help resolve anemia*
4. administer whole blood or packed red cells if ordered
5. increase client's activity gradually as allowed and tolerated; explain to client that a progressive and gradual increase in activity is necessary *in order to strengthen the myocardium without causing a sudden increase in cardiac workload.*

## 5. NURSING DIAGNOSIS: Altered thought processes

related to:
a. cerebral ischemia associated with factors such as inadequate cerebral perfusion while on heart-lung machine, decreased cardiac output, hypotensive episodes, and embolization;
b. sleep deprivation and/or sensory overload associated with fear, anxiety, pain, and frequent assessments and treatments.

| Desired Outcome | Nursing Actions and ***Selected Purposes/Rationales*** |
|---|---|
| 5. The client will regain usual thought processes as evidenced by:<br>a. usual memory, reasoning ability, and judgment<br>b. absence of agitation, confusion, hallucinations, and combativeness. | 5.a. Assess client for altered thought processes (e.g. impaired memory, reasoning ability, and judgment; agitation; confusion; hallucinations; combativeness).<br>b. Ascertain from significant others client's usual level of intellectual and emotional functioning.<br>c. Implement measures *to maintain optimal thought processes:*<br>1. perform actions *to reduce fear and anxiety* (e.g. explain treatments; keep monitor out of client's view; be readily available to client; project a calm, confident manner)<br>2. perform actions to promote sleep (see Standardized Postoperative Care Plan, Nursing Diagnosis 15, action c [pp. 127-128])<br>3. perform actions to maintain an adequate cardiac output (see Postoperative Nursing Diagnosis 1, action c) *in order to promote optimal cerebral blood flow*<br>4. perform actions *to minimize environmental stimuli:*<br>a. organize care to allow for periods of uninterrupted rest<br>b. dim lights in room<br>c. keep auditory level on monitors as low as possible<br>d. avoid unnecessary conversations in or directly outside of client's room<br>e. restrict the number of visitors and their length of stay.<br>d. If client shows evidence of altered thought processes:<br>1. initiate appropriate safety precautions (e.g. side rails up, accompany when out of bed)<br>2. reorient client to person, place, and time as necessary<br>3. address client by name<br>4. place familiar objects, clock, and calendar within client's view<br>5. approach client in a slow, calm manner; allow adequate time for communication<br>6. repeat instructions as necessary using clear, simple language and short sentences<br>7. maintain a consistent and fairly structured routine when possible<br>8. have client perform only one activity at a time and allow adequate time for performance of activities<br>9. encourage client to make lists of planned activities, questions, and concerns |

| Desired Outcome | Nursing Actions and ***Selected Purposes/Rationales*** |
|---|---|
| | 10. assist client to problem solve if necessary<br>11. maintain realistic expectations of client's ability to learn, comprehend, and remember information provided; provide client with a written copy of instructions<br>12. encourage significant others to be supportive of client; instruct them in methods of dealing with client's altered thought processes<br>13. inform client and significant others that symptoms client is experiencing are not unusual and should gradually subside<br>14. consult physician if altered thought processes persist or worsen. |

## 6.A. COLLABORATIVE DIAGNOSES:

**Potential complications: cardiac**

1. **myocardial infarction (MI)** related to insufficient coronary blood flow associated with hypovolemia, decreased cardiac output, and increased myocardial oxygen demands;
2. **cardiac arrhythmias** related to impaired nodal function and/or altered myocardial conductivity associated with trauma to the heart during surgery, hypoxia, sympathetic stimulation (can result from anxiety, volume depletion, and pain), and electrolyte and acid-base imbalances;
3. **heart failure** related to pre-existing myocardial dilation or hypertrophy and decreased cardiac output postoperatively associated with damage to and further stress on the heart;
4. **postpericardiotomy syndrome (pericarditis)** related to an immune response to pericardial injury and residual blood in the pericardial sac;
5. **cardiac tamponade** related to accumulation of fluid (usually blood) in the pericardial sac and/or mediastinum associated with excessive bleeding, malposition or malfunction of the mediastinal tube, and postpericardiotomy syndrome.

| Desired Outcomes | Nursing Actions and ***Selected Purposes/Rationales*** |
|---|---|
| 6.A.1. The client will not experience an MI as evidenced by:<br>a. no episodes of sudden and persistent chest pain<br>b. stable vital signs<br>c. cardiac enzyme levels declining toward normal range<br>d. absence of ST segment elevation, T wave changes, and pathological Q wave on ECG reading. | 6.A.1.a. Assess for and report signs and symptoms of a myocardial infarction (e.g. sudden and persistent chest pain; significant change in vital signs; further increase in cardiac enzymes; ST segment elevation, T wave changes, and/or pathological Q wave on ECG reading).<br>b. Implement measures to maintain adequate cardiac output (see Postoperative Nursing Diagnosis 1, action c) *in order to improve myocardial blood supply and reduce the risk of myocardial infarction.*<br>c. If signs and symptoms of a myocardial infarction occur:<br>1. initiate cardiac monitoring if not still being done<br>2. maintain client on strict bed rest in a semi- to high Fowler's position<br>3. maintain oxygen therapy as ordered<br>4. administer the following medications if ordered:<br>a. morphine sulfate *to reduce pain and anxiety and decrease cardiac workload*<br>b. nitrates *to improve coronary blood flow and reduce myocardial oxygen requirements*<br>c. beta-adrenergic blocking agents *to reduce myocardial oxygen requirements by decreasing heart rate and myocardial contractility*<br>5. provide emotional support to client and significant others<br>6. refer to Care Plan on Myocardial Infarction for additional care measures. |
| 6.A.2. The client will not experience cardiac | 6.A.2.a. Assess for and report signs and symptoms of cardiac arrhythmias (e.g. irregular apical pulse; pulse rate below 60 or above 100 beats/ |

arrhythmias as evidenced by:
a. regular apical pulse at 60-100 beats/minute
b. equal apical and radial pulses
c. absence of syncope and palpitations
d. ECG reading showing normal sinus rhythm.

minute; apical-radial pulse deficit; syncope; palpitations; abnormal rate, rhythm, or configurations on ECG).

b. Implement measures *to prevent cardiac arrhythmias:*
   1. perform actions to maintain adequate cardiac output and myocardial blood flow (see Postoperative Nursing Diagnosis 1, action c)
   2. maintain oxygen therapy as ordered
   3. perform actions to maintain fluid and electrolyte balance (see Postoperative Nursing Diagnosis 3)
   4. perform actions to improve breathing pattern (see Postoperative Nursing Diagnosis 2) and promote effective airway clearance (see Standardized Postoperative Care Plan, Nursing Diagnosis 3, action b [pp. 115-116]), *in order to improve tissue oxygenation and prevent respiratory acidosis or alkalosis (myocardial conductivity is altered by hypoxia and acid-base imbalance).*
c. If cardiac arrhythmias occur:
   1. initiate cardiac monitoring if not still being done
   2. administer the following medications if ordered:
      a. Class I antiarrhythmics (e.g. lidocaine, quinidine, procainamide, moricizine) *to delay the rate of depolarization*
      b. Class II antiarrhythmics (e.g. esmolol, propranolol) *to block effects of beta-adrenergic stimulation on the heart*
      c. Class III antiarrhythmics (e.g. bretylium, amiodarone) *to prolong repolarization and the duration of the action potential*
      d. Class IV antiarrhythmics (e.g. verapamil) *to block the slow calcium channels, which then prolongs conduction and refractory period in the AV node and depresses automaticity in SA and AV nodes*
      e. anticholinergic agents (e.g. atropine) *to increase the heart rate*
      f. cardiac glycosides (e.g. digitalis) *to decrease the heart rate*
   3. restrict client's activity based on his/her tolerance and severity of arrhythmia
   4. maintain oxygen therapy as ordered
   5. assess cardiovascular status frequently and report signs and symptoms of inadequate tissue perfusion (e.g. decline in B/P; cool, clammy, mottled skin; cyanosis; diminished peripheral pulses; declining urine output; restlessness and agitation; shortness of breath)
   6. maintain temporary pacemaker function as ordered
   7. have emergency cart readily available for cardioversion, defibrillation, or cardiopulmonary resuscitation.

6.A.3. The client will not develop heart failure as evidenced by:
a. pulse 60-100 beats/minute
b. absence of an $S_3$ heart sound or summation gallop
c. usual mental status
d. absence of adventitious breath sounds
e. absence of dyspnea, orthopnea, and cough

6.A.3.a. Assess for and report signs and symptoms of heart failure:
   1. significant increase in pulse rate
   2. presence of an $S_3$ heart sound or summation gallop
   3. restlessness, anxiousness, confusion
   4. crackles (rales)
   5. dyspnea, orthopnea
   6. cough
   7. diminished or absent peripheral pulses
   8. increased weakness and fatigue
   9. cool, diaphoretic skin
   10. oliguria
   11. weight gain
   12. peripheral edema
   13. distended neck veins
   14. enlarged, tender liver.
b. Monitor chest x-ray results. Report findings of cardiomegaly, pleural effusion, or pulmonary edema.
c. Implement measures *to prevent heart failure:*
   1. perform actions to maintain adequate cardiac output (see

Desired Outcomes | Nursing Actions and ***Selected Purposes/Rationales***

f. palpable peripheral pulses
g. increased strength and activity tolerance
h. skin warm and dry
i. urine output at least 30 ml/hour
j. stable weight
k. absence of peripheral edema; distended neck veins; and enlarged, tender liver.

Postoperative Nursing Diagnosis 1, action c)
2. perform actions to prevent and treat cardiac arrhythmias (see actions 2.b and c in this diagnosis) *because arrhythmias contribute to the development of heart failure.*

d. If signs and symptoms of heart failure occur:
1. continue with above actions
2. administer the following medications if ordered:
   a. positive inotropic agents (e.g. dobutamine, amrinone, digitalis preparations) *to increase myocardial contractility*
   b. diuretics and vasodilators *to decrease cardiac workload*
   c. morphine sulfate *to reduce preload and anxiety* (used primarily in clients with pulmonary edema)
3. refer to Care Plan on Heart Failure for additional care measures.

6.A.4. The client will experience resolution of postpericardiotomy syndrome if it occurs as evidenced by:
a. fewer complaints of precordial pain
b. absence of pericardial friction rub
c. unlabored respirations at 14-20/minute
d. temperature declining toward normal
e. WBC count and sedimentation rate declining toward normal range.

6.A.4.a. Assess for and report signs and symptoms of postpericardiotomy syndrome:
1. precordial pain that frequently radiates to shoulder, neck, back, and arm (usually left); is intensified during deep inspiration, movement, and coughing; and is usually relieved by sitting up and leaning forward
2. pericardial friction rub (may be transient)
3. dyspnea, tachypnea
4. persistent temperature elevation
5. further increase in WBC count and sedimentation rate (both will be elevated as a result of the surgery)
6. chest x-ray and echocardiography results showing cardiomegaly and pericardial effusion.

b. If signs and symptoms of postpericardiotomy syndrome occur:
1. allay client's anxiety (client may believe that symptoms indicate a "heart attack")
2. assist client to assume position of comfort (usually sitting up and leaning forward on overbed table)
3. maintain activity restrictions as ordered (usually bed rest until symptoms subside)
4. administer the following medications if ordered:
   a. nonsteroidal anti-inflammatory agents (e.g. aspirin, ibuprofen)
   b. analgesics
   c. corticosteroids
5. assess for and immediately report signs of cardiac tamponade (see action 5.a.3 in this diagnosis)
6. prepare client for pericardiocentesis or surgical drainage of pericardial fluid if indicated (may be performed if signs of cardiac tamponade are present).

6.A.5. The client will not experience cardiac tamponade as evidenced by:
a. stable vital signs
b. absence of dyspnea
c. audible heart sounds
d. absence of jugular vein distention

6.A.5.a. Assess for and immediately report:
1. a sudden decrease in chest tube drainage
2. chest x-ray reports showing widening of the mediastinum
3. signs and symptoms of cardiac tamponade (e.g. significant decline in B/P, narrowed pulse pressure, pulsus paradoxus, dyspnea, distant or muffled heart sounds, jugular vein distention, increased CVP).

b. Implement measures *to reduce the risk of cardiac tamponade:*
1. administer medications to treat postpericardiotomy syndrome if it occurs (see action 4.b.4 in this diagnosis) *in order to reduce inflammation and fluid accumulation in the pericardial sac*

e. CVP within normal limits.

2. perform actions to maintain patency and integrity of chest drainage system (see Postoperative Collaborative Diagnosis 6.B, action 6.d.1)
3. if chest tube becomes obstructed, assist with clearing of existing tube and/or insertion of a new tube
4. when removing the pacemaker catheter(s), do it carefully *to avoid trauma to the surrounding vessels and subsequent bleeding.*

c. If signs and symptoms of cardiac tamponade occur, prepare client for:
1. echocardiography
2. pericardiocentesis or surgical drainage of pericardial fluid if indicated.

---

**6.B. COLLABORATIVE DIAGNOSES:**

**Potential complications: extracardiac**

1. **bleeding** related to:
   a. impaired platelet and clotting factor function (can result from mechanical damage to platelets and clotting factors by heart-lung machine, effects of hypothermia, relative decrease in levels associated with hemodilution, and consumption coagulopathy that can occur with major trauma)
   b. incomplete neutralization of the heparin used to prime the heart-lung machine
   c. anticoagulant therapy (relevant primarily for clients who have had valve replacement);
2. **thromboembolism** related to:
   a. trauma to the coronary arteries and donor vessels during grafting procedure
   b. thrombi formation at the prosthetic valve site
   c. incomplete filtration of air by heart-lung machine
   d. formation of microemboli associated with incomplete emptying of cardiac chambers if atrial fibrillation occurs
   e. venous stasis associated with diminished cardiac output and decreased activity
   f. hypercoagulability associated with increased release of tissue thromboplastin into the blood (occurs as a result of surgical trauma)
   g. decreased fibrinolytic activity (occurs in response to surgical trauma);
3. **cerebral ischemia** related to inadequate cerebral perfusion during surgery, low cardiac output, or an embolus;
4. **impaired renal function** related to deposit of hemolyzed red blood cells in renal tubules or inadequate renal blood flow associated with low cardiac output, hypovolemia, an embolus, or effects of vasopressor drugs;
5. **atelectasis** related to:
   a. partial collapse of alveoli and decreased surfactant production while on heart-lung machine
   b. hypoventilation associated with depressant effects of anesthesia and some medications, weakness, chest incision pain, and fear of dislodging chest tube
   c. obstruction of the bronchioles with retained secretions;
6. **pneumothorax** related to the accumulation of air in the pleural space if the pleura was opened during surgery.

| Desired Outcomes | Nursing Actions and ***Selected Purposes/Rationales*** |
|---|---|
| 6.B.1. The client will not experience unusual bleeding as evidenced by:<br>a. gradual decline in amount of bloody drainage from chest tube | 6.B.1.a. Assess client for and report signs and symptoms of unusual bleeding:<br>1. excessive amount of bloody drainage from chest tube (200 ml/hour is maximum amount expected in first 4-6 hours; drainage should then markedly decline)<br>2. continuous oozing of blood from incisions<br>3. prolonged bleeding from puncture sites<br>4. gingival bleeding<br>5. petechiae, purpura, ecchymoses |

| Desired Outcomes | Nursing Actions and ***Selected Purposes/Rationales*** |
|---|---|
| b. skin and mucous membranes free of active bleeding, petechiae, purpura, and ecchymoses<br>c. absence of unusual joint pain<br>d. no increase in abdominal girth<br>e. absence of frank and occult blood in stool, urine, and vomitus<br>f. usual menstrual flow<br>g. vital signs within normal range for client<br>h. stable or improved Hct and Hb. | 6. epistaxis, hemoptysis<br>7. unusual joint pain<br>8. increase in abdominal girth<br>9. frank or occult blood in stool, urine, or vomitus<br>10. menorrhagia<br>11. restlessness, confusion<br>12. significant drop in B/P accompanied by an increased pulse rate<br>13. decline in Hct and Hb levels.<br>b. Monitor platelet count and coagulation test results (e.g. prothrombin time, activated partial thromboplastin time, bleeding time). Report abnormal values.<br>c. If platelet count is low, coagulation test results are abnormal, or Hct and Hb levels decline, test all stools, urine, and vomitus for occult blood. Report positive results.<br>d. Implement measures *to prevent bleeding:*<br>1. use the smallest gauge needle possible when giving injections and performing venous and arterial punctures<br>2. apply gentle, prolonged pressure to puncture sites after injections and venous and arterial punctures<br>3. when taking B/P, avoid overinflating the cuff<br>4. caution client to avoid activities that increase the risk for trauma (e.g. shaving with a straight-edge razor, using stiff-bristle toothbrush or dental floss)<br>5. pad side rails if client is confused or restless<br>6. perform actions *to reduce the risk for falls* (e.g. keep bed in low position with side rails up when client is in bed, avoid unnecessary clutter in room, instruct client to wear shoes with nonslip soles when ambulating)<br>7. instruct client to avoid blowing nose forcefully or straining to have a bowel movement; consult physician regarding order for a decongestant, stool softener, and/or laxative if indicated<br>8. administer the following if ordered:<br>a. vitamin K (e.g. phytonadione, menadione)<br>b. protamine sulfate<br>c. platelets<br>d. plasma or whole blood.<br>e. If bleeding occurs and does not subside spontaneously:<br>1. apply firm, prolonged pressure to bleeding area(s) if possible<br>2. if epistaxis occurs, place client in a high Fowler's position and apply pressure and ice pack to nasal area<br>3. maintain oxygen therapy as ordered<br>4. perform gastric lavage as ordered *to control gastric bleeding*<br>5. administer vitamin K (e.g. phytonadione), protamine sulfate, and/or blood products (e.g. fresh frozen plasma, whole blood, platelets) as ordered<br>6. assess for and report signs and symptoms of hypovolemic shock (e.g. restlessness; confusion; significant decrease in B/P; rapid, thready pulse; rapid respirations; cool, pale skin; urine output less than 30 ml/hour)<br>7. prepare client for return to surgery if planned<br>8. provide emotional support to client and significant others. |
| 6.B.2. The client will not develop a thromboembolism as evidenced by:<br>a. absence of pain, tenderness, heaviness, | 6.B.2.a. Assess for and report signs and symptoms of:<br>1. deep vein thrombus (e.g. pain, tenderness, heaviness, swelling, unusual warmth, and/or positive Homan's sign in extremity)<br>2. arterial embolus (e.g. diminished or absent peripheral pulses; pallor, coolness, numbness, and/or pain in extremity)<br>3. cerebral ischemia (see action 3.a in this diagnosis for a list of signs and symptoms) |

numbness, and swelling in extremities
b. usual temperature and color of extremities
c. palpable peripheral pulses
d. usual mental status
e. usual sensory and motor function
f. absence of sudden chest pain and dyspnea.

4. pulmonary embolism (e.g. sudden chest pain, dyspnea, restlessness and apprehension).

b. Implement measures to prevent and treat deep vein thrombus and pulmonary embolism (see Standardized Postoperative Care Plan, Collaborative Diagnosis 19, actions c.1.b and c and c.2.b and c [pp. 132-133]).

c. Implement measures *to prevent thrombi and microemboli formation in the heart:*
   1. perform actions *to prevent stasis of blood in the heart:*
      a. implement measures to prevent and treat cardiac arrhythmias (see Postoperative Collaborative Diagnosis 6.A, actions 2.b and c)
      b. implement measures to improve cardiac output (see Postoperative Nursing Diagnosis 1, action c)
   2. administer anticoagulants (e.g. heparin, warfarin) or antiplatelet agents (e.g. low-dose aspirin, dipyridamole) if ordered.

d. If signs and symptoms of an arterial embolus occur:
   1. maintain client on strict bed rest with affected extremity in a level or slightly dependent position *to improve arterial blood flow*
   2. prepare client for diagnostic studies (e.g. Doppler ultrasound, arteriography)
   3. administer anticoagulants (e.g. continuous intravenous heparin, warfarin) if ordered
   4. prepare client for surgical intervention (e.g. embolectomy, revascularization) if planned
   5. refer to action 3.c in this diagnosis for additional care measures if signs and symptoms of cerebral ischemia occur
   6. provide emotional support to client and significant others.

6.B.3. The client will maintain adequate cerebral blood flow as evidenced by:
a. absence of dizziness, syncope, and visual disturbances
b. mentally alert and oriented
c. normal sensory and motor function.

6.B.3.a. Assess for and report signs and symptoms of cerebral ischemia:
   1. dizziness, syncope
   2. visual disturbances
   3. decreased level of consciousness
   4. paresthesias, motor weakness, paralysis.

b. Implement measures *to promote adequate cerebral blood flow:*
   1. keep head of bed flat until B/P is stabilized at a satisfactory level (at least 100 mm Hg systolic)
   2. keep head and neck in proper alignment
   3. perform actions to maintain adequate cardiac output (see Postoperative Nursing Diagnosis 1, action c)
   4. perform actions to prevent thrombi and microemboli formation in the heart (see action 2.c in this diagnosis).

c. If signs and symptoms of cerebral ischemia occur:
   1. continue with above measures
   2. maintain client on bed rest with head of bed flat unless contraindicated
   3. provide emotional support to client and significant others
   4. refer to Care Plan on Cerebrovascular Accident for additional care measures if signs and symptoms persist.

6.B.4. The client will maintain adequate renal function as evidenced by:
a. urine output at least 30 ml/hour
b. urine specific gravity, BUN, serum creatinine, and creatinine clearance within normal range.

6.B.4.a. Assess for and report signs and symptoms of impaired renal function (e.g. urine output less than 30 ml/hour, urine specific gravity fixed at or less than 1.010, elevated BUN and serum creatinine levels).

b. Collect a 24-hour urine specimen if ordered. Report decreased creatinine clearance.

c. Implement measures *to maintain adequate renal blood flow:*
   1. maintain a minimum fluid intake of 1000 ml/day unless ordered otherwise
   2. perform actions to maintain adequate cardiac output (see Postoperative Nursing Diagnosis 1, action c)
   3. perform actions to prevent thrombi and microemboli formation in the heart (see action 2.c in this diagnosis).

Desired Outcomes | Nursing Actions and ***Selected Purposes/Rationales***

d. If signs and symptoms of impaired renal function occur:
   1. continue with above actions
   2. administer diuretics if ordered *to increase urine output*
   3. assess for and report signs of acute renal failure (e.g. oliguria or anuria; weight gain; edema; elevated B/P; lethargy and confusion; increasing BUN and serum creatinine, phosphorus, and potassium levels)
   4. prepare client for dialysis if indicated
   5. refer to Care Plan on Renal Failure for additional care measures.

6.B.5. The client will not develop atelectasis (see Standardized Postoperative Care Plan, Collaborative Diagnosis 19, outcome b [p. 132], for outcome criteria).

6.B.5.a. Refer to Standardized Postoperative Care Plan, Collaborative Diagnosis 19, action b (p. 132), for measures related to assessment, prevention, and treatment of atelectasis.

b. Assure client that chest tube is sutured in place and that coughing and deep breathing should not dislodge the tube or disrupt the incision.

6.B.6. The client will experience normal lung re-expansion as evidenced by:
   a. normal breath sounds and percussion note by 3rd-4th postoperative day
   b. unlabored respirations at 14-20/minute
   c. blood gases returning toward normal
   d. chest x-ray showing lung re-expansion.

6.B.6.a. Assess for and immediately report signs and symptoms of:
   1. malfunction of chest drainage system (e.g. respiratory distress, sudden cessation of drainage, excessive bubbling in water seal chamber, significant increase in subcutaneous emphysema)
   2. further lung collapse (e.g. extended area of absent breath sounds with hyperresonant percussion note; further increase in pulse rate; rapid, shallow, and/or labored respirations; increased chest pain; restlessness; confusion).

b. Monitor blood gases. Report values that have worsened.

c. Monitor chest x-ray results. Report findings of delayed lung re-expansion or further lung collapse.

d. Implement measures *to promote lung re-expansion and prevent further lung collapse:*
   1. perform actions *to maintain patency and integrity of chest drainage system:*
      a. maintain water seal and suction levels as ordered
      b. maintain air occlusive dressing over chest tube insertion site
      c. tape all connections securely
      d. milk chest tube if ordered
      e. keep chest drainage and suction tubing free of kinks
      f. keep drainage system below level of client's chest at all times
   2. perform actions to improve breathing pattern (see Postoperative Nursing Diagnosis 2) and promote effective airway clearance (see Standardized Postoperative Care Plan, Nursing Diagnosis 3, action b [pp. 115-116]).

e. If signs and symptoms of further lung collapse occur:
   1. maintain client on bed rest in a semi- to high Fowler's position
   2. maintain oxygen therapy as ordered
   3. assess for and immediately report signs and symptoms of tension pneumothorax (e.g. severe dyspnea, increased restlessness and agitation, rapid and/or irregular pulse rate, hypotension, neck vein distention, shift in trachea toward unaffected side)
   4. assist with clearing of existing chest tube and/or insertion of a new tube
   5. provide emotional support to client and significant others.

## 7. NURSING DIAGNOSIS: Knowledge deficit

regarding follow-up care.

| Desired Outcomes | Nursing Actions and ***Selected Purposes/Rationales*** |
|---|---|
| 7.a. The client will identify modifiable cardiovascular risk factors and ways to reduce these factors. | 7.a.1. Inform client that the following modifiable factors have been shown to contribute to cardiovascular disease:<br>a. obesity<br>b. hyperlipidemia<br>c. sedentary life style<br>d. smoking<br>e. stressful life style<br>f. hypertension.<br>2. Inform client that alcohol intake should not exceed 1 oz of ethanol (i.e. 2 oz of 100-proof whiskey, 8 oz of wine, 24 oz of beer) a day on a regular basis because there is evidence that excessive alcohol intake contributes to the development of hypertension and some forms of heart disease.<br>3. Assist the client to identify ways he/she can make appropriate changes in life style to reduce above factors. Provide information about stress management classes and weight loss, cardiovascular fitness, smoking cessation, and alcohol rehabilitation programs. Initiate a referral if indicated. |
| 7.b. The client will verbalize an understanding of the rationale for and components of a diet restricted in sodium, saturated fat, and cholesterol. | 7.b.1. Explain the rationale for a diet restricting sodium, saturated fat, and cholesterol intake.<br>2. Provide the following information about decreasing sodium intake:<br>a. be aware that the terms salt and sodium are often used interchangeably but are not synonymous; there is 40% sodium in table salt<br>b. read food labels and calculate sodium content of items (often expressed in milligrams [1 gm is 1000 mg])<br>c. do not add salt when cooking foods or to prepared foods; use low-sodium herbs and spices if desired<br>d. avoid canned soups and vegetables<br>e. avoid processed convenience foods and commercial sauces<br>f. avoid cured and smoked foods<br>g. avoid salty snack foods.<br>3. Provide the following instructions on ways to reduce intake of saturated fat and cholesterol:<br>a. trim visible fat off meat and remove all skin from poultry<br>b. eat no more than 2 whole eggs/week<br>c. avoid commercial baked goods<br>d. avoid dairy products containing more than 1% fat<br>e. reduce intake of red meat once anemia has resolved.<br>4. Obtain a dietary consult to assist client in planning meals that will meet the prescribed restrictions of sodium, saturated fat, and cholesterol. |
| 7.c. The client will verbalize an understanding of activity restrictions and the rate of activity progression. | 7.c. Reinforce physician's instructions regarding activity. Instruct client to:<br>1. gradually rebuild activity level by adhering to a planned exercise program (often begins with walking and light household activities)<br>2. take frequent rest periods for 4-6 weeks following surgery<br>3. avoid lifting heavy objects in order to allow incision to heal and prevent a sudden increase in cardiac workload<br>4. avoid driving for 4-6 weeks<br>5. stop any activity that causes chest pain, shortness of breath, palpitations, dizziness, or extreme fatigue or weakness |

| Desired Outcomes | Nursing Actions and ***Selected Purposes/Rationales*** |
|---|---|
| | 6. begin a cardiovascular fitness program when allowed by physician. |
| 7.d. The client will verbalize an understanding of medications ordered including rationale, side effects, schedule for taking, and importance of taking as prescribed. | 7.d.1. Explain the rationale for, side effects of, and importance of taking medications prescribed.<br>2. If client has had a valve replacement and is discharged on a coumarin derivative (e.g. warfarin), instruct to:<br>a. keep scheduled appointments for periodic blood studies to monitor coagulation times<br>b. take medication at the same time each day, do not stop taking medication abruptly, and do not attempt to make up for missed doses<br>c. avoid regular and/or excessive intake of alcohol *(may alter responsiveness to coumarins)*<br>d. avoid taking over-the-counter products containing aspirin or other salicylates *(these products enhance the action of coumarins)*<br>e. avoid eating large amounts of foods high in vitamin K (e.g. green leafy vegetables)<br>f. take the following precautions to minimize risk of bleeding:<br>1. use an electric rather than a straight-edge razor<br>2. floss and brush teeth gently<br>3. avoid putting sharp objects (e.g. toothpicks) in mouth<br>4. do not walk barefoot<br>5. cut nails carefully<br>6. avoid situations that could result in injury (e.g. contact sports)<br>7. avoid blowing nose forcefully<br>8. avoid straining to have a bowel movement<br>g. report prolonged or excessive bleeding from skin, nose, or mouth; blood in urine, vomitus, sputum, or stools; prolonged or excessive menses; excessive bruising; severe headache; or sudden abdominal or back pain<br>h. apply firm, prolonged pressure to any bleeding area if possible<br>i. wear a Medic-Alert band identifying self as being on anticoagulant therapy<br>j. inform physician immediately if pregnancy is suspected *(coumarin crosses the placental barrier)*.<br>3. Instruct client to inform physician before taking other prescription and nonprescription medications.<br>4. Instruct client to inform all health care providers of medications being taken. |
| 7.e. The client will state signs and symptoms to report to the health care provider. | 7.e.1. Refer to Standardized Postoperative Care Plan, Nursing Diagnosis 21, action c (p. 135), for signs and symptoms to report to the health care provider.<br>2. Instruct client to report these additional signs and symptoms:<br>a. chest pain that seems unrelated to incisional discomfort<br>b. development of or increased shortness of breath<br>c. dizziness, fainting<br>d. increased fatigue and weakness<br>e. weight gain of more than 2 pounds a day<br>f. swelling of feet or ankles<br>g. persistent cough, especially if productive of yellow, green, rust-colored, or frothy sputum<br>h. significant change in pulse rate or rhythm (check with physician about client's need to monitor pulse at home)<br>i. temperature above 101° F (38.4° C) that lasts more than 1 day<br>j. depression or problems with concentration or memory that last more than 6 weeks. |
| 7.f. The client will identify community resources | 7.f. 1. Provide information about community resources that can assist client with cardiac rehabilitation and adjustment to having had heart surgery |

| | |
|---|---|
| that can assist with cardiac rehabilitation and adjustment to having had heart surgery. | (e.g. American Heart Association, Mended Hearts Club, counseling services).<br>2. Initiate a referral if indicated. |
| 7.g. The client will verbalize an understanding of and a plan for adhering to recommended follow-up care including future appointments with health care provider, wound care, and pain management. | 7.g.1. Refer to Standardized Postoperative Care Plan, Nursing Diagnosis 21 (pp. 135-136), for routine postoperative instructions and measures to improve client compliance.<br>2. If client had a valve replacement, instruct him/her to:<br>a. not have dental work for 6 months<br>b. inform health care providers of valve surgery so prophylactic antimicrobials may be started before any dental work, invasive diagnostic procedures, or surgery<br>c. perform good oral hygiene but avoid flossing in order to reduce the risk for infective endocarditis. |

# Hypertension

Hypertension is defined as a sustained elevation of arterial blood pressure at a level of 140/90 mm Hg or higher. Isolated systolic hypertension refers to a systolic pressure greater than 140 mm Hg with a diastolic pressure less than 90 mm Hg. Hypertension is classified as primary (essential or idiopathic) or secondary. Primary hypertension, which constitutes approximately 90% of the cases, has an unknown etiology. Secondary hypertension has identifiable causes, which include renal disease, Cushing's syndrome, certain neurological disorders, pheochromocytoma, hyperaldosteronism, coarctation of the aorta, and use of certain drugs (e.g. oral contraceptives, amphetamines, sympathomimetics). Hypertension is also classified according to severity. The current classification schema for hypertension includes systolic as well as diastolic pressure levels and divides hypertension into four stages. Stage 1 (mild) hypertension is an average blood pressure of 140-159/90-99 mm Hg, whereas stage 4 (very severe) hypertension includes blood pressure readings of 210/120 mm Hg or greater. Accelerated hypertension is a term used to describe a rapidly progressive increase in blood pressure with a diastolic pressure greater than 120 mm Hg and evidence of Grade III-IV retinopathy. Hypertensive urgency or emergency are terms used to describe a situation in which the pressure elevation poses an immediate threat to the client's life.

The most common pathological finding in hypertension is an increase in peripheral vascular resistance. In order to sustain adequate tissue perfusion when vascular resistance is increased, the heart must pump harder. A prolonged increase in cardiac workload eventually leads to ventricular hypertrophy and heart failure. The prolonged increase in vascular pressure causes widespread pathological changes in the large and small blood vessels. The end result of all the changes in the cardiovascular system is a decreased blood supply to the tissues with end-organ damage occurring most often in the eyes, kidneys, brain, and heart.

Initial treatment of hypertension is usually nonpharmacological and consists of life-style modifications such as weight reduction, increased physical activity, and moderation of dietary sodium and alcohol intake. If a conservative approach does not achieve the desired control of blood pressure, pharmacological therapy is initiated utilizing a stepped-care approach. This approach progresses from use of a diuretic, beta-adrenergic blocking agent, calcium-channel blocking agent, angiotensin converting enzyme (ACE) inhibitor, $alpha_1$-receptor blocker, or combination alpha-beta blocker in the first step to use of other types of antihypertensive agents and/or combinations of drugs until the desired control of blood pressure is achieved with a minimum of side effects.

**This care plan focuses on the adult client hospitalized with severe hypertension that is either newly diagnosed or uncontrolled.** The goals of care are to lower the blood pressure to a safe level, reduce fear and anxiety, prevent complications, and educate the client regarding follow-up care.

## DIAGNOSTIC TESTS

Renal arteriography
Renal ultrasound
Renal radionuclide imaging
Excretory urography (intravenous pyelography)
Chest x-ray
Urine studies (e.g. urinalysis, catecholamine level, creatinine clearance, cortisol level)
Blood studies (e.g. chemistry screen, lipoprotein profile, cortisol level, catecholamine level, renin level)

## DISCHARGE CRITERIA

Prior to discharge, the client will:

- ❖ have blood pressure within a safe range
- ❖ verbalize a basic understanding of hypertension and its effects on the body
- ❖ identify modifiable risk factors for hypertension and ways to reduce these factors
- ❖ verbalize an understanding of medications ordered including rationale, side effects, schedule for taking, and importance of taking as prescribed
- ❖ verbalize an understanding of the rationale for and components of the recommended diet
- ❖ demonstrate accuracy in taking, reading, and recording blood pressure
- ❖ state signs and symptoms to report to the health care provider
- ❖ identify community resources that can assist in making life-style changes necessary for effective control of hypertension
- ❖ verbalize an understanding of and a plan for adhering to recommended follow-up care including future appointments with health care provider and activity level.

## NURSING/COLLABORATIVE DIAGNOSES



## 1. NURSING DIAGNOSIS: Altered tissue perfusion

related to decreased peripheral blood flow associated with increased peripheral vascular resistance.

| Desired Outcome | Nursing Actions and ***Selected Purposes/Rationales*** |
|---|---|
| 1. The client will maintain adequate tissue perfusion as evidenced by:<br>a. B/P declining toward normal range for client<br>b. usual mental status<br>c. extremities warm with absence of pallor and cyanosis<br>d. palpable peripheral pulses<br>e. capillary refill time less than 3 seconds<br>f. absence of exercise-induced pain<br>g. balanced intake and output. | 1.a. Assess for and report the following:<br>1. further increase in B/P or failure of B/P to decline in response to antihypertensive agents<br>2. signs and symptoms of diminished tissue perfusion (e.g. restlessness, confusion, cool extremities, pallor or cyanosis of extremities, diminished or absent peripheral pulses, slow capillary refill, angina, oliguria).<br>b. Implement measures *to reduce blood pressure in order to improve tissue perfusion:*<br>1. administer the following medications if ordered:<br>a. adrenergic inhibiting agents:<br>1. central-acting adrenergic inhibitors (e.g. clonidine, methyldopa, guanabenz, guanfacine)<br>2. alpha$_1$-receptor blockers (e.g. prazosin, terazosin, doxozosin)<br>3. peripheral-acting adrenergic inhibitors (e.g. reserpine, guanethidine, guanadrel)<br>4. beta-adrenergic blockers (e.g. propranolol, metoprolol, atenolol, nadolol, acebutolol)<br>5. combined alpha- and beta-adrenergic blockers (e.g. labetalol)<br>b. vasodilators (e.g. minoxidil, hydralazine, nitroprusside, diazoxide); this group of medications is most often used when immediate reduction of B/P is necessary<br>c. angiotensin-converting enzyme inhibitors (e.g. captopril, lisinopril, enalapril)<br>d. calcium-channel blocking agents (e.g. nifedipine, verapamil, isradipine, nicardipine, diltiazem)<br>e. diuretics<br>2. perform actions *to reduce sympathetic nervous system stimulation:*<br>a. implement measures to reduce fear and anxiety (see Nursing Diagnosis 5, action b)<br>b. implement measures to relieve headache (see Nursing Diagnosis 2, action e)<br>c. implement measures to promote rest (see Nursing Diagnosis 3, action b.1)<br>3. discourage excessive intake of fluids high in caffeine such as coffee, tea, and colas<br>4. discourage smoking *(smoke causes vasoconstriction; it also contributes to decreased tissue oxygenation by reducing oxygen availability)*<br>5. maintain dietary sodium restrictions as ordered *to reduce fluid retention.*<br>c. Consult physician if signs and symptoms of diminished tissue perfusion persist or worsen. |

## 2. NURSING DIAGNOSIS: Pain: headache

related to distention of the cerebral blood vessels associated with increased vascular pressure.

| Desired Outcome | Nursing Actions and ***Selected Purposes/Rationales*** |
|---|---|
| 2. The client will obtain relief of headache as evidenced by:<br>a. verbalization of headache relief | 2.a. Determine how the client usually responds to pain.<br>b. Assess client's perception of headache including location, intensity, and type. Utilize a numerical scale to rate intensity.<br>c. Assess for nonverbal signs of headache (e.g. wrinkled brow, reluctance to |

| Desired Outcome | Nursing Actions and ***Selected Purposes/Rationales*** |
|---|---|
| b. relaxed facial expression and body positioning<br>c. increased participation in activities. | move head, rubbing head, avoidance of bright lights and noises, clenched fists).<br>d. Assess for factors that seem to aggravate and alleviate the headache.<br>e. Implement measures *to relieve headache:*<br>1. perform actions to reduce blood pressure (see Nursing Diagnosis 1, action b)<br>2. perform actions *to minimize environmental stimuli* (e.g. provide a calm environment, restrict visitors, dim lights)<br>3. avoid jarring bed or startling client *to minimize risk of sudden movements*<br>4. provide or assist with nonpharmacological measures for headache relief (e.g. cool cloth to forehead, back and neck rubs, elevation of head, relaxation techniques, diversional activities)<br>5. administer analgesics if ordered.<br>f. Consult physician if above measures fail to relieve headache. |

## 3. NURSING DIAGNOSIS: Activity intolerance

related to:
a. decreased tissue oxygenation associated with inadequate tissue perfusion;
b. difficulty resting and sleeping associated with fear, anxiety, frequent assessments, and headache.

| Desired Outcome | Nursing Actions and ***Selected Purposes/Rationales*** |
|---|---|
| 3. The client will demonstrate an increased tolerance for activity as evidenced by:<br>a. verbalization of feeling less fatigued and weak<br>b. ability to perform activities of daily living without exertional dyspnea, chest pain, diaphoresis, dizziness, and a significant change in vital signs. | 3.a. Assess for signs and symptoms of activity intolerance:<br>1. statements of fatigue and weakness<br>2. exertional dyspnea, chest pain, diaphoresis, or dizziness<br>3. abnormal heart rate response to activity (e.g. increase in rate of 20 beats/minute above resting rate, decrease in rate, rate not returning to preactivity level within 3 minutes after stopping activity, change from regular to irregular rate)<br>4. decreased systolic B/P or a significant further increase (10-15 mm Hg) in systolic or diastolic pressure with activity.<br>b. Implement measures *to improve activity tolerance:*<br>1. perform actions *to promote rest and/or conserve energy:*<br>a. maintain activity restrictions as ordered<br>b. minimize environmental activity and noise<br>c. organize nursing care to allow for periods of uninterrupted rest<br>d. limit the number of visitors and their length of stay<br>e. assist client with self-care activities as needed<br>f. keep supplies and personal articles within easy reach<br>g. instruct client in energy-saving techniques (e.g. using shower chair when showering, sitting to brush teeth or comb hair)<br>h. implement measures to reduce fear and anxiety (see Nursing Diagnosis 5, action b)<br>i. implement measures to relieve headache (see Nursing Diagnosis 2, action e)<br>2. perform actions to reduce blood pressure and improve tissue perfusion (see Nursing Diagnosis 1, action b)<br>3. increase client's activity gradually as allowed and tolerated.<br>c. Instruct client to:<br>1. report a decreased tolerance for activity |

2. stop any activity that causes chest pain, shortness of breath, dizziness, or extreme fatigue or weakness.

d. Consult physician if signs and symptoms of activity intolerance persist or worsen.

---

## 4. COLLABORATIVE DIAGNOSES:

**Potential complications:**

a. **cerebrovascular accident** related to cerebral hemorrhage, thrombosis, or embolism associated with injury to the arterial walls resulting from atherosclerosis and/or a prolonged increase in pressure in the cerebral vessels;
b. **hypertensive encephalopathy** related to excessive cerebral blood flow (results from decompensation of usual autoregulatory mechanisms in response to markedly elevated blood pressure) and the subsequent increase in intracranial pressure;
c. **ischemic heart disease (angina and/or myocardial infarction)** related to myocardial oxygen deficiency associated with increased myocardial oxygen utilization resulting from an increased cardiac workload (a result of increased vascular resistance);
d. **impaired renal function** related to vascular changes in the kidneys associated with effects of prolonged or severe hypertension;
e. **heart failure** related to the prolonged increase in cardiac workload associated with increased peripheral vascular resistance;
f. **aortic dissection** related to weakening of the muscularis layer of the aorta associated with effects of a prolonged increase in vascular pressure.

| Desired Outcomes | Nursing Actions and ***Selected Purposes/Rationales*** |
|---|---|
| 4.a. The client will not experience a cerebrovascular accident or hypertensive encephalopathy as evidenced by:<br>1. absence of dizziness, syncope, and visual disturbances<br>2. absence or resolution of headache<br>3. absence of vomiting<br>4. mentally alert and oriented<br>5. pupils equal and normally reactive to light<br>6. normal sensory and motor function. | 4.a.1. Assess for and report signs and symptoms of a cerebrovascular accident and/or hypertensive encephalopathy:<br>a. dizziness, syncope<br>b. visual disturbances (e.g. diplopia, scotoma, blurred vision, loss of vision)<br>c. persistent or increasing headache<br>d. vomiting<br>e. decreased level of consciousness<br>f. unequal pupils or a sluggish or absent pupillary reaction to light<br>g. paresthesias, facial ptosis, motor weakness, paralysis<br>h. seizures.<br>2. Implement measures *to reduce the risk of a cerebrovascular accident and hypertensive encephalopathy:*<br>a. perform actions to reduce blood pressure (see Nursing Diagnosis 1, action b)<br>b. instruct client to avoid activities that create a Valsalva response (e.g. straining to have a bowel movement, holding breath while moving) *in order to prevent a sudden increase in intracranial pressure*<br>c. keep head of bed elevated at least 30° and encourage client to keep head and neck in proper alignment *in order to promote adequate venous return from the cerebral vessels.*<br>3. If signs and symptoms of a cerebrovascular accident or hypertensive encephalopathy occur:<br>a. continue with above measures<br>b. maintain client on bed rest with head of bed elevated 20-30°<br>c. initiate appropriate safety measures (e.g. side rails up, seizure precautions)<br>d. administer osmotic diuretics (e.g. mannitol) and corticosteroids (e.g. |

| Desired Outcomes | Nursing Actions and ***Selected Purposes/Rationales*** |
|---|---|
| | dexamethasone, methylprednisolone) if ordered *to decrease cerebral edema*<br>e. provide emotional support to client and significant others<br>f. refer to Care Plan on Cerebrovascular Accident for additional care measures if signs and symptoms persist. |
| 4.b. The client will not experience episodes of myocardial ischemia as evidenced by:<br>1. absence of chest pain<br>2. unlabored respirations at 14-20/minute<br>3. normal cardiac enzymes<br>4. normal ECG readings. | 4.b.1. Assess for signs and symptoms of myocardial ischemia (e.g. chest pain, dyspnea).<br>2. Implement measures *to prevent myocardial ischemia:*<br>a. perform actions to reduce blood pressure (see Nursing Diagnosis 1, action b)<br>b. instruct client to avoid activities that create a Valsalva response (e.g. straining to have a bowel movement, holding breath while moving)<br>c. increase activity gradually as allowed and tolerated.<br>3. If signs and symptoms of myocardial ischemia occur:<br>a. consult physician about an order for cardiac enzyme/isoenzyme levels and ECG; report significant elevation of cardiac enzymes and a significant ST segment elevation, T wave changes, and/or pathological Q wave on ECG reading<br>b. maintain client on strict bed rest in a semi- to high Fowler's position<br>c. maintain oxygen therapy as ordered<br>d. administer the following medications if ordered:<br>1. nitrates *to improve coronary blood flow and reduce myocardial oxygen requirements*<br>2. morphine sulfate *to reduce pain and anxiety and decrease cardiac workload*<br>3. beta-adrenergic blocking agents *to reduce myocardial oxygen requirements by decreasing heart rate and myocardial contractility*<br>e. provide emotional support to client and significant others<br>f. refer to Care Plans on Angina Pectoris and Myocardial Infarction for additional care measures. |
| 4.c. The client will maintain adequate renal function as evidenced by:<br>1. urine output at least 30 ml/hour<br>2. urine specific gravity, BUN, serum creatinine, and creatinine clearance within normal range. | 4.c.1. Assess for and report signs and symptoms of impaired renal function (e.g. urine output less than 30 ml/hour, urine specific gravity fixed at or less than 1.010, elevated BUN and serum creatinine levels).<br>2. Collect a 24-hour urine specimen if ordered. Report decreased creatinine clearance.<br>3. Implement measures *to maintain adequate renal blood flow:*<br>a. perform actions to reduce blood pressure (see Nursing Diagnosis 1, action b)<br>b. maintain an adequate fluid intake *to reduce risk of dehydration.*<br>4. If signs and symptoms of impaired renal function occur:<br>a. continue with above actions<br>b. administer diuretics if ordered *to increase urine output*<br>c. assess for and report signs of acute renal failure (e.g. oliguria or anuria; weight gain; edema; increasing B/P; lethargy and confusion; increasing BUN and serum creatinine, phosphorous, and potassium levels)<br>d. prepare client for dialysis if indicated<br>e. refer to Care Plan on Renal Failure for additional care measures. |
| 4.d. The client will not develop heart failure as evidenced by:<br>1. pulse 60-100 beats/minute<br>2. absence of an $S_3$ heart sound or summation gallop<br>3. usual mental status | 4.d.1. Assess for and report signs and symptoms of heart failure:<br>a. tachycardia<br>b. presence of an $S_3$ heart sound or summation gallop<br>c. restlessness, agitation, confusion<br>d. crackles (rales)<br>e. dyspnea, orthopnea<br>f. cough<br>g. development of or increased weakness and fatigue<br>h. cool, diaphoretic skin<br>i. diminished or absent peripheral pulses |

| Desired Outcome | Nursing Actions and *Selected Purposes/Rationales* |
|---|---|
| 4. normal breath sounds<br>5. absence of dyspnea, orthopnea, and cough<br>6. increased strength and activity tolerance<br>7. skin warm and dry<br>8. palpable peripheral pulses<br>9. balanced intake and output<br>10. stable weight<br>11. absence of peripheral edema; distended neck veins; and enlarged, tender liver. | j. oliguria<br>k. weight gain<br>l. peripheral edema<br>m. distended neck veins<br>n. enlarged, tender liver.<br>2. Monitor chest x-ray results. Report findings of cardiomegaly, pleural effusion, or pulmonary edema.<br>3. Implement measures to reduce blood pressure (see Nursing Diagnosis 1, action b) *in order to reduce cardiac workload and prevent heart failure.*<br>4. If signs and symptoms of heart failure occur:<br>a. continue with above actions<br>b. maintain oxygen therapy as ordered<br>c. administer the following medications if ordered:<br>1. positive inotropic agents (e.g. digitalis preparations, dobutamine, amrinone) *to increase myocardial contractility*<br>2. diuretics and vasodilators *to decrease cardiac workload*<br>3. morphine sulfate *to reduce preload and anxiety* (used primarily in clients with pulmonary edema)<br>d. provide emotional support to client and significant others<br>e. refer to Care Plan on Heart Failure for additional care measures. |
| 4.e. The client will not experience dissection of the aorta as evidenced by:<br>1. absence of sudden, severe chest pain<br>2. palpable peripheral pulses with no change in pulse pattern<br>3. usual sensory and motor function<br>4. usual mental status<br>5. stable vital signs<br>6. skin warm, dry, and usual color. | 4.e.1. Assess for and immediately report the following:<br>a. signs and symptoms of aortic dissection (e.g. sudden, severe chest pain that may radiate to back; abnormal pulse pattern [discrepancies in character, timing, and magnitude] in extremities; hemianesthesia; hemiplegia; paraplegia)<br>b. signs and symptoms of hypovolemic shock (e.g. restlessness; agitation; significant decline in B/P; rapid, thready pulse; cool, moist skin; pallor; diminished or absent pulses).<br>2. Implement measures *to prevent aortic dissection:*<br>a. perform actions to reduce blood pressure (see Nursing Diagnosis 1, action b)<br>b. instruct client to avoid activities that create a Valsalva response (e.g. straining to have a bowel movement, holding breath while moving).<br>3. If signs and symptoms of aortic dissection occur:<br>a. maintain client on strict bed rest<br>b. monitor vital signs frequently<br>c. administer oxygen as ordered<br>d. prepare client for diagnostic studies (e.g. aortogram, computerized tomography) if planned<br>e. administer antihypertensive agents (e.g. nitroprusside, propranolol) if ordered<br>f. prepare client for surgery if planned<br>g. provide emotional support to client and significant others. |

## 5. NURSING DIAGNOSIS: Anxiety

related to necessity for urgent treatment; possibility of severe disability or sudden death; unfamiliar environment; persistent or severe headache; and lack of understanding of diagnostic tests, diagnosis, and treatment plan.

| Desired Outcome | Nursing Actions and ***Selected Purposes/Rationales*** |
|---|---|
| 5. The client will experience a reduction in anxiety as evidenced by: | 5.a. Assess client for signs and symptoms of anxiety (e.g. verbalization of fears and concerns, insomnia, tenseness, tremors, irritability, restlessness, diaphoresis, tachypnea, tachycardia, further elevation of blood pressure, |

| Desired Outcome | Nursing Actions and ***Selected Purposes/Rationales*** |
|---|---|
| a. verbalization of feeling less anxious and fearful<br>b. usual sleep pattern<br>c. relaxed facial expression and body movements<br>d. vital signs returning to normal range for client<br>e. usual perceptual ability and interactions with others. | facial pallor or flushing, narrowed perceptual field, withdrawal, noncompliance with treatment plan). Validate perceptions carefully, remembering that some behaviors may result from decreased tissue perfusion and neurological changes.<br>b. Implement measures *to reduce fear and anxiety:*<br>1. orient client to hospital environment, equipment, and routines<br>2. provide a calm, restful environment<br>3. introduce staff who will be participating in his/her care; if possible, maintain consistency in staff assigned to his/her care *to provide feelings of stability and comfort with the environment*<br>4. assure client that staff members are nearby; respond to call signal as soon as possible<br>5. maintain a calm, supportive, confident manner when interacting with client<br>6. encourage verbalization of fear and anxiety; provide feedback<br>7. explain all diagnostic tests<br>8. reinforce physician's explanations and clarify misconceptions the client has about hypertension, the treatment plan, and prognosis<br>9. perform actions to relieve headache (see Nursing Diagnosis 2, action e)<br>10. instruct client in relaxation techniques and encourage participation in diversional activities<br>11. assist client to identify specific stressors and ways to cope with them<br>12. encourage significant others to project a caring, concerned attitude without obvious anxiousness<br>13. administer antianxiety agents if ordered.<br>c. Include significant others in orientation and teaching sessions and encourage their continued support of client.<br>d. Provide information based on current needs of client and significant others at a level they can understand. Encourage questions and clarification of information provided.<br>e. Consult physician if above actions fail to control fear and anxiety. |

## 6. NURSING DIAGNOSIS: Ineffective management of therapeutic regimen

related to:

a. lack of understanding of the implications of not following the prescribed treatment plan;
b. difficulty modifying personal habits (e.g. smoking, alcohol intake, dietary preferences);
c. undesirable side effects of some antihypertensive agents;
d. insufficient financial resources.

| Desired Outcome | Nursing Actions and ***Selected Purposes/Rationales*** |
|---|---|
| 6. The client will demonstrate the probability of effective | 6.a. Assess for indications that the client may be unable to effectively manage the therapeutic regimen:<br>1. statements reflecting that he/she was unable to manage care at home |

management of the therapeutic regimen as evidenced by:

a. willingness to learn about and participate in treatments and care
b. statements reflecting ways to modify personal habits
c. statements reflecting an understanding of the implications of not following the prescribed treatment plan.

2. failure to adhere to treatment plan while in hospital (e.g. not adhering to dietary modifications, refusing medications)
3. statements reflecting a lack of understanding of factors that may cause progression of hypertension
4. statements reflecting an unwillingness or inability to modify personal habits
5. statements reflecting view that hypertension will reverse itself or that the situation is hopeless and efforts to comply with the therapeutic regimen are useless
6. statements reflecting that the side effects of medications are too uncomfortable and that he/she feels better when not taking medication
7. statements reflecting that medications are too expensive.

b. Implement measures *to promote effective management of the therapeutic regimen:*
   1. explain hypertension in terms the client can understand; stress the fact that hypertension is a chronic condition and that adherence to the treatment plan is necessary in order to delay and/or prevent complications
   2. encourage questions and clarify misconceptions client has about hypertension and its effects and the side effects of medications
   3. provide instructions on and encourage client to participate in the treatment plan (e.g. calculating sodium intake, monitoring blood pressure); determine areas of misunderstanding and reinforce teaching as necessary
   4. provide client with written instructions about dietary modifications, signs and symptoms to report, medication therapy, blood pressure monitoring, and exercise regimen
   5. assist client to identify ways he/she can incorporate medication regimen, exercise, and dietary modifications into life style; focus on modifications of life style rather than complete change
   6. assist client to identify a reward system for self that will assist him/her to effect necessary change(s)
   7. initiate and reinforce discharge teaching outlined in Nursing Diagnosis 7 *in order to promote a sense of control*
   8. provide information about and encourage utilization of community resources that can assist client to make necessary life-style changes (e.g. cardiovascular fitness, weight loss, and smoking cessation programs)
   9. encourage client to discuss his/her concerns regarding the cost of medications and visits with health care provider; obtain a social service consult to assist with financial planning and to obtain financial aid if indicated
   10. encourage client to attend follow-up educational classes
   11. reinforce behaviors suggesting future compliance with the therapeutic regimen (e.g. statements reflecting plans for adhering to treatment plan, statements reflecting an understanding of hypertension and its long-term effects)
   12. include significant others in explanations and teaching sessions and encourage their support; reinforce the need for client to assume responsibility for managing as much of care as possible.

c. Consult physician regarding referrals to community health agencies if continued instruction or support is needed.

## 7. NURSING DIAGNOSIS: Knowledge deficit

regarding follow-up care.

| Desired Outcomes | Nursing Actions and ***Selected Purposes/Rationales*** |
|---|---|
| 7.a. The client will verbalize a basic understanding of hypertension and its effects on the body. | 7.a.1. Explain hypertension and its effects in terms client can understand. Utilize available teaching aids (e.g. pamphlets, videotapes).<br>2. Inform client that hypertension is often asymptomatic and that absence of symptoms is not a reliable indication that blood pressure is within a safe range. |
| 7.b. The client will identify modifiable risk factors for hypertension and ways to reduce these factors. | 7.b.1. Inform client that the following modifiable factors have been shown to contribute to hypertension:<br>a. obesity<br>b. sedentary life style<br>c. smoking<br>d. daily alcohol intake exceeding 1 oz of ethanol (i.e. 2 oz of 100-proof whiskey, 8 oz of wine, 24 oz of beer) on a regular basis<br>e. excessive sodium intake<br>f. stressful life style.<br>2. Assist the client to identify ways he/she can make appropriate changes in life style to reduce modifiable risk factors. Provide information about weight reduction plans, stress management classes, and smoking cessation and alcohol rehabilitation programs. Initiate a referral if indicated.<br>3. Instruct client to participate in a regular isotonic exercise program (e.g. walking, swimming) and avoid isometric exercise (e.g. weight training). Caution client to consult physician before beginning an exercise program.<br>4. If client is taking an oral contraceptive, instruct her to consult physician regarding other methods of birth control. |
| 7.c. The client will verbalize an understanding of medications ordered including rationale, side effects, schedule for taking, and importance of taking as prescribed. | 7.c.1. Explain the rationale for, side effects of, and importance of taking medications prescribed.<br>2. If client is discharged on a diuretic, instruct to:<br>a. take once-daily dose or the larger dose in the morning to minimize nighttime urination<br>b. weigh self daily and keep a record of daily weights<br>c. change from a lying to a standing position slowly if experiencing dizziness or lightheadedness with position change<br>d. increase intake of foods/fluids high in potassium (e.g. orange juice, bananas, figs, dates, cantaloupe, potatoes, raisins, apricots) if taking a potassium-depleting diuretic<br>e. notify physician if unable to tolerate food or fluids (dehydration can develop rapidly if intake is poor and client continues to take a diuretic)<br>f. avoid salt substitutes with a high potassium content if discharged on a potassium-sparing diuretic (e.g. triamterene, spironolactone)<br>g. report the following signs and symptoms:<br>1. weight loss of more than 5 pounds a week<br>2. excessive thirst<br>3. severe dizziness or episodes of fainting<br>4. muscle weakness or cramping, nausea, vomiting, irregular pulse, or increased pulse rate.<br>3. If client is discharged on an antihypertensive such as an adrenergic inhibiting agent, vasodilator, or angiotensin-converting enzyme inhibitor, instruct to:<br>a. change from a lying to standing position slowly if experiencing dizziness or lightheadedness with position change<br>b. avoid strenuous exercise (especially in hot weather), hot baths and showers, steam room, and sauna<br>c. limit alcohol intake<br>d. report continued dizziness, lightheadedness, or fainting<br>e. report side effects such as impotence, dry mouth, and unusual mood changes if they persist more than a few weeks. |

4. Instruct client to take medication on a regular basis and avoid skipping doses, altering prescribed dose, making up for missed doses, and discontinuing medication without permission of health care provider.
5. Instruct the client to consult health care provider before taking other prescription and nonprescription medications.

7.d. The client will verbalize an understanding of the rationale for and components of the recommended diet.

7.d.1. Explain the rationale for the recommended dietary modifications.
2. Depending on the physician's recommendations:
   a. provide the following information about decreasing sodium intake:
      1. be aware that the terms salt and sodium are often used interchangeably but are not synonymous; there is 40% sodium in table salt
      2. read food labels and calculate sodium content of items (often expressed in milligrams [2 gm is 2000 mg])
      3. do not add salt when cooking foods or to prepared foods; use low-sodium seasonings such as herbs and spices if desired
      4. avoid canned soups and vegetables
      5. avoid processed convenience foods and commercial sauces
      6. avoid cured and smoked foods
      7. avoid salty snack foods
   b. provide the following instructions on ways to reduce intake of saturated fat and cholesterol:
      1. reduce intake of red meat
      2. trim visible fat off meat and remove all skin from poultry
      3. eat no more than 2 whole eggs/week
      4. avoid commercial baked goods
      5. avoid dairy products containing more than 1% fat.
3. Instruct client to avoid restricting intake of dairy products to lower sodium intake (there is some evidence that a low calcium intake may contribute to hypertension).
4. Instruct client to include the recommended daily allowances of potassium, calcium, and magnesium in diet.

7.e. The client will demonstrate accuracy in taking, reading, and recording blood pressure.

7.e.1. Teach client to take, read, and record blood pressure.
2. Allow time for return demonstration and accuracy check.
3. Instruct client to monitor and record blood pressure weekly (or more often if directed by physician) and bring record of pressures to visits with health care provider.

7.f. The client will state signs and symptoms to report to the health care provider.

7.f. Instruct the client to report:
1. persistent headache or headache present upon awakening
2. sudden and continued increase in B/P (if B/P is monitored at home)
3. chest pain
4. shortness of breath
5. significant weight gain or swelling of feet or ankles
6. changes in vision
7. frequent or uncontrollable nosebleeds
8. severe depression or emotional lability
9. persistent dizziness, lightheadedness, or fainting
10. persistent side effects experienced from use of antihypertensive medications (e.g. impotence, dry mouth)
11. side effects of diuretic therapy (see action c.2.g in this diagnosis).

7.g. The client will identify community resources that can assist in making life-style changes necessary for effective control of hypertension.

7.g.1. Provide information regarding community resources and support groups that can assist client in making life-style changes that are necessary for effective control of hypertension (e.g. cardiovascular fitness, weight loss, and smoking cessation programs; stress management classes).
2. Initiate a referral if indicated.

7.h. The client will verbalize an understanding of and

7.h.1. Reinforce the importance of keeping follow-up appointments with health care provider and continuing lifelong medical supervision.
2. Reinforce the physician's instructions regarding activity level.

| Desired Outcomes | Nursing Actions and ***Selected Purposes/Rationales*** |
|---|---|
| a plan for adhering to recommended follow-up care including future appointments with health care provider and activity level. | 3. Refer to Nursing Diagnosis 6, action b, for measures to promote client's ability to effectively manage the therapeutic regimen. |

# Myocardial Infarction

A myocardial infarction (MI) is a result of prolonged ischemia of the heart muscle and occurs when blood flow to an area of the myocardium is insufficient to meet the myocardial oxygen requirements. Sustained ischemia causes tissue necrosis and irreversible cellular damage, which results in disturbances in mechanical, biochemical, and electrical function in the necrotic or infarcted area. The degree of altered function depends on the area of the heart involved and the size of the infarct. Infarctions are sometimes classified as transmural (involving the full thickness of the myocardium) or subendocardial (involving only a partial thickness of the myocardium). MIs are also classified as Q wave or non–Q wave infarctions. An MI is most frequently caused by thrombosis of an atherosclerotic coronary artery. Other less common causes include spasm of a coronary artery, severe or prolonged hypotension, a rapid ventricular rate, and cocaine use.

The classic symptom of an MI is intense chest pain that is described as a squeezing, viselike, or crushing sensation; may radiate to the left arm, neck, or jaw; lasts longer than 30 minutes; and is unrelieved by nitroglycerin and rest. However 15% to 25% of infarctions go unrecognized because clients have only mild or no chest discomfort. Other signs and symptoms may include shortness of breath, diaphoresis, anxiousness, weakness, dizziness, pallor, nausea, and vomiting. Prognosis is largely influenced by size and location of the infarct, concurrent cardiovascular status, and promptness and effectiveness of treatment.

**This care plan focuses on the adult client hospitalized during an episode of intense chest pain for definitive diagnosis and management of a myocardial infarction.** The goals of care are to relieve pain, improve cardiac output, reduce fear and anxiety, prevent complications, and educate the client regarding follow-up care.

## DIAGNOSTIC TESTS

Electrocardiogram (ECG)
Cardiac enzymes/isoenzymes
Radionuclide imaging
Coronary angiography
Echocardiography
Vectorcardiography
Blood gases and chemistry
Oximetry
WBC count
Serum cholesterol and triglyceride levels and lipoprotein profile

## DISCHARGE CRITERIA

Prior to discharge, the client will:

- tolerate prescribed activity without a significant change in vital signs, chest pain, dyspnea, dizziness, or extreme fatigue or weakness
- verbalize a basic understanding of a myocardial infarction
- demonstrate accuracy in counting pulse
- identify modifiable cardiovascular risk factors and ways to reduce these factors

- verbalize an understanding of the rationale for and components of a diet restricted in sodium, saturated fat, and cholesterol
- verbalize an understanding of medications ordered including rationale, side effects, schedule for taking, and importance of taking as prescribed
- verbalize an understanding of activity restrictions and the rate at which activity can be progressed
- state signs and symptoms to report to the health care provider
- identify community resources that can assist with cardiac rehabilitation and adjustment to the effects of a myocardial infarction
- share feelings and concerns about changes in body functioning and usual roles and life style
- verbalize an understanding of and a plan for adhering to recommended follow-up care including future appointments with health care provider.

**NURSING/ COLLABORATIVE DIAGNOSES**



## 1. NURSING DIAGNOSIS: Decreased cardiac output

related to decreased myocardial contractility and altered conductivity of the heart associated with myocardial damage.

| Desired Outcome | Nursing Actions and ***Selected Purposes/Rationales*** |
|---|---|
| 1. The client will have improved cardiac output as evidenced by:<br>a. B/P within normal range for client<br>b. apical pulse between 60-100 beats/minute and regular<br>c. resolution of gallop rhythms<br>d. increased strength and activity tolerance | 1.a. Assess for and report the following:<br>1. diagnostic findings indicative of an MI:<br>a. elevated CK (CPK)-MB<br>b. elevated LDH with an $LDH_1$ level that is higher than the $LDH_2$ (a reliable indicator of an acute MI)<br>c. elevated WBC count and/or AST (SGOT); these tests are not specific for myocardial injury but support the diagnosis when CK-MB and LDH are elevated<br>d. temperature elevation (reflects tissue destruction and resulting inflammation)<br>e. ECG showing ST segment elevation, T wave inversion, and/or presence of pathological Q wave (there may be no Q waves and the |

| Desired Outcome | Nursing Actions and ***Selected Purposes/Rationales*** |
|---|---|

e. unlabored respirations at 14-20/ minute
f. normal breath sounds
g. usual mental status
h. absence of vertigo and syncope
i. palpable peripheral pulses
j. improved skin temperature and color
k. capillary refill time less than 3 seconds
l. balanced intake and output
m. absence of peripheral edema and jugular vein distention
n. hemodynamic measurements such as cardiac output (CO), pulmonary artery pressure (PAP), pulmonary capillary wedge pressure (PCWP), and central venous pressure (CVP) within or returning toward normal range.

ST segment may be depressed if client has had a subendocardial infarction)

f. presence of an $S_4$ heart sound

2. signs and symptoms of decreased cardiac output:
   a. variations in B/P (may be increased because of pain or compensatory vasoconstriction; may be decreased when compensatory mechanisms and pump fail)
   b. tachycardia, irregular pulse
   c. presence of gallop rhythm
   d. fatigue and weakness
   e. dyspnea, tachypnea
   f. crackles (rales)
   g. restlessness, anxiousness, confusion
   h. vertigo, syncope
   i. diminished or absent peripheral pulses
   j. cool, clammy skin
   k. pallor, mottling, or cyanosis of skin
   l. capillary refill time greater than 3 seconds
   m. oliguria
   n. peripheral edema
   o. jugular vein distention (JVD)
   p. hemodynamic changes such as decreased CO and increased PAP and PCWP or CVP (use internal jugular vein pulsation method to estimate CVP if monitoring device not present).

b. Monitor for and report the following:
   1. chest x-ray results showing pulmonary vascular congestion, pulmonary edema, or pleural effusion
   2. abnormal blood gases
   3. significant change in oximetry results.

c. Implement measures *to improve cardiac output:*
   1. prepare client for procedures that may be performed *to improve coronary blood flow:*
      a. injection of a thrombolytic agent (e.g. streptokinase, tissue plasminogen activator [tPA], anistreplase [APSAC, Eminase])
      b. percutaneous transluminal coronary angioplasty (PTCA)
      c. insertion of an intra-aortic balloon pump (IABP)
   2. perform actions *to reduce cardiac workload:*
      a. maintain activity restrictions as ordered
      b. place client in a semi- to high Fowler's position
      c. instruct client to avoid activities that create a Valsalva response (e.g. straining to have a bowel movement, holding breath while moving) *in order to prevent the marked increase in venous return and preload that occurs with exhalation*
      d. implement measures to promote rest and conserve energy (see Nursing Diagnosis 3, action b.1)
      e. maintain oxygen therapy as ordered
      f. discourage smoking *(smoke has a cardiostimulatory effect, causes vasoconstriction, and reduces oxygen availability)*
      g. provide small meals rather than large ones *(large meals require an increase in blood supply to gastrointestinal tract for digestion)*
      h. discourage excessive intake of fluids high in caffeine such as coffee, tea, and colas *(caffeine is a myocardial stimulant and increases myocardial oxygen consumption)*
      i. implement measures *to prevent fluid volume excess:*
         1. restrict sodium intake as ordered
         2. administer diuretics if ordered
      j. increase activity gradually as allowed and tolerated

3. administer the following medications if ordered:
    a. nitrates (e.g. nitroglycerin) *to dilate the coronary and peripheral (primarily venous) blood vessels and subsequently improve coronary blood flow and reduce cardiac workload and myocardial oxygen requirements*
    b. beta-adrenergic blocking agents (e.g. atenolol, metoprolol, propranolol) *to reduce myocardial oxygen requirements by decreasing heart rate and myocardial contractility*
    c. calcium-channel blocking agents (e.g. diltiazem) *to increase coronary blood flow and reduce cardiac workload by decreasing afterload and the force of myocardial contractility*
    d. antiarrhythmics (e.g. quinidine, procainamide) if arrhythmias are present *to improve cardiac output by prolonging the diastolic filling time and thereby increasing stroke volume*
    e. anticoagulants (e.g. intravenous heparin) and antiplatelet agents (e.g. low-dose aspirin) *to prevent occlusion of the coronary artery(ies) by thrombosis.*

d. Consult physician if signs and symptoms of decreased cardiac output persist or worsen.

## 2. NURSING DIAGNOSIS: Pain: chest pain that may radiate to arm, neck, jaw, or back

related to myocardial ischemia (a decreased oxygen supply forces the myocardium to convert to anaerobic metabolism; the end products of anaerobic metabolism act as irritants to myocardial neural receptors).

| Desired Outcome | Nursing Actions and ***Selected Purposes/Rationales*** |
|---|---|
| 2. The client will experience diminished pain as evidenced by:<br>a. verbalization of pain relief<br>b. relaxed facial expression and body positioning<br>c. increased participation in activities<br>d. stable vital signs. | 2.a. Determine how the client usually responds to pain.<br>b. Assess client's perception of pain including location, intensity, and type. Utilize a numerical scale to rate intensity.<br>c. Assess for nonverbal signs of pain (e.g. wrinkled brow; rubbing neck, jaw, or arm; clenched fists; reluctance to move; clutching chest; restlessness; shallow, guarded respirations; diaphoresis; facial pallor; increase in B/P and pulse).<br>d. Assess for factors that seem to aggravate and alleviate pain.<br>e. Implement measures *to reduce pain:*<br>1. maintain oxygen therapy as ordered *to increase the myocardial oxygen supply*<br>2. maintain client on bed rest in a semi- to high Fowler's position<br>3. administer the following medications if ordered:<br>a. narcotic analgesics (an intravenous rather than an intramuscular route should be used *because intramuscular injections are poorly absorbed if tissue perfusion is decreased; intramuscular injections also elevate serum enzyme levels, which may interfere with assessment of myocardial damage*)<br>b. nitrates (e.g. nitroglycerin)<br>4. provide or assist with nonpharmacological measures for pain relief (e.g. position change, relaxation techniques, restful environment).<br>f. Consult physician if above measures fail to provide adequate pain relief. |

## 3. NURSING DIAGNOSIS: Activity intolerance

related to:
a. tissue hypoxia associated with decreased cardiac output;
b. difficulty resting and sleeping associated with pain, frequent assessments and treatments, fear, and anxiety.

| Desired Outcome | Nursing Actions and ***Selected Purposes/Rationales*** |
|---|---|
| 3. The client will demonstrate an increased tolerance for activity as evidenced by:<br>a. verbalization of feeling less fatigued and weak<br>b. ability to perform activities of daily living without exertional dyspnea, chest pain, diaphoresis, dizziness, and a significant change in vital signs. | 3.a. Assess for signs and symptoms of activity intolerance:<br>1. statements of fatigue and weakness<br>2. exertional dyspnea, chest pain, diaphoresis, or dizziness<br>3. abnormal heart rate response to activity (e.g. increase in rate of 20 beats/minute above resting rate, decrease in rate, rate not returning to preactivity level within 3 minutes after stopping activity, change from regular to irregular rate)<br>4. decreased systolic B/P or a significant increase (10-15 mm Hg) in systolic or diastolic pressure with activity.<br>b. Implement measures *to improve activity tolerance:*<br>1. perform actions *to promote rest and/or conserve energy:*<br>a. maintain activity restrictions as ordered<br>b. minimize environmental activity and noise<br>c. organize nursing care to allow for periods of uninterrupted rest<br>d. limit the number of visitors and their length of stay<br>e. assist client with self-care activities as needed<br>f. keep supplies and personal articles within easy reach<br>g. instruct client in energy-saving techniques (e.g. using shower chair when showering, sitting to brush teeth or comb hair)<br>h. implement measures to reduce fear and anxiety (see Nursing Diagnosis 6, action b)<br>i. implement measures to promote sleep (see Nursing Diagnosis 4, action c)<br>j. implement measures to reduce pain (see Nursing Diagnosis 2, action e)<br>2. perform actions to improve cardiac output (see Nursing Diagnosis 1, action c)<br>3. maintain oxygen therapy as ordered<br>4. increase client's activity gradually as allowed and tolerated.<br>c. Instruct client to:<br>1. report a decreased tolerance for activity<br>2. stop any activity that causes chest pain, shortness of breath, dizziness, or extreme fatigue or weakness.<br>d. Consult physician if signs and symptoms of activity intolerance persist or worsen. |

## 4. NURSING DIAGNOSIS: Sleep pattern disturbance

related to pain, frequent assessments and treatments, fear, and anxiety.

| Desired Outcome | Nursing Actions and ***Selected Purposes/Rationales*** |
|---|---|
| 4. The client will attain optimal amounts of sleep within the parameters of the treatment regimen as evidenced by:<br>a. statements of feeling well rested<br>b. usual mental status<br>c. absence of frequent yawning, dark circles under eyes, and hand tremors. | 4.a. Assess for signs and symptoms of a sleep pattern disturbance (e.g. verbal complaints of difficulty falling asleep, sleep interruptions, or not feeling well rested; irritability; lethargy; disorientation; frequent yawning; dark circles under eyes; slight hand tremors).<br>b. Determine the client's usual sleep habits.<br>c. Implement measures *to promote sleep:*<br>1. discourage long periods of sleep during the day unless signs and symptoms of sleep deprivation exist or daytime sleep is usual for client<br>2. perform actions to reduce pain (see Nursing Diagnosis 2, action e)<br>3. perform actions to reduce fear and anxiety (see Nursing Diagnosis 6, action b)<br>4. encourage participation in relaxing diversional activities during the evening<br>5. discourage intake of fluids high in caffeine (e.g. coffee, tea, colas), especially in the evening<br>6. offer client a high-protein evening snack unless contraindicated<br>7. allow client to continue usual sleep practices (e.g. position, time, bedtime rituals such as reading and meditating) if possible<br>8. satisfy basic needs such as comfort and warmth before sleep<br>9. have client empty bladder just before bedtime<br>10. maintain a quiet, restful atmosphere; have earplugs available for client if needed<br>11. utilize relaxation techniques (e.g. progressive relaxation exercises, back massage, meditation, soft music) before sleep<br>12. ensure good room ventilation<br>13. administer sedative-hypnotics if ordered<br>14. perform actions *to reduce interruptions during sleep (80-100 minutes of uninterrupted sleep are usually needed to complete one sleep cycle):*<br>a. restrict visitors<br>b. group care (e.g. medications, treatments, physical care, assessments) whenever possible.<br>d. Consult physician if signs and symptoms of sleep deprivation persist or worsen. |

## 5. COLLABORATIVE DIAGNOSES:

**Potential complications:**

a. **cardiac arrhythmias** related to impaired nodal function and/or altered myocardial conductivity associated with damage to the myocardium, hypoxia, and possible electrolyte and acid-base imbalances;

b. **heart failure** related to decreased myocardial contractility and inability of heart to pump an adequate supply of blood to meet the body's metabolic needs;

c. **thromboembolism** related to:
   1. stasis of blood in the cardiac chambers associated with incomplete emptying
   2. formation of mural thrombi on the infarcted endocardium
   3. venous stasis associated with peripheral pooling of blood if activity restrictions are prolonged;

d. **rupture of a portion of the heart (e.g. ventricular free wall, interventricular septum, papillary muscle)** related to thinning and weakening of the necrotic area in the myocardium;

e. **pericarditis** related to an inflammatory response to myocardial necrosis;

f. **infarct extension or recurrence** related to insufficient myocardial blood supply to meet the myocardial oxygen requirements associated with decreased cardiac output or reocclusion of coronary artery(ies);

g. **cardiogenic shock** related to inability of damaged heart, intrinsic compensatory mechanisms, and treatment measures to maintain adequate tissue perfusion to vital organs associated with extensive damage to the left ventricle, severe heart failure, severe or prolonged arrhythmias, or rupture of the ventricle wall.

| Desired Outcomes | Nursing Actions and ***Selected Purposes/Rationales*** |
|---|---|
| 5.a. The client will not experience cardiac arrhythmias as evidenced by:<br>1. regular apical pulse at 60-100 beats/minute<br>2. equal apical and radial pulses<br>3. absence of syncope and palpitations<br>4. ECG reading showing normal sinus rhythm. | 5.a.1. Assess for and report signs and symptoms of cardiac arrhythmias (e.g. irregular apical pulse; pulse rate below 60 or above 100 beats/minute; apical-radial pulse deficit; syncope; palpitations; abnormal rate, rhythm, or configurations on ECG).<br>2. Implement measures to improve cardiac output (see Nursing Diagnosis 1, action c) *in order to promote adequate myocardial tissue perfusion and oxygenation and reduce the risk of cardiac arrhythmias.*<br>3. If cardiac arrhythmias occur:<br>a. initiate cardiac monitoring if not still being done<br>b. administer the following medications if ordered:<br>1. Class I antiarrhythmics (e.g. lidocaine, quinidine, procainamide, tocainide, moricizine) *to delay the rate of depolarization*<br>2. Class II antiarrhythmics (e.g. esmolol, propranolol) *to block the effects of beta-adrenergic stimulation on the heart*<br>3. Class III antiarrhythmics (e.g. bretylium, amiodarone) *to prolong repolarization and the duration of the action potential*<br>4. Class IV antiarrhythmics (e.g. verapamil) *to block the slow calcium channels, which then prolongs conduction and refractory period in AV node and depresses automaticity in SA and AV nodes*<br>5. anticholinergic agents (e.g. atropine) *to increase heart rate if bradycardia is present*<br>c. restrict client's activity based on his/her tolerance and severity of arrhythmia<br>d. maintain oxygen therapy as ordered<br>e. prepare client for electrophysiological studies (EPS) if planned *to diagnose the conduction problem or evaluate the effectiveness of antiarrhythmic agents*<br>f. assess cardiovascular status frequently and report signs and symptoms of inadequate tissue perfusion (e.g. decline in B/P; cool, clammy, mottled skin; cyanosis; diminished peripheral pulses; declining urine output; increased restlessness and agitation; shortness of breath)<br>g. prepare client for the following if planned:<br>1. cardioversion<br>2. insertion of a pacemaker or automatic implantable cardioverter defibrillator (AICD)<br>3. electrode catheter ablation or surgical resection of irritable site<br>h. have emergency cart readily available for defibrillation or cardiopulmonary resuscitation. |
| 5.b. The client will not develop heart failure as evidenced by:<br>1. pulse 60-100 beats/minute<br>2. absence of an $S_3$ heart sound and summation gallop<br>3. usual mental status<br>4. normal breath sounds<br>5. absence of or no | 5.b.1. Assess for and report signs and symptoms of heart failure:<br>a. tachycardia<br>b. presence of an $S_3$ heart sound or summation gallop<br>c. increased restlessness or anxiousness, confusion<br>d. crackles (rales)<br>e. development of or increased shortness of breath<br>f. cough<br>g. diminished or absent peripheral pulses<br>h. increased weakness and fatigue<br>i. cool, diaphoretic skin<br>j. oliguria<br>k. weight gain<br>l. peripheral edema |

increase in dyspnea and orthopnea
6. absence of cough
7. palpable peripheral pulses
8. increased strength and activity tolerance
9. skin warm and dry
10. balanced intake and output
11. stable weight
12. absence of peripheral edema; distended neck veins; and enlarged, tender liver.

m. distended neck veins
n. enlarged, tender liver.

2. Monitor chest x-ray results. Report findings of cardiomegaly, pleural effusion, or pulmonary edema.
3. Implement measures *to prevent heart failure:*
   a. perform actions to improve cardiac output (see Nursing Diagnosis 1, action c)
   b. perform actions to treat cardiac arrhythmias if present (see action a.3 in this diagnosis) *because arrhythmias contribute to the development of heart failure.*
4. If signs and symptoms of heart failure occur:
   a. continue with above actions
   b. administer the following medications if ordered:
      1. diuretics and vasodilators *to decrease cardiac workload*
      2. morphine sulfate *to reduce preload and anxiety* (used primarily in clients with pulmonary edema)
   c. refer to Care Plan on Heart Failure for additional care measures.

5.c. The client will not develop a thromboembolism as evidenced by:
1. absence of pain, tenderness, heaviness, numbness, and swelling in extremities
2. usual temperature and color of extremities
3. palpable peripheral pulses
4. usual mental status
5. usual sensory and motor function
6. absence of sudden chest pain and dyspnea.

5.c.1. Assess for and report signs and symptoms of:
   a. deep vein thrombus (e.g. pain, tenderness, heaviness, swelling, unusual warmth, and/or positive Homan's sign in extremity)
   b. arterial embolus (e.g. diminished or absent peripheral pulses; pallor, coolness, numbness, and/or pain in extremity)
   c. cerebral ischemia (e.g. decreased level of consciousness, alteration in usual sensory and motor function)
   d. pulmonary embolism (e.g. sudden chest pain, dyspnea, increased restlessness and apprehension).
2. Implement measures *to prevent the development of thromboemboli:*
   a. perform actions *to reduce the risk of thrombus formation in the heart:*
      1. implement measures to improve cardiac output (see Nursing Diagnosis 1, action c)
      2. implement measures to treat arrhythmias if present (see action a.3 in this diagnosis)
      3. implement measures to treat heart failure if it occurs (see action b.4 in this diagnosis)
   b. if client remains on bed rest or activity is severely limited for longer than 48 hours, refer to Care Plan on Immobility, Collaborative Diagnosis 12, actions a.1.b and c and a.2.b and c (pp. 149-150) for measures to prevent and treat a deep vein thrombus and pulmonary embolism
   c. administer anticoagulants (e.g. warfarin, heparin) or antiplatelet agents (e.g. low-dose aspirin) if ordered.
3. If signs and symptoms of an arterial embolus occur:
   a. maintain client on bed rest with affected extremity in a level or slightly dependent position *to improve arterial blood flow*
   b. prepare client for diagnostic studies (e.g. Doppler ultrasound, arteriography) if planned
   c. prepare client for the following if planned:
      1. injection of a thrombolytic agent (e.g. streptokinase)
      2. embolectomy
   d. administer anticoagulants (e.g. continuous intravenous heparin, warfarin) if ordered
   e. provide emotional support to client and significant others.
4. If signs and symptoms of cerebral ischemia occur:
   a. maintain client on bed rest with head of bed flat unless contraindicated
   b. provide emotional support to client and significant others

| Desired Outcomes | Nursing Actions and ***Selected Purposes/Rationales*** |
|---|---|
| | c. refer to Care Plan on Cerebrovascular Accident for additional care measures if signs and symptoms persist. |
| 5.d. The client will not experience rupture of any portion of the heart as evidenced by absence of signs of acute heart failure and/or cardiogenic shock (see outcomes b and g in this diagnosis for outcome criteria). | 5.d.1. Assess for and report signs and symptoms of the following:<br>a. papillary muscle rupture (e.g. holosystolic murmur, dyspnea, finding of papillary muscle rupture on echocardiography)<br>b. ventricular septal defect (e.g. holosystolic murmur, parasternal thrill, finding of septal defect on echocardiography and cardiac catheterization)<br>c. cardiac tamponade resulting from ventricular wall rupture (e.g. significant decline in B/P, narrowed pulse pressure, pulsus paradoxus, increased dyspnea, distant or muffled heart sounds, jugular vein distention, increased CVP).<br>2. Assess for and immediately report signs and symptoms of acute heart failure and/or cardiogenic shock (see actions b.1 and 2 and g.1 in this diagnosis) that may occur as a result of rupture of a portion of the heart.<br>3. Implement measures to reduce cardiac workload (see Nursing Diagnosis 1, action c.2) *in order to reduce risk of rupture of the papillary muscle and ventricular free wall or septum.*<br>4. If signs and symptoms of rupture of a portion of the heart occur:<br>a. maintain client on bed rest<br>b. assist with pericardiocentesis if performed<br>c. assist with measures to treat heart failure or cardiogenic shock (see actions b.4 and g.3 in this diagnosis)<br>d. prepare client for surgical intervention (e.g. valve replacement, repair of ventricular septal defect) if planned<br>e. provide emotional support to client and significant others. |
| 5.e. The client will experience resolution of pericarditis if it develops as evidenced by:<br>1. fewer complaints of precordial pain<br>2. absence of pericardial friction rub<br>3. unlabored respirations at 14-20/minute<br>4. temperature declining toward normal<br>5. WBC count and sedimentation rate declining toward normal range. | 5.e.1. Assess for and report signs and symptoms of pericarditis:<br>a. precordial pain that frequently radiates to shoulder, neck, back, and arm (usually left); is intensified during deep inspiration, movement, and coughing; and usually is relieved by sitting up and leaning forward<br>b. pericardial friction rub (may be transient)<br>c. increased dyspnea, tachypnea<br>d. persistent temperature elevation<br>e. further increase in WBC count and sedimentation rate (both can be elevated as a result of the infarction)<br>f. chest x-ray and echocardiography results showing cardiomegaly and pericardial effusion.<br>2. If signs and symptoms of pericarditis occur:<br>a. allay client's anxiety (client may believe that symptoms indicate recurrent MI)<br>b. assist client to assume position of comfort (usually sitting up and leaning forward on overbed table)<br>c. maintain activity restrictions as ordered<br>d. administer nonsteroidal anti-inflammatory agents (e.g. aspirin) if ordered<br>e. assess for and immediately report signs of cardiac tamponade (e.g. significant decline in B/P, narrowed pulse pressure, pulsus paradoxus, increased dyspnea, distant or muffled heart sounds, jugular vein distention, increased CVP)<br>f. prepare client for and assist with pericardiocentesis if indicated (may be performed if signs of cardiac tamponade are present). |
| 5.f. The client will not experience infarct extension or recurrence as evidenced by: | 5.f. 1. Assess for and report signs and symptoms of infarct extension or recurrence (e.g. recurrent episode of persistent chest pain; significant change in vital signs; further increase in cardiac enzymes; recurrent or further increase in ST segment elevation, T wave changes, and development of a Q wave [if not already present] on ECG). |

1. no further episodes of persistent chest pain
2. stable vital signs
3. cardiac enzyme levels declining toward normal range
4. improved ECG readings.

2. Implement measures to improve cardiac output (see Nursing Diagnosis 1, action c) *in order to reduce risk of infarct extension or recurrence.*
3. If signs and symptoms of myocardial infarction persist, intensify, or recur, continue with measures identified in this care plan.

5.g. The client will not develop cardiogenic shock as evidenced by:
1. stable or improved mental status
2. stable vital signs
3. palpable peripheral pulses
4. stable or improved skin temperature and color
5. urine output at least 30 ml/hour
6. PCWP within normal range.

5.g.1. Assess for and immediately report signs and symptoms of cardiogenic shock:
   a. increased restlessness, lethargy, or confusion
   b. systolic B/P below 90 mm Hg
   c. rapid, thready pulse
   d. diminished or absent peripheral pulses
   e. increased coolness and duskiness or cyanosis of skin
   f. urine output less than 30 ml/hour
   g. elevated PCWP.

2. Implement measures *to prevent cardiogenic shock:*
   a. perform actions to improve cardiac output (see Nursing Diagnosis 1, action c)
   b. perform actions to treat cardiac arrhythmias if present (see action a.3 in this diagnosis)
   c. perform actions to treat heart failure if it occurs (see action b.4 in this diagnosis)
   d. perform actions to treat rupture of any portion of the heart if it occurs (see action d.4 in this diagnosis).
3. If signs and symptoms of cardiogenic shock occur:
   a. continue with above actions
   b. maintain client on bed rest
   c. maintain oxygen therapy as ordered
   d. prepare client for diagnostic studies (e.g. echocardiography)
   e. administer the following if ordered:
      1. sympathomimetics (e.g. dopamine, dobutamine, norepinephrine) *to increase cardiac output and maintain arterial pressure*
      2. vasodilators (e.g. nitroprusside, nitroglycerin) *to decrease cardiac workload* (sympathomimetics are given in conjunction with vasodilators *to maintain arterial pressure)*
      3. intravenous fluids (may be given if PCWP is low)
      4. intravenous sodium bicarbonate *to correct acidosis* (reserved for use in severe acidosis when the pH is less than 7.1)
   f. assist with intubation and insertion of hemodynamic monitoring device (e.g. Swan-Ganz catheter) and intra-aortic balloon pump (IABP) if indicated
   g. provide emotional support to client and significant others.

## 6. NURSING DIAGNOSIS: Anxiety

related to severe pain; feeling of suffocation; possibility of severe disability or impending death; unfamiliar environment; and lack of understanding of diagnostic tests, the diagnosis, and treatment plan.

| Desired Outcome | Nursing Actions and ***Selected Purposes/Rationales*** |
|---|---|
| 6. The client will experience a reduction in anxiety as evidenced by:<br>a. verbalization of feeling less anxious and fearful<br>b. usual sleep pattern<br>c. relaxed facial expression and body movements<br>d. stable vital signs<br>e. usual perceptual ability and interactions with others. | 6.a. Assess client for signs and symptoms of anxiety (e.g. verbalization of fears and concerns, insomnia, tenseness, tremors, irritability, restlessness, diaphoresis, tachycardia, tachypnea, facial pallor or flushing, narrowed perceptual field, withdrawal, noncompliance with treatment plan). Validate perceptions carefully, remembering that some behaviors may result from hypoxia.<br>b. Implement measures *to reduce fear and anxiety:*<br>1. provide care in a calm, supportive, confident manner<br>2. if client is having severe pain:<br>a. do not leave alone during period of acute distress<br>b. perform actions to reduce pain (see Nursing Diagnosis 2, action e)<br>3. encourage significant others to project a caring, concerned attitude without obvious anxiousness<br>4. once the period of acute distress has subsided:<br>a. orient client to hospital environment, equipment, and routines; include an explanation of cardiac monitoring devices<br>b. introduce staff who will be participating in client's care; if possible, maintain consistency in staff assigned to his/her care *to provide feelings of stability and comfort with the environment*<br>c. assure client that staff members are nearby; respond to call signal as soon as possible<br>d. keep cardiac monitor out of client's view and the sound turned as low as possible<br>e. encourage verbalization of fear and anxiety; provide feedback<br>f. explain all diagnostic tests<br>g. reinforce physician's explanation of invasive measures that may be performed to improve coronary blood flow (e.g. streptokinase, tissue plasminogen activator [tPA], or anistreplase [APSAC, Eminase] infusion; percutaneous transluminal coronary angioplasty [PTCA]; intra-aortic balloon pump [IABP]) if planned<br>h. reinforce physician's explanations and clarify misconceptions client has about an MI, the treatment plan, and prognosis<br>i. provide a calm, restful environment<br>j. instruct client in relaxation techniques and encourage participation in diversional activities<br>k. assist client to identify specific stressors and ways to cope with them<br>l. administer antianxiety agents if ordered.<br>c. Include significant others in orientation and teaching sessions and encourage their continued support of the client.<br>d. Provide information based on current needs of client and significant others at a level they can understand. Encourage questions and clarification of information provided.<br>e. Consult physician if above actions fail to control fear and anxiety. |

## 7. NURSING DIAGNOSIS: Grieving*

related to loss of normal function of the heart; possible changes in life style, occupation, and roles; and uncertainty of prognosis.

*This diagnostic label includes anticipatory grieving and grieving following the actual losses.

| Desired Outcome | Nursing Actions and ***Selected Purposes/Rationales*** |
|---|---|
| 7. The client will demonstrate beginning progression through the grieving process as evidenced by:<br>a. verbalization of feelings about having had an MI<br>b. expression of grief<br>c. participation in treatment plan and self-care activities<br>d. utilization of available support systems<br>e. verbalization of a plan for integrating prescribed follow-up care into life style. | 7.a. Assess for signs and symptoms of grieving (e.g. change in eating habits, inability to concentrate, insomnia, anger, noncompliance, withdrawal from significant others, denial of MI). Be aware that client's response to the MI will be affected by factors such as previous experience with loss, age, developmental stage, available support systems, spiritual and cultural background, current health status, and significance of MI on his/her future.<br>b. Implement measures *to facilitate the grieving process:*<br>1. assist the client to acknowledge the loss of normal heart function and the need to alter usual life style *so grief work can begin;* assess for factors that may hinder and facilitate acknowledgment<br>2. discuss the grieving process and assist client to accept the phases of grieving as an expected response to an MI<br>3. allow time for client to progress through the phases of grieving (phases vary among theorists but progress from shock and alarm to acceptance); be aware that not every phase is expressed by all individuals, that recurrence of phases is common, and that the grieving process may take months to years<br>4. assist client to identify personal strengths that have helped him/her to cope in previous situations of loss<br>5. perform actions *to promote trust* (e.g. answer questions honestly, provide requested information)<br>6. provide an atmosphere of care and concern (e.g. provide privacy, be available and nonjudgmental, display empathy and respect) *so that client will feel free to verbalize feelings*<br>7. encourage the verbal expression of anger and sadness about having had an MI; recognize displacement of anger and assist client to see the actual cause of angry feelings and resentment<br>8. encourage client to express his/her feelings in whatever ways are comfortable (e.g. writing, drawing, conversation)<br>9. support realistic hope regarding the prognosis<br>10. support behaviors suggesting successful grief work (e.g. verbalizing feelings about loss of normal heart function, expressing sorrow, focusing on ways to adapt to changes)<br>11. explain the phases of the grieving process to significant others; encourage their support and understanding<br>12. facilitate communication between the client and significant others; be aware that they may be in different phases of the grieving process<br>13. provide information regarding counseling services and support groups that might assist client in working through grief<br>14. arrange for a visit from clergy if desired by client.<br>c. Consult physician regarding referral for counseling if signs of dysfunctional grieving (e.g. persistent denial of losses, excessive anger or sadness, hysteria, suicidal behaviors) occur. |

## 8. NURSING DIAGNOSIS: Knowledge deficit

regarding follow-up care.

| Desired Outcomes | Nursing Actions and ***Selected Purposes/Rationales*** |
|---|---|
| 8.a. The client will verbalize a basic | 8.a. Explain a myocardial infarction in terms the client can understand. Utilize appropriate teaching aids (e.g. pictures, videotapes, heart models). Inform |

| Desired Outcomes | Nursing Actions and ***Selected Purposes/Rationales*** |
|---|---|
| understanding of a myocardial infarction. | models). Inform client that it takes approximately 6-8 weeks for the heart to heal after a myocardial infarction. |
| 8.b. The client will demonstrate accuracy in counting pulse. | 8.b.1. Teach client how to count his/her pulse, being alert to the regularity of the rhythm.<br>2. Allow time for return demonstration and accuracy check. |
| 8.c. The client will identify modifiable cardiovascular risk factors and ways to reduce these factors. | 8.c.1. Inform client that the following modifiable factors have been shown to contribute to cardiovascular disease:<br>a. obesity<br>b. hyperlipidemia<br>c. sedentary life style<br>d. smoking<br>e. hypertension<br>f. stressful life style.<br>2. Inform client that alcohol intake should not exceed 1 oz of ethanol (i.e. 2 oz of 100-proof whiskey, 8 oz of wine, 24 oz of beer) a day on a regular basis because there is evidence that excessive alcohol intake contributes to the development of hypertension and some forms of heart disease.<br>3. Assist the client to identify ways he/she can make appropriate changes in life style to reduce the above factors. Provide information about weight reduction plans; stress management classes; and cardiovascular fitness, smoking cessation, and alcohol rehabilitation programs. Initiate a referral if indicated. |
| 8.d. The client will verbalize an understanding of the rationale for and components of a diet restricted in sodium, saturated fat, and cholesterol. | 8.d.1. Explain the rationale for restricting sodium, saturated fat, and cholesterol intake.<br>2. Provide the following information about decreasing sodium intake:<br>a. be aware that the terms salt and sodium are often used interchangeably but are not synonymous; there is 40% sodium in table salt<br>b. read food labels and calculate sodium content of items (often expressed in milligrams [2 gm is 2000 mg])<br>c. do not add salt when cooking foods or to prepared foods; use low-sodium herbs and spices if desired<br>d. avoid canned soups and vegetables<br>e. avoid processed convenience foods and commercial sauces<br>f. avoid cured and smoked foods<br>g. avoid salty snack foods.<br>3. Provide the following instructions on ways to reduce intake of saturated fat and cholesterol:<br>a. reduce intake of red meat<br>b. trim visible fat off meat and remove all skin from poultry<br>c. eat no more than 2 whole eggs/week<br>d. avoid commercial baked goods<br>e. avoid dairy products containing more than 1% fat.<br>4. Obtain a dietary consult to assist client in planning meals that will meet the prescribed limitations of sodium, saturated fat, and cholesterol. |
| 8.e. The client will verbalize an understanding of medications ordered including rationale, side effects, schedule for taking, and importance of taking as prescribed. | 8.e.1. Explain the rationale for, side effects of, and importance of taking the medications prescribed.<br>2. If client is discharged on nitroglycerin, instruct to:<br>a. avoid drinking alcoholic beverages<br>b. have tablets readily available at all times<br>c. take a tablet before strenuous activity and in emotionally stressful situations<br>d. take one tablet when chest pain occurs and another every 5 minutes up to a total of 3 times if necessary; notify physician if pain persists<br>e. place tablet under tongue and allow it to dissolve thoroughly before swallowing<br>f. store tablets in a cool place in a light-resistant, airtight container; |

when opening bottle for initial use, remove cotton plug and do not replace it
   g. replace tablets every 5 months or sooner if they do not relieve discomfort or do not cause a slight tingling/stinging sensation at sublingual site
   h. avoid rising to a standing position quickly after taking nitroglycerin in order to reduce dizziness associated with its vasodilatory effect
   i. recognize that dizziness, flushing, and mild headache may occur after taking nitroglycerin; instruct client to notify physician if fainting occurs or headache persists more than a few days.
3. If nitroglycerin skin patches are prescribed:
   a. provide instructions about correct application, skin care, need to rotate sites, and frequency of change
   b. caution client that activities that increase blood flow to the skin (e.g. hot bath or shower, sauna) can cause a sudden reduction in blood pressure.
4. If client is discharged on a beta-adrenergic blocking agent (e.g. propranolol, metoprolol, atenolol), instruct to:
   a. take the medication at the same time every day
   b. check pulse before taking medication; consult physician before taking medication if pulse rate is unusually slow (it is expected that pulse will be lower than normal)
   c. avoid skipping doses, altering the prescribed dose, trying to make up for missed doses, and discontinuing medication without physician's permission
   d. change from a lying to a sitting or standing position slowly if dizziness is a problem
   e. limit intake of alcoholic beverages
   f. take medication 1 hour after meals if gastrointestinal distress occurs and report continued problems
   g. monitor blood glucose on a regular basis if a diabetic (beta blockers may affect blood sugar).
5. Instruct client to take antilipemic agents (e.g. lovastatin, gemfibrozil, pravastatin, simvastatin) and antiplatelet agents (e.g. aspirin) as prescribed.
6. Instruct client to consult physician before taking other prescription and nonprescription medications.
7. Instruct client to inform all health care providers of medications being taken.

8.f. The client will verbalize an understanding of activity restrictions and the rate at which activity can be progressed.

8.f. 1. Reinforce physician's instructions about activity. Instruct client to:
   a. gradually increase activity tolerance by adhering to a regular exercise program (often begins with walking)
   b. take frequent rest periods for about 4-8 weeks after discharge
   c. avoid physical conditioning programs such as jogging and aerobic dancing until advised by physician
   d. avoid isometric exercise/activities (e.g. weight lifting, pushing, straining)
   e. avoid activity immediately after meals and in extreme heat or cold
   f. stop any activity that causes chest pain, shortness of breath, palpitations, dizziness, or extreme fatigue or weakness
   g. begin cardiovascular fitness program when approved by physician.
2. Reinforce instructions regarding sexual activity:
   a. sexual activity with usual partner can be resumed after the prescribed length of time (many physicians consider a client ready to resume sexual activity when he/she is able to climb 2 flights of stairs briskly without dyspnea or angina)
   b. assume a comfortable and unstrenuous position for intercourse (e.g. side-lying, partner on top)
   c. a new sexual relationship can be started but may result in greater

| Desired Outcomes | Nursing Actions and ***Selected Purposes/Rationales*** |
|---|---|
| | energy expenditure until it becomes a more familiar or usual experience<br>d. take nitroglycerin before sexual activity in order to prevent angina<br>e. avoid intercourse for 1-2 hours after a heavy meal or alcohol consumption<br>f. avoid sexual activity when fatigued or stressed<br>g. avoid hot or cold showers just before and after intercourse. |
| 8.g. The client will state signs and symptoms to report to the health care provider. | 8.g. Instruct the client to report:<br>1. chest, arm, neck, or jaw pain unrelieved by nitroglycerin<br>2. shortness of breath<br>3. significant weight gain or swelling of feet or ankles<br>4. irregular pulse or a significant unexpected change in the pulse rate<br>5. persistent impotence or decreased libido (can be a side effect of certain medications or result from anxiety, depression, or fatigue)<br>6. inability to tolerate prescribed activity. |
| 8.h. The client will identify community resources that can assist with cardiac rehabilitation and adjustment to the effects of a myocardial infarction. | 8.h.1. Provide information on community resources and support groups that can assist client with cardiac rehabilitation and adjustment to the effects of an MI (e.g. American Heart Association, "coronary clubs," counseling services).<br>2. Initiate a referral if indicated. |
| 8.i. The client will verbalize an understanding of and a plan for adhering to recommended follow-up care including future appointments with health care provider. | 8.i. 1. Reinforce the importance of keeping follow-up appointments with health care provider and for stress testing.<br>2. Implement measures to improve client compliance:<br>a. include significant others in teaching sessions if possible<br>b. encourage questions and allow time for reinforcement and clarification of information provided<br>c. provide written instructions on future appointments with health care provider, dietary modifications, activity progression, medications prescribed, and signs and symptoms to report. |

# Pacemaker Insertion

A pacemaker is an electrical device used to stimulate the heart to beat regularly when a person has symptomatic SA-AV node conduction disturbances. Pacemakers are implanted to treat bradyarrhythmias, particularly complete heart block, sick sinus syndrome, and certain tachyarrhythmias that have been refractory to medical treatment and are resulting in diminished cardiac output.

Pacemakers are either temporary or permanent. Temporary pacemakers are used in emergency situations to regulate the heart rate. Temporary pacing can be done externally by using transcutaneous pacing electrodes or, more frequently, by implanting a temporary pacemaker catheter via a transvenous or transthoracic approach and regulating it with an external pacemaker device.

Permanent pacemakers are utilized for long-term management of certain arrhythmias. There are a number of permanent programmable pacemakers available. They are described by a 3- or 5-letter code established by the Inter-Society Commission for Heart Disease (ICHD). The code specifies the chamber being paced, the chamber being sensed, mode of response (triggered or inhibited), programmability, and antitachycardia functions.

The two components of a permanent pacemaker are the pacemaker electrode catheter and a pulse generator. Permanent pacemakers can be single- or dual-chambered. With a single-chambered pacemaker, the pacing catheter is placed in one chamber (usually the ventricle), whereas dual-chambered pacemakers have electrodes placed in both the atrium and the ventricle and a programmed AV interval. The pulse generator is implanted in the subcutaneous tissue in the chest or the abdomen. Insertion of a permanent pacemaker is most commonly performed using local anesthesia and a transvenous approach. Most pacemakers implanted at this time have a lithium battery that lasts 7 to 10 years.

**This care plan focuses on the adult client hospitalized for transvenous insertion of a permanent pacemaker under local anesthesia.** Preoperative goals of care are to maintain adequate cardiac output and assist the client to adjust psychologically to the idea of having a permanent pacemaker. Postoperatively, the goals of care are to prevent complications and educate the client regarding follow-up care.

## DIAGNOSTIC TESTS

Electrocardiogram (ECG)
Electrophysiological studies (EPS)

## DISCHARGE CRITERIA

Prior to discharge, the client will:

- ❖ have adequate cardiac output
- ❖ have no signs and symptoms of complications
- ❖ verbalize a basic understanding of the rationale for and function of a permanent pacemaker
- ❖ demonstrate knowledge of how to monitor pacemaker function
- ❖ demonstrate the ability to correctly perform range of motion exercises of arm and shoulder on the side of pacemaker insertion
- ❖ identify appropriate safety precautions associated with having a permanent pacemaker
- ❖ state signs and symptoms to report to the health care provider
- ❖ verbalize an understanding of and a plan for adhering to recommended follow-up care including future appointments with health care provider, medications prescribed, wound care, and activity restrictions.

## NURSING/COLLABORATIVE DIAGNOSES

**Preoperative**

1. Decreased cardiac output△ *399*
2. Anxiety△ *400*

**Postoperative**

1. Potential complications:
   - **a.** pacemaker malfunction: failure to capture, fire, or sense
   - **b.** myocardial perforation△ *401*
2. Knowledge deficit△ *402*

**See Standardized Preoperative and Postoperative Care Plans for additional diagnoses.**

## PREOPERATIVE

**Use in conjunction with the Standardized Preoperative Care Plan.**

### 1. NURSING DIAGNOSIS: Decreased cardiac output

related to abnormal heart rate and/or rhythm associated with altered myocardial conductivity.

**Desired Outcome**

1. The client will maintain adequate cardiac output as evidenced by:
   a. systolic B/P of at least 90 mm Hg
   b. palpable peripheral pulses
   c. no increase in number or duration of syncopal episodes
   d. no further decline in mental status
   e. absence of mottling and cyanosis
   f. urine output at least 30 ml/hour.

**Nursing Actions and *Selected Purposes/Rationales***

1.a. Assess client upon admission for baseline data regarding status of cardiac output. Expect that many of the following signs and symptoms of arrhythmias and low cardiac output will be present:
   1. B/P less than 110/70 mm Hg or below normal for client
   2. irregular pulse
   3. pulse rate less than 60 or greater than 100 beats/minute
   4. fatigue and weakness
   5. diminished peripheral pulses
   6. vertigo, syncope
   7. restlessness, change in mental status
   8. tachypnea, exertional dyspnea
   9. cool, pale skin
   10. capillary refill time greater than 3 seconds.

b. Monitor ECG readings and report worsening of or additional arrhythmias.

c. Reassess cardiac status frequently and report the following signs and symptoms that may indicate the need for emergency pacemaker insertion:
   1. systolic B/P below 90 mm Hg
   2. absent peripheral pulses
   3. prolonged or increased frequency of syncopal episodes
   4. persistent decline in mental status
   5. mottling, cyanosis
   6. urine output less than 30 ml/hour.

d. Implement measures *to maintain an adequate cardiac output before surgery:*
   1. perform actions *to reduce cardiac workload:*
      a. maintain activity restrictions as ordered
      b. place client in a semi- to high Fowler's position
      c. implement measures *to promote emotional rest* (e.g. reduce fear and anxiety)
      d. maintain oxygen therapy as ordered
      e. discourage smoking *(smoke has a cardiostimulatory effect, causes vasoconstriction, and reduces oxygen availability)*
   2. instruct client to avoid activities that create a Valsalva response (e.g. straining to have a bowel movement, holding breath while moving) *in order to reduce vagal stimulation and the subsequent slowing of heart rate and prevent the sudden increase in cardiac workload that occurs with exhalation*
   3. administer the following medications if ordered:
      a. antiarrhythmics (e.g. procainamide, disopyramide, quinidine, lidocaine) *to treat tachyarrhythmias*
      b. anticholinergic agents (e.g. atropine) or sympathomimetics (e.g. isoproterenol) *to increase heart rate*
   4. notify physician if serum potassium level is abnormal *(abnormal potassium levels affect myocardial conductivity)*
   5. if client has heart block, consult physician before giving prescribed digitalis preparations *(digitalis preparations delay AV node conductivity)*
   6. maintain transcutaneous external pacing if ordered.

## 2. NURSING DIAGNOSIS: Anxiety

related to unfamiliar environment, lack of understanding of surgical procedure, anticipated postoperative discomfort, possibility of pacemaker malfunction, and possible changes in life style as a result of having a pacemaker.

| Desired Outcome | Nursing Actions and ***Selected Purposes/Rationales*** |
|---|---|
| 2. The client will experience a reduction in anxiety (see Standardized Preoperative Care Plan, Nursing Diagnosis 1 [pp. 108-109], for outcome criteria). | 2.a. Refer to Standardized Preoperative Care Plan, Nursing Diagnosis 1 (pp. 105-109), for measures related to assessment and reduction of fear and anxiety.<br>b. Implement additional measures *to reduce fear and anxiety:*<br>1. explain the rationale for and function of a pacemaker; utilize diagrams, pamphlets, and a pacemaker unit if available<br>2. explain that procedure will be performed using local anesthesia<br>3. inform client that pacemakers are electrically safe and are not harmed during usual daily activities<br>4. inform client of the expected life span of the particular pacemaker he/she is to have implanted; depending on the kind to be implanted, explain that only the generator will need to be replaced when the battery gets weak<br>5. discuss the client's concerns regarding whether his/her occupation and hobbies can be continued safely with a pacemaker in place; if the occupation or interests involve contact sports or contact with high-voltage electrical equipment, large running gas or electric motors, magnetic force machines, television or radio transmitters, radiation, or radar equipment, instruct him/her to consult physician about the safety of continuing these activities. |

## POSTOPERATIVE

**Use in conjunction with the Standardized Postoperative Care Plan.**

### 1. COLLABORATIVE DIAGNOSES:

**Potential complications:**

a. **pacemaker malfunction: failure to capture, fire, or sense** related to break in lead wire, pulse generator malfunction, or dislodgment of the pacemaker catheter;

b. **myocardial perforation** related to displacement of the pacemaker catheter associated with excessive arm and shoulder movement in the immediate postoperative period.

| Desired Outcomes | Nursing Actions and ***Selected Purposes/Rationales*** |
|---|---|
| 1.a. The client will experience normal pacemaker function as evidenced by:<br>1. regular pulse at a rate within 2-3 beats of the preset level<br>2. stable B/P<br>3. absence of dizziness, syncope, and dyspnea<br>4. ECG readings showing pacer spikes before the P wave and/or QRS complex when the pulse rate falls | 1.a.1. Ascertain the method of pacing being used and the rate set by the physician in surgery. Use this information when assessing pacemaker function.<br>2. Assess for and report signs and symptoms of pacemaker malfunction:<br>a. apical pulse less than preset pacemaker rate<br>b. significant decline in B/P<br>c. dizziness, syncope<br>d. dyspnea<br>e. ECG readings showing any of the following:<br>1. absence of pacer spikes when heart rate falls below the preset level<br>2. pacer spikes present with normal P waves and QRS complexes<br>3. absence of P wave (if an atrial pacer) or QRS complex following a pacer spike<br>4. presence of premature beats.<br>3. Implement measures *to prevent pacemaker catheter breakage and dislodgment and subsequent pacemaker malfunction:* |

| Desired Outcomes | Nursing Actions and ***Selected Purposes/Rationales*** |
|---|---|
| below the preset rate. | a. maintain activity restrictions as ordered<br>b. instruct client to limit movement of the arm and shoulder on the side of pacemaker insertion for the first 48 hours after surgery.<br>4. If signs and symptoms of pacemaker malfunction or dislodgment occur:<br>a. turn client to either side *(helps achieve placement of the electrode against the endocardium)*<br>b. follow manufacturer's suggestions for problem solving (e.g. have a pacemaker magnet readily available to test function and convert sensing mechanism to fixed rate mode if necessary)<br>c. prepare client for chest x-ray to check pacemaker catheter placement<br>d. prepare client for surgical repair or replacement of pacemaker if indicated<br>e. provide emotional support to client and significant others. |
| 1.b. The client will not experience myocardial perforation as evidenced by:<br>1. absence of hiccoughing and intercostal muscle twitching<br>2. stable vital signs<br>3. audible heart sounds<br>4. absence of jugular vein distention. | 1.b.1. Assess for and report signs and symptoms of perforation of the myocardium by the pacemaker catheter:<br>a. hiccoughs and/or twitching of the intercostal muscles<br>b. significant decline in B/P, narrowed pulse pressure, pulsus paradoxus, dyspnea, distant or muffled heart sounds, jugular vein distention *(indicative of cardiac tamponade)*.<br>2. Implement measures to prevent pacemaker dislodgment (see action a.3 in this diagnosis) *in order to prevent myocardial perforation.*<br>3. If signs and symptoms of myocardial perforation occur:<br>a. prepare client for chest x-ray<br>b. prepare client for repositioning or replacement of pacemaker catheter, repair of perforation, and/or pericardiocentesis if planned<br>c. provide emotional support to client and significant others. |

## 2. NURSING DIAGNOSIS: Knowledge deficit

regarding follow-up care.

| Desired Outcomes | Nursing Actions and ***Selected Purposes/Rationales*** |
|---|---|
| 2.a. The client will verbalize a basic understanding of the rationale for and function of a permanent pacemaker. | 2.a. Reinforce preoperative teaching regarding the rationale for and basic function of a permanent pacemaker. |
| 2.b. The client will demonstrate knowledge of how to monitor pacemaker function. | 2.b.1. Teach the client how to count his/her pulse, being alert to the regularity of the rhythm. Allow time for return demonstration and accuracy check.<br>2. Inform client of pacemaker's set rate.<br>3. Instruct client to check resting pulse at least once a week or more frequently if experiencing prepacemaker symptoms.<br>4. Instruct client to have pulse generator function checked regularly per physician's instructions or if experiencing prepacemaker symptoms. Inform client that monitoring may be done at the physician's office or by a telephone monitoring device. |
| 2.c. The client will demonstrate the ability to correctly perform range of motion | 2.c.1. Teach client range of motion exercises for arm and shoulder on the side of pacemaker insertion. Instruct client to perform range of motion exercises at least 3 times/day and to do the exercises slowly and gently in order to prevent dislodgment of the pacemaker catheter. |

| Outcome | Nursing Actions |
|---|---|
| exercises of arm and shoulder on the side of pacemaker insertion. | 2. Allow adequate time for questions, clarification, and return demonstration. |
| 2.d. The client will identify appropriate safety precautions associated with having a permanent pacemaker. | 2.d. Instruct client to adhere to the following safety precautions:<br>1. avoid activities that may cause blunt trauma to the pulse generator (e.g. contact sports, firing rifle with butt end of a gun against affected shoulder)<br>2. avoid pressure on the insertion site and pulse generator (e.g. do not wear constrictive clothing or purse strap over the shoulder on operative side)<br>3. avoid close proximity with high-voltage electrical equipment, television and radio transmitters, radar equipment, large running gas or electric motors, radiation, and magnetic force machines<br>4. do not place any electrical device directly over pacemaker<br>5. move away from any electrical device if dizziness, lightheadedness, or decline in pulse rate occurs; caution client that some store antitheft devices may also affect pacemaker function<br>6. if planning to travel, obtain name of a physician and/or pacemaker clinic at point(s) of destination<br>7. alert airport personnel to pacemaker (the pacemaker may set off the security alarm) and request a seat away from the galley since most meals are heated in a large microwave oven<br>8. always wear a Medic-Alert tag and carry a pacemaker identification card; identification card should have insertion date, model and serial number of pacemaker, ICHD code, and rate setting. |
| 2.e. The client will state signs and symptoms to report to the health care provider. | 2.e.1. Refer to Standardized Postoperative Care Plan, Nursing Diagnosis 21, action c (p. 135), for signs and symptoms to report to the health care provider.<br>2. Instruct client to report these additional signs and symptoms:<br>a. irregular pulse<br>b. pulse rate lower than the pacemaker's preset rate<br>c. unexplained fatigue<br>d. lightheadedness, dizziness, fainting spell<br>e. shortness of breath<br>f. swelling of feet and ankles<br>g. chest pain<br>h. hiccoughing lasting more than 2 hours. |
| 2.f. The client will verbalize an understanding of and a plan for adhering to recommended follow-up care including future appointments with health care provider, medications prescribed, wound care, and activity restrictions. | 2.f. 1. Refer to Standardized Postoperative Care Plan, Nursing Diagnosis 21 (pp. 135-136), for routine postoperative instructions and measures to improve client compliance.<br>2. Instruct client to progress activity as tolerated.<br>3. Instruct client to limit vigorous movement of arms and shoulders and avoid heavy lifting the first 6 weeks after surgery. |

UNIT

# X

# *Nursing Care of the Client with Disturbances of Peripheral Vascular Function*

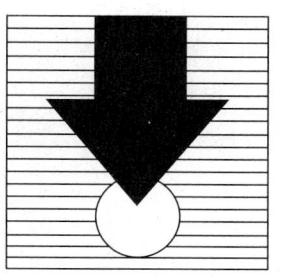

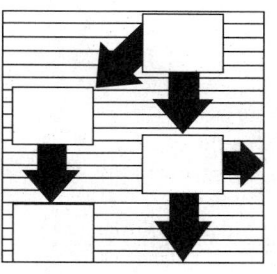

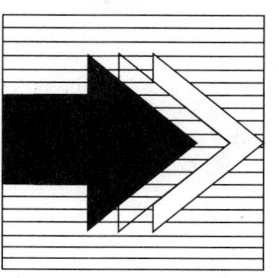

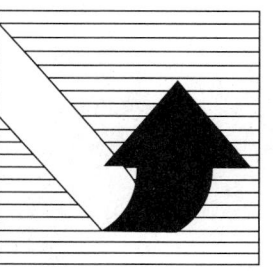

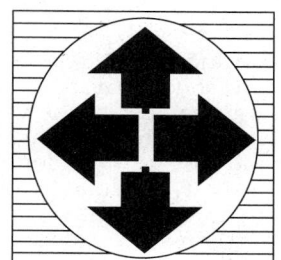

# Abdominal Aortic Aneurysm Repair

An abdominal aortic aneurysm is an abnormal dilation of the wall of the abdominal aorta. The aneurysm usually develops in the segment of the vessel that is between the renal arteries and the iliac branches of the aorta. The most common cause of an abdominal aortic aneurysm is atherosclerosis. The plaque that forms on the wall of the artery causes degenerative changes in the medial layer of the vessel, which leads to weakening and eventual dilation of the affected segment. Some other causes of abdominal aortic aneurysm include trauma, cystic medial necrosis, and bacterial infection. Surgical repair of the aneurysm is usually performed when the aneurysm reaches a size of 5 cm or larger or when the client experiences symptoms such as mild to severe abdominal or low back pain and/or lower extremity arterial insufficiency.

**This care plan focuses on the adult client hospitalized for surgical repair of an abdominal aortic aneurysm.** Preoperatively, goals of care are to reduce fear and anxiety and decrease the risk of aneurysm rupture. The goals of postoperative care are to maintain comfort, prevent complications, and educate the client regarding follow-up care.

## DIAGNOSTIC TESTS

Abdominal x-ray
Abdominal ultrasound
Abdominal aortography
Computed tomography (CT)
Magnetic resonance imaging (MRI)

## DISCHARGE CRITERIA

Prior to discharge, the client will:

- have no signs and symptoms of complications
- identify modifiable factors that increase the risk of vascular disease and ways to reduce these factors
- state signs and symptoms to report to the health care provider
- verbalize an understanding of and a plan for adhering to recommended follow-up care including future appointments with health care provider, medications prescribed, activity level, and wound care.

## NURSING/ COLLABORATIVE DIAGNOSES

**Preoperative**

**1.** Anxiety△ *407*
**2.** Potential complications:
  **a.** hypovolemic shock
  **b.** distal arterial embolization△ *407*

**Postoperative**

**1.** Altered fluid and electrolyte balance:
  **a.** third-spacing of fluid
  **b.** fluid volume excess or water intoxication
  **c.** fluid volume deficit
  **d.** hypokalemia, hypochloremia, and/or metabolic alkalosis△ *409*
**2.** Potential complications:
  **a.** hypovolemic shock
  **b.** lower extremity arterial embolization
  **c.** bowel ischemia
  **d.** impaired renal function△ *410*
**3.** Sexual dysfunction△ *412*
**4.** Knowledge deficit△ *413*

**See Standardized Preoperative and Postoperative Care Plans for additional diagnoses.**

## PREOPERATIVE

**Use in conjunction with the Standardized Preoperative Care Plan.**

### 1. NURSING DIAGNOSIS: Anxiety

related to:
a. unfamiliar environment and separation from significant others;
b. lack of understanding of diagnostic tests, surgical procedure, and postoperative care;
c. anticipated loss of control, effects of anesthesia, and postoperative discomfort;
d. risk of disease if blood transfusions are necessary;
e. potential change in sexual functioning;
f. possibility of death.

| Desired Outcome | Nursing Actions and ***Selected Purposes/Rationales*** |
|---|---|
| 1. The client will experience a reduction in anxiety (see Standardized Preoperative Care Plan, Nursing Diagnosis 1 [pp. 108-109], for outcome criteria). | 1.a. Refer to Standardized Preoperative Care Plan, Nursing Diagnosis 1 (pp. 108-109), for measures related to the assessment and reduction of fear and anxiety.<br>b. Implement additional measures *to reduce fear and anxiety:*<br>1. explain all diagnostic tests<br>2. orient client to intensive care unit if appropriate<br>3. describe and explain the rationale for equipment and tubes that may be present postoperatively (e.g. cardiac monitor, ventilator, intravenous and intra-arterial lines, nasogastric tube, urinary catheter)<br>4. explain that B/P may be taken in both arms and thighs in order to better evaluate circulatory status<br>5. establish an alternative method of communicating with client (e.g. paper and pencil, magic slate) if he/she is expected to be on a ventilator postoperatively (mechanical ventilatory support is occasionally needed for 1-2 days following this major surgery)<br>6. reinforce physician's explanations and clarify misconceptions client has about effects of the surgery on sexual functioning (impotence can result from diminished blood flow in the internal iliac arteries during or after surgery and/or damage to the inferior mesenteric plexus during surgery). |

### 2. COLLABORATIVE DIAGNOSES: Potential complications:

a. **hypovolemic shock** related to excessive blood loss if the aneurysm ruptures;
b. **distal arterial embolization** related to mobilization of a thrombus from the aneurysm site.

| Desired Outcomes | Nursing Actions and ***Selected Purposes/Rationales*** |
|---|---|
| 2.a. The client will not develop hypovolemic shock as evidenced by:<br>1. usual mental status<br>2. stable vital signs | 2.a.1. Assess for and immediately report signs and symptoms of conditions that indicate impending aneurysm rupture:<br>a. leaking aneurysm:<br>1. increasing abdominal girth<br>2. ecchymosis of scrotum, perineum, or penis |

| Desired Outcomes | Nursing Actions and ***Selected Purposes/Rationales*** |
|---|---|
| 3. skin warm, dry, and usual color<br>4. palpable peripheral pulses<br>5. urine output at least 30 ml/hour. | 3. frank or occult gastrointestinal bleeding *(occurs if there is erosion into the duodenum)*<br>4. declining RBC, Hct, and Hb levels<br>5. new or increased complaints of lumbar, abdominal, pelvic, or groin pain *(accumulation of blood causes irritation of and pressure on the tissues and nerves)*<br>6. diminishing peripheral pulses<br>7. further decline in thigh B/P as compared with B/P in arm (thigh B/P is usually slightly lower than B/P in arm of a client with an abdominal aortic aneurysm)<br>b. expanding aneurysm:<br>1. new or increased complaints of lumbar, flank, or groin pain *(results from pressure on lumbar nerves)*<br>2. increased size of pulsating mass in abdomen<br>3. increasing sense of abdominal and/or gastric fullness *(results from pressure on duodenum)*<br>4. decreasing motor or sensory function of lower extremities *(results from pressure on lumbar and/or sacral nerves).*<br>2. Assess for and report signs and symptoms of hypovolemic shock:<br>a. restlessness, agitation, confusion<br>b. significant decrease in B/P<br>c. postural hypotension<br>d. rapid, thready pulse<br>e. rapid respirations<br>f. cool, moist skin<br>g. pallor, cyanosis<br>h. diminished or absent peripheral pulses<br>i. urine output less than 30 ml/hour.<br>3. Implement measures *to decrease risk of aneurysm rupture:*<br>a. instruct client to avoid elevating legs when in bed, using knee gatch, sitting for prolonged periods, and crossing legs *in order to prevent restriction of peripheral blood flow and subsequent increase in pressure on aneurysm site*<br>b. perform actions *to prevent an increase in blood pressure:*<br>1. limit client's activity as ordered<br>2. instruct client to avoid activities that create a Valsalva response (e.g. straining to have a bowel movement, holding breath while moving, lifting heavy objects)<br>3. implement measures to reduce fear and anxiety (see Preoperative Nursing Diagnosis 1)<br>c. administer antihypertensives if ordered *to reduce pressure in the dilated vessel.*<br>4. If signs and symptoms of hypovolemic shock occur:<br>a. place client flat in bed unless contraindicated<br>b. monitor vital signs frequently<br>c. administer oxygen as ordered<br>d. administer blood products and/or volume expanders as ordered (these need to be used with caution *since increased vascular pressure can extend a tear at site of rupture)*<br>e. prepare client for insertion of hemodynamic monitoring devices (e.g. central venous catheter, intra-arterial catheter) if indicated<br>f. prepare client for emergency surgical repair of aneurysm if indicated<br>g. provide emotional support to client and significant others. |
| 2.b. The client will not experience distal arterial embolization as evidenced by: | 2.b.1. Assess for and report signs and symptoms of distal arterial embolization (e.g. diminished or absent peripheral pulses; cool, pale, or mottled extremities; colicky or diffuse abdominal pain; new or increased lumbar, groin, or lower extremity pain). |

| Desired Outcomes | Nursing Actions and *Selected Purposes/Rationales* |
|---|---|
| 1. palpable peripheral pulses<br>2. usual temperature and color of lower extremities<br>3. absence of or no increase in abdominal, lumbar, groin, or lower extremity pain. | 2. Implement measures to prevent an increase in or reduce B/P (see actions a.3.b and c in this diagnosis) *in order to reduce risk of embolization.*<br>3. If signs and symptoms of distal arterial embolization occur:<br>a. maintain client on bed rest<br>b. prepare client for diagnostic studies (e.g. Doppler ultrasound, arteriography) if planned<br>c. administer anticoagulants (e.g. continuous intravenous heparin, warfarin) if ordered<br>d. prepare client for embolectomy if planned<br>e. provide emotional support to client and significant others. |

## POSTOPERATIVE

**Use in conjunction with the Standardized Postoperative Care Plan.**

### 1. NURSING/COLLABORATIVE DIAGNOSIS:

### Altered fluid and electrolyte balance:

a. **third-spacing of fluid** related to increased capillary permeability in surgical area associated with extensive dissection of tissue during major abdominal surgery;
b. **fluid volume excess or water intoxication** related to:
   1. vigorous fluid replacement
   2. increased secretion of antidiuretic hormone (output of ADH is stimulated by trauma, pain, anesthetic agents, and narcotic analgesics)
   3. reabsorption of third-space fluid (occurs about the 3rd postoperative day)
   4. fluid retention associated with renal insufficiency (can occur if there is inadequate blood flow to the kidneys during or after surgery);
c. **fluid volume deficit** related to blood loss, loss of fluid associated with nasogastric tube drainage, and inadequate fluid replacement;
d. **hypokalemia, hypochloremia, and/or metabolic alkalosis** related to loss of electrolytes and hydrochloric acid associated with nasogastric tube drainage.

| Desired Outcomes | Nursing Actions and *Selected Purposes/Rationales* |
|---|---|
| 1.a. The client will experience resolution of third-spacing as evidenced by:<br>1. absence of ascites<br>2. B/P and pulse within normal range for client and stable with position change. | 1.a.1. Assess for and report signs and symptoms of third-spacing:<br>a. ascites<br>b. evidence of vascular depletion (e.g. postural hypotension; weak, rapid pulse).<br>2. Monitor serum albumin levels. Report below-normal levels *(albumin maintains plasma colloid osmotic pressure).*<br>3. Implement measures *to prevent further third-spacing and/or promote mobilization of fluid back into the vascular space:*<br>a. perform actions to reduce fluid volume excess (see Standardized Postoperative Care Plan, Nursing Diagnosis 4, action b.3 [p. 117])<br>b. administer salt-poor albumin if ordered *to increase colloid osmotic pressure.*<br>4. Consult physician if signs and symptoms of third-spacing worsen or fail to resolve within expected length of time (reabsorption usually begins on 3rd postoperative day). |
| 1.b. The client will not experience fluid volume excess or water intoxication (see Standardized Postoperative Care | 1.b. Refer to Standardized Postoperative Care Plan, Nursing Diagnosis 4, action b (p. 117), for measures related to assessment, prevention, and treatment of fluid volume excess and water intoxication. |

| Desired Outcomes | Nursing Actions and ***Selected Purposes/Rationales*** |
|---|---|
| Plan, Nursing Diagnosis 4, outcome b [p. 117], for outcome criteria). | |
| 1.c. The client will maintain fluid and electrolyte balance (see Standardized Postoperative Care Plan, Nursing Diagnosis 4, outcome a [pp. 116-117], for outcome criteria). | 1.c. Refer to Standardized Postoperative Care Plan, Nursing Diagnosis 4, action a (pp. 116-117), for measures related to assessment, prevention, and treatment of fluid and electrolyte imbalance. |

## 2. COLLABORATIVE DIAGNOSES:

**Potential complications:**

a. **hypovolemic shock** related to hypovolemia associated with blood loss during surgery, third-space fluid shift, nasogastric tube drainage, inadequate fluid replacement, and hemorrhage if graft separation occurs;
b. **lower extremity arterial embolization** related to dislodgment of necrotic debris or clot from surgical site;
c. **bowel ischemia** related to diminished blood supply to bowel associated with ligation of the inferior mesenteric artery during surgery, hypovolemia, and embolization;
d. **impaired renal function** related to insufficient blood flow to the kidneys associated with hypovolemia and prolonged aortic clamp time.

| Desired Outcomes | Nursing Actions and ***Selected Purposes/Rationales*** |
|---|---|
| 2.a. The client will not develop hypovolemic shock (see Standardized Postoperative Care Plan, Collaborative Diagnosis 19, outcome a [pp. 131-132], for outcome criteria). | 2.a.1. Assess for and report signs and symptoms of leakage at graft site:<br>a. new or expanding hematoma at incision site and/or ecchymosis of the scrotum, perineum, or penis<br>b. increased abdominal girth (can also occur with third-spacing)<br>c. new or increased complaints of lumbar, abdominal, pelvic, or groin pain<br>d. increasing feeling of abdominal and/or gastric fullness unrelated to oral intake<br>e. diminishing or absent peripheral pulses<br>f. decreased motor or sensory function in lower extremities<br>g. declining B/P, increasing pulse<br>h. decreasing RBC, Hct, and Hb values.<br>2. Assess for and report signs and symptoms of hypovolemic shock (see Standardized Postoperative Care Plan, Collaborative Diagnosis 19, action a.3 [p. 132]).<br>3. Implement measures *to prevent hypovolemic shock:*<br>a. perform actions *to prevent or treat hypovolemia:*<br>1. provide maximum fluid intake allowed (a fluid restriction may be ordered *to prevent fluid overload and subsequent pressure on the graft sites)*<br>2. administer blood and/or volume expanders as ordered<br>3. administer salt-poor albumin if ordered *to promote mobilization of fluid back into the vascular space and reduce further third-spacing*<br>b. perform actions *to reduce stress on graft sites in order to prevent graft separation:*<br>1. instruct client to avoid positions that compromise peripheral blood |

flow (e.g. elevating legs when in bed, use of knee gatch, sitting for prolonged periods, crossing legs)
2. implement measures to reduce the accumulation of gastrointestinal gas and fluid, prevent nausea and vomiting, and prevent or control hiccoughs (see Standardized Postoperative Care Plan, Nursing Diagnoses 7.A, action 3; 7.B, action 2; and 7.C [pp. 119-121])
3. implement measures to prevent or treat fluid volume excess and water intoxication (see Standardized Postoperative Care Plan, Nursing Diagnosis 4, action b.3 [p. 117])
4. instruct client to avoid activities that create a Valsalva response (e.g. straining to have a bowel movement, holding breath while moving)
5. instruct client to avoid vigorous coughing; consult physician about an order for an antitussive if indicated
6. administer antihypertensives if ordered *to reduce vascular pressure.*

4. If signs and symptoms of hypovolemic shock occur:
   a. place client flat in bed unless contraindicated
   b. monitor vital signs frequently
   c. administer oxygen as ordered
   d. administer blood products and/or volume expanders if ordered (these need to be used with caution if graft separation is suspected)
   e. prepare client for surgical repair of the graft if indicated
   f. provide emotional support to client and significant others.

2.b. The client will not experience lower extremity arterial embolization as evidenced by:
1. no complaints of pain or diminished sensation in lower extremities
2. palpable peripheral pulses
3. usual temperature and color of extremities.

2.b.1. Assess for and report signs and symptoms of lower extremity arterial embolization:
   a. complaints of pain and/or numbness in lower extremity(ies)
   b. diminishing or absent peripheral pulses (pulses can be absent for 4-12 hours after surgery *as a result of vasospasm)*
   c. cool, pale, or mottled extremities.
2. Implement measures *to reduce risk of embolization:*
   a. limit client's activity as ordered
   b. instruct client to avoid activities that create a Valsalva response (e.g. straining to have a bowel movement, holding breath while moving) *in order to prevent dislodgment of clot.*
3. If signs and symptoms of lower extremity arterial embolization occur:
   a. maintain client on bed rest
   b. prepare client for the following if planned:
      1. diagnostic studies (e.g. Doppler ultrasound, arteriography)
      2. embolectomy
   c. provide emotional support to client and significant others.

2.c. The client will not develop bowel ischemia as evidenced by:
1. absence of blood in stools
2. absence of diarrhea
3. absence of colicky or diffuse abdominal pain
4. soft, nontender abdomen.

2.c.1. Assess for and report signs and symptoms of bowel ischemia (e.g. blood in stools, diarrhea, complaints of colicky or diffuse abdominal pain, distended abdomen).
2. Implement measures to prevent hypovolemic shock and embolization (see actions a.3 and b.2 in this diagnosis) *in order to maintain adequate blood supply to the bowel.*
3. If signs and symptoms of bowel ischemia occur:
   a. administer antimicrobials if ordered
   b. prepare client for the following if planned:
      1. bowel resection (usually performed if client has extensive bowel tissue necrosis or gangrenous patches have developed)
      2. embolectomy
   c. provide emotional support to client and significant others.

2.d. The client will maintain adequate renal function as evidenced by:
1. urine output at least 30 ml/hour

2.d.1. Assess for and report signs and symptoms of impaired renal function (e.g. urine output less than 30 ml/hour, urine specific gravity fixed at or less than 1.010, elevated BUN and serum creatinine levels).
2. Collect a 24-hour urine specimen if ordered. Report decreased creatinine clearance.

| Desired Outcomes | Nursing Actions and ***Selected Purposes/Rationales*** |
|---|---|
| 2. urine specific gravity, BUN, serum creatinine, and creatinine clearance within normal range. | 3. Implement measures to prevent hypovolemic shock (see action a.3 in this diagnosis) *in order to maintain adequate renal blood flow.*<br>4. If signs and symptoms of impaired renal function occur:<br>a. continue with above actions<br>b. administer diuretics if ordered *to increase urine output*<br>c. assess for and report signs of acute renal failure (e.g. oliguria or anuria; weight gain; edema; elevated B/P; lethargy and confusion; increasing BUN and serum creatinine, phosphorus, and potassium levels)<br>d. prepare client for dialysis if indicated<br>e. refer to Care Plan on Renal Failure for additional care measures. |

## 3. NURSING DIAGNOSIS: Sexual dysfunction

related to:

a. decreased libido associated with operative site discomfort and fear of graft site bleeding;
b. impotence associated with:
   1. prolonged reduction in blood flow in the internal iliac arteries (can occur as a result of prolonged aortic clamp time during surgery, persistent hypovolemia, embolization, or graft occlusion)
   2. damage to the inferior mesenteric plexus (can occur during surgery).

| Desired Outcome | Nursing Actions and ***Selected Purposes/Rationales*** |
|---|---|
| 3. The client will demonstrate beginning acceptance of changes in sexual functioning as evidenced by:<br>a. verbalization of a perception of self as sexually acceptable and adequate<br>b. statements reflecting beginning adjustment to the effects of surgery on sexual functioning<br>c. maintenance of relationship with significant other. | 3.a. Assess for signs and symptoms of sexual dysfunction (e.g. verbalization of sexual concerns, alteration in relationship with significant other, limitations imposed by the surgery).<br>b. Provide accurate information about the effects of the surgery on sexual functioning. Encourage questions and clarify misconceptions.<br>c. Implement measures *to promote optimal sexual functioning:*<br>1. facilitate communication between client and his/her partner; focus on feelings the couple share and assist them to identify changes that may affect their sexual relationship<br>2. discuss ways to be creative in expressing sexuality (e.g. massage, fantasies, cuddling)<br>3. arrange for uninterrupted privacy during hospital stay if desired by the couple<br>4. if impotence is a problem:<br>a. encourage client to discuss it and various treatment options (e.g. penile prosthesis) with physician<br>b. suggest alternative methods of sexual gratification if appropriate<br>c. discuss alternative methods of parenting (e.g. adoption) if of concern to client<br>5. if client is concerned that operative site discomfort will interfere with usual sexual activity:<br>a. assure him/her that the discomfort is temporary and will diminish as incision heals<br>b. encourage alternatives to intercourse or use of positions that decrease pressure on the surgical site (e.g. side-lying)<br>6. reinforce the physician's instructions regarding when client can safely resume sexual activity; inform client that the suture line and graft sites should be secure when healing is complete. |

d. Include partner in above discussions and encourage his/her continued support of the client.
e. Consult physician if counseling appears indicated.

**4. NURSING DIAGNOSIS: Knowledge deficit**
regarding follow-up care.

| Desired Outcomes | Nursing Actions and ***Selected Purposes/Rationales*** |
|---|---|
| 4.a. The client will identify modifiable factors that increase the risk of vascular disease and ways to reduce these factors. | 4.a.1. Inform the client of modifiable factors that have been shown to increase the risk of vascular disease:<br>a. obesity<br>b. hyperlipidemia<br>c. sedentary life style<br>d. smoking<br>e. hypertension<br>f. stressful life style.<br>2. Inform client that alcohol intake should not exceed 1 oz of ethanol (i.e. 2 oz of 100-proof whiskey, 8 oz of wine, 24 oz of beer) a day because there is evidence that excessive alcohol intake contributes to the development of hypertension.<br>3. Assist the client to identify ways he/she can make appropriate changes in life style. Provide information about stress management classes and weight loss, smoking cessation, cardiovascular fitness, and alcohol rehabilitation programs if appropriate. Initiate a referral if indicated.<br>4. Provide the following instructions on ways to reduce intake of saturated fat and cholesterol:<br>a. reduce intake of red meat<br>b. trim visible fat off meat and remove all skin from poultry<br>c. eat no more than 2 whole eggs/week<br>d. avoid commercial baked goods<br>e. avoid dairy products containing more than 1% fat.<br>5. Instruct client to take antilipemic agents (e.g. lovastatin, gemfibrozil, pravastatin, simvastatin) if prescribed. |
| 4.b. The client will state signs and symptoms to report to the health care provider. | 4.b.1. Refer to Standardized Postoperative Care Plan, Nursing Diagnosis 21, action c (p. 135), for signs and symptoms to report to the health care provider.<br>2. Instruct client to report these additional signs and symptoms:<br>a. sudden or gradual increase in lower back, flank, groin, or abdominal pain<br>b. coolness or pallor of lower extremities<br>c. increased weakness and fatigue<br>d. decreased urine output<br>e. dark brown, bloody, or persistent diarrhea<br>f. increased bruising of incision site, perineum, scrotum, or penis<br>g. impotence. |
| 4.c. The client will verbalize an understanding of and a plan for adhering to recommended follow-up care including future appointments | 4.c.1. Refer to Standardized Postoperative Care Plan, Nursing Diagnosis 21 (pp. 135-136), for routine postoperative instructions and measures to improve client compliance.<br>2. Reinforce the physician's instructions regarding:<br>a. importance of scheduling adequate rest periods<br>b. ways to prevent constipation and subsequent straining to have a bowel movement (e.g. drink at least 10 glasses of liquid/day unless |

| Desired Outcomes | Nursing Actions and ***Selected Purposes/Rationales*** |
|---|---|
| with health care provider, medications prescribed, activity level, and wound care. | contraindicated, increase intake of foods high in fiber, take stool softeners if necessary)<br>c. the need to avoid prolonged sitting, sexual intercourse, isometric exercise/activity (e.g. lifting objects over 10 pounds, pushing heavy objects), and strenuous exercise for specified length of time (usually 6-12 weeks depending on the activity). |

# Carotid Endarterectomy

Carotid endarterectomy is the surgical removal of atherosclerotic plaque from the intima of the carotid artery. The most common site of plaque formation in the carotid artery is the bifurcation. Access to this extracranial area is gained through an incision along the anterior sternocleidomastoid muscle. Surgery is performed to improve carotid artery blood flow and to reduce the risk of cerebral embolization and stroke.

**This care plan focuses on the adult client hospitalized for a carotid endarterectomy.** Preoperatively, the goals of care are to reduce fear and anxiety and maintain adequate cerebral tissue perfusion. Postoperative goals of care are to prevent complications and educate the client regarding follow-up care.

## DIAGNOSTIC TESTS

Carotid duplex scan
Cerebral angiography
Ocular pneumoplethysmography

## DISCHARGE CRITERIA

Prior to discharge, the client will:

- have adequate cerebral blood flow
- identify ways to prevent or slow the progression of atherosclerosis
- identify ways to manage signs and symptoms resulting from cranial nerve damage if it has occurred
- state signs and symptoms to report to the health care provider
- verbalize an understanding of and a plan for adhering to recommended follow-up care including future appointments with health care provider, medications prescribed, activity level, and wound care.

## NURSING/COLLABORATIVE DIAGNOSES

**Preoperative**



**Postoperative**

**1.** Potential complications:
  **a.** cerebral ischemia
  **b.** respiratory distress

c. cranial nerve injury (particularly the facial, hypoglossal, glossopharyngeal, vagus, and/or accessory nerves)△ *416*

2. Knowledge deficit△ *418*

**See Standardized Preoperative and Postoperative Care Plans for additional diagnoses.**

## PREOPERATIVE

**Use in conjunction with the Standardized Preoperative Care Plan.**

### 1. NURSING DIAGNOSIS: Altered cerebral tissue perfusion

related to:
a. partial or complete occlusion of the carotid artery by atherosclerotic plaque and/or a thrombus;
b. a cerebral embolus.

| Desired Outcome | Nursing Actions and ***Selected Purposes/Rationales*** |
|---|---|
| 1. The client will maintain adequate cerebral tissue perfusion as evidenced by:<br>a. mentally alert and oriented<br>b. absence of dizziness, visual disturbances, and speech impairments<br>c. normal motor and sensory function. | 1.a. Assess client upon admission for baseline data regarding status of cerebral tissue perfusion including:<br>1. level of consciousness<br>2. complaints of dizziness<br>3. presence of visual disturbances<br>4. presence of speech impairments<br>5. motor and sensory function.<br>b. Implement measures *to maintain adequate cerebral tissue perfusion:*<br>1. administer anticoagulants (e.g. heparin, warfarin) or antiplatelet agents (e.g. low-dose aspirin) if ordered *to prevent new or extended thrombus formation and further occlusion of the carotid artery* (these medications might be discontinued before surgery *to reduce the risk of intraoperative and postoperative hemorrhage*)<br>2. perform actions *to prevent hypertension in order to reduce the risk of cerebral embolism:*<br>a. implement measures *to reduce stress* (e.g. reduce fear and anxiety)<br>b. administer antihypertensives as ordered (these medications are sometimes discontinued before surgery *to reduce the risk of a critical drop in B/P during and immediately following surgery*).<br>c. Reassess neurological status frequently and report signs and symptoms of carotid artery occlusion and/or cerebral embolization (e.g. agitation, lethargy, confusion, dizziness, diplopia, ipsilateral blindness, homonymous hemianopsia, slurred speech, expressive aphasia, paresthesias, contralateral hemiparesis or hemiplegia).<br>d. If signs and symptoms of altered cerebral tissue perfusion occur:<br>1. maintain client on bed rest with head of bed flat unless contraindicated<br>2. administer anticoagulants (e.g. continuous intravenous heparin, warfarin) if ordered<br>3. provide emotional support to client and significant others; be aware that presence of signs and symptoms usually necessitates postponement or cancellation of planned surgery<br>4. refer to Care Plan on Cerebrovascular Accident for additional care measures if signs and symptoms persist. |

## POSTOPERATIVE

**Use in conjunction with the Standardized Postoperative Care Plan.**

### 1. COLLABORATIVE DIAGNOSES:

**Potential complications:**

a. **cerebral ischemia** related to:
   1. prolonged carotid artery clamp time during surgery and/or vasospasm associated with clamping and manipulation of cerebral vessels
   2. hypovolemia associated with intraoperative and/or postoperative blood loss
   3. compression of carotid vessels associated with edema and/or development of a hematoma in the operative area
   4. hypotension associated with stimulation of the carotid sinus baroreceptors resulting from surgical manipulation and/or improved blood flow in the carotid artery following surgery
   5. embolization during or after surgery;

b. **respiratory distress** related to airway obstruction associated with tracheal compression (can occur as a result of hematoma formation and/or edema in the surgical area);

c. **cranial nerve injury (particularly the facial, hypoglossal, glossopharyngeal, vagus, and/or accessory nerves)** related to surgical trauma and/or compression of the nerves (can occur as a result of hematoma formation and/or edema).

| Desired Outcomes | Nursing Actions and ***Selected Purposes/Rationales*** |
|---|---|
| 1.a. The client will maintain adequate cerebral blood flow as evidenced by:<br>1. mentally alert and oriented<br>2. absence of dizziness, visual disturbances, and speech impairments<br>3. normal sensory and motor function. | 1.a.1. Assess for and report signs and symptoms of:<br>a. excessive operative site bleeding (e.g. new or expanding hematoma; continued bright red bleeding from incision or drain [a drain is sometimes in place for about 24 hours after surgery]; decreasing RBC, Hct, and Hb levels)<br>b. hypovolemic shock (see Standardized Postoperative Care Plan, Collaborative Diagnosis 19, action a.3 [p. 132])<br>c. cerebral ischemia:<br>1. agitation, irritability, lethargy, confusion<br>2. dizziness<br>3. visual disturbances (e.g. blurred or dimmed vision, diplopia, ipsilateral blindness, homonymous hemianopsia)<br>4. speech impairments (e.g. slurred speech, expressive aphasia)<br>5. paresthesias, paresis, paralysis.<br>2. Implement measures *to prevent cerebral ischemia:*<br>a. perform actions to prevent or treat hypovolemic shock (see Standardized Postoperative Care Plan, Collaborative Diagnosis 19, actions a.4 and 5 [p. 132])<br>b. perform actions *to reduce pressure on carotid vessels:*<br>1. implement measures *to reduce operative site edema:*<br>a. keep head of bed elevated 30° unless contraindicated<br>b. apply ice pack to incisional area as ordered<br>c. administer corticosteroids if ordered<br>2. implement measures *to reduce stress on the suture line and prevent subsequent bleeding and hematoma formation:*<br>a. maintain patency of drain (e.g. keep tubing free of kinks, empty collection device as often as necessary) if present<br>b. instruct client to support head and neck with hands during position changes and to avoid turning head abruptly or hyperextending neck |

c. administer the following medications if ordered *to maintain blood pressure within a safe range:*
   1. antihypertensives *to prevent rupture of the operative vessel or reduce the risk of dislodgment of any existing thrombus* (hypertension may occur *as a result of the underlying disease process or damage to the carotid sinus baroreceptors during surgery*)
   2. sympathomimetics (e.g. dopamine) *to treat hypotension resulting from carotid sinus baroreceptor stimulation.*

3. If signs and symptoms of cerebral ischemia occur:
   a. continue with above measures
   b. maintain client on bed rest with head of bed flat unless contraindicated
   c. provide emotional support to client and significant others
   d. refer to Care Plan on Cerebrovascular Accident for additional care measures if signs and symptoms persist.

1.b. The client will not experience respiratory distress as evidenced by:
1. usual mental status
2. unlabored respirations at 14-20/minute
3. absence of stridor and sternocleidomastoid muscle retraction
4. blood gases within normal range.

1.b.1. Assess for and report:
   a. increased edema or expanding hematoma in surgical area
   b. deviation of trachea from midline
   c. new or increased difficulty swallowing
   d. signs and symptoms of respiratory distress (e.g. restlessness, agitation, rapid and/or labored respirations, stridor, sternocleidomastoid muscle retraction)
   e. abnormal blood gases
   f. significant change in oximetry results.

2. Have tracheostomy and suction equipment readily available.
3. Implement measures *to prevent compression of the trachea and subsequent respiratory distress:*
   a. perform actions to prevent edema and hematoma formation in the operative area (see action a.2.b in this diagnosis)
   b. administer antihypertensives if ordered *(increased B/P can cause excessive pressure in the operative vessel and result in bleeding and hematoma formation).*
4. If signs and symptoms of respiratory distress occur:
   a. place client in a high Fowler's position unless contraindicated
   b. loosen neck dressing if it appears tight
   c. administer oxygen as ordered
   d. assist with intubation or tracheostomy if indicated
   e. prepare client for evacuation of hematoma or surgical repair of the bleeding vessel if indicated
   f. provide emotional support to client and significant others.

1.c. The client will experience beginning resolution of cranial nerve damage if it occurs as evidenced by:
1. gradual return of facial symmetry and usual taste sensation
2. increased ability to chew and swallow
3. improved speech
4. return of usual shoulder movements.

1.c.1. Assess for signs and symptoms of the following:
   a. facial nerve damage (e.g. facial ptosis on affected side, impaired sense of taste)
   b. vagus and glossopharyngeal nerve damage (e.g. loss of gag reflex, difficulty swallowing, hoarseness, inability to speak clearly, asymmetrical movement of soft palate when saying "ah")
   c. hypoglossal nerve damage (e.g. tongue biting when chewing, tongue deviation toward affected side, difficulty swallowing and speaking)
   d. accessory nerve damage (e.g. unilateral shoulder sag, difficulty raising shoulder against resistance).

2. Implement measures to prevent compression of the cranial nerves at the operative site (see actions a.2.b and b.3.b in this diagnosis).
3. If signs and symptoms of cranial nerve damage occur:
   a. if the facial, hypoglossal, vagus, and/or glossopharyngeal nerves are affected:
      1. withhold oral foods/fluids until gag reflex returns and client is better able to chew and swallow *in order to reduce the risk of aspiration;* provide parenteral nutrition or tube feeding if indicated

| Desired Outcomes | Nursing Actions and ***Selected Purposes/Rationales*** |
|---|---|
| | 2. when oral intake is allowed and tolerated:<br>a. implement measures *to improve client's ability to chew and/or swallow:*<br>1. place client in high Fowler's position for meals and snacks<br>2. assist client to select foods that require little or no chewing and are easily swallowed (e.g. custard, eggs, canned fruits, mashed potatoes)<br>3. avoid serving foods that are sticky (e.g. peanut butter, soft bread, bananas)<br>4. serve thick fluids or thicken thin fluids with substances such as "Thick-it," gelatin, or baby cereal<br>5. moisten dry foods with gravy or sauces (e.g. catsup, sour cream, salad dressing)<br>b. instruct client to add extra sweeteners or seasonings to foods/fluids if desired *in order to compensate for impaired sense of taste*<br>3. implement measures *to facilitate communication* (e.g. maintain quiet environment; provide pad and pencil, magic slate, or word cards; listen carefully when client speaks)<br>4. consult speech pathologist about additional ways to facilitate swallowing and communication<br>b. if the accessory nerve is affected, instruct client in and assist with exercises *to prevent atrophy of trapezius and sternocleidomastoid muscles* (e.g. range of motion of affected shoulder, wall climbing with fingers, shoulder shrugs)<br>c. provide emotional support to client and significant others; assure them that the nerve damage is usually not permanent but caution them that the symptoms may take months to resolve. |

## 2. NURSING DIAGNOSIS: Knowledge deficit

regarding follow-up care.

| Desired Outcomes | Nursing Actions and ***Selected Purposes/Rationales*** |
|---|---|
| 2.a. The client will identify ways to prevent or slow the progression of atherosclerosis. | 2.a.1. Inform the client that certain modifiable factors such as hyperlipidemia and hypertension have been shown to increase the risk of atherosclerosis.<br>2. Assist client to identify ways he/she can make appropriate changes in life style to reduce modifiable factors.<br>3. Provide the following instructions on ways to reduce intake of saturated fat and cholesterol:<br>a. reduce intake of red meat<br>b. trim visible fat off meat and remove all skin from poultry<br>c. eat no more than 2 whole eggs/week<br>d. avoid commercial baked goods<br>e. avoid dairy products containing more than 1% fat.<br>4. Instruct client to take antilipemic agents (e.g. lovastatin, colestipol, pravastatin, simvastatin) as prescribed. |
| 2.b. The client will identify ways to manage signs and symptoms | 2.b.1. If signs and symptoms of hypoglossal, facial, vagus, and/or glossopharyngeal nerve damage are present:<br>a. reinforce techniques to improve swallowing and speaking |

| | |
|---|---|
| resulting from cranial nerve damage if it has occurred. | b. assist client in identifying foods that are nutritious and easy to chew and swallow; obtain a dietary consult if needed<br>c. instruct client to increase the amount of sweeteners and seasonings he/she usually uses and/or to try different seasonings in foods and beverages if sense of taste is altered.<br>2. If signs and symptoms of accessory nerve damage are present, reinforce exercises that should be performed to maintain shoulder muscle tone and prevent contractures.<br>3. Allow time for questions, clarification, and return demonstration. |
| 2.c. The client will state signs and symptoms to report to the health care provider. | 2.c.1. Refer to Standardized Postoperative Care Plan, Nursing Diagnosis 21, action c (p. 135), for signs and symptoms to report to the health care provider.<br>2. Instruct client to report these additional signs and symptoms:<br>a. increased swelling or purple discoloration at wound site<br>b. new or increased difficulty chewing, swallowing, or speaking<br>c. any loss of or change in vision<br>d. dizziness<br>e. numbness, tingling, or weakness of arm(s) or leg(s)<br>f. increasing irritability<br>g. lethargy, confusion<br>h. failure of signs and symptoms of cranial nerve damage to resolve as expected. |
| 2.d. The client will verbalize an understanding of and a plan for adhering to recommended follow-up care including future appointments with health care provider, medications prescribed, activity level, and wound care. | 2.d. Refer to Standardized Postoperative Care Plan, Nursing Diagnosis 21 (pp. 135-136), for routine postoperative instructions and measures to improve client compliance. |

# Deep Vein Thrombosis

Venous thrombosis occurs when a thrombus forms in a superficial or deep vein. This condition is often called thrombophlebitis because of the associated inflammation in the involved vessel wall. The predisposing factors for venous thrombus formation are venous stasis, trauma to the endothelium of the vein wall, and/or hypercoagulability. Conditions/factors associated with a high risk for venous thrombosis are surgery (especially orthopedic and urologic surgery), immobility, age (over 40), heart failure, malignancy, fractures or other injuries of lower extremities, varicose veins, severe infections, obesity, and oral contraceptive use.

Deep vein thrombosis usually develops in a lower extremity. Clinical manifestations of deep vein thrombosis are often not distinctive and, in many cases, the client is asymptomatic. Signs and symptoms that may be present include pain, tenderness, feeling of heaviness, swelling, unusual warmth, and/or positive Homan's sign in the involved extremity. The greatest danger associated with deep vein thrombosis is that the clot, or parts of it, will detach and cause embolic occlusion of a pulmonary vessel. Persons with deep vein thrombosis are usually treated medically rather than surgically unless there is massive occlusion of a vessel and it is refractory to medical treatment.

**This care plan focuses on the adult client hospitalized for treatment of deep vein thrombosis in a lower extremity.** The goals of care are to reduce discomfort, promote adequate peripheral circulation, prevent complications, and educate the client regarding follow-up care.

## DIAGNOSTIC TESTS

Duplex ultrasound
Impedance plethysmography
Venography
Coagulation studies

## DISCHARGE CRITERIA

Prior to discharge, the client will:

- ❖ have adequate tissue perfusion in affected extremity
- ❖ identify ways to promote venous blood flow and reduce the risk of chronic venous insufficiency and recurrent thrombus formation
- ❖ verbalize an understanding of medications ordered including rationale, side effects, schedule for taking, and importance of taking as prescribed
- ❖ identify precautions necessary to prevent bleeding associated with anticoagulant therapy
- ❖ state signs and symptoms to report to the health care provider
- ❖ verbalize an understanding of and a plan for adhering to recommended follow-up care including future appointments with health care provider and activity level.

---

**Use in conjunction with the Care Plan on Immobility.**

**NURSING/ COLLABORATIVE DIAGNOSES**



**See Care Plan on Immobility for additional diagnoses.**

---

## 1. NURSING DIAGNOSIS: Altered peripheral tissue perfusion

related to:
a. obstructed venous blood flow in affected extremity associated with the presence of a thrombus and inflammation of the vessel;
b. venous stasis associated with decreased mobility.

| Desired Outcome | Nursing Actions and ***Selected Purposes/Rationales*** |
|---|---|
| 1. The client will have improved venous blood flow in the affected extremity as evidenced by:<br>a. diminished pain, | 1.a. Assess for signs and symptoms of deep vein thrombosis and impaired venous blood flow in the affected extremity:<br>1. pain, tenderness, or heavy feeling in extremity<br>2. increase in circumference of extremity<br>3. distention of superficial blood vessels in extremity<br>4. unusual warmth of extremity. |

tenderness, feeling of heaviness, swelling, and distended superficial blood vessels in extremity
b. usual temperature of extremity.

b. In the acute phase, implement measures *to treat deep vein thrombosis and improve venous blood flow:*
   1. maintain activity restrictions as ordered (client is usually on bed rest for 5-7 days)
   2. elevate affected leg as ordered (some physicians oppose extremity elevation *because they believe it may increase the risk for thrombus dislodgment)*
   3. discourage positions that compromise venous blood flow (e.g. crossing legs, pillows under knees, sitting for long periods)
   4. maintain a minimum fluid intake of 2500 ml/day (unless contraindicated) *to maintain adequate hydration and prevent increased blood viscosity, which leads to venous stasis*
   5. administer anticoagulants (e.g. continuous intravenous heparin, warfarin) as ordered
   6. prepare client for the following if planned:
      a. injection of a thrombolytic agent (e.g. streptokinase, urokinase, tissue plasminogen activator [tPA])
      b. thrombectomy.
c. When ambulation is allowed, implement additional measures *to prevent venous stasis and promote adequate venous blood flow:*
   1. consult physician about an order for elastic stockings; apply before client gets out of bed
   2. instruct client to avoid prolonged sitting or standing.
d. Consult physician if signs and symptoms of deep vein thrombosis and impaired venous blood flow in affected extremity persist or worsen.

---

## 2. NURSING DIAGNOSIS: Pain: affected extremity

related to:
a. decreased tissue perfusion and swelling associated with obstructed venous blood flow;
b. inflammation of vein.

| Desired Outcome | Nursing Actions and ***Selected Purposes/Rationales*** |
|---|---|
| 2. The client will experience diminished pain in the affected extremity as evidenced by:<br>a. verbalization of pain relief<br>b. relaxed facial expression and body positioning<br>c. increased participation in activities when allowed. | 2.a. Determine how the client usually responds to pain.<br>b. Assess client's perception of pain including location, intensity, and type. Utilize a numerical scale to rate intensity.<br>c. Assess for nonverbal signs of pain (e.g. wrinkled brow, rubbing affected area, restlessness, reluctance to move).<br>d. Assess for factors that seem to aggravate and alleviate pain.<br>e. Implement measures *to reduce pain:*<br>1. perform actions to treat deep vein thrombosis and improve venous blood flow (see Nursing Diagnosis 1, actions b and c)<br>2. apply heat to affected area if ordered<br>3. perform actions *to protect the affected extremity from trauma, pressure, or excessive movement:*<br>a. avoid jarring the bed<br>b. use a bed cradle or footboard *to relieve pressure from bed linens*<br>c. support extremity during position changes<br>d. maintain activity restrictions as ordered<br>e. instruct client to move affected extremity slowly and cautiously<br>4. provide or assist with nonpharmacological measures for pain relief (e.g. position change, relaxation techniques, quiet conversation, restful |

| Desired Outcome | Nursing Actions and ***Selected Purposes/Rationales*** |
|---|---|
| | environment, diversional activities); caution client and significant others that the painful extremity should not be rubbed to relieve pain *(rubbing could dislodge the thrombus)*<br>5. administer analgesics and anti-inflammatory agents if ordered.<br>f. Consult physician if above measures fail to provide adequate pain relief. |

## 3. NURSING DIAGNOSIS: High risk for impaired skin integrity

related to:

a. ischemia of the skin and subcutaneous tissue associated with prolonged pressure on tissues as a result of decreased mobility;
b. damage to the skin and/or subcutaneous tissue associated with friction or shearing;
c. increased skin fragility in affected extremity associated with insufficient blood flow and edema.

| Desired Outcome | Nursing Actions and ***Selected Purposes/Rationales*** |
|---|---|
| 3. The client will maintain skin integrity as evidenced by:<br>a. absence of redness and irritation<br>b. no skin breakdown. | 3.a. Inspect the skin (especially bony prominences, dependent areas, and affected extremity) for pallor, redness, and breakdown.<br>b. Refer to Care Plan on Immobility, Nursing Diagnosis 4, action b (pp. 141-142), for measures to prevent skin breakdown.<br>c. Implement measures *to prevent skin breakdown in involved extremity:*<br>1. perform actions to treat deep vein thrombosis and improve venous blood flow (see Nursing Diagnosis 1, actions b and c)<br>2. perform actions *to protect affected extremity from trauma and/or excessive pressure:*<br>a. use a bed cradle or footboard *to relieve pressure from bed linens*<br>b. keep heel off bed by elevating extremity on foam block or pillows or using heel protector<br>c. instruct and assist client to move affected extremity cautiously<br>d. remove elastic stockings for 30-60 minutes at least twice daily<br>e. use caution when applying heat to extremity.<br>d. If skin breakdown occurs:<br>1. notify physician<br>2. continue with above measures to prevent further irritation and breakdown<br>3. perform decubitus care as ordered or per standard hospital procedure<br>4. implement measures to treat stasis ulcers (e.g. debriding ointments, Unna boot, wet-to-dry dressings)<br>5. assess client closely and report signs and symptoms of infection (e.g. elevated temperature; redness, warmth, and edema around area of breakdown; unusual drainage from site). |

## 4. COLLABORATIVE DIAGNOSES: Potential complications:

a. **pulmonary embolism** related to dislodgment of thrombus;
b. **bleeding** related to prolonged coagulation time associated with anticoagulant therapy.

Desired Outcomes | Nursing Actions and ***Selected Purposes/Rationales***

4.a. The client will not experience a pulmonary embolism as evidenced by:
1. absence of sudden chest pain
2. unlabored respirations at 14-20/minute
3. pulse 60-100 beats/minute
4. usual mental status
5. blood gases within normal range.

4.a.1. Assess for and report signs and symptoms of a pulmonary embolism (e.g. sudden chest pain, dyspnea, tachypnea, tachycardia, restlessness, apprehension, low $PaO_2$).
2. Implement measures *to prevent a pulmonary embolism:*
   a. perform actions *to prevent dislodgment of thrombus:*
      1. maintain client on bed rest as ordered
      2. do not exercise or check for Homan's sign in affected extremity during acute phase of deep vein thrombosis
      3. never massage affected extremity and caution client not to allow significant others to massage extremity
      4. caution client to avoid activities that create a Valsalva response (e.g. straining to have a bowel movement, holding breath while moving)
   b. administer anticoagulants (e.g. continuous intravenous heparin, warfarin) as ordered
   c. prepare client for a vena caval interruption (e.g. insertion of an intracaval filtering device) if planned.
3. If signs and symptoms of a pulmonary embolism occur:
   a. maintain client on strict bed rest in a semi- to high Fowler's position
   b. maintain oxygen therapy as ordered
   c. prepare client for diagnostic tests (e.g. blood gases, ventilation-perfusion lung scan, pulmonary angiography)
   d. administer anticoagulants (e.g. continuous intravenous heparin, warfarin) as ordered
   e. prepare client for the following if planned:
      1. injection of a thrombolytic agent (streptokinase, urokinase, tissue plasminogen activator [tPA])
      2. vena caval interruption (e.g. insertion of an intracaval filtering device) *to prevent further pulmonary emboli*
      3. embolectomy
   f. provide emotional support to client and significant others
   g. refer to Care Plan on Pulmonary Embolism for additional care measures.

4.b. The client will not experience unusual bleeding as evidenced by:
1. skin and mucous membranes free of petechiae, purpura, ecchymoses, and active bleeding
2. absence of unusual joint pain
3. no increase in abdominal girth
4. absence of frank and occult blood in stool, urine, and vomitus
5. usual menstrual flow
6. vital signs within normal range for client
7. stable Hct and Hb.

4.b.1. Assess client for and report signs and symptoms of unusual bleeding:
   a. petechiae, purpura, ecchymoses
   b. gingival bleeding
   c. prolonged bleeding from puncture sites
   d. epistaxis, hemoptysis
   e. unusual joint pain
   f. increase in abdominal girth
   g. frank or occult blood in stool, urine, or vomitus
   h. menorrhagia
   i. restlessness, confusion
   j. declining B/P and increased pulse rate
   k. decline in Hct and Hb levels.
2. Monitor platelet count and coagulation test results (e.g. prothrombin time, activated partial thromboplastin time, partial thromboplastin time). Report a low platelet count and coagulation test results that exceed the therapeutic range.
3. If platelet count is low, coagulation test results are abnormal, or Hct and Hb levels decline, test all stool, urine, and vomitus for occult blood. Report positive results.
4. Implement measures *to prevent bleeding:*
   a. use the smallest gauge needle possible when giving injections and performing venous and arterial punctures
   b. apply gentle, prolonged pressure after injections and venous and arterial punctures

| Desired Outcomes | Nursing Actions and ***Selected Purposes/Rationales*** |
|---|---|
| | c. take B/P only when necessary and avoid overinflating the cuff<br>d. caution client to avoid activities that increase the risk for trauma (e.g. shaving with a straight-edge razor, using stiff-bristle toothbrush or dental floss)<br>e. pad side rails if client is confused or restless<br>f. avoid procedures that can cause injury to rectal mucosa (e.g. inserting a rectal suppository or tube, administering an enema)<br>g. perform actions *to reduce the risk for falls* (e.g. keep bed in low position with side rails up when client is in bed, avoid unnecessary clutter in room, instruct client to wear shoes with nonslip soles when ambulating)<br>h. instruct client to avoid blowing nose forcefully or straining to have a bowel movement; consult physician about an order for a decongestant, stool softener, and/or laxative if indicated.<br>5. If bleeding occurs and does not subside spontaneously:<br>a. apply firm, prolonged pressure to bleeding area(s) if possible<br>b. if epistaxis occurs, place client in a high Fowler's position and apply pressure and ice pack to nasal area<br>c. maintain oxygen therapy as ordered<br>d. perform gastric lavage as ordered *to control gastric bleeding*<br>e. administer protamine sulfate (antidote for heparin), vitamin K (e.g. phytonadione), and plasma or whole blood as ordered<br>f. assess for and report signs and symptoms of hypovolemic shock (e.g. restlessness; confusion; significant decrease in B/P; rapid, thready pulse; rapid respirations; cool, pale skin; urine output less than 30 ml/hour)<br>g. prepare client for surgical repair of bleeding vessels if indicated<br>h. provide emotional support to client and significant others. |

## 5. NURSING DIAGNOSIS: Knowledge deficit

regarding follow-up care.

| Desired Outcomes | Nursing Actions and ***Selected Purposes/Rationales*** |
|---|---|
| 5.a. The client will identify ways to promote venous blood flow and reduce the risk of chronic venous insufficiency and recurrent thrombus formation. | 5.a. Provide the following instructions on ways to promote venous blood flow and reduce the risk for chronic venous insufficiency (can result from residual vein damage) and recurrent thrombus development:<br>1. avoid wearing constrictive clothing (e.g. garters, girdles, narrow-banded knee-high hose)<br>2. avoid sitting and standing in one position for long periods of time<br>3. wear graduated compression stockings or support hose during the day<br>4. avoid crossing legs and lying or sitting with pillows under knees<br>5. engage in regular aerobic exercise (e.g. swimming, walking, bicycling)<br>6. elevate legs periodically, especially when sitting<br>7. dorsiflex feet regularly<br>8. maintain an ideal body weight for age, height, and body frame<br>9. avoid smoking and use of oral contraceptives (these are risk factors for thrombus formation). |
| 5.b. The client will verbalize an | 5.b.1. Explain the rationale for, side effects of, and importance of taking medications prescribed. |

| | |
|---|---|
| understanding of medications ordered including rationale, side effects, schedule for taking, and importance of taking as prescribed. | 2. If client is discharged on a coumarin derivative (e.g. warfarin), instruct to:<br>a. keep scheduled appointments for periodic blood studies to monitor coagulation times<br>b. take medication at the same time each day, do not stop taking medication abruptly, and do not attempt to make up for missed doses<br>c. avoid taking over-the-counter products containing aspirin or other salicylates (these products enhance the action of coumarins)<br>d. avoid regular and/or excessive intake of alcohol (may alter responsiveness to coumarins)<br>e. avoid eating large amounts of foods high in vitamin K (e.g. green leafy vegetables)<br>f. report prolonged or excessive bleeding from skin, nose, or mouth; blood in urine, vomitus, sputum, or stool; prolonged or excessive menses; excessive bruising; severe headache; or sudden abdominal or back pain<br>g. inform physician immediately if pregnancy is suspected (coumarin crosses the placental barrier)<br>h. wear a Medic-Alert band identifying self as being on anticoagulant therapy.<br>3. Instruct client to inform physician of any other prescription and nonprescription medications he/she is taking.<br>4. Instruct client to inform all health care providers of medications being taken. |
| 5.c. The client will identify precautions necessary to prevent bleeding associated with anticoagulant therapy. | 5.c.1. Instruct client about ways to minimize risk of bleeding:<br>a. use an electric rather than straight-edge razor<br>b. floss and brush teeth gently<br>c. avoid putting sharp objects (e.g. toothpicks) in mouth<br>d. do not walk barefoot<br>e. cut nails carefully<br>f. avoid situations that could result in injury (e.g. contact sports)<br>g. avoid blowing nose forcefully<br>h. avoid straining to have a bowel movement.<br>2. Instruct client to control any bleeding by applying firm, prolonged pressure to the area if possible. |
| 5.d. The client will state signs and symptoms to report to the health care provider. | 5.d. Instruct client to report:<br>1. recurrent tenderness, pain, or swelling in extremity<br>2. sudden chest pain accompanied by shortness of breath<br>3. unusual bleeding (see action b.2.f in this diagnosis)<br>4. discoloration, unusual dryness, or itching of affected extremity<br>5. skin breakdown on affected extremity. |
| 5.e. The client will verbalize an understanding of and a plan for adhering to recommended follow-up care including future appointments with health care provider and activity level. | 5.e.1. Reinforce importance of keeping follow-up appointments with health care provider.<br>2. Reinforce physician's instructions regarding activity limitations.<br>3. Implement measures to improve client compliance:<br>a. include significant others in teaching sessions if possible<br>b. encourage questions and allow time for reinforcement and clarification of information provided<br>c. provide written instructions regarding future appointments with health care provider, medications prescribed, activity restrictions, signs and symptoms to report, and future laboratory studies. |

# Femoropopliteal Bypass

Lower extremity arterial bypass is performed to treat peripheral artery insufficiency that has not responded well to conservative management. Signs and symptoms that usually indicate the need for surgical intervention include intermittent claudication that has become disabling, foot pain that is present at rest, and/or the presence of lower extremity ischemic ulcers. The impaired blood flow can occur as a result of acute conditions (e.g. trauma, embolization) but most often is caused by atherosclerotic changes in the vessels. The femoropopliteal arterial segment is the most common site of occlusion in persons with lower extremity arterial disease, although significant narrowing of other vascular segments (e.g. aortoiliac, popliteal-tibial, peroneal) can also occur. The diseased femoropopliteal arterial segment can be removed and replaced with a synthetic graft, but the usual procedure is to bypass the segment using a synthetic or, more frequently, an autogenous vein graft. The saphenous vein is the preferred graft for femoropopliteal bypass because it is thick walled and has an adequate lumen diameter. Prior to grafting the saphenous vein proximal and distal to the occluded arterial segment, reversal of the vein or division of its valve cusps is done to allow unimpeded arterial blood flow.

**This care plan focuses on the adult client with atherosclerotic occlusion of the femoropopliteal arterial segment who has been hospitalized for a femoropopliteal bypass.** Preoperatively, goals of care are to reduce fear and anxiety, control pain, and maintain optimal tissue perfusion in the affected lower extremity. The goals of postoperative care are to maintain comfort, prevent complications, and educate the client regarding follow-up care.

## DIAGNOSTIC TESTS

Duplex ultrasound
Plethysmography
Arteriography of affected lower extremity
Magnetic resonance imaging (MRI)
Segmental limb pressure measurements

## DISCHARGE CRITERIA

Prior to discharge, the client will:

- have adequate circulation in the operative extremity
- identify ways to prevent or slow the progression of atherosclerosis
- identify ways to promote blood flow in the operative extremity
- state signs and symptoms to report to the health care provider
- verbalize an understanding of and a plan for adhering to recommended follow-up care including future appointments with health care provider, medications prescribed, activity level, and wound care.

## NURSING/ COLLABORATIVE DIAGNOSES

**Preoperative**

1. Altered peripheral tissue perfusion△ *427*
2. Pain: intermittent claudication and rest pain△ *427*

**Postoperative**

1. Altered peripheral tissue perfusion△ *428*
2. Potential complications:
   a. graft occlusion
   b. compartment syndrome
   c. saphenous nerve damage△ *429*
3. Knowledge deficit△ *431*

**See Standardized Preoperative and Postoperative Care Plans for additional diagnoses.**

## PREOPERATIVE

**Use in conjunction with the Standardized Preoperative Care Plan.**

### 1. NURSING DIAGNOSIS: Altered peripheral tissue perfusion

related to diminished blood flow in the affected lower extremity associated with atherosclerotic changes in the femoral and popliteal arteries.

| Desired Outcome | Nursing Actions and ***Selected Purposes/Rationales*** |
|---|---|
| 1. The client will not experience further reduction in arterial blood flow in the affected lower extremity as evidenced by:<br>a. no increase in lower extremity pain<br>b. no further decrease in or absence of peripheral pulses<br>c. no increase in capillary refill time<br>d. usual temperature and color of extremity. | 1.a. Assess for signs and symptoms of a further reduction in arterial blood flow in the affected lower extremity:<br>1. intermittent claudication occurring with increased intensity and/or with less activity than previously<br>2. development of or increase in intensity of rest pain (the foot and toe pain that occurs when the client is resting in a horizontal position results from decreased blood flow to the skin and subcutaneous tissue; because it occurs in the absence of lower extremity muscle activity, it reflects a severe reduction in the femoropopliteal arterial blood flow)<br>3. diminishing peripheral pulses<br>4. increase in usual capillary refill time<br>5. increased coolness and cyanosis of foot and lower leg<br>6. higher level of and/or more rapid appearance of rubor when affected extremity is in a dependent position.<br>b. Implement measures *to prevent further reduction in and/or improve blood flow in the affected lower extremity:*<br>1. discourage positions that compromise blood flow in lower extremities (e.g. crossing legs, pillows under knees, use of knee gatch, elevating legs when in bed, sitting for long periods)<br>2. perform actions *to prevent vasoconstriction:*<br>a. implement measures *to reduce stress* (e.g. maintain a calm environment, control pain, explain preoperative and postoperative care)<br>b. discourage smoking<br>c. implement measures *to keep client from getting cold* (e.g. maintain a comfortable room temperature; provide adequate clothing, warm socks, and blankets)<br>3. encourage short walks as tolerated<br>4. administer pentoxifylline (Trental) if ordered *to improve capillary blood flow.*<br>c. Consult physician if signs and symptoms of further reduction in lower extremity tissue perfusion occur. |

### 2. NURSING DIAGNOSIS: Pain: intermittent claudication and rest pain

related to diminished arterial blood flow in the affected lower extremity (ischemia results in the release of anaerobic metabolites that irritate the nerve endings of the affected lower extremity).

| Desired Outcome | Nursing Actions and ***Selected Purposes/Rationales*** |
|---|---|
| 2. The client will experience diminished lower extremity pain as evidenced by:<br>a. verbalization of same<br>b. relaxed facial expression and body positioning. | 2.a. Determine how the client usually responds to pain.<br>b. Assess for signs and symptoms of pain in the affected lower extremity:<br>1. intermittent claudication (e.g. complaints of pain, aching, and/or cramping [usually in the calf muscle] during ambulation)<br>2. rest pain (e.g. awakening at night with complaints of severe burning or aching in foot or toes)<br>3. wrinkled brow, restlessness, reluctance to move, and/or rubbing lower leg or foot.<br>c. Assess for factors that aggravate and alleviate pain.<br>d. Implement measures *to reduce pain in the affected extremity:*<br>1. perform actions to prevent further reduction in and/or improve blood flow in the affected lower extremity (see Preoperative Nursing Diagnosis 1, action b)<br>2. perform actions *to reduce the number of episodes of intermittent claudication:*<br>a. encourage client to stop activity minutes before he/she usually experiences symptoms (intermittent claudication is predictable and the client is often aware of how far or how long he/she can ambulate before the discomfort begins or intensifies)<br>b. maintain client on bed rest if he/she is experiencing severe intermittent claudication *(limiting activity decreases muscle contractions in and subsequent ischemia of the affected lower extremity)*<br>3. if client is experiencing rest pain in the affected extremity, perform actions *to facilitate gravity flow of arterial blood to the ischemic area:*<br>a. allow client to sleep in a recliner with legs in a dependent position or, if in bed, to hang affected lower leg over the side of bed<br>b. instruct client to avoid horizontal positioning and elevation of affected extremity for prolonged periods<br>4. provide or assist with nonpharmacological measures for relief of pain (e.g. relaxation techniques, position change, quiet conversation, diversional activity)<br>5. administer analgesics if ordered.<br>e. Consult physician if above measures fail to provide adequate pain relief. |

## POSTOPERATIVE

**Use in conjunction with the Standardized Postoperative Care Plan.**

### 1. NURSING DIAGNOSIS: Altered peripheral tissue perfusion

related to diminished blood flow in the operative extremity associated with:

a. trauma to the surrounding vessels during surgery;
b. inflammation of the femoral and popliteal arteries at the sites of graft anastomosis;
c. pressure on vessels in the operative extremity resulting from edema that can occur as a result of decreased venous return and dissection around perivascular lymphatics;
d. venous stasis resulting from decreased mobility and decreased venous return if the saphenous vein was used for the bypass graft (can result in impaired venous return until collateral venous circulation improves).

| Desired Outcome | Nursing Actions and ***Selected Purposes/Rationales*** |
|---|---|
| 1. The client will maintain adequate tissue perfusion in the operative extremity as evidenced by:<br>a. resolution of leg and foot pain<br>b. palpable peripheral pulses<br>c. adequate Doppler flow readings in operative extremity<br>d. absence of coolness and cyanosis in foot and lower leg<br>e. resolution of edema in operative extremity<br>f. capillary refill time less than 3 seconds. | 1.a. Assess for and report signs and symptoms of diminished tissue perfusion in operative extremity:<br>1. pain unrelieved by prescribed analgesics<br>2. diminished or absent pulses (the pulses may be difficult to palpate *because of vasospasm that can occur for 4-12 hours after surgery and edema in the operative extremity)*<br>3. diminished or absent Doppler flow readings over operative extremity<br>4. coolness or cyanosis of foot and lower leg<br>5. increase in edema in the operative extremity<br>6. capillary refill time greater than 3 seconds.<br>b. Implement measures *to promote adequate tissue perfusion in operative extremity:*<br>1. avoid 90° flexion of the hip as much as possible (e.g. place client in high Fowler's position for meals only, limit length of time that client is in straight-back chair, provide recliner for client's use when sitting up)<br>2. limit length of time that operative leg is in dependent position (e.g. allow client to sit up for meals only; encourage short, frequent walks rather than long walks)<br>3. maintain knee in a neutral or slightly flexed position<br>4. if lower extremity edema is present, elevate foot of bed 15° as ordered *to promote venous return without compromising arterial flow*<br>5. place a bed cradle over lower extremities *to minimize pressure from bed linens*<br>6. instruct client to perform active foot and leg exercises every 1-2 hours while awake<br>7. perform actions *to prevent vasoconstriction:*<br>a. implement measures *to reduce stress* (e.g. control pain, maintain a calm environment, explain postoperative care)<br>b. discourage smoking<br>c. implement measures *to keep client from getting cold* (e.g. maintain a comfortable room temperature; provide adequate clothing, warm socks, and blankets).<br>c. Consult physician if signs and symptoms of diminished tissue perfusion in the operative extremity persist or worsen. |

## 2. COLLABORATIVE DIAGNOSES:

**Potential complications:**

a. **graft occlusion** related to thrombus formation, kink in graft, or inadequate vessel diameter at sites of anastomosis;
b. **compartment syndrome** related to leg edema associated with surgical site inflammation resulting from surgical trauma, reperfusion of the ischemic muscles, or dissection around the perivascular lymphatics;
c. **saphenous nerve damage** related to surgical trauma or actual nerve dissection during surgery.

| Desired Outcomes | Nursing Actions and ***Selected Purposes/Rationales*** |
|---|---|
| 2.a. The client will not experience graft | 2.a.1. Assess for and report signs and symptoms of graft occlusion in the operative extremity (e.g. sudden, severe pain in toes or foot; |

| Desired Outcomes | Nursing Actions and ***Selected Purposes/Rationales*** |
|---|---|
| occlusion in the operative extremity as evidenced by:<br>1. no complaints of sudden, severe toe or foot pain<br>2. palpable peripheral pulses<br>3. capillary refill time less than 3 seconds<br>4. absence of cyanosis, coolness, and diminishing sensation in the foot. | diminishing or absent peripheral pulses; capillary refill time greater than 3 seconds; cyanosis, coolness, or diminished sensation in the foot).<br>2. Avoid prolonged flexion of the knee (e.g. limit sitting as ordered, do not place pillows under knees when in bed) *to prevent kinking of graft and thrombus formation.*<br>3. If signs and symptoms of graft occlusion occur:<br>a. maintain client on bed rest with operative leg in horizontal position<br>b. prepare client for surgical intervention (e.g. thrombectomy, straightening of graft, widening of lumen at site[s] of anastomosis) if planned<br>c. provide emotional support to client and significant others. |
| 2.b. The client will not experience compartment syndrome in the operative extremity as evidenced by:<br>1. no complaints of increasing leg pain<br>2. no statements of new or increasing numbness and tingling in foot or leg or tightness and tenseness of thigh or calf muscle<br>3. ability to move leg and foot<br>4. no decrease in or absence of peripheral pulses<br>5. absence of cyanosis and coldness of leg and foot. | 2.b.1. Assess for and report signs and symptoms of compartment syndrome in the operative extremity:<br>a. complaints of increasing leg pain<br>b. statements of new or increasing numbness and tingling in foot or leg or tightness and tenseness of thigh or calf muscle<br>c. difficulty moving foot<br>d. diminishing or absent peripheral pulses<br>e. cyanotic, cold foot and leg.<br>2. Implement measures *to prevent or treat edema in operative leg in order to reduce the risk of development of compartment syndrome:*<br>a. limit length of time that operative leg is in a dependent position (e.g. limit sitting and walking as ordered)<br>b. elevate operative extremity 15° if ordered<br>c. administer osmotic diuretics (e.g. mannitol) if ordered.<br>3. If signs and symptoms of compartment syndrome occur:<br>a. maintain client on bed rest<br>b. assess for and report brown discoloration of urine *(could indicate myoglobinuria resulting from the release of myoglobin from the damaged muscle cells; if an excessive amount of myoglobin is released, it can get trapped in the renal tubules and cause renal failure)*<br>c. prepare client for a fasciotomy if planned<br>d. provide emotional support to client and significant others. |
| 2.c. The client will have resolution of or adapt to operative extremity saphenous nerve damage if it has occurred. | 2.c.1. Assess for and report signs and symptoms of saphenous nerve damage (e.g. numbness, tingling, or hypersensitivity of the operative extremity).<br>2. If signs and symptoms of saphenous nerve damage are present:<br>a. adhere to and instruct client in the following safety precautions:<br>1. wear shoes or slippers whenever out of bed<br>2. do not apply heat or cold to the affected extremity<br>3. test temperature of bath water before use<br>4. protect operative extremity from trauma<br>b. reinforce information from physician regarding permanence of numbness, tingling, or hypersensitivity (these symptoms are permanent if the nerve was severed intentionally or inadvertently during surgery; if the nerve was just traumatized, the symptoms are temporary and expected to resolve within 1 year)<br>c. consult physician if signs and symptoms increase in severity. |

## 3. NURSING DIAGNOSIS: Knowledge deficit

regarding follow-up care.

| Desired Outcomes | Nursing Actions and ***Selected Purposes/Rationales*** |
|---|---|
| 3.a. The client will identify ways to prevent or slow the progression of atherosclerosis. | 3.a.1. Inform the client that certain modifiable factors such as hyperlipidemia and hypertension have been shown to increase the risk of atherosclerosis.<br>2. Assist client to identify ways he/she can make appropriate changes in life style to reduce modifiable factors.<br>3. Provide the following instructions on ways to reduce intake of saturated fat and cholesterol:<br>a. reduce intake of red meat<br>b. trim visible fat off meat and remove all skin from poultry<br>c. eat no more than 2 whole eggs/week<br>d. avoid commercial baked goods<br>e. avoid dairy products containing more than 1% fat.<br>4. Instruct client to take antilipemic agents (e.g. pravastatin, colestipol) as prescribed. |
| 3.b. The client will identify ways to promote blood flow in the operative extremity. | 3.b. Provide the following instructions about ways to promote blood flow in the operative extremity:<br>1. avoid wearing constrictive clothing (e.g. garters, girdles, narrow-banded knee-high stockings)<br>2. avoid positions that compromise blood flow (e.g. pillows under knees, crossing legs, sitting or standing for prolonged periods)<br>3. do active foot and leg exercises for 5 minutes every hour while awake<br>4. maintain a regular exercise program (walking and swimming are recommended)<br>5. stop smoking<br>6. drink at least 10 glasses of liquid/day. |
| 3.c. The client will state signs and symptoms to report to the health care provider. | 3.c.1. Refer to Standardized Postoperative Care Plan, Nursing Diagnosis 21, action c (p. 135), for signs and symptoms to report to the health care provider.<br>2. Instruct client to report these additional signs and symptoms:<br>a. sudden or gradual increase in operative leg or foot pain<br>b. increased swelling or purple discoloration at incision sites<br>c. pallor, coldness, or bluish color of the operative extremity<br>d. diminishing or sudden absence of peripheral pulses (client may be instructed to monitor his/her peripheral pulses)<br>e. significant increase in swelling of operative extremity (edema is expected to resolve gradually in 1-6 weeks)<br>f. difficulty moving foot<br>g. increasing numbness and/or tingling sensation of lower leg or foot. |
| 3.d. The client will verbalize an understanding of and a plan for adhering to recommended follow-up care including future appointments with health care provider, medications prescribed, activity level, and wound care. | 3.d.1. Refer to Standardized Postoperative Care Plan, Nursing Diagnosis 21 (pp. 135-136), for routine postoperative instructions and measures to improve client compliance.<br>2. Reinforce the physician's instructions regarding:<br>a. importance of scheduling adequate rest periods<br>b. need to avoid sitting or standing for long periods. |

UNIT

# XI

# *Nursing Care of the Client with Disturbances of Respiratory Function*

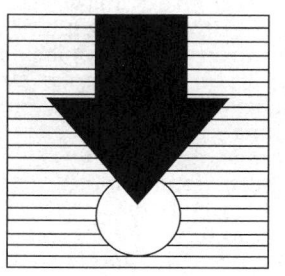

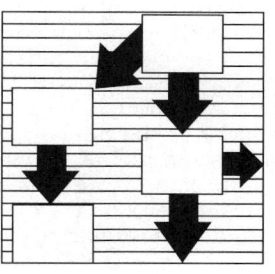

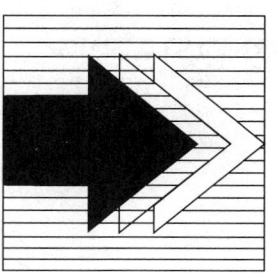

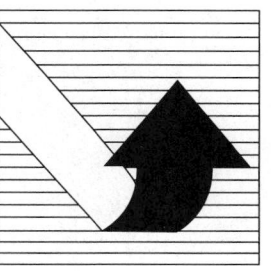

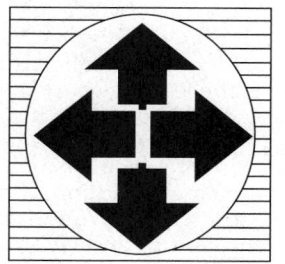

# Cancer of the Lung

Cancer of the lung, a malignant neoplasm involving lung tissue, is the leading cause of cancer-related deaths in the United States today. The rising incidence of cancer of the lung in both men and women is related to several factors, the chief of which is smoking. Other factors include environmental pollution; exposure to carcinogens such as asbestos, radioactive substances, arsenic, nickel, iron oxide, chromium, and chloromethyl ether; genetic factors; and lung scarring from previous inflammatory processes.

Cancer of the lung can occur as a primary tumor or as a metastasis from a primary site elsewhere in the body. The World Health Organization has identified 12 categories of primary lung neoplasms. Over 90% of these arise from the bronchoalveolar surface epithelium and from bronchial mucous glands and can be grouped into small cell lung cancer (SCLC) or one of the three non–small cell types of lung cancer (NSCLC), which include squamous cell (epidermoid) carcinoma, adenocarcinoma, and large cell cancer. These four histological types vary in relation to where they arise in the lung, responsiveness to the major modes of treatment, pattern of spread, clinical course, and prognosis. Squamous cell carcinoma and adenocarcinoma are the most common types. Squamous cell carcinoma is almost always associated with smoking, usually occurs as a central tumor, and produces early symptoms of local disease because of bronchial obstruction. It generally spreads by direct extension to surrounding tissue and has the best 5-year survival rate. Adenocarcinoma occurs most frequently in the periphery of the lungs, has a slow growth rate, tends to invade the pleura, typically does not produce symptoms until late in the course of the disease, and occurs more frequently in women and nonsmokers. Large cell tumors are similar to the squamous cell type, although they tend to arise in the peripheral area of the lung and frequently present with necrotic or cavitary surfaces. Small cell lung carcinoma tends to occur in the hilar or perihilar area, is a systemic disease at the time of diagnosis, and has a very poor prognosis. It is the type most frequently associated with paraneoplastic syndromes, which may predate x-ray evidence of the lung tumor by many months. The regional lymph nodes, bones, brain, liver, and adrenal glands are common sites of metastasis of lung cancer.

The treatment selected depends on the type of tumor and whether or not metastasis has occurred. The treatment of choice for NSCLC is surgical resection of the tumor if feasible. External radiation therapy and brachytherapy may be used as an adjunct to surgery or alone for cure or palliation. Clients who present with metastasis at diagnosis are candidates for chemotherapy. This treatment modality is also used preoperatively to improve the resectability of the tumor. Biotherapy has been used with limited success. The usual treatment for SCLC is aggressive combination chemotherapy because of the systemic nature of the disease at diagnosis. Response of the client primarily depends on the extensiveness of the disease.

**This care plan focuses on care of the adult client with cancer of the lung hospitalized either for staging and initiation of treatment or for management of complications that have developed as a result of the disease process or its treatment.** The goals of care are to reduce fear and anxiety, relieve symptoms associated with the disease process and its treatment, and educate the client regarding follow-up care. If surgery is planned, this care plan should be used in conjunction with the Care Plan on Thoracic Surgery.

## DIAGNOSTIC/STAGING TESTS*

Chest x-ray
Magnetic resonance imaging (MRI)
Computed tomography (CT)
Blood chemistry
Serial sputum cytology
Pulmonary function studies
Blood gases
Bronchoscopy, Mediastinoscopy
Biopsies (may include peripheral nodular lesions; lymph nodes such as scalene, mediastinal, and supraclavicular; pleura; bone marrow)
Barium esophography
Thoracentesis
Radionuclide bone, brain, and liver scans
Pulmonary angiography

*Tests will vary according to the histological type of the tumor and the client's symptoms.

## DISCHARGE CRITERIA

Prior to discharge, the client will:

- have an adequate respiratory status
- have no signs and symptoms of complications
- identify ways to improve oxygenation status and maximize pulmonary health
- demonstrate proper chest physiotherapy techniques and the ability to use the equipment recommended to maximize pulmonary health
- identify ways to minimize the risk of infection
- verbalize ways to improve appetite and maintain an adequate nutritional status
- verbalize ways to manage chronic syndrome of inappropriate antidiuretic hormone (SIADH)
- state signs and symptoms to report to the health care provider
- share thoughts and feelings about the diagnosis of lung cancer, the prognosis, and the effects of the disease process and its treatment on self-concept, life style, and roles
- identify community resources that can assist with home management and adjustment to changes resulting from the diagnosis and the effects of treatment
- verbalize an understanding of and a plan for adhering to recommended follow-up care including future appointments with health care provider, medications prescribed, activity level, and plans for subsequent treatment.

---

**Use in conjunction with the Care Plans on Chemotherapy and External Radiation Therapy if appropriate.**

## NURSING/ COLLABORATIVE DIAGNOSES

**See Care Plans on Chemotherapy and External Radiation Therapy for additional diagnoses.**

## 1. NURSING DIAGNOSIS: Anxiety

related to current signs and symptoms; lack of understanding of the diagnosis, diagnostic tests, and treatment plan; unfamiliar environment; financial concerns; anticipated effects of cancer and its treatment on body functioning and usual life style and roles; and probability of premature death.

| Desired Outcome | Nursing Actions and ***Selected Purposes/Rationales*** |
|---|---|
| 1. The client will experience a reduction in anxiety as evidenced by:<br>a. verbalization of feeling less anxious and fearful<br>b. usual sleep pattern<br>c. relaxed facial expression and body movements<br>d. stable vital signs<br>e. usual perceptual ability and interactions with others. | 1.a. Assess client on admission for:<br>1. fears, misconceptions, and level of understanding about lung cancer, tests to stage the disease, and possible treatment modes<br>2. perception of anticipated results of diagnostic tests and planned treatment<br>3. significance of the diagnosis of lung cancer to client<br>4. availability of an adequate support system<br>5. past experiences with cancer and its treatment<br>6. signs and symptoms of anxiety (e.g. verbalization of fears and concerns, insomnia, tenseness, tremors, irritability, restlessness, diaphoresis, tachycardia, tachypnea, elevated blood pressure, facial pallor or flushing, narrowed perceptual field, withdrawal, noncompliance with treatment plan).<br>b. Refer to Nursing Diagnosis 1, action b (pp. 192 and 219-220), in Care Plans on Chemotherapy and External Radiation Therapy for measures to reduce fear and anxiety associated with the diagnosis and planned treatment program.<br>c. Implement additional measures *to reduce fear and anxiety:*<br>1. explain all diagnostic tests performed to stage lung cancer<br>2. perform actions to reduce pain (see Nursing Diagnosis 5)<br>3. perform actions to improve respiratory status (see Nursing Diagnosis 2, action c) *in order to reduce dyspnea*<br>4. inform client that the amount of blood in sputum does not necessarily correlate with severity of the disease; provide an opaque, covered container for sputum collection *to reduce anxiety associated with hemoptysis*<br>5. perform actions to assist client to cope with the diagnosis and its implications (see Nursing Diagnosis 15).<br>d. Include significant others in orientation and teaching sessions and encourage their continued support of client.<br>e. Provide information based on current needs of client and significant others at a level they can understand. Encourage questions and clarification of information provided.<br>f. Consult physician if above actions fail to control fear and anxiety. |

**2. NURSING DIAGNOSIS: Impaired respiratory function*:**

a. **ineffective breathing pattern** related to:
   1. fear, anxiety, and pain
   2. respiratory depressant effects of some medications (e.g. narcotic analgesics)
   3. restricted lung expansion associated with:
      a. paralysis and/or elevation of hemidiaphragm if the tumor involves the phrenic nerve
      b. pleural effusion if present
      c. weakness
      d. compression of lung tissue by tumor;

b. **ineffective airway clearance** related to:
   1. excessive mucus production associated with inflammation of lung tissue resulting from the disease process
   2. stasis of secretions associated with poor cough effort and decreased activity
   3. airway obstruction associated with the presence of tumor;

c. **impaired gas exchange** related to:
   1. decrease in effective lung surface associated with compression and/or replacement of lung tissue by neoplastic cells
   2. pulmonary shunting associated with extensive pneumonitis or atelectasis if present.

---

*This diagnostic label includes the following nursing diagnoses: ineffective breathing pattern, ineffective airway clearance, and impaired gas exchange.

| Desired Outcome | Nursing Actions and ***Selected Purposes/Rationales*** |
|---|---|
| 2. The client will experience adequate respiratory function as evidenced by:<br>a. normal rate, rhythm, and depth of respirations<br>b. decreased dyspnea<br>c. usual or improved breath sounds<br>d. usual mental status<br>e. usual skin color<br>f. blood gases within normal range. | 2.a. Assess for and report signs and symptoms of impaired respiratory function:<br>1. rapid, shallow, slow, or irregular respirations<br>2. dyspnea, orthopnea<br>3. use of accessory muscles when breathing<br>4. adventitious breath sounds (e.g. crackles [rales], wheezes)<br>5. diminished or absent breath sounds<br>6. restlessness, irritability<br>7. confusion, somnolence<br>8. central cyanosis (a late sign).<br>b. Monitor for and report the following:<br>1. abnormal blood gases<br>2. significant changes in oximetry and chest x-ray results.<br>c. Implement measures *to improve respiratory status:*<br>1. place client in a semi- to high Fowler's position unless contraindicated; position overbed table so client can lean on it if desired<br>2. perform actions to reduce fear and anxiety (see Nursing Diagnosis 1, actions b and c)<br>3. perform actions to reduce pain (see Nursing Diagnosis 5)<br>4. perform actions to increase strength and activity tolerance (see Nursing Diagnosis 7, action b)<br>5. instruct client to breathe slowly if he/she is hyperventilating<br>6. maintain oxygen therapy as ordered<br>7. assist client to turn from side at least every 2 hours while in bed<br>8. instruct client to deep breathe or use incentive spirometer at least every 2 hours<br>9. perform actions *to facilitate removal of pulmonary secretions:*<br>a. instruct and assist client to cough or "huff" every 1-2 hours<br>b. implement measures *to liquefy tenacious secretions:*<br>1. maintain a fluid intake of 2500 ml/day unless contraindicated<br>2. humidify inspired air as ordered |

| Desired Outcome | Nursing Actions and ***Selected Purposes/Rationales*** |
|---|---|
| | c. assist with administration of diluent and mucolytic agents via nebulizer or IPPB treatments as ordered<br>d. assist with or perform postural drainage, percussion, and vibration if ordered<br>e. perform tracheal suctioning if needed<br>10. instruct client to avoid intake of gas-forming foods (e.g. beans, cauliflower, cabbage, onions), carbonated beverages, and large meals *in order to prevent gastric distention and increased pressure on the diaphragm*<br>11. discourage smoking *(smoke causes bronchoconstriction, increases mucus production, impairs ciliary function, and decreases oxygen availability)*<br>12. protect client from exposure to irritants such as smoke, flowers, and perfume *(can cause bronchospasm and increased mucus production)*<br>13. maintain activity restrictions; increase activity as allowed and tolerated<br>14. administer central nervous system depressants judiciously; hold medication and consult physician if respiratory rate is less than 12/minute<br>15. administer the following medications if ordered:<br>a. bronchodilators (e.g. methylxanthines, sympathomimetics)<br>b. corticosteroids *to decrease airway inflammation and thereby improve bronchial airflow*<br>c. chemotherapeutic agents *to reduce the tumor mass*<br>16. assist with thoracentesis if performed *to remove excessive pleural fluid and improve lung expansion*<br>17. prepare client for laser photoresection if planned *to reduce the size of an obstructing central tumor and subsequently relieve dyspnea.*<br>d. Consult physician if signs and symptoms of impaired respiratory function persist or worsen. |

## 3. NURSING DIAGNOSIS: Altered nutrition: less than body requirements

related to:

a. decreased oral intake associated with:
   1. impaired swallowing resulting from oral, pharyngeal, or esophageal pain; esophageal invasion or compression by tumor; or dry mouth and viscous oral secretions
   2. anorexia resulting from factors such as depression, fear, anxiety, fatigue, discomfort, dyspnea, early satiety, and altered sense of taste;

b. loss of nutrients associated with vomiting resulting from administration of cytotoxic agents;

c. impaired utilization of nutrients associated with:
   1. accelerated and inefficient metabolism of proteins, carbohydrates, and fats resulting from the disease process
   2. decreased absorption of nutrients resulting from loss of intestinal absorptive surface if mucositis has developed with the administration of cytotoxic agents
   3. utilization of available nutrients by the malignant cells rather than the host.

| Desired Outcome | Nursing Actions and ***Selected Purposes/Rationales*** |
|---|---|
| 3. The client will maintain an adequate nutritional status (see Care Plan on Chemotherapy, Nursing | 3.a. Refer to Care Plan on Chemotherapy, Nursing Diagnosis 2 (pp. 193-194), for measures related to assessment and maintenance of an adequate nutritional status.<br>b. Place client in a high Fowler's position for meals and provide |

| Desired Outcome | Nursing Actions and ***Selected Purposes/Rationales*** |
|---|---|
| Diagnosis 2 [p. 193], for outcome criteria). | supplemental oxygen therapy during meals if indicated *to help relieve dyspnea.* |

## 4. NURSING DIAGNOSIS: Impaired swallowing

related to:

a. esophageal invasion or compression by tumor;
b. oral, pharyngeal, and esophageal pain (can occur if mucositis develops as a result of administration of cytotoxic agents or radiation therapy to upper chest);
c. dry mouth and viscous oral secretions associated with decreased oral intake and changes in the quantity and quality of saliva resulting from stomatitis if present (can occur as a result of treatment with cytotoxic agents).

| Desired Outcome | Nursing Actions and ***Selected Purposes/Rationales*** |
|---|---|
| 4. The client will experience an improvement in swallowing (see Care Plan on Chemotherapy, Nursing Diagnosis 3 [p. 194], for outcome criteria). | 4. Refer to Care Plan on Chemotherapy, Nursing Diagnosis 3 (p. 194), for measures related to assessment and improvement of impaired swallowing. |

## 5. NURSING DIAGNOSIS: Pain:

a. **tissue and skeletal pain** related to pressure from tumor and enlarged lymph nodes, nerve involvement, excessive coughing episodes, and metastasis to the bone (particularly the ribs, spine, and pelvis) or other organs if it has occurred;
b. **chest pain** related to inflammation and tumor involvement of the parietal pleura and chest wall;
c. **pain within the irradiated area** related to inflammation and exposure of nerve endings associated with moist desquamation if it occurs;
d. **pharyngeal and esophageal pain** related to inflammation and/or ulceration of the mucosa associated with radiation to upper chest and/or side effects of cytotoxic drugs;
e. **oral pain** related to stomatitis associated with the side effects of cytotoxic drugs.

| Desired Outcome | Nursing Actions and ***Selected Purposes/Rationales*** |
|---|---|
| 5. The client will experience diminished pain (see Care Plan on External Radiation Therapy, Nursing Diagnosis 4 [p. 222], for outcome criteria). | 5.a. Refer to Care Plan on External Radiation Therapy, Nursing Diagnosis 4 (pp. 222-223), for measures related to assessment and management of pain.<br>b. Implement additional measures *to reduce pain:*<br>1. perform actions *to reduce skeletal pain:*<br>a. move client carefully; obtain adequate assistance when needed<br>b. when turning client, logroll and support all extremities<br>c. utilize smooth motions when moving client; avoid pushing or pulling on body parts<br>d. caution client to avoid sudden twisting and turning<br>e. provide a firm mattress or place a bed board under mattress for added support |

| Desired Outcome | Nursing Actions and ***Selected Purposes/Rationales*** |
|---|---|
| | f. utilize a bed cradle *to protect affected extremities from excessive weight of bed linens*<br>g. administer anti-inflammatory agents if ordered<br>h. prepare client for radiation therapy to painful skeletal areas if planned *to shrink metastatic tumor and reduce bone pressure*<br>2. perform actions *to reduce chest pain:*<br>a. instruct and assist client to splint chest with hands or pillow when deep breathing, coughing, and changing position<br>b. position on affected side for 2-hour periods *to reduce stretching of the inflamed pleura*<br>c. assist with an intercostal nerve block if performed *for intractable pain*<br>3. perform actions to control excessive coughing (see Nursing Diagnosis 9, action b.4). |

## 6. NURSING DIAGNOSIS: Impaired verbal communication

related to entrapment of the recurrent laryngeal nerve if the tumor has extended into the mediastinal area.

| Desired Outcome | Nursing Actions and ***Selected Purposes/Rationales*** |
|---|---|
| 6. The client will successfully communicate needs and desires. | 6.a. Assess client for impaired verbal communication (e.g. hoarseness, difficulty speaking).<br>b. Implement measures *to facilitate communication:*<br>1. maintain a patient, calm approach; listen attentively and allow ample time for communication<br>2. maintain a calm, quiet environment *so that client does not have to speak loudly*<br>3. ask questions that require short answers or nod of head if client is having difficulty speaking and/or is fatigued<br>4. provide materials such as magic slate, pad and pencil, and/or word cards if appropriate; try to ensure that placement of intravenous line does not interfere with use of these communication aids<br>5. answer call signal in person rather than using intercommunication system.<br>c. Inform significant others and health care personnel of techniques being used to facilitate client's ability to communicate.<br>d. Consult physician if client experiences increasing impairment of verbal communication. |

## 7. NURSING DIAGNOSIS: Activity intolerance

related to:

a. tissue hypoxia associated with impaired alveolar gas exchange;
b. possible loss of muscle mass, tone, and strength associated with malnutrition and decreased physical activity;
c. difficulty resting and sleeping associated with discomfort, fear, anxiety, depression, and unfamiliar environment;
d. increased energy expenditure associated with dyspnea and an increase in the metabolic rate resulting from continuous, active tumor growth.

| Desired Outcome | Nursing Actions and ***Selected Purposes/Rationales*** |
|---|---|
| 7. The client will demonstrate an increased tolerance for activity as evidenced by:<br>a. verbalization of feeling less fatigued and weak<br>b. ability to perform activities of daily living without exertional dyspnea, chest pain, diaphoresis, dizziness, and a significant change in vital signs. | 7.a. Assess for signs and symptoms of activity intolerance:<br>1. statements of fatigue and weakness<br>2. exertional dyspnea, chest pain, diaphoresis, or dizziness<br>3. abnormal heart rate response to activity (e.g. increase in rate of 20 beats/minute above resting rate, decrease in rate, rate not returning to preactivity level within 3 minutes after stopping activity, change from regular to irregular rate)<br>4. decreased systolic B/P or a significant increase (10-15 mm Hg) in systolic or diastolic pressure with activity.<br>b. Implement measures *to improve activity tolerance:*<br>1. perform actions *to promote rest and/or conserve energy:*<br>a. maintain activity restrictions as ordered<br>b. minimize environmental activity and noise<br>c. organize nursing care to allow for periods of uninterrupted rest<br>d. limit the number of visitors and their length of stay<br>e. assist client with self-care activities as needed<br>f. keep supplies and personal articles within easy reach<br>g. instruct client in energy-saving techniques (e.g. using shower chair when showering, sitting to brush teeth or comb hair)<br>h. implement measures to reduce fear and anxiety (see Nursing Diagnosis 1, actions b and c)<br>i. implement measures to promote sleep (see Nursing Diagnosis 9)<br>j. implement measures to reduce pain (see Nursing Diagnosis 5)<br>2. discourage smoking and excessive intake of beverages high in caffeine such as coffee, tea, and colas *(nicotine and caffeine increase cardiac workload and myocardial oxygen utilization, thereby decreasing oxygen availability)*<br>3. perform actions to improve respiratory status (see Nursing Diagnosis 2, action c) *in order to help relieve dyspnea and improve tissue oxygenation*<br>4. if oxygen therapy is necessary during activity, keep portable oxygen equipment readily available for client's use<br>5. perform actions to maintain an adequate nutritional status (see Nursing Diagnosis 3)<br>6. increase client's activity gradually as allowed and tolerated.<br>c. Instruct client to:<br>1. report a decreased tolerance for activity<br>2. stop any activity that causes chest pain, increased shortness of breath, dizziness, or extreme fatigue or weakness.<br>d. Consult physician if signs and symptoms of activity intolerance persist or worsen. |

## 8. NURSING DIAGNOSIS: Self-care deficit

related to:
a. altered thought processes if present;
b. weakness, fatigue, and discomfort associated with the disease process, diagnostic tests, and/or the side effects of radiation therapy or treatment with cytotoxic drugs.

| Desired Outcome | Nursing Actions and ***Selected Purposes/Rationales*** |
|---|---|
| 8. The client will demonstrate increased | 8.a. Refer to Care Plan on Chemotherapy, Nursing Diagnosis 9 (pp. 199-200), for measures related to planning for and meeting client's self-care needs. |

| Desired Outcome | Nursing Actions and ***Selected Purposes/Rationales*** |
|---|---|
| participation in self-care activities within limitations imposed by the disease process and treatment plan. | b. Implement measures to increase strength and improve activity tolerance (see Nursing Diagnosis 7, action b) *in order to further facilitate client's ability to perform self-care.* |

## 9. NURSING DIAGNOSIS: Sleep pattern disturbance

related to:
a. fear, anxiety, and depression;
b. decreased activity, unfamiliar environment, and frequent assessments and treatments;
c. persistent cough and inability to assume usual sleep position associated with orthopnea;
d. discomfort associated with the disease process and side effects of treatment.

| Desired Outcome | Nursing Actions and ***Selected Purposes/Rationales*** |
|---|---|
| 9. The client will attain optimal amounts of sleep within the parameters of the treatment regimen (see Care Plan on Chemotherapy, Nursing Diagnosis 11 [p. 201], for outcome criteria). | 9.a. Refer to Care Plan on Chemotherapy, Nursing Diagnosis 11 (p. 201), for measures related to assessment and promotion of sleep.<br>b. Implement additional measures *to promote sleep:*<br>1. perform actions to reduce fear and anxiety (see Nursing Diagnosis 1, actions b and c)<br>2. perform actions to improve respiratory status (see Nursing Diagnosis 2, action c) *in order to relieve orthopnea*<br>3. perform actions to reduce pain (see Nursing Diagnosis 5)<br>4. perform actions *to control excessive coughing:*<br>a. instruct client to avoid intake of very hot or cold foods/fluids *(these can stimulate cough)*<br>b. protect client from irritants such as flowers, smoke, and powder<br>c. encourage client not to smoke *(smoke irritates the respiratory tract)*<br>d. humidify inspired air as ordered<br>e. administer antitussives if ordered<br>5. if client has orthopnea, assist him/her to assume a position *that facilitates breathing* (e.g. head of bed elevated with arms supported on pillows, resting forward on overbed table with good pillow support, sitting in chair)<br>6. maintain oxygen therapy during sleep. |

## 10. NURSING DIAGNOSIS: Altered thought processes

related to:
a. cerebral hypoxia associated with impaired alveolar gas exchange;
b. central nervous system depressant effects of hypercalcemia if present.

| Desired Outcome | Nursing Actions and ***Selected Purposes/Rationales*** |
|---|---|
| 10. The client will experience an | 10.a. Assess client for altered thought processes (e.g. slowed verbal responses, impaired memory, shortened attention span, confusion). |

improvement in thought processes as evidenced by:
a. improved verbal response time
b. improved memory
c. longer attention span
d. improved level of orientation.

b. Ascertain from significant others client's usual level of intellectual functioning.
c. Implement measures *to maintain optimal thought processes:*
   1. perform actions to improve respiratory status (see Nursing Diagnosis 2, action c) *in order to reduce cerebral hypoxia*
   2. perform actions to prevent or treat hypercalcemia (see Collaborative Diagnosis 13.C, action 2.b).
d. If client shows evidence of altered thought processes:
   1. reorient client to person, place, and time as necessary
   2. address client by name
   3. place familiar objects, clock, and calendar within client's view
   4. approach client in a slow, calm, manner; allow adequate time for communication
   5. repeat instructions as necessary using clear, simple language and short sentences
   6. maintain a consistent and fairly structured routine and write out a schedule of activities for client to refer to if desired
   7. have client perform only one activity at a time and allow adequate time for performance of activities
   8. encourage client to make lists of planned activities, questions, and concerns
   9. encourage significant others to be supportive of client; instruct them in methods of dealing with client's altered thought processes
   10. discuss physiological basis for altered thought processes with client and significant others; inform them that intellectual and emotional functioning usually improve once serum calcium levels have returned to normal and oxygenation has improved
   11. consult physician if altered thought processes persist or worsen.

## 11. NURSING DIAGNOSIS: High risk for infection

related to:
a. stasis of pulmonary secretions associated with airway obstruction, poor cough effort, and decreased activity;
b. decreased resistance to infection associated with malnutrition, general debilitation, stress, and immunosuppressive side effects of cytotoxic drugs;
c. break in skin integrity associated with radiation-induced desquamation if it has occurred;
d. break in mucosal surfaces associated with effects of cytotoxic drugs.

| Desired Outcome | Nursing Actions and ***Selected Purposes/Rationales*** |
|---|---|
| 11. The client will not develop infection (see Care Plan on Chemotherapy, Nursing Diagnosis 12 [p. 202], for outcome criteria). | 11.a. Refer to Care Plan on Chemotherapy, Nursing Diagnosis 12 (pp. 202-203), for measures related to assessment and prevention of infection.<br>b. Implement measures to facilitate removal of pulmonary secretions (see Nursing Diagnosis 2, action c.9) *in order to prevent pneumonia.* |

## 12. NURSING DIAGNOSIS: High risk for trauma

related to falls associated with:
a. confusion and lethargy resulting from impaired gas exchange and hypercalcemia if present;

b. weakness resulting from nutritional and sleep deficits, impaired alveolar gas exchange, hypercalcemia, and side effects of radiation therapy and/or chemotherapy.

| Desired Outcome | Nursing Actions and ***Selected Purposes/Rationales*** |
|---|---|
| 12. The client will not experience falls. | 12.a. Implement measures *to prevent falls:*<br>1. keep bed in low position with side rails up when client is in bed<br>2. keep needed items within easy reach<br>3. encourage client to request assistance whenever needed; have call signal within easy reach<br>4. use lap belt when client is in chair if indicated<br>5. instruct client to wear well-fitting slippers/shoes with nonslip soles and low heels when ambulating<br>6. keep floor free of clutter and wipe up spills promptly<br>7. carefully position tubings and equipment so that they will not interfere with ambulation<br>8. accompany client during ambulation utilizing a transfer safety belt if he/she is weak or dizzy<br>9. provide ambulatory aids (e.g. walker, cane) if client is weak or unsteady on feet<br>10. instruct client to ambulate in well-lit areas and to utilize handrails if needed<br>11. do not rush client; allow adequate time for ambulation to the bathroom and in hallway<br>12. make sure that bathtub and shower have nonslip bottom surfaces and that shower chair, secure bath mat, call light, hand grips, and adequate lighting are present<br>13. administer central nervous system depressants judiciously<br>14. perform actions to prevent or treat hypercalcemia (see Collaborative Diagnosis 13.C, action 2.b) *in order to help maintain mental alertness and normal neuromuscular function*<br>15. perform actions to improve respiratory status (see Nursing Diagnosis 2, action c) *in order to facilitate gas exchange and reduce cerebral hypoxia*<br>16. perform actions to increase strength and improve activity tolerance (see Nursing Diagnosis 7, action b)<br>17. if client is confused or irrational:<br>a. reorient frequently to surroundings and necessity of adhering to safety precautions<br>b. provide constant supervision (e.g. staff member, significant other) if indicated<br>c. consult physician about the temporary use of jacket or wrist restraints if necessary<br>d. administer antianxiety and antipsychotic medications if ordered.<br>b. Include client and significant others in planning and implementing measures to prevent falls.<br>c. If client falls, initiate first aid if appropriate and notify physician. |

## 13.A. COLLABORATIVE DIAGNOSES:

**Potential pulmonary complications:**

1. **atelectasis** related to:
   a. stasis of secretions in the alveoli and bronchioles associated with poor cough effort, decreased activity, and obstruction by tumor
   b. restricted lung expansion associated with weakness, presence of tumor, and/or pleural effusion if present

   c. obstructed airflow associated with tumor involvement of major airways;
2. **lung abscess** related to necrosis of tissue within and around tumor;
3. **pleural effusion** related to:
   a. increased capillary permeability associated with presence of malignant cells in the pleura
   b. increased capillary hydrostatic pressure in the visceral pleura associated with obstruction of the pulmonary veins by the tumor
   c. increased pulmonary and pleural lymphatic pressures associated with lymph node obstruction
   d. increased colloid osmotic pressure in the pleural space associated with the presence of necrotic malignant cells.

| Desired Outcomes | Nursing Actions and ***Selected Purposes/Rationales*** |
|---|---|
| 13.A.1. The client will not develop atelectasis or will experience resolution of atelectasis if it occurs as evidenced by:<br>a. usual or improved breath sounds for client<br>b. resonant percussion note over lungs<br>c. no increase in dyspnea<br>d. pulse rate within normal range for client<br>e. afebrile status. | 13.A.1.a. Assess for and report signs and symptoms of atelectasis (e.g. diminished or absent breath sounds, dull percussion note over affected area, increased respiratory rate, increased dyspnea, tachycardia, elevated temperature).<br>b. Monitor chest x-ray results. Report findings of atelectasis.<br>c. Implement measures to improve respiratory status (see Nursing Diagnosis 2, action c) *in order to reduce the risk of or help resolve atelectasis.*<br>d. If signs and symptoms of atelectasis occur:<br>1. increase frequency of turning, coughing or "huffing," deep breathing, and use of incentive spirometer<br>2. increase activity as allowed and tolerated<br>3. consult physician if signs and symptoms of atelectasis persist or worsen. |
| 13.A.2. The client will have resolution of a lung abscess if it occurs as evidenced by:<br>a. absence of chills and fever<br>b. vital signs within normal range for client<br>c. usual breath sounds for client<br>d. resonant percussion note over lungs<br>e. cough productive of clear mucus only<br>f. no increase in chest pain. | 13.A.2.a. Assess for and report signs and symptoms of a lung abscess (e.g. chills; fever; tachycardia; tachypnea; diminished or absent breath sounds; dull percussion note over a particular lung area; cough productive of purulent, foul-smelling sputum; increased chest pain).<br>b. Monitor chest x-ray and lung scan results. Report findings of lung abscess.<br>c. If signs and symptoms of a lung abscess occur:<br>1. prepare client for surgical drainage of abscess if indicated<br>2. administer antimicrobials if ordered<br>3. provide emotional support to client and significant others. |
| 13.A.3. The client will experience resolution of | 13.A.3.a. Assess for and report signs and symptoms of pleural effusion (e.g. increased dyspnea; tracheal deviation; decreased chest excursion; dull percussion note and diminished or absent breath sounds over |

| Desired Outcomes | Nursing Actions and ***Selected Purposes/Rationales*** |
|---|---|
| pleural effusion if it occurs as evidenced by:<br>a. decreased dyspnea<br>b. trachea in midline position<br>c. usual chest excursion<br>d. resonant percussion note throughout lung fields<br>e. improved breath sounds<br>f. decrease in chest pain and cough. | affected area; increase in pleuritic or dull, aching chest pain; development of or increase in nonproductive cough).<br>b. Monitor chest x-ray and computed tomography results. Report findings of pleural fluid.<br>c. Assist with aspiration of pleural fluid if performed *to confirm the presence of malignant cells and rule out other causes.*<br>d. Implement measures *to treat pleural effusion and/or prevent recurrence:*<br>1. administer cytotoxic agents as ordered *to treat underlying malignancy*<br>2. prepare client for and assist with thoracentesis and insertion of chest tube if indicated<br>3. prepare client for the following if planned:<br>a. instillation of a sclerosing agent (e.g. bleomycin, tetracycline)<br>b. pleural stripping (if life expectancy is long)<br>c. talc poudrage and pleurectomy<br>d. pleuroperitoneal shunt<br>e. radiation therapy (may be used if pleural effusion is caused by mediastinal lymph node obstruction or invasion of the pleura by malignant cells). |

## 13.B. COLLABORATIVE DIAGNOSES:

**Potential metastatic extrapulmonary manifestations of cancer of the lung:**

1. **Pancoast's and Horner's syndromes** related to invasion of adjacent structures and involvement of the eighth cervical and first and second thoracic nerves by a superior sulcus tumor (occurs most frequently with squamous cell carcinoma);
2. **superior vena cava syndrome (SVCS)** related to obstruction of the superior vena cava associated with extrinsic pressure by tumor or enlarged lymph nodes, intraluminal thrombosis, or invasion of venous wall by tumor cells (occurs most frequently with a superior mediastinal or hilar mass);
3. **spinal cord compression** related to metastasis to the vertebrae and epidural space if it has occurred.

| Desired Outcomes | Nursing Actions and ***Selected Purposes/Rationales*** |
|---|---|
| 13.B.1. The client will experience optimal relief of signs and symptoms associated with Pancoast's and Horner's syndromes if they occur as evidenced by:<br>a. reduced pain in affected shoulder and along ulnar distribution in arm<br>b. absence of ipsilateral | 13.B.1.a. Assess for and report signs and symptoms of:<br>1. Pancoast's syndrome (e.g. pain in shoulder on affected side radiating along ulnar distribution in arm)<br>2. Horner's syndrome (e.g. ipsilateral miosis, ptosis, enophthalmos, and inability to sweat).<br>b. If signs and symptoms of Pancoast's and/or Horner's syndromes occur:<br>1. administer analgesics as ordered<br>2. prepare client for external radiation therapy and en bloc resection of the tumor and involved chest wall if indicated<br>3. provide emotional support to client and significant others. |

miosis, ptosis, enophthalmos, and ability to sweat.

13.B.2. The client will experience optimal relief of signs and symptoms associated with SVCS if it occurs as evidenced by:
a. decreased dyspnea
b. absence of edema of face, arms, and hands
c. absence of plethora and cyanosis
d. absence of hoarseness, increased chest pain, headache, vertigo, and blurred vision.

13.B.2.a. Assess for and report signs and symptoms of SVCS (e.g. increased dyspnea; edema of the face, arms, or hands; erythema of face, neck, or upper trunk [plethora]; cyanosis; prominent superficial veins over upper body; hoarseness; increased chest pain; headache; vertigo; blurred vision). Symptoms may become more pronounced if client bends forward or lies flat for an extended period.

b. If signs and symptoms of SVCS occur:
1. prepare client for chest x-ray, computed tomography, and/or radionuclide venography if planned
2. implement measures to improve respiratory status (see Nursing Diagnosis 2, action c) *in order to decrease dyspnea*
3. maintain client on bed rest with head of bed elevated
4. elevate arms on pillows *to reduce edema*
5. assist client to remove rings and other constrictive jewelry
6. avoid performing venipunctures and taking B/P in upper extremities
7. prepare client for the following if planned (intervention depends on etiology and severity of symptoms):
   a. external radiation therapy (treatment of choice for NSCLC with a reduction of symptoms usually occurring within 7-10 days after initiation of treatment)
   b. chemotherapy alone or in conjunction with external radiation therapy if histological diagnosis is SCLC (drugs are usually administered via lower extremity vein *because of impaired blood flow in arms)*
   c. surgery such as superior vena cava bypass or radical excision of superior vena cava with grafting if SVCS is caused by thrombosis or if symptoms are severe and have not been relieved by radiation therapy and/or chemotherapy
8. administer the following medications if ordered:
   a. corticosteroids (e.g. dexamethasone) *to decrease inflammation and edema at site of obstruction of superior vena cava*
   b. diuretics *to reduce edema,* particularly if client is experiencing respiratory distress (diuretics provide only temporary relief and are used cautiously *because they can further decrease venous return)*
   c. thrombolytic agents (e.g. urokinase, streptokinase) if etiology is intraluminal thrombosis
9. initiate appropriate emergency care if severe respiratory distress occurs
10. provide emotional support to client and significant others.

13.B.3. The client will experience optimal relief of signs and symptoms of spinal cord compression if it occurs as evidenced by:
a. reduction in back pain
b. improved motor and sensory function
c. normal bowel

13.B.3.a. Assess for and report signs and symptoms of spinal cord compression (e.g. central back pain that may or may not radiate and is not relieved by lying down, motor weakness, sensory deficits, loss of bowel and bladder control). Signs and symptoms manifested depend on the area of spinal cord involved and extent of compression.

b. If signs and symptoms of spinal cord compression occur:
1. prepare client for diagnostic tests (e.g. x-ray of spine, myelogram, computed tomography, magnetic resonance imaging, bone scan)
2. prepare client for the following if planned:
   a. external radiation therapy (a fractionated dose of 3000-4000 cGy is given over a few weeks)
   b. surgical decompression and spine stabilization if neurological

| Desired Outcomes | Nursing Actions and ***Selected Purposes/Rationales*** |
|---|---|
| and bladder control. | deterioration is rapid and relief is not achieved with radiation to affected area<br>3. administer corticosteroids (e.g. dexamethasone) as ordered *to reduce spinal cord edema*<br>4. assist client with activities of daily living as needed<br>5. provide emotional support to client and significant others<br>6. refer to Care Plan on Spinal Cord Injury for additional care measures. |

## 13.C. COLLABORATIVE DIAGNOSES: Potential nonmetastatic extrapulmonary manifestations of lung cancer:

1. **syndrome of inappropriate antidiuretic hormone (SIADH)** related to:
   a. ectopic production and secretion of antidiuretic hormone (ADH) by tumor cells (occurs most frequently with SCLC)
   b. administration of some antineoplastic agents found to be associated with the occurrence of SIADH (e.g. cisplatin, cyclophosphamide, vincristine)
   c. stimulation of ADH output associated with pain, stress, and the use of some narcotic analgesics (e.g. morphine);
2. **hypercalcemia** related to:
   a. increased bone resorption associated with the release of several mediators such as PTH-related protein, transforming growth factor alpha, cytokines, and/or tumor necrosis factor by tumor cells (particularly squamous cell)
   b. increased renal tubular reabsorption of calcium associated with the release of mediators such as PTH-related protein by the tumor cells;
3. **atypical Cushing's syndrome** related to bilateral adrenocortical hyperplasia associated with ectopic adrenocorticotropic hormone (ACTH) production by tumor cells.

| Desired Outcomes | Nursing Actions and ***Selected Purposes/Rationales*** |
|---|---|
| 13.C.1. The client will experience resolution of SIADH if it develops as evidenced by:<br>a. decline in weight toward normal<br>b. balanced intake and output<br>c. usual mental status<br>d. absence of headache, muscle weakness, cellular edema, abdominal | 13.C.1.a. Assess for and report signs and symptoms of SIADH:<br>1. sudden weight gain<br>2. intake greater than output<br>3. lethargy, confusion<br>4. complaints of persistent headache<br>5. muscle weakness<br>6. fingerprint edema over sternum (indicative of cellular edema)<br>7. abdominal cramping, nausea, vomiting<br>8. seizures<br>9. urine specific gravity greater than 1.012<br>10. elevated urine sodium and osmolality levels<br>11. low serum sodium and osmolality levels.<br>b. If signs and symptoms of SIADH occur:<br>1. maintain fluid restrictions if ordered (usually 500-1000 ml/day) *to prevent further fluid retention*<br>2. implement measures *to prevent further ADH stimulation:*<br>a. perform actions to reduce pain (see Nursing Diagnosis 5)<br>b. perform actions to reduce fear and anxiety (see Nursing Diagnosis 1, actions b and c) |

cramping, nausea, vomiting, and seizure activity
e. urine specific gravity within normal range
f. serum and urine sodium and osmolality levels within normal limits.

3. encourage intake of foods/fluids high in sodium (e.g. cured meats, processed cheese, canned soups, catsup, dill pickles, salty snacks, tomato juice, canned vegetables, bouillon)
4. initiate seizure precautions
5. administer the following if ordered:
   a. diuretics (usually furosemide) *to promote water excretion*
   b. intravenous infusions of isotonic or hypertonic saline solutions *to treat hyponatremia*
   c. demeclocycline *to promote water excretion (inhibits effect of ADH at the renal tubular level)*
6. prepare client for treatment of the underlying malignancy if planned
7. provide emotional support to client and significant others.

13.C.2. The client will maintain a safe serum calcium level as evidenced by:
a. usual mental status
b. usual muscle strength and tone and reflex responses
c. absence of nausea, vomiting, and anorexia
d. regular pulse at 60-100 beats/minute
e. serum calcium within normal range.

13.C.2.a. Assess for and report signs and symptoms of hypercalcemia (e.g. change in mental status, muscle weakness, depressed reflexes, nausea, vomiting, anorexia, constipation, polyuria, cardiac arrhythmias, elevated serum calcium level).

b. Implement measures *to prevent or treat hypercalcemia:*
1. prepare client for treatment of underlying malignancy
2. consult physician prior to administering calcium-containing antacids (e.g. Tums, Titralac), vitamin D preparations, or thiazide diuretics *(these may all increase serum calcium levels)*
3. encourage mobility as tolerated *(weight-bearing reduces calcium loss from the bones)*
4. maintain a minimum fluid intake of 2500 ml/day unless contraindicated *(hydrating the client lowers serum calcium by dilution)*
5. administer the following if ordered:
   a. saline infusions *to increase urinary calcium excretion*
   b. calcitonin *to inhibit bone resorption and increase renal clearance of calcium*
   c. loop diuretics (e.g. ethacrynic acid, furosemide) *to increase renal excretion of calcium*
   d. plicamycin (mithramycin) *to inhibit calcium loss from bones*
   e. diphosphonates (e.g. etidronate disodium) *to decrease bone resorption.*

c. Consult physician if serum calcium levels remain above a safe level.

13.C.3. The client will experience a reduction in signs and symptoms associated with atypical Cushing's syndrome if it occurs as evidenced by:
a. increased muscle strength
b. resolution of edema
c. B/P within normal range for client
d. usual mental status
e. serum glucose, potassium, ACTH, and cortisol levels

13.C.3.a. Assess for and report signs and symptoms of atypical Cushing's syndrome (e.g. muscle weakness, edema, mild hypertension, psychosis, hyperglycemia, decreased serum potassium, high serum ACTH and cortisol levels, increased urinary cortisol and 17-hydroxycorticoid levels, increased pH and $CO_2$ content).

b. If signs and symptoms of atypical Cushing's syndrome occur:
1. administer metyrapone or aminoglutethimide if ordered *to inhibit adrenal cortisol synthesis*
2. prepare client for treatment of the underlying malignancy if planned
3. provide emotional support to client and significant others.

| Desired Outcomes | Nursing Actions and ***Selected Purposes/Rationales*** |
|---|---|
| within normal range<br>f. normal urinary cortisol and 17-hydroxycorticoid levels<br>g. blood gases within normal range for client. | |

## 14 . NURSING DIAGNOSIS: Self-concept disturbance*

related to:

a. loss of normal lung function;
b. change in appearance (e.g. excessive weight loss, hair loss associated with chemotherapy, skin changes associated with radiation therapy, gynecomastia associated with ectopic hormone production by tumor cells);
c. temporary or permanent infertility associated with gonadal dysfunction resulting from cytotoxic drug therapy;
d. changes in sexual functioning associated with weakness, fatigue, dyspnea, pain, and anxiety;
e. dependence on others to meet self-care needs;
f. stigma associated with the diagnosis of cancer;
g. anticipated changes in life style and roles associated with effects of the disease process and its treatment.

*This diagnostic label includes the nursing diagnoses of body image disturbance, self-esteem disturbance, and altered role performance.

| Desired Outcome | Nursing Actions and ***Selected Purposes/Rationales*** |
|---|---|
| 14. The client will demonstrate beginning adaptation to changes in appearance, body functioning, life style, and roles (see Care Plan on Chemotherapy, Nursing Diagnosis 14 [p. 209], for outcome criteria). | 14. Refer to Care Plan on Chemotherapy, Nursing Diagnosis 14 (pp. 209-210), for measures related to assessment and promotion of a positive self-concept. |

## 15. NURSING DIAGNOSIS: Ineffective individual coping

related to:

a. persistent discomfort associated with the disease process and the side effects of chemotherapy and/or external radiation therapy;
b. guilt associated with the diagnosis of lung cancer if a personal habit such as smoking was the major cause;
c. fear, anxiety, and depression associated with the diagnosis of lung cancer, effects of treatment, and poor prognosis;
d. inadequate support system.

| Desired Outcome | Nursing Actions and ***Selected Purposes/Rationales*** |
|---|---|
| 15. The client will demonstrate the use of effective coping skills (see Care Plan on Chemotherapy, Nursing Diagnosis 15 [pp. 210-211], for outcome criteria). | 15.a. Refer to Care Plan on Chemotherapy, Nursing Diagnosis 15 (pp. 210-211), for measures related to assessment and management of ineffective coping.<br>b. Assist the client to work through feelings of guilt about factors that contributed to the development of lung cancer (e.g. smoking, occupation). |

## 16. NURSING DIAGNOSIS: Grieving*

related to:

a. loss of normal function of the lung;
b. changes in body image associated with extrapulmonary manifestations of the disease and existing and anticipated side effects of radiation therapy and/or chemotherapy;
c. alteration in usual life style and roles resulting from the disease process and its treatment;
d. diagnosis of cancer with probability of premature death.

*This diagnostic label includes anticipatory grieving and grieving following the actual losses.

| Desired Outcome | Nursing Actions and ***Selected Purposes/Rationales*** |
|---|---|
| 16. The client will demonstrate beginning progression through the grieving process (see Care Plan on Chemotherapy, Nursing Diagnosis 16 [pp. 211-212], for outcome criteria). | 16. Refer to Care Plan on Chemotherapy, Nursing Diagnosis 16 (pp. 211-212), for measures related to assessment and facilitation of grieving. |

## 17. NURSING DIAGNOSIS: Knowledge deficit

regarding follow-up care.

| Desired Outcomes | Nursing Actions and ***Selected Purposes/Rationales*** |
|---|---|
| 17.a. The client will identify ways to improve oxygenation status and maximize pulmonary health. | 17.a. Instruct client in ways to improve oxygenation status and maximize pulmonary health:<br>1. schedule adequate rest periods<br>2. avoid exposure to respiratory irritants such as tobacco smoke, dust, perfume, aerosol sprays, paint fumes, and solvents whenever possible<br>3. stop smoking<br>4. remain indoors when temperature is extremely hot or cold<br>5. wear a mask or scarf over nose and mouth if exposure to high levels of irritants such as smoke, fumes, and dust is unavoidable<br>6. avoid high altitudes<br>7. minimize risk of respiratory tract infections:<br>a. avoid contact with persons who have respiratory tract infections |

| Desired Outcomes | Nursing Actions and ***Selected Purposes/Rationales*** |
|---|---|
| | b. avoid crowds and poorly ventilated areas<br>c. maintain good oral hygiene<br>d. adhere to prescribed chest physiotherapy (e.g. postural drainage, vibration, percussion, breathing exercises)<br>e. take medications such as bronchodilators, antimicrobials, and mucolytics as prescribed<br>f. cleanse all respiratory care equipment properly<br>g. drink at least 10 glasses of liquid/day. |
| 17.b. The client will demonstrate proper chest physiotherapy techniques and ability to use the equipment recommended to maximize pulmonary health. | 17.b.1. Reinforce instructions about chest physiotherapy and equipment recommended to maximize pulmonary health including:<br>a. postural drainage, percussion, and vibration techniques<br>b. oxygen, IPPB machine, incentive spirometer, and humidifier.<br>2. Allow time for questions, clarification, and return demonstration. |
| 17.c. The client will identify ways to minimize the risk of infection. | 17.c. Refer to Care Plan on Chemotherapy, Nursing Diagnosis 17, action a (pp. 212-213), for instructions related to preventing infection. |
| 17.d. The client will verbalize ways to improve appetite and maintain an adequate nutritional status. | 17.d. Refer to Care Plan on Chemotherapy, Nursing Diagnosis 17, action e (p. 214), for instructions related to improving appetite and maintaining an adequate nutritional status. |
| 17.e. The client will verbalize ways to manage chronic SIADH. | 17.e. Provide the following instructions related to home management of chronic SIADH:<br>1. continue fluid restriction (usually 1 quart/day) if recommended by physician<br>2. take medications (e.g. furosemide, demeclocycline) as prescribed<br>3. increase intake of foods/fluids high in sodium (e.g. tomato juice, cured meats, processed cheese, canned vegetables and soups, catsup, dill pickles, salty snacks, bouillon)<br>4. increase intake of foods/fluids high in potassium (e.g. bananas, orange juice, potatoes, raisins, figs, apricots, dates, tomato juice, white beans) if discharged on a potassium-depleting diuretic<br>5. report an increase in signs and symptoms of SIADH (e.g. sudden weight gain, intake persistently greater than output, drowsiness, confusion, weakness, headache, nausea, vomiting, abdominal cramping, seizures). |
| 17.f. The client will state signs and symptoms to report to the health care provider. | 17.f. 1. Instruct client to report the following:<br>a. drainage from and/or persistent redness of biopsy site(s)<br>b. signs and symptoms of hypercalcemia (e.g. nausea, vomiting, increased urination, muscle weakness, confusion)<br>c. persistent fever<br>d. development of or persistent difficulty swallowing<br>e. excessive weight loss<br>f. increasing fatigue, weakness, or shortness of breath<br>g. pain in shoulder, arm, or neck<br>h. swollen, painful joints (may indicate the development of hypertrophic pulmonary osteoarthropathy)<br>i. swelling of upper body<br>j. persistent headache<br>k. increasing cough productive of purulent, foul-smelling, or blood-tinged sputum<br>l. weakness of proximal muscles, numbness or tingling or loss of motor function in extremities, or uncoordinated movements (may indicate development of a neuromuscular syndrome) |

m. irritability, drowsiness, or confusion
n. signs and symptoms of SIADH (see action e.5 in this diagnosis)
o. excessive depression or difficulty coping with the diagnosis.

2. If appropriate, refer to the Care Plan on Chemotherapy, Nursing Diagnosis 17, action l (p. 216) and/or the Care Plan on External Radiation Therapy, Nursing Diagnosis 16, action i (p. 242), for additional signs and symptoms client should report if he/she is receiving chemotherapy and/or radiation therapy.

17.h. The client will identify community resources that can assist with home management and adjustment to changes resulting from the diagnosis and the effects of treatment.

17.h.1. Provide information about and encourage utilization of community resources that can assist client and significant others with home management and adjustment to the diagnosis of lung cancer and effects of prescribed treatment (e.g. American Cancer Society, counselors, social service agencies, I Can Cope, Meals on Wheels, local support groups, Hospice).
2. Initiate a referral if indicated.

17.i. The client will verbalize an understanding of and a plan for adhering to recommended follow-up care including future appointments with health care provider, medications prescribed, activity level, and plans for subsequent treatment.

17.i. 1. Reinforce physician's explanation of planned radiation therapy and/or chemotherapy schedule if appropriate. Stress importance of strictly following the prescribed protocol for radiation therapy and/or chemotherapy and keeping all appointments for follow-up supervision and laboratory work.
2. Explain rationale for, side effects of, and importance of taking medications prescribed.
3. Emphasize need for planned rest periods and for gauging activity according to tolerance.
4. Implement measures to improve client compliance:
a. include significant others in teaching sessions if possible
b. encourage questions and allow time for reinforcement and clarification of information provided
c. provide written instructions regarding scheduled appointments with health care provider and for chemotherapy, radiation therapy, and laboratory work; medications prescribed; and signs and symptoms to report.

# Chronic Obstructive Pulmonary Disease

Chronic obstructive pulmonary disease (COPD) is a disorder characterized by lower airway obstruction and a reduction in expiratory flow rate. Signs and symptoms include a productive cough and dyspnea that progressively worsen. The two major diseases that comprise COPD are chronic bronchitis and emphysema. Chronic bronchitis is characterized by a cough that persists at least 3 months of the year for 2 consecutive years and an excessive production of mucus in the bronchi due to inflammation of the bronchioles and hypertrophy and hyperplasia of the mucous glands. In contrast, emphysema is characterized by dyspnea and a mild cough. The impaired airflow that occurs with emphysema is related to loss of lung elasticity and narrowed bronchioles. Both chronic bronchitis and emphysema are usually present to some degree in the person with COPD, although one of the two conditions usually predominates.

Causative factors of COPD include chronic irritation of the lungs by cigarette smoke, exposure to air pollution and chemical irritants, and recurrent respiratory tract infections. In a small percentage of cases of emphysema, the destruction of lung tissue by proteolytic enzymes is a result of a genetic deficiency of alpha$_1$-antitrypsin.

**This care plan focuses on care of the adult client with COPD who is hospitalized during an acute exacerbation.** Goals of care are to improve respiratory function, prevent complications, and educate the client regarding ways to manage existing symptoms and slow the progression of the disease process.

## DIAGNOSTIC TESTS

Chest x-ray
Pulmonary function studies
Arterial blood gases
Oximetry

## DISCHARGE CRITERIA

Prior to discharge, the client will:

- have improved respiratory function
- have no signs and symptoms of complications
- identify ways to prevent or minimize respiratory problems
- demonstrate proper breathing techniques, chest physiotherapy, and use of respiratory equipment
- verbalize an understanding of medications ordered including rationale, side effects, method of administering, and importance of taking as prescribed
- identify appropriate safety measures related to COPD and its treatment
- state signs and symptoms to report to the health care provider
- share feelings and thoughts about the effects of COPD on life style and roles
- identify community resources that can assist with home management and adjustment to changes resulting from COPD
- verbalize an understanding of and a plan for adhering to recommended follow-up care including future appointments with health care provider and graded exercise program.

## NURSING/COLLABORATIVE DIAGNOSES



## 1. NURSING DIAGNOSIS: Impaired respiratory function*:

a. **ineffective breathing pattern** related to:
   1. fear and anxiety
   2. decreased lung/chest wall expansion associated with weakness, fatigue, and presence of a flattened diaphragm (a result of prolonged hyperinflation of the lungs);

b. **ineffective airway clearance** related to:
   1. narrowing of the bronchioles associated with:

---

*This diagnostic label includes the following nursing diagnoses: ineffective breathing pattern, ineffective airway clearance, and impaired gas exchange.

a. presence of excessive mucus
b. inflammation and hyperplasia of the bronchial walls (especially with chronic bronchitis)
c. bronchospasm resulting from irritation of the bronchioles by excessive mucus
2. collapse of the alveoli associated with destruction of lung tissue by proteolytic enzymes (occurs primarily with emphysema)
3. stasis of secretions associated with:
a. poor cough effort resulting from fatigue and weakness
b. impaired ciliary function resulting from loss of ciliated epithelium (occurs with inflammation and destruction and fibrosis of bronchial walls)
c. decreased mobility if present;

c. **impaired gas exchange** related to narrowing or obstruction of the small airways and a decrease in effective lung surface resulting from collapse, destruction, and fibrosis of alveolar walls.

| Desired Outcome | Nursing Actions and ***Selected Purposes/Rationales*** |
|---|---|
| 1. The client will experience adequate respiratory function as evidenced by:<br>a. usual rate, rhythm, and depth of respirations<br>b. decreased dyspnea<br>c. usual or improved breath sounds<br>d. usual mental status<br>e. usual skin color<br>f. blood gases within normal range for client. | 1.a. Assess for signs and symptoms of impaired respiratory function:<br>1. shallow, rapid, or irregular respirations<br>2. dyspnea, orthopnea<br>3. use of accessory muscles when breathing<br>4. adventitious breath sounds (e.g. rhonchi)<br>5. diminished or absent breath sounds<br>6. restlessness, irritability<br>7. confusion, somnolence<br>8. central cyanosis (a late sign).<br>b. Monitor for and report significant abnormalities of and/or changes in blood gases, oximetry results, and chest x-ray reports.<br>c. Assist with pulmonary function studies. Report results that worsen or do not improve after treatment begins.<br>d. Implement measures *to improve respiratory status:*<br>1. perform actions to increase strength and improve activity tolerance (see Nursing Diagnosis 3, action b)<br>2. perform actions to reduce fear and anxiety (see Nursing Diagnosis 8, action b)<br>3. place client in a semi- to high Fowler's position; position overbed table so client can lean on it if desired<br>4. maintain oxygen therapy as ordered (question any order for high oxygen concentration *since many persons with COPD are dependent on hypoxemia as the stimulus to breathe)*<br>5. assist client to turn from side to side every 2 hours while in bed<br>6. instruct client in and assist with diaphragmatic and pursed-lip breathing techniques<br>7. instruct client to deep breathe or use incentive spirometer at least every 2 hours<br>8. perform actions *to facilitate removal of pulmonary secretions:*<br>a. instruct and assist client to cough or "huff" every 1-2 hours<br>b. implement measures *to liquefy tenacious secretions:*<br>1. maintain a fluid intake of at least 2500 ml/day unless contraindicated<br>2. humidify inspired air as ordered<br>c. assist with administration of diluent and mucolytic agents via nebulizer as ordered<br>d. assist with or perform postural drainage, percussion, and vibration if ordered<br>e. perform tracheal suctioning if needed<br>f. administer expectorants if ordered<br>9. instruct client to avoid intake of large meals, gas-forming foods (e.g. |

| Desired Outcome | Nursing Actions and ***Selected Purposes/Rationales*** |
|---|---|
| | beans, cauliflower, cabbage, onions), and carbonated beverages *in order to prevent gastric distention and increased pressure on the diaphragm*<br>10. discourage smoking *(smoke decreases oxygen availability, increases mucus production, causes bronchoconstriction, and impairs ciliary function)*<br>11. protect client from exposure to irritants such as smoke, flowers, and perfume *(can cause bronchospasm and increased mucus production)*<br>12. maintain activity restrictions; increase activity as allowed and tolerated<br>13. avoid use of central nervous system depressants *(these further depress respiratory status)*<br>14. administer the following medications if ordered:<br>a. bronchodilators:<br>1. methylxanthines (e.g. theophylline)<br>2. sympathomimetics (e.g. isoproterenol, metaproterenol, albuterol)<br>3. anticholinergics (e.g. ipratropium)<br>b. corticosteroids (e.g. methylprednisolone) *to decrease airway inflammation and thereby improve bronchial air flow.*<br>e. Consult physician if signs and symptoms of impaired respiratory function persist or worsen. |

## 2. NURSING DIAGNOSIS: Altered nutrition: less than body requirements

related to:
a. decreased oral intake associated with:
   1. dyspnea, weakness, fatigue, and depression
   2. nausea (can occur in response to noxious stimuli such as sight of expectorated sputum)
   3. early satiety resulting from compression of the stomach by flattened diaphragm;
b. increased metabolic needs associated with increased energy expenditure resulting from strenuous breathing efforts and persistent coughing.

| Desired Outcome | Nursing Actions and ***Selected Purposes/Rationales*** |
|---|---|
| 2. The client will maintain an adequate nutritional status as evidenced by:<br>a. weight within normal range for client's age, height, and body frame<br>b. normal BUN and serum albumin, transferrin, and lymphocyte levels<br>c. triceps skinfold thickness within normal range<br>d. usual strength and activity tolerance<br>e. healthy oral mucous membrane. | 2.a. Assess for and report signs and symptoms of malnutrition:<br>1. weight below normal for client's age, height, and body frame<br>2. abnormal BUN and low serum albumin, transferrin, and lymphocyte levels<br>3. triceps skinfold thickness less than normal<br>4. increased weakness and fatigue<br>5. stomatitis.<br>b. Monitor percentage of meals and snacks client consumes. Report a pattern of inadequate intake.<br>c. Implement measures *to maintain an adequate nutritional status:*<br>1. perform actions *to improve oral intake:*<br>a. implement measures to improve respiratory status (see Nursing Diagnosis 1, action d) *in order to help relieve dyspnea*<br>b. implement measures to facilitate psychological adjustment (see Nursing Diagnoses 9, actions c-t and 10, actions c-l) *in order to reduce depression*<br>c. schedule treatments that assist in mobilizing mucus (e.g. aerosol treatments, postural drainage) at least 1 hour before or after meals *to prevent nausea*<br>d. increase activity as allowed and tolerated *(activity stimulates appetite)* |

e. obtain a dietary consult if necessary to assist client in selecting foods/fluids that meet nutritional needs as well as personal and cultural preferences whenever possible
f. encourage a rest period before meals *to minimize fatigue*
g. eliminate noxious sights and odors from the environment; provide client with an opaque, covered container for expectorated sputum; empty container frequently and remove it from the table during mealtime if it is not needed *(noxious stimuli can cause nausea)*
h. maintain a clean environment and a relaxed, pleasant atmosphere
i. provide oral care before meals and after respiratory treatments
j. if client is quite dyspneic, assist him/her to select foods that require little or no chewing
k. serve small portions of nutritious foods/fluids that are appealing to the client
l. place client in a high Fowler's position for meals and provide supplemental oxygen therapy during meals if indicated *to help relieve dyspnea*
m. allow adequate time for meals; reheat food if necessary
n. limit fluid intake (unless it has a high nutritional value) with meals *to reduce early satiety and subsequent decreased food intake*

2. ensure that meals are well balanced and high in essential nutrients; offer dietary supplements between meals if indicated
3. administer vitamins and minerals if ordered.

d. Perform a 72-hour calorie count if ordered. Report totals to dietitian and physician.
e. Consult physician about alternative methods of providing nutrition (e.g. parenteral nutrition, tube feedings) if client does not consume enough food or fluids to meet nutritional needs.

## 3. NURSING DIAGNOSIS: Activity intolerance

related to:
a. tissue hypoxia associated with impaired gas exchange;
b. inadequate nutritional status;
c. difficulty resting and sleeping associated with dyspnea, excessive coughing (especially with chronic bronchitis), fear, anxiety, frequent assessments and treatments, and side effects of medication therapy (e.g. some bronchodilators);
d. increased energy expenditure associated with strenuous breathing efforts and persistent coughing.

| Desired Outcome | Nursing Actions and ***Selected Purposes/Rationales*** |
|---|---|
| 3. The client will demonstrate an increased tolerance for activity as evidenced by:<br>a. verbalization of feeling less fatigued and weak<br>b. ability to perform activities of daily living without increased shortness of breath, chest pain, diaphoresis, | 3.a. Assess for signs and symptoms of activity intolerance:<br>1. statements of fatigue and weakness<br>2. exertional dyspnea, chest pain, diaphoresis, or dizziness<br>3. abnormal heart rate response to activity (e.g. increase in rate of 20 beats/minute above resting rate, decrease in rate, rate not returning to preactivity level within 3 minutes after stopping activity, change from regular to irregular rate)<br>4. decreased systolic B/P or a significant increase (10-15 mm Hg) in systolic or diastolic pressure with activity.<br>b. Implement measures *to improve activity tolerance:*<br>1. perform actions *to promote rest and/or conserve energy:*<br>a. maintain activity restrictions as ordered<br>b. minimize environmental activity and noise |

| Desired Outcome | Nursing Actions and ***Selected Purposes/Rationales*** |
|---|---|
| dizziness, and a significant change in vital signs. | c. organize nursing care to allow for periods of uninterrupted rest<br>d. limit the number of visitors and their length of stay<br>e. assist client with self-care activities as needed<br>f. keep supplies and personal articles within easy reach<br>g. instruct client in energy-saving techniques (e.g. using shower chair when showering, sitting to brush teeth or comb hair)<br>h. implement measures to reduce fear and anxiety (see Nursing Diagnosis 8, action b)<br>i. implement measures to promote sleep (see Nursing Diagnosis 5, action c)<br>j. implement measures *to control cough:*<br>1. instruct client to avoid intake of very hot or cold foods/fluids *(these can stimulate cough)*<br>2. protect client from exposure to irritants such as flowers, smoke, and powder<br>3. administer antitussives if ordered *to suppress cough* (usually only ordered if cough is nonproductive and persistent)<br>2. perform actions to improve respiratory status (see Nursing Diagnosis 1, action d) *in order to improve tissue oxygenation and help relieve dyspnea*<br>3. perform actions to maintain an adequate nutritional status (see Nursing Diagnosis 2, action c)<br>4. reinforce use of controlled breathing techniques (e.g. inhaling through nose and exhaling slowly through pursed lips) during activity<br>5. if oxygen therapy is necessary during activity, keep portable oxygen equipment readily available for client's use<br>6. increase client's activity gradually as allowed and tolerated.<br>c. Instruct client to:<br>1. report a decreased tolerance for activity<br>2. stop any activity that causes chest pain, increased shortness of breath, dizziness, or extreme fatigue or weakness.<br>d. Consult physician if signs and symptoms of activity intolerance persist or worsen. |

## 4. NURSING DIAGNOSIS: Self-care deficit

related to weakness, fatigue, and dyspnea.

| Desired Outcome | Nursing Actions and ***Selected Purposes/Rationales*** |
|---|---|
| 4. The client will demonstrate increased participation in self-care activities within physical limitations. | 4.a. With client, develop a realistic plan for meeting daily physical needs.<br>b. Encourage maximum independence within limitations imposed by dyspnea, weakness, and fatigue.<br>c. Implement measures *to facilitate client's ability to perform self-care activities:*<br>1. schedule care at a time when client is most likely to be able to participate:<br>a. a couple of hours after arising *(bronchial secretions and inflammation are greater immediately upon awakening because of client's inactivity through the night)*<br>b. after rest periods<br>c. not immediately after meals or treatments<br>2. keep needed objects within easy reach<br>3. perform actions to increase strength and improve activity tolerance (see Nursing Diagnosis 3, action b) |

4. perform actions to improve respiratory status (see Nursing Diagnosis 1, action d) *in order to reduce dyspnea*
5. consult occupational therapist about assistive devices available (e.g. long-handled hairbrush and shoehorn); reinforce use of these devices if indicated
6. allow adequate time for accomplishment of self-care activities.

d. Provide positive feedback for all efforts and accomplishments of self-care.
e. Assist client with activities he/she is unable to perform independently.
f. Inform significant others of client's abilities to perform own care. Explain the importance of encouraging and allowing client to maintain an optimal level of independence within his/her activity tolerance level.

## 5. NURSING DIAGNOSIS: Sleep pattern disturbance

related to fear, anxiety, unfamiliar environment, excessive coughing, frequent assessments and treatments, side effects of some medications (e.g. some bronchodilators), and inability to assume usual sleep position associated with orthopnea.

### Desired Outcome

5. The client will attain optimal amounts of sleep within the parameters of the treatment regimen as evidenced by:
   a. statements of feeling well rested
   b. usual mental status
   c. absence of frequent yawning, dark circles under eyes, and hand tremors.

### Nursing Actions and ***Selected Purposes/Rationales***

5.a. Assess for signs and symptoms of a sleep pattern disturbance (e.g. verbal complaints of difficulty falling asleep, sleep interruptions, or not feeling well rested; irritability; lethargy; disorientation; frequent yawning; dark circles under eyes; slight hand tremors).

b. Determine the client's usual sleep habits.

c. Implement measures *to promote sleep:*
1. discourage long periods of sleep during the day unless signs and symptoms of sleep deprivation exist or daytime sleep is usual for client
2. perform actions to reduce fear and anxiety (see Nursing Diagnosis 8, action b)
3. perform actions to improve respiratory status (see Nursing Diagnosis 1, action d) *in order to relieve orthopnea*
4. encourage participation in relaxing diversional activities during the evening
5. discourage intake of fluids high in caffeine (e.g. coffee, tea, colas), especially in the evening
6. offer client a high-protein evening snack (e.g. cheese) unless contraindicated
7. allow client to continue usual sleep practices (e.g. position, time, bedtime rituals such as reading and meditating) if possible
8. satisfy basic needs such as comfort and warmth before sleep
9. have client empty bladder just before bedtime
10. perform actions to control cough (see Nursing Diagnosis 3, action b.1.j)
11. maintain a quiet, restful atmosphere; have earplugs available for client if needed
12. utilize relaxation techniques (e.g. progressive relaxation exercises, back massage, meditation, soft music) before sleep
13. ensure good room ventilation
14. assist client to assume a position *that facilitates breathing* (e.g. head of bed elevated with arms supported on pillows, resting forward on overbed table with good pillow support, sitting in a chair)
15. maintain oxygen therapy during sleep

| Desired Outcome | Nursing Actions and ***Selected Purposes/Rationales*** |
|---|---|
| | 16. perform actions *to reduce interruptions during sleep (80-100 minutes of uninterrupted sleep are usually needed to complete one sleep cycle):*<br>a. restrict visitors<br>b. group care (e.g. medications, treatments, physical care, assessments) whenever possible.<br>d. Consult physician if signs and symptoms of sleep deprivation persist or worsen. |

## 6. NURSING DIAGNOSIS: High risk for infection: pneumonia

related to stasis of secretions in the lungs (secretions provide a good medium for bacterial growth).

| Desired Outcome | Nursing Actions and ***Selected Purposes/Rationales*** |
|---|---|
| 6. The client will not develop pneumonia as evidenced by:<br>a. usual breath sounds and percussion note over lungs<br>b. absence of tachypnea<br>c. cough productive of clear mucus only<br>d. afebrile status<br>e. absence of pleuritic pain<br>f. WBC count within normal range<br>g. blood gases returning to normal range for client<br>h. negative sputum culture. | 6.a. Assess for and report signs and symptoms of pneumonia:<br>1. abnormal breath sounds (e.g. crackles [rales], pleural friction rub, bronchial breath sounds, diminished or absent breath sounds)<br>2. dull percussion note over affected lung area<br>3. increase in respiratory rate<br>4. cough productive of purulent, green, or rust-colored sputum<br>5. chills and fever<br>6. pleuritic pain<br>7. elevated WBC count.<br>b. Monitor oximetry and blood gas results. Report values that have worsened.<br>c. Obtain sputum specimen for culture if ordered. Report abnormal results.<br>d. Monitor chest x-ray results. Report findings indicative of pneumonia.<br>e. Implement measures *to prevent pneumonia:*<br>1. perform actions to improve respiratory status (see Nursing Diagnosis 1, action d)<br>2. protect client from persons with respiratory tract infections<br>3. encourage and assist client to perform good oral hygiene *in order to reduce the colonization of bacteria in the oropharynx and subsequent aspiration of these microorganisms.*<br>f. If signs and symptoms of pneumonia occur:<br>1. continue with above measures<br>2. administer antimicrobials if ordered<br>3. refer to Care Plan on Pneumonia for additional care measures. |

## 7. COLLABORATIVE DIAGNOSES: Potential complications:

a. **right-sided heart failure (cor pulmonale)** related to increased cardiac workload associated with:
   1. pulmonary hypertension resulting from pulmonary vasoconstriction that occurs in response to hypoxia
   2. compensatory response to the decreased pulmonary blood flow that results

from loss of large portions of the pulmonary vascular bed (occurs as a result of destruction and fibrosis of lung tissue);

b. **respiratory failure** related to severe ventilation-perfusion imbalance.

| Desired Outcomes | Nursing Actions and ***Selected Purposes/Rationales*** |
|---|---|
| 7.a. The client will not develop right-sided heart failure as evidenced by:<br>1. pulse 60-100 beats/minute<br>2. no increase in intensity of $S_2$ heart sound or development of summation gallop<br>3. usual mental status<br>4. no increase in dyspnea, weakness, and fatigue<br>5. balanced intake and output<br>6. stable weight<br>7. CVP within normal range<br>8. absence of peripheral edema; distended neck veins; and enlarged, tender liver. | 7.a.1. Assess for and report signs and symptoms of right-sided heart failure:<br>a. increase in pulse rate<br>b. development of a loud $S_2$ heart sound and/or summation gallop<br>c. restlessness, anxiousness, confusion<br>d. increased dyspnea, weakness, and/or fatigue<br>e. oliguria<br>f. weight gain<br>g. elevated CVP<br>h. peripheral edema<br>i. distended neck veins<br>j. enlarged, tender liver.<br>2. Monitor chest x-ray results. Report findings of cardiomegaly.<br>3. Implement measures to improve respiratory status (see Nursing Diagnosis 1, action d) *in order to reduce cardiac workload and the subsequent risk for right-sided heart failure.*<br>4. If signs and symptoms of right-sided heart failure occur:<br>a. maintain oxygen therapy as ordered<br>b. maintain fluid and sodium restrictions as ordered<br>c. maintain client on strict bed rest in a semi- to high Fowler's position<br>d. administer medications that may be ordered *to reduce vascular congestion and/or cardiac workload* (e.g. diuretics, cardiotonics, vasodilators)<br>e. provide emotional support to client and significant others<br>f. refer to Care Plan on Heart Failure for additional care measures. |
| 7.b. The client will not experience respiratory failure as evidenced by:<br>1. usual skin color<br>2. usual mental status<br>3. $Pa_{O_2}$ above 50 mm Hg and $Pa_{CO_2}$ below 50 mm Hg. | 7.b.1. Assess for and report signs and symptoms of severe respiratory distress (e.g. increased sternocleidomastoid and intercostal muscle retraction, dusky or cyanotic skin color, drowsiness, confusion).<br>2. Monitor blood gas and oximetry results. Report values that have worsened.<br>3. Implement measures *to prevent respiratory failure:*<br>a. perform actions to improve respiratory status (see Nursing Diagnosis 1, action d)<br>b. perform actions to prevent and treat pneumonia (see Nursing Diagnosis 6, actions e and f) *in order to prevent a further compromise in respiratory status.*<br>4. If signs and symptoms of respiratory failure occur:<br>a. continue with above actions<br>b. assist with intubation, mechanical ventilation, and transfer to intensive care unit if indicated<br>c. continue with comfort measures such as keeping upper airway free of mucus and wiping face with cool cloth if life-saving measures are not indicated; refer to Care Plan on Terminal Care if appropriate<br>d. provide emotional support to client and significant others. |

## 8. NURSING DIAGNOSIS: Anxiety

related to dyspnea and feeling of suffocation, unfamiliar environment, financial concerns, prognosis, and feeling of lack of control over progression of the disease.

| Desired Outcome | Nursing Actions and ***Selected Purposes/Rationales*** |
|---|---|
| 8. The client will experience a reduction in anxiety as evidenced by:<br>a. verbalization of feeling less anxious and fearful<br>b. usual sleep pattern<br>c. relaxed facial expression and body movements<br>d. stable vital signs<br>e. usual perceptual ability and interactions with others. | 8.a. Assess client for signs and symptoms of anxiety (e.g. verbalization of fears and concerns, insomnia, tenseness, tremors, irritability, restlessness, diaphoresis, elevated blood pressure, increased respiratory rate, tachycardia, facial pallor or flushing, narrowed perceptual field, withdrawal, noncompliance with treatment plan). Validate perceptions carefully, remembering that some behavior may result from tissue hypoxia.<br>b. Implement measures *to reduce fear and anxiety:*<br>1. maintain a calm, supportive, confident manner when interacting with client<br>2. do not leave client alone during period of acute respiratory distress<br>3. perform actions to improve respiratory status (see Nursing Diagnosis 1, action d) *in order to reduce dyspnea*<br>4. perform actions *to decrease client's feeling of suffocation:*<br>a. open curtains and doors<br>b. approach client from the side rather than face-on *(close face-on contact may make client feel closed in)*<br>c. limit number of visitors in room at any one time<br>d. remove unnecessary equipment from room<br>e. administer oxygen via nasal cannula rather than mask if possible<br>5. encourage significant others to project a caring, concerned attitude without obvious anxiousness<br>6. once the period of acute respiratory distress has subsided:<br>a. orient client to hospital environment, equipment, and routines<br>b. introduce staff who will be participating in his/her care; if possible, maintain consistency in staff assigned to his/her care *to provide feelings of stability and comfort with the environment*<br>c. assure client that staff members are nearby; respond to call signal as soon as possible<br>d. provide a calm, restful environment<br>e. encourage verbalization of fear and anxiety; provide feedback<br>f. reinforce physician's explanations and clarify misconceptions the client has about COPD, the treatment plan, and prognosis<br>g. explain all diagnostic tests<br>h. instruct client in relaxation techniques and encourage participation in diversional activities<br>i. assist client to identify specific stressors and ways to cope with them<br>j. perform actions to reduce client's feeling of powerlessness (see Nursing Diagnosis 10, actions c-l)<br>k. initiate financial and/or social service referrals if indicated<br>l. administer antianxiety agents if ordered.<br>c. Include significant others in orientation and teaching sessions and encourage their continued support of the client.<br>d. Provide information based on current needs of client and significant others at a level they can understand. Encourage questions and clarification of information provided.<br>e. Consult physician if above actions fail to control fear and anxiety. |

## 9. NURSING DIAGNOSIS: Self-concept disturbance*

related to:

a. change in appearance (e.g. "barrel" chest, clubbing of fingers, retraction of tissues around the neck and supraclavicular spaces);

*This diagnostic label includes the nursing diagnoses of body image disturbance, self-esteem disturbance, and altered role performance.

b. dependence on others to meet self-care needs;
c. possible alterations in sexual functioning (may result from dyspnea, weakness, fatigue, and persistent cough);
d. stigma of having a chronic illness;
e. possible changes in life style and roles.

| Desired Outcome | Nursing Actions and ***Selected Purposes/Rationales*** |
|---|---|
| 9. The client will demonstrate beginning adaptation to changes in appearance, body functioning, level of independence, life style, and roles as evidenced by:<br>a. verbalization of feelings of self-worth<br>b. maintenance of relationships with significant others<br>c. active participation in activities of daily living<br>d. active interest in personal appearance<br>e. verbalization of a plan for adapting life style to meet restrictions imposed by the effects of COPD. | 9.a. Assess for signs and symptoms of a self-concept disturbance (e.g. verbal or nonverbal cues denoting a negative response to changes in body functioning or appearance such as denial of or preoccupation with changes that have occurred or withdrawal from significant others).<br>b. Determine the meaning of changes in appearance, body functioning, life style, and roles to the client by encouraging him/her to verbalize feelings and by noting nonverbal responses to changes experienced.<br>c. Be aware that client will grieve the progressive loss of respiratory function. Assist client through his/her present phase of grieving (e.g. shock, disbelief, denial, anger, sadness, depression). Do not reinforce maladaptive denial of situation.<br>d. Discuss with client realistic expectations of improvements in body functioning and ability to resume usual activities.<br>e. Implement measures *to assist client to increase self-esteem* (e.g. limit negative self-assessment, encourage positive comments about self, assist to identify strengths, give positive feedback about accomplishments and behaviors that are indicative of high self-esteem).<br>f. Assist client to identify and utilize coping techniques that have been helpful in the past.<br>g. If client is self-conscious about appearance, suggest clothing styles that make physical changes less apparent (e.g. loose-fitting shirts, shirts with high collars).<br>h. Assist client with usual grooming and makeup habits if necessary.<br>i. Reinforce measures that can help client improve his/her activity tolerance (e.g. resting prior to activity, maintaining a good nutritional status, sitting rather than standing when performing tasks, adhering to a graded exercise program, taking medications as prescribed, using portable oxygen as prescribed).<br>j. If appropriate, discuss with client ways in which he/she can reduce dyspnea during sexual activity (e.g. obtain adequate rest and use inhaled bronchodilators before sexual activity, use oxygen before and during sexual activity, assume positions such as side-lying that reduce energy expenditure).<br>k. Consult occupational therapist if indicated about a home evaluation before discharge to identify assistive devices and environmental modifications that could help the client to be more independent in his/her living situation.<br>l. Encourage significant others to allow client to do as much as he/she is able *so that independence can be reestablished and/or self-esteem redeveloped.*<br>m. Implement measures to reduce client's feelings of powerlessness (see Nursing Diagnosis 10, actions c-l).<br>n. Assess for and support behaviors suggesting positive adaptation to changes that have occurred (e.g. compliance with treatment plan, verbalization of feelings of self-worth, maintenance of relationships with significant others).<br>o. Assist client's and significant others' adjustment by listening, facilitating communication, and providing information.<br>p. Assist client and significant others to have similar expectations and understanding of future life style and to identify ways that personal and family goals can be adjusted rather than abandoned. |

| Desired Outcome | Nursing Actions and ***Selected Purposes/Rationales*** |
|---|---|
| | q. Encourage visits and support from significant others.<br>r. Encourage client to pursue usual roles and interests and to continue involvement in social activities. If previous roles, interests, and hobbies cannot be pursued, encourage development of new ones.<br>s. Provide information about and encourage utilization of community agencies and support groups (e.g. vocational rehabilitation; family, individual, and/or financial counseling).<br>t. Consult physician about psychological counseling if client desires or if he/she seems unwilling or unable to adapt to changes resulting from COPD. |

## 10. NURSING DIAGNOSIS: Powerlessness

related to physical limitations; disease progression despite efforts to comply with treatment plan; dependence on others to meet self-care needs; and alterations in roles, life style, and future plans.

| Desired Outcome | Nursing Actions and ***Selected Purposes/Rationales*** |
|---|---|
| 10. The client will demonstrate increased feelings of control over his/her situation as evidenced by:<br>a. verbalization of same<br>b. active participation in planning of care<br>c. participation in self-care activities within physical limitations. | 10.a. Assess for behaviors that may indicate feelings of powerlessness (e.g. verbalization of lack of control over self-care or current situation, anger, apathy, hostility, excessive dependency, lack of participation in care planning or self-care).<br>b. Obtain information from client and significant others regarding client's usual response to situations in which he/she has had limited control (e.g. loss of job, financial stress).<br>c. Evaluate with client his/her perceptions of current situation, strengths, weaknesses, expectations, and parts of current situation that are under his/her control. Correct misinformation and inaccurate perceptions and encourage discussion of feelings about areas in which he/she perceives a lack of control.<br>d. Assist client to establish realistic short- and long-term goals.<br>e. Reinforce physician's explanations about COPD and the importance of adhering to the treatment plan as a way to slow disease progression and prevent or delay the development of complications. Clarify misconceptions.<br>f. Support realistic hope about the client's ability to slow the progression of COPD and adapt to changes that have occurred as a result of it.<br>g. Remind client of his/her right to ask questions about current condition and the prescribed treatment plan.<br>h. Support client's efforts to increase knowledge of and control over condition. Provide relevant pamphlets and audiovisual materials.<br>i. Include client in the planning of care, encourage maximum participation in the treatment plan, and allow choices whenever possible *to promote a sense of control.*<br>j. Inform client of scheduled procedures and tests *so that unpredictability is eliminated as much as possible and feeling of control is promoted.*<br>k. Encourage client to be as active as possible in making decisions about his/her living situation.<br>l. Encourage client's participation in self-help groups if indicated. |

## 11. NURSING DIAGNOSIS: Ineffective management of therapeutic regimen

related to:
a. lack of understanding of the implications of not following the prescribed treatment plan;
b. feeling of lack of control over disease progression;
c. difficulty modifying personal habits (e.g. smoking) and integrating necessary treatments into life style;
d. insufficient financial resources.

**Desired Outcome**

11. The client will demonstrate the probability of effective management of the therapeutic regimen as evidenced by:
    a. willingness to learn about and participate in treatments and care
    b. statements reflecting ways to modify personal habits and integrate treatments into life style
    c. statements reflecting an understanding of the implications of not following the prescribed treatment plan.

**Nursing Actions and *Selected Purposes/Rationales***

11.a. Assess for indications that the client may be unable to effectively manage the therapeutic regimen:
1. statements reflecting that he/she was unable to manage care at home
2. failure to adhere to treatment plan while in hospital (e.g. refusing to use proper breathing techniques, refusing medications)
3. statements reflecting a lack of understanding of factors that may cause further progression of COPD
4. statements reflecting an unwillingness or inability to modify personal habits and integrate necessary treatments into life style
5. statement reflecting view that COPD is curable or that the situation is hopeless and efforts to comply with the treatment plan are useless.

b. Implement measures *to promote effective management of the therapeutic regimen:*
1. explain COPD in terms the client can understand; stress the fact that adherence to the treatment program is necessary in order to delay and/or prevent complications
2. encourage questions and clarify misconceptions client has about COPD and its effects
3. encourage client to participate in treatment plan (e.g. chest physiotherapy, breathing exercises)
4. provide instruction regarding respiratory care (e.g. use of nebulizers and metered-dose devices, pursed-lip and diaphragmatic breathing techniques); allow time for return demonstration; determine areas of difficulty and misunderstanding and reinforce teaching as necessary
5. perform actions to promote a positive self-concept and reduce feelings of powerlessness (see Nursing Diagnoses 9, actions c-t and 10, actions c-l) *in order to promote a sense of self-reliance and control over the effects of COPD*
6. initiate and reinforce the discharge teaching outlined in Nursing Diagnosis 12 *in order to promote a sense of control over disease progression*
7. provide client with written instructions about breathing techniques, chest physiotherapy, ways to prevent further respiratory problems, prescribed medications, signs and symptoms to report, and future appointments with health care provider
8. assist client to identify ways he/she can incorporate treatments into life style; focus on modifications of life style rather than complete change
9. encourage client to discuss his/her concerns regarding cost of hospitalization, medications, oxygen equipment, and follow-up care; obtain a social service consult to assist with financial planning and to obtain financial aid if indicated
10. provide information about and encourage utilization of community resources that can assist client to make necessary life-style changes (e.g. American Lung Association; pulmonary rehabilitation groups;

| Desired Outcome | Nursing Actions and ***Selected Purposes/Rationales*** |
|---|---|
| | Better Breather's Club; counseling, vocational, and social services; smoking cessation programs)<br>11. reinforce behaviors suggesting future compliance with prescribed treatments (e.g. statements reflecting plans for integrating treatments into life style, active participation in treatment plan, changes in personal habits)<br>12. include significant others in explanations and teaching sessions and encourage their support; reinforce the need for client to assume responsibility for managing as much of care as possible.<br>c. Consult physician about referrals to community health agencies if continued instruction, support, or supervision is needed. |

## 12. NURSING DIAGNOSIS: Knowledge deficit

regarding follow-up care.

| Desired Outcomes | Nursing Actions and ***Selected Purposes/Rationales*** |
|---|---|
| 12.a. The client will identify ways to prevent or minimize further respiratory problems. | 12.a.1. Instruct client in ways to prevent or minimize further respiratory problems:<br>a. maintain overall general good health:<br>1. eat a well-balanced diet<br>2. schedule adequate rest periods to avoid undue fatigue<br>3. adhere to prescribed graded exercise program<br>4. control or eliminate factors that cause stress<br>b. stop smoking<br>c. avoid exposure to respiratory irritants such as tobacco smoke, dust, perfumes, aerosol sprays, paint fumes, and solvents<br>d. remain indoors when air pollution levels and/or pollen counts are high and/or outdoor temperatures are extremely hot or cold<br>e. avoid high altitudes<br>f. wear a mask or scarf over nose and mouth if exposure to high levels of irritants such as smoke, fumes, and dust is unavoidable<br>g. decrease the risk of respiratory tract infections:<br>1. avoid contact with persons who have respiratory tract infections<br>2. avoid crowds and poorly ventilated areas<br>3. receive immunizations against influenza and pneumococcal pneumonia<br>4. take antimicrobials as prescribed (many physicians instruct clients to begin antimicrobial therapy if sputum color becomes yellow or green)<br>5. adhere to chest physiotherapy (e.g. postural drainage, vibration, percussion, breathing exercises) as ordered<br>6. take medications such as bronchodilators and mucolytics as prescribed<br>7. cleanse all respiratory care equipment properly<br>8. drink at least 10 glasses of liquid/day.<br>2. Assist client in identifying ways he/she can make appropriate changes in personal habits and life style to reduce modifiable risk factors. |
| 12.b. The client will | 12.b.1. Reinforce instructions about proper breathing techniques and chest |

| | |
|---|---|
| demonstrate proper breathing techniques, chest physiotherapy, and use of respiratory equipment. | physiotherapy including:<br>a. diaphragmatic breathing<br>b. pursed lip breathing<br>c. postural drainage, percussion, and vibration.<br>2. Reinforce instructions about use of respiratory equipment (e.g. oxygen, incentive spirometer).<br>3. Allow time for questions, clarification, and return demonstration. |
| 12.c. The client will verbalize an understanding of medications ordered including rationale, side effects, methods of administering, and importance of taking as prescribed. | 12.c.1. Explain the rationale for, side effects of, and importance of taking medications prescribed.<br>2. Instruct in proper use of nebulizers and metered-dose inhalers (MDI) if prescribed. Allow time for client to practice the techniques.<br>3. If client is discharged on theophylline, instruct to:<br>a. take it with food to minimize nausea, vomiting, and epigastric pain<br>b. take it on a regular basis as ordered to maintain therapeutic blood levels<br>c. report signs and symptoms that could indicate overdose (e.g. persistent nausea, vomiting, dizziness, insomnia, rapid pulse, profuse diaphoresis, muscle twitching, seizures)<br>d. have blood theophylline levels evaluated periodically.<br>4. Reinforce the need to consult health care provider before taking additional prescription and nonprescription medications. |
| 12.d. The client will identify appropriate safety measures related to COPD and its treatment. | 12.d. Instruct client regarding the following safety measures:<br>1. do not smoke when using oxygen therapy<br>2. do not set oxygen flow rate at a level higher than prescribed by physician<br>3. do not allow any source of spark or flame within 10 feet of the oxygen source<br>4. ensure that all electrical equipment in the area of the oxygen source is grounded<br>5. always wear a Medic-Alert tag to ensure that proper medications and appropriate oxygen flow rate are administered in emergency situations<br>6. notify health care providers of the disease condition and current therapy. |
| 12.e. The client will state signs and symptoms to report to the health care provider. | 12.e. Instruct client to report:<br>1. changes in sputum characteristics (e.g. increase in volume or consistency, yellow or green color)<br>2. sputum that does not return to usual color after 3 days of antimicrobial therapy<br>3. cough that becomes worse<br>4. increased fatigue, weakness, and shortness of breath<br>5. increased need for medications and/or oxygen therapy<br>6. elevated temperature<br>7. drowsiness, confusion<br>8. chest pain<br>9. persistent weight loss or sudden weight gain<br>10. swelling in ankles and/or feet<br>11. signs and symptoms of theophylline overdose (see action c.3.c in this diagnosis). |
| 12.f. The client will identify community resources that can assist with home management and adjustment to changes resulting from COPD. | 12.f.1. Provide information regarding community resources that can assist client and significant others with home management and adjustment to changes resulting from COPD (e.g. American Lung Association; respiratory equipment companies; Better Breather's Club; pulmonary rehabilitation groups; counseling, vocational, and social services; Meals on Wheels; transportation services; home health agencies).<br>2. Initiate a referral if indicated. |
| 12.g. The client will | 12.g.1. Reinforce importance of lifelong follow-up care. |

| Desired Outcomes | Nursing Actions and ***Selected Purposes/Rationales*** |
|---|---|
| verbalize an understanding of and a plan for adhering to recommended follow-up care including future appointments with health care provider and graded exercise program. | 2. Reinforce physician's instructions about a graded exercise program (e.g. walking for 20 minutes 3 times a week, stationary bicycling).<br>3. Implement measures to promote effective management of the therapeutic regimen (see Nursing Diagnosis 11, action b). |

# Pneumonia

Pneumonia is an acute inflammation of lung tissue resulting from exposure to environmental irritants such as toxic chemicals, gases, and dust or pathogenic organisms (e.g. bacteria, viruses, fungi). Pneumonia can also result from aspiration of body secretions, food, fluid, and foreign objects.

Pneumonia is usually classified according to the causative organism or etiological factor. It may also be classified as community-acquired, hospital-acquired, or atypical. The types differ in relation to the mechanism of lung invasion (i.e. inhalation, aspiration, vascular system, direct extension), incubation period, signs and symptoms experienced by the client, complications that can result, and mortality rate. The most common type of bacterial pneumonia is community-acquired pneumococcal pneumonia. It occurs most often in winter and early spring, has an abrupt onset, and usually follows an upper respiratory infection. Persons at greatest risk for development of pneumococcal pneumonia are those who have impaired pulmonary defense mechanisms (e.g. the immunosuppressed, the very young or old, persons with chronic pulmonary disease or alcoholism, those with neurological deficits that result in a decreased level of consciousness or swallowing impairments, smokers). The majority of cases result from aspiration of "normal" oropharyngeal secretions containing pneumococci into the terminal bronchioles and alveoli and the subsequent inability to clear these secretions adequately from the respiratory tract. Pneumococcal pneumonia may involve segments of one or more lobes of the lung.

**This care plan focuses on the adult client hospitalized for treatment of pneumococcal pneumonia.** Goals of care are to improve respiratory function, relieve discomfort, prevent complications, and educate the client regarding follow-up care.

## DIAGNOSTIC TESTS

Chest x-ray
White blood cell count and differential
Serum studies (e.g. viral or *Legionella* titers, cold agglutinins)
Sputum studies for Gram's stain, culture, and sensitivity
Oximetry
Blood gases

## DISCHARGE CRITERIA

Prior to discharge, the client will:

- have no signs and symptoms of complications
- identify ways to maintain respiratory health
- state signs and symptoms to report to the health care provider
- verbalize an understanding of and a plan for adhering to recommended follow-up care including future appointments with health care provider, medications prescribed, and activity limitations.

**NURSING/ COLLABORATIVE DIAGNOSES**



## 1. NURSING DIAGNOSIS: Impaired respiratory function*:

a. **ineffective breathing pattern** related to:
   1. impaired lung/chest wall expansion associated with weakness, fatigue, chest pain, and pleural effusion if present
   2. increase in the metabolic rate associated with the infectious process;

b. **ineffective airway clearance** related to:
   1. increased production of secretions associated with the inflammatory process
   2. stasis of secretions associated with decreased activity, impaired ciliary function (results from the increased viscosity and volume of mucus with the infectious process), and poor cough effort resulting from fatigue and chest pain;

c. **impaired gas exchange** related to a decrease in effective lung surface associated with the accumulation of secretions and consolidation of lung tissue.

*This diagnostic label includes the following nursing diagnoses: ineffective breathing pattern, ineffective airway clearance, and impaired gas exchange.

| Desired Outcome | Nursing Actions and ***Selected Purposes/Rationales*** |
|---|---|
| 1. The client will experience adequate respiratory function as evidenced by:<br>a. normal rate, rhythm, and depth of respirations<br>b. decreased dyspnea<br>c. improved breath sounds<br>d. usual mental status<br>e. usual skin color<br>f. blood gases within normal range. | 1.a. Assess for and report signs and symptoms of impaired respiratory function:<br>1. rapid, shallow, or irregular respirations<br>2. dyspnea, orthopnea<br>3. use of accessory muscles when breathing<br>4. abnormal breath sounds (e.g. diminished, bronchial, crackles [rales], wheezes)<br>5. restlessness, irritability<br>6. confusion, somnolence<br>7. central cyanosis (a late sign).<br>b. Monitor for and report the following:<br>1. abnormal blood gases<br>2. significant changes in oximetry results<br>3. abnormal chest x-ray results. |

| Desired Outcome | Nursing Actions and ***Selected Purposes/Rationales*** |
|---|---|

c. Implement measures *to improve respiratory status:*
   1. maintain client on bed rest as ordered during the acute phase *to reduce oxygen needs*
   2. place client in a semi- to high Fowler's position unless contraindicated; position with pillows *to prevent slumping*
   3. instruct client to breathe slowly if he/she is hyperventilating
   4. assist client to turn from side to side at least every 2 hours while in bed
   5. instruct client to deep breathe or use incentive spirometer at least every 2 hours
   6. assist with IPPB treatments as ordered
   7. perform actions *to facilitate removal of pulmonary secretions:*
      a. instruct and assist client to cough or "huff" every 1-2 hours
      b. implement measures *to liquefy tenacious secretions:*
         1. maintain a fluid intake of at least 2500 ml/day unless contraindicated
         2. humidify inspired air as ordered
      c. assist with administration of diluent and mucolytic agents via nebulizer or IPPB treatment if ordered
      d. assist with or perform postural drainage, percussion, and vibration if ordered
      e. perform tracheal suctioning if ordered
      f. administer expectorants if ordered
   8. perform actions to reduce chest pain (see Nursing Diagnosis 4, action e)
   9. maintain oxygen therapy as ordered
   10. instruct client to avoid intake of gas-forming foods (e.g. beans, cauliflower, cabbage, onions), carbonated beverages, and large meals *in order to prevent gastric distention and increased pressure on the diaphragm*
   11. discourage smoking *(smoke causes bronchoconstriction, increases mucus production, impairs ciliary function, and decreases oxygen availability)*
   12. protect client from exposure to irritants such as smoke, flowers, and perfume *(can cause bronchospasm and increased mucus production)*
   13. when activity is allowed, perform actions to increase strength and activity tolerance (see Nursing Diagnosis 7, action b)
   14. administer central nervous system depressants judiciously; hold medication and consult physician if respiratory rate is less than 12/minute
   15. administer the following medications if ordered:
      a. bronchodilators (e.g. theophylline)
      b. antimicrobials.

d. Consult physician if signs and symptoms of impaired respiratory function persist or worsen.

## 2. NURSING DIAGNOSIS: High risk for fluid volume deficit

related to decreased oral intake and excessive fluid loss (occurs with profuse diaphoresis and hyperventilation if present).

| Desired Outcome | Nursing Actions and ***Selected Purposes/Rationales*** |
|---|---|
| 2. The client will not experience a fluid | 2.a. Assess for and report signs and symptoms of fluid volume deficit:<br>1. decreased skin turgor |

volume deficit as evidenced by:
a. normal skin turgor
b. moist mucous membranes
c. stable weight
d. B/P and pulse within normal range for client and stable with position change
e. small vein filling time less than 3-5 seconds
f. BUN and Hct within normal range
g. balanced intake and output.

2. dry mucous membranes, thirst
3. sudden weight loss of 2% or greater
4. low B/P and/or postural hypotension
5. weak, rapid pulse
6. delayed small vein filling time (longer than 3-5 seconds)
7. elevated BUN and Hct
8. decreased urine output (reflects an actual rather than potential fluid volume deficit).

b. Implement measures *to prevent fluid volume deficit:*
1. perform actions to improve oral intake (see Nursing Diagnosis 3, action c.1)
2. perform actions to reduce fever (see Nursing Diagnosis 6, action b) *in order to reduce fluid loss resulting from the diaphoresis and hyperventilation that may accompany an increase in temperature*
3. maintain a fluid intake of at least 2500 ml/day unless contraindicated; if oral intake is inadequate or contraindicated, maintain intravenous therapy as ordered.

## 3. NURSING DIAGNOSIS: Altered nutrition: less than body requirements

related to:
a. decreased oral intake associated with fatigue, excessive coughing, the foul odor and taste of sputum and some aerosol treatments, nausea, chest pain, and dyspnea;
b. increased nutritional needs associated with the increase in metabolic rate that occurs with an infectious process.

| Desired Outcome | Nursing Actions and ***Selected Purposes/Rationales*** |
|---|---|

3. The client will maintain an adequate nutritional status as evidenced by:
a. weight within normal range for client's age, height, and body frame
b. normal BUN and serum albumin, Hct, Hb, and transferrin levels
c. triceps skinfold thickness within normal range
d. usual strength and activity tolerance
e. healthy oral mucous membrane.

3.a. Assess for and report signs and symptoms of malnutrition:
1. weight below normal for client's age, height, and body frame
2. abnormal BUN and low serum albumin, Hct, Hb, and transferrin levels
3. triceps skinfold thickness less than normal
4. increased weakness and fatigue
5. stomatitis.

b. Monitor percentage of meals and snacks client consumes. Report a pattern of inadequate intake.

c. Implement measures *to maintain an adequate nutritional status:*
1. perform actions *to improve oral intake:*
   a. implement measures to prevent or treat nausea (see Nursing Diagnosis 5.B, action 2)
   b. implement measures to reduce pain (see Nursing Diagnosis 4, action e)
   c. schedule respiratory therapy 1 hour before or after meals if possible
   d. increase activity as allowed and tolerated *(activity stimulates appetite)*
   e. obtain a dietary consult if necessary to assist client in selecting foods/fluids that meet nutritional needs as well as personal and cultural preferences whenever possible
   f. encourage a rest period before meals *to minimize fatigue*
   g. maintain a clean environment and a relaxed, pleasant atmosphere
   h. assist with oral hygiene before meals and after respiratory therapy
   i. serve small portions of nutritious foods/fluids that are appealing to the client
   j. place client in a high Fowler's position for meals and provide supplemental oxygen therapy during meals if indicated *to help relieve dyspnea*

| Desired Outcome | Nursing Actions and ***Selected Purposes/Rationales*** |
|---|---|
| | k. allow adequate time for meals; reheat food if necessary<br>2. ensure that meals are well balanced and high in essential nutrients; offer dietary supplements between meals if indicated<br>3. administer vitamins and minerals if ordered.<br>d. Perform a 72-hour calorie count if ordered. Report totals to dietitian and physician.<br>e. Consult physician about alternative methods of providing nutrition (e.g. parenteral nutrition, tube feedings) if client does not consume enough food or fluids to meet nutritional needs. |

## 4. NURSING DIAGNOSIS: Pain: chest

related to:

a. irritation of the parietal pleura and lung parenchyma associated with the inflammatory process;
b. muscle strain associated with excessive coughing.

| Desired Outcome | Nursing Actions and ***Selected Purposes/Rationales*** |
|---|---|
| 4. The client will experience diminished chest pain as evidenced by:<br>a. verbalization of pain relief<br>b. relaxed facial expression and body positioning<br>c. increased participation in activities<br>d. stable vital signs. | 4.a. Determine how the client usually responds to pain.<br>b. Assess client's perception of pain including location, intensity, and type. Utilize a numerical scale to rate intensity.<br>c. Assess for nonverbal signs of pain (e.g. wrinkled brow, clenched fists, reluctance to move, restlessness, guarding of affected side of chest, diaphoresis, facial pallor, increased B/P, further increase in pulse).<br>d. Assess for factors that seem to aggravate and alleviate pain.<br>e. Implement measures *to reduce chest pain:*<br>1. perform actions *to reduce fear and anxiety about the pain experience* (e.g. assure client that his/her need for pain relief will be met)<br>2. medicate prior to any painful procedures (e.g. transtracheal sputum aspiration) and before pain becomes severe<br>3. instruct and assist client to splint chest with hands or pillow when deep breathing, coughing, and changing position<br>4. assist client to assume a position of comfort (usually lying on affected side, *which minimizes stretching of the inflamed pleura*)<br>5. provide or assist with nonpharmacological measures for pain relief (e.g. back rub, position change, relaxation techniques, quiet conversation, restful environment, diversional activities)<br>6. perform actions to decrease excessive coughing (see Nursing Diagnosis 7, action b.1.j)<br>7. administer analgesics if ordered.<br>f. Consult physician if above actions fail to provide adequate relief of chest pain. |

## 5.A. NURSING DIAGNOSIS: Altered comfort: chills and excessive diaphoresis

related to persistent fever associated with the infectious process.

| Desired Outcome | Nursing Actions and ***Selected Purposes/Rationales*** |
|---|---|
| 5.A. The client will not experience discomfort associated with chills and excessive diaphoresis as evidenced by:<br>1. verbalization of comfort<br>2. ability to rest. | 5.A.1. Assess client for chills and excessive diaphoresis.<br>2. Implement measures to reduce fever (see Nursing Diagnosis 6, action b).<br>3. Implement measures *to promote comfort if client is having chills:*<br>a. maintain a room temperature that is comfortable for client<br>b. protect client from drafts<br>c. provide extra blankets and clothing as needed<br>d. provide warm liquids to drink as tolerated.<br>4. Implement measures *to promote comfort if excessive diaphoresis is present:*<br>a. change linen and clothing whenever damp<br>b. bathe client and sponge his/her face as needed.<br>5. Consult physician if client continues to have chills and excessive diaphoresis. |

## 5.B. NURSING DIAGNOSIS: Altered comfort: nausea

related to cortical stimulation of the vomiting center associated with the foul odor and taste of sputum and some aerosol treatments.

| Desired Outcome | Nursing Actions and ***Selected Purposes/Rationales*** |
|---|---|
| 5.B. The client will verbalize relief of nausea. | 5.B.1. Assess client for nausea.<br>2. Implement measures *to prevent or treat nausea:*<br>a. encourage client to take deep, slow breaths when nauseated<br>b. eliminate noxious sights and odors from the environment; provide client with an opaque, covered container for expectorated sputum; empty container frequently and remove it from the table during mealtime if it is not needed *(noxious stimuli cause cortical stimulation of the vomiting center)*<br>c. provide oral hygiene after chest physiotherapy and aerosol treatments and before meals<br>d. schedule treatments that assist in mobilizing mucus (e.g. aerosol treatments, postural drainage, percussion, vibration) at least 1 hour before or after meals<br>e. provide small, frequent meals; instruct client to ingest foods and fluids slowly<br>f. avoid serving foods with an overpowering aroma; remove lids from hot foods before entering room<br>g. encourage client to eat dry foods (e.g. toast, crackers) and avoid drinking liquids with meals if nauseated<br>h. administer antiemetics if ordered.<br>3. Consult physician if above measures fail to control nausea. |

## 6. NURSING DIAGNOSIS: Hyperthermia

related to stimulation of the thermoregulatory center in the hypothalamus by endogenous pyrogens that are released in an infectious process.

**Desired Outcome** | **Nursing Actions and *Selected Purposes/Rationales***

**Desired Outcome**

6. The client will experience resolution of hyperthermia as evidenced by:
   a. skin usual temperature and color
   b. pulse rate between 60-100 beats/minute
   c. respirations 14-20/minute
   d. normal body temperature.

**Nursing Actions and *Selected Purposes/Rationales***

6.a. Assess for signs and symptoms of hyperthermia (e.g. warm, flushed skin; tachycardia; tachypnea; elevated temperature).
  b. Implement measures *to reduce fever:*
    1. perform actions *to resolve the infectious process:*
      a. implement measures to facilitate removal of pulmonary secretions (see Nursing Diagnosis 1, action c.7)
      b. implement measures to promote rest and/or conserve energy (see Nursing Diagnosis 7, action b.1)
      c. implement measures to maintain an adequate nutritional status (see Nursing Diagnosis 3, action c)
      d. administer antimicrobials if ordered
    2. administer tepid sponge bath and/or apply cool cloths to groin and axillae
    3. apply cooling blanket as ordered
    4. utilize a room fan *to provide cool circulating air and increase heat loss through conduction*
    5. administer antipyretics if ordered.
  c. Consult physician if temperature remains elevated.

## 7. NURSING DIAGNOSIS: Activity intolerance

related to:
a. tissue hypoxia associated with impaired gas exchange;
b. difficulty resting and sleeping associated with excessive coughing, dyspnea, discomfort, unfamiliar environment, and frequent assessments and treatments;
c. inadequate nutritional status;
d. increased energy expenditure associated with persistent coughing and the increased metabolic rate that is present in an infectious process.

**Desired Outcome**

7. The client will demonstrate an increased tolerance for activity as evidenced by:
   a. verbalization of feeling less fatigued and weak
   b. ability to perform activities of daily living without dizziness; increased dyspnea, chest pain, and diaphoresis; and a significant change in vital signs.

**Nursing Actions and *Selected Purposes/Rationales***

7.a. Assess for signs and symptoms of activity intolerance:
    1. statements of fatigue and weakness
    2. exertional dyspnea, chest pain, diaphoresis, or dizziness
    3. abnormal heart rate response to activity (e.g. increase in rate of 20 beats/minute above resting rate, decrease in rate, rate not returning to preactivity level within 3 minutes after stopping activity, change from regular to irregular rate)
    4. decreased systolic B/P or a significant increase (10-15 mm Hg) in systolic or diastolic pressure with activity.
  b. Implement measures *to improve activity tolerance:*
    1. perform actions *to promote rest and/or conserve energy:*
      a. maintain activity restrictions as ordered
      b. minimize environmental activity and noise
      c. organize nursing care to allow for periods of uninterrupted rest
      d. limit the number of visitors and their length of stay
      e. assist client with self-care activities as needed
      f. keep supplies and personal articles within easy reach
      g. instruct client in energy-saving techniques (e.g. using shower chair when showering, sitting to brush teeth or comb hair)
      h. implement measures to promote sleep (see Nursing Diagnosis 8, action c)

i. implement measures to reduce discomfort (see Nursing Diagnoses 4, action e; 5.A, actions 3 and 4; and 5.B, action 2)
j. implement measures *to decrease excessive coughing:*
   1. protect client from exposure to irritants such as smoke, flowers, and powder
   2. instruct client to avoid intake of extremely hot or cold foods/fluids *(these can stimulate cough)*
   3. administer antitussives if ordered (may be prescribed during the acute phase when the cough is usually nonproductive)

2. perform actions to reduce fever (see Nursing Diagnosis 6, action b)
3. discourage smoking and excessive intake of beverages high in caffeine such as coffee, tea, and colas *(nicotine and caffeine increase cardiac workload and myocardial oxygen utilization, thereby decreasing oxygen availability)*
4. perform actions to improve respiratory status (see Nursing Diagnosis 1, action c) *in order to relieve dyspnea and improve tissue oxygenation*
5. if oxygen therapy is necessary during activity, keep portable oxygen equipment readily available for client's use
6. perform actions to maintain an adequate nutritional status (see Nursing Diagnosis 3, action c)
7. increase client's activity gradually as allowed and tolerated.

c. Instruct client to:
   1. report a decreased tolerance for activity
   2. stop any activity that causes increased chest pain, increased shortness of breath, dizziness, or extreme fatigue or weakness.

d. Consult physician if signs and symptoms of activity intolerance persist or worsen.

## 8. NURSING DIAGNOSIS: Sleep pattern disturbance

related to unfamiliar environment, discomfort, excessive coughing, inability to assume usual sleep position because of dyspnea, and frequent assessments and treatments.

| Desired Outcome | Nursing Actions and ***Selected Purposes/Rationales*** |
|---|---|
| 8. The client will attain optimal amounts of sleep within the parameters of the treatment regimen as evidenced by:<br>a. statements of feeling well rested<br>b. usual mental status<br>c. absence of frequent yawning, dark circles under eyes, and hand tremors. | 8.a. Assess for signs and symptoms of a sleep pattern disturbance (e.g. verbal complaints of difficulty falling asleep, sleep interruptions, or not feeling well rested; irritability; lethargy; disorientation; frequent yawning; dark circles under eyes; slight hand tremors).<br>b. Determine the client's usual sleep habits.<br>c. Implement measures *to promote sleep:*<br>1. discourage long periods of sleep during the day unless signs and symptoms of sleep deprivation exist or daytime sleep is usual for client<br>2. perform actions to reduce discomfort (see Nursing Diagnoses 4, action e; 5.A, actions 3 and 4; and 5.B, action 2)<br>3. perform actions to reduce excessive coughing (see Nursing Diagnosis 7, action b.1.j)<br>4. encourage participation in relaxing diversional activities during the evening<br>5. discourage intake of fluids high in caffeine (e.g. coffee, tea, colas), especially in the evening<br>6. offer client a high-protein evening snack (e.g. cheese) unless contraindicated |

| Desired Outcome | Nursing Actions and ***Selected Purposes/Rationales*** |
|---|---|
| | 7. allow client to continue usual sleep practices (e.g. time, bedtime rituals such as reading and meditating) if possible<br>8. satisfy basic needs such as comfort and warmth before sleep<br>9. have client empty bladder just before bedtime<br>10. maintain a quiet, restful atmosphere; have earplugs available for client if needed<br>11. utilize relaxation techniques (e.g. back massage, meditation, soft music) before sleep<br>12. ensure good room ventilation<br>13. if client has orthopnea, assist him/her to assume a position *that facilitates breathing* (e.g. head of bed elevated with arms supported on pillows, resting forward on overbed table with good pillow support, sitting in a chair)<br>14. maintain oxygen therapy during sleep<br>15. administer sedative-hypnotics if ordered<br>16. perform actions *to reduce interruptions during sleep (80-100 minutes of uninterrupted sleep are usually needed to complete one sleep cycle):*<br>a. restrict visitors<br>b. group care (e.g. medications, treatments, physical care, assessments) whenever possible.<br>d. Consult physician if signs and symptoms of sleep deprivation persist or worsen. |

## 9. NURSING DIAGNOSIS: High risk for infection: extrapulmonary (e.g. bacteremia, pericarditis, endocarditis, meningitis, septic arthritis) and/or superinfection (e.g. candidiasis)

related to:
a. spread of pneumococcus via the blood stream associated with inadequate host defenses;
b. resistance of pneumococcus to antimicrobial agents;
c. interruption in the balance of usual endogenous microbial flora associated with the administration of antimicrobial agents.

| Desired Outcome | Nursing Actions and ***Selected Purposes/Rationales*** |
|---|---|
| 9. The client will not develop an extrapulmonary infection or a superinfection as evidenced by:<br>a. gradual return of vital signs to normal<br>b. improved breath sounds<br>c. usual mental status<br>d. absence of joint pain and swelling<br>e. absence of unusual drainage from any body cavity | 9.a. Assess for and report signs and symptoms of an extrapulmonary infection or a superinfection:<br>1. increase in temperature above previous levels<br>2. increase in dyspnea and pulse rate<br>3. cardiac arrhythmias<br>4. breath sounds that worsen or fail to improve<br>5. change in mental status<br>6. swollen, red, painful joints<br>7. unusual color, amount, and odor of vaginal drainage; perineal itching; white patches or ulcerated areas in the mouth or vagina *(fungal infections are common superinfections with antimicrobial therapy)*<br>8. stiff neck, headache<br>9. increase in WBC count above previous levels and/or significant change in differential.<br>b. Obtain specimens (e.g. blood, urine, mouth, sputum, vaginal) for culture as ordered. Report positive results. |

f. absence of unusual lesions
g. absence of stiff neck and headache
h. WBC and differential counts returning toward normal range for client
i. negative results of cultured specimens.

c. Implement measures *to prevent an extrapulmonary infection and/or a superinfection:*
   1. perform actions to resolve the infectious process (see Nursing Diagnosis 6, action b.1)
   2. use good handwashing technique and encourage client to do the same
   3. maintain meticulous aseptic technique during all invasive procedures (e.g. catheterizations, venous and arterial punctures, injections)
   4. change intravenous tubings and solutions and rotate insertion sites according to hospital policy
   5. protect client from others with infection
   6. perform actions *to prevent the introduction of microorganisms into the urinary tract* (e.g. assist client with perineal care as needed, instruct and assist female client to wipe from front to back after urinating and defecating)
   7. reinforce importance of good oral hygiene.
d. If signs and symptoms of an extrapulmonary infection or a superinfection occur:
   1. continue with above measures
   2. prepare client for and/or assist with diagnostic tests (e.g. spinal tap, echocardiography) if planned
   3. implement appropriate comfort measures for symptoms experienced
   4. implement measures *to ensure client safety* (e.g. raise side rails, assist client with ambulation) if changes in mental status are present
   5. administer antimicrobials as ordered.

## 10. COLLABORATIVE DIAGNOSES:

**Potential complications:**

a. **pleural effusion** related to an increase in pulmonary capillary permeability associated with the inflammatory process;
b. **atelectasis** related to shallow respirations, stasis of secretions in the alveoli and bronchioles, and decreased surfactant production (results from inadequate deep breathing and changes in regional blood flow in the lungs that can occur when mobility is decreased).

| Desired Outcomes | Nursing Actions and ***Selected Purposes/Rationales*** |
|---|---|
| 10.a. The client will not develop pleural effusion as evidenced by:<br>1. no increase in chest pain<br>2. unlabored respirations at 14-20/minute<br>3. usual chest excursion<br>4. improved breath sounds and percussion note throughout lung fields. | 10.a.1. Assess for and report signs and symptoms of pleural effusion:<br>a. increase in chest pain<br>b. increased dyspnea<br>c. decreased chest excursion on affected side<br>d. dull percussion note and diminished or absent breath sounds over affected area.<br>2. Monitor chest x-ray, ultrasound, and computed tomography results. Report findings of pleural effusion.<br>3. Implement measures to resolve the infectious process (see Nursing Diagnosis 6, action b.1) *in order to reduce the risk for the development of pleural effusion.*<br>4. If signs and symptoms of pleural effusion occur:<br>a. continue with actions to improve respiratory status (see Nursing Diagnosis 1, action c)<br>b. prepare client for a thoracentesis and/or insertion of chest tube if planned. |
| 10.b. The client will not | 10.b.1. Assess for and report signs and symptoms of atelectasis (e.g. |

| Desired Outcomes | Nursing Actions and ***Selected Purposes/Rationales*** |
|---|---|
| develop atelectasis as evidenced by:<br>1. improved breath sounds and percussion note over lungs<br>2. unlabored respirations at 14-20/minute<br>3. no increase in dyspnea, pulse rate, or temperature. | diminished or absent breath sounds; dull percussion note over affected area; further increase in respiratory rate, dyspnea, and temperature).<br>2. Monitor chest x-ray results. Report findings of atelectasis.<br>3. Implement measures to improve respiratory status (see Nursing Diagnosis 1, action c) *in order to reduce the risk of atelectasis.*<br>4. If signs and symptoms of atelectasis occur:<br>a. increase frequency of turning, coughing or "huffing," deep breathing, and use of incentive spirometer<br>b. increase activity as allowed and tolerated<br>c. consult physician if signs and symptoms of atelectasis persist or worsen. |

## 11. NURSING DIAGNOSIS: Knowledge deficit regarding follow-up care.

| Desired Outcomes | Nursing Actions and ***Selected Purposes/Rationales*** |
|---|---|
| 11.a. The client will identify ways to maintain respiratory health. | 11.a. Instruct client in ways to maintain respiratory health:<br>1. consume a well-balanced diet<br>2. drink at least 10 glasses of liquid/day<br>3. maintain a balanced program of rest and exercise<br>4. avoid crowds during flu and cold season<br>5. avoid contact with persons who have respiratory infections<br>6. consult physician about vaccinations available if at high risk for recurrent pneumonia<br>7. continue coughing and deep breathing exercises for at least 6-8 weeks after discharge and during any period of decreased physical activity or respiratory infection<br>8. maintain good oral hygiene in order to reduce the number of organisms in the oropharynx<br>9. avoid excessive alcohol intake and stop smoking to prevent depression of pulmonary antimicrobial defenses. |
| 11.b. The client will state signs and symptoms to report to the health care provider. | 11.b. Instruct client to report the following signs and symptoms:<br>1. persistent or recurrent temperature elevation<br>2. chills<br>3. difficulty breathing<br>4. restlessness, irritability, drowsiness, or confusion<br>5. persistent or increased chest pain or irregular heart rate<br>6. persistent weight loss<br>7. persistent fatigue<br>8. persistent cough productive of purulent or rust-colored sputum<br>9. unusual color, amount, and odor of vaginal secretions<br>10. white patches or ulcerated areas in the mouth or vagina<br>11. stiff neck or headache<br>12. swollen, red, painful joints. |
| 11.c. The client will verbalize an understanding of and a plan for adhering | 11.c. 1. Reinforce the importance of keeping follow-up appointments with health care provider.<br>2. Explain the rationale for, side effects of, and importance of taking medications prescribed (e.g. antimicrobials, mucolytics).<br>3. Implement measures to improve client compliance: |

to recommended follow-up care including future appointments with health care provider, medications prescribed, and activity limitations.

a. include significant others in all discharge teaching sessions if possible
b. encourage questions and allow time for reinforcement and clarification of information provided
c. provide written instructions regarding scheduled appointments with health care provider, medications prescribed, fluid requirements, respiratory care, and signs and symptoms to report.

# Pneumothorax

Pneumothorax is an accumulation of air in the pleural space that results in complete or partial collapse of the lung. Pneumothorax is typically classified as spontaneous or traumatic. A spontaneous pneumothorax is one that occurs in the absence of accidental or intentional trauma. This type may be further classified as primary (simple) or secondary. A primary spontaneous pneumothorax most commonly occurs in tall, thin, young men between the ages of 20 and 40 years. The cause is usually unknown, but it is thought in many cases to be the result of rupture of subpleural blebs at the apex of the lung directly into the pleural space. A secondary spontaneous pneumothorax occurs as a result of preexisting lung disease such as emphysema, asthma, or a malignancy. In a traumatic pneumothorax, air enters the pleural space as a result of a penetrating or nonpenetrating chest injury. This type frequently is surgically induced or occurs as a complication of a diagnostic or therapeutic measure (e.g. insertion of a central venous catheter, transtracheal biopsy, positive-pressure mechanical ventilation).

Symptoms experienced by the client with a pneumothorax depend on the degree of lung collapse. If the pneumothorax involves less than 20% of the hemithorax and the client is asymptomatic, no treatment is necessary and the air in the pleural space is usually reabsorbed in 7 to 14 days. In the majority of situations, however, intervention is needed to re-establish negative intrapleural pressure and re-expand the lung. Establishment of a chest drainage system is the treatment of choice. Resection of lung blebs and/or pleural scarification may also be indicated for the client who has experienced recurrent episodes of spontaneous pneumothorax.

**This care plan focuses on the adult client hospitalized for diagnosis and treatment of a primary spontaneous pneumothorax.** Goals of care are to maintain an adequate respiratory status, relieve pain, prevent complications, and educate the client regarding follow-up care.

## DIAGNOSTIC TESTS

Chest x-ray
Blood gas analysis
Oximetry

## DISCHARGE CRITERIA

Prior to discharge, the client will:

- experience re-expansion of affected lung
- demonstrate the ability to perform appropriate wound care
- identify ways to reduce the risk of recurrent spontaneous pneumothorax
- state signs and symptoms to report to the health care provider
- verbalize an understanding of and plan for adhering to recommended follow-up care including future appointments with health care provider, medications prescribed, and activity restrictions.

**NURSING/ COLLABORATIVE DIAGNOSES**



## 1. NURSING DIAGNOSIS: Ineffective breathing pattern

related to chest pain, fear, and anxiety.

| Desired Outcome | Nursing Actions and ***Selected Purposes/Rationales*** |
|---|---|
| 1. The client will maintain an effective breathing pattern as evidenced by:<br>a. normal rate and depth of respirations<br>b. decreased dyspnea<br>c. blood gases within normal range. | 1.a. Assess for signs and symptoms of an ineffective breathing pattern (e.g. shallow respirations, tachypnea, dyspnea, use of accessory muscles when breathing).<br>b. Monitor for and report the following:<br>1. abnormal blood gases<br>2. significant changes in oximetry results.<br>c. Implement measures *to improve breathing pattern:*<br>1. perform actions to reduce chest pain (see Nursing Diagnosis 3, action e)<br>2. perform actions to reduce fear and anxiety (see Nursing Diagnosis 5, action b)<br>3. place client in a semi- to high Fowler's position unless contraindicated<br>4. assist client to turn at least every 2 hours while in bed<br>5. instruct client to deep breathe or use incentive spirometer at least every 2 hours<br>6. instruct client to breathe slowly if he/she is hyperventilating<br>7. increase activity as allowed and tolerated<br>8. administer central nervous system depressants judiciously; hold medication and consult physician if respiratory rate is less than 12/minute.<br>d. Consult physician if ineffective breathing pattern continues. |

## 2. NURSING DIAGNOSIS: Impaired gas exchange

related to a decrease in effective surface area of lung associated with lung collapse.

| Desired Outcome | Nursing Actions and ***Selected Purposes/Rationales*** |
|---|---|
| 2. The client will experience adequate $O_2/CO_2$ exchange as evidenced by:<br>a. usual mental status<br>b. decreased dyspnea | 2.a. Assess for and report signs and symptoms of impaired gas exchange:<br>1. restlessness, irritability<br>2. confusion, somnolence<br>3. tachypnea, dyspnea<br>4. decreased $PaO_2$ and increased $PaCO_2$.<br>b. Monitor for and report significant changes in oximetry results. |

c. blood gases within normal range.

c. Implement measures *to improve gas exchange:*
   1. perform actions *to promote lung re-expansion and prevent recurrent pneumothorax:*
      a. prepare client for and assist with needle aspiration of air or insertion of chest tube if planned
      b. if chest tube is inserted:
         1. perform actions *to maintain patency and integrity of chest drainage system:*
            a. maintain water seal and suction levels as ordered
            b. maintain air occlusive dressing over chest tube insertion site
            c. tape all connections securely
            d. keep chest drainage and suction tubing free of kinks
            e. keep drainage system below level of client's chest at all times
         2. assess for and report signs and symptoms that may indicate malfunction of chest drainage system (e.g. respiratory distress, sudden cessation of drainage, excessive bubbling in water seal chamber, subcutaneous emphysema)
   2. perform actions to improve breathing pattern (see Nursing Diagnosis 1, action c)
   3. maintain oxygen therapy as ordered
   4. discourage smoking *(smoke decreases oxygen availability)*
   5. maintain activity restrictions as ordered; increase activity gradually as allowed and tolerated.

d. Consult physician if signs and symptoms of impaired gas exchange persist or worsen.

---

## 3. NURSING DIAGNOSIS: Pain: chest

related to:
a. irritation of the parietal pleura associated with:
   1. stretching of the pleura resulting from air in the pleural space
   2. inflammatory process if pleural scarification is performed;
b. tissue irritation associated with insertion and presence of chest tube.

| Desired Outcome | Nursing Actions and ***Selected Purposes/Rationales*** |
|---|---|
| 3. The client will experience diminished chest pain as evidenced by:<br>a. verbalization of pain relief<br>b. relaxed facial expression and body positioning<br>c. improved breathing pattern<br>d. increased participation in activities<br>e. stable vital signs. | 3.a. Determine how client usually responds to pain.<br>b. Assess client's perception of pain including location, intensity, and type. Utilize a numerical scale to rate intensity.<br>c. Assess for nonverbal signs of pain (e.g. wrinkled brow, clenched fists, reluctance to move, guarding of affected side of chest, diaphoresis, shallow respirations, increased blood pressure, tachycardia).<br>d. Assess for factors that seem to aggravate and alleviate pain.<br>e. Implement measures *to reduce chest pain:*<br>1. perform actions *to reduce fear and anxiety about the pain experience* (e.g. assure client that his/her need for pain relief will be met, perform preprocedure teaching)<br>2. medicate prior to any painful treatments or procedures (e.g. insertion of chest tube, pleural scarification, thoracentesis) and before pain becomes severe<br>3. instruct and assist client to splint chest with hands or pillow when deep breathing, coughing, and changing position<br>4. provide or assist with nonpharmacological measures for pain relief (e.g. position change, relaxation techniques, quiet conversation, restful environment, diversional activities) |

| Desired Outcome | Nursing Actions and ***Selected Purposes/Rationales*** |
|---|---|
| | 5. securely anchor chest tube *to limit its movement and resulting tissue irritation*<br>6. administer analgesics if ordered<br>7. assist with intercostal nerve block if performed.<br>f. Consult physician if the above measures fail to provide adequate pain relief. |

## 4. COLLABORATIVE DIAGNOSIS: Potential complication: tension pneumothorax with mediastinal shift

related to a further increase in pressure in the pleural space associated with inability of air to leave pleural space during expiration (can occur as a result of chest tube malfunction).

| Desired Outcome | Nursing Actions and ***Selected Purposes/Rationales*** |
|---|---|
| 4. The client will not develop tension pneumothorax with mediastinal shift as evidenced by:<br>a. no sudden increase in dyspnea<br>b. vital signs within normal range for client<br>c. usual mental status<br>d. absence of neck vein distention<br>e. trachea in midline position<br>f. usual skin color<br>g. blood gases returning toward normal<br>h. chest x-ray showing re-expansion of lung on affected side. | 4.a. Assess for and immediately report signs and symptoms of tension pneumothorax with mediastinal shift (e.g. increased dyspnea, rapid and/or irregular heart rate, hypotension, restlessness, agitation, neck vein distention, shift in trachea toward unaffected side, cyanosis).<br>b. Monitor blood gases. Report values that have worsened.<br>c. Monitor chest x-ray results. Report findings of tension pneumothorax with mediastinal shift.<br>d. Implement measures to maintain patency and integrity of chest drainage system (see Nursing Diagnosis 2, action c.1.b.1) *in order to reduce the risk of tension pneumothorax with mediastinal shift.*<br>e. If signs and symptoms of tension pneumothorax with mediastinal shift occur:<br>1. maintain client on bed rest in a semi- to high Fowler's position<br>2. maintain oxygen therapy as ordered<br>3. assist with clearing of existing chest tube, insertion of new tube, and/or needle aspiration of air from the pleural space *to reduce intrapleural pressure*<br>4. provide emotional support to client and significant others. |

## 5. NURSING DIAGNOSIS: Anxiety

related to difficulty breathing; chest pain; unfamiliar environment; and lack of understanding of diagnostic tests, diagnosis, treatment measures, and prognosis.

| Desired Outcome | Nursing Actions and ***Selected Purposes/Rationales*** |
|---|---|
| 5. The client will experience a reduction in anxiety as evidenced by:<br>a. verbalization of | 5.a. Assess client for signs and symptoms of anxiety (e.g. verbalization of fears and concerns, insomnia, tenseness, tremors, irritability, restlessness, diaphoresis, tachypnea, tachycardia, elevated blood pressure, facial pallor or flushing, narrowed perceptual field, withdrawal, noncompliance with |

feeling less anxious and fearful
b. usual sleep pattern
c. relaxed facial expression and body movements
d. stable vital signs
e. usual perceptual ability and interactions with others.

treatment plan). Validate perceptions carefully, remembering that some behaviors may be the result of tissue hypoxia and respiratory distress.

b. Implement measures *to reduce fear and anxiety:*
   1. orient client to hospital environment, equipment, and routines
   2. introduce staff who will be participating in client's care; if possible, maintain consistency in staff assigned to his/her care *to provide feelings of stability and comfort with the environment*
   3. assure client that staff members are nearby; respond to call signal as soon as possible
   4. maintain a calm, supportive, confident manner when interacting with client
   5. encourage verbalization of fear and anxiety; provide feedback
   6. reinforce the physician's explanations and clarify misconceptions the client has about the pneumothorax, treatment plan, and prognosis
   7. explain all diagnostic tests
   8. perform actions to reduce chest pain (see Nursing Diagnosis 3, action e)
   9. perform actions to improve gas exchange (see Nursing Diagnosis 2, action c) *in order to relieve respiratory distress*
   10. provide a calm, restful environment
   11. instruct client in relaxation techniques and encourage participation in diversional activities once the period of acute pain and respiratory distress has subsided
   12. assist client to identify specific stressors and ways to cope with them
   13. encourage significant others to project a caring, concerned attitude without obvious anxiousness
   14. if surgical intervention is indicated, begin preoperative teaching
   15. administer antianxiety agents if ordered.
c. Include significant others in orientation and teaching sessions and encourage their continued support of the client.
d. Provide information based on current needs of client and significant others at a level they can understand. Encourage questions and clarification of information provided.
e. Consult physician if above actions fail to control fear and anxiety.

## 6. NURSING DIAGNOSIS: Knowledge deficit

regarding follow-up care.

| Desired Outcomes | Nursing Actions and ***Selected Purposes/Rationales*** |
|---|---|
| 6.a. The client will demonstrate the ability to perform appropriate wound care. | 6.a.1. Instruct client on care of chest tube insertion site (e.g. occlusive dressing).<br>2. Allow time for questions, clarification, and return demonstration. |
| 6.b. The client will identify ways to reduce the risk of recurrent spontaneous pneumothorax. | 6.b.1. Caution client to avoid situations and activities that would expose him/her to marked changes in atmospheric pressure (e.g. scuba diving, flying in unpressurized aircraft).<br>2. Encourage client to stop smoking. |
| 6.c. The client will state signs and symptoms to report to the health care provider. | 6.c. Instruct client to report the following signs and symptoms:<br>1. difficulty breathing<br>2. chest pain<br>3. elevated temperature<br>4. chills |

| Desired Outcomes | Nursing Actions and ***Selected Purposes/Rationales*** |
|---|---|
| | 5. increased redness and warmth at chest tube insertion site<br>6. purulent drainage from chest tube insertion site. |
| 6.d. The client will verbalize an understanding of and plan for adhering to recommended follow-up care including future appointments with health care provider, medications prescribed, and activity restrictions. | 6.d.1. Reinforce importance of keeping follow-up appointments with health care provider.<br>2. Instruct client to avoid excessive physical exertion and lifting objects over 10 pounds until permitted by physician.<br>3. Reinforce physician's explanation about the possibility of recurrent spontaneous pneumothorax (occurs in approximately 30-50% of clients after initial episode). Assist client to develop a plan for obtaining emergency assistance should spontaneous pneumothorax recur.<br>4. Encourage client to continue with deep breathing exercises and use of incentive spirometer for time period recommended by physician.<br>5. Explain the rationale for, side effects of, and importance of taking medications prescribed.<br>6. Implement measures to improve client compliance:<br>a. include significant others in teaching sessions if possible<br>b. encourage questions and allow time for reinforcement and clarification of information provided<br>c. provide written instructions about care of chest tube insertion site, signs and symptoms to report, future appointments with health care provider, medications prescribed, and activity restrictions. |

# Pulmonary Embolism

Pulmonary embolism is the partial or complete occlusion of one of the pulmonary arteries or its branches by an embolus. The most common source of the embolism is a thrombus that originates in the deep veins of the lower extremities or the pelvis. Less frequently, the embolism can result from a thrombus originating in the right atrium or from a nonthrombic source such as air, fat, amniotic fluid, neoplastic cells, and foreign material (e.g. talc or cornstarch [may occur with intravenous drug abuse], a piece of intravenous catheter).

The clinical manifestations of pulmonary embolism are varied and nonspecific. They can range from absence of symptoms to shock. The extensiveness of the signs and symptoms depends on the size and number of emboli, size of the vessel that is occluded, extent of vessel occlusion, and presence of pre-existing cardiac or pulmonary disease. The classic signs and symptoms of a moderate-size pulmonary embolism are sudden onset of dyspnea, tachypnea, tachycardia, and a feeling of apprehension. The person may also experience chest pain.

Medical treatment varies depending on the source of the embolism and its effect on cardiopulmonary function. When the source is a thrombus, treatment usually consists of bed rest and initiation of intravenous anticoagulant therapy. A thrombolytic agent might also be administered if the thromboembolus is occluding a large vessel and/or cardiopulmonary status is severely compromised. Oral anticoagulant therapy begins during hospitalization and often continues for 3-6 months following discharge. If thrombolytic agents and anticoagulant therapy are contraindicated or unsuccessful or the source of the embolism is nonthrombic, surgical removal of the embolus may be indicated.

**This care plan focuses on the adult client hospitalized for treatment of pulmonary embolism resulting from a deep vein thrombus.** The goals of care are to reduce fear and anxiety, maintain optimal respiratory function, prevent complications, and educate the client regarding follow-up care.

## DIAGNOSTIC TESTS

Chest x-ray
Lung scan (ventilation-perfusion [V/Q] scan or perfusion scan)
Pulmonary angiography
Arterial blood gases

**DISCHARGE CRITERIA**

Prior to discharge, the client will:

- ❖ have adequate respiratory function
- ❖ have no signs and symptoms of complications
- ❖ identify ways to reduce the risk of recurrent thrombus formation and pulmonary embolism
- ❖ verbalize an understanding of medications ordered including rationale, side effects, schedule for taking, and importance of taking as prescribed
- ❖ identify ways to prevent bleeding associated with anticoagulant therapy
- ❖ state signs and symptoms to report to the health care provider
- ❖ verbalize an understanding of and a plan for adhering to recommended follow-up care including future appointments with health care provider and activity level.

**Use in conjunction with the Care Plan on Immobility.**

**NURSING/ COLLABORATIVE DIAGNOSES**

1. Ineffective breathing pattern△ 485
2. Impaired gas exchange△ 486
3. Pain: chest△ 487
4. Potential complications:
   a. right-sided heart failure
   b. extended or recurrent pulmonary embolism
   c. atelectasis
   d. bleeding△ 487
5. Anxiety△ 490
6. Knowledge deficit△ 490

**See Care Plan on Immobility for additional diagnoses.**

**1. NURSING DIAGNOSIS:**  **Ineffective breathing pattern**

related to fear, anxiety, chest pain, depressant effects of some medications (e.g. narcotic analgesics), and stimulant effects of hypoxia.

| Desired Outcome | Nursing Actions and *Selected Purposes/Rationales* |
|---|---|
| 1. The client will maintain an effective breathing pattern as evidenced by:<br>a. normal rate and depth of respirations<br>b. decreased dyspnea<br>c. blood gases within normal range. | 1.a. Assess for signs and symptoms of an ineffective breathing pattern (e.g. rapid, shallow respirations; dyspnea; use of accessory muscles when breathing).<br>b. Monitor for and report the following:<br>  1. abnormal blood gases<br>  2. significant changes in oximetry results.<br>c. Implement measures *to improve breathing pattern:*<br>  1. perform actions to reduce pain (see Nursing Diagnosis 3, action e)<br>  2. perform actions to reduce fear and anxiety (see Nursing Diagnosis 5)<br>  3. perform actions to improve gas exchange (see Nursing Diagnosis 2, action c) *in order to reduce hypoxia and subsequent stimulation of the respiratory center* |

| Desired Outcome | Nursing Actions and ***Selected Purposes/Rationales*** |
|---|---|
| | 4. place client in a semi- to high Fowler's position unless contraindicated<br>5. instruct client to breathe slowly if he/she is hyperventilating<br>6. instruct client to deep breathe or use incentive spirometer at least every 2 hours<br>7. administer central nervous system depressants judiciously; hold medication and consult physician if respiratory rate is less than 12/minute<br>8. increase activity when allowed.<br>d. Consult physician if ineffective breathing pattern persists or worsens. |

## 2. NURSING DIAGNOSIS: Impaired gas exchange

related to:

a. decreased pulmonary perfusion associated with partial or complete occlusion of pulmonary arterial blood flow by the embolus and vasoconstriction resulting from the release of vasoactive substances (e.g. serotonin, thromboxane $A_2$) from the clot;

b. decreased bronchial airflow associated with bronchoconstriction resulting from:
   1. the release of substances such as serotonin and thromboxane $A_2$ from the clot
   2. a compensatory response to an increase in the amount of dead space in the underperfused lung area (the compensatory bronchoconstriction also affects airways in perfused lung areas);

c. alveolar collapse associated with atelectasis if it occurs.

| Desired Outcome | Nursing Actions and ***Selected Purposes/Rationales*** |
|---|---|
| 2. The client will experience adequate $O_2$/$CO_2$ exchange as evidenced by:<br>a. usual mental status<br>b. unlabored respirations at 14-20/minute<br>c. blood gases within normal range. | 2.a. Assess for and report signs and symptoms of impaired gas exchange:<br>1. restlessness, irritability<br>2. confusion, somnolence<br>3. tachypnea, dyspnea.<br>b. Monitor for and report the following:<br>1. abnormal blood gases<br>2. significant changes in oximetry results.<br>c. Implement measures *to improve gas exchange:*<br>1. maintain client on bed rest *to reduce oxygen demand during acute respiratory distress;* increase activity gradually as allowed and tolerated<br>2. maintain oxygen therapy as ordered<br>3. perform actions to improve breathing pattern (see Nursing Diagnosis 1, action c)<br>4. discourage smoking *(smoke decreases oxygen availability and causes vasoconstriction)*<br>5. perform actions *to improve pulmonary blood flow:*<br>a. administer anticoagulants (e.g. continuous intravenous heparin, warfarin) if ordered<br>b. prepare client for the following if planned: |

1. injection of a thrombolytic agent (e.g. streptokinase, urokinase, tissue plasminogen activator [tPA])
2. embolectomy.

d. Consult physician if signs and symptoms of impaired gas exchange persist or worsen.

---

## 3. NURSING DIAGNOSIS: Pain: chest

related to:

a. decreased pulmonary tissue perfusion associated with obstructed pulmonary blood flow;

b. inflammation of the lung parenchyma or overlying pleura associated with tissue damage in the infarcted area.

| Desired Outcome | Nursing Actions and ***Selected Purposes/Rationales*** |
|---|---|
| 3. The client will experience diminished chest pain as evidenced by:<br>a. verbalization of pain relief<br>b. relaxed facial expression and body positioning<br>c. increased participation in activities when allowed<br>d. improved breathing pattern<br>e. pulse and B/P within normal range for client. | 3.a. Determine how the client usually responds to pain.<br>b. Assess client's perception of pain including location, intensity, and type. Utilize a numerical scale to rate intensity.<br>c. Assess for nonverbal signs of pain (e.g. wrinkled brow, rubbing chest, clenched fists, reluctance to move, restlessness, diaphoresis, facial pallor, shallow respirations, tachycardia, increased B/P).<br>d. Assess for factors that seem to aggravate and alleviate pain.<br>e. Implement measures *to reduce pain:*<br>1. perform actions *to reduce fear and anxiety about the pain experience* (e.g. assure client that his/her need for pain relief will be met)<br>2. perform actions to improve gas exchange (see Nursing Diagnosis 2, action c) *in order to reduce tissue hypoxia in the involved lung area*<br>3. instruct and assist client to splint chest with hands or pillow when deep breathing, coughing, and changing position<br>4. provide or assist with nonpharmacological measures for pain relief (e.g. position change, relaxation techniques, restful environment, diversional activities)<br>5. administer analgesics if ordered.<br>f. Consult physician if above actions fail to provide adequate pain relief. |

---

## 4. COLLABORATIVE DIAGNOSES: Potential complications:

a. **right-sided heart failure** related to increased cardiac workload associated with pulmonary hypertension (can result from pulmonary vasoconstriction that occurs in response to the decrease in pulmonary arterial blood flow);

b. **extended or recurrent pulmonary embolism** related to inadequate response to treatment and/or continued presence of predisposing conditions;

c. **atelectasis** related to:
   1. shallow respirations associated with chest pain, fear, and anxiety
   2. stasis of secretions in the alveoli and bronchioles associated with bronchoconstriction and decreased mobility during time that activity is restricted
   3. decreased surfactant production associated with reduced pulmonary blood flow and inadequate deep breathing;

d. **bleeding** related to prolonged coagulation time associated with anticoagulant therapy.

| Desired Outcomes | Nursing Actions and ***Selected Purposes/Rationales*** |
|---|---|
| 4.a. The client will not develop right-sided heart failure as evidenced by:<br>1. pulse 60-100 beats/minute<br>2. no increase in intensity of $S_2$ heart sound or development of summation gallop<br>3. usual mental status<br>4. decreased dyspnea<br>5. usual strength and activity tolerance<br>6. balanced intake and output<br>7. stable weight<br>8. CVP within normal range<br>9. absence of peripheral edema; distended neck veins; and enlarged, tender liver. | 4.a.1. Assess for and report signs and symptoms of right-sided heart failure:<br>a. further increase in pulse<br>b. development of a loud $S_2$ heart sound and/or summation gallop<br>c. restlessness, anxiousness, confusion<br>d. increased shortness of breath<br>e. development of or increased weakness and fatigue<br>f. oliguria<br>g. weight gain<br>h. elevated CVP<br>i. peripheral edema<br>j. distended neck veins<br>k. enlarged, tender liver.<br>2. Monitor chest x-ray results. Report findings of cardiomegaly.<br>3. Implement measures to improve pulmonary blood flow (see Nursing Diagnosis 2, action c.5) *in order to reduce the risk for pulmonary hypertension and subsequent right-sided heart failure.*<br>4. If signs and symptoms of right-sided heart failure occur:<br>a. maintain oxygen therapy as ordered<br>b. maintain client on strict bed rest in a semi- to high Fowler's position<br>c. maintain fluid and sodium restrictions as ordered<br>d. administer medications that may be ordered *to reduce vascular congestion and/or cardiac workload* (e.g. diuretics, cardiotonics, vasodilators)<br>e. provide emotional support to client and significant others<br>f. refer to Care Plan on Heart Failure for additional care measures. |
| 4.b. The client will not experience extension or recurrence of a pulmonary embolism as evidenced by:<br>1. absence of or diminishing chest pain<br>2. decreased dyspnea<br>3. pulse 60-100 beats/minute<br>4. usual mental status<br>5. absence of cough and hemoptysis<br>6. blood gases returning toward normal. | 4.b.1. Assess for and report signs and symptoms of extended or recurrent pulmonary embolism (e.g. development of, persistent, or increased chest pain, dyspnea, tachypnea, tachycardia, restlessness, cough, or hemoptysis; declining $Pa_{O_2}$).<br>2. Monitor WBC count. Report levels that increase or fail to return to normal *(this may indicate tissue necrosis resulting from pulmonary infarction).*<br>3. Administer heparin and/or assist with administration of thrombolytic agents (e.g. urokinase, tissue plasminogen activator [tPA], streptokinase) if ordered *to prevent extension of the embolism.*<br>4. Implement measures *to prevent recurrence of a pulmonary embolism:*<br>a. perform actions to prevent and treat a deep vein thrombus (see Care Plan on Immobility, Collaborative Diagnosis 12, actions a.1.b and c [pp. 149-150])<br>b. perform actions *to prevent dislodgment of thrombus:*<br>1. maintain client on bed rest as ordered<br>2. do not exercise, check for Homan's sign in, or massage any extremity known to have a thrombus<br>3. caution client to avoid activities that create a Valsalva response (e.g. straining to have a bowel movement, holding breath while moving).<br>5. If signs and symptoms of extended or recurrent pulmonary embolism occur:<br>a. maintain client on strict bed rest in a semi- to high Fowler's position<br>b. maintain oxygen therapy as ordered<br>c. prepare client for diagnostic tests (e.g. ventilation-perfusion lung scan, blood gases, pulmonary angiography) if indicated<br>d. prepare client for surgical intervention (e.g. embolectomy) if indicated<br>e. provide emotional support to client and significant others. |
| 4.c. The client will not | 4.c.1. Refer to Care Plan on Immobility, Collaborative Diagnosis 12, action b |

develop atelectasis (see Care Plan on Immobility, Collaborative Diagnosis 12, outcome b [p. 150], for outcome criteria).

(p. 150), for measures related to assessment, prevention, and treatment of atelectasis.

2. Implement measures to improve breathing pattern and gas exchange (see Nursing Diagnoses 1, action c and 2, action c) *in order to decrease the risk for atelectasis.*

4.d. The client will not experience unusual bleeding as evidenced by:
1. skin and mucous membranes free of petechiae, purpura, ecchymoses, and active bleeding
2. absence of unusual joint pain
3. no increase in abdominal girth
4. absence of frank and occult blood in stool, urine, and vomitus
5. usual menstrual flow
6. vital signs within normal range for client
7. stable Hct and Hb.

4.d.1. Assess client for and report signs and symptoms of unusual bleeding:
a. petechiae, purpura, ecchymoses
b. gingival bleeding
c. prolonged bleeding from puncture sites
d. epistaxis, hemoptysis
e. unusual joint pain
f. increase in abdominal girth
g. frank or occult blood in stool, urine, or vomitus
h. menorrhagia
i. restlessness, confusion
j. declining B/P and increased pulse rate
k. decline in Hct and Hb levels.

2. Monitor platelet count and coagulation test results (e.g. prothrombin time, activated partial thromboplastin time, bleeding time). Report a low platelet count and coagulation test results that exceed the therapeutic range.
3. If platelet count is low, coagulation test results are abnormal, or Hct and Hb levels decline, test all stools, urine, and vomitus for occult blood. Report positive results.
4. Implement measures *to prevent bleeding:*
   a. use the smallest gauge needle possible when giving injections and performing venous and arterial punctures
   b. apply gentle, prolonged pressure to puncture sites after injections and venous and arterial punctures
   c. avoid overinflating the cuff when taking BP
   d. caution client to avoid activities that increase the risk for trauma (e.g. shaving with a straight-edge razor, using stiff-bristle toothbrush or dental floss)
   e. avoid procedures that can cause injury to the rectal mucosa (e.g. taking temperature rectally, inserting a rectal suppository, administering an enema)
   f. perform actions *to reduce the risk for falls* (e.g. keep bed in low position with side rails up when client is in bed, avoid unnecessary clutter in room, instruct client to wear slippers/shoes with nonslip soles when ambulating)
   g. pad side rails if client is confused or restless
   h. instruct client to avoid blowing nose forcefully or straining to have a bowel movement; consult physician about an order for a decongestant, stool softener, and/or laxative if indicated.
5. If bleeding occurs and does not subside spontaneously:
   a. apply firm, prolonged pressure to bleeding area(s) if possible
   b. if epistaxis occurs, place client in a high Fowler's position and apply pressure and ice pack to nasal area
   c. maintain oxygen therapy as ordered
   d. perform gastric lavage as ordered *to control gastric bleeding*
   e. administer protamine sulfate (antidote for heparin), vitamin K (e.g. phytonadione), and plasma or whole blood as ordered
   f. assess for and report signs and symptoms of hypovolemic shock (e.g. restlessness; confusion; significant decrease in B/P; rapid, thready pulse; rapid respirations; cool, pale skin; urine output less than 30 ml/hour)
   g. prepare client for surgical repair of bleeding vessels if indicated
   h. provide emotional support to client and significant others.

## 5. NURSING DIAGNOSIS: Anxiety

related to dyspnea; chest pain; lack of understanding of diagnostic tests, diagnosis, and treatments; unfamiliar environment; possibility of recurrent embolism; and threat of death.

| Desired Outcome | Nursing Actions and ***Selected Purposes/Rationales*** |
|---|---|
| 5. The client will experience a reduction in anxiety (see Care Plan on Immobility, Nursing Diagnosis 13 [p. 153], for outcome criteria). | 5.a. Refer to Care Plan on Immobility, Nursing Diagnosis 13 (p. 153), for measures related to assessment and reduction of fear and anxiety.<br>b. Implement additional measures *to reduce fear and anxiety:*<br>1. do not leave client alone during period of acute respiratory distress<br>2. perform actions to improve gas exchange (see Nursing Diagnosis 2, action c) *in order to relieve dyspnea*<br>3. perform actions to reduce chest pain (see Nursing Diagnosis 3, action e)<br>4. explain all diagnostic tests<br>5. reassure client that his/her extreme apprehension or "sense of doom" is a common symptom of pulmonary embolism and will diminish as condition stabilizes. |

## 6. NURSING DIAGNOSIS: Knowledge deficit

regarding follow-up care.

| Desired Outcomes | Nursing Actions and ***Selected Purposes/Rationales*** |
|---|---|
| 6.a. The client will identify ways to reduce the risk of recurrent thrombus formation and pulmonary embolism. | 6.a.1. Provide the following instructions on ways to promote venous blood flow and reduce the risk of thrombus recurrence:<br>a. avoid wearing constrictive clothing (e.g. garters, girdles, narrow-banded knee-high hose)<br>b. avoid sitting and standing in one position for long periods of time<br>c. wear graduated compression stockings or support hose during the day<br>d. avoid crossing legs and lying or sitting with pillows under knees<br>e. engage in regular aerobic exercise (e.g. swimming, walking, cycling)<br>f. elevate legs periodically, especially when sitting<br>g. dorsiflex feet regularly<br>h. maintain an ideal body weight for age, height, and body frame<br>i. avoid smoking and use of oral contraceptives (these are risk factors for thrombus formation).<br>2. Instruct client to avoid trauma to or massage of any area of suspected thrombus formation in order to decrease risk of pulmonary embolism.<br>3. Provide information regarding exercise programs and support groups that can assist the client to stop smoking and/or lose weight. |
| 6.b. The client will verbalize an understanding of medications ordered including rationale, side effects, schedule | 6.b.1. Explain the rationale for, side effects of, and importance of taking medications prescribed.<br>2. If client is discharged on a coumarin derivative (e.g. warfarin), instruct to:<br>a. keep scheduled appointments for periodic blood studies to monitor coagulation times |

for taking, and importance of taking as prescribed.

b. take medication at the same time each day, do not stop taking medication abruptly, and do not attempt to make up for missed doses
c. avoid taking over-the-counter products containing aspirin or other salicylates (these products enhance the action of coumarin)
d. avoid regular and/or excessive intake of alcohol (may alter responsiveness to coumarin)
e. avoid eating large amounts of foods high in vitamin K (e.g. green leafy vegetables)
f. report prolonged or excessive bleeding from skin, nose, or mouth; blood in urine, vomitus, sputum, or stool; prolonged or excessive menses; excessive bruising; severe headache; or sudden abdominal or back pain
g. inform physician immediately if pregnancy is suspected (coumarin crosses the placental barrier)
h. wear a Medic-Alert band identifying self as being on anticoagulant therapy.

3. Instruct client to inform physician of any other prescription and nonprescription medications he/she is taking.
4. Instruct client to inform all health care providers of medications being taken.

6.c. The client will identify ways to prevent bleeding associated with anticoagulant therapy.

6.c.1. Instruct client about ways to minimize the risk of bleeding while on anticoagulant therapy:
a. use an electric rather than straight-edge razor
b. floss and brush teeth gently
c. avoid putting sharp objects (e.g. toothpicks) in mouth
d. do not walk barefoot
e. cut nails carefully
f. avoid situations that could result in injury (e.g. contact sports)
g. do not blow nose forcefully
h. avoid straining to have a bowel movement.

2. Instruct client to control any bleeding by applying firm, prolonged pressure to the area if possible.

6.d. The client will state signs and symptoms to report to the health care provider.

6.d. Stress the importance of reporting the following signs and symptoms:
1. redness, swelling, or pain in extremity
2. sudden chest pain accompanied by shortness of breath
3. extreme anxiousness or restlessness
4. cough productive of blood-tinged sputum
5. unusual bleeding (see action b.2.f in this diagnosis).

6.e. The client will verbalize an understanding of and a plan for adhering to recommended follow-up care including future appointments with health care provider and activity level.

6.e.1. Reinforce the importance of keeping follow-up appointments with health care provider.
2. Reinforce the physician's instructions regarding activity limitations.
3. Implement measures to improve client compliance:
a. include significant others in teaching sessions if possible
b. encourage questions and allow time for reinforcement and clarification of information provided
c. provide written instructions regarding future appointments with health care provider, medications prescribed, activity restrictions, signs and symptoms to report, and future laboratory studies.

# Thoracic Surgery

Thoracic surgery is a term used to encompass a variety of procedures that involve entry into the thoracic cavity. It includes procedures such as thoracotomy, pulmonary decortication, and surgery on the lung itself. Lung surgery may consist of a pneumonectomy (removal of the entire lung), a lobectomy (removal of a lobe), a segmental resection, or a wedge resection. A pneumonectomy is typically performed for treatment of cancer, extensive unilateral tuberculosis or bronchiectasis, or lung abscesses. A lobectomy (the most common type of lung surgery) or a segmental resection is indicated when the disease process is confined to a limited area of the lung. Either may be performed to remove benign or malignant tumors, small areas of bronchiectasis, and blebs or bullae. A wedge resection is performed to biopsy lung tissue or to excise a small, well-defined lesion or nodule.

**This care plan focuses on the adult client hospitalized for thoracic surgery to remove a portion or all of a lung.** Preoperative goals of care are to reduce fear and anxiety and assist the client to maintain an optimal respiratory status. The goals of postoperative care are to prevent and detect complications, maintain comfort, and educate the client regarding follow-up care. The care plan will need to be individualized according to the client's diagnosis, prognosis, and plans for subsequent treatment.

## DIAGNOSTIC TESTS

Pulmonary function studies
Chest x-ray
Lung scan
Lung biopsy
Sputum for cytology and/or acid-fast bacilli
Blood gases
Electrocardiogram (ECG)
Bronchoscopy
Cardiac catheterization (if pneumonectomy is planned)

## DISCHARGE CRITERIA

Prior to discharge, the client will:

- have optimal respiratory function
- have no signs and symptoms of complications
- demonstrate the ability to perform prescribed arm and shoulder exercises
- state signs and symptoms to report to the health care provider
- identify community resources that can assist with home management and adjustment to the diagnosis, effects of surgery, and adjuvant treatment if planned
- verbalize an understanding of and a plan for adhering to recommended follow-up care including future appointments with health care provider, medications prescribed, activity level, pain management, wound care, and subsequent treatment of the underlying disorder.

## NURSING/COLLABORATIVE DIAGNOSES

**Preoperative**



**Postoperative**

**1.** Impaired respiratory function:
  **a.** ineffective breathing pattern
  **b.** ineffective airway clearance

   **c.** impaired gas exchange△ *495*
2. Potential complications:
   **a.** extended pneumothorax
   **b.** hemothorax
   **c.** mediastinal shift
   **d.** acute pulmonary edema
   **e.** bronchopleural fistula
   **f.** restricted arm and shoulder movement△ *496*
3. Grieving△ *499*
4. Knowledge deficit△ *500*

**See Standardized Preoperative and Postoperative Care Plans for additional diagnoses.**

## PREOPERATIVE

**Use in conjunction with the Standardized Preoperative Care Plan.**

### 1. NURSING DIAGNOSIS: Anxiety

related to:

a. lack of understanding of diagnostic tests, diagnosis, surgical procedure, and postoperative management;
b. unfamiliar environment and financial concerns;
c. anticipated loss of control, effects of anesthesia, and postoperative discomfort;
d. possible changes in usual activities associated with loss of all or part of a lung.

| Desired Outcome | Nursing Actions and ***Selected Purposes/Rationales*** |
|---|---|
| 1. The client will experience a reduction in anxiety (see Standardized Preoperative Care Plan, Nursing Diagnosis 1 [pp. 108-109], for outcome criteria). | 1.a. Refer to Standardized Preoperative Care Plan, Nursing Diagnosis 1 (pp. 108-109), for measures related to assessment and reduction of fear and anxiety.<br>b. Implement additional measures *to reduce fear and anxiety:*<br>1. reinforce physician's explanations about anticipated effect of loss of lung tissue on activity tolerance<br>2. provide instruction about the purpose of chest drainage system that will be present after partial removal of a lung (chest tubes are usually not inserted during a pneumonectomy)<br>3. inform client that he/she will receive supplemental oxygen following surgery if needed. |

### 2. NURSING DIAGNOSIS: Ineffective airway clearance

related to:

a. excessive or tenacious pulmonary secretions associated with the underlying disease process;
b. ineffective cough effort associated with weakness and pain (may occur as a result of underlying disease process).

| Desired Outcome | Nursing Actions and ***Selected Purposes/Rationales*** |
|---|---|
| 2. The client will maintain clear, open airways as evidenced by:<br>a. usual breath sounds<br>b. usual rate and depth of respirations<br>c. absence of dyspnea<br>d. absence of cyanosis. | 2.a. Assess for signs and symptoms of ineffective airway clearance (e.g. abnormal breath sounds; rapid, shallow respirations; dyspnea; cyanosis).<br>b. Implement measures *to promote effective airway clearance:*<br>1. instruct and assist client to turn, cough or "huff," and deep breathe every 1-2 hours<br>2. perform actions *to facilitate removal of pulmonary secretions:*<br>a. implement measures *to liquefy tenacious secretions:*<br>1. maintain a fluid intake of at least 2500 ml/day unless contraindicated<br>2. humidify inspired air as ordered<br>b. assist with administration of diluent and mucolytic agents via nebulizer or IPPB treatment as ordered<br>c. assist with or perform postural drainage, percussion, and vibration if ordered<br>d. perform tracheal suctioning if ordered<br>e. administer expectorants if ordered<br>3. increase activity as allowed and tolerated<br>4. discourage smoking *(smoke causes bronchoconstriction, increases mucus production, and impairs ciliary function)*<br>5. protect client from exposure to irritants such as smoke, flowers, and perfume *(can cause bronchospasm and increased mucus production)*<br>6. reinforce correct use of incentive spirometer and assist with IPPB treatments if ordered *to promote bronchodilation and movement of secretions*<br>7. administer bronchodilators (e.g. theophylline) if ordered *to improve bronchial airflow.*<br>c. Consult physician if signs and symptoms of ineffective airway clearance persist or worsen. |

## 3. NURSING DIAGNOSIS: Impaired gas exchange

related to loss of effective lung surface associated with the underlying disease process.

| Desired Outcome | Nursing Actions and ***Selected Purposes/Rationales*** |
|---|---|
| 3. The client will experience adequate $O_2$/$CO_2$ exchange as evidenced by:<br>a. usual mental status<br>b. unlabored respirations at 14-20/minute<br>c. blood gases within normal range for client. | 3.a. Assess for and report signs and symptoms of impaired gas exchange:<br>1. restlessness, irritability<br>2. confusion, somnolence<br>3. tachypnea, dyspnea<br>4. decreased $PaO_2$ and increased $PaCO_2$.<br>b. Monitor for and report significant changes in oximetry results.<br>c. Implement measures *to improve gas exchange:*<br>1. perform actions to promote effective airway clearance (see Preoperative Nursing Diagnosis 2, action b)<br>2. place client in a semi- to high Fowler's position unless contraindicated; position overbed table so client can rest on it if desired<br>3. maintain oxygen therapy as ordered<br>4. discourage smoking *(smoke decreases oxygen availability)*<br>5. administer central nervous system depressants judiciously; hold medication and consult physician if respiratory rate is less than 12/minute.<br>d. Consult physician if signs and symptoms of impaired gas exchange persist or worsen. |

## POSTOPERATIVE

**Use in conjunction with the Standardized Postoperative Care Plan.**

### 1. NURSING DIAGNOSIS: Impaired respiratory function*:

a. **ineffective breathing pattern** related to:
   1. fear, anxiety, and pain
   2. depressant effects of anesthesia and some medications (e.g. narcotic analgesics)
   3. reluctance to breathe deeply associated with incisional pain and fear of dislodging chest tube(s) if in place
   4. restricted expansion of remaining lung tissue associated with positioning, weakness, and pressure on the diaphragm if abdominal distention occurs;

b. **ineffective airway clearance** related to:
   1. blockage of the pharynx by the base of the tongue associated with muscular flaccidity resulting from the effects of anesthesia and some medications (e.g. narcotic analgesics)
   2. stasis of secretions associated with decreased activity and poor cough effort resulting from depressant effects of anesthesia and some medications (e.g. narcotic analgesics), pain, weakness, and fatigue
   3. increased secretions associated with irritation of the respiratory tract (can result from inhalation anesthetics and endotracheal intubation)
   4. tenacious secretions associated with fluid loss and decreased fluid intake;

c. **impaired gas exchange** related to inability of pulmonary system to compensate fully for the decrease in alveolar surface associated with the extensive removal of lung tissue.

*This diagnostic label includes the following nursing diagnoses: ineffective breathing pattern, ineffective airway clearance, and impaired gas exchange.

| Desired Outcome | Nursing Actions and ***Selected Purposes/Rationales*** |
|---|---|
| 1. The client will experience adequate respiratory function as evidenced by:<br>a. improved rate, rhythm, and depth of respirations<br>b. absence of dyspnea<br>c. normal breath sounds over remaining lung tissue<br>d. usual mental status<br>e. usual skin color<br>f. blood gases returning toward normal range. | 1.a. Assess for and report signs and symptoms of impaired respiratory function:<br>1. rapid, shallow, slow, or irregular respirations<br>2. dyspnea, orthopnea<br>3. use of accessory muscles when breathing<br>4. adventitious breath sounds (e.g. crackles [rales], rhonchi)<br>5. diminished or absent breath sounds over remaining lung tissue<br>6. restlessness, irritability<br>7. confusion, somnolence<br>8. central cyanosis (a late sign).<br>b. Monitor for and report significant changes in blood gases and oximetry and chest x-ray results.<br>c. Implement measures *to improve respiratory status:*<br>1. perform actions to improve breathing pattern and promote effective airway clearance (see Standardized Postoperative Care Plan, Nursing Diagnoses 2, action c and 3, action b [pp. 114-116])<br>2. perform actions to reduce pain (see Standardized Postoperative Care Plan, Nursing Diagnosis 6, action e [p. 119])<br>3. perform actions to maintain patency and integrity of chest drainage system (see Postoperative Collaborative Diagnosis 2, action a.4.a) *in order to promote lung re-expansion*<br>4. if chest tube(s) present, assure client that deep breathing and coughing will not dislodge the tube(s)<br>5. position client as ordered (e.g. on back or on operative side after |

| Desired Outcome | Nursing Actions and ***Selected Purposes/Rationales*** |
|---|---|
| | pneumonectomy, on back or either side following removal of a portion of the lung) *to allow full expansion of remaining lung tissue*<br>6. keep head of bed elevated *to facilitate lung expansion and promote drainage of fluid and residual air via chest tubes*<br>7. maintain oxygen therapy as ordered<br>8. administer bronchodilators (e.g. theophylline) if ordered.<br>d. Consult physician if signs and symptoms of impaired respiratory function persist or worsen. |

## 2. COLLABORATIVE DIAGNOSES:

**Potential complications:**

a. **extended pneumothorax** related to an increase in intrapleural pressure on operative side following a lobectomy associated with accumulation of air in pleural space as a result of chest tube malfunction;
b. **hemothorax** related to intraoperative or postoperative bleeding and/or chest tube malfunction;
c. **mediastinal shift** related to:
   1. increase in intrapleural pressure on the operative side following a lobectomy associated with an accumulation of fluid and air in the pleural space
   2. excessive negative pressure on operative side following pneumonectomy associated with inadequate serous fluid accumulation in the empty thoracic space (the position of the mediastinum is maintained by accumulation of serous fluid in the empty thoracic space);
d. **acute pulmonary edema** related to:
   1. increased pulmonary capillary permeability associated with hypoxia
   2. excessive hydrostatic pressure in the remaining pulmonary vessels associated with removal of a large portion of the pulmonary vascular system if a pneumonectomy was performed;
e. **bronchopleural fistula** related to:
   1. inadequate bronchial closure and healing following a partial or complete resection of the lung
   2. presence of empyema in residual lung tissue (can occur following removal of a portion of the lung);
f. **restricted arm and shoulder movement** related to decreased activity of the arm and shoulder on the operative side associated with pain and adhesion formation between incised muscles.

| Desired Outcomes | Nursing Actions and ***Selected Purposes/Rationales*** |
|---|---|
| 2.a. The client will experience normal lung re-expansion as evidenced by:<br>1. normal breath sounds and percussion note over remaining lung tissue by 3rd-4th postoperative day<br>2. unlabored respirations at 14-20/minute<br>3. blood gases | 2.a.1. Assess for and immediately report signs and symptoms of:<br>a. malfunction of chest drainage system (e.g. respiratory distress, sudden cessation of drainage, excessive bubbling in water seal chamber, significant increase in subcutaneous emphysema)<br>b. extended pneumothorax (e.g. extended area of absent breath sounds with hyperresonant percussion note; rapid, shallow, and/or labored respirations; increased chest pain; restlessness; confusion).<br>2. Monitor blood gases. Report values that have worsened.<br>3. Monitor chest x-ray results. Report findings of delayed lung re-expansion or further lung collapse.<br>4. Implement measures *to promote lung re-expansion and prevent extended pneumothorax:*<br>a. perform actions *to maintain patency and integrity of chest drainage system if present:*<br>1. maintain water seal and suction levels as ordered |

returning toward normal
4. chest x-ray showing lung re-expansion.

2. maintain air occlusive dressing over chest tube insertion site(s)
3. tape all connections securely
4. milk chest tube(s) routinely if ordered
5. keep chest drainage and suction tubing free of kinks; place a rolled towel around chest tube(s) when client is turned to operative side *in order to prevent pressure on the tube(s)*
6. keep drainage system below level of client's chest at all times

b. perform actions to improve respiratory status (see Postoperative Nursing Diagnosis 1, action c).

5. If signs and symptoms of extended pneumothorax occur:
a. maintain client on bed rest in a semi- to high Fowler's position
b. maintain oxygen therapy as ordered
c. assess for and immediately report signs and symptoms of mediastinal shift (see action c.1 in this diagnosis)
d. assist with clearing of existing chest tube(s) and/or insertion of a new tube
e. provide emotional support to client and significant others.

2.b. The client will not develop hemothorax as evidenced by:
1. normal breath sounds and percussion note over remaining lung tissue by 3rd-4th postoperative day
2. unlabored respirations at 14-20/minute
3. blood gases returning toward normal range.

2.b.1. Assess for and immediately report signs and symptoms of:
a. thoracic bleeding (e.g. unexpected increase in the amount of bloody drainage from chest tube[s], increase in bloody drainage on dressing, further decrease in Hct and Hb)
b. hemothorax (e.g. diminished or absent breath sounds with dull percussion note over affected area, dyspnea).

2. Monitor blood gases. Report values that have worsened.
3. Implement measures to maintain patency and integrity of chest drainage system (see action a.4.a in this diagnosis) *in order to reduce risk of hemothorax.*
4. If signs and symptoms of hemothorax occur:
a. maintain client on bed rest in a semi- to high Fowler's position
b. maintain oxygen therapy as ordered
c. assess for and report signs and symptoms of a mediastinal shift (see action c.1 in this diagnosis)
d. assess for and report signs and symptoms of shock (e.g. hypotension; increased pulse and respirations; urine output less than 30 ml/hour; cool, clammy skin; change in mental status)
e. administer blood products and/or volume expanders if ordered
f. assist with clearing of existing chest tube(s), thoracentesis, or insertion of chest tube if not already present
g. prepare client for surgical intervention to ligate bleeding vessels if indicated
h. provide emotional support to client and significant others.

2.c. The client will not develop a mediastinal shift as evidenced by:
1. absence of or no sudden increase in dyspnea
2. vital signs within normal range for client
3. usual mental status
4. trachea in midline position
5. absence of neck vein distention
6. blood gases returning toward normal range.

2.c. 1. Assess for and immediately report signs and symptoms of mediastinal shift (e.g. severe dyspnea, rapid and/or irregular pulse rate, hypotension, restlessness and agitation, shift in trachea from midline, neck vein distention).
2. Monitor blood gases and report values that have worsened.
3. Implement measures *to reduce risk of mediastinal shift:*
a. keep chest tube clamped if one is in place after a pneumonectomy *(serous fluid accumulation is essential to maintain proper pressure gradient on operative side)*
b. position client as ordered (e.g. on back or on operative side after pneumonectomy)
c. perform actions to prevent and treat pneumothorax and hemothorax (see actions a.4 and 5 and b.3 and 4 in this diagnosis).
4. If signs and symptoms of mediastinal shift occur:
a. maintain client on bed rest in a semi- to high Fowler's position
b. maintain oxygen therapy as ordered
c. if chest tube(s) malfunctioning or not present, assist with clearing of existing tube(s), thoracentesis, or insertion of new tube(s) if indicated

| Desired Outcomes | Nursing Actions and ***Selected Purposes/Rationales*** |
|---|---|
| | d. provide emotional support to client and significant others. |
| 2.d. The client will not develop pulmonary edema as evidenced by:<br>1. unlabored respirations at 14-20/minute<br>2. pulse 60-100 beats/minute<br>3. clear breath sounds and resonant percussion note over unoperative area<br>4. absence of productive, persistent cough<br>5. usual skin color<br>6. blood gases returning toward normal range. | 2.d.1. Assess for and report signs and symptoms of pulmonary edema (e.g. severe dyspnea, tachycardia, adventitious breath sounds, dull percussion note over remaining lung tissue, persistent cough productive of frothy and/or blood-tinged sputum, cyanosis).<br>2. Monitor for and report the following:<br>a. decline in $Pa_{O_2}$ or increase in $Pa_{CO_2}$<br>b. significant change in oximetry results.<br>3. Monitor chest x-ray results. Report findings of pulmonary edema.<br>4. Implement measures *to prevent hypoxia and reduce the risk of pulmonary edema:*<br>a. perform actions to improve respiratory status (see Postoperative Nursing Diagnosis 1, action c)<br>b. perform actions to maintain patency and integrity of chest drainage system if present (see action a.4.a in this diagnosis) *in order to promote lung re-expansion.*<br>5. If signs and symptoms of pulmonary edema occur:<br>a. continue with above measures<br>b. administer the following medications if ordered:<br>1. bronchodilators (e.g. theophylline) *to increase bronchial airflow*<br>2. agents *to reduce pulmonary vascular congestion* (e.g. diuretics, morphine sulfate). |
| 2.e. The client will experience resolution of a bronchopleural fistula if it occurs as evidenced by:<br>1. afebrile status<br>2. cough productive of clear mucus only<br>3. absence of continuous bubbling in water seal chamber of chest drainage system<br>4. normal rate and depth of respirations<br>5. WBC and differential counts returning toward normal. | 2.e.1. Assess for and report signs and symptoms of a bronchopleural fistula (e.g. fever, cough productive of serosanguinous or purulent sputum, continuous bubbling in water seal chamber of chest drainage system, respiratory distress).<br>2. Monitor for and report the following:<br>a. persistent elevation of WBC count and significant change in differential<br>b. chest x-ray results showing probable bronchopleural fistula.<br>3. If signs and symptoms of a bronchopleural fistula occur:<br>a. turn client to operative side if he/she has had a pneumonectomy until adequate thoracotomy drainage has been achieved *(this will reduce the risk for aspiration of pleural fluid into the remaining lung)*<br>b. administer antimicrobial agents if ordered<br>c. prepare client for surgery *to repair bronchial stump or to resect additional lung tissue*<br>d. provide emotional support to client and significant others. |
| 2.f. The client will maintain normal arm and shoulder function as evidenced by ability to move arm and shoulder on operative side through usual range of motion. | 2.f. 1. Assess for and report signs and symptoms of restricted arm and shoulder movement on operative side (e.g. inability to move arm and shoulder through usual range of motion, inability to use arm in activities of daily living).<br>2. Implement measures *to prevent restriction of arm and shoulder movement on operative side:*<br>a. instruct client in and assist with arm and shoulder exercises as ordered<br>b. perform actions to reduce pain (see Standardized Postoperative Care Plan, Nursing Diagnosis 6, action e [p. 119]) *in order to increase client's ability and willingness to move arm and shoulder*<br>c. encourage client to use arm on operative side to perform self-care activities<br>d. place frequently used articles and bed stand on operative side *so that client will be encouraged to reach with affected arm* |

e. anchor pull rope at foot of bed; encourage client to use arm on operative side to pull self to sitting position.

3. If signs and symptoms of restricted arm and shoulder movement occur:
   a. continue with above actions
   b. assist with planned physical therapy program
   c. provide emotional support to client and significant others.

## 3. NURSING DIAGNOSIS: Grieving*

related to loss of all or part of a lung and anticipated changes in usual life style as a result of altered lung capacity.

*This diagnostic label includes anticipatory grieving and grieving following the actual losses.

| Desired Outcome | Nursing Actions and ***Selected Purposes/Rationales*** |
|---|---|
| 3. The client will demonstrate beginning progression through the grieving process as evidenced by:<br>a. verbalization of feelings about the loss of all or part of a lung and its anticipated effects on life style<br>b. expression of grief<br>c. participation in treatment plan and self-care activities<br>d. utilization of available support systems<br>e. verbalization of ways to modify current life style to compensate for altered lung capacity. | 3.a. Assess for signs and symptoms of grieving (e.g. change in eating habits, inability to concentrate, insomnia, anger, noncompliance, withdrawal from significant others, denial of loss). Be aware that client's response to a loss will be affected by factors such as previous experience with loss, age, developmental stage, available support systems, spiritual and cultural background, current health status, and significance of the loss.<br>b. Implement measures *to facilitate the grieving process:*<br>1. assist client to acknowledge the changes resulting from loss of lung function *so grief work can begin;* assess for factors that may hinder and facilitate acknowledgment<br>2. discuss the grieving process and assist client to accept the phases of grieving as an expected response to his/her actual and/or anticipated loss<br>3. allow time for client to progress through the phases of grieving (phases vary among theorists but progress from shock and alarm to acceptance); be aware that not every phase is expressed by all individuals, that recurrence of phases is common, and that the grieving process may take months to years<br>4. provide an atmosphere of care and concern (e.g. provide privacy, be available and nonjudgmental, display empathy and respect) *so client will feel free to verbalize feelings*<br>5. perform actions *to promote trust* (e.g. answer questions honestly, provide requested information)<br>6. encourage the verbal expression of anger and sadness about the loss of the lung; recognize displacement of anger and assist client to see the actual cause of angry feelings and resentment<br>7. encourage client to express his/her feelings in whatever ways are comfortable (e.g. writing, drawing, conversation)<br>8. assist client to identify personal strengths that have helped him/her to cope in previous situations of loss<br>9. support realistic hope about client's ability to resume usual activities<br>10. support behaviors suggesting successful grief work (e.g. verbalizing feelings about the loss of a lung, expressing sorrow, focusing on ways to adapt to altered lung capacity)<br>11. explain the phases of the grieving process to significant others; encourage their support and understanding<br>12. facilitate communication between client and significant others<br>13. provide information regarding counseling services and support groups that might assist client in working through grief |

| Desired Outcome | Nursing Actions and ***Selected Purposes/Rationales*** |
|---|---|
| | 14. arrange for visit from clergy if desired by client.<br>c. Consult physician regarding referral for counseling if signs of dysfunctional grieving (e.g. persistent denial of loss and necessary changes in life style, excessive anger or sadness, hysteria, suicidal behaviors) occur. |

## 4. NURSING DIAGNOSIS: Knowledge deficit

regarding follow-up care.

| Desired Outcomes | Nursing Actions and ***Selected Purposes/Rationales*** |
|---|---|
| 4.a. The client will demonstrate the ability to perform prescribed arm and shoulder exercises. | 4.a.1. Instruct client regarding importance of exercising the arm and shoulder on operative side. Emphasize that the exercises should be performed at least 5 times/day for several weeks.<br>2. Demonstrate appropriate arm and shoulder exercises (e.g. shoulder shrugs, arm circles).<br>3. Allow time for questions, clarification, and return demonstration. |
| 4.b. The client will state signs and symptoms to report to the health care provider. | 4.b.1. Refer to Standardized Postoperative Care Plan, Nursing Diagnosis 21, action c (p. 135), for signs and symptoms to report to the health care provider.<br>2. Instruct the client to report these additional signs and symptoms:<br>a. increased discomfort in or decreased ability to move arm and shoulder on operative side<br>b. increased shortness of breath<br>c. persistent cough. |
| 4.c. The client will identify community resources that can assist with home management and adjustment to the diagnosis, effects of surgery, and adjuvant treatment if planned. | 4.c.1. Provide information about community resources that can assist the client and significant others with home management and adjustment to the diagnosis, effects of surgery, and adjuvant treatment if planned (e.g. American Lung Association, American Cancer Society, Meals on Wheels, counselors, support groups, home health agencies).<br>2. Initiate a referral if indicated. |
| 4.d. The client will verbalize an understanding of and a plan for adhering to recommended follow-up care including future appointments with health care provider, medications prescribed, activity level, pain management, wound care, and subsequent treatment of the underlying disorder. | 4.d.1. Refer to Standardized Postoperative Care Plan, Nursing Diagnosis 21 (pp. 135-136), for routine postoperative instructions and measures to improve client compliance.<br>2. Reinforce physician's instructions about activity restrictions:<br>a. gauge activity according to tolerance and ensure adequate rest periods<br>b. stop any activity that causes excessive fatigue, dyspnea, or chest pain<br>c. avoid lifting heavy objects until complete healing of chest muscles has occurred.<br>3. Inform client that numbness and discomfort in the operative area will persist for several weeks but are usually temporary. Explain that application of heat is sometimes helpful in relieving the discomfort.<br>4. Clarify plans for subsequent treatment of underlying disorder (e.g. chemotherapy, radiation therapy) if appropriate. |

UNIT

# XII

# *Nursing Care of the Client with Disturbances of the Kidney and Urinary Tract*

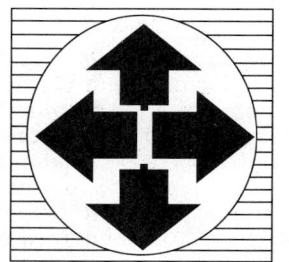

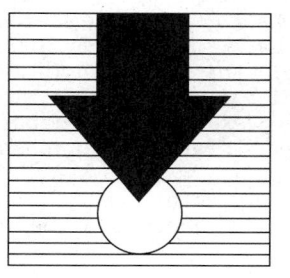

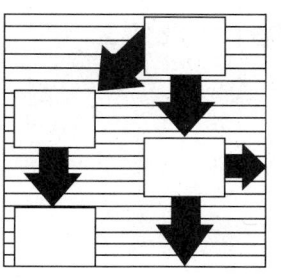

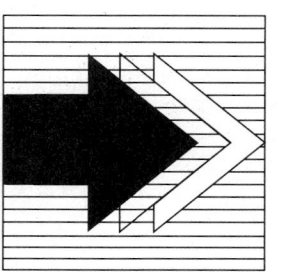

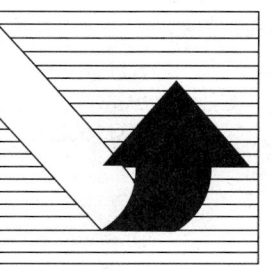

# Bladder Suspension

A bladder suspension is a surgical procedure to restore the bladder neck and proximal urethra to a high, fixed retropubic position from a dependent one in the pelvis by resuspension of the urethropelvic ligaments. It is performed to correct anatomic stress incontinence (the loss of urine from the urethra during an elevation of intra-abdominal pressure without true detrusor muscle contractions). Anatomic stress incontinence is caused by the abnormally low position of the urethrovesical junction that occurs because of loss of pelvic support of the bladder and urethra as a result of trauma during childbirth or surgery, pelvic denervation (can occur with conditions such as multiple sclerosis), and/or hormonal changes that occur with menopause.

A bladder suspension is indicated when conservative measures for treating anatomic stress incontinence (e.g. pelvic floor exercises, biofeedback, estrogen therapy) have failed. It can be accomplished by an abdominal approach (e.g. Marshall-Marchetti-Krantz, Burch) or vaginal approach (e.g. Gittes, Stamey, Raz). The approach selected depends on the physiological condition of the client, the severity of the incontinence, the presence of associated pelvic floor abnormalities (e.g. enterocele, uterine prolapse, cystocele, rectocele), and the need for additional abdominal surgery.

The most common approach used today is the vaginal one. In this procedure, a special transferring needle is used to resuspend the bladder neck and proximal urethra with sutures that anchor tissue adjacent to the bladder neck to the abdominal fascia.

**This care plan focuses on the adult client hospitalized for a bladder suspension using a vaginal approach.** Preoperative goals of care are to reduce fear and anxiety and prepare the client for the surgical experience. Postoperatively, goals of care are to maintain comfort, prevent complications, and educate the client regarding follow-up care. If repair of a cystocele and/or rectocele is planned concurrently, use this care plan in conjunction with the Care Plan on Colporrhaphy.

## DIAGNOSTIC TESTS

Excretory urography (intravenous pyelography)
Cystoscopy
Urine studies (e.g. urinalysis, culture)
Uroflowmetry
Cystometry
Urethral pressure profile
Bladder stress test

## DISCHARGE CRITERIA

Prior to discharge, the client will:

- have no signs and symptoms of complications
- demonstrate care of a suprapubic catheter if in place
- demonstrate the ability to perform self-catheterization if planned
- demonstrate the ability to measure residual urine
- state signs and symptoms to report to the health care provider
- verbalize an understanding of and a plan for adhering to recommended follow-up care including future appointments with health care provider and medications prescribed.

## NURSING/ COLLABORATIVE DIAGNOSES

**Postoperative**

3. Potential complication: bladder, urethral, or ureteral injury△ *504*
4. Knowledge deficit△ *504*

**See Standardized Preoperative and Postoperative Care Plans for additional diagnoses.**

## PREOPERATIVE

**Refer to the Standardized Preoperative Care Plan.**

## POSTOPERATIVE

**Use in conjunction with the Standardized Postoperative Care Plan.**

### 1. NURSING DIAGNOSIS: Urinary retention

related to:
a. obstruction of the urethral and/or suprapubic catheters if present;
b. difficulty urinating following removal of the catheter(s) associated with:
   1. edema of the bladder neck and urethra resulting from surgical trauma and irritation of tissue by the urethral catheter
   2. sympathetic nervous system stimulation of the bladder and urinary sphincters resulting from pain, fear, and anxiety
   3. decreased bladder muscle tone and perception of bladder fullness resulting from the depressant effects of some medications (e.g. anesthetic agents, narcotic analgesics).

| Desired Outcome | Nursing Actions and ***Selected Purposes/Rationales*** |
|---|---|
| 1. The client will not experience urinary retention as evidenced by:<br>a. no complaints of bladder fullness and suprapubic discomfort<br>b. absence of bladder distention<br>c. balanced intake and output within 48 hours after surgery<br>d. voiding adequate amounts at expected intervals after removal of the catheter(s). | 1.a. Assess for and report the following:<br>1. urinary retention when suprapubic and/or urethral catheters are present (e.g. complaints of bladder fullness or suprapubic discomfort, bladder distention, absence of fluid in urinary drainage tubing, output that continues to be less than intake 48 hours after surgery)<br>2. urinary retention following catheter removal (e.g. complaints of bladder fullness or suprapubic discomfort, bladder distention, output that continues to be less than intake 48 hours after surgery, frequent voiding of small amounts [25-60 ml] of urine).<br>b. Implement measures *to prevent urinary retention:*<br>1. perform actions *to maintain patency of urinary catheter(s):*<br>a. keep drainage tubing free of kinks<br>b. keep collection container below level of bladder<br>c. tape catheter tubing securely (suprapubic to abdomen, urethral to thigh) *in order to prevent inadvertent removal*<br>d. irrigate suprapubic catheter gently if ordered<br>2. after urethral catheter is removed, open suprapubic catheter if client is unable to void voluntarily and as scheduled<br>3. when both urethral and suprapubic catheters have been removed, refer to Standardized Postoperative Care Plan, Nursing Diagnosis 13, actions d and e (p. 126), for measures related to prevention and treatment of urinary retention. |

## 2. NURSING DIAGNOSIS: High risk for infection: urinary tract

related to:
a. increased bacterial growth associated with urinary stasis;
b. introduction of pathogens associated with the presence of vaginal drainage, urethral and/or suprapubic catheters, or intermittent catheterizations for post-void residuals.

| Desired Outcome | Nursing Actions and ***Selected Purposes/Rationales*** |
|---|---|
| 2. The client will remain free of urinary tract infection (see Standardized Postoperative Care Plan, Nursing Diagnosis 16, outcome c [p. 129], for outcome criteria). | 2.a. Refer to Standardized Postoperative Care Plan, Nursing Diagnosis 16, action c (p. 129), for measures related to assessment, prevention, and treatment of urinary tract infection.<br>b. Implement measures to prevent urinary retention (see Postoperative Nursing Diagnosis 1, action b) *in order to further reduce the risk of urinary stasis and subsequent urinary tract infection.* |

## 3. COLLABORATIVE DIAGNOSIS: Potential complication: bladder, urethral, or ureteral injury

related to accidental tear or ligation during the surgical procedure.

| Desired Outcome | Nursing Actions and ***Selected Purposes/Rationales*** |
|---|---|
| 3. The client will experience healing of bladder, urethral, or ureteral injury if it occurs as evidenced by:<br>a. gradual resolution of hematuria and backache<br>b. output greater than 200 ml within 6-8 hours after surgery. | 3.a. Assess for and report signs and symptoms of bladder, urethral, or ureteral injury (e.g. persistent or increasing hematuria or backache, urine output less than 200 ml in first 6-8 hours after surgery).<br>b. If signs and symptoms of bladder, urethral, or ureteral injury are present:<br>1. continue to monitor output carefully<br>2. prepare client for surgical repair if indicated<br>3. provide emotional support to client and significant others. |

## 4. NURSING DIAGNOSIS: Knowledge deficit

regarding follow-up care.

| Desired Outcomes | Nursing Actions and ***Selected Purposes/Rationales*** |
|---|---|
| 4.a. The client will demonstrate care of a suprapubic catheter if in place. | 4.a.1. Provide the following instructions about care of suprapubic catheter if client is discharged with one in place:<br>a. tape catheter securely to abdomen<br>b. keep drainage tubing free of kinks |

| | |
|---|---|
| | c. keep collection bag below level of bladder.<br>2. Allow time for questions, clarification, and return demonstration. |
| 4.b. The client will demonstrate the ability to perform self-catheterization if planned. | 4.b.1. Provide the following instructions on self-catheterization using clean technique if client is to catheterize self at home:<br>a. position self on bed or toilet<br>b. separate labia to expose urinary meatus<br>c. wash area thoroughly with soap and water, wiping from front to back<br>d. lubricate the tip of the catheter with water-soluble lubricant<br>e. while keeping the labia separated, slowly insert the catheter into the urinary meatus about 3-4 inches or until urine starts to flow; allow urine to drain into measuring container<br>f. remove catheter slowly when urine stops draining<br>g. wash catheter in warm, soapy water; rinse it thoroughly; and dry it with a clean towel<br>h. store catheter in a plastic storage bag or container.<br>2. Allow time for questions, clarification, and return demonstration. |
| 4.c. The client will demonstrate the ability to measure residual urine. | 4.c.1. Provide the following instructions about how to measure residual urine:<br>a. wait for a fairly strong urge to urinate before attempting to do so<br>b. if attempt to urinate is unsuccessful after trying for a full minute, drain bladder by opening suprapubic catheter or performing self-catheterization<br>c. if voluntary urination occurs, open the suprapubic catheter or perform self-catheterization as instructed to drain residual urine after urination is complete<br>d. measure and record amount of urine voided and the amount of residual urine.<br>2. Allow time for questions, clarification, and return demonstration. |
| 4.d. The client will state signs and symptoms to report to the health care provider. | 4.d.1. Refer to Standardized Postoperative Care Plan, Nursing Diagnosis 21, action c (p. 135), for signs and symptoms to report to the health care provider.<br>2. Instruct client to report these additional signs and symptoms:<br>a. unusual, odorous vaginal discharge<br>b. stress incontinence<br>c. excessive perineal edema or pain<br>d. persistent bright red vaginal bleeding<br>e. persistent inability to void voluntarily<br>f. persistent residual urine amounts in excess of 100 ml. |
| 4.e. The client will verbalize an understanding of and a plan for adhering to recommended follow-up care including future appointments with health care provider and medications prescribed. | 4.e.1. Refer to Standardized Postoperative Care Plan, Nursing Diagnosis 21 (pp. 135-136), for routine postoperative instructions and measures to improve client compliance.<br>2. Instruct client not to have sexual intercourse until permitted by physician (usually 6 weeks).<br>3. Emphasize the importance of good perineal hygiene, particularly after defecation.<br>4. Instruct client to avoid taking tub baths and lifting heavy objects until healing is complete (about 6 weeks). |

# Chronic Renal Failure

Chronic renal failure (CRF) is a progressive, irreversible loss of kidney function that usually develops gradually over many years. Some of the more common causes of CRF include glomerulonephritis, diabetic nephropathy, hypertension, systemic lupus erythematosus, polycystic kidney disease, renal calculi, prostatic hypertrophy, and analgesic abuse. It can also develop following acute renal failure that has resulted in irreversible renal damage.

Chronic renal failure is usually divided into three stages. The glomerular filtration rate (GFR), which is measured by creatinine clearance, is used as the basis for this staging. The lower the GFR, the greater the loss of kidney function. In the first stage, decreased renal reserve, clients can have a GFR as low as 30% of normal, but because homeostatic mechanisms are able to maintain fluid balance and keep serum electrolytes, urea nitrogen, and creatinine within normal ranges, the renal dysfunction usually goes undiagnosed. The client has no clinical manifestations of renal dysfunction at this point. Renal insufficiency, the second stage, starts when the GFR is about 25% of normal. In this stage, creatinine clearance continues to decline and azotemia (the retention of nitrogenous substances in the blood) begins. Even though the blood urea nitrogen and serum creatinine are elevated in this stage, they are not high enough to cause symptoms that are problematic for the client. During the renal insufficiency stage, the client progresses from a nonoliguric phase in which the kidneys are unable to concentrate the urine to an oliguric phase. In this oliguric phase, symptoms become more evident and result mainly from a decreased ability of the kidneys to excrete fluid and electrolytes. The third stage of CRF is uremia or end-stage renal disease (ESRD). It occurs when the GFR is less than 10% of normal and nitrogenous substances (e.g. urea, creatinine, phenols) accumulate to levels high enough to cause toxic effects on other body systems. Typical signs and symptoms of ESRD can include lethargy, irritability, extreme fatigue and weakness, pruritus, nausea and vomiting, muscle cramping, and stomatitis. Fluid, electrolyte, and acid-base imbalances also worsen and, in this stage, dialysis or kidney transplantation is necessary for survival.

**This care plan focuses on the adult client with renal insufficiency who has progressed from the nonoliguric to the oliguric phase and is hospitalized for treatment and further evaluation of renal function.** The goals of care are to reduce fear and anxiety, control symptoms, prevent complications, and educate the client regarding follow-up care.

## DIAGNOSTIC TESTS

Urine studies (e.g. creatinine clearance, osmolality, electrolytes, protein)
Blood studies (e.g. BUN, creatinine, CBC, electrolytes, $CO_2$ content, protein, osmolality)
Computed tomography of the kidneys (nephrotomography)
Renal ultrasonography (nephrosonography)
Excretory urography (intravenous pyelogram)
X-ray of the kidneys, ureters, and bladder (KUB)
Renal angiography
Renal biopsy

## DISCHARGE CRITERIA

Prior to discharge, the client will:

- not have signs and symptoms of uremic syndrome
- have blood pressure within a safe range
- have fluid and electrolyte balance stabilized within a safe range
- verbalize a basic understanding of CRF
- identify ways to slow the progression of kidney damage
- verbalize an understanding of fluid restrictions and dietary modifications
- demonstrate the ability to accurately weigh self, measure fluid intake and output, and monitor own blood pressure
- identify ways to reduce the risk of infection
- identify ways to manage conditions that often occur as a result of CRF
- share feelings and concerns about the effects of CRF on life style and roles
- state signs and symptoms to report to the health care provider

- ❖ identify community resources that can assist with adjustment to changes resulting from CRF
- ❖ verbalize an understanding of and a plan for adhering to recommended follow-up care including future appointments with health care provider and medications prescribed.

**NURSING/ COLLABORATIVE DIAGNOSES**



## 1. NURSING/ COLLABORATIVE DIAGNOSIS:

### Altered fluid and electrolyte balance:

a. **fluid volume excess** related to retention of sodium and water associated with:
   1. decrease in number of functioning nephrons and subsequent decreased GFR
   2. activation of the renin-angiotension-aldosterone mechanism resulting from decreased renal blood flow (can occur as a result of the underlying disease process);

b. **hyponatremia** related to excessive fluid intake in relation to output (causes a relative hyponatremia), restricted dietary intake of sodium, and loss of sodium associated with diuretic therapy;

c. **hypernatremia** related to:
   1. decreased ability of the kidneys to excrete sodium
   2. increased aldosterone output associated with activation of the renin-angiotension-aldosterone mechanism if decreased renal blood flow has occurred as a result of the underlying disease process
   3. dietary sodium intake in excess of prescribed restrictions;

d. **hyperkalemia** related to:
   1. decreased ability of the kidneys to excrete potassium
   2. increased cellular release of potassium associated with progressive renal tissue damage and metabolic acidosis
   3. dietary potassium intake in excess of prescribed restrictions
   4. use of potassium-sparing diuretics or salt substitutes containing potassium;

e. **hypocalcemia** related to:
   1. decreased absorption of calcium associated with inability of the kidneys to

activate vitamin D (the active metabolite of vitamin D is needed to stimulate calcium absorption from the small intestine)
2. hyperphosphatemia (calcium binds with excess serum phosphate);

f. **hyperphosphatemia** related to decreased ability of the kidneys to excrete phosphorus and hypocalcemia (an inverse relationship exists between phosphorus and calcium);

g. **hypermagnesemia** related to:
1. decreased ability of the kidneys to excrete magnesium
2. excessive intake of magnesium-containing antacids;

h. **metabolic acidosis** related to:
1. decreased ability of the kidneys to excrete hydrogen ions and reabsorb bicarbonate
2. hyperkalemia (high serum potassium levels cause hydrogen ions to shift into the vascular space).

| Desired Outcomes | Nursing Actions and ***Selected Purposes/Rationales*** |
|---|---|
| 1.a. The client will experience resolution of fluid volume excess as evidenced by:<br>1. decline in weight toward client's normal<br>2. B/P within normal range for client<br>3. absence of an $S_3$ heart sound<br>4. balanced intake and output<br>5. usual mental status<br>6. normal breath sounds<br>7. absence of dyspnea, orthopnea, peripheral edema, and distended neck veins<br>8. small vein emptying time less than 3-5 seconds<br>9. CVP within normal range. | 1.a.1. Assess for and report signs and symptoms of fluid volume excess:<br>a. weight gain<br>b. elevated B/P (B/P may not be elevated if fluid has shifted out of vascular space)<br>c. presence of an $S_3$ heart sound<br>d. intake greater than output<br>e. change in mental status<br>f. crackles (rales) and diminished or absent breath sounds<br>g. dyspnea, orthopnea<br>h. peripheral edema<br>i. distended neck veins<br>j. delayed small vein emptying time (longer than 3-5 seconds)<br>k. elevated CVP (use internal jugular vein pulsation method to estimate CVP if monitoring device not present).<br>2. Monitor chest x-ray results. Report findings of pulmonary vascular congestion, pleural effusion, or pulmonary edema.<br>3. Implement measures *to reduce fluid volume excess:*<br>a. maintain fluid restrictions as ordered (intake allowed is usually 500-700 ml plus the amount of urine output in the previous 24 hours)<br>b. restrict sodium intake as ordered<br>c. administer the following medications if ordered:<br>1. diuretics *to increase excretion of water*<br>2. arterial vasodilators *to improve renal blood flow (reduced renal perfusion stimulates the renin-angiotension-aldosterone mechanism).*<br>4. Consult physician if signs and symptoms of fluid volume excess persist or worsen. |
| 1.b. The client will maintain a safe serum sodium level as evidenced by:<br>1. absence of nausea, abdominal cramps, and thirst<br>2. moist mucous membranes<br>3. usual mental status<br>4. usual muscle strength<br>5. absence of tremors and seizure activity<br>6. serum sodium | 1.b.1. Assess for and report signs and symptoms of:<br>a. hyponatremia (e.g. nausea, abdominal cramps, lethargy, confusion, weakness, tremors, seizures)<br>b. hypernatremia (e.g. thirst; dry, sticky mucous membranes; restlessness; lethargy; weakness; elevated temperature; seizures).<br>2. Monitor serum sodium results. Report values that are not within a safe range for client.<br>3. Implement measures *to prevent or treat hyponatremia:*<br>a. maintain fluid restrictions as ordered *to prevent dilutional hyponatremia*<br>b. increase dietary allotment of sodium if ordered<br>c. administer loop diuretics (e.g. furosemide) if ordered *to treat dilutional hyponatremia (loop diuretics induce a fairly isotonic diuresis so that water loss can occur without further hyponatremia).*<br>4. Implement measures *to prevent or treat hypernatremia:*<br>a. maintain maximum fluid intake allowed |

within a safe range for client.

b. maintain dietary sodium restrictions if ordered
c. administer thiazide diuretics if ordered.
5. Consult physician if unsafe serum sodium levels persist.

1.c. The client will maintain a safe serum potassium level as evidenced by:
1. regular pulse at 60-100 beats/minute
2. absence of paresthesias
3. usual muscle tone and strength
4. normal bowel sounds
5. absence of diarrhea and intestinal colic
6. normal ECG reading
7. serum potassium within a safe range for client.

1.c.1. Assess for and report signs and symptoms of hyperkalemia (e.g. slow or irregular pulse; paresthesias; twitching or cramps progressing to muscle weakness and flaccidity; hyperactive bowel sounds with diarrhea and intestinal colic; ECG reading showing peaked T wave, prolonged PR interval, and/or widened QRS; elevated serum potassium level).
2. Implement measures *to prevent or treat hyperkalemia:*
   a. maintain dietary restrictions of potassium as ordered
   b. instruct client to consult physician or dietitian about which salt substitute he/she can safely use *(most salt substitutes contain potassium)*
   c. perform actions *to reduce the cellular release of potassium:*
      1. implement measures *to spare body proteins and prevent excessive tissue breakdown:*
         a. encourage client to consume the amount of dietary protein allotted
         b. provide allotted amount of carbohydrates *(spares the protein by providing a quick energy source)*
         c. perform actions to prevent infection (see Nursing Diagnosis 5, action c) *in order to prevent an increase in metabolic rate and subsequent increase in protein catabolism*
      2. implement measures to prevent or treat metabolic acidosis (see action g.2 in this diagnosis)
   d. if signs and symptoms of hyperkalemia are present, consult physician before administering prescribed potassium supplements and other medications that can increase potassium levels (e.g. potassium penicillin G, potassium-sparing diuretics)
   e. if transfusions are necessary:
      1. request fresh blood *(the potassium content of blood stored longer than 48-72 hours is higher than that of fresh blood)*
      2. follow recommended precautions *to prevent damage to cells* (e.g. fill drip chamber above filter top, use 18 gauge needle)
   f. administer the following medications if ordered:
      1. loop diuretics (e.g. ethacrynic acid, furosemide) *to increase renal excretion of potassium*
      2. cation-exchange resins (e.g. sodium polystyrene sulfonate [Kayexalate]) *to increase potassium excretion via the intestines (act by exchanging sodium for potassium)*
      3. intravenous insulin and hypertonic glucose solutions *to enhance transport of potassium back into cells.*
3. If signs and symptoms of hyperkalemia persist or worsen:
   a. consult physician
   b. have intravenous calcium preparation (e.g. calcium gluconate) readily available *(may be ordered to counteract the effect of a high potassium level on the heart).*

1.d. The client will maintain a safe serum calcium level as evidenced by:
1. usual mental status
2. regular pulse at 60-100 beats/minute
3. negative Chvostek's and Trousseau's signs
4. absence of numbness and tingling in fingers,

1.d.1. Assess for and report signs and symptoms of hypocalcemia (e.g. anxiousness; irritability; cardiac arrhythmias; positive Chvostek's and Trousseau's signs; numbness or tingling of fingers, toes, or circumoral area; hyperactive reflexes; tetany; seizures; serum calcium level that is lower than normal for client).
2. Implement measures *to prevent or treat hypocalcemia:*
   a. provide sources of calcium (e.g. milk, milk products) in diet unless contraindicated
   b. administer activated vitamin D (e.g. calcitriol, calcifediol) and calcium supplements if ordered
   c. avoid rapid transfusion of citrated blood *(the citrate that is added to blood to prevent clotting binds calcium; the liver normally removes citrate unless it is infused too rapidly)*

| Desired Outcomes | Nursing Actions and ***Selected Purposes/Rationales*** |
|---|---|
| toes, and circumoral area; hyperreflexia; tetany; and seizure activity<br>5. serum calcium within a safe range for client. | d. perform actions to prevent or treat hyperphosphatemia (see action e.2 in this diagnosis)<br>e. avoid rapid or aggressive treatment of acidosis *(rapidly reversing acidosis can result in decreased ionization of calcium).*<br>3. If signs and symptoms of hypocalcemia occur:<br>a. institute seizure precautions<br>b. have intravenous calcium preparation (e.g. calcium gluconate) readily available. |
| 1.e. The client will maintain a safe serum phosphorus level as evidenced by:<br>1. absence of paresthesias, tetany, and seizure activity<br>2. serum phosphorus within a safe range for client. | 1.e.1. Assess for and report signs and symptoms of hyperphosphatemia (e.g. paresthesias, tetany, seizures, higher than normal serum phosphorus level for client).<br>2. Implement measures *to prevent or treat hyperphosphatemia:*<br>a. restrict dietary intake of phosphorus if ordered by limiting foods/fluids such as organ meats, poultry, milk, milk products, eggs, and legumes<br>b. administer phosphate-binding medications such as aluminum hydroxide (e.g. Amphojel), aluminum carbonate (e.g. Basaljel), and calcium carbonate (e.g. Tums) if ordered.<br>3. Consult physician if signs and symptoms of hyperphosphatemia persist or worsen. |
| 1.f. The client will maintain a safe serum magnesium level as evidenced by:<br>1. absence of flushing, nausea, vomiting, and muscle weakness<br>2. usual mental status<br>3. vital signs within normal range for client<br>4. serum magnesium within a safe range for client. | 1.f. 1. Assess for and report signs and symptoms of hypermagnesemia (e.g. flushed, warm skin; nausea; vomiting; muscle weakness; drowsiness; lethargy; hypotension; bradypnea; bradycardia; higher than normal serum magnesium level for client).<br>2. Implement measures *to prevent or treat hypermagnesemia:*<br>a. avoid giving laxatives and antacids that contain magnesium (e.g. Milk of Magnesia, Gelusil, Mylanta, Maalox)<br>b. maintain dietary restrictions of magnesium if ordered by limiting intake of foods/fluids such as nuts, whole-grain breads and cereals, and legumes.<br>3. Consult physician if signs and symptoms of hypermagnesemia persist or worsen. |
| 1.g. The client will maintain acid-base balance as evidenced by:<br>1. usual mental status<br>2. unlabored respirations at 14-20/minute<br>3. absence of headache, nausea, vomiting, and cardiac arrhythmias<br>4. blood gases within a safe range for client<br>5. anion gap within normal range. | 1.g.1. Assess for and report signs and symptoms of metabolic acidosis (e.g. drowsiness; disorientation; stupor; rapid, deep respirations; headache; nausea; vomiting; cardiac arrhythmias; lower than usual pH and $CO_2$ content; increased anion gap).<br>2. Implement measures *to prevent or treat metabolic acidosis:*<br>a. perform actions to prevent or treat hyperkalemia (see action c.2 in this diagnosis)<br>b. administer sodium bicarbonate if ordered (usually reserved for treatment of severe acidosis [pH less than 7.1-7.2]).<br>3. Consult physician if signs and symptoms of acidosis persist or worsen. |

**2. NURSING DIAGNOSIS: Altered nutrition: less than body requirements**

related to decreased oral intake associated with:
a. dislike of prescribed diet;
b. prescribed dietary modifications (especially protein restrictions that are necessary in order to control the serum levels of nitrogenous substances).

| Desired Outcome | Nursing Actions and ***Selected Purposes/Rationales*** |
|---|---|
| 2. The client will maintain an adequate nutritional status as evidenced by:<br>a. weight within normal range for client's age, height, and body frame<br>b. serum albumin, Hct, Hb, transferrin, and lymphocyte levels within normal range<br>c. triceps skinfold thickness within normal range<br>d. usual or improved strength and activity tolerance<br>e. healthy oral mucous membrane. | 2.a. Assess for and report signs and symptoms of malnutrition:<br>1. weight below normal for client's age, height, and body frame<br>2. low serum albumin, Hct, Hb, transferrin, and lymphocyte levels (some of these values may be abnormal as a result of decreased renal function)<br>3. triceps skinfold thickness less than normal<br>4. weakness and fatigue (may also be a reflection of decreasing renal function)<br>5. stomatitis.<br>b. Monitor percentage of meals and snacks client consumes. Report a pattern of inadequate intake.<br>c. Implement measures *to maintain an adequate nutritional status:*<br>1. perform actions *to improve oral intake:*<br>a. increase activity as tolerated *(activity stimulates appetite)*<br>b. obtain a dietary consult if necessary to assist client in selecting foods/fluids that meet nutritional needs and dietary restrictions as well as personal and cultural preferences whenever possible<br>c. encourage a rest period before meals *to minimize fatigue*<br>d. maintain a clean environment and a relaxed, pleasant atmosphere<br>e. provide oral care before meals<br>f. serve small portions of nutritious foods/fluids that are appealing to client<br>g. allow adequate time for meals; reheat food if necessary<br>2. encourage client to eat the maximum amount of protein allowed; instruct him/her to satisfy protein requirements with foods/fluids that are complete proteins and contain essential amino acids (e.g. eggs, milk, meat, poultry)<br>3. offer dietary supplements between meals if indicated<br>4. administer vitamins and minerals if ordered.<br>d. Perform a 72-hour calorie count if ordered. Report totals to dietitian and physician.<br>e. Consult physician regarding alternative methods of providing nutrition (e.g. parenteral nutrition, tube feedings) if client does not consume enough food or fluids to meet nutritional needs. |

**3. NURSING DIAGNOSIS: Altered oral mucous membrane: dryness**

related to restricted fluid intake.

| Desired Outcome | Nursing Actions and ***Selected Purposes/Rationales*** |
|---|---|
| 3. The client will maintain a moist, intact oral mucous membrane. | 3.a. Assess client for dryness of the oral mucosa.<br>b. Implement measures *to relieve dryness of the oral mucous membrane:*<br>1. maintain the maximum fluid intake allowed (usually 500-700 ml plus the amount of urine output for the previous 24 hours); encourage client to space fluid intake evenly throughout the hours he/she is awake<br>2. instruct and assist client to perform good oral hygiene as often as needed<br>3. instruct client to avoid products such as lemon-glycerin swabs and commercial mouthwashes containing alcohol *(these products have a drying or irritating effect on the oral mucous membrane)*<br>4. encourage client to rinse mouth frequently with water or dilute mouthwash<br>5. encourage client to lubricate lips frequently with K-Y jelly, ChapStick, Blistex, or mineral oil<br>6. encourage client to breathe through nose rather than his/her mouth<br>7. encourage client not to smoke *(smoking irritates and dries the mucosa)*<br>8. perform actions *to increase salivary flow:*<br>a. encourage client to chew gum or suck on sour, hard candy<br>b. offer small amounts of hot tea with lemon or warm lemonade at regular intervals unless contraindicated.<br>c. Consult physician if dryness worsens and/or cracking or breakdown of oral mucous membrane occurs. |

## 4. NURSING DIAGNOSIS: Activity intolerance

related to:

a. inadequate tissue oxygenation associated with anemia resulting from:
   1. decreased secretion of erythropoietin as a result of impaired renal function (erythropoietin stimulates the bone marrow to produce RBCs)
   2. decreased production and shortened life span of RBCs (as renal failure progresses, the nitrogenous substances in the blood increase and suppress the bone marrow's production of RBCs and reduce the life span of the RBCs that are released);

b. inadequate nutritional status.

| Desired Outcome | Nursing Actions and ***Selected Purposes/Rationales*** |
|---|---|
| 4. The client will demonstrate an increased tolerance for activity as evidenced by:<br>a. verbalization of feeling less fatigued and weak<br>b. ability to perform activities of daily living without exertional dyspnea, chest pain, diaphoresis, dizziness, and a significant change in vital signs. | 4.a. Assess for signs and symptoms of activity intolerance:<br>1. statements of fatigue and weakness<br>2. exertional dyspnea, chest pain, diaphoresis, or dizziness<br>3. abnormal heart rate response to activity (e.g. increase in rate of 20 beats/minute above resting rate, decrease in rate, rate not returning to preactivity level within 3 minutes after stopping activity, change from regular to irregular rate)<br>4. decreased systolic B/P or a significant increase (10-15 mm Hg) in systolic or diastolic pressure with activity.<br>b. Implement measures *to improve activity tolerance:*<br>1. perform actions *to promote rest and/or conserve energy:*<br>a. maintain activity restrictions if ordered<br>b. minimize environmental activity and noise<br>c. organize nursing care to allow for periods of uninterrupted rest<br>d. limit the number of visitors and their length of stay<br>e. assist client with self-care activities as needed |

f. keep supplies and personal articles within easy reach
g. instruct client in energy-saving techniques (e.g. using shower chair when showering, sitting to brush teeth or comb hair)
2. perform actions to reduce the levels of serum nitrogenous substances (see Collaborative Diagnosis 6, action a.4) *in order to prevent the suppression of RBC production and RBC hemolysis*
3. perform actions to maintain an adequate nutritional status (see Nursing Diagnosis 2, action c)
4. administer hematopoietic agents (e.g. epoetin alfa) and/or androgens (e.g. testosterone propionate, fluoxymesterone) if ordered *to stimulate RBC production*
5. increase client's activity gradually as tolerated.

c. Instruct client to:
1. report a decreased tolerance for activity
2. stop any activity that causes chest pain, shortness of breath, dizziness, or extreme fatigue or weakness.

d. Consult physician if signs and symptoms of activity intolerance persist or worsen.

## 5. NURSING DIAGNOSIS: High risk for infection

related to:
a. lowered natural resistance associated with:
1. depressed immune response resulting from increasing levels of nitrogenous substances as a result of diminished renal function
2. malnutrition;

b. stasis of respiratory secretions and urinary stasis if mobility is decreased.

| Desired Outcome | Nursing Actions and ***Selected Purposes/Rationales*** |
|---|---|
| 5. The client will remain free of infection as evidenced by:<br>a. absence of fever and chills<br>b. pulse within normal limits<br>c. normal breath sounds<br>d. voiding clear urine without complaints of frequency, urgency, and burning<br>e. absence of heat, pain, redness, swelling, and unusual drainage in any area<br>f. no complaints of increased weakness and fatigue<br>g. WBC and differential counts within normal range<br>h. negative results of cultured specimens. | 5.a. Assess for and report signs and symptoms of infection:<br>1. elevated temperature<br>2. chills<br>3. increased pulse<br>4. abnormal breath sounds<br>5. cloudy, foul-smelling urine<br>6. complaints of frequency, urgency, or burning when urinating<br>7. presence of WBCs, bacteria, and/or nitrites in urine<br>8. heat, pain, redness, swelling, or unusual drainage in any area<br>9. complaints of increased weakness or fatigue<br>10. elevated WBC count and/or significant change in differential.<br>b. Obtain specimens (e.g. urine, vaginal, mouth, sputum, blood) for culture as ordered. Report positive results.<br>c. Implement measures *to prevent infection:*<br>1. perform actions to reduce the levels of serum nitrogenous substances (see Collaborative Diagnosis 6, action a.4)<br>2. maintain the maximum fluid intake allowed<br>3. use good handwashing technique and encourage client to do the same<br>4. maintain meticulous aseptic technique during all invasive procedures (e.g. catheterizations, venous and arterial punctures, injections)<br>5. change intravenous tubings and solutions and rotate insertion sites according to hospital policy<br>6. protect client from others who have an infection and instruct him/her to continue this after discharge |

**Desired Outcome** | **Nursing Actions and *Selected Purposes/Rationales***

7. perform actions to maintain an adequate nutritional status (see Nursing Diagnosis 2, action c)
8. perform actions to reduce stress (see Nursing Diagnosis 7, action b) *in order to prevent excessive secretion of cortisol (cortisol inhibits the immune response)*
9. reinforce importance of good oral hygiene
10. perform actions *to prevent stasis of respiratory secretions* (e.g. instruct and assist client to turn, cough, and deep breathe; increase activity as tolerated)
11. perform actions to prevent urinary retention (e.g. instruct client to urinate when the urge is first felt, promote relaxation during voiding attempts) *in order to prevent urinary stasis*
12. perform actions *to prevent the introduction of microorganisms into the urinary tract* (e.g. assist client with perineal care as needed, instruct and assist female client to wipe from front to back after urinating and defecating, maintain sterile technique during urinary catheterization).

## 6. COLLABORATIVE DIAGNOSES:

**Potential complications:**

a. **uremic syndrome** related to accumulation of serum nitrogenous substances (e.g. creatinine, urea, phenols) associated with extensive loss of renal function (uremic syndrome develops when GFR falls to less than 10% of normal);
b. **hypertension** related to retention of fluid and sodium and increased plasma renin levels (occurs when there is diminished renal blood flow).

**Desired Outcomes** | **Nursing Actions and *Selected Purposes/Rationales***

6.a. The client will not experience uremic syndrome as evidenced by:
1. pulse regular at 60-100 beats/minute
2. usual mental status
3. usual skin color
4. improved strength and activity tolerance
5. no complaints of nausea, insomnia, itching, muscle cramping, paresthesias, and taste alterations
6. intact oral mucous membrane
7. absence of vomiting, unusual bleeding, pericarditis, asterixis, and seizure activity.

6.a.1. Assess for signs and symptoms of uremic syndrome:
- a. cardiac arrhythmias
- b. difficulty concentrating, lethargy, confusion, or hallucinations
- c. sallow or grayish-bronze skin color
- d. increased weakness and fatigue
- e. complaints of nausea, insomnia, itching, muscle cramps, paresthesias, or metallic or bitter taste in mouth
- f. stomatitis
- g. vomiting
- h. unusual bleeding (e.g. ecchymoses; prolonged bleeding from puncture sites; gingival bleeding; frank or occult blood in stool, urine, or vomitus)
- i. pericarditis (e.g. precordial pain, pericardial friction rub, dyspnea, tachypnea, elevated temperature)
- j. asterixis, seizures.

2. Monitor BUN and serum creatinine results. Report levels that increase or fail to return to a safe level.
3. Collect a 24-hour urine specimen if ordered. Report creatinine clearance levels that decrease or fail to return to a safe level.
4. Implement measures *to reduce the levels of serum nitrogenous substances in order to prevent uremic syndrome:*
   - a. perform actions to maintain an adequate nutritional status (see Nursing Diagnosis 2, action c) *in order to reduce catabolism of body proteins*
   - b. maintain dietary protein restrictions

c. perform actions to prevent infection (see Nursing Diagnosis 5, action c) *in order to prevent an increase in metabolic rate and subsequent cellular catabolism*
d. perform actions *to prevent further renal damage:*
    1. implement measures as ordered to control disease conditions such as diabetes that have caused or contributed to CRF
    2. consult the physician before administering medications that are known to be nephrotoxic (e.g. gentamicin, streptomycin, salicylates, ibuprofen).

5. If signs and symptoms of uremic syndrome occur:
    a. consult physician
    b. continue with above measures
    c. maintain a safe environment for client (e.g. side rails up while in bed, assistance with ambulation as needed, constant supervision if indicated, seizure precautions)
    d. perform actions *to treat cardiac arrhythmias if present* (e.g. administer antiarrhythmics as ordered, restrict activity if indicated)
    e. perform actions *to control nausea and vomiting if present* (e.g. administer antiemetics as ordered; provide small, frequent meals; instruct client to ingest foods/fluids slowly)
    f. perform actions *to reduce pruritus if present* (e.g. use tepid water and mild soap for bathing, apply emollient creams or ointments frequently, administer antihistamines if ordered)
    g. perform actions *to control muscle cramps if they occur* (e.g. instruct client to push feet against footboard when leg cramps occur, apply warm packs to affected areas)
    h. perform actions *to reduce the severity of stomatitis if present* (e.g. instruct client to avoid substances such as extremely hot, spicy, or acidic foods/fluids; assist with frequent oral hygiene; apply topical anesthetics or oral protective pastes as ordered)
    i. perform actions *to prevent bleeding* (e.g. apply gentle, prolonged pressure after injections and venous and arterial punctures; instruct client to use an electric rather than a straight-edge razor and to use a soft-bristle toothbrush and low-pressure power spray for oral care)
    j. perform actions *to control bleeding if it occurs* (e.g. apply firm, prolonged pressure to bleeding area if possible; administer clotting factors, vitamin K, or hemostatic agent if ordered)
    k. perform actions *to treat pericarditis if present* (e.g. maintain activity restrictions as ordered, administer an anti-inflammatory agent and analgesics if ordered)
    l. prepare client for dialysis if planned (often initiated when serum creatinine level is around 10 mg/dL or BUN is around 100 mg/dL)
    m. provide emotional support to client and significant others.

6.b. The client will maintain B/P within a safe range as evidenced by:
1. systolic pressure of 140 mm Hg or less and diastolic pressure of 90 mm Hg or less
2. no complaints of headache and dizziness.

6.b.1. Assess for and report signs and symptoms of hypertension (e.g. systolic pressure of 140 mm Hg or greater, diastolic pressure of 90 mm Hg or greater, headache, dizziness).
2. Implement measures *to prevent or control hypertension:*
    a. perform actions to reduce fluid volume excess and prevent or treat hypernatremia (see Nursing Diagnosis 1, actions a.3 and b.4)
    b. perform actions to reduce fear and anxiety (see Nursing Diagnosis 7, action b)
    c. administer antihypertensives (e.g. propranolol, captopril).
3. If hypertension persists or worsens:
    a. consult physician
    b. continue with above actions
    c. refer to Care Plan on Hypertension for additional care measures.

## 7. NURSING DIAGNOSIS: Anxiety

related to lack of understanding of diagnosis, diagnostic tests, and treatment plan; uncertainty regarding extensiveness of disease progression; prognosis; financial concerns; unfamiliar environment; and the effects of CRF on life style and roles.

**Desired Outcome**

7. The client will experience a reduction in anxiety as evidenced by:
   a. verbalization of feeling less anxious and fearful
   b. usual sleep pattern
   c. relaxed facial expression and body movements
   d. stable vital signs
   e. usual perceptual ability and interactions with others.

**Nursing Actions and *Selected Purposes/Rationales***

7.a. Assess client for signs and symptoms of anxiety (e.g. verbalization of fears and concerns, insomnia, tenseness, tremors, irritability, restlessness, diaphoresis, tachypnea, tachycardia, elevated blood pressure, facial pallor or flushing, narrowed perceptual field, withdrawal, noncompliance with treatment plan). Validate perceptions carefully, remembering that some behavior may result from fluid and electrolyte imbalances.

b. Implement measures *to reduce fear and anxiety:*
   1. orient client to hospital environment, equipment, and routines
   2. introduce staff who will be participating in his/her care; if possible, maintain consistency in staff assigned to his/her care *to provide feelings of stability and comfort with the environment*
   3. assure client that staff members are nearby; respond to call signal as soon as possible
   4. maintain a calm, supportive, confident manner when interacting with client
   5. encourage verbalization of fear and anxiety; provide feedback
   6. reinforce physician's explanations and clarify misconceptions the client has about CRF, diagnostic tests, the treatment plan, and prognosis
   7. explain all diagnostic tests performed to assess the level of renal function
   8. provide a calm, restful environment
   9. instruct client in relaxation techniques and encourage participation in diversional activities
   10. initiate financial and/or social service referrals if indicated
   11. assist client to identify specific stressors and ways to cope with them
   12. encourage significant others to project a caring, concerned attitude without obvious anxiousness
   13. administer antianxiety agents if ordered.

c. Include significant others in orientation and teaching sessions and encourage their continued support of the client.

d. Provide information based on current needs of client and significant others at a level they can understand. Encourage questions and clarification of information provided.

e. Consult physician if above measures fail to control fear and anxiety.

## 8. NURSING DIAGNOSIS: Grieving*

related to progressive loss of kidney function and the effects of this on life style and roles.

*This diagnostic label includes anticipatory grieving and grieving following the actual losses.

| Desired Outcome | Nursing Actions and ***Selected Purposes/Rationales*** |
|---|---|
| 8. The client will demonstrate beginning progression through the grieving process as evidenced by:<br>a. verbalization of feelings about having chronic renal failure<br>b. expression of grief<br>c. participation in treatment plan and self-care activities<br>d. utilization of available support systems<br>e. verbalization of a plan for integrating prescribed follow-up care into life style. | 8.a. Assess for signs and symptoms of grieving (e.g. change in eating habits, inability to concentrate, insomnia, anger, noncompliance, withdrawal from significant others, denial of progressive loss of kidney function). Be aware that client's response to a loss will be affected by factors such as previous experience with loss, age, developmental stage, available support systems, spiritual and cultural background, current health status, and significance of the loss.<br>b. Implement measures *to facilitate the grieving process:*<br>1. assist client to acknowledge the progressive loss of kidney function *so grief work can begin;* assess for factors that may hinder and facilitate acknowledgment<br>2. discuss the grieving process and assist client to accept the phases of grieving as an expected response to an actual and/or anticipated loss; support the realization that grief may recur because of the chronic, progressive nature of the disease<br>3. allow time for client to progress through the phases of grieving (phases vary among theorists but progress from shock and alarm to acceptance); be aware that not every phase is expressed by all individuals, that recurrence of phases is common, and that the grieving process may take months to years<br>4. provide an atmosphere of care and concern (e.g. provide privacy, be available and nonjudgmental, display empathy and respect) *so that client will feel free to verbalize feelings*<br>5. perform actions *to promote trust* (e.g. answer questions honestly, provide requested information)<br>6. encourage the verbal expression of anger and sadness about the loss experienced; recognize displacement of anger and assist client to see the actual cause of angry feelings and resentment; establish limits on abusive behavior if demonstrated<br>7. encourage client to express his/her feelings in whatever ways are comfortable (e.g. writing, drawing, conversation)<br>8. assist client to identify personal strengths that have helped him/her to cope in previous situations of loss<br>9. support realistic hope about the effect that adherence to the treatment plan has on prognosis<br>10. support behaviors suggesting successful grief work (e.g. verbalizing feelings about loss, focusing on ways to adapt to progressive loss of kidney function)<br>11. explain the phases of the grieving process to significant others; encourage their support and understanding<br>12. facilitate communication between the client and significant others; be aware that they may be in different phases of the grieving process<br>13. provide information regarding counseling services and support groups that might assist client in working through grief<br>14. arrange for visit from clergy if desired by client.<br>c. Consult physician regarding referral for counseling if signs of dysfunctional grieving (e.g. persistent denial of loss, excessive anger or sadness, hysteria, suicidal behaviors) occur. |

## 9. NURSING DIAGNOSIS: Ineffective management of therapeutic regimen

related to lack of understanding of the implications of not following the prescribed treatment plan, difficulty integrating necessary treatments into life style, and lack of financial resources.

| Desired Outcome | Nursing Actions and ***Selected Purposes/Rationales*** |
|---|---|
| 9. The client will demonstrate the probability of effective management of the therapeutic regimen as evidenced by:<br>a. willingness to learn about and participate in treatments and care<br>b. statements reflecting ways to modify personal habits and integrate prescribed care into life style<br>c. statements reflecting an understanding of the implications of not following the prescribed treatment plan. | 9.a. Assess for indications that the client may be unable to effectively manage the therapeutic regimen:<br>1. statements reflecting that he/she was unable to manage care at home<br>2. failure to adhere to treatment plan while in the hospital (e.g. not adhering to dietary modifications and fluid restrictions, refusing medications)<br>3. statements reflecting a lack of understanding of factors that will cause further renal damage<br>4. statements reflecting an unwillingness or inability to modify personal habits and integrate necessary treatments into life style<br>5. statements reflecting view that kidney damage will reverse itself or that the situation is hopeless and efforts to comply with prescribed care are useless.<br>b. Implement measures *to promote effective management of the therapeutic regimen:*<br>1. explain renal failure in terms client can understand; stress the fact that it is a chronic disease and that adherence to treatment plan is necessary in order to delay and/or prevent complications<br>2. initiate and reinforce discharge teaching outlined in Nursing Diagnosis 10 *in order to promote a sense of control and self-reliance*<br>3. encourage client to participate in prescribed care (e.g. monitoring intake and output, calculating allowed fluid intake, selecting foods and fluids within dietary restrictions)<br>4. assist client to identify ways he/she can incorporate care into life style; focus on modifications of life style rather than complete change<br>5. obtain a dietary consult to assist client in planning a dietary program based on prescribed modifications and client's likes, dislikes, and daily routines<br>6. encourage questions and clarify misconceptions the client has about CRF and its effects<br>7. perform actions to facilitate the grieving process (see Nursing Diagnosis 8, action b)<br>8. provide client with verbal and written instructions about future appointments with health care provider, ways to prevent further kidney damage, dietary modifications, fluid restrictions, medications, and signs and symptoms to report; determine areas of difficulty and misunderstanding and reinforce teaching as necessary<br>9. encourage client to discuss his/her concerns about the cost of medications and follow-up medical care; obtain a social service consult to assist with financial planning and to obtain financial aid if indicated<br>10. provide information about and encourage utilization of community resources that can assist client to make necessary life-style changes (e.g. local chapter of the American Kidney Association, vocational rehabilitation, counseling services)<br>11. reinforce behaviors suggesting future compliance with the therapeutic regimen (e.g. statements reflecting plans for integrating care into life style, active participation in treatment plan, changes in personal habits)<br>12. include significant others in explanations and teaching sessions and encourage their support; reinforce the need for client to assume responsibility for managing as much of care as possible.<br>c. Consult physician regarding referrals to community health agencies if continued instruction, support, or supervision is needed. |

## 10. NURSING DIAGNOSIS: Knowledge deficit

regarding follow-up care.

| Desired Outcomes | Nursing Actions and ***Selected Purposes/Rationales*** |
|---|---|
| 10.a. The client will verbalize a basic understanding of CRF. | 10.a. Explain renal failure in terms that client can understand. Utilize appropriate teaching aids (e.g. pictures, videotapes, kidney models). |
| 10.b. The client will identify ways to slow the progression of kidney damage. | 10.b.1. Provide instructions regarding ways to slow the progression of kidney damage:<br>a. control hypertension by adhering to dietary modifications and taking medications as prescribed<br>b. reduce the risk of urinary tract infection by:<br>1. cleaning perianal area thoroughly after each bowel movement<br>2. maintaining allowed fluid intake<br>3. wiping from front to back after urination and defecation (if female)<br>c. reduce the risk of nephrotoxic reactions by:<br>1. consulting the health care provider before:<br>a. taking any additional prescription and nonprescription drugs<br>b. receiving any vaccines<br>c. resuming any occupation or hobby involving exposure to chemicals or fumes<br>2. avoiding contact with products such as antifreeze, pesticides, carbon tetrachloride, mercuric chloride, lead, arsenic, and creosote.<br>2. With client and significant others, discuss ways in which above health care measures can be incorporated into life style. |
| 10.c. The client will verbalize an understanding of fluid restrictions and dietary modifications. | 10.c.1. Reinforce the importance of adhering to prescribed fluid restrictions and dietary modifications.<br>2. Reinforce physician's instructions about specific fluid restrictions and dietary modifications.<br>3. Reinforce dietitian's instructions on how to calculate and measure dietary allotments. Have client develop sample menus.<br>4. If client is on a protein- and sodium-restricted diet, inform him/her that numerous salt-free and protein-free products are available. Provide names of local stores that carry these products.<br>5. If client is on fluid restrictions, instruct to:<br>a. take oral medications with soft foods (e.g. applesauce, pudding) rather than liquids<br>b. reduce thirst by:<br>1. sucking on sour, hard candy or ice cubes made with favorite juices (caution client that the fluid volume of the ice cubes must be considered as oral fluid intake)<br>2. spacing fluids evenly throughout the hours he/she is awake<br>c. set out the 24-hour allotment of liquids in the morning in order to visualize the amount allowed for the day. |
| 10.d. The client will demonstrate the ability to accurately weigh self, measure fluid intake and | 10.d.1. If client needs to monitor weight, instruct him/her to weigh at the same time, on the same scale, and with similar amounts of clothing on.<br>2. Demonstrate how to measure and record fluid intake and urinary output if indicated. Stress that any substance that is liquid at room temperature is counted as fluid intake. |

| Desired Outcomes | Nursing Actions and ***Selected Purposes/Rationales*** |
|---|---|
| output, and monitor own blood pressure. | 3. If client needs to monitor B/P, instruct him/her how to take, read, and record it.<br>4. Allow time for questions, clarification, practice, and accuracy checks. Instruct client to take record of weights, fluid intake and urinary output, and B/P readings to appointments with health care provider. |
| 10.e. The client will identify ways to reduce the risk of infection. | 10.e. Instruct client in ways to reduce the risk of infection:<br>1. avoid contact with persons who have an infection<br>2. avoid crowds during the flu or cold season<br>3. decrease or stop smoking<br>4. drink allotted amounts of liquids<br>5. maintain good personal hygiene<br>6. maintain a good nutritional status<br>7. take antimicrobials as prescribed before scheduled dental work or surgical procedures. |
| 10.f. The client will identify ways to manage conditions that often occur as a result of CRF. | 10.f. Provide instructions regarding ways to manage the following conditions that often occur as a result of CRF:<br>1. weakness and fatigue:<br>a. schedule frequent rest periods throughout the day<br>b. maintain a good nutritional status<br>2. dry mouth:<br>a. space fluid allotments evenly throughout waking hours<br>b. perform oral hygiene frequently<br>3. decreased libido (can occur as a result of weakness and fatigue, depression, and side effects of some medications):<br>a. schedule rest periods before and after sexual activity<br>b. explore creative ways of expressing sexuality (e.g. massage, fantasies, cuddling). |
| 10.g. The client will state signs and symptoms to report to the health care provider. | 10.g. Instruct client to report the following:<br>1. weight gain of more than 0.5 kg (1 pound)/day or a continued weight loss<br>2. uncontrolled nausea or vomiting<br>3. increasing fatigue and weakness<br>4. difficulty concentrating and making decisions<br>5. confusion<br>6. persistent or severe headache<br>7. palpitations or chest pain<br>8. blood in stools, urine, or vomitus; persistent bleeding from nose, mouth, or any cut; prolonged or excessive menses; excessive bruising; or sudden abdominal or back pain<br>9. fever or chills<br>10. numbness or tingling in extremities<br>11. impotence (could indicate electrolyte imbalances and/or increasing serum levels of nitrogenous substances)<br>12. amenorrhea (could indicate hormonal imbalances caused by increasing serum levels of nitrogenous substances)<br>13. increasing blood pressure (if B/P is monitored at home)<br>14. swelling of feet, ankles, or hands<br>15. diarrhea or constipation (either can occur as a side effect of some antacid therapy; physicians generally recommend alternating antacids containing magnesium with those containing aluminum or calcium to prevent these bowel problems)<br>16. persistent dizziness, lightheadedness, or fainting<br>17. itching<br>18. oral pain or breakdown of oral mucous membrane<br>19. shortness of breath<br>20. muscle cramping<br>21. twitching, tremors, or seizures. |

| | |
|---|---|
| 10.h. The client will identify community resources that can assist with adjustment to changes resulting from CRF. | 10.h.1. Provide information about community resources that can assist the client and significant others to adjust to changes resulting from chronic renal failure (e.g. local chapter of the American Kidney Association, vocational rehabilitation, social services, counseling services).<br>2. Initiate a referral if indicated. |
| 10.i. The client will verbalize an understanding of and a plan for adhering to recommended follow-up care including future appointments with health care provider and medications prescribed. | 10.i. 1. Reinforce the importance of keeping follow-up appointments with health care provider.<br>2. Explain the rationale for, side effects of, and importance of taking prescribed medications (e.g. antihypertensives, antacids, vitamins, electrolyte supplements, diuretics, hematopoietic agents).<br>3. Refer to Nursing Diagnosis 9, action b, for measures to promote the client's ability to effectively manage the therapeutic regimen. |

# Cystectomy with Urinary Diversion

Cystectomy is the removal of the bladder and is accompanied by a procedure to divert urinary flow. It may be performed to treat a malignancy of the bladder (particularly if it involves the trigone), congenital bladder anomalies, neurogenic bladder, and strictures of or irreparable trauma to the urethra and/or ureters. A cystectomy may also be performed to prevent further deterioration of renal function associated with chronic bladder infection. In some cases, the cystectomy includes just removal of the bladder (simple cystectomy); in others, such as with an invasive malignancy, a more radical procedure is performed. In men, a radical cystectomy includes removal of the bladder, prostate, seminal vesicles, the pelvic vas deferens and its ampulla, and the pelvic lymph nodes. The urethra is also removed unless a bladder replacement or substitution is planned. In women, a radical cystectomy includes removal of the bladder, urethra and external meatus, uterus, fallopian tubes, ovaries, a portion of the anterior vaginal wall, and the pelvic lymph nodes.

There are several ways to accomplish urinary diversion. The most common surgical method is the appliance-dependent ("wet") ileal or colon conduit. In this procedure, the ureters are implanted in the proximal end of an isolated piece of the terminal ileum or the colon, and the distal end is then brought through the abdominal wall to create the stoma. Alternatives to this are the continent urinary diversions in which the urine is diverted to the rectum and through the anal sphincter (e.g. ureteroileocecosigmoidostomy, augmented and valved rectum) and the continent abdominal wall stoma (e.g. Kock pouch, Gilchrist ileocecal reservoir, Mainz pouch, Indiana pouch). In the latter procedures, segments of the bowel (e.g. right colon, ileum and colon, ileum) are detubularized and remodeled to create a nonrefluxing reservoir into which the ureters are anastomosed. The volume of the pouch varies depending on the technique utilized, but most will remain continent with a 4 to 6 hour catheterization program. Orthotopic bladder replacement (e.g. Camey procedure, orthotopic Kock) is a type of diversion that may be an option for the male client undergoing a radical cystectomy, depending on the involvement of his urethra in the underlying disease process and the effectiveness of his urinary sphincters. Most clients will achieve daytime continence with orthotopic bladder replacement, but enuresis is a common problem. In clients who are not able to tolerate prolonged surgery, ureters can be implanted directly into the abdominal wall (cutaneous ureterostomy). Since there is a high rate of stomal stenosis with this procedure, it is usually reserved for clients whose life expectancy is very short. The type of urinary diversion selected depends on the preference and life expectancy of the client, his/her ability to perform intermittent self-catheterization, availability of a sufficient quantity of healthy large and small bowel to create the appropriate size reservoir and valves to maintain continence and prevent reflux, ability of the client to undergo a lengthy surgical procedure, and expertise of the surgeon.

**This care plan focuses on the adult client hospitalized for a cystectomy with urinary diversion by means of an ileal conduit.** The goals of preoperative care are to reduce fear and anxiety and prepare the client for the change in body image and function. Postoperatively, goals of care are to maintain peristomal skin integrity, prevent complications, facilitate psychological adjustment to the changes experienced, and educate the client regarding management of the urinary diversion and follow-up care.

## DIAGNOSTIC TESTS

Excretory urography (intravenous pyelogram)
Bladder ultrasonography
Bowel contrast studies
Urinalysis
Cystography
Urodynamic studies

## DISCHARGE CRITERIA

Prior to discharge, the client will:

- ❖ have no signs and symptoms of complications
- ❖ verbalize a basic understanding of the anatomical changes that have occurred as a result of the surgery
- ❖ demonstrate the ability to change ostomy appliance and maintain stomal and peristomal skin integrity
- ❖ demonstrate proper technique for cleansing reusable ostomy equipment
- ❖ verbalize ways to prevent excessive skin growth over the stoma and peristomal area
- ❖ identify ways to control odor of ostomy drainage and pouch
- ❖ identify ways to prevent urinary tract infection
- ❖ state signs and symptoms to report to the health care provider
- ❖ share thoughts and feelings about altered urinary function and its effect on body image and life style
- ❖ identify appropriate community resources that can assist with home management and adjustment to changes resulting from the urinary diversion
- ❖ verbalize an understanding of and a plan for adhering to recommended follow-up care including future appointments with health care provider, wound care, activity level, and medications prescribed.

## NURSING/ COLLABORATIVE DIAGNOSES

**See Standardized Preoperative and Postoperative Care Plans for additional diagnoses.**

## PREOPERATIVE

**Use in conjunction with the Standardized Preoperative Care Plan.**

### 1. NURSING DIAGNOSIS: Anxiety

related to:
a. unfamiliar environment and separation from significant others;
b. lack of understanding of diagnostic tests, surgical procedure, and care required for the urinary diversion;
c. anticipated loss of control, effects of anesthesia, and postoperative discomfort;
d. anticipated changes in body image and functioning and effects of urinary diversion on future life style;
e. economic factors associated with hospitalization;
f. ability to independently care for urinary diversion following discharge;
g. uncertain prognosis if the reason for the diversion is a malignancy.

| Desired Outcome | Nursing Actions and ***Selected Purposes/Rationales*** |
|---|---|
| 1. The client will experience a reduction in anxiety (see Standardized Preoperative Care Plan, Nursing Diagnosis 1 [pp. 108-109]), for outcome criteria. | 1.a. Refer to Standardized Preoperative Care Plan, Nursing Diagnosis 1 (pp. 108-109), for measures related to assessment and reduction of fear and anxiety.<br>b. Implement additional measures *to reduce fear and anxiety:*<br>1. show client and significant others a diagram of how the diversion is accomplished and a picture of a stoma *so that they will know what to expect;* explain that the stoma will shrink in size during the first 6 weeks postoperatively and that every attempt will be made to place the stoma in an area where the appliance will lie flat and be unobtrusive (usually right side of abdomen)<br>2. assure client that stoma has no pain receptors and will not be painful when touched<br>3. explain that current ostomy collection devices are odorproof and available in sizes to fit various body contours<br>4. explain that the stoma will begin to function immediately upon implantation of the ureters into the bowel segment and that a pouch connected to a drainage system will be applied in the operating room<br>5. assure client that no dietary changes are necessary after the initial postoperative period<br>6. if desired by client, arrange for a visit with a person of similar age and same sex who has successfully adapted to a urinary diversion<br>7. assure client that an ostomy need not alter life style (only contact sports are contraindicated). |

## 2. NURSING DIAGNOSIS: Knowledge deficit

regarding hospital routines associated with surgery, physical preparation for the cystectomy with urinary diversion, sensations that normally occur following surgery and anesthesia, and postoperative care and management of the ileal conduit.

| Desired Outcomes | Nursing Actions and ***Selected Purposes/Rationales*** |
|---|---|
| 2.a. The client will verbalize an understanding of usual preoperative care and postoperative sensations and care. | 2.a.1. Refer to Standardized Preoperative Care Plan, Nursing Diagnosis 4, actions a.1-4 (pp. 111-112), for information to include in preoperative teaching.<br>2. Explain measures utilized preoperatively to ensure that the bowel is adequately prepared (e.g. low-residue or clear liquid diet, enemas, cathartics, antimicrobial therapy).<br>3. Inform client that a tentative stoma site will be mapped out preoperatively by the physician or enterostomal therapist. Explain that an optimal stoma site allows proper fit of an appliance, freedom of movement, and good visualization by client.<br>4. Explain that a urethral catheter will be in place (if the urethra has not been removed) to drain excessive fluid from the space that had been occupied by the bladder.<br>5. Explain that ureteral stents (small, firm catheters) will be inserted in surgery to maintain patency of the ureters and protect the anastomoses between the ureters and the bowel segment. The stents will extend from the stoma and are usually removed 5-10 days after surgery.<br>6. Allow time for questions and clarification of information provided. |
| 2.b. The client will demonstrate the ability to perform activities designed to prevent postoperative complications. | 2.b. Refer to Standardized Preoperative Care Plan, Nursing Diagnosis 4, action b (p. 112), for instructions on ways to prevent postoperative complications. |
| 2.c. The client will verbalize an understanding of the function, appearance, and management of the ostomy. | 2.c.1. Arrange for a visit with enterostomal therapist.<br>2. Reinforce basic information provided by physician and/or enterostomal therapist regarding:<br>a. expected location of stoma<br>b. expected appearance of stoma postoperatively (red, initially edematous)<br>c. expected drainage (slight bleeding of stoma, blood in urine for 24-48 hours, mucus in urine [occurs because the bowel mucosa normally secretes mucus])<br>d. management of ostomy (e.g. skin care, odor control, use of various types of appliances)<br>e. ostomy appliances that client will be using in the immediate postoperative period.<br>3. Provide visual aids and allow client to handle appliances if he/she desires.<br>4. Encourage client to try wearing an appliance partially filled with water in order to experience how it feels and to validate if site will be adequate for successful adhesion of appliance.<br>5. Allow time for questions and clarification of information provided. |

## POSTOPERATIVE

**Use in conjunction with the Standardized Postoperative Care Plan.**

## 1. NURSING DIAGNOSIS: Actual/High risk for impaired skin integrity

related to:

a. disruption of skin associated with the surgical procedure;
b. delayed wound healing associated with decreased nutritional status, inadequate blood supply to wound area, infection, stress on wound area, and preoperative radiation therapy (may have been done if the underlying disease process is a malignancy);
c. irritation of skin around suture lines and wound drains associated with contact with wound drainage, pressure from drainage tubes, and use of tape;
d. irritation of peristomal area associated with:
   1. chemical irritation resulting from prolonged contact with urine (particularly alkaline urine), soap residue and perspiration under the appliance, and allergic reaction to substances used to secure the appliance
   2. mechanical irritation resulting from frequent and/or improper removal of adhesives, skin cements, and tape; aggressive cleansing of peristomal area; and pressure from appliance belt and drainage valve or clamp.

| Desired Outcomes | Nursing Actions and ***Selected Purposes/Rationales*** |
|---|---|
| 1.a. The client will experience normal healing of surgical wounds (see Standardized Postoperative Care Plan, Nursing Diagnosis 9, outcome a [p. 122], for outcome criteria). | 1.a. Refer to Standardized Postoperative Care Plan, Nursing Diagnosis 9, action a (pp. 122-123), for measures related to assessment and promotion of wound healing. |
| 1.b. The client will maintain skin integrity (see Standardized Postoperative Care Plan, Nursing Diagnosis 9, outcome b [p. 123], for outcome criteria). | 1.b.1. Inspect skin areas that are in contact with wound drainage, tape, and drainage tubings for signs of irritation and breakdown.<br>2. Assess for signs and symptoms of peristomal irritation and breakdown (e.g. redness, inflammation, and/or excoriation of peristomal skin; complaints of itching and burning under the appliance; inability to keep appliance on).<br>3. Refer to Standardized Postoperative Care Plan, Nursing Diagnosis 9, actions b.2 and 3 (p. 123), for measures to prevent and treat skin irritation and breakdown resulting from wound drainage, tape, and drainage tubings.<br>4. Implement measures *to prevent peristomal irritation and breakdown:*<br>a. patch test all adhesives, sprays, solvents, sealants, and skin barriers before initial use; do not use products that cause redness, itching, or burning<br>b. change appliance only when necessary (e.g. as ordered, if appliance or seal is leaking, if client complains of burning or itching under seal); appliance is typically changed every 3 days in the early postoperative period and then should be able to remain in place for 5-7 days<br>c. use a 2-piece appliance (barrier and pouch) *so that collection bag can be changed without having to remove adhesive from the skin* (a 1-piece appliance [stoma pouch] is commonly used once the stents are removed)<br>d. perform actions *to reduce peristomal irritation during removal of appliance:*<br>1. place drops of warm water or solvent at edge of barrier or |

| Desired Outcomes | Nursing Actions and ***Selected Purposes/Rationales*** |
|---|---|

adhesive disc if necessary *to loosen adhesive* (allow time for adhesive to dissolve before pulling appliance off)
2. remove appliance gently and in the direction of hair growth

e. perform actions *to prevent urine from coming in contact with the skin when changing appliance:*
1. change appliance when the ostomy is least active (in the morning before drinking liquids or when fluid intake has been reduced for a few hours)
2. place a "wick" (rolled gauze pad), vaginal tampon, or tissue on the stoma opening when the appliance is off

f. cleanse peristomal skin thoroughly with a no-residue skin cleanser (e.g. Peri-wash, UniWash) or mild soap and water, rinse completely, and pat dry; use tepid rather than hot water *to prevent burns*

g. apply skin sealant (e.g. Skin-Prep, Sween Prep, Skin Gel) before application of barrier or stoma pouch

h. use skin barriers composed of synthetic material (e.g. Premium Skin Barrier, Stomahesive); avoid the use of hydrophilic barriers (e.g. karaya) *because they attract and hold water and will dissolve when in contact with urine*

i. perform actions *to prevent urine from contacting the skin when appliance is on:*
1. ensure that skin barrier opening is exactly the same size as the stoma
2. measure diameter of stoma and select a pouch with an opening that is no more than 0.15-0.3 cm (1/16-1/8 inch) larger than stoma (it may be necessary to create a pattern to use for cutting pouch opening if stoma has an irregular shape and cannot be measured using appliance manufacturer's standard measuring guide)
3. instruct and assist client to remeasure the stoma size frequently during first 6 weeks after surgery and to alter barrier and pouch openings as stomal edema decreases
4. implement measures *to achieve an adequate seal:*
   a. avoid use of ointments, lotions, or creams on peristomal skin *(these can interfere with adequate adhesive bonding)*
   b. follow manufacturer's instructions carefully when applying skin products such as barriers or sealants and appliance
   c. use ostomy paste (e.g. Stomahesive paste, Premium paste) to fill in irregularities around stoma site (e.g. body folds, previous scars, retention sutures) before applying barrier or stoma pouch
   d. apply firm pressure and remove all air pockets when applying barrier or stoma pouch; place client in a supine position *to increase tautness of skin surface during application*
   e. use products with a flexible or convex backing or medical adhesive if needed
5. use a pouch with an antireflux valve
6. empty pouch every 2-3 hours or when it is about 1/3 full *(the weight of pouch could cause it to separate from the skin)*
7. position pouch so gravity flow facilitates drainage away from stoma and skin
8. close valve or clamp tightly after emptying pouch *to prevent leakage*

j. if a belted appliance is used, fasten the belt so that 2 fingers can easily slip between belt and skin *to prevent excessive pressure on the skin*

k. instruct and assist client to check appliance periodically to ensure that clamp or valve is not pressing on the skin.

5. If signs and symptoms of peristomal skin irritation and breakdown occur:
   a. identify irritant *so that appropriate treatment can be instituted*
   b. cleanse area gently with warm water

c. expose affected area to air for 20-30 minutes when flange or stoma pouch is removed
d. perform skin care according to enterostomal therapist's or physician's order or hospital procedure (usual care may include exposing affected area to heat source such as a hairdryer on low or cool setting; covering all irritated skin with a properly fitted, hypoallergenic, solid skin barrier; and avoiding appliance changes unless there are signs of leakage)
e. consult physician and/or enterostomal therapist if:
   1. condition of peristomal skin does not improve within 48 hours
   2. signs and symptoms of infection (e.g. elevated temperature; redness, warmth, and edema around area of breakdown; unusual drainage or odor from site) are present.

## 2. NURSING DIAGNOSIS: High risk for infection: urinary tract

related to:
a. increased bacterial growth associated with stasis of urine resulting from:
   1. continuous presence of urine (about 5 ml) in conduit
   2. reflux and obstruction of urine flow associated with edema or collection of mucus at stoma or ureteroileal junction or malfunction of stents;
b. introduction of pathogens via the stoma or urethral catheter (if present).

| Desired Outcome | Nursing Actions and ***Selected Purposes/Rationales*** |
|---|---|
| 2. The client will remain free of urinary tract infection as evidenced by:<br>a. no increase in sediment in urine<br>b. no unusual odor of urine<br>c. absence of chills and fever<br>d. absence of bacteria, nitrites, and WBCs in urine<br>e. negative urine culture. | 2.a. Assess for and report signs and symptoms of urinary tract infection (e.g. increased sediment in urine; cloudy, foul-smelling urine; chills; elevated temperature).<br>b. Monitor urinalysis and report presence of bacteria, nitrites, and/or WBCs.<br>c. Obtain a urine specimen for culture and sensitivity if ordered. Report abnormal results.<br>d. Implement measures *to prevent urinary tract infection:*<br>1. perform actions *to prevent urinary reflux and/or stasis:*<br>a. implement measures to prevent urinary obstruction (see Postoperative Collaborative Diagnosis 3, action b.2)<br>b. use a pouch with an antireflux valve<br>c. instruct and assist client to empty pouch when it is 1/3 full *in order to prevent reflux and reduce risk of bacterial growth resulting from stasis of urine in pouch*<br>d. instruct and assist client to change to a bedside collection system before lying down for an extended period<br>e. increase activity as tolerated<br>2. ensure that any reusable pouch is cleansed thoroughly, rinsed, and allowed to dry completely between applications<br>3. perform actions *to maintain urine acidity:*<br>a. encourage client to increase intake of foods/fluids that form an acid ash (e.g. cranberry juice, prune juice, plums, meat, eggs, poultry, fish, whole grains)<br>b. instruct client to decrease intake of milk, most fruits and vegetables, and carbonated beverages *(these tend to alkalinize urine)*<br>c. administer medications such as ascorbic acid if ordered<br>4. if a urethral catheter is in place, perform catheter care as often as needed *to prevent accumulation of mucus around the meatus*<br>5. administer antimicrobial agents if ordered prophylactically. |

## 3. COLLABORATIVE DIAGNOSES:

**Potential complications:**

a. **stomal changes:**
   1. **prolapse** related to pressure around the stoma, poor tissue turgor, and loss of integrity of suture line
   2. **excessive bleeding** related to irritation associated with aggressive cleansing techniques and/or improper fit or application of appliance
   3. **necrosis** related to intraoperative and/or postoperative interruption of blood supply to the stoma;

b. **urinary obstruction** related to:
   1. malfunctioning ureteral stents
   2. edema of stoma and/or ureteroileal junction associated with surgical trauma
   3. collection of mucus at stoma and/or ureteral openings;

c. **peritonitis** related to:
   1. leakage of urine and/or intestinal contents into the peritoneum associated with failure of the surgical anastomoses
   2. leakage of urine into and/or exposure of the peritoneum associated with retraction of peristomal skin from stoma (mucocutaneous separation) resulting from slippage of the sutures or impaired healing of surgical site.

| Desired Outcomes | Nursing Actions and ***Selected Purposes/Rationales*** |
| --- | --- |
| 3.a. The client will maintain integrity of the stoma as evidenced by:<br>1. dark pink or red coloring of stoma<br>2. expected stomal height<br>3. absence of excessive bleeding and increasing edema of the stoma. | 3.a.1. Assess for and report signs and symptoms of impaired stomal integrity (e.g. pale, dark red, or blue-black color of stoma; increased stomal height; increased stomal edema or bleeding). Use only clear appliances during immediate postoperative period *to allow easy visibility of stoma.*<br>2. Implement measures *to maintain integrity of stoma:*<br>a. perform actions *to maintain adequate stomal circulation:*<br>1. ensure that the openings of the skin barrier and pouch are the right size; be careful to center stoma in the openings *in order to prevent pressure on stoma*<br>2. use properly fitted flange and belt *to reduce peristomal pressure*<br>b. anchor flange and pouch securely *to prevent a shearing action across stoma*<br>c. cleanse stoma gently using a soft cloth, gauze, or tissue.<br>3. If signs and symptoms of impaired stomal integrity occur:<br>a. perform wound care as ordered<br>b. prepare client for surgical revision of stoma if indicated<br>c. provide emotional support to client and significant others. |
| 3.b. The client will not experience urinary obstruction as evidenced by:<br>1. balanced intake and output beginning 48 hours postoperatively<br>2. gradual resolution of abdominal tenderness and distention<br>3. expected volume of drainage from abdominal wound. | 3.b.1. Assess for and report signs and symptoms of ureteral or stomal obstruction (e.g. significant decrease in urinary output from stoma or ureteral stents, increasing abdominal tenderness and distention, increase in drainage from abdominal wound).<br>2. Implement measures *to prevent urinary obstruction:*<br>a. encourage a fluid intake of 2500 ml/day unless contraindicated *to keep urine dilute and maintain adequate urine flow (helps flush conduit and prevent mucus from congealing)*<br>b. flush ureteral stents if ordered *to maintain patency* (should be done with very little fluid and gently)<br>c. change pouch carefully *in order to avoid dislodgment of the ureteral stents* (stents usually remain in place for 5-10 days postoperatively).<br>3. If signs and symptoms of urinary obstruction occur:<br>a. prepare client for dilation of the stoma, surgical revision of stoma or sites of anastomoses, and/or replacement of ureteral stents<br>b. provide emotional support to client and significant others. |
| 3.c. The client will not develop peritonitis as evidenced by:<br>1. gradual resolution | 3.c.1. Assess for and report signs and symptoms of peritonitis (e.g. increase in severity of abdominal pain; rebound tenderness; tense, rigid abdomen; increase in temperature; tachycardia; tachypnea; hypotension; nausea; vomiting; failure of bowel sounds to return to normal). |

of abdominal pain
2. soft, nondistended abdomen
3. temperature declining toward normal
4. stable vital signs
5. absence of nausea and vomiting
6. gradual return of normal bowel sounds
7. WBC count declining toward normal.

2. Monitor WBC counts. Report levels that increase or fail to decline toward normal.
3. Implement measures *to prevent peritonitis:*
   a. perform actions to prevent and treat wound infection (see Standardized Postoperative Care Plan, Nursing Diagnosis 16, actions b.4 and 5 [p. 129])
   b. perform actions *to maintain patency of wound drain if present:*
      1. keep tubing free of kinks
      2. empty collection device as often as necessary
      3. maintain suction as ordered
   c. perform actions *to prevent inadvertent removal of wound drain if present:*
      1. use caution when changing dressings surrounding drain
      2. provide extension tubing if necessary *to enable client to move without placing tension on the drain*
      3. instruct client not to pull on drain and drainage tubing
   d. perform actions *to prevent urinary obstruction* (see action b.2 in this diagnosis) *in order to prevent resultant strain on and leakage from the suture line*
   e. if separation of stoma from peristomal skin occurs:
      1. perform wound care as ordered *to facilitate the formation of granulation tissue in retracted area*
      2. prepare client for surgical intervention if planned.
4. If signs and symptoms of peritonitis occur:
   a. withhold all food and fluid as ordered
   b. place client on bed rest in a semi-Fowler's position *to assist in pooling or localizing gastrointestinal contents and urine in the pelvis rather than under the diaphragm*
   c. insert a nasogastric tube if not already present and maintain suction as ordered
   d. administer antimicrobials if ordered
   e. administer intravenous fluids and/or blood volume expanders if ordered *to prevent or treat shock (can result from the increased capillary permeability that occurs with inflammation and the subsequent escape of protein, fluid, and electrolytes from the vascular space into the peritoneal cavity)*
   f. prepare client for surgical intervention (e.g. repair of sites of anastomoses or retracted peristomal skin) if indicated
   g. provide emotional support to client and significant others.

## 4. NURSING DIAGNOSIS: Sexual dysfunction

related to:
a. decreased libido associated with feelings of loss of femininity/masculinity and sexual attractiveness, fear of offensive odor or leakage of urine from the pouch, fear of rejection by partner, discomfort resulting from surgical incision, and depression;
b. impotence (can occur as a result of nerve damage during a radical cystectomy);
c. change in sensation experienced and decreased potential for orgasm in the female client associated with clitoral injury (can occur with radical cystectomy);
d. dyspareunia associated with decreased diameter of the vaginal introitus and shortening of the vaginal canal resulting from removal of a portion of the anterior vaginal wall if a radical cystectomy was performed.

| Desired Outcome | Nursing Actions and ***Selected Purposes/Rationales*** |
|---|---|
| 4. The client will demonstrate beginning acceptance of changes in sexual functioning as evidenced by:<br>a. verbalization of a perception of self as sexually acceptable and adequate<br>b. statements reflecting beginning adjustment to the effects of the urinary diversion on sexuality<br>c. maintenance of relationship with significant other. | 4.a. Assess for signs and symptoms of sexual dysfunction (e.g. verbalization of sexual concerns; alteration in relationship with significant other, limitations imposed by nerve damage and structural changes incurred during surgery).<br>b. Provide accurate information about effects of the cystectomy and urinary diversion on sexual functioning. Encourage questions and clarify misconceptions.<br>c. Implement measures *to promote optimal sexual functioning:*<br>1. facilitate communication between client and his/her partner; focus on the feelings the couple share and assist them to identify changes that may affect their sexual relationship<br>2. perform actions to facilitate psychological adjustment to the changes that have occurred (see Postoperative Nursing Diagnoses 5, actions d-r; 6, action c; and 7, action b)<br>3. instruct client in ways *to reduce risk of leakage of urine from the pouch during sexual activity:*<br>a. empty appliance before sexual activity<br>b. secure appliance seal with tape for added security<br>4. if client is concerned about odor, instruct him/her to:<br>a. shower or bathe before sexual activity<br>b. use an odorproof pouch or pouch deodorant<br>c. use cologne or perfume if desired<br>d. keep room well ventilated<br>5. perform actions *to decrease possibility of rejection by partner:*<br>a. assist the partner to acknowledge feelings about changes in the client<br>b. if appropriate, involve partner in ostomy care *to facilitate adjustment to the changes in client's appearance and body functioning*<br>6. if client is concerned about the presence of the stoma and appliance, discuss the possibility of:<br>a. using opaque or patterned pouches or decorative pouch covers<br>b. wearing underwear with the crotch removed (for females), boxer shorts (for males), or large elastic wraps around abdomen during sexual activity<br>7. arrange for uninterrupted privacy during hospital stay if desired by the couple<br>8. if client is concerned that operative site discomfort will interfere with usual sexual activity:<br>a. assure him/her that discomfort is temporary and will diminish as the incision heals<br>b. encourage alternatives to intercourse or use of positions that decrease pressure on surgical site (e.g. side-lying)<br>9. if impotence is a problem:<br>a. encourage client to discuss it and various treatment options (e.g. penile prosthesis) with physician<br>b. explain that desire, penile sensation, and orgasmic capabilities are not diminished<br>c. suggest alternative methods of sexual gratification if appropriate<br>d. discuss alternative methods of parenting (e.g. artificial insemination, adoption) if of concern to client<br>10. discuss ways to be creative in expressing sexuality (e.g. massage, fantasies, cuddling)<br>11. if appropriate, discuss with female client the need for vaginal dilatation after healing has occurred *to prevent further contraction and shortening of the vaginal canal*<br>12. encourage client to obtain written information regarding sexual activity from the United Ostomy Association and from manufacturers of ostomy appliances. |

d. Include partner in above discussion and encourage his/her continued support of the client.
e. Consult physician if counseling appears indicated.

## 5. NURSING DIAGNOSIS: Self-concept disturbance*

related to:
a. loss of bladder and ability to urinate normally;
b. temporary or permanent dependence on others to assist with ostomy management;
c. feeling of loss of control associated with altered urinary elimination;
d. change in appearance associated with the presence of a stoma;
e. changes in usual sexual functioning;
f. embarrassment associated with odor of ostomy drainage;
g. sterility associated with:
   1. loss of ejaculatory function in the male client resulting from removal of the prostate and seminal vesicles if a radical cystectomy was performed
   2. removal of the ovaries, uterus, and fallopian tubes in the female client if a radical cystectomy was performed.

*This diagnostic label includes the nursing diagnoses of body image disturbance, self-esteem disturbance, and altered role performance.

| Desired Outcome | Nursing Actions and ***Selected Purposes/Rationales*** |
|---|---|
| 5. The client will demonstrate beginning adaptation to changes in appearance, body functioning, and life style as evidenced by:<br>a. verbalization of feelings of self-worth and sexual adequacy<br>b. maintenance of relationships with significant others<br>c. active participation in activities of daily living<br>d. active interest in personal appearance<br>e. willingness to pursue usual roles and participate in social activities<br>f. verbalization of a beginning plan for integrating changes in appearance and urinary elimination into life style. | 5.a. Assess for signs and symptoms of a self-concept disturbance (e.g. verbal or nonverbal cues denoting a negative response to changes in body functioning or appearance such as denial of or preoccupation with changes that have occurred, refusal to look at or touch stoma, or withdrawal from significant others).<br>b. Determine the meaning of changes in appearance, body functioning, and life style to the client by encouraging him/her to verbalize feelings and by noting nonverbal responses to the changes experienced.<br>c. Implement measures to facilitate the grieving process (see Postoperative Nursing Diagnosis 7, action b).<br>d. Discuss with client improvements in body functioning and appearance that can realistically be expected.<br>e. Implement measures *to assist client to increase self-esteem* (e.g. limit negative self-assessment, encourage positive comments about self, assist to identify strengths, give positive feedback about accomplishments and behaviors that are indicative of high self-esteem).<br>f. Reinforce actions to assist client to cope with effects of the urinary diversion (see Postoperative Nursing Diagnosis 6, action c).<br>g. Implement measures to promote optimal sexual functioning (see Postoperative Nursing Diagnosis 4, action c).<br>h. Instruct and assist client in ways *to decrease odor of ostomy drainage and pouch:*<br>1. use odorproof pouches and change appliance regularly<br>2. use disposable appliances or clean reusable items thoroughly<br>3. empty appliance regularly<br>4. perform actions to achieve an adequate pouch seal (see Postoperative Nursing Diagnosis 1, action b.4.i.4)<br>5. instruct client to avoid foods that cause urine to have a strong odor (e.g. asparagus, onions)<br>6. use room or pouch deodorizers<br>7. change bed linens and clothing as soon as they become soiled. |

| Desired Outcome | Nursing Actions and ***Selected Purposes/Rationales*** |
|---|---|
| | i. Assure client that once the edema and discomfort associated with the surgery have resolved, he/she will be able to dress as before with minor, if any, modifications.<br>j. Show client and significant others some of the attractive ostomy appliances (e.g. opaque or patterned pouches, pouch covers) that are available.<br>k. Assist client with usual grooming and makeup habits if necessary.<br>l. Promote activities that require client to confront the body changes that have occurred (e.g. active participation in ostomy care). Be aware that the integration of the change in body image does not usually occur until 2-6 months after the actual physical change has occurred.<br>m. Demonstrate acceptance of client using techniques such as touch and frequent visits. Encourage significant others to do the same.<br>n. Assess for and support behaviors suggesting positive adaptation to changes that have occurred (e.g. willingness to care for ostomy, compliance with the treatment plan, verbalization of feelings of self-worth, maintenance of relationships with significant others).<br>o. Encourage significant others to allow client to do what he/she is able *so that independence can be re-established and/or self-esteem redeveloped.*<br>p. Assist client's and significant others' adjustment by listening, facilitating communication, and providing information.<br>q. Encourage visits and support from significant others.<br>r. Encourage client to pursue usual roles and interests and to continue involvement in social activities. Assure him/her that an ostomy need not alter life style (only contact sports are contraindicated).<br>s. Consult physician about psychological counseling if client desires or if he/she seems unwilling or unable to adapt to changes resulting from the urinary diversion. |

## 6. NURSING DIAGNOSIS: Ineffective individual coping

related to:
a. fear, anxiety, and depression associated with the diagnosis, prognosis, loss of control over urinary elimination, and possibility of rejection by significant others;
b. difficulty caring for ostomy;
c. need for lifelong medical supervision;
d. inadequate support system.

| Desired Outcome | Nursing Actions and ***Selected Purposes/Rationales*** |
|---|---|
| 6. The client will demonstrate the use of effective coping skills as evidenced by:<br>a. verbalization of ability to cope with the urinary diversion and its effects<br>b. utilization of appropriate problem-solving techniques | 6.a. Assess for and report signs and symptoms of ineffective individual coping (e.g. verbalization of inability to cope; inability to ask for help, problem solve, or meet basic needs; reluctance to participate in treatment plan; destructive behavior toward self or others; inappropriate use of defense mechanisms; inability to meet role expectations).<br>b. Assess client's perception of current situation including precipitating factors and effectiveness of coping mechanisms.<br>c. Implement measures *to promote effective coping:*<br>1. allow time for client to adjust psychologically to the urinary diversion<br>2. assist client to recognize and manage inappropriate denial if it is present |

c. willingness to participate in treatment plan and meet basic needs
d. absence of destructive behavior toward self and others
e. appropriate use of defense mechanisms
f. recognition and utilization of available support systems.

3. arrange for a visit with an ostomate of similar age and same sex who has successfully adjusted to a urinary diversion
4. perform actions to reduce fear and anxiety (see Standardized Postoperative Care Plan, Nursing Diagnosis 20, action b [p. 134])
5. encourage verbalization about current situation
6. assist client to identify personal strengths and resources that can be utilized to facilitate coping with the current situation
7. demonstrate acceptance of client but set limits on inappropriate behavior
8. create an atmosphere of trust and support
9. maintain consistency of approaches and explanations
10. do not overload client with information irrelevant to present stage of ostomy management unless client is questioning or expressing an interest
11. encourage participation in ostomy care as soon as possible
12. use appliances that client is expected to use when discharged
13. ensure adequate time for and privacy during ostomy care
14. include client in planning of care, encourage maximum participation in ostomy care, and allow choices when possible *to enable him/her to maintain a sense of control*
15. instruct client in effective problem-solving techniques (e.g. accurate identification of stressors, determination of various options to solve problem)
16. assist client to maintain usual daily routines whenever possible
17. discuss with significant others the fear of rejection client may be experiencing and encourage their support
18. administer antianxiety and/or antidepressant agents if ordered
19. assist client to identify and utilize available support systems; provide information about available community resources that can assist client and significant others in coping with effects of urinary diversion and the underlying disease process (e.g. United Ostomy Association, American Cancer Society, counseling services, local ostomy support groups, community health agencies)
20. encourage the client to share with significant others the kind of support that would be most beneficial (e.g. listening, inspiring hope, providing reassurance and accurate information)
21. support behaviors suggesting positive adaptation to changes experienced (e.g. willingness to participate in treatment plan, verbalization of ability to cope, utilization of effective problem-solving strategies).

d. Consult physician about psychological counseling if appropriate. Initiate a referral if necessary.

## 7. NURSING DIAGNOSIS: Grieving*

related to loss of bladder and the ability to urinate normally, change in appearance, and possible effects of the surgery on sexual functioning.

*This diagnostic label includes anticipatory grieving and grieving following the actual losses.

| Desired Outcome | Nursing Actions and ***Selected Purposes/Rationales*** |
| --- | --- |
| 7. The client will demonstrate beginning progression through the | 7.a. Assess for signs and symptoms of grieving (e.g. change in eating habits, inability to concentrate, insomnia, anger, noncompliance, withdrawal from significant others, denial of loss). Be aware that client's response to a loss |

| Desired Outcome | Nursing Actions and ***Selected Purposes/Rationales*** |
|---|---|
| grieving process as evidenced by:<br>a. verbalization of feelings about the urinary diversion and its effects<br>b. expression of grief<br>c. participation in treatment plan and self-care activities<br>d. utilization of available support systems<br>e. verbalization of a plan for integrating ostomy care into life style. | will be affected by factors such as previous experience with loss, age, developmental stage, available support systems, spiritual and cultural background, current health status, and significance of the loss.<br>b. Implement measures *to facilitate the grieving process:*<br>1. assist client to acknowledge the losses experienced *so grief work can begin;* assess for factors that may hinder and facilitate acknowledgment<br>2. discuss the grieving process and assist client to accept the phases of grieving as an expected response to actual and anticipated losses; support the realization that grief may recur because of the extended period of adjustment to the urinary diversion and, if diversion was performed for cancer, subsequent treatment<br>3. allow time for client to progress through the phases of grieving (phases vary among theorists but progress from shock and alarm to acceptance); be aware that not every phase is expressed by all individuals, that recurrence of phases is common, and that the grieving process may take months to years<br>4. provide an atmosphere of care and concern (e.g. provide privacy, be available and nonjudgmental, display empathy and respect) *so that client will feel free to verbalize feelings*<br>5. perform actions *to promote trust* (e.g. answer questions honestly, provide requested information)<br>6. encourage the verbal expression of anger and sadness about the losses experienced; recognize displacement of anger and assist client to see the actual cause of angry feelings and resentment<br>7. encourage client to express his/her feelings in whatever ways are comfortable (e.g. writing, drawing, conversation)<br>8. perform actions to promote effective coping (see Postoperative Nursing Diagnosis 6, action c)<br>9. support realistic hope about the effects of the surgery on his/her life (e.g. increased comfort, improved urinary elimination ability)<br>10. support behaviors suggesting successful grief work (e.g. verbalizing feelings about the urinary diversion, focusing on ways to adapt to losses that have occurred, learning to care for ostomy)<br>11. explain the phases of the grieving process to significant others; encourage their support and understanding<br>12. facilitate communication between the client and significant others; be aware that they may be in different phases of the grieving process<br>13. provide information regarding counseling services and support groups that might assist client in working through grief<br>14. arrange for visit from clergy if desired by client.<br>c. Consult physician about referral for counseling if signs of dysfunctional grieving (e.g. persistent denial of losses, excessive anger or sadness, hysteria, suicidal behaviors) occur. |

## 8. NURSING DIAGNOSIS: Knowledge deficit

regarding follow-up care.

| Desired Outcomes | Nursing Actions and ***Selected Purposes/Rationales*** |
|---|---|
| 8.a. The client will verbalize a basic understanding of the | 8.a. Reinforce teaching about the anatomical changes that have occurred as a result of the cystectomy and urinary diversion. Use appropriate teaching aids (e.g. pictures, videotapes, anatomical models). |

anatomical changes that have occurred as a result of the surgery.

8.b. The client will demonstrate the ability to change ostomy appliance and maintain stomal and peristomal skin integrity.

8.b.1. Demonstrate correct application of the ostomy appliance.
2. Provide instructions on ways to maintain stomal and peristomal skin integrity:
   a. patch test all adhesives, sprays, solvents, and skin sealants and barriers before using for the first time; avoid any product that causes redness, itching, or burning
   b. change appliance only when necessary (should be able to remain in place for 5-7 days after the initial postoperative period)
   c. shave peristomal skin regularly with an electric razor
   d. remove appliance carefully (e.g. loosen adhesive with warm water or solvent, remove appliance in direction of hair growth)
   e. prevent skin contact with urine (e.g. change appliance when the ostomy is least active; place a wick [rolled gauze pad], vaginal tampon, or tissue on stoma when appliance is off; utilize skin sealants; accurately fit and apply pouch; ensure an adequate appliance seal; empty pouch when 1/3 full; position pouch properly; utilize a bedside collection system when lying down for extended periods)
   f. prevent urine crystals from forming on stoma and peristomal skin:
      1. maintain acidity of urine (see action d.2.c in this diagnosis)
      2. apply a white vinegar soak to stoma and peristomal skin when appliance is changed (vinegar may cause stoma to blanch temporarily)
      3. replace reusable equipment from which urine crystals cannot be completely removed
      4. be sure that barrier opening is same size as stoma and that opening on pouch is only 1/16–1/8 inch larger than diameter of stoma
   g. if urine crystals form on stoma and peristomal skin:
      1. apply white vinegar soaks to affected area with each pouch change
      2. if a 2-piece appliance is being used, remove pouch and apply white vinegar soaks to stoma 3-4 times a day
   h. follow special precautions for products used (e.g. inert, moldable skin barriers must be kept in airtight container; skin sealants should be used only on healthy peristomal skin because they can further irritate reddened and excoriated skin).
3. Allow time for questions, clarification, practice, and return demonstration of appliance application and appropriate care of the stoma and peristomal skin.

8.c. The client will demonstrate proper technique for cleansing reusable ostomy equipment.

8.c.1. Discuss recommended method of cleansing reusable ostomy equipment based on manufacturer's recommendations.
2. Demonstrate appropriate cleansing technique. Emphasize importance of:
   a. washing and rinsing pouch thoroughly upon removal
   b. soaking pouch according to manufacturer's instructions
   c. allowing pouch to dry thoroughly
   d. storing pouch according to manufacturer's instructions (e.g. apply powder or cornstarch to inside and store in a clean, dry place).
3. Allow time for questions, clarification, and return demonstration.

8.d. The client will verbalize ways to prevent excessive skin growth over the stoma and peristomal area.

8.d.1. Explain that excessive skin growth over the stoma and peristomal area is thought to be caused by prolonged skin contact with urine (particularly alkaline urine).
2. Instruct client in ways to prevent excessive skin growth over the stoma and peristomal area:
   a. check pH of urine as directed to be sure acidity is being maintained
   b. reduce contact of stoma and peristomal area with urine by:

| Desired Outcomes | Nursing Actions and ***Selected Purposes/Rationales*** |
|---|---|
| | 1. using a pouch with an antireflux value<br>2. utilizing skin barriers that fit properly<br>3. fitting and applying pouch correctly<br>c. maintain urine acidity by:<br>1. increasing intake of foods/fluids that form an acid ash (e.g. cranberry juice, prune juice, plums, meat, eggs, poultry, fish, whole grains)<br>2. limiting intake of milk, carbonated beverages, and citrus fruit<br>3. taking medications such as ascorbic acid as prescribed<br>4. preventing urinary tract infection (see action f in this diagnosis). |
| 8.e. The client will identify ways to control odor of ostomy drainage and pouch. | 8.e. Provide instructions on ways to control odor of ostomy drainage and pouch:<br>1. drink at least 10 glasses of liquid/day; increase volume of liquid if urine appears concentrated<br>2. avoid foods that cause urine to have a strong odor (e.g. asparagus, onions)<br>3. place a small amount of deodorizer or white vinegar in bottom of pouch<br>4. change appliance at appropriate intervals and cleanse it thoroughly<br>5. rinse appliance with a white vinegar and water solution<br>6. prevent urinary tract infection (see action f in this diagnosis)<br>7. use odorproof pouch and empty appliance regularly. |
| 8.f. The client will identify ways to prevent urinary tract infection. | 8.f. Provide instructions on ways to prevent urinary tract infection:<br>1. drink at least 10 glasses of liquid/day<br>2. prevent reflux of urine by:<br>a. emptying pouch when it is 1/3 full (approximately every 2-3 hours)<br>b. attaching a bedside collection system when lying down for an extended period<br>c. using a pouch with an antireflux valve<br>3. maintain urine acidity (see action d.2.c.1-3 in this diagnosis)<br>4. clean reusable equipment thoroughly (see action c.2 in this diagnosis)<br>5. take prophylactic antimicrobials as prescribed. |
| 8.g. The client will state signs and symptoms to report to the health care provider. | 8.g.1. Refer to Standardized Postoperative Care Plan, Nursing Diagnosis 21, action c (p. 135), for signs and symptoms to report to the health care provider.<br>2. Instruct client to also report:<br>a. dark red, blue-black, or pale stoma<br>b. absence of or reduction in urinary output despite an adequate fluid intake<br>c. excessive bleeding of stoma or bloody drainage from ostomy<br>d. excessive mucus drainage from urinary meatus (some drainage should be expected for several weeks postoperatively)<br>e. change in contour of stoma (use diagrams and descriptive terms so client does not confuse decreasing stomal size due to resolving edema with actual stomal retraction)<br>f. persistent skin irritation or breakdown of peristomal skin<br>g. persistent presence of urine crystals on stoma or peristomal skin<br>h. persistent leakage of ostomy appliance<br>i. inability to maintain an acidic urine<br>j. signs and symptoms of urinary tract infection (e.g. fever; chills; cloudy, foul-smelling urine; increased sediment in urine [emphasize that some mucous shreds in urine are normal with an ileal conduit])<br>k. signs and symptoms of renal calculi (e.g. dull, aching or severe, colicky flank pain; blood in urine; nausea; vomiting); stone formation, a late complication of a urinary diversion, may result from persistent urinary stasis, urinary tract infection, or inadequate fluid intake |

| | |
|---|---|
| | l. signs and symptoms of bowel obstruction (e.g. abdominal pain and distention, vomiting)<br>m. difficulty coping with ostomy care or altered urinary elimination. |
| 8.h. The client will identify appropriate community resources that can assist with home management and adjustment to changes resulting from the urinary diversion. | 8.h.1. Provide information about community resources that can assist the client and significant others with home management and adjustment to changes resulting from urinary diversion (e.g. local ostomy support groups; American Cancer Society; community health agencies; enterostomal therapist; home health agencies; financial, individual, and family counseling services).<br>2. Initiate a referral if indicated. |
| 8.i. The client will verbalize an understanding of and a plan for adhering to recommended follow-up care including future appointments with health care provider, wound care, activity level, and medications prescribed. | 8.i. 1. Refer to Standardized Postoperative Care Plan, Nursing Diagnosis 21 (pp. 135-136), for routine postoperative instructions and measures to improve client compliance.<br>2. Reinforce the physician's instructions regarding activity limitations:<br>a. avoid lifting heavy objects until permitted by physician<br>b. avoid participating in contact sports to prevent stomal damage.<br>3. Explain the rationale for, side effects of, and importance of taking medications prescribed (e.g. antimicrobials, ascorbic acid). |

# Nephrectomy

Nephrectomy is the surgical removal of the kidney. Renal conditions that are commonly treated by nephrectomy include malignancy and irreparable kidney damage caused by trauma, hypertension, polycystic disease, or calculi. The kidney may also be removed for the purpose of donation.

The approach used depends on the extensiveness of the surgery planned, age and physiological status of the client (particularly cardiopulmonary function), underlying pathology, and prior surgical incisions. The most common approach utilized for a simple nephrectomy (removal of kidney and upper ureter) is the subcostal flank approach. Other approaches (e.g. thoracoabdominal, transabdominal, dorsolumbar) may be utilized when greater visualization, improved access, or a more radical procedure is necessary.

**This care plan focuses on the adult client hospitalized for a simple unilateral nephrectomy.** Preoperatively, the goals of care are to reduce fear and anxiety and prepare the client for the surgical experience. Postoperative goals of care are to maintain comfort, prevent complications, and educate the client regarding follow-up care. The care plan will need to be individualized according to the client's diagnosis, prognosis, and plans for subsequent treatment.

## DIAGNOSTIC TESTS

Excretory urography (intravenous pyelography)
Magnetic resonance imaging (MRI)
Ultrasonography
Computed tomography (CT)
Radionuclide renal scan
Renal angiography
X-ray of kidneys, ureters, and bladder (KUB)
Complete blood count (CBC)
Blood chemistry
Urinalysis
Creatinine clearance

**DISCHARGE CRITERIA**

Prior to discharge, the client will:

❖ have no signs and symptoms of complications
❖ have adequate urine output
❖ verbalize ways to maintain health of the remaining kidney
❖ state signs and symptoms to report to the health care provider
❖ share thoughts and feelings about the loss of the kidney
❖ verbalize an understanding of and a plan for adhering to recommended follow-up care including future appointments with health care provider, medications prescribed, activity level, wound care, and plans for subsequent treatment of the underlying disorder.

---

**NURSING/**
**COLLABORATIVE**
**DIAGNOSES**

**Postoperative**
1. Ineffective breathing pattern△ 538
2. Potential complications:
   a. hypovolemic shock
   b. pneumothorax△ 539
3. Grieving△ 540
4. Knowledge deficit△ 541

**See Standardized Preoperative and Postoperative Care Plans for additional diagnoses.**

---

**PREOPERATIVE**

**Refer to the Standardized Preoperative Care Plan.**

---

**POSTOPERATIVE**

**Use in conjunction with the Standardized Postoperative Care Plan.**

---

**1. NURSING DIAGNOSIS:**  **Ineffective breathing pattern**

related to:
a. reluctance to breathe deeply associated with incisional pain (particularly if a thoracoabdominal or subcostal approach was used) and fear of dislodging chest tube if one is in place following a thoracoabdominal approach;
b. respiratory depressant effects of anesthesia and some medications (e.g. narcotic analgesics);
c. fear, anxiety, weakness, and fatigue.

| Desired Outcome | Nursing Actions and *Selected Purposes/Rationales* |
|---|---|
| 1. The client will maintain an effective breathing pattern (see Standardized Postoperative Care Plan, Nursing Diagnosis 2 [p. 114], for outcome criteria). | 1.a. Refer to Standardized Postoperative Care Plan, Nursing Diagnosis 2 (pp. 114-115), for measures related to assessment and management of an ineffective breathing pattern.<br>b. Implement additional measures *to improve breathing pattern:*<br>   1. assure client that deep breathing will not dislodge chest tube if present<br>   2. provide pillow support between lower costal margin and iliac crest when client is lying on operative side *in order to decrease strain on flank incision and subsequently increase ease of deep breathing.* |

**2. COLLABORATIVE DIAGNOSES:**

**Potential complications:**

a. **hypovolemic shock** related to:
   1. massive blood loss (the renal area is highly vascular)
   2. fluid volume deficit associated with excessive fluid loss and inadequate fluid replacement;

b. **pneumothorax** related to surgical opening of pleura and/or malfunction of chest tube if thoracoabdominal approach was used.

| Desired Outcomes | Nursing Actions and ***Selected Purposes/Rationales*** |
|---|---|
| 2.a. The client will not develop hypovolemic shock (see Standardized Postoperative Care Plan, Collaborative Diagnosis 19, outcome a [pp. 131-132], for outcome criteria). | 2.a.1. Refer to Standardized Postoperative Care Plan, Collaborative Diagnosis 19, action a (pp. 131-132), for measures related to assessment, prevention, and treatment of hypovolemic shock.<br>2. Implement additional measures *to prevent hypovolemic shock:*<br>a. perform actions *to reduce strain on the suture line in order to prevent hemorrhage:*<br>1. instruct client to splint incisional area with hands or pillow when turning, coughing, and deep breathing<br>2. maintain patency of wound drain if present<br>3. implement measures to prevent nausea and vomiting (see Standardized Postoperative Care Plan, Nursing Diagnosis 7.B, action 2 [p. 120]).<br>b. prepare client for immediate surgical ligation of bleeding vessels if indicated. |
| 2.b. The client will experience normal lung re-expansion if pneumothorax occurs as evidenced by:<br>1. normal breath sounds and percussion note by the 3rd-4th postoperative day<br>2. unlabored respirations at 14-20/minute<br>3. blood gases returning toward normal<br>4. chest x-ray showing lung re-expansion. | 2.b.1. Assess for and immediately report signs and symptoms of:<br>a. malfunction of the chest drainage system (e.g. respiratory distress, sudden cessation of drainage, excessive bubbling in water seal chamber, significant increase in subcutaneous emphysema)<br>b. further lung collapse (e.g. extended area of absent breath sounds with hyperresonant percussion note; rapid, shallow and/or labored respirations; tachycardia; increased chest pain; restlessness; confusion).<br>2. Monitor blood gases. Report values that have worsened.<br>3. Monitor chest x-ray results. Report findings of delayed lung re-expansion or further lung collapse.<br>4. Implement measures *to promote lung re-expansion and prevent further lung collapse:*<br>a. perform actions *to maintain patency and integrity of chest drainage system:*<br>1. maintain water seal and suction levels as ordered<br>2. maintain air occlusive dressing over chest tube insertion site<br>3. tape all connections securely<br>4. milk chest tube routinely if ordered<br>5. keep chest drainage and suction tubing free of kinks<br>6. keep drainage system below level of client's chest at all times<br>b. perform actions to improve breathing pattern (see Postoperative Nursing Diagnosis 1) and facilitate airway clearance (see Standardized Postoperative Care Plan, Nursing Diagnosis 3, action b [pp. 115-116]).<br>5. If signs and symptoms of further lung collapse occur:<br>a. maintain client on bed rest in a semi- to high Fowler's position<br>b. maintain oxygen therapy as ordered<br>c. assess for and immediately report signs and symptoms of tension pneumothorax with mediastinal shift (e.g. severe dyspnea, increased restlessness and agitation, rapid and/or irregular pulse rate, hypotension, neck vein distention, shift in trachea toward unaffected side) |

| Desired Outcomes | Nursing Actions and ***Selected Purposes/Rationales*** |
|---|---|
| | d. assist with clearing of existing chest tube and/or insertion of a new tube<br>e. provide emotional support to client and significant others. |

## 3. NURSING DIAGNOSIS: Grieving*

related to loss of the kidney.

*This diagnostic label includes anticipatory grieving and grieving following the actual loss.

| Desired Outcome | Nursing Actions and ***Selected Purposes/Rationales*** |
|---|---|
| 3. The client will demonstrate beginning progression through the grieving process as evidenced by:<br>a. verbalization of feelings about the loss of a kidney<br>b. expression of grief<br>c. participation in treatment plan and self-care activities<br>d. utilization of available support systems. | 3.a. Assess for signs and symptoms of grieving (e.g. change in eating habits, inability to concentrate, insomnia, anger, noncompliance, withdrawal from significant others, denial of loss). Be aware that client's response to a loss will be affected by factors such as previous experience with loss, age, developmental stage, available support systems, spiritual and cultural background, current health status, and significance of the loss.<br>b. Implement measures *to facilitate the grieving process:*<br>1. assist client to acknowledge the loss of the kidney *so grief work can begin;* assess for factors that may hinder and facilitate acknowledgment<br>2. discuss the grieving process and assist client to accept the phases of grieving as an expected response to his/her loss<br>3. allow time for client to progress through the phases of grieving (phases vary among theorists but progress from shock and alarm to acceptance); be aware that not every phase is expressed by all individuals, that recurrence of phases is common, and that the grieving process may take months to years<br>4. provide an atmosphere of care and concern (e.g. provide privacy, be available and nonjudgmental, display empathy and respect) *so client will feel free to verbalize feelings*<br>5. perform actions *to promote trust* (e.g. answer questions honestly, provide requested information)<br>6. encourage the verbal expression of anger and sadness about the loss of the kidney; recognize displacement of anger and assist client to see the actual cause of angry feelings and resentment<br>7. encourage client to express his/her feelings in whatever ways are comfortable (e.g. writing, drawing, conversation)<br>8. assist client to identify personal strengths that have helped him/her to cope in previous situations of loss<br>9. support realistic hope about the ability to resume his/her usual activities; reassure client that one functional kidney is sufficient to meet body needs<br>10. support behaviors suggesting successful grief work (e.g. verbalizing feelings about loss of the kidney, expressing sorrow)<br>11. explain the phases of the grieving process to significant others; encourage their support and understanding<br>12. facilitate communication between the client and significant others; be aware that they may be in different phases of the grieving process<br>13. provide information regarding counseling services and support groups that might assist client in working through grief<br>14. arrange for visit from clergy if desired by client. |

c. Consult physician about referral for counseling if signs of dysfunctional grieving (e.g. persistent denial of loss, excessive anger or sadness, hysteria, suicidal behaviors) occur.

## 4. NURSING DIAGNOSIS: Knowledge deficit

regarding follow-up care.

| Desired Outcomes | Nursing Actions and ***Selected Purposes/Rationales*** |
|---|---|
| 4.a. The client will verbalize ways to maintain health of the remaining kidney. | 4.a. Instruct client regarding ways to maintain health of the remaining kidney:<br>1. adhere to precautions to prevent a urinary tract infection:<br>a. perform actions to prevent urinary stasis:<br>1. drink at least 10 glasses of liquid/day<br>2. urinate whenever the urge is felt<br>3. avoid long periods of inactivity (if unable to maintain a program of moderate activity, be sure to change positions frequently)<br>b. modify diet to maintain acidic urine if prescribed:<br>1. include foods/fluids in diet that form an acid ash (e.g. cranberry and prune juice, plums, meat, eggs, poultry, fish, whole-grain products)<br>2. limit intake of milk, carbonated beverages, and most fruits<br>c. wipe from front to back after urinating and defecating (if female)<br>d. keep perineal area clean and dry<br>2. immediately report signs and symptoms of a urinary tract infection (e.g. chills; fever; urgency, frequency, or burning on urination; cloudy, foul-smelling urine)<br>3. notify physician if a cold or other infection persists for more than 3 days or if unable to maintain an adequate fluid intake<br>4. inform other health care providers about the nephrectomy so that prophylactic antimicrobials may be initiated before dental work and invasive procedures such as cystoscopy and minor surgeries<br>5. avoid activities that might cause trauma to the remaining kidney (e.g. contact sports, horseback riding)<br>6. consult health care provider before taking any prescription and nonprescription medications that may be toxic to the remaining kidney (e.g. aminoglycosides, salicylates, ibuprofen, sulfonamides)<br>7. if nephrectomy was performed because of renal calculi, reinforce physician's instructions on diet, drug therapy, and daily fluid requirements to prevent formation of stones in the remaining kidney<br>8. if surgery was necessary because of renal hypertension, reinforce the physician's instructions about methods of controlling B/P (e.g. dietary modifications, medications, stress management). |
| 4.b. The client will state signs and symptoms to report to the health care provider. | 4.b.1. Refer to Standardized Postoperative Care Plan, Nursing Diagnosis 21, action c (p. 135), for signs and symptoms to report to the health care provider.<br>2. Instruct client to report these additional signs and symptoms:<br>a. unexplained weight gain<br>b. decreased urine output<br>c. flank pain on the unoperative side<br>d. blood in the urine. |
| 4.c. The client will verbalize an understanding of and | 4.c.1. Refer to Standardized Postoperative Care Plan, Nursing Diagnosis 21 (pp. 135-136), for routine postoperative instructions and measures to improve client compliance. |

| Desired Outcomes | Nursing Actions and ***Selected Purposes/Rationales*** |
|---|---|
| a plan for adhering to recommended follow-up care including future appointments with health care provider, medications prescribed, activity level, wound care, and plans for subsequent treatment of the underlying disorder. | 2. Reinforce physician's instructions regarding activity:<br>a. gauge activity according to tolerance and allow adequate rest periods<br>b. avoid lifting heavy objects for 3-6 months to allow complete healing of incised muscles.<br>3. Clarify plans for subsequent treatment of the underlying disorder (e.g. chemotherapy, radiation therapy) if appropriate. |

UNIT XIII

# *Nursing Care of the Client with Disturbances of Hematopoietic and Lymphatic Function*

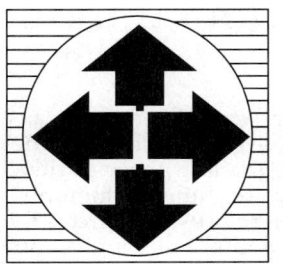

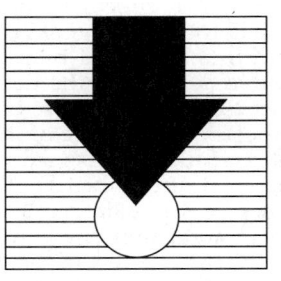

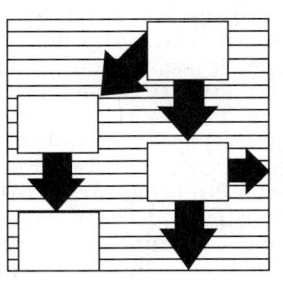

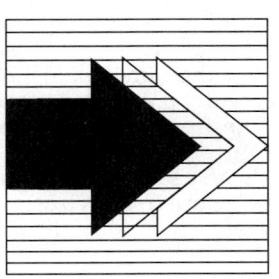

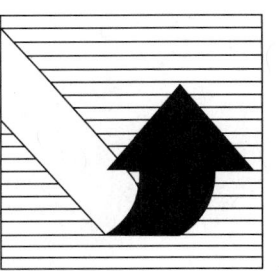

# Acquired Immune Deficiency Syndrome: Human Immunodeficiency Virus Infection

Acquired immune deficiency syndrome (AIDS) is an infectious disease of the immune system and is considered to be the last phase of the clinical spectrum of infection by the human immunodeficiency virus (HIV). HIV is a retrovirus that affects the cells in the body that have a CD4 molecule (a glycoprotein) on their surface. The largest group of these cells in the body are the CD4+ T lymphocytes (also called the $T_4$ or T-helper lymphocytes). Other body cells that have this molecule are macrophages and their precursor (monocytes) and tissue-dendritic cells found in the skin, mucous membranes, lymph nodes, spleen, and brain. The behavior of the virus seems to depend on the host cell and other cofactors such as competency of the client's immune system prior to exposure to HIV, age of the client, and the presence of other viruses and sexually transmitted diseases. HIV ultimately destroys the CD4+ T lymphocytes which results in severely impaired cell-mediated immunity in the host. Humoral immune function is also impaired because of the direct effect of the virus on B lymphocyte function and because the B cells are unable to respond appropriately to the presence of a new antigen without the help of normal CD4+ T lymphocytes. The effect of the virus itself and altered CD4+ T lymphocyte function on macrophage activity further depresses immune system function. It is also thought that macrophages serve as reservoirs for HIV within the body and may be responsible for its dissemination to the lungs and brain.

The virus has been isolated from blood, semen, vaginal secretions, saliva, tears, breast milk, cerebrospinal and amniotic fluid, and urine. At this point, however, transmission has only been associated with blood, semen, vaginal secretions, and possibly breast milk. HIV is transmitted sexually and parenterally and tends to occur in distinct groups of people: homosexual/bisexual males, recreational intravenous drug users, recipients of blood/blood products from HIV-infected individuals, sexual partners of those infected, and infants born to infected mothers. Serum conversion typically occurs 8-12 weeks after the initial exposure.

Infection with HIV tends to follow a particular course of action. The Centers for Disease Control (CDC) has identified four groups within this progression. The disease begins with acute HIV infection (group 1) 2-3 weeks following exposure to the virus. The client may develop an acute, transitory, flu-like illness with symptoms such as fever, chills, myalgias, arthralgias, abdominal cramps, diarrhea, lymphadenopathy, and sometimes a rash which may persist for a week or longer. Following resolution of the initial symptoms and seroconversion, the client enters an asymptomatic or latent phase (group 2), which may last as long as 13 years depending on the rapidity with which the CD4+ T lymphocytes are destroyed. Conversion to group 3 disease is manifested by the development of various nonspecific symptoms such as chronically enlarged lymph nodes; persistent viral, bacterial, or fungal infections; unexplained fever and weight loss; malaise; night sweats; and persistent diarrhea. AIDS (group 4) is the end-stage manifestation of HIV infection and is heralded by the development of certain symptoms and/or specific disease processes for which there is no other explanation. These include symptoms such as progressive weight loss or wasting despite adequate caloric intake and persistent fever and diarrhea; neurologic disease (e.g. dementia, myelopathy); opportunistic infections (e.g. *Pneumocystis carinii* pneumonia [PCP], candidiasis, tuberculosis, *Mycobacterium avium* complex [MAC]); AIDS-related cancers (e.g. Kaposi's sarcoma, primary central nervous system lymphoma); and/or other HIV-related conditions such as lymphoid interstitial pneumonitis. At this time there is no cure for HIV infection or the underlying immunodeficiency. Treatment is aimed primarily at controlling replication of HIV in the host with antiviral agents such as zidovudine (AZT), dideoxycytidine (ddC), and didanosine (ddI, Videx) and preventing and controlling the potentially fatal opportunistic diseases to which the infected person is particularly susceptible.

**This care plan focuses on the adult client hospitalized with signs and symptoms of an opportunistic infection and probable AIDS.** Goals of care are to assist with measures to treat the infection, reduce fear and anxiety, maintain comfort, assist the client to cope with the diagnosis, and educate him/her regarding follow-up care. A major concern while caring for the client with AIDS is prevention of the spread of infection to others. It is the responsibility of each health care provider to adhere to appropriate precautions to prevent disease transmission. If the client is admitted with an opportunistic infection involving the respiratory system, this care plan should be used in conjunction with the Care Plan on Pneumonia.

## DIAGNOSTIC TESTS

Enzyme-linked immunosorbent assay (ELISA)
Enzyme immunoassay (EIA)
Western blot assay
Immunofluorescence assay (IFA)
Complete blood count (CBC)
Polymerase chain reaction (PCR)
P24-antigen

Absolute CD4+ T lymphocyte count
Percentage of CD4+ T lymphocytes
Lymph node biopsy
Skin lesion biopsy
Cerebrospinal fluid analysis
Magnetic resonance imaging (MRI)
Chest x-ray
Transbronchial lung biopsy
Bronchoalveolar lavage

## DISCHARGE CRITERIA

Prior to discharge, the client will:

- have current signs and symptoms controlled
- identify ways to prevent the spread of HIV
- identify ways to decrease the risk for developing opportunistic infections
- state signs and symptoms to report to the health care provider
- share feelings about change in self-concept and the social isolation that may result from the diagnosis
- identify resources that can assist in adjustment to changes resulting from the diagnosis of AIDS
- verbalize an understanding of and a plan for adhering to recommended follow-up care including future appointments with health care provider and medications prescribed.

## NURSING DIAGNOSES



## 1. NURSING DIAGNOSIS: Anxiety

related to:

a. current signs and symptoms, unfamiliar environment, lack of understanding of diagnostic tests, and financial concerns;

b. diagnosis of a fatal disease with the potential for a rapid decline to death;
c. probability of disfigurement, pain, and disability;
d. possible loss of job and change in intimate relationship(s) associated with disclosure of diagnosis;
e. possibility of having transmitted HIV infection to others and the need to inform them;
f. likelihood of being publically identified with a highly stigmatized group (e.g. homosexual, bisexual, intravenous drug user) once diagnosis is known.

**Desired Outcome**

1. The client will experience a reduction in anxiety as evidenced by:
   a. verbalization of feeling less anxious and fearful
   b. usual sleep pattern
   c. relaxed facial expression and body movements
   d. stable vital signs
   e. usual perceptual ability and interactions with others.

**Nursing Actions and *Selected Purposes/Rationales***

1.a. Assess client for signs and symptoms of anxiety (e.g. verbalization of fears and concerns, insomnia, tenseness, tremors, irritability, restlessness, diaphoresis, tachypnea, tachycardia, elevated blood pressure, facial pallor or flushing, narrowed perceptual field, withdrawal, noncompliance with treatment plan). Validate perceptions carefully, remembering that some behavior may be caused by neurological changes resulting from HIV infection.

b. Implement measures *to reduce fear and anxiety:*
   1. orient client to hospital environment, equipment, and routines
   2. introduce staff who will be participating in his/her care; if possible, maintain consistency in staff assigned to his/her care *to provide feelings of stability and comfort with the environment*
   3. assure client that staff members are nearby; respond to call signal as soon as possible
   4. maintain a calm, supportive, confident manner when interacting with client
   5. encourage verbalization of fear and anxiety; provide feedback
   6. explain all tests that may be performed to diagnose HIV infection and/or concurrent diseases
   7. reinforce physician's explanation about HIV infection including mode of transmission, effects on immune system, concurrent diseases, and prognosis; encourage questions and clarify misconceptions
   8. provide a calm, restful environment
   9. instruct client in relaxation techniques and encourage participation in diversional activities
   10. perform actions to assist client to cope with the diagnosis and its implications (see Nursing Diagnosis 15, action c)
   11. initiate financial and/or social service referrals if indicated
   12. encourage significant others to project a caring, concerned attitude without obvious anxiousness
   13. administer antianxiety agents if ordered.

c. Include significant others in orientation and teaching sessions and encourage their continued support of the client. Assist them to understand the client's fears and to express theirs. Explain that the client's high level of anxiety may persist for 2-3 months following the diagnosis of AIDS.

d. Provide information based on current needs of client and significant others at a level they can understand. Encourage questions and clarification of information provided.

e. Consult physician if above actions fail to control fear and anxiety.

## 2. NURSING DIAGNOSIS: Altered nutrition: less than body requirements

related to:

a. decreased oral intake associated with:
   1. anorexia resulting from malaise, fatigue, fear, anxiety, and depression

2. oral pain and/or dysphagia resulting from stomatitis and pharyngitis;
b. increased metabolic needs associated with infection;
c. malabsorption of nutrients if primary intestinal infection or opportunistic gastrointestinal infection is present;
d. loss of nutrients associated with persistent diarrhea.

**Desired Outcome**

2. The client will maintain an adequate nutritional status as evidenced by:
   a. weight within normal range for client's age, height, and body frame
   b. normal BUN and serum albumin, Hct, Hb, and transferrin levels
   c. triceps skinfold thickness within normal range
   d. usual strength and activity tolerance
   e. healthy oral mucous membrane.

**Nursing Actions and *Selected Purposes/Rationales***

2.a. Assess for and report signs and symptoms of malnutrition:
   1. weight below normal for client's age, height, and body frame
   2. abnormal BUN and low serum albumin, Hct, Hb, and transferrin levels
   3. triceps skinfold thickness less than normal
   4. weakness and fatigue
   5. stomatitis.

b. Monitor percentage of meals and snacks client consumes. Report a pattern of inadequate intake.

c. Implement measures *to maintain an adequate nutritional status:*
   1. perform actions *to improve oral intake:*
      a. implement measures to reduce discomfort associated with altered oral mucous membrane (see Nursing Diagnosis 5, actions d and e)
      b. implement measures to reduce fear and anxiety (see Nursing Diagnosis 1, action b) and assist client to adjust psychologically to the diagnosis of AIDS (see Nursing Diagnoses 15, action c; 16, actions c-m; and 17, action b)
      c. obtain a dietary consult if necessary to assist client in selecting foods/fluids that meet nutritional needs as well as personal and cultural preferences whenever possible
      d. assist client to select foods that are easily chewed and swallowed
      e. encourage a rest period before meals *to minimize fatigue*
      f. maintain a clean environment and a relaxed, pleasant atmosphere
      g. provide oral care before meals
      h. serve small portions of nutritious foods/fluids that are appealing to the client
      i. encourage significant others to bring in client's favorite foods and eat with him/her *to make eating more of a familiar social experience*
      j. allow adequate time for meals; reheat food if necessary
      k. increase activity as allowed and tolerated *(activity stimulates appetite)*
   2. perform actions to control diarrhea (see Nursing Diagnosis 9, action f)
   3. ensure that meals are well balanced and high in essential nutrients; offer high-protein, high-calorie dietary supplements between meals if indicated
   4. administer the following if ordered:
      a. vitamins and minerals
      b. megestrol acetate *to stimulate appetite.*

d. Perform a 72-hour calorie count if ordered. Report totals to dietitian and physician.

e. Consult physician about alternative methods of providing nutrition (e.g. parenteral nutrition, tube feedings) if client does not consume enough food or fluids to meet nutritional needs.

---

## 3.A. NURSING DIAGNOSIS: Altered comfort: chills and excessive diaphoresis

related to persistent or recurrent fever associated with HIV and opportunistic infections.

| Desired Outcome | Nursing Actions and ***Selected Purposes/Rationales*** |
|---|---|
| 3.A. The client will not experience discomfort associated with chills and diaphoresis as evidenced by:<br>1. verbalization of comfort<br>2. ability to rest. | 3.A.1. Assess client for chills and excessive diaphoresis.<br>2. Implement measures to reduce fever (see Nursing Diagnosis 4, action b) *in order to decrease chills and excessive diaphoresis.*<br>3. Implement measures *to promote comfort if client is having chills:*<br>a. maintain a room temperature that is comfortable for client<br>b. protect client from drafts<br>c. provide extra blankets and clothing as needed<br>d. provide warm liquids to drink as tolerated.<br>4. Implement measures *to promote comfort if excessive diaphoresis is present:*<br>a. change linen and clothing whenever damp<br>b. bathe client and sponge his/her face as needed.<br>5. Consult physician if client continues to have chills and excessive diaphoresis. |

## 3.B. NURSING DIAGNOSIS: Altered comfort: pruritus

related to:
1. dry skin associated with fluid volume deficit (can occur as a result of decreased oral intake, excessive diaphoresis, and/or persistent diarrhea);
2. cutaneous infection (e.g. staphylococcal folliculitis), seborrheic dermatitis, and/or photodermatitis if present;
3. reaction to some antimicrobials (e.g. trimethoprim-sulfamethoxazole) administered to prevent or treat infection;
4. skin eruptions of unknown etiology (a common occurrence in the client with AIDS).

| Desired Outcome | Nursing Actions and ***Selected Purposes/Rationales*** |
|---|---|
| 3.B. The client will experience relief of pruritus as evidenced by:<br>1. verbalization of same<br>2. no scratching or rubbing of skin. | 3.B. 1. Assess client's pruritus including onset, characteristics, location, and factors that aggravate and alleviate it.<br>2. Instruct client in and/or implement measures *to reduce pruritus:*<br>a. apply cool, moist compresses to pruritic areas<br>b. perform actions *to reduce skin dryness:*<br>1. use tepid water and mild soaps for bathing<br>2. apply oil-based agents to skin immediately after bathing when skin is hydrated unless contraindicated<br>3. apply emollient creams or ointments frequently<br>4. encourage a fluid intake of 2500 ml/day unless contraindicated<br>5. utilize a room humidifier *to maintain moisture in the air and reduce fluid loss by evaporation*<br>c. add emollients, cornstarch, baking soda, or oatmeal preparations to bath water unless contraindicated<br>d. pat skin dry, making sure to dry thoroughly<br>e. encourage participation in diversional activity<br>f. utilize relaxation techniques<br>g. utilize cutaneous stimulation techniques (e.g. pressure, massage, vibration, stroking with a soft brush) at sites of itching or acupressure points<br>h. encourage client to wear loose, cotton garments; launder clothing in mild soap<br>i. administer the following if ordered:<br>1. antihistamines<br>2. topical corticosteroids (e.g. triamcinolone, hydrocortisone, desonide) |

3. topical or oral ketoconazole *to treat seborrheic dermatitis.*
3. Consult physician if above measures fail to reduce pruritus or if the skin becomes excoriated.

## 4. NURSING DIAGNOSIS: Hyperthermia

related to stimulation of the thermoregulatory center in the hypothalamus by endogenous pyrogens that are released in an infectious process.

| Desired Outcome | Nursing Actions and ***Selected Purposes/Rationales*** |
|---|---|
| 4. The client will experience resolution of hyperthermia as evidenced by:<br>a. skin usual temperature and color<br>b. pulse rate between 60-100 beats/minute<br>c. respirations 14-20/minute<br>d. normal body temperature. | 4.a. Assess for signs and symptoms of hyperthermia (e.g. warm, flushed skin; tachycardia; tachypnea; elevated temperature).<br>b. Implement measures *to reduce fever:*<br>1. perform actions *to resolve the opportunistic infection:*<br>a. implement measures to promote rest (see Nursing Diagnosis 7, action b.1)<br>b. implement measures to maintain an adequate nutritional status (see Nursing Diagnosis 2, action c)<br>c. administer antimicrobials if ordered<br>2. administer tepid sponge bath and/or apply cool cloths to groin and axillae if indicated<br>3. use a room fan *to provide cool circulating air and increase heat loss through conduction*<br>4. apply cooling blanket as ordered<br>5. administer antipyretics if ordered.<br>c. Consult physician if temperature remains higher than 38.5° C. |

## 5. NURSING DIAGNOSIS: Altered oral mucous membrane

related to:
a. malnutrition;
b. HIV-associated periodontal disease;
c. infections such as *Candida albicans*, herpes simplex, herpes zoster, oral hairy leukoplakia, histoplasmosis, and/or cryptococcosis;
d. Kaposi's sarcoma or lymphoma in the oral cavity or pharynx.

| Desired Outcome | Nursing Actions and ***Selected Purposes/Rationales*** |
|---|---|
| 5. The client will have a healthy oral cavity as evidenced by:<br>a. absence of inflammation<br>b. pink, moist, intact mucosa<br>c. absence of lesions<br>d. absence of halitosis | 5.a. Assess client for and report signs and symptoms of altered oral mucous membrane (e.g. inflamed and/or ulcerated oral mucosa; corrugated, white projections, particularly on sides of tongue; groups of vesicles; reddened and retracted gingivae; red or purple macules, papules, or nodules; leukoplakia; halitosis; complaints of oral or pharyngeal dryness and pain; dysphagia).<br>b. Culture oral lesions as ordered. Report positive results.<br>c. Prepare client for and assist with biopsy of oral lesions if planned. Report positive results. |

| Desired Outcome | Nursing Actions and ***Selected Purposes/Rationales*** |
|---|---|
| e. no complaints of oral and pharyngeal dryness and pain<br>f. ability to swallow without discomfort. | d. Implement measures *to maintain or regain integrity of oral mucous membrane:*<br>1. reinforce importance of and assist client with oral hygiene after meals and snacks; avoid products such as lemon-glycerin swabs and commercial mouthwashes containing alcohol *(these products have a drying or irritating effect on the oral mucous membrane)*<br>2. have client rinse mouth frequently with warm saline; baking soda and water; or a solution of salt, baking soda, and water<br>3. use a soft-bristle brush, sponge-tipped applicator, or low-pressure power spray for oral hygiene<br>4. lubricate client's lips frequently with K-Y jelly, ChapStick, Blistex, or mineral oil<br>5. encourage client to breathe through nose rather than his/her mouth *in order to reduce mouth dryness*<br>6. encourage a fluid intake of at least 2500 ml/day unless contraindicated<br>7. perform actions to maintain an adequate nutritional status (see Nursing Diagnosis 2, action c)<br>8. encourage client not to smoke *(smoking irritates and dries the mucosa)*<br>9. assist client with selection of soft, bland foods<br>10. instruct client to avoid foods/fluids that are extremely hot<br>11. administer antifungal agents (e.g. amphotericin B, clotrimazole troches, nystatin suspension, ketoconazole) and antiviral agents (e.g. acyclovir) if ordered<br>12. if periodontal disease is present, administer the following if ordered:<br>a. oral rinses of chlorhexidene gluconate<br>b. metronidazole<br>13. if Kaposi's sarcoma or lymphoma lesions are present in the oral cavity or pharynx, prepare client for radiation therapy, chemotherapy, and/or laser treatments if planned<br>14. if stomatitis is not controlled:<br>a. increase frequency of oral hygiene<br>b. if client has dentures, remove and replace only for meals.<br>e. Administer topical anesthetics, oral protective pastes or coating agents, and topical and systemic analgesics if ordered.<br>f. Consult physician if signs and symptoms of altered oral mucous membrane persist or worsen. |

## 6. NURSING DIAGNOSIS: Actual/High risk for impaired skin integrity

related to:

a. presence of cutaneous infections such as folliculitis, herpes zoster or simplex, bullous impetigo, disseminated histoplasmosis or cryptococcosis, and/or abscesses (it is common for the client with AIDS to have 2 or more types of skin disorders concurrently and for a skin lesion to have more than 1 infectious agent in it);
b. presence of eczematous dermatitis (e.g. seborrheic dermatitis, atopic dermatitis, photodermatitis) and/or papulosquamous skin conditions (e.g. psoriasis);
c. skin lesions associated with Kaposi's sarcoma if present;
d. excessive scratching associated with pruritus;
e. increased skin fragility associated with dryness and malnutrition;
f. persistent contact with irritants associated with diarrhea;
g. damage to the skin and/or subcutaneous tissue associated with prolonged pressure on tissues, friction, or shearing if mobility is decreased.

| Desired Outcome | Nursing Actions and ***Selected Purposes/Rationales*** |
|---|---|

6. The client will maintain and/or regain skin integrity as evidenced by:
   a. absence of redness and irritation
   b. no skin breakdown.

6.a. Assess the skin for:
   1. signs of infection (e.g. pustules, superficial erosions or ulcers, groups of vesicles with reddened bases, subcutaneous nodules)
   2. signs of eczematous and/or papulosquamous skin conditions (e.g. papules; vesicles; erythematous plaques with fine, white scale; erythematous areas with indistinct margins and yellow, greasy scale; plaques with sharp margins and silver scale).

b. Assess bony prominences, perineum, and dependent and pruritic areas for pallor, redness, and breakdown.

c. Administer systemic antimicrobials (e.g. dicloxacillin, acyclovir) and/or apply topical corticosteroids as ordered *to treat existing cutaneous conditions.*

d. Implement measures *to prevent additional skin breakdown:*
   1. assist client to turn at least every 2 hours; use all 4 sides (prone, lateral, dorsal) unless contraindicated
   2. gently massage around reddened areas at least every 2 hours
   3. perform actions *to prevent shearing* (shearing occurs when one tissue layer slides past another) *and skin surface abrasion:*
      a. apply a thin layer of powder or cornstarch to bottom sheet or skin *to absorb moisture (moist skin is more likely to adhere to sheet) and reduce friction*
      b. lift and move client carefully using a turn sheet and adequate assistance
      c. limit length of time client is in semi-Fowler's position to 30 minutes *(in this position, client tends to slide down in bed)*
   4. instruct client to shift weight every 30 minutes
   5. if fade time (length of time it takes for reddened area to fade after pressure is removed) is greater than 15 minutes, increase frequency of position changes
   6. keep skin clean and dry
   7. apply a thin layer of powder or cornstarch to areas with opposing skin surfaces (e.g. axillae, perineum, beneath breasts) if indicated *to absorb moisture and/or reduce friction*
   8. keep bed linens dry and wrinkle-free
   9. increase activity as allowed and tolerated
   10. provide devices to reduce pressure on the skin, decrease shearing, and/or prevent moisture buildup (e.g. alternating pressure mattress or pad, flotation pad, sheepskin)
   11. perform actions to maintain an adequate nutritional status (see Nursing Diagnosis 2, action c)
   12. perform actions to prevent skin dryness (see Nursing Diagnosis 3.B, action 2.b)
   13. perform actions *to prevent skin irritation resulting from diarrhea:*
      a. implement measures to reduce diarrhea (see Nursing Diagnosis 9, action f)
      b. assist client to thoroughly cleanse and dry perineal area with soft tissue or cloth after each bowel movement; apply a protective ointment or cream (e.g. Desitin, A&D ointment, Vaseline)
      c. apply a drainable fecal collector if diarrhea is severe
      d. provide incontinence pads if needed to absorb moisture; do not allow skin to come in contact with plastic portion of pads
   14. perform actions *to prevent skin irritation resulting from scratching:*
      a. implement measures to relieve pruritus (see Nursing Diagnosis 3.B, action 2)
      b. keep nails trimmed and/or apply mittens if necessary
      c. instruct client to apply firm pressure to pruritic areas rather than scratching.

| Desired Outcome | Nursing Actions and ***Selected Purposes/Rationales*** |
|---|---|
| | e. If skin breakdown occurs or existing breakdown progresses:<br>1. notify physician<br>2. continue with above measures to treat existing skin disorders and prevent further irritation, inflammation, and breakdown<br>3. perform wound and/or decubitus care as ordered or per standard hospital procedure<br>4. assess client closely and report signs and symptoms of further infection (e.g. further elevation in temperature; redness, warmth, and edema around area of breakdown; unusual drainage from site). |

## 7. NURSING DIAGNOSIS: Activity intolerance

related to:

a. difficulty resting and sleeping;
b. increased energy utilization associated with the elevated metabolic rate that is present in infection;
c. malnutrition;
d. tissue hypoxia associated with:
   1. impaired alveolar gas exchange if respiratory infection is present
   2. anemia resulting from HIV infection that involves the bone marrow and/or treatment with medications that can cause bone marrow suppression (e.g. AZT);
e. deconditioning if activity is significantly limited for a week or longer.

| Desired Outcome | Nursing Actions and ***Selected Purposes/Rationales*** |
|---|---|
| 7. The client will demonstrate an increased tolerance for activity as evidenced by:<br>a. verbalization of feeling less fatigued and weak<br>b. ability to perform activities of daily living without exertional dyspnea, chest pain, increased diaphoresis, dizziness, and a significant change in vital signs. | 7.a. Assess for signs and symptoms of activity intolerance:<br>1. statements of fatigue and weakness<br>2. exertional dyspnea, chest pain, increased diaphoresis, or dizziness<br>3. abnormal heart rate response to activity (e.g. increase in rate of 20 beats/minute above resting rate, decrease in rate, rate not returning to preactivity level within 3 minutes after stopping activity, change from regular to irregular rate)<br>4. decreased systolic B/P or a significant increase (10-15 mm Hg) in systolic or diastolic pressure with activity.<br>b. Implement measures *to improve activity tolerance:*<br>1. perform actions *to promote rest and/or conserve energy:*<br>a. maintain activity restrictions if ordered<br>b. minimize environmental activity and noise<br>c. organize nursing care to allow for periods of uninterrupted rest<br>d. limit the number of visitors and their length of stay<br>e. assist client with self-care activities as needed<br>f. keep supplies and personal articles within easy reach<br>g. instruct client in energy-saving techniques (e.g. using shower chair when showering, sitting to brush teeth or comb hair)<br>h. implement measures to reduce fear and anxiety (see Nursing Diagnosis 1, action b)<br>i. implement measures to promote sleep (see Nursing Diagnosis 11, action c)<br>2. perform actions to resolve the opportunistic infection (see Nursing Diagnosis 4, action b.1)<br>3. perform actions to maintain an adequate nutritional status (see Nursing Diagnosis 2, action c)<br>4. discourage smoking and excessive intake of beverages high in caffeine |

such as coffee, tea, and colas *(nicotine and caffeine increase cardiac workload and myocardial oxygen utilization, thereby decreasing oxygen availability)*
5. administer the following if ordered:
   a. whole blood or packed red cells
   b. hematopoietic agents (e.g. epoetin alpha) *to stimulate RBC production*
6. maintain oxygen therapy if ordered
7. increase client's activity gradually as allowed and tolerated.

c. Instruct client to:
   1. report a decreased tolerance for activity
   2. stop any activity that causes chest pain, shortness of breath, dizziness, or extreme fatigue or weakness.

d. Consult physician if signs and symptoms of activity intolerance persist or worsen.

## 8. NURSING DIAGNOSIS: Self-care deficit

related to:
a. cognitive and/or motor impairments associated with HIV encephalopathy if present;
b. activity intolerance and activity restrictions imposed by the treatment plan;
c. depression.

| Desired Outcome | Nursing Actions and ***Selected Purposes/Rationales*** |
|---|---|
| 8. The client will demonstrate increased participation in self-care activities within physical limitations and activity restrictions imposed by the treatment plan. | 8.a. With client, develop a realistic plan for meeting daily physical needs.<br>b. Encourage maximum independence within physical limitations and prescribed activity restrictions.<br>c. Implement measures *to facilitate client's ability to perform self-care activities:*<br>1. perform actions to improve activity tolerance (see Nursing Diagnosis 7, action b)<br>2. schedule care at a time when client is most likely to be able to participate (e.g. after rest periods, not immediately after meals or treatments)<br>3. keep needed objects within easy reach<br>4. allow adequate time for accomplishment of self-care activities<br>5. perform actions to facilitate adjustment to the diagnosis of AIDS (see Nursing Diagnoses 15, action c; 16, actions c-m; and 17, action b).<br>d. Provide positive feedback for all efforts and accomplishments of self-care.<br>e. Assist the client with activities he/she is unable to perform independently.<br>f. Inform significant others of client's abilities to perform own care. Explain the importance of encouraging and allowing client to maintain an optimal level of independence within prescribed activity restrictions and his/her activity tolerance level and level of orientation. |

## 9. NURSING DIAGNOSIS: Diarrhea

related to:
a. enterocolitis associated with opportunistic infection(s);
b. increased gastrointestinal motility associated with extreme fear and anxiety;
c. AIDS enteropathy (a condition of unknown etiology involving the small bowel).

| Desired Outcome | Nursing Actions and ***Selected Purposes/Rationales*** |
|---|---|
| 9. The client will have fewer bowel movements and more formed stool. | 9.a. Ascertain client's usual bowel elimination habits.<br>b. Assess for signs and symptoms of diarrhea (e.g. frequent, loose stools; urgency; abdominal pain and cramping).<br>c. Assess bowel sounds regularly. Report an increase in frequency of bowel sounds.<br>d. Obtain stool specimens for culture and/or examination for parasites. Report positive results.<br>e. Prepare client for endoscopy if planned *to examine intestinal mucosa, obtain specimens for culture, and/or perform biopsies.*<br>f. Implement measures *to control diarrhea:*<br>1. perform actions *to rest the bowel:*<br>a. restrict oral intake if ordered<br>b. when oral intake is allowed:<br>1. gradually progress from fluids to small meals<br>2. instruct client to avoid foods/fluids that may stimulate or irritate the inflamed bowel:<br>a. those high in fiber (e.g. whole-grain cereals, raw fruits and vegetables)<br>b. gas producers (e.g. cabbage, beans, onions, cauliflower)<br>c. those that are spicy or extremely hot or cold<br>d. those high in lactose (e.g. milk, milk products)<br>e. those high in fat (e.g. butter, cream, fried foods)<br>c. implement measures to reduce fear and anxiety (see Nursing Diagnosis 1, action b)<br>d. encourage client to rest<br>e. discourage smoking *(nicotine has a stimulant effect on the gastrointestinal tract)*<br>2. administer the following medications if ordered:<br>a. opiate or opiate-like substances (e.g. loperamide, diphenoxylate hydrochloride) *to decrease gastrointestinal motility*<br>b. antimicrobial agents (e.g. acyclovir, ganciclovir, AZT, ampicillin, amoxicillin, amphotericin B, metronidazole, ketoconazole, trimethoprim-sulfamethoxazole) *to treat the infectious process.*<br>g. Consult physician if:<br>1. diarrhea persists or worsens<br>2. signs and symptoms of fluid volume deficit (e.g. decreased skin turgor, significant weight loss, dry mucous membranes, decreased B/P, increased pulse) and/or electrolyte imbalances (e.g. confusion, muscle or abdominal cramps, irregular pulse, muscle twitching or spasms, paresthesias, abdominal distention, hypoactive or absent bowel sounds) occur. |

## 10. NURSING DIAGNOSIS: Altered thought processes

related to:

a. HIV encephalopathy (AIDS dementia complex) associated with the direct effect of HIV on the central nervous system (encephalopathy may begin soon after seroconversion but more typically is characteristic of later phases of HIV infection);

b. opportunistic infections and/or neoplasms involving the central nervous system (e.g. cerebral toxoplasmosis, cryptococcal meningitis, progressive multifocal leukoencephalopathy, cytomegalovirus [CMV] encephalitis, primary central nervous system lymphoma);

c. depression and severe anxiety.

| Desired Outcome | Nursing Actions and ***Selected Purposes/Rationales*** |
|---|---|
| 10. The client will experience improvement in thought processes as evidenced by:<br>a. improved verbal response time<br>b. longer attention span<br>c. improved memory<br>d. improved reasoning ability and judgment<br>e. decreased apathy<br>f. improved level of orientation<br>g. absence of hallucinations. | 10.a. Assess client for altered thought processes (e.g. slowed verbal responses, decreased ability to concentrate, impaired memory, poor reasoning ability or judgment, apathy, disorientation, hallucinations).<br>b. Ascertain from significant others client's usual level of intellectual and emotional functioning.<br>c. Prepare client for computed tomography (CT) or magnetic resonance imaging (MRI) of the brain, cerebrospinal fluid analysis, EEG, and/or neuropsychiatric testing if indicated *to determine specific cause of mental decline.*<br>d. Administer the following medications if ordered *to treat conditions that can alter thought processes:*<br>1. antimicrobials (e.g. clindamycin, vidarabine, pyrimethamine, sulfadiazine, amphotericin B, acyclovir, ganciclovir, AZT) *to treat infectious processes*<br>2. cytotoxic agents *to treat neoplastic conditions affecting nervous system*<br>3. psychoactive drugs such as antipsychotic agents (e.g. haloperidol, thioridazine) *to reduce restlessness, agitation, or hallucinations* or central nervous system stimulants (e.g. dextroamphetamine sulfate) *to reduce apathy and withdrawn behavior* (psychoactive drugs should be used very cautiously and in small, titrated doses *because of their potential to initiate or aggravate delirium in the client with HIV encephalopathy).*<br>e. If client shows evidence of altered thought processes:<br>1. reorient client to person, place, and time as necessary<br>2. address client by name<br>3. place familiar objects, clock, and calendar within client's view<br>4. approach client in a slow, calm manner; allow adequate time for communication<br>5. repeat instructions as necessary using clear, simple language and short sentences<br>6. keep environmental stimuli to a minimum<br>7. maintain a consistent and fairly structured routine and write out schedule of activities for client to refer to if desired<br>8. have client perform only one activity at a time and allow adequate time for performance of activities<br>9. encourage client to make lists of planned activities, questions, and concerns<br>10. assist client to problem solve if necessary<br>11. maintain realistic expectations of client's ability to learn, comprehend, and remember information provided; provide client with a written copy of instructions<br>12. if client is experiencing hallucinations, allow significant others to remain with client *in order to provide constant reassurance*<br>13. encourage significant others to be supportive of client; instruct them in methods of dealing with client's altered thought processes<br>14. discuss physiological basis for altered thought processes with client and significant others; inform them that intellectual and emotional functioning may improve with drug therapy<br>15. consult physician if altered thought processes persist or worsen. |

## 11. NURSING DIAGNOSIS: Sleep pattern disturbance

related to fear, anxiety, depression, frequent assessments and treatments, diarrhea, pruritus, chills, night sweats, coughing and dyspnea (may occur if respiratory infection is present), and unfamiliar environment.

| Desired Outcome | Nursing Actions and ***Selected Purposes/Rationales*** |
|---|---|
| 11. The client will attain optimal amounts of sleep within the parameters of the treatment regimen as evidenced by:<br>a. statements of feeling well rested<br>b. usual mental status<br>c. absence of frequent yawning, dark circles under eyes, and hand tremors. | 11.a. Assess for signs and symptoms of a sleep pattern disturbance (e.g. verbal complaints of difficulty falling asleep, sleep interruptions, or not feeling well rested; irritability; lethargy; disorientation; frequent yawning; dark circles under eyes; slight hand tremors).<br>b. Determine the client's usual sleep habits.<br>c. Implement measures *to promote sleep:*<br>1. discourage long periods of sleep during the day unless signs and symptoms of sleep deprivation exist or daytime sleep is usual for client<br>2. perform actions to reduce fear and anxiety (see Nursing Diagnosis 1, action b)<br>3. perform actions to reduce discomfort associated with chills and excessive diaphoresis and pruritus (see Nursing Diagnoses 3.A, actions 3 and 4 and 3.B, action 2)<br>4. perform actions to control diarrhea (see Nursing Diagnosis 9, action f)<br>5. encourage participation in relaxing diversional activities during the evening<br>6. discourage intake of fluids high in caffeine (e.g. coffee, tea, colas), especially in the evening<br>7. offer client a high-protein evening snack unless contraindicated<br>8. allow client to continue usual sleep practices (e.g. position, time, bedtime rituals such as reading and meditating) if possible<br>9. satisfy basic needs such as comfort and warmth before sleep<br>10. have client empty bladder just before bedtime<br>11. maintain a quiet, restful atmosphere; have earplugs available for client if needed<br>12. utilize relaxation techniques (e.g. progressive relaxation exercises, back massage, meditation, soft music) before sleep<br>13. ensure good room ventilation<br>14. if client has orthopnea:<br>a. assist him/her to assume a position *that facilitates breathing* (e.g. head of bed elevated with arms supported on pillows, resting forward on overbed table with good pillow support, sitting in a chair)<br>b. maintain oxygen therapy during sleep<br>15. if client has a persistent cough, perform actions *to control coughing:*<br>a. instruct client to avoid intake of very hot or cold foods/fluids *(these can stimulate cough)*<br>b. protect client from irritants such as flowers, smoke, and powder<br>c. encourage client not to smoke *(smoking irritates the respiratory tract)*<br>d. humidify inspired air as ordered<br>e. administer antitussives if ordered<br>16. administer sedative-hypnotics if ordered<br>17. perform actions *to reduce interruptions during sleep (80-100 minutes of uninterrupted sleep are usually needed to complete one sleep cycle):*<br>a. restrict visitors<br>b. group care (e.g. medications, treatments, physical care, assessments) whenever possible.<br>d. Consult physician if signs and symptoms of sleep deprivation persist or worsen. |

## 12. NURSING DIAGNOSIS: High risk for infection: opportunistic

related to decreased resistance to infection associated with:

a. cellular and humoral immune deficiencies present in HIV infection;

b. inadequate nutritional status;
c. depletion of immune mechanisms resulting from presenting infection and treatment with antimicrobial agents;
d. stasis of respiratory secretions and/or urinary stasis if mobility is decreased.

| Desired Outcome | Nursing Actions and ***Selected Purposes/Rationales*** |
|---|---|

**Desired Outcome**

12. The client will remain free of additional opportunistic infection(s) as evidenced by:
    a. return of temperature toward normal
    b. decrease in episodes of chills and diaphoresis
    c. pulse returning toward normal range
    d. normal or improved breath sounds
    e. absence or resolution of dyspnea
    f. voiding clear urine without complaints of frequency, urgency, and burning
    g. absence or resolution of painful, pruritic skin lesions
    h. stable or gradual increase in body weight
    i. no complaints of increased weakness and fatigue
    j. absence of visual disturbances
    k. absence of heat, pain, redness, swelling, and unusual drainage in any area
    l. absence or resolution of oral mucous membrane irritation and ulceration
    m. ability to swallow without difficulty
    n. WBC and differential counts returning toward normal range

**Nursing Actions and *Selected Purposes/Rationales***

12.a. Assess for and report signs and symptoms of additional opportunistic infection(s):
   1. increase in temperature above client's usual level
   2. increase in episodes of chills and diaphoresis
   3. increased pulse
   4. development or worsening of abnormal breath sounds
   5. development or worsening of dyspnea
   6. cloudy, foul-smelling urine
   7. complaints of frequency, urgency, or burning when urinating
   8. presence of WBCs, bacteria, and/or nitrites in urine
   9. extensive vesicular lesions particularly on face, lips, and perianal area
   10. new or increased complaints of pain in and/or itching of skin lesions and surrounding tissue
   11. further increase in weight loss, fatigue, or weakness
   12. visual disturbances
   13. heat, pain, redness, swelling, or unusual drainage in any area
   14. new or increased irritation or ulceration of oral mucous membrane
   15. development of or increased dysphagia
   16. significant change in WBC count and/or differential.

b. Obtain specimens (e.g. urine, vaginal, stool, mouth, sputum, blood, skin lesions) for culture as ordered. Report positive results.

c. Implement measures *to prevent further infection:*
   1. administer the following medications if ordered:
      a. antibiotic and antifungal agents
      b. immune system stimulators (e.g. interleukin-2, interferon alpha-2a)
      c. antiviral agents (e.g. acyclovir or ganciclovir *to treat opportunistic infection,* AZT *to prevent replication of HIV*)
      d. granulocyte colony-stimulating factor (G-CSF) *to stimulate neutrophil production*
   2. maintain a fluid intake of at least 2500 ml/day unless contraindicated
   3. use good handwashing technique and encourage client to do the same
   4. protect client from others with infection
   5. perform actions to maintain an adequate nutritional status (see Nursing Diagnosis 2, action c)
   6. perform actions to reduce stress (see Nursing Diagnosis 1, action b) *in order to prevent excessive secretion of cortisol (cortisol inhibits the immune response)*
   7. perform actions to maintain or regain integrity of oral mucous membrane (see Nursing Diagnosis 5, action d)
   8. maintain meticulous aseptic technique during all invasive procedures (e.g. catheterization, venous and arterial punctures, injections)
   9. change intravenous tubings and solutions and rotate insertion sites according to hospital policy
   10. perform actions to promote rest (see Nursing Diagnosis 7, action b.1)
   11. perform actions *to prevent stasis of respiratory secretions* (e.g. assist client to turn, cough, and deep breathe; increase activity as allowed and tolerated)
   12. perform actions to prevent or treat skin breakdown (see Nursing Diagnosis 6, actions c-e)
   13. perform actions to prevent urinary retention (e.g. instruct client to

| Desired Outcome | Nursing Actions and ***Selected Purposes/Rationales*** |
|---|---|
| o. negative results of cultured specimens. | urinate when the urge is first felt, promote relaxation during voiding attempts) *in order to prevent urinary stasis*<br>14. perform actions *to prevent the introduction of microorganisms into the urinary tract* (e.g. assist client with perineal care as needed, instruct and assist female client to wipe from front to back after urinating and defecating, maintain sterile technique during urinary catheterization). |

## 13. NURSING DIAGNOSIS: High risk for trauma

related to falls associated with:

a. weakness and fatigue;

b. confusion, dizziness, and/or impaired motor function resulting from the direct effect of HIV on the brain and spinal cord (e.g. AIDS dementia complex, vacuolar myelopathy), opportunistic nervous system infections (e.g. cerebral toxoplasmosis, cryptococcal meningitis, cytomegalovirus encephalitis), and/or opportunistic neoplasms involving the nervous system (e.g. primary central nervous system lymphoma).

| Desired Outcome | Nursing Actions and ***Selected Purposes/Rationales*** |
|---|---|
| 13. The client will not experience falls. | 13.a. Implement measures *to prevent falls:*<br>1. keep bed in low position with side rails up when client is in bed<br>2. keep needed items within easy reach<br>3. encourage client to request assistance whenever needed; have call signal within easy reach<br>4. use lap belt when client is in chair if indicated<br>5. instruct client to wear well-fitting slippers/shoes with nonslip soles and low heels when ambulating<br>6. keep floor free of clutter and wipe up spills promptly<br>7. accompany client during ambulation utilizing a transfer safety belt if he/she is weak or dizzy<br>8. provide ambulatory aids (e.g. walker, cane) if client is weak or unsteady on feet<br>9. reinforce instructions from physical therapist regarding correct transfer and ambulation techniques<br>10. instruct client to ambulate in well-lit areas and to use handrails if needed<br>11. do not rush client; allow adequate time for ambulation to the bathroom and in hallway<br>12. make sure that bathtub and shower have nonslip bottom surfaces and that shower chair, secure bath mat, call light, hand grips, and adequate lighting are present<br>13. perform actions to improve strength and activity tolerance (see Nursing Diagnosis 7, action b)<br>14. administer central nervous system depressants judiciously<br>15. if client is confused or irrational:<br>a. reorient frequently to surroundings and necessity of adhering to safety precautions<br>b. provide constant supervision (e.g. staff member, significant other) if indicated<br>c. consult physician about the temporary use of jacket or wrist restraints if necessary<br>d. administer antianxiety and antipsychotic medications if ordered<br>16. administer medications (e.g. antimicrobials, cytotoxic agents) as |

ordered *to treat the underlying disease condition and subsequently improve mental status and motor function.*

b. Include client and significant others in planning and implementing measures to prevent falls.

c. If client falls, initiate first aid if appropriate and notify physician.

## 14. NURSING DIAGNOSIS: Altered sexuality patterns

related to:

a. rejection by desired partner associated with his/her fear of contracting HIV;
b. need to disclose to new partner(s) the diagnosis of AIDS;
c. decreased sexual desire associated with fatigue, weakness, anxiety, depression, and fear of transmitting or contracting disease.

| Desired Outcome | Nursing Actions and ***Selected Purposes/Rationales*** |
|---|---|
| 14. The client will perceive self as sexually adequate and acceptable as evidenced by:<br>a. verbalization of same<br>b. maintenance of relationship with significant other<br>c. statements reflecting beginning adjustment to effects of AIDS on sexuality. | 14.a. Assess for signs and symptoms of altered sexuality patterns (e.g. verbalization of sexual concerns, failure to maintain relationship with significant other).<br>b. Determine attitudes, knowledge, and concerns about AIDS in relation to sexual functioning.<br>c. Communicate interest, understanding, and respect for the values of the client and his/her partner.<br>d. Implement measures *to promote optimal sexual functioning:*<br>1. facilitate communication between client and his/her partner; focus on the feelings they share and assist them to identify factors that may affect their sexual relationship<br>2. provide accurate information about the transmission of HIV during intimate contact; encourage questions, clarify misconceptions and fears, and encourage client and significant other to keep current on information about how HIV is spread<br>3. discuss ways to be creative in expressing sexuality (e.g. massage, fantasies, cuddling)<br>4. discuss various options for meeting sexual needs (e.g. masturbation, safe sexual activity with partner that takes into consideration the type[s] of opportunistic infection present)<br>5. arrange for uninterrupted privacy during hospital stay if desired by couple<br>6. instruct client to allow for adequate rest periods before sexual activity<br>7. perform actions to reduce fear and anxiety (see Nursing Diagnosis 1, action b) and facilitate adjustment to the diagnosis of AIDS (see Nursing Diagnoses 15, action c; 16, actions c-m; and 17, action b)<br>8. provide information about support groups and professional counselors that can assist client in adjusting to the effects of AIDS on sexuality.<br>e. Include partner in above discussions and encourage his/her continued support of the client.<br>f. Consult physician if counseling appears indicated. |

## 15. NURSING DIAGNOSIS: Ineffective individual coping

related to:

a. depression, fear, and anxiety associated with the diagnosis of AIDS and poor prognosis;

b. need for permanent change in life style and possibly roles associated with impaired immune system functioning and potential for disease transmission to others;
c. uncertainty of disease course;
d. need for disclosure of diagnosis and possibly life style with possibility of subsequent rejection and/or distancing by others and loss of employment and health benefits;
e. guilt associated with past behavior (if it was a factor in contracting HIV) and/or possibility of having transmitted HIV to others;
f. lack of personal resources to deal with disability and premature death associated with youth (the majority of clients are in their twenties or thirties and are not developmentally prepared to acknowledge and cope with disability and their own mortality);
g. multiple losses (e.g. death of close friends with AIDS; loss of normal body functioning, family support, financial security, and/or usual life style and roles);
h. inadequate support system.

| Desired Outcome | Nursing Actions and ***Selected Purposes/Rationales*** |
|---|---|
| 15. The client will demonstrate the use of effective coping skills as evidenced by:<br>a. verbalization of ability to cope with the diagnosis and its implications<br>b. utilization of appropriate problem-solving techniques<br>c. willingness to participate in treatment plan and meet basic needs<br>d. absence of destructive behavior toward self and others<br>e. appropriate use of defense mechanisms<br>f. recognition and utilization of available support systems. | 15.a. Assess for and report signs and symptoms of ineffective individual coping (e.g. verbalization of inability to cope; inability to ask for help, problem solve, or meet basic needs; reluctance to participate in treatment plan; destructive behavior toward self or others; inappropriate use of defense mechanisms; inability to meet role expectations).<br>b. Assess client's perception of current situation including precipitating factors and effectiveness of coping mechanisms.<br>c. Implement measures *to promote effective coping:*<br>1. allow time for client to adjust psychologically to diagnosis and its implications, planned treatment, and anticipated changes in life style and roles<br>2. assist client to recognize and manage inappropriate denial if it is present<br>3. perform actions to reduce fear and anxiety (see Nursing Diagnosis 1, action b)<br>4. encourage verbalization about current situation<br>5. assist client to identify personal strengths and resources that can be utilized to facilitate coping with the current situation<br>6. demonstrate acceptance of client but set limits on inappropriate behavior<br>7. create an atmosphere of trust and support<br>8. arrange for a visit from another individual who is successfully living with AIDS<br>9. include client in planning care, encourage maximum participation in treatment plan, and allow choices when possible *to enable him/her to maintain a sense of control*<br>10. instruct client in effective problem-solving techniques (e.g. accurate identification of stressors, determination of various options to solve problem)<br>11. assist client to maintain usual daily routines whenever possible<br>12. assist client as he/she starts to plan for necessary life-style and role changes after discharge; help client identify priorities and attainable goals<br>13. assist client and significant others to identify ways that personal and family goals can be adjusted rather than abandoned<br>14. discuss ways to maintain optimal health; focus on methods of altering rather than changing life style<br>15. assist client through methods such as role playing to prepare for negative reactions from others because of diagnosis of AIDS |

16. administer antianxiety and/or antidepressant agents if ordered
17. assist client to identify and utilize available support systems; provide information about resources and support groups that can assist client and significant others in coping with effects of AIDS (e.g. American Foundation for AIDS Research, National AIDS Clearinghouse, National Association of People with AIDS, Women's AIDS Network, hospice programs, Cascade AIDS Project, drug abuse programs)
18. encourage continued emotional support from significant others; provide them with current, accurate information about HIV infection *in order to reduce risk of their rejection of the client*
19. encourage client to share with significant others the kind of support that would be most beneficial (e.g. listening, inspiring hope, providing reassurance and accurate information)
20. support behaviors suggesting positive adaptation to changes experienced (e.g. participation in treatment plan, verbalization of the ability to cope with diagnosis of AIDS, utilization of effective problem-solving strategies).

d. Consult physician about psychological counseling if appropriate. Initiate a referral if necessary.

## 16. NURSING DIAGNOSIS: Powerlessness

related to:
a. the disabling and terminal nature of AIDS;
b. increasing dependence on others to meet basic needs;
c. changes in roles, relationships, and future plans.

| Desired Outcome | Nursing Actions and ***Selected Purposes/Rationales*** |
|---|---|
| 16. The client will demonstrate increased feelings of control over his/her situation as evidenced by:<br>a. verbalization of same<br>b. active participation in planning of care<br>c. participation in self-care activities within physical limitations. | 16.a. Assess client for behaviors that may indicate feelings of powerlessness (e.g. verbalization of lack of control over current situation, anger, apathy, hostility, excessive dependency, lack of participation in care planning or self-care).<br>b. Obtain information from client and significant others regarding client's usual response to situations in which he/she has had limited control (e.g. loss of job, financial stress).<br>c. Evaluate with client his/her perceptions of current situation, strengths, weaknesses, expectations, and parts of current situation which are under his/her control. Correct misinformation and inaccurate perceptions and encourage discussion of feelings about areas in which he/she perceives a lack of control.<br>d. Assist client to establish realistic short- and long-term goals.<br>e. Reinforce physician's explanation about AIDS and the treatment plan. Clarify misconceptions.<br>f. Implement measures to promote effective coping (see Nursing Diagnosis 15, action c) *in order to promote an increased sense of control over his/her situation.*<br>g. Support realistic hope about the possibility of future independence, effectiveness of drugs in controlling conditions that can result from an impaired immune system, and the possibility of a cure for AIDS.<br>h. Remind client of his/her right to ask questions about current condition, prognosis, and treatment regimen.<br>i. Support client's efforts to increase knowledge of and control over condition. Provide relevant pamphlets, audiovisual materials, and |

| Desired Outcome | Nursing Actions and ***Selected Purposes/Rationales*** |
|---|---|
| | information about available community support for persons with HIV infection.<br>j. Inform client of scheduled procedures and tests *so that unpredictability is eliminated as much as possible and feeling of control is promoted.*<br>k. Consult occupational therapist (if indicated) about assistive devices and environmental modifications that would allow client more independence in performing activities of daily living.<br>l. Encourage significant others to allow client to do as much as he/she is able *so that a feeling of independence can be maintained.*<br>m. Encourage client's participation in support groups if indicated. |

## 17. NURSING DIAGNOSIS: Grieving*

related to:
a. diagnosis of an incurable illness with an uncertain course and a high probability of premature death;
b. changes in body functioning, appearance, life style, and roles associated with the disease process.

*This diagnostic label includes anticipatory grieving and grieving following the actual losses.

| Desired Outcome | Nursing Actions and ***Selected Purposes/Rationales*** |
|---|---|
| 17. The client will demonstrate beginning progression through the grieving process as evidenced by:<br>a. verbalization of feelings about AIDS and its implications<br>b. expression of grief<br>c. participation in treatment plan and self-care activities<br>d. utilization of available support systems<br>e. verbalization of a plan for integrating prescribed follow-up care into life style. | 17.a. Assess for signs and symptoms of grieving (e.g. change in eating habits, inability to concentrate, insomnia, anger, noncompliance, withdrawal from significant others, denial of loss). Be aware that client's response to a loss will be affected by factors such as previous experience with loss, age, developmental stage, available support systems, spiritual and cultural background, current health status, and significance of the loss.<br>b. Implement measures *to facilitate the grieving process:*<br>1. assist client to acknowledge the losses resulting from the diagnosis of AIDS *so grief work can begin;* assess for factors that may hinder and facilitate acknowledgment<br>2. discuss the grieving process and assist client to accept the phases of grieving as an expected response to actual and/or anticipated losses<br>3. allow time for client to progress through the phases of grieving (phases vary among theorists but progress from shock and alarm to acceptance); be aware that not every phase is expressed by all individuals, that recurrence of phases is common, and that the grieving process may take months to years<br>4. provide an atmosphere of care and concern (e.g. provide privacy, be available and nonjudgmental, display empathy and respect) *so that client will feel free to verbalize feelings*<br>5. perform actions *to promote trust* (e.g. answer questions honestly, provide requested information)<br>6. encourage the verbal expression of anger and sadness about the diagnosis of AIDS; recognize displacement of anger and assist client to see actual cause of angry feelings and resentment; establish limits on abusive behavior if demonstrated<br>7. encourage client to express his/her feelings in whatever ways are comfortable (e.g. writing, drawing, conversation)<br>8. perform actions to promote effective coping (see Nursing Diagnosis 15, action c)<br>9. support realistic hope by providing accurate information about |

research currently being done on HIV infection and the possibility of more effective treatment and discovery of a cure
10. support behaviors suggesting successful grief work (e.g. verbalizing feelings about the diagnosis of AIDS and changes in body functioning, learning needed skills, developing or renewing relationships, focusing on ways to adapt to losses)
11. explain the phases of the grieving process to significant others; encourage their support, understanding, and presence
12. facilitate communication between the client and significant others; be aware that they may be in different phases of the grieving process
13. provide information regarding counseling services and support groups that might assist client in working through grief
14. arrange for a visit from clergy if desired by client.

c. Consult physician about referral for counseling if signs of dysfunctional grieving (e.g. persistent denial of losses, excessive anger or sadness, hysteria, suicidal behaviors) occur.

## 18. NURSING DIAGNOSIS: Social isolation

related to:
a. fear of associating with others because of possibility of contracting an infection;
b. stigma and discrimination associated with the diagnosis of AIDS and others' fear of contracting HIV;
c. precautions necessary to prevent spread of HIV;
d. anger towards others responsible for disease transmission to him/her.

| Desired Outcome | Nursing Actions and ***Selected Purposes/Rationales*** |
|---|---|
| 18. The client will experience a decreased sense of isolation as evidenced by:<br>a. maintenance of relationships with significant others<br>b. verbalization of decreasing feelings of aloneness and rejection. | 18.a. Ascertain client's usual degree of social interaction.<br>b. Assess for indications of social isolation (e.g. absence of supportive significant others; uncommunicative; withdrawn; expression of feelings of rejection, being different from others, or aloneness imposed by others; hostility; sad, dull affect).<br>c. Implement measures *to decrease social isolation:*<br>1. assist client to identify reasons for feeling isolated and alone; aid him/her in developing a plan of action to reduce these feelings<br>2. reinforce physician's explanation about the immune deficiency; assure client that continued social contact with healthy people will not cause disease or infection<br>3. provide information to client and significant others about how HIV is known to be transmitted; assure them that HIV does not spread through ordinary physical contact<br>4. demonstrate acceptance of client using techniques such as touch and frequent visits<br>5. encourage significant others to visit<br>6. encourage client to maintain telephone contact with significant others<br>7. schedule time each day to sit and talk with client<br>8. assist client to identify a few persons he/she feels comfortable with and encourage interactions with them<br>9. encourage contact with those who are not likely to reject client (e.g. AIDS volunteers and support groups, clergy)<br>10. encourage client to allow friends and family to share their feelings and fears *in order to reduce the possibility of their distancing from client*<br>11. make items such as telephone, TV, radio, and newspapers accessible to client |

| Desired Outcome | Nursing Actions and ***Selected Purposes/Rationales*** |
|---|---|
| | 12. have significant others bring client's favorite objects from home and place in room. |

## 19. NURSING DIAGNOSIS: Altered family processes

related to:
a. diagnosis of terminal, communicable disease in family member;
b. fear of disclosure of diagnosis with subsequent rejection of family unit;
c. change in family roles and structure associated with progressive disability and eventual death of family member;
d. financial burden associated with extended illness and progressive disability of client;
e. fear of contracting disease from client;
f. decisions made by client and his/her partner about such issues as treatment plan, life support, and disposition of property that may be in conflict with the client's family of origin;
g. anticipatory grief.

| Desired Outcome | Nursing Actions and ***Selected Purposes/Rationales*** |
|---|---|
| 19. The family members* will demonstrate beginning adjustment to diagnosis of AIDS in client and changes in functioning of family member and family roles and structure as evidenced by:<br>a. meeting client's needs<br>b. verbalization of ways to adapt to required role and life-style changes<br>c. active participation in decision making and client's care<br>d. positive interactions with one another. | 19.a. Assess for signs and symptoms of altered family processes (e.g. inability to meet client's needs, statements of not being able to accept client's diagnosis or make necessary role and life-style changes, inability to make decisions, inability or refusal to participate in client's care, negative family interactions).<br>b. Identify components of the family and their patterns of communication and role expectations.<br>c. Implement measures *to facilitate family members' adjustment to client's diagnosis, changes in his/her functioning within the family system, and altered family roles and structure:*<br>1. encourage and assist family members to verbalize feelings about client's diagnosis and its effect on their life style and family structure; actively listen to each family member and maintain a nonjudgmental attitude about feelings shared<br>2. reinforce physician's explanation about AIDS, how HIV is transmitted, and planned treatment program<br>3. assist family to gain a realistic perspective of client's situation, conveying as much hope as appropriate<br>4. provide privacy *so that family members and client can share their feelings with one another;* stress the importance of and facilitate the use of good communication techniques<br>5. assist family members to progress through their own grieving process; explain that they may encounter times when they need to focus on meeting their own rather than the client's needs<br>6. emphasize the need for family members to obtain adequate rest and nutrition and to identify and utilize stress management techniques *so that they are better able to emotionally and physically deal with the changes that are being experienced, physical care of the client, and reactions of others when diagnosis is known*<br>7. encourage and assist family members to identify coping strategies for dealing with the client's diagnosis and its effect on the family<br>8. assist family to identify realistic goals and ways of reaching these goals |

*The term "family members" is being used here to include client's significant others.

9. include family members in decision making about client and his/her care; convey appreciation for their input and continued support of the client
10. encourage and allow family members to participate in client's care as appropriate
11. assist family members to identify resources that can assist them in coping with their feelings and meeting their immediate and long-term needs (e.g. counseling and social services; pastoral care; service, church, and AIDS support groups); initiate a referral if indicated.

d. Consult physician if family members continue to demonstrate difficulty adjusting to client's diagnosis and change in client's functioning, roles, and family structure.

## 20. NURSING DIAGNOSIS: Knowledge deficit

regarding follow-up care.

| Desired Outcomes | Nursing Actions and ***Selected Purposes/Rationales*** |
|---|---|
| 20.a. The client will identify ways to prevent the spread of HIV. | 20.a. Instruct client in ways to prevent spread of HIV to others:<br>1. wash hands before handling food<br>2. cleanse hands carefully after using bathroom and after contact with body fluids such as semen, mucus, and blood<br>3. wash dishes in very hot, soapy water (disinfectant is not necessary)<br>4. if a spill of urine or other body fluids occurs, cleanse area with hot, soapy water and then disinfect with a solution of 1 part bleach to 10 parts water (this solution is sufficient to kill HIV and other organisms)<br>5. do not rinse mops and sponges used to clean up body fluid spills in sinks where food is prepared; dirty mop water should be disposed of in the toilet<br>6. do not share eating utensils, towels, washcloths, toothbrushes, razors, enema equipment, or sexual devices<br>7. cover mouth when coughing and sneezing<br>8. if sexually active with a partner, instruct to:<br>a. avoid getting pregnant<br>b. avoid multiple sexual partners and sexual contact with promiscuous persons<br>c. choose healthy partners<br>d. be honest with desired partner about HIV infection<br>e. modify techniques so that body fluids are not shared<br>f. avoid unsafe sexual practices (e.g. urinating in mouth or anus or on skin; sharing dildos and sex toys; allowing ejaculate to come in contact with broken skin or mucous membranes; unprotected anal sex; any activity that could cause tears in lining of vagina, anus, or penis; combining oral and anal sexual activity)<br>g. use the following guidelines in relation to condom use:<br>1. always use a condom during anal, vaginal, and oral penetration (condom should be applied every time a body orifice is entered because HIV is found in preseminal fluid)<br>2. use only latex condoms (HIV can penetrate other types of materials)<br>3. use only condoms with a receptacle tip to reduce the risk of spillage of semen; if that type is unavailable, create a receptacle |

| Desired Outcomes | Nursing Actions and ***Selected Purposes/Rationales*** |
|---|---|
| | for ejaculate by pinching tip of condom as it is rolled on erect penis<br>4. lubricate outside of condom and area to be penetrated to minimize possibility of condom breakage; use a water-based lubricant such as K-Y jelly or a spermicidal compound containing nonoxynol-9 (nonoxynol-9 is known to have some antiviral activity)<br>5. avoid lubricants made of mineral oil or petroleum distillates such as Vaseline or baby oil (these products weaken latex)<br>6. hold condom at base of penis during withdrawal and use caution during removal of condom to prevent spillage of semen (penis should be withdrawn and condom removed before the penis has totally relaxed)<br>7. dispose of condom immediately after use (a new one should be used for subsequent sexual activity)<br>8. if participating in anal receptive sex, use condoms made specifically for that purpose<br>9. store condoms in a cool place to prevent them from drying out and breaking during use<br>9. do not donate blood, sperm, or body organs<br>10. if an intravenous drug user, encourage and/or instruct to:<br>a. get involved in a drug treatment program<br>b. not share drug paraphernalia with others<br>c. clean skin and equipment well (needles should be cleaned with household bleach)<br>d. avoid "shooting galleries." |
| 20.b. The client will identify ways to decrease the risk for developing opportunistic infections. | 20.b. Instruct client in ways to decrease risk for developing an opportunistic infection:<br>1. cleanse kitchen and bathroom surfaces (particularly floor of shower) regularly with a disinfectant to prevent fungal growth<br>2. use a 1:10 solution of household bleach and water for cleaning and/or disinfecting areas soiled with blood or other body fluids<br>3. avoid contact with pet excreta; if unavoidable, wear gloves when performing activities such as cleaning litter boxes, bird cages, and aquariums<br>4. use liquid soap from a pump dispenser rather than bar soap<br>5. cleanse hands carefully after contact with body fluids such as semen, mucus, and blood<br>6. do not share eating utensils, towels, washcloths, toothbrushes, razors, enema equipment, or sexual devices<br>7. keep living quarters well ventilated to reduce exposure to airborne disease<br>8. change furnace filters regularly<br>9. avoid contact with persons who have an infection (particularly viral) and those who have been recently vaccinated<br>10. maintain an adequate balance between activity and rest<br>11. inform all health care providers of HIV infection so that drugs that further suppress the immune system (e.g. corticosteroids, immunosuppressants) will not be prescribed unnecessarily<br>12. maintain an optimal nutritional status<br>13. avoid eating raw fish or eggs, rare meat, and foods that have molded or are beyond expiration date<br>14. drink at least 10 glasses of liquid/day. |
| 20.c. The client will state signs and symptoms to report to the health care provider. | 20.c. Stress importance of notifying the health care provider if the following signs and symptoms occur:<br>1. persistent fever or chills<br>2. night sweats<br>3. persistent headache |

4. swollen glands
5. painful, itchy skin lesions
6. reddish-purple patches or nodules on any body area
7. white patches or ulcerations in the mouth
8. difficulty swallowing
9. persistent diarrhea
10. perianal itching and/or pain
11. frequency, urgency, or burning on urination
12. cloudy, foul-smelling urine
13. dry cough or a cough productive of purulent, green, or rust-colored sputum
14. progressive shortness of breath
15. increasing weakness, unexplained fatigue or weight loss
16. change in vision
17. dizziness
18. numbness or tingling in extremities.

20.d. The client will identify resources that can assist in adjustment to changes resulting from the diagnosis of AIDS.

20.d.1. Provide information to client and significant others about resources that can assist in adjustment to the diagnosis of AIDS (e.g. American Foundation for AIDS Research, National Association of People with AIDS, hospice programs, community support groups, Women's AIDS Network, AIDS hotlines, Public Health Service, Centers for Disease Control, counselors).
2. Initiate a referral if indicated.

20.e. The client will verbalize an understanding of and a plan for adhering to recommended follow-up care including future appointments with health care provider and medications prescribed.

20.e.1. Reinforce the importance of keeping scheduled follow-up appointments with health care provider.
2. Explain the rationale for, side effects of, and importance of taking medications prescribed.
3. If trimethoprim-sulfamethoxazole is prescribed prophylactically to prevent PCP, provide the following instructions:
   a. take the medication with a large glass of water at least 1 hour before or 2 hours after a meal
   b. drink at least 10 glasses of liquid/day
   c. report development of a rash, sore throat, fever, or yellowing of skin
   d. report a sudden reduction in daily urine output.
4. If aerosol pentamidine is prescribed to prevent PCP, provide instructions regarding use:
   a. reconstitute the prescribed dose (usually 300 mg) in 6 ml of sterile water (the drug will precipitate in a saline solution)
   b. do not mix with any other drug
   c. administer only with the specified nebulizer equipment (e.g. Respirgard II) and maintain a flow rate of 5-7 liters/minute from a 40-50 psi air or oxygen source
   d. use the aerosol device until the chamber is empty (this can take as long as 45 minutes)
   e. report persistent nausea, vomiting, diarrhea, and/or difficulty breathing.
5. If client is discharged on AZT, instruct him/her to:
   a. follow schedule of drug administration carefully (every 4 hours around the clock is usually preferred or it may be prescribed 3 times/day to improve compliance)
   b. avoid taking any other medications for AIDS unless approved by physician
   c. report immediately any signs and symptoms of bone marrow depression such as unusual bleeding and excessive fatigue (it is not uncommon for clients taking this drug to require blood transfusions as a result of the drug's bone marrow depressant effects).
6. If client is discharged on didanosine, instruct to:
   a. take 1 hour before or 2-3 hours after eating

| Desired Outcomes | Nursing Actions and ***Selected Purposes/Rationales*** |
|---|---|
| | b. take 2 pills at a time and thoroughly chew them or dissolve them in water in order to ensure release of buffering agent in the pills<br>c. avoid intake of alcohol because of the increased risk of pancreatitis with this drug<br>d. report abdominal pain; nausea; vomiting; or pain, numbness, or tingling in extremities.<br>7. Stress the importance of taking hematopoietic agents (e.g. epoetin alpha [Epogen], granulocyte colony-stimulating factor [G-CSF]) as prescribed.<br>8. Implement measures to improve client compliance:<br>a. include significant others in discharge teaching sessions if possible<br>b. encourage questions and allow time for reinforcement and clarification of information provided<br>c. provide written instructions regarding scheduled appointments with health care provider, medications prescribed, signs and symptoms to report, and ways to prevent infection. |

# Anemia

Anemia is a hematological disorder characterized by a reduction in the number of red blood cells, the amount of hemoglobin, or the volume of packed red cells (hematocrit). The main consequence of anemia is hypoxia, with signs and symptoms being a result of the decreased oxygen-carrying capacity of the blood and compensatory responses to the hypoxia. Dyspnea, palpitations, and diaphoresis following exercise are usually the only symptoms the client experiences until the hemoglobin drops to 7-8 g/dl. The onset of signs and symptoms often depends on how rapidly the anemia developed and the client's age.

Anemia is usually classified by pathophysiologic or morphologic criteria. Anemias based on pathophysiologic criteria include those caused by blood loss, increased red cell destruction, or defective or decreased red blood cell production (e.g. iron deficiency anemia, vitamin $B_{12}$ or folate deficiency, aplastic anemia). Morphologic classification of anemia is commonly based on cell size (i.e. macrocytic, microcytic, normocytic). Some anemias are secondary to chronic systemic conditions such as cirrhosis, renal failure, certain endocrine disorders, and connective tissue disorders and are often referred to as secondary anemias.

**This care plan focuses on the adult client with symptoms of anemia hospitalized for definitive diagnosis and initiation of treatment for probable nutritional/absorptive or chronic blood loss anemia.** Although many of the signs and symptoms of common types of anemia are addressed in this care plan, it will need to be individualized based on the cause of the anemia and the extensiveness of the neuropsychiatric manifestations (these occur mainly with vitamin $B_{12}$ deficiency). The goals of care are to ensure adequate rest, initiate replacement therapy, improve nutritional status, and educate the client regarding follow-up care.

## DIAGNOSTIC TESTS

Red blood cell (RBC) count
Hematocrit (Hct)
Hemoglobin (Hb)
Red blood cell indices
Serum iron and total iron-binding capacity (TIBC)
Serum ferritin
Transferrin saturation
Free erythrocyte protoporphyrin (FEP)
Serum folate and vitamin $B_{12}$ (cobalamin)
Reticulocyte count

Blood smear examination (stained red blood cell examination)
Bone marrow examination
Stool examination for occult blood
Schilling test
Gastric analysis

## DISCHARGE CRITERIA

Prior to discharge, the client will:

- ❖ perform activities of daily living without extreme fatigue or dyspnea
- ❖ have an increased red blood cell count, hemoglobin, and hematocrit
- ❖ verbalize an understanding of the rationale for and components of the recommended diet
- ❖ verbalize an understanding of medications ordered including rationale, side effects, and importance of taking as prescribed
- ❖ identify ways to prevent injury associated with neurological deficits if present
- ❖ state signs and symptoms to report to the health care provider
- ❖ verbalize an understanding of and a plan for adhering to recommended follow-up care including activity level and future appointments with health care provider and for laboratory studies.

## NURSING/ COLLABORATIVE DIAGNOSES



## 1. NURSING DIAGNOSIS: Altered nutrition: less than body requirements

related to inadequate intake; malabsorption; or impaired utilization of iron, vitamin $B_{12}$, or folate.

| Desired Outcome | Nursing Actions and ***Selected Purposes/Rationales*** |
|---|---|
| 1. The client will experience an improved nutritional status as evidenced by:<br>a. weight within or approaching normal | 1.a. Assess for and report signs and symptoms of malnutrition:<br>1. weight below normal for client's age, height, and body frame<br>2. abnormal BUN and low serum albumin, Hct, Hb, $B_{12}$, folate, transferrin, lymphocyte, and ferritin levels<br>3. triceps skinfold thickness less than normal<br>4. weakness and fatigue |

| Desired Outcome | Nursing Actions and ***Selected Purposes/Rationales*** |
|---|---|
| range for client's age, height, and body frame<br>b. improved BUN and serum albumin, Hct, Hb, $B_{12}$, folate, transferrin, lymphocyte, and ferritin levels<br>c. triceps skinfold thickness within or approaching normal range<br>d. improved strength and activity tolerance<br>e. healthy oral mucous membrane. | 5. stomatitis.<br>b. Monitor percentage of meals and snacks client consumes. Report a pattern of inadequate intake.<br>c. Implement measures *to improve nutritional status:*<br>1. perform actions *to improve oral intake:*<br>a. implement measures to reduce dyspepsia (see Nursing Diagnosis 3.A, action 3)<br>b. implement measures to reduce pain (see Nursing Diagnosis 2, action e)<br>c. increase activity as allowed and tolerated *(activity stimulates appetite)*<br>d. obtain a dietary consult if necessary to assist client in selecting foods/fluids that meet nutritional needs as well as personal and cultural preferences whenever possible<br>e. encourage a rest period before meals *to minimize fatigue*<br>f. maintain a clean environment and a relaxed, pleasant atmosphere<br>g. provide oral care before meals<br>h. serve small portions of nutritious foods/fluids that are appealing to the client and easy to chew<br>i. encourage significant others to bring in client's favorite foods unless contraindicated<br>j. allow adequate time for meals; reheat food if necessary<br>2. instruct and assist client to select meals that are well balanced and that meet his/her specific dietary needs (determined by the cause of the anemia and the specific deficiency):<br>a. foods high in iron (e.g. organ meats, dried fruit, dark green leafy vegetables, whole-grain or iron-enriched breads and cereals); inform client that iron is poorly absorbed from most food sources unless taken with a source of vitamin C (e.g. citrus fruits or juices)<br>b. foods high in vitamin $B_{12}$ (e.g. meat, milk and milk products, eggs)<br>c. foods high in folate (e.g. raw, dark green leafy vegetables; legumes; whole-grain breads and cereals)<br>3. administer the following medications if ordered:<br>a. iron preparations (e.g. iron dextran, ferrous sulfate, ferrous gluconate)<br>b. vitamin $B_{12}$ (e.g. cyanocobalamin); if client has pernicious anemia, vitamin $B_{12}$ must be given parenterally or in combination with intrinsic factor *in order to be absorbed*<br>c. folic acid (e.g. Folvite).<br>d. Perform a 72-hour calorie count if ordered. Report totals to dietitian and physician.<br>e. Consult physician about alternative methods of providing nutrition (e.g. parenteral nutrition, tube feedings) if client does not consume enough food or fluids to meet nutritional needs. |

## 2. NURSING DIAGNOSIS: Pain:

a. **oral pain** related to inflammation and fissures of the tongue and lips (particularly at the corners of the mouth) associated with glossitis and cheilosis that develop as a result of a deficiency of iron, vitamin $B_{12}$, or folate;
b. **headache** related to dilation of the cerebral arteries associated with cerebral hypoxia.

| Desired Outcome | Nursing Actions and ***Selected Purposes/Rationales*** |
|---|---|
| 2. The client will experience diminished pain as evidenced by:<br>a. verbalization of pain relief<br>b. relaxed facial expression and body positioning<br>c. increased participation in activities. | 2.a. Determine how the client usually responds to pain.<br>b. Assess client's perception of pain including location, severity, and type. Use a numerical scale to rate intensity.<br>c. Assess for nonverbal signs of:<br>1. headache (e.g. wrinkled brow, reluctance to move head, rubbing head, restlessness)<br>2. oral pain (e.g. reluctance to eat).<br>d. Assess for factors that seem to aggravate and alleviate pain.<br>e. Implement measures *to reduce pain:*<br>1. perform actions *to relieve oral pain:*<br>a. implement measures to reduce the severity of glossitis and cheilosis (see Nursing Diagnosis 5, action b)<br>b. have client rinse mouth frequently with a warm saline solution *to soothe the oral mucous membrane*<br>c. instruct client to avoid substances that might irritate the oral mucosa (e.g. spicy, acidic, or extremely hot foods/fluids; dry or hard foods)<br>d. offer cool, soothing items such as nonacidic juices, ices, and ice cream<br>e. use a soft-bristle brush, sponge-tipped applicator, or low-pressure power spray for oral hygiene<br>f. lubricate client's lips frequently with K-Y jelly, ChapStick, Blistex, or mineral oil<br>g. apply topical anesthetics, oral protective pastes or coating agents, and topical analgesics if ordered<br>2. perform actions *to relieve headache:*<br>a. implement measures *to minimize environmental stimuli* (e.g. provide a calm environment, restrict visitors, dim lights)<br>b. avoid jarring bed or startling client *to minimize risk of sudden movements*<br>c. provide or assist with nonpharmacologic measures for pain relief (e.g. cool cloth to forehead, relaxation techniques, restful environment, diversional activities)<br>3. administer analgesics if ordered.<br>f. Consult physician if above measures fail to provide adequate pain relief. |

## 3.A. NURSING DIAGNOSIS: Altered comfort: dyspepsia

related to atrophy of the gastrointestinal mucosa associated with diminished proliferation and function of epithelial tissue resulting from a deficiency of iron, vitamin $B_{12}$, or folate (occurs most frequently with vitamin $B_{12}$ and folate deficiency anemias).

| Desired Outcome | Nursing Actions and ***Selected Purposes/Rationales*** |
|---|---|
| 3.A. The client will verbalize relief of dyspepsia. | 3.A.1. Assess client for verbal complaints of dyspepsia (e.g. gnawing pain in epigastric area, feeling of fullness or bloating, indigestion, nausea).<br>2. Determine if particular foods/fluids contribute to dyspepsia.<br>3. Implement measures *to reduce dyspepsia:*<br>a. provide small, frequent meals rather than 3 large ones<br>b. instruct client to ingest foods and fluids slowly<br>c. instruct client to avoid foods/fluids that may irritate the gastric |

| Desired Outcome | Nursing Actions and ***Selected Purposes/Rationales*** |
|---|---|
| | mucosa (e.g. spicy foods; caffeine-containing beverages such as coffee, tea, and colas; decaffeinated coffee)<br>d. instruct client to eat dry foods (e.g. toast, crackers) and avoid drinking liquids with meals if nauseated<br>e. instruct client to rest with head of bed elevated after eating<br>f. administer oral iron preparations with or immediately after meals *to reduce gastric irritation*<br>g. encourage client not to smoke<br>h. administer the following medications if ordered *to protect the gastric mucosa:*<br>1. antacids (be aware that antacids may reduce iron absorption if they are given at the same time)<br>2. cytoprotective agents (e.g. sucralfate)<br>3. histamine$_2$ receptor antagonists (e.g. ranitidine, famotidine, cimetidine).<br>4. Consult physician if above measures fail to control dyspepsia. |

## 3.B. NURSING DIAGNOSIS: Altered comfort: coldness and chills

related to a compensatory decrease in blood flow to the skin in an attempt to adequately perfuse and oxygenate the major organs.

| Desired Outcome | Nursing Actions and ***Selected Purposes/Rationales*** |
|---|---|
| 3.B. The client will not experience chills and a feeling of being cold. | 3.B. 1. Assess client for chills, cool skin, and statements of feeling cold.<br>2. Implement measures *to prevent chills and feeling of being cold:*<br>a. protect client from drafts<br>b. maintain a room temperature that is comfortable for client<br>c. provide client with extra blankets and clothing as needed<br>d. provide warm liquids for client to drink.<br>3. Consult physician if client continues to have chills or complaints of being cold. |

## 4. NURSING DIAGNOSIS: High risk for impaired skin integrity

related to:

a. increased skin fragility associated with malnutrition;
b. damage to the skin and/or subcutaneous tissue associated with prolonged pressure on the tissues, friction, or shearing if mobility is decreased;
c. increased susceptibility to injury associated with diminished sensation if neurological deficits are present.

| Desired Outcome | Nursing Actions and ***Selected Purposes/Rationales*** |
|---|---|
| 4. The client will maintain skin integrity as evidenced by:<br>a. absence of redness and irritation | 4.a. Inspect the skin (especially bony prominences, dependent areas, and areas of decreased sensation) for pallor, redness, and breakdown.<br>b. Implement measures *to prevent skin breakdown:*<br>1. assist client to turn every 2 hours if activity is limited<br>2. gently massage around reddened areas at least every 2 hours |

b. no skin breakdown.

3. perform actions *to prevent shearing* (shearing occurs when one tissue layer slides past another) *and skin surface abrasion:*
   a. apply a thin layer of powder or cornstarch to bottom sheet or skin *to absorb moisture (moist skin is more likely to adhere to sheet) and reduce friction*
   b. limit length of time client is in semi-Fowler's position to 30 minutes *(in this position, client tends to slide down in bed)*
4. instruct or assist client to shift weight every 30 minutes
5. if fade time (length of time it takes for reddened area to fade after pressure is removed) is greater than 15 minutes, increase frequency of position changes
6. keep skin lubricated, clean, and dry
7. apply a thin layer of powder or cornstarch to areas with opposing skin surfaces (e.g. axillae, perineum, beneath breasts) if indicated *to absorb moisture and/or reduce friction*
8. keep bed linens dry and wrinkle-free
9. increase activity as allowed and tolerated
10. provide devices to reduce pressure on the skin, decrease shearing, and/or prevent moisture buildup (e.g. alternating pressure mattress or pad, flotation pad, sheepskin)
11. perform actions to improve nutritional status (see Nursing Diagnosis 1, action c).

c. If skin breakdown occurs:
1. notify physician
2. continue with above measures to prevent further irritation and breakdown
3. perform decubitus care as ordered or per standard hospital procedure
4. assess client closely and report signs and symptoms of infection (e.g. elevated temperature; redness, warmth, and edema around area of breakdown; unusual drainage from site).

---

## 5. NURSING DIAGNOSIS: Altered oral mucous membrane: glossitis and cheilosis

related to atrophy of the oral epithelium associated with iron, vitamin $B_{12}$, or folate deficiency.

| Desired Outcome | Nursing Actions and ***Selected Purposes/Rationales*** |
|---|---|
| 5. The client will maintain a healthy oral mucous membrane as evidenced by:<br>a. normal-appearing tongue<br>b. absence of tongue pain<br>c. absence of inflamed, painful fissures in lips and at corners of mouth. | 5.a. Assess client for and report signs and symptoms of glossitis and cheilosis (e.g. glossy, beefy red tongue; complaints of a sore, burning tongue; painful, reddened fissures in lips or at corners of mouth).<br>b. Implement measures *to prevent or reduce the severity of glossitis and cheilosis:*<br>1. reinforce importance of and assist client with oral hygiene after meals and snacks; avoid products such as lemon-glycerin swabs and commercial mouthwashes containing alcohol *(these products have a drying or irritating effect on the oral mucous membrane)*<br>2. perform actions to improve nutritional status (see Nursing Diagnosis 1, action c)<br>3. encourage client not to smoke *(smoking irritates and dries the mucosa)*<br>4. lubricate client's lips with K-Y jelly, ChapStick, Blistex, or mineral oil frequently<br>5. instruct client to avoid substances that might further irritate the oral mucosa (e.g. extremely hot, spicy, or acidic foods/fluids).<br>c. Consult physician if signs and symptoms of glossitis or cheilosis persist or worsen. |

## 6. NURSING DIAGNOSIS: Activity intolerance

related to tissue hypoxia associated with decreased oxygen-carrying capacity of the blood resulting from a decrease in erythrocytes and/or hemoglobin concentration.

| Desired Outcome | Nursing Actions and ***Selected Purposes/Rationales*** |
|---|---|
| 6. The client will demonstrate an increased tolerance for activity as evidenced by:<br>a. verbalization of feeling less fatigued and weak<br>b. ability to perform activities of daily living without exertional dyspnea, chest pain, diaphoresis, dizziness, and a significant change in vital signs. | 6.a. Assess for signs and symptoms of activity intolerance:<br>1. statements of fatigue and weakness<br>2. exertional dyspnea, chest pain, diaphoresis, or dizziness<br>3. abnormal heart rate response to activity (e.g. increase in rate of 20 beats/minute above resting rate, decrease in rate, rate not returning to preactivity level within 3 minutes after stopping activity, change from regular to irregular rate)<br>4. decreased systolic B/P or a significant increase (10-15 mm Hg) in systolic or diastolic pressure with activity.<br>b. Implement measures *to improve activity tolerance:*<br>1. perform actions *to promote rest and/or conserve energy:*<br>a. maintain activity restrictions as ordered<br>b. minimize environmental activity and noise<br>c. organize nursing care to allow for periods of uninterrupted rest<br>d. limit the number of visitors and their length of stay<br>e. assist client with self-care activities as needed<br>f. keep supplies and personal articles within easy reach<br>g. instruct client in energy-saving techniques (e.g. using shower chair when showering, sitting to brush teeth or comb hair)<br>2. discourage smoking and excessive intake of beverages high in caffeine such as coffee, tea, and colas *(nicotine and caffeine increase cardiac workload and myocardial oxygen utilization, thereby decreasing oxygen availability)*<br>3. maintain oxygen therapy as ordered<br>4. perform actions to improve nutritional status (see Nursing Diagnosis 1, action c)<br>5. administer whole blood or packed red cells if ordered (blood should be administered slowly if any evidence of cardiac decompensation or fluid overload is present)<br>6. increase client's activity gradually as allowed and tolerated.<br>c. Instruct client to:<br>1. report a decreased tolerance for activity<br>2. stop any activity that causes chest pain, increased shortness of breath, dizziness, or extreme fatigue or weakness.<br>d. Consult physician if signs and symptoms of activity intolerance persist or worsen. |

## 7. NURSING DIAGNOSIS: Altered thought processes

related to:

a. cerebral hypoxia associated with decreased oxygen-carrying capacity of the blood;
b. degenerative changes in the cerebral cortex (can occur with vitamin $B_{12}$ deficiency).

| Desired Outcome | Nursing Actions and ***Selected Purposes/Rationales*** |
|---|---|
| 7. The client will experience an improvement in thought processes as evidenced by:<br>a. improved verbal response time<br>b. improved memory<br>c. longer attention span<br>d. absence of personality changes, paranoia, and confusion. | 7.a. Assess client for altered thought processes (e.g. slowed verbal response time, impaired memory, shortened attention span, personality changes, paranoia, confusion).<br>b. Ascertain from significant others client's usual level of intellectual and emotional functioning and whether personality changes have occurred.<br>c. Implement measures *to maintain optimal thought processes:*<br>1. perform actions to improve nutritional status (see Nursing Diagnosis 1, action c) *and subsequently resolve the anemia and vitamin deficiencies*<br>2. administer vitamin $B_{12}$ (e.g. cyanocobalamin) injections if ordered<br>3. maintain oxygen therapy as ordered.<br>d. If client shows evidence of altered thought processes:<br>1. reorient client to person, place, and time as necessary<br>2. address client by name<br>3. place familiar objects, clock, and calendar within client's view<br>4. approach client in a slow, calm manner; allow adequate time for communication<br>5. repeat instructions as necessary using clear, simple language and short sentences<br>6. keep environmental stimuli to a minimum<br>7. maintain a consistent and fairly structured routine and write out a schedule of activities for client to refer to if desired<br>8. have client perform only one activity at a time and allow adequate time for performance of activities<br>9. encourage client to make lists of planned activities, questions, and concerns<br>10. maintain realistic expectations of client's ability to learn, comprehend, and remember information provided; provide client with a written copy of instructions<br>11. encourage significant others to be supportive of client; instruct them in methods of dealing with the client's altered thought processes<br>12. discuss physiological basis for altered thought processes with client and significant others; inform them that intellectual and emotional functioning usually improve once the anemia has been adequately treated<br>13. consult physician if altered thought processes persist or worsen. |

## 8. NURSING DIAGNOSIS: High risk for infection

related to lowered resistance to infection associated with:
a. inadequate nutritional status;
b. possible abnormal leukopoiesis and/or defective cell-mediated immunity associated with a deficiency of vitamin $B_{12}$, folate, or iron.

| Desired Outcome | Nursing Actions and ***Selected Purposes/Rationales*** |
|---|---|
| 8. The client will remain free of infection as evidenced by:<br>a. absence of fever and chills<br>b. pulse within normal limits<br>c. normal breath sounds | 8.a. Assess for and report signs and symptoms of infection:<br>1. elevated temperature<br>2. chills<br>3. increased pulse<br>4. abnormal breath sounds<br>5. cloudy, foul-smelling urine<br>6. complaints of frequency, urgency, or burning when urinating<br>7. presence of WBCs, bacteria, and/or nitrites in urine |

| Desired Outcome | Nursing Actions and ***Selected Purposes/Rationales*** |
|---|---|
| d. voiding clear urine without complaints of frequency, urgency, and burning<br>e. absence of heat, pain, redness, swelling, and unusual drainage in any area<br>f. no complaints of increased weakness and fatigue<br>g. WBC and differential counts within normal range<br>h. negative results of cultured specimens. | 8. heat, pain, redness, swelling, or unusual drainage in any area<br>9. complaints of increased weakness or fatigue<br>10. elevated WBC count and/or significant change in differential.<br>b. Obtain specimens (e.g. urine, vaginal, mouth, sputum, blood) for culture as ordered. Report positive results.<br>c. Implement measures *to prevent infection:*<br>1. maintain a fluid intake of at least 2500 ml/day unless contraindicated<br>2. use good handwashing technique and encourage client to do the same<br>3. maintain meticulous aseptic technique during all invasive procedures (e.g. catheterization, venous and arterial punctures, injections)<br>4. change intravenous tubings and solutions and rotate insertion sites according to hospital policy<br>5. protect client from others with infection<br>6. perform actions to improve nutritional status (see Nursing Diagnosis 1, action c)<br>7. perform actions to prevent or reduce the severity of glossitis and cheilosis (see Nursing Diagnosis 5, action b)<br>8. perform actions *to prevent stasis of respiratory secretions* (e.g. assist client to turn, cough, and deep breathe; increase activity as allowed and tolerated)<br>9. perform actions to prevent skin breakdown (see Nursing Diagnosis 4, action b)<br>10. perform actions to prevent urinary retention (e.g. instruct client to urinate when the urge is first felt, promote relaxation during voiding attempts) *in order to prevent urinary stasis*<br>11. perform actions *to prevent the introduction of microorganisms into the urinary tract* (e.g. assist client with perineal care as needed, instruct and assist female client to wipe from front to back after urinating and defecating, maintain sterile technique during urinary catheterization). |

## 9. NURSING DIAGNOSIS: High risk for trauma

related to:

a. falls associated with:
   1. dizziness and lightheadedness resulting from cerebral hypoxia
   2. impaired proprioception resulting from neurological changes that can occur with vitamin $B_{12}$ deficiency
   3. weakness
   4. altered thought processes if present
   5. gait disturbances resulting from the demyelinating neuropathy that can occur with a vitamin $B_{12}$ deficiency;

b. cuts and burns associated with:
   1. altered thought processes if present
   2. paresthesias and uncoordinated movements resulting from the demyelinating neuropathy that can occur with vitamin $B_{12}$ deficiency.

| Desired Outcome | Nursing Actions and ***Selected Purposes/Rationales*** |
|---|---|
| 9. The client will not experience falls, burns, or cuts. | 9.a. Implement measures *to reduce the risk for trauma:*<br>1. perform actions *to prevent falls:*<br>a. keep bed in low position with side rails up when client is in bed<br>b. keep needed items within easy reach<br>c. encourage client to request assistance whenever needed; have call signal within easy reach |

d. use lap belt when client is in chair if indicated
e. instruct client to wear well-fitting slippers/shoes with nonslip soles and low heels when ambulating
f. keep floor free of clutter and wipe up spills promptly
g. accompany client during ambulation using a transfer safety belt if he/she is weak or dizzy
h. provide ambulatory aids (e.g. walker, cane) if client is weak or unsteady on feet
i. reinforce instructions from physical therapist on correct ambulation techniques if gait disturbances are present
j. instruct client to ambulate in well-lit areas and to use handrails if needed
k. do not rush client; allow adequate time for ambulation to the bathroom and in hallway
l. make sure that bathtub and shower have nonslip bottom surfaces and that shower chair, secure bath mat, call light, hand grips, and adequate lighting are present
m. implement actions to improve strength and activity tolerance (see Nursing Diagnosis 6, action b)

2. perform actions *to prevent burns:*
   a. let hot foods and fluids cool slightly before serving
   b. supervise client while smoking if indicated
   c. assess temperature of bath water and heating pad before and during use
3. assist client with tasks that require fine motor skills (e.g. shaving) *in order to prevent cuts*
4. administer central nervous system depressants judiciously
5. if client is confused or irrational:
   a. reorient frequently to surroundings and necessity of adhering to safety precautions
   b. provide constant supervision (e.g. staff member, significant other) if indicated
   c. consult physician about the temporary use of jacket or wrist restraints if necessary
   d. administer antianxiety and antipsychotic medications if ordered.

b. Include client and significant others in planning and implementing measures to prevent trauma.
c. If injury does occur, initiate appropriate first aid and notify physician.

---

**10. COLLABORATIVE DIAGNOSIS:** **Potential complication: heart failure**

related to a prolonged increase in cardiac workload resulting from the heart's attempt to compensate for tissue hypoxia.

| Desired Outcome | Nursing Actions and ***Selected Purposes/Rationales*** |
|---|---|
| 10. The client will not develop heart failure as evidenced by:<br>a. pulse 60-100 beats/minute<br>b. absence of an $S_3$ heart sound or summation gallop<br>c. usual mental status | 10.a. Assess for and report signs and symptoms of heart failure:<br>1. tachycardia<br>2. presence of an $S_3$ heart sound or summation gallop<br>3. restlessness, anxiousness, confusion<br>4. crackles (rales)<br>5. development of or increase in dyspnea and orthopnea<br>6. cough<br>7. increased weakness and fatigue<br>8. diminished or absent peripheral pulses |

| Desired Outcome | Nursing Actions and ***Selected Purposes/Rationales*** |
|---|---|
| d. normal breath sounds<br>e. absence of or no increase in dyspnea and orthopnea<br>f. absence of cough<br>g. no further decline in strength and activity tolerance<br>h. palpable peripheral pulses<br>i. skin warm and dry<br>j. balanced intake and output<br>k. stable weight<br>l. absence of peripheral edema; distended neck veins; and enlarged, tender liver. | 9. cool, diaphoretic skin<br>10. oliguria<br>11. weight gain<br>12. peripheral edema<br>13. distended neck veins<br>14. enlarged, tender liver.<br>b. Monitor chest x-ray results. Report findings of cardiomegaly, pleural effusion, or pulmonary edema.<br>c. Implement measures *to reduce cardiac workload in order to prevent heart failure:*<br>1. perform actions to promote rest and/or conserve energy (see Nursing Diagnosis 6, action b.1)<br>2. place client in a semi- to high Fowler's position<br>3. maintain oxygen therapy as ordered<br>4. instruct client to avoid activities that create a Valsalva response (e.g. straining to have a bowel movement, holding breath while moving) *in order to prevent the marked increase in venous return and preload that occurs with exhalation*<br>5. discourage smoking *(smoke has a cardiostimulatory effect, causes vasoconstriction, and reduces myocardial oxygen availability)*<br>6. discourage excessive intake of beverages high in caffeine such as coffee, tea, and colas *(caffeine is a myocardial stimulant and increases myocardial oxygen consumption)*<br>7. increase activity gradually as allowed and tolerated.<br>d. If signs and symptoms of heart failure occur:<br>1. continue with above actions<br>2. administer the following medications if ordered:<br>a. positive inotropic agents (e.g. digitalis preparations, dobutamine, amrinone) *to increase myocardial contractility*<br>b. diuretics and vasodilators *to decrease cardiac workload*<br>c. morphine sulfate *to reduce preload and anxiety* (used primarily in clients with pulmonary edema)<br>3. refer to Care Plan on Heart Failure for additional care measures. |

## 11. NURSING DIAGNOSIS: Knowledge deficit

regarding follow-up care.

| Desired Outcomes | Nursing Actions and ***Selected Purposes/Rationales*** |
|---|---|
| 11.a. The client will verbalize an understanding of the rationale for and components of the recommended diet. | 11.a.1. Explain the importance of diet therapy in the treatment of anemia.<br>2. Reinforce appropriate dietary instructions (see Nursing Diagnosis 1, action c.2). Instructions will vary according to the type of anemia.<br>3. Obtain a dietary consult to assist client in menu planning if appropriate. |
| 11.b. The client will verbalize an understanding of medications ordered | 11.b.1. Explain the rationale for, side effects of, and importance of taking medications prescribed.<br>2. If client is discharged on an iron preparation, instruct to:<br>a. take medication between meals if tolerated to promote maximum |

including rationale, side effects, and importance of taking as prescribed.

absorption; if gastric upset occurs, take iron with or immediately after meals
b. take iron with a source of vitamin C (e.g. citrus fruits or juices) in order to increase iron absorption
c. dilute liquid preparations, drink solution through a straw, and rinse mouth well after taking to avoid staining teeth
d. expect stools to be dark green or black
e. report persistent gastric upset, diarrhea, or constipation
f. continue to take iron for the length of time prescribed (it is usually recommended that iron be taken for 3-6 months to replenish iron stores).

3. If client is discharged on parenteral vitamin $B_{12}$:
a. demonstrate appropriate injection technique and location of possible injection sites
b. allow time for questions, clarification, and return demonstration.

4. If client is discharged on a folic acid preparation:
a. instruct client to restrict alcohol intake to a minimum because it impairs folic acid utilization
b. instruct the client to inform physician if taking any other medications (some medications such as phenytoin, triamterene, methotrexate, and trimethoprim interfere with folic acid utilization)
c. reinforce the need to continue intake of foods high in folic acid content; caution that excessive cooking of vegetables destroys folic acid content.

11.c. The client will identify ways to prevent injury associated with neurological deficits if present.

11.c. Provide the following instructions on ways to reduce risk of injury until existing neurological deficits have resolved:
1. obtain assistance or use a cane or walker when ambulating until steadiness has returned
2. wear shoes or slippers with nonslip soles and low heels to prevent falls
3. use an electric rather than straight-edge razor for shaving to prevent cuts
4. reduce risk of burns by:
   a. letting hot foods and fluids cool slightly before consuming
   b. testing bath water with thermometer before use
   c. avoiding use of heating pads and hot water bottles
5. do not hurry; allow ample time for all activities.

11.d. The client will state signs and symptoms to report to the health care provider.

11.d. Instruct client to report the following signs and symptoms:
1. increased weakness and fatigue
2. development of or increased shortness of breath
3. chest pain
4. persistent headache, dizziness, or lightheadedness
5. increased or persistent epigastric pain, heartburn, indigestion, or nausea
6. progressive loss of sensation or motor function
7. increasing loss of memory, difficulty concentrating or making decisions, or behavior changes
8. cracked, painful lips and/or tongue.

11.e. The client will verbalize an understanding of and a plan for adhering to recommended follow-up care including activity level and future appointments with health care provider and for laboratory studies.

11.e.1. Reinforce the importance of keeping follow-up appointments with health care provider and for laboratory studies.
2. Reinforce the need to adhere to planned rest periods and avoid strenuous activity until anemia has improved.
3. Implement measures to improve client compliance:
a. include significant others in teaching sessions if possible
b. encourage questions and allow time for reinforcement and clarification of information provided
c. provide written instructions on future appointments with health care provider, medications prescribed, diet therapy, signs and symptoms to report, and future laboratory studies.

# Splenectomy

Splenectomy is the surgical removal of the spleen. The most common indication for the surgery is rupture of the spleen. Causes of rupture include trauma to the spleen, accidental tearing of the splenic capsule during surgery on nearby organs, and softening of or damage to the spleen as a result of disease (e.g. infectious mononucleosis). A splenectomy may also be indicated if the spleen is removing excessive quantities of platelets, erythrocytes, or granulocytes from the circulation (hypersplenism). Conditions associated with hypersplenism include hairy cell leukemia, idiopathic thrombocytopenia purpura, Felty's syndrome, thalassemia major, and sickle cell disease. Additionally, splenectomy may be the treatment of choice for splenic aneurysm, cysts, and neoplasm. When feasible, a partial splenectomy or splenic autotransplantation (transplantation of a small portion of the spleen into another area of the abdomen) is performed so that some of the spleen's immunological function is maintained.

**This care plan focuses on the adult client hospitalized with a suspected splenic rupture resulting from trauma.** Preoperatively, goals of care are to prevent hypovolemic shock and prepare the client for surgery. Postoperative goals of care are to maintain comfort, prevent complications, and educate the client regarding follow-up care.

## DIAGNOSTIC TESTS

Computed tomography (CT)
Ultrasonography

## DISCHARGE CRITERIA

Prior to discharge, the client will:

- have surgical pain controlled
- have no signs and symptoms of complications
- identify appropriate safety measures to follow because of increased risk for infection
- state signs and symptoms to report to the health care provider
- verbalize an understanding of and a plan for adhering to recommended follow-up care including future appointments with health care provider, medications prescribed, wound care, and activity level.

## NURSING/COLLABORATIVE DIAGNOSES



**See Standardized Preoperative and Postoperative Care Plans for additional diagnoses.**

## PREOPERATIVE

**Use in conjunction with the Standardized Preoperative Care Plan.**

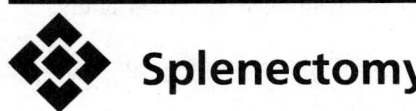

**1. COLLABORATIVE DIAGNOSIS:** **Potential complication: hypovolemic shock**

related to excessive blood loss associated with trauma to the spleen (the spleen is a highly vascular organ).

| Desired Outcome | Nursing Actions and ***Selected Purposes/Rationales*** |
|---|---|
| 1. The client will not develop hypovolemic shock as evidenced by:<br>a. usual mental status<br>b. stable vital signs<br>c. skin warm, dry, and usual color<br>d. palpable peripheral pulses<br>e. urine output at least 30 ml/hour. | 1.a. Assess for and report:<br>1. signs and symptoms of splenic rupture (e.g. left upper abdominal pain and tenderness, generalized abdominal pain, pain in left shoulder [a result of diaphragmatic irritation and referred to as Kehr's sign])<br>2. declining RBC, Hct, and Hb levels<br>3. signs and symptoms of hypovolemic shock:<br>a. restlessness, agitation, confusion<br>b. significant decrease in B/P<br>c. postural hypotension<br>d. rapid, thready pulse<br>e. rapid respirations<br>f. cool, moist skin<br>g. pallor, cyanosis<br>h. diminished or absent peripheral pulses<br>i. urine output less than 30 ml/hour.<br>b. Administer blood products and/or volume expanders if ordered *to prevent hypovolemic shock.*<br>c. If signs and symptoms of hypovolemic shock occur:<br>1. continue to administer blood products and/or volume expanders as ordered<br>2. place client flat in bed with legs elevated unless contraindicated<br>3. monitor vital signs frequently<br>4. administer oxygen as ordered<br>5. prepare client for splenectomy (surgery may need to be performed before scheduled time)<br>6. provide emotional support to client and significant others. |

## POSTOPERATIVE

**Use in conjunction with the Standardized Postoperative Care Plan.**

**1. NURSING DIAGNOSIS:** **High risk for infection**

related to decreased resistance to infection associated with removal of the spleen (the macrophages and lymphocytes in the spleen are responsible for phagocytizing infectious organisms and producing antibodies).

| Desired Outcome | Nursing Actions and ***Selected Purposes/Rationales*** |
|---|---|
| 1. The client will remain free of infection as evidenced by:<br>a. absence of fever and chills | 1.a. Assess for and report signs and symptoms of infection:<br>1. elevated temperature<br>2. chills<br>3. increased pulse<br>4. abnormal breath sounds |

| Desired Outcome | Nursing Actions and ***Selected Purposes/Rationales*** |
|---|---|
| b. pulse within normal limits<br>c. normal breath sounds<br>d. voiding clear urine without complaints of frequency, urgency, and burning<br>e. absence of heat, redness, swelling, and unusual drainage in any area<br>f. no further increase in WBC count or significant change in differential<br>g. negative results of cultured specimens. | 5. cloudy, foul-smelling urine<br>6. complaints of frequency, urgency, or burning when urinating<br>7. presence of WBCs, bacteria, and/or nitrites in urine<br>8. heat, redness, swelling, or unusual drainage in any area<br>9. WBC count that continues to increase and/or a significant change in differential (a transient leukocytosis is expected for 1-2 weeks after surgery).<br>b. Obtain specimens (e.g. wound, urine, vaginal, mouth, sputum, blood) for culture as ordered. Report positive results.<br>c. Implement measures *to prevent infection:*<br>1. maintain a fluid intake of at least 2500 ml/day unless contraindicated<br>2. use good handwashing technique and encourage client to do the same<br>3. maintain meticulous aseptic technique during all invasive procedures (e.g. catheterizations, venous and arterial punctures, injections)<br>4. change intravenous tubings and solutions and rotate insertion sites according to hospital policy<br>5. protect client from others with infection and instruct him/her to continue this after discharge<br>6. perform actions to maintain an adequate nutritional status (see Standardized Postoperative Care Plan, Nursing Diagnosis 5, action d [p. 118])<br>7. reinforce importance of good oral hygiene<br>8. perform actions *to prevent stasis of respiratory secretions* (e.g. assist client to turn, cough, and deep breathe; increase activity as allowed and tolerated)<br>9. perform actions to prevent urinary retention (e.g. instruct client to urinate when the urge is first felt, promote relaxation during voiding attempts, administer bethanechol as ordered) *in order to prevent urinary stasis*<br>10. perform actions *to prevent the introduction of microorganisms into the urinary tract* (e.g. assist client with perineal care as needed, instruct and assist female client to wipe from front to back after urinating and defecating, maintain sterile technique during urinary catheterization)<br>11. perform actions *to prevent wound infection* (e.g. maintain aseptic technique during wound care, instruct client to avoid touching wound, maintain patency of wound drain)<br>12. administer antimicrobials if ordered. |

## 2. COLLABORATIVE DIAGNOSES:

### Potential complications:

a. **pancreatitis** related to trauma to the pancreas during surgery;
b. **subphrenic abscess** related to suppuration in the surgical area and increased susceptibility to infection;
c. **thromboembolism** related to:
   1. hypercoagulability associated with:
      a. increase in the number of circulating erythrocytes and platelets (occurs because the spleen is no longer available to destroy the cells that are old or damaged and to store blood [usually stores 150-300 ml of blood including about 30% of the platelet mass])
      b. increased release of tissue thromboplastin into the blood (occurs as a result of trauma from the injury and surgery)
   2. venous stasis associated with decreased activity, fluid volume deficit, and abdominal distention (the distended intestine can put pressure on the abdominal vessels)

3. decreased fibrinolytic activity (occurs in response to trauma from the injury and surgery)
4. trauma to vein walls during surgery;

d. **postsplenectomy sepsis** related to decreased resistance to infection.

| Desired Outcomes | Nursing Actions and ***Selected Purposes/Rationales*** |
|---|---|
| 2.a. The client will experience resolution of pancreatitis if it occurs as evidenced by:<br>1. gradual resolution of abdominal pain<br>2. temperature declining toward normal<br>3. stable B/P and pulse<br>4. serum amylase and lipase levels declining toward normal<br>5. renal amylase/creatinine clearance ratio returning toward normal<br>6. WBC count declining toward normal. | 2.a.1. Assess for and report signs and symptoms of pancreatitis (e.g. extension of abdominal pain to back, increased midepigastric or left upper quadrant pain, increase in temperature, hypotension, tachycardia, elevated serum amylase and lipase levels).<br>2. Collect a timed (usually 2-hour) urine specimen if ordered. Report an elevated renal amylase/creatinine clearance ratio.<br>3. Monitor WBC counts. Report levels that increase or fail to decline toward normal.<br>4. If signs and symptoms of pancreatitis occur:<br>a. assist client to assume position of greatest comfort (e.g. side-lying, sitting with trunk and knees flexed, sitting and leaning forward)<br>b. maintain food and fluid restrictions as ordered<br>c. insert nasogastric tube and maintain suction as ordered *(removal of gastric secretions reduces pancreatic stimulation)*<br>d. administer the following medications if ordered:<br>1. analgesics<br>2. antacids and/or histamine$_2$ receptor antagonists (e.g. famotidine, ranitidine, cimetidine) *to decrease the acidity of gastric contents and thereby reduce stimulation of the pancreas (when acidic gastric contents enter the duodenum and jejunum, secretin is released; secretin stimulates pancreatic secretion)*<br>e. refer to Care Plan on Pancreatitis for additional care measures. |
| 2.b. The client will experience resolution of a subphrenic abscess if it develops as evidenced by:<br>1. decrease in abdominal pain<br>2. temperature declining toward normal<br>3. WBC count declining toward normal. | 2.b.1. Assess for and report signs and symptoms of a subphrenic abscess (e.g. increased, persistent abdominal pain; increase in temperature and pulse rate).<br>2. Monitor WBC count and report levels that increase or fail to decline toward normal.<br>3. If signs and symptoms of subphrenic abscess occur:<br>a. administer antimicrobials if ordered<br>b. prepare client for surgical intervention (e.g. incision and drainage of abscess) if planned<br>c. assess for and report signs and symptoms of peritonitis (e.g. tense, rigid abdomen; increased severity of abdominal pain; rebound tenderness; continued diminished or absent bowel sounds; nausea; vomiting; further increase in temperature; tachycardia, tachypnea; hypotension)<br>d. provide emotional support to client and significant others. |
| 2.c. The client will not experience signs and symptoms of a deep vein thrombus or pulmonary embolism (see Standardized Postoperative Care Plan, Collaborative Diagnosis 19, outcomes c.1 and 2 [pp. 132-133], for outcome criteria). | 2.c.1. Refer to Standardized Postoperative Nursing Care Plan, Collaborative Diagnosis 19, actions c.1 and 2 (pp. 132-133), for measures related to assessment, prevention, and treatment of a deep vein thrombus and pulmonary embolism.<br>2. Assess for and report increasing abdominal distention and pain *(may indicate portal vein or mesenteric venous thrombus)*. |

| Desired Outcomes | Nursing Actions and ***Selected Purposes/Rationales*** |
|---|---|
| 2.d. The client will not experience postsplenectomy sepsis as evidenced by:<br>1. absence of nausea, vomiting, and headache<br>2. usual mental status<br>3. stable vital signs. | 2.d.1. Assess for and report signs and symptoms of postsplenectomy sepsis (e.g. nausea, vomiting, headache, confusion, hypotension, tachycardia, tachypnea). Be aware that client's condition can progress to shock, coma, and death within 12-24 hours of the onset of symptoms.<br>2. Implement measures *to reduce the risk for postsplenectomy sepsis:*<br>a. perform actions to prevent infection (see Postoperative Nursing Diagnosis 1, action c)<br>b. assess for and immediately report signs and symptoms of infection (see Postoperative Nursing Diagnosis 1, action a) *so that orders for treatment can be obtained and initiated promptly (a mild infection can develop into sepsis within hours).*<br>3. If signs and symptoms of postsplenectomy sepsis occur:<br>a. maintain intravenous fluid therapy as ordered<br>b. monitor vital signs frequently<br>c. obtain cultures from all possible sites of infection (e.g. urine, infusion sites, wound, blood, sputum) as ordered<br>d. administer antimicrobials as ordered<br>e. prepare client for transfer to intensive care unit and insertion of hemodynamic monitoring devices (e.g. central venous catheter, intra-arterial catheter) if planned<br>f. provide emotional support to client and significant others. |

## 3. NURSING DIAGNOSIS: Knowledge deficit

regarding follow-up care.

| Desired Outcomes | Nursing Actions and ***Selected Purposes/Rationales*** |
|---|---|
| 3.a. The client will identify appropriate safety measures to follow because of increased risk for infection. | 3.a.1. Explain to client that he/she is more prone to infection because the rest of the lymphoid system cannot completely compensate for the loss of the spleen.<br>2. Instruct client to:<br>a. continue to adhere to measures to prevent infection (see Standardized Postoperative Care Plan, Nursing Diagnosis 21, action a [p. 135])<br>b. consult health care provider about receiving vaccinations to reduce the risk of pneumonia and influenza<br>c. inform all health care providers of being asplenic so that prophylactic antimicrobials can be started before any dental work, invasive diagnostic procedure, or surgery is performed<br>d. carry an identification card and wear a Medic-Alert tag identifying self as being asplenic and at increased risk for infection. |
| 3.b. The client will state signs and symptoms to report to the health care provider. | 3.b.1. Refer to Standardized Postoperative Care Plan, Nursing Diagnosis 21, action c (p. 135), for signs and symptoms to report to the health care provider.<br>2. Instruct client to report these additional signs and symptoms:<br>a. nausea, vomiting, headache, and/or confusion (could indicate postsplenectomy sepsis)<br>b. any febrile illness<br>c. any minor infection. |

| | |
|---|---|
| 3.c. The client will verbalize an understanding of and a plan for adhering to recommended follow-up care including future appointments with health care provider, medications prescribed, wound care, and activity level. | 3.c. Refer to Standardized Postoperative Care Plan, Nursing Diagnosis 21 (pp. 135-136), for routine postoperative instructions and measures to improve client compliance. |

UNIT

# XIV

# *Nursing Care of the Client with Disturbances of the Gastrointestinal Tract*

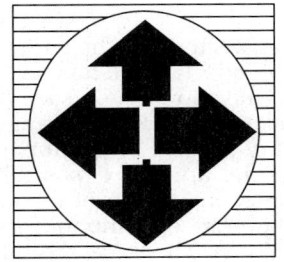

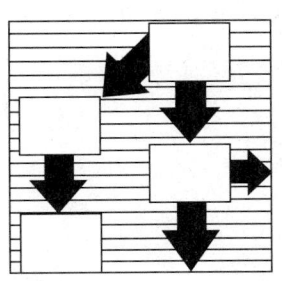

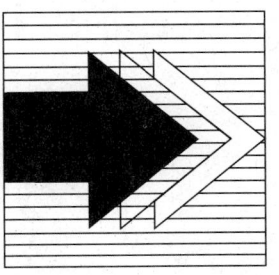

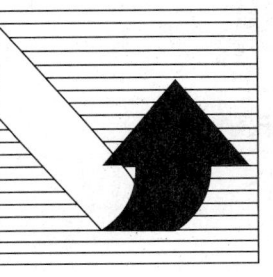

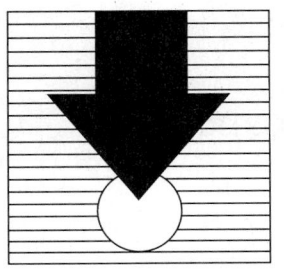

# Appendectomy

An appendectomy is the surgical removal of the vermiform appendix (a small tubular projection of unknown function at the end of the cecum just below the ileocecal valve). It is performed to treat appendicitis which occurs as a result of kinking of the appendix; ulceration of the mucosa of the appendix (possibly due to a virus); or obstruction of the lumen of the appendix by a fecalith, parasites, tumor, or lymphoid hyperplasia (can occur with infections). The increased intraluminal pressure in the appendix that occurs as a result of obstruction and/or inflammation eventually exceeds venous pressure. This results in a decreased blood supply to the area with new or increased mucosal ulceration and possible bacterial invasion. Infection causes further inflammation which leads to increased ischemia. If untreated, the appendix will rupture and peritonitis will result.

**This care plan focuses on the adult client with suspected appendicitis who is hospitalized for a possible appendectomy.** Preoperative goals of care are to reduce fear and anxiety, control discomfort, and prevent rupture of the appendix. The goals of postoperative care are to maintain comfort, prevent complications, and educate the client regarding follow-up care.

## DIAGNOSTIC TESTS

White blood cell (WBC) count and differential
Ultrasonography
Computed tomography (CT)
Abdominal x-ray
Urinalysis

## DISCHARGE CRITERIA

Prior to discharge, the client will:

- have no signs and symptoms of complications
- state signs and symptoms to report to the health care provider
- verbalize an understanding of and a plan for adhering to recommended follow-up care including future appointments with health care provider, medications prescribed, activity level, and wound care.

## NURSING/COLLABORATIVE DIAGNOSES

**Preoperative**

1. Pain: abdominal (particularly in the periumbilical area or right lower quadrant)△ *589*
2. Altered comfort: nausea and vomiting△ *589*
3. Hyperthermia△ *590*
4. Potential complication: peritonitis△ *590*

**Postoperative**

1. Potential complications:
   a. abscess formation
   b. peritonitis△ *591*
2. Knowledge deficit△ *592*

**See Standardized Preoperative and Postoperative Care Plans for additional diagnoses.**

## PREOPERATIVE

**Use in conjunction with the Standardized Preoperative Care Plan.**

**1. NURSING DIAGNOSIS: Pain: abdominal (particularly in the periumbilical area or right lower quadrant)**

related to stretching of the appendix associated with obstruction and inflammation of the appendix and subsequent irritation of the peritoneum (occurs with extension of the inflammatory process).

| Desired Outcome | Nursing Actions and ***Selected Purposes/Rationales*** |
|---|---|
| 1. The client will experience diminished abdominal pain as evidenced by:<br>a. verbalization of reduction of pain<br>b. relaxed facial expression and body positioning<br>c. stable vital signs. | 1.a. Determine how client usually responds to pain.<br>b. Assess client's perception of pain including location, intensity, and type. Use a numerical scale to rate intensity.<br>c. Assess for nonverbal signs of pain (e.g. wrinkled brow, guarding or rubbing of abdomen, clenched fists, reluctance to move, restlessness, diaphoresis, facial pallor, increased B/P, tachycardia).<br>d. Assess for factors that seem to aggravate and alleviate pain.<br>e. Implement measures *to reduce abdominal pain:*<br>1. perform actions *to reduce fear and anxiety about the pain experience* (e.g. assure client that his/her need for pain relief will be met once a definitive diagnosis is made)<br>2. apply ice pack to painful area if ordered *in order to reduce inflammation*<br>3. assist client to assume a comfortable position (e.g. side-lying with right knee flexed)<br>4. administer analgesics if ordered (analgesics may be held until the diagnosis is established).<br>f. Consult physician if above measures fail to provide adequate pain relief. |

**2. NURSING DIAGNOSIS: Altered comfort: nausea and vomiting**

related to stimulation of the vomiting center associated with:

a. stimulation of the afferent vagal and/or sympathetic pathways resulting from visceral irritation associated with inflammation of the appendix and abdominal distention (can result from decreased gastrointestinal motility);
b. cortical stimulation resulting from pain and stress.

| Desired Outcome | Nursing Actions and ***Selected Purposes/Rationales*** |
|---|---|
| 2. The client will experience relief of nausea and vomiting as evidenced by:<br>a. verbalization of relief of nausea<br>b. absence of vomiting. | 2.a. Assess client for nausea and vomiting.<br>b. Implement measures *to reduce nausea and vomiting:*<br>1. perform actions to reduce abdominal pain (see Preoperative Nursing Diagnosis 1, action e)<br>2. perform actions to reduce fear and anxiety (see Standardized Preoperative Care Plan, Nursing Diagnosis 1, action c [p. 109])<br>3. eliminate noxious sights and odors from the environment *(noxious stimuli cause cortical stimulation of the vomiting center)*<br>4. encourage client to take deep, slow breaths when nauseated<br>5. encourage client to change positions slowly *(rapid movement stimulates the afferent vestibulocerebellar pathway with resultant stimulation of the chemoreceptor trigger zone)*<br>6. provide oral hygiene every 2 hours and after each emesis |

| Desired Outcome | Nursing Actions and ***Selected Purposes/Rationales*** |
|---|---|
| | 7. maintain food and fluid restrictions as ordered<br>8. administer antiemetics if ordered.<br>c. If above measures fail to control nausea and vomiting:<br>1. consult physician<br>2. be prepared to insert a nasogastric tube and maintain suction as ordered. |

## 3. NURSING DIAGNOSIS: Hyperthermia

related to stimulation of the thermoregulatory center in the hypothalamus by endogenous pyrogens that are released in an infectious process.

| Desired Outcome | Nursing Actions and ***Selected Purposes/Rationales*** |
|---|---|
| 3. The client will experience resolution of hyperthermia as evidenced by:<br>a. skin usual temperature and color<br>b. pulse rate between 60-100 beats/minute<br>c. respirations 14-20/minute<br>d. normal body temperature. | 3.a. Assess for signs and symptoms of hyperthermia (e.g. warm, flushed skin; tachycardia; tachypnea; elevated temperature).<br>b. Implement measures *to reduce fever:*<br>1. administer tepid sponge bath and/or apply cool cloths to groin and axillae<br>2. administer the following if ordered:<br>a. antipyretics<br>b. antimicrobials *to resolve the infectious process.*<br>c. Consult physician if temperature remains higher than 38.5° C. |

## 4. COLLABORATIVE DIAGNOSIS: Potential complication: peritonitis

related to release of intestinal contents into the peritoneal cavity associated with rupture of the appendix.

| Desired Outcome | Nursing Actions and ***Selected Purposes/Rationales*** |
|---|---|
| 4. The client will not develop peritonitis as evidenced by:<br>a. no further increase in temperature<br>b. soft, nondistended abdomen<br>c. no increase in abdominal pain and tenderness, nausea, and vomiting<br>d. normal bowel sounds<br>e. stable vital signs | 4.a. Assess for and report signs and symptoms of peritonitis (e.g. further increase in temperature; tense, rigid abdomen; increase in severity of abdominal pain; rebound tenderness; increased nausea and vomiting; diminished or absent bowel sounds; tachycardia; tachypnea; hypotension).<br>b. Monitor WBC counts. Report increasing levels.<br>c. Implement measures *to prevent rupture of the appendix and subsequent peritonitis:*<br>1. perform actions *to prevent a further increase in intraluminal pressure:*<br>a. maintain food and fluid restrictions as ordered<br>b. insert a nasogastric tube and maintain suction if ordered<br>c. do not administer an enema<br>2. avoid use of laxatives *(may cause excessive peristalsis)*<br>3. do not apply heat to abdomen *(may speed up the suppurative process and precipitate rupture).* |

f. no further increase in WBC count.

d. If signs and symptoms of peritonitis occur:
   1. withhold all food and fluid as ordered
   2. place client on bed rest in a semi-Fowler's position *to assist in pooling or localizing gastrointestinal contents in the pelvis rather than under the diaphragm*
   3. insert nasogastric tube and maintain suction as ordered
   4. administer antimicrobials if ordered
   5. administer intravenous fluids and/or blood volume expanders if ordered *to prevent or treat shock (can result from the increased capillary permeability that occurs with inflammation and the subsequent escape of protein, fluid, and electrolytes from the vascular space into the peritoneal cavity)*
   6. provide emotional support to client and significant others.

## POSTOPERATIVE

**Use in conjunction with the Standardized Postoperative Care Plan.**

### 1. COLLABORATIVE DIAGNOSES:

**Potential complications:**

a. **abscess formation** related to suppuration in the inflamed or infected area;
b. **peritonitis** related to entrance of pathogens/irritants into peritoneal cavity associated with wound infection, leakage from an abscess, and/or release of intestinal contents into the peritoneal cavity resulting from preoperative or intraoperative rupture of the appendix and leakage of suture lines postoperatively.

| Desired Outcomes | Nursing Actions and ***Selected Purposes/Rationales*** |
|---|---|
| 1.a. The client will experience resolution of an abscess if it occurs as evidenced by:<br>1. temperature declining toward normal<br>2. absence of abdominal cramping<br>3. gradual resolution of abdominal pain<br>4. WBC count declining toward normal. | 1.a.1. Assess for and report signs and symptoms of abscess formation (e.g. increase in temperature, abdominal cramping, increased or more constant abdominal pain, further increase in WBC count).<br>2. If signs and symptoms of an abscess occur:<br>a. prepare client for rectal exam and/or abdominal ultrasonography *to determine location of abscess*<br>b. administer antimicrobials if ordered<br>c. prepare client for surgical drainage of the abscess if planned<br>d. provide emotional support to client and significant others. |
| 1.b. The client will not develop or will have resolution of peritonitis as evidenced by:<br>1. gradual resolution of abdominal pain<br>2. soft, nondistended abdomen<br>3. temperature | 1.b.1. Refer to Preoperative Collaborative Diagnosis 4, actions a and d, for measures related to assessment and treatment of peritonitis.<br>2. Monitor WBC counts. Report levels that increase or fail to return to normal.<br>3. Implement measures *to prevent peritonitis:*<br>a. perform actions to treat an abscess if it occurs (see action a.2 in this diagnosis)<br>b. perform actions *to maintain patency of wound drain(s) if present in order to prevent increased pressure on the suture line:*<br>1. keep tubing free of kinks |

| Desired Outcomes | Nursing Actions and ***Selected Purposes/Rationales*** |
|---|---|
| declining toward normal<br>4. stable vital signs<br>5. gradual return of normal bowel sounds<br>6. WBC count declining toward normal. | 2. empty collection device as often as necessary<br>3. maintain suction as ordered<br>c. perform actions *to prevent inadvertent removal of wound drain(s) if present:*<br>1. use caution when changing dressings surrounding drain(s)<br>2. provide extension tubing if necessary *to enable client to move without placing tension on the drain(s)*<br>3. instruct client not to pull on drain(s) and drainage tubing<br>d. maintain aseptic technique during dressing changes and wound care<br>e. keep abdominal dressing clean and dry<br>f. administer antimicrobials if ordered. |

## 2. NURSING DIAGNOSIS: Knowledge deficit

regarding follow-up care.

| Desired Outcomes | Nursing Actions and ***Selected Purposes/Rationales*** |
|---|---|
| 2.a. The client will state signs and symptoms to report to the health care provider. | 2.a. Refer to Standardized Postoperative Care Plan, Nursing Diagnosis 21, action c (p. 135), for signs and symptoms to report to the health care provider. |
| 2.b. The client will verbalize an understanding of and a plan for adhering to recommended follow-up care including future appointments with health care provider, medications prescribed, activity level, and wound care. | 2.b. Refer to Standardized Postoperative Care Plan, Nursing Diagnosis 21 (pp. 135-136), for routine postoperative instructions and measures to improve client compliance. |

# Bowel Diversion: Ileostomy

An ileostomy is the diversion of the ileum from the abdominal cavity through an opening created in the abdominal wall. It may be performed following abdominal trauma or to treat conditions such as familial polyposis, intestinal cancer, and, most commonly, inflammatory bowel disease that is refractory to conservative management. An ileostomy can be temporary or permanent.

A temporary ileostomy is usually established to allow the bowel to heal following traumatic abdominal injury or to permit healing of a newly constructed ileoanal reservoir. The ileoanal reservoir or pouch is a treatment option for some persons with chronic ulcerative colitis or familial polyposis. In the initial surgery, the diseased portion of the intestine is removed, a temporary loop ileostomy is performed, and a pouch or reservoir is created in the rectal area using a portion of the ileum. After 2-4 months, the ileostomy is closed and intestinal continuity is established between the remaining intestine and the ileoanal pouch.

There are 2 types of permanent ileostomies. The conventional type (end ileostomy, Brooke ileostomy) is the most common one. The ileostomy is made by bringing a portion of the terminal ileum through an opening created in the abdominal wall, usually the right lower quadrant. The ileostomy drains intermittently but because it cannot be regulated, a collection device needs to be worn over the stoma at all times. Another type of permanent ileal diversion is the continent ileostomy in which the terminal ileum is used to construct an intra-abdominal reservoir (Kock pouch). Initially, the reservoir drains via a catheter that is placed in the stoma and through the surgically constructed one-way valve. After the surgical area heals, the catheter is removed and the reservoir only needs to be drained periodically using a catheter. The type of permanent ileostomy constructed depends on the client's age, underlying disease process, and preference and expertise of the surgeon. A proctocolectomy (removal of the colon and rectum) may be done at the same time as a permanent ileostomy to treat the disease process or to prevent future bowel changes that could occur with recurrent inflammatory bowel disease or cancer of the colon. If a proctocolectomy is not performed, the rectum stays intact and the rectal stump is sutured across the top. This internal pouch (Hartmann's pouch) secretes mucus that is expelled via the anus.

**This care plan focuses on the adult client with inflammatory bowel disease hospitalized for bowel diversion with creation of a permanent ileostomy.** Preoperatively, goals of care are to reduce fear and anxiety and begin to prepare the client for the changes in body image and function. The postoperative goals of care are to maintain integrity of the peristomal and perianal skin, prevent complications, facilitate psychological adjustment to the ileostomy, and educate the client regarding follow-up care.

## DIAGNOSTIC TESTS

**Refer to Care Plan on Inflammatory Bowel Disease.**

## DISCHARGE CRITERIA

Prior to discharge, the client will:

- have no signs and symptoms of complications
- verbalize a basic understanding of the anatomical changes that have occurred as a result of the bowel diversion
- identify ways to maintain fluid and electrolyte balance
- verbalize ways to maintain an optimal nutritional status
- identify methods of controlling odor and sound associated with ostomy drainage and gas
- demonstrate the ability to change the pouch system, maintain integrity of the peristomal and perianal skin, and maintain adequate stomal circulation and integrity
- demonstrate proper use and care of ostomy products
- demonstrate proper techniques for draining and irrigating a continent ileostomy if present
- identify ways to prevent and treat blockage of the stoma
- state signs and symptoms to report to the health care provider
- share thoughts and feelings about the effect of altered bowel function on self-concept and life style

- identify appropriate community resources that can assist with home management and adjustment to changes resulting from the bowel diversion
- verbalize an understanding of and a plan for adhering to recommended follow-up care including future appointments with health care provider, wound care, activity level, and medications prescribed.

## NURSING/COLLABORATIVE DIAGNOSES



**See Care Plan on Inflammatory Bowel Disease and the Standardized Preoperative and Postoperative Care Plans for additional diagnoses.**

## PREOPERATIVE

**Use in conjunction with the Care Plan on Inflammatory Bowel Disease and the Standardized Preoperative Care Plan.**

### 1. NURSING DIAGNOSIS: Anxiety

related to:
a. unfamiliar environment and separation from significant others;
b. anticipated loss of control, effects of anesthesia, and postoperative discomfort;
c. lack of understanding of diagnostic tests, surgical procedure, and care required for the ileostomy;
d. economic factors associated with hospitalization;
e. anticipated changes in body image and functioning and effects of ileostomy on future life style;
f. ability to independently perform ileostomy care following discharge.

| Desired Outcome | Nursing Actions and ***Selected Purposes/Rationales*** |
|---|---|
| 1. The client will experience a reduction in anxiety (see Standardized Preoperative Care Plan, Nursing Diagnosis 1 [pp. 108-109], for outcome criteria). | 1.a. Refer to Standardized Preoperative Care Plan, Nursing Diagnosis 1 (pp. 108-109), for measures related to assessment and reduction of fear and anxiety.<br>b. Implement additional measures *to reduce fear and anxiety:*<br>1. show client a diagram of how the ileostomy is accomplished and a picture of a stoma *so that he/she will know what to expect*<br>2. explain that every attempt will be made to place the stoma in an area that will be easily accessible for self-care and enable the appliance to lie flat and be unobtrusive (the tentative stoma site is mapped out preoperatively by the physician and/or enterostomal therapist)<br>3. assure client that the stoma has no pain receptors and will not be painful when touched<br>4. initiate and reinforce the teaching outlined in Preoperative Nursing Diagnosis 2<br>5. stress that usual effluent (intestinal drainage from the stoma) has a weakly acidic or sweet odor that is not unpleasant<br>6. assure client that ostomy pouches are odorproof and available in sizes that fit various body contours<br>7. emphasize the positive effects of the surgery on future life style (the discomfort and frequent diarrhea associated with inflammatory bowel disease and the side effects of medications such as corticosteroids usually have had a disruptive effect on many aspects of the client's life)<br>8. if desired by client, arrange for a visit with a person of similar age and same sex who has successfully adjusted to his/her ileostomy. |

## 2. NURSING DIAGNOSIS: Knowledge deficit

regarding hospital routines associated with the surgery, physical preparation for the bowel diversion, sensations that normally occur following surgery and anesthesia, and postoperative care and management of the ileostomy.

| Desired Outcomes | Nursing Actions and ***Selected Purposes/Rationales*** |
|---|---|
| 2.a. The client will verbalize an understanding of usual preoperative care and postoperative sensations and care. | 2.a.1. Refer to Standardized Preoperative Care Plan, Nursing Diagnosis 4, actions a.1-4 (pp. 111-112), for information to include in preoperative teaching.<br>2. Provide additional information regarding specific preoperative and postoperative care for clients having a bowel diversion with ileostomy:<br>a. explain the preoperative bowel preparation (e.g. low-residue or clear liquid diet, enemas, antimicrobial therapy)<br>b. if proctocolectomy is planned, inform client that:<br>1. a perineal wound drain will be present after surgery<br>2. occasional feelings of pressure in the perineal area are expected after surgery and that these will subside as edema decreases<br>c. if a continent ileostomy is planned, inform client that:<br>1. a temporary drainage catheter will be in the stoma for at least 10-14 days after surgery and an external collection device will need to be worn during this time<br>2. an intermittent catheter clamping regimen will begin 10-14 days after surgery and catheter irrigations will be done periodically; when the surgical area has healed, the catheter will be removed and one will be inserted for short periods (usually 10-15 minutes) at scheduled intervals to drain the internal reservoir<br>d. offer basic information regarding postoperative care of the stoma and |

| Desired Outcomes | Nursing Actions and ***Selected Purposes/Rationales*** |
|---|---|
| | peristomal and perianal skin, ways to control intestinal gas and odor of the effluent, and use of various types of ostomy products.<br>3. Allow time for questions and clarification of information provided. |
| 2.b. The client will demonstrate the ability to perform activities designed to prevent postoperative complications. | 2.b. Refer to Standardized Preoperative Care Plan, Nursing Diagnosis 4, action b (p. 112), for instructions on ways to prevent postoperative complications. |
| 2.c. The client will verbalize an understanding of the appearance, function, and management of the ileostomy. | 2.c.1. Arrange for a visit with an enterostomal therapist if available.<br>2. Reinforce information provided by physician and/or enterostomal therapist about the appearance and function of the ileostomy:<br>a. the stoma will be pinkish-red and moist (similar in appearance to healthy oral mucous membrane)<br>b. the stoma will shrink in size as edema resolves during the first 6 weeks after surgery (final stoma height is usually 1.5-2.5 cm [about ½-1 inch] from the skin surface)<br>c. slight bleeding of the stoma is expected when it is wiped with tissue<br>d. for the first day or two after surgery, the stoma will drain a small amount of clear to white, blood-tinged fluid containing some mucus; after a few days, the color of the drainage will change to green and then to light to medium brown as the diet progresses<br>e. when the ileostomy begins to function (usually 2-3 days after surgery), the drainage will be watery and high-volume (up to 1-2 liters/day) but within a couple of weeks the amount will begin to decrease (expected amount of output after 2-3 months is 400-800 ml/day) and develop a thicker, paste-like consistency.<br>3. Allow client to see and handle ostomy products he/she will be using in the immediate postoperative period. Provide a pouch clamp so that client can practice putting it on and taking it off of an empty pouch.<br>4. Encourage client to try wearing a pouch system partially filled with water in order to experience how it feels and to validate if planned stoma site will be adequate for successful adhesion of the pouch.<br>5. Allow time for questions and clarification of information provided. |

## POSTOPERATIVE

**Use in conjunction with the Standardized Postoperative Care Plan.**

### 1. NURSING/COLLABORATIVE DIAGNOSIS:

**Altered fluid and electrolyte balance:**

a. **fluid volume deficit, hypokalemia, hypomagnesemia, and hypochloremia** related to excessive loss of fluid and electrolytes associated with vomiting, nasogastric tube drainage, and/or ileostomy output (effluent contains fluid and electrolytes that would normally be absorbed throughout the intestine);
b. **metabolic alkalosis** related to excessive loss of hydrochloric acid associated with vomiting and nasogastric tube drainage;
c. **metabolic acidosis** related to loss of bicarbonate ions associated with excessive ileostomy output (effluent contains bicarbonate ions that would normally be absorbed throughout the large intestine).

| Desired Outcome | Nursing Actions and ***Selected Purposes/Rationales*** |
|---|---|
| 1. The client will maintain fluid and electrolyte balance as evidenced by:<br>a. normal skin turgor<br>b. moist mucous membranes<br>c. stable weight<br>d. B/P and pulse within normal range for client and stable with position change<br>e. small vein filling time less than 3-5 seconds<br>f. balanced intake and output within 48 hours after surgery<br>g. urine specific gravity within normal range<br>h. return of peristalsis within expected time<br>i. usual mental status<br>j. absence of cardiac arrhythmias, twitching, muscle weakness, paresthesias, dizziness, headache, nausea, and vomiting<br>k. negative Chvostek's and Trousseau's signs<br>l. BUN, serum electrolytes, and blood gases within normal range. | 1.a. Assess for and report:<br>1. signs and symptoms of fluid volume deficit, hypokalemia, hypochloremia, and metabolic alkalosis (see Standardized Postoperative Care Plan, Nursing Diagnosis 4, action a.1 [p. 116])<br>2. signs and symptoms of hypomagnesemia (e.g. anxiousness, irritability, cardiac arrhythmias, hyperactive reflexes, positive Chvostek's and Trousseau's signs, seizures)<br>3. signs and symptoms of metabolic acidosis (e.g. drowsiness; disorientation; stupor; rapid, deep respirations; headache; nausea; vomiting; cardiac arrhythmias)<br>4. elevated BUN and abnormal serum electrolyte and blood gas values.<br>b. Monitor for and report excessive ileostomy output (after bowel activity returns, expected output may be as high as 2000 ml/day and then in 10-14 days it should begin to gradually decrease to 400-800 ml/day within 2-3 months).<br>c. Refer to Standardized Postoperative Care Plan, Nursing Diagnosis 4, action a.3 (pp. 116-117), for measures to prevent or treat fluid and electrolyte imbalances.<br>d. Implement additional measures *to prevent or treat fluid and electrolyte imbalances:*<br>1. administer additional electrolyte replacements (e.g. magnesium sulfate, sodium bicarbonate) if ordered<br>2. as diet advances, perform actions *to prevent or control excessive ileostomy output:*<br>a. instruct client to avoid excessive intake of foods/fluids that may cause diarrhea (e.g. most raw fruits; highly spiced or extremely hot or cold items; coffee; fried, greasy foods; rich sauces)<br>b. encourage intake of bulk-forming foods (e.g. applesauce, bananas, boiled rice)<br>c. administer antidiarrheal agents (e.g. loperamide, diphenoxylate hydrochloride) if ordered.<br>e. Consult physician if signs and symptoms of fluid and electrolyte imbalances persist or worsen. |

## 2. NURSING DIAGNOSIS: Altered nutrition: less than body requirements

related to:

a. decreased oral intake associated with prescribed dietary modifications; discomfort; fatigue; nausea; and fear of excessive ileostomy output, gas, and/or odor;
b. inadequate nutritional replacement therapy;
c. loss of nutrients associated with vomiting and excessive ileostomy output;
d. decreased absorption of nutrients associated with loss of absorptive surface of the bowel resulting from resection;
e. increased nutritional needs associated with the increased metabolic rate that occurs during wound healing.

| Desired Outcome | Nursing Actions and ***Selected Purposes/Rationales*** |
|---|---|
| 2. The client will maintain an adequate nutritional status (see Standardized | 2.a. Refer to Standardized Postoperative Care Plan, Nursing Diagnosis 5 (p. 118), for measures related to assessment and maintenance of an adequate nutritional status. |

| Desired Outcome | Nursing Actions and ***Selected Purposes/Rationales*** |
|---|---|
| Postoperative Care Plan, Nursing Diagnosis 5 [p. 118], for outcome criteria). | b. Implement additional measures *to maintain an adequate nutritional status:*<br>1. perform actions to prevent or control excessive ileostomy output (see Postoperative Nursing Diagnosis 1, action d.2)<br>2. reinforce methods of reducing gas and odor of effluent (see Postoperative Nursing Diagnosis 6, actions g and h) *so that this concern does not cause client to limit oral intake*<br>3. instruct client to chew food thoroughly *in order to enhance digestion and subsequent absorption of nutrients.* |

## 3. NURSING DIAGNOSIS: Actual/High risk for impaired skin integrity

related to:

a. disruption of skin associated with the surgical procedure;
b. delayed wound healing associated with decreased nutritional status and inadequate blood supply to wound area;
c. irritation of skin associated with:
   1. contact with wound drainage, ileostomy output (effluent is rich in proteolytic enzymes), soap residue and perspiration under the pouch, and/or mucous drainage from the anus (occurs if rectum was left intact)
   2. frequent and/or improper removal of tape and adhesives or other substances used to secure pouch to the skin
   3. aggressive cleansing of peristomal area
   4. sensitivity to tape, pouch material, and/or substances used to secure pouch to the skin (e.g. adhesive disk, skin barrier, skin cement, adhesive spray)
   5. pressure from drainage tubes, appliance belt, and/or pouch drainage valve or clamp.

| Desired Outcomes | Nursing Actions and ***Selected Purposes/Rationales*** |
|---|---|
| 3.a. The client will experience normal healing of surgical wounds (see Standardized Postoperative Care Plan, Nursing Diagnosis 9, outcome a [p. 122], for outcome criteria). | 3.a. Refer to Standardized Postoperative Care Plan, Nursing Diagnosis 9, action a (pp. 122-123), for measures related to assessment and promotion of wound healing. |
| 3.b. The client will maintain skin integrity as evidenced by:<br>1. absence of redness and irritation<br>2. no skin breakdown. | 3.b.1. Inspect skin areas that are in contact with wound drainage, tape, and drainage tubings for signs of irritation and breakdown.<br>2. Assess for signs and symptoms of:<br>a. peristomal irritation or breakdown (e.g. redness or excoriation of peristomal skin, complaints of itching or burning of peristomal skin; inability to keep pouch on)<br>b. perianal irritation or breakdown (e.g. redness or excoriation of perianal skin, complaints of itching or burning in perianal area).<br>3. Refer to Standardized Postoperative Care Plan, Nursing Diagnosis 9, actions b.2 and 3 (p. 123), for measures to prevent and treat skin irritation and breakdown resulting from wound drainage, tape, and drainage tubings.<br>4. Implement measures *to prevent peristomal irritation and breakdown:*<br>a. remove hair from peristomal skin using an electric razor *to help* |

*maintain an adequate seal and to reduce irritation when the pouch system is removed*

b. patch test all products that will come in contact with the skin (e.g. sealant, barrier, adhesive, solvent) before initial use; do not use products that cause redness, rash, itching, or burning
c. do not change entire pouch system more frequently than every 3-7 days unless stoma size changes, pouch seal is leaking, or client complains of itching or burning of the peristomal skin
d. use a 2-piece pouch system (e.g. faceplate and pouch, wafer with flange and pouch) during the initial postoperative period *so that pouch can be removed to assess the stoma without having to remove the faceplate or wafer from the skin*
e. perform actions *to reduce peristomal irritation during removal of the pouch system:*
   1. place drops of warm water or mild solvent where the pouch system adheres to the skin *in order to facilitate removal;* allow time for adhesive to loosen before removing pouch system from the skin
   2. remove pouch system gently and in direction of hair growth; hold skin adjacent to faceplate taut *to provide support as it is removed* and push down on skin slightly *to facilitate separation*
f. perform actions *to prevent effluent from coming in contact with the skin when changing the pouch system or pouch:*
   1. perform the change when the ostomy is least active (e.g. upon awakening in the morning, before meals, 2-4 hours after eating, before retiring at night)
   2. place a "wick" (rolled gauze pad), vaginal tampon, or tissue on the stoma opening when the pouch system or pouch is off
g. cleanse peristomal skin thoroughly with a no-residue skin cleanser (e.g. Peri-Wash, UniWash) or mild soap and water, rinse completely, and pat dry; use tepid rather that hot water *to prevent burns*
h. apply skin sealant to the clean, dry peristomal skin before applying adhesive or barrier *so that when the pouch system is removed, the adhesive lifts the sealant rather than the top layer of the skin*
i. if using skin adhesive, allow it to dry thoroughly before applying the pouch system *in order to prevent chemical burns*
j. always use a skin barrier (e.g. Stomahesive, ReliaSeal) *to protect skin from the proteolytic enzymes that are in the effluent*
k. perform actions *to prevent effluent from contacting the skin when the pouch system is on:*
   1. measure the diameter of the stoma; cut skin barrier the same size as stoma and select a pouch with an opening that is not more than 0.3 cm (⅛ inch) larger than the stoma (it may be necessary to create a pattern to use for cutting barrier and pouch openings if stoma has an irregular shape and cannot be measured using appliance manufacturer's standard measuring guide)
   2. instruct and assist client to remeasure the stoma frequently during the first 6 weeks after surgery and to alter size of skin barrier and pouch openings as stomal edema decreases
   3. implement measures *to achieve an adequate seal:*
      a. avoid use of oil-based ointments or lotions on peristomal skin *(these can interfere with adequate adhesive bonding)*
      b. follow manufacturer's instructions carefully when applying skin products and pouch system
      c. use products such as ostomy paste (e.g. Stomahesive paste, Premium paste) to fill in irregularities around stoma site (e.g. body folds, scars) before applying pouch system
      d. apply firm pressure and remove air pockets when applying

Desired Outcomes | Nursing Actions and ***Selected Purposes/Rationales***

pouch system; place client in a supine position *to increase tautness of skin surface during application*

e. use products with a flexible or convex backing if needed

4. empty pouch when it is ⅓ to ½ full of effluent or inflated with gas *(a heavy or inflated pouch can cause a disruption in the pouch seal)*
5. position pouch so gravity flow facilitates drainage away from stoma and skin
6. cleanse bottom of drainable pouch after emptying it and close it securely *to prevent leakage*
7. use drainable pouch, 2-piece pouch system, and/or pouch with release valve if gas is a problem; never puncture or cut the pouch to release gas *because effluent can seep out of the opening*

l. if a belted pouch system is used, fasten the belt so that 2 fingers can slip easily between belt and skin *to prevent excessive pressure on skin*

m. instruct and assist client to check pouch periodically to ensure that clamp or valve is not placing pressure on the skin.

5. Implement measures *to prevent perianal irritation and breakdown:*
   a. keep perianal area clean and dry
   b. instruct client to perform perineal exercises (e.g. relaxing and tightening perineal and gluteal muscles) regularly *to increase anal sphincter tone and reduce the risk of mucus leakage*
   c. place absorbent pads in client's underwear if needed and change pads when they become damp
   d. expose perianal area to air for 20-30 minutes 1-4 times/day if possible
   e. apply petroleum-based ointment to perianal area as ordered *to protect skin.*
6. If signs and symptoms of peristomal and/or perianal skin irritation or breakdown occur:
   a. cleanse areas gently with warm water
   b. avoid use of any product that can further irritate affected skin (e.g. karaya powder, plain tincture of benzoin)
   c. perform skin care according to physician's order, enterostomal therapist's instructions, or hospital procedure
   d. apply corticosteroid cream or spray if ordered *to reduce inflammation associated with severe skin reactions*
   e. consult physician and/or enterostomal therapist if:
      1. areas of irritation or breakdown worsen or do not improve within 48 hours
      2. signs and symptoms of infection (e.g. elevated temperature; redness, warmth, and edema around area of breakdown; unusual drainage from site) are present.

## 4. COLLABORATIVE DIAGNOSES:

### Potential complications:

a. **peritonitis** related to:
   1. wound infection (preoperative immunosuppression associated with long-term corticosteroid use and/or malnutrition results in increased risk for infection)
   2. leakage of bowel contents into the peritoneum during surgery or postoperatively associated with failure of the surgical anastomosis or retraction of the peristomal skin and/or stoma (retraction can occur with slippage of the sutures or shrinkage of the supporting tissues);

b. **stoma changes:**
   1. **necrosis** related to intraoperative and/or postoperative interruption of blood supply to the stoma associated with trauma or edema
   2. **excessive bleeding** related to irritation associated with aggressive cleansing and/or improper fit or application of pouch system
   3. **prolapse** related to loss of integrity of the sutures or weak abdominal muscles around the stoma;

c. **stomal obstruction** related to edema and/or blockage by food.

| Desired Outcomes | Nursing Actions and ***Selected Purposes/Rationales*** |
|---|---|

**Desired Outcomes**

4.a. The client will not develop peritonitis as evidenced by:
1. gradual resolution of abdominal pain
2. soft, nondistended abdomen
3. temperature declining toward normal
4. stable vital signs
5. absence of nausea and vomiting
6. gradual return of normal bowel sounds
7. WBC count declining toward normal.

**Nursing Actions and *Selected Purposes/Rationales***

4.a.1. Assess for and report signs and symptoms of peritonitis (e.g. increase in severity of abdominal pain; generalized abdominal pain; rebound tenderness; tense, rigid abdomen; increase in temperature; tachycardia; tachypnea; hypotension; nausea; vomiting; continued absent or diminished bowel sounds).

2. Monitor WBC counts. Report levels that increase or fail to decline toward normal.

3. Implement measures *to prevent peritonitis:*
   a. perform actions to prevent and treat wound infection (see Standardized Postoperative Care Plan, Nursing Diagnosis 16, actions b.4 and 5 [p. 129])
   b. perform actions *to prevent distention of the intestine and resultant strain on and leakage from the suture line:*
      1. implement measures to prevent obstruction of the stoma (see action c.2 in this diagnosis)
      2. instruct client to avoid activities that can cause air swallowing (e.g. chewing gum, sucking on hard candy, smoking)
   c. perform actions *to maintain patency of wound drain if present:*
      1. keep tubing free of kinks
      2. empty collection device as often as necessary
      3. maintain suction as ordered
   d. perform actions *to prevent inadvertent removal of wound drain if present:*
      1. use caution when changing dressings surrounding drain
      2. provide extension tubing if necessary *to enable client to move without placing tension on drain*
      3. instruct client not to pull on drain and drainage tubing
   e. if client has a continent ileostomy:
      1. perform actions *to prevent distention of the reservoir and resultant strain on and leakage from the suture line:*
         a. maintain stomal catheter suction as ordered *to keep the reservoir decompressed*
         b. when suction is discontinued, keep stomal catheter and drainage bag below level of reservoir *to maintain gravity drainage*
         c. keep stomal catheter free of kinks and dependent loops
         d. irrigate the reservoir as ordered using only the prescribed amount of irrigating solution (usually 20-30 ml of normal saline)
      2. do not reposition the stomal catheter *(repositioning may damage or disrupt the suture line)*
   f. if peristomal skin is retracted, perform wound care as ordered *to facilitate the formation of granulation tissue in retracted area*
   g. prepare client for surgical reconstruction of stoma if planned (may be indicated if retraction of stoma occurs).

4. If signs and symptoms of peritonitis occur:
   a. withhold all food and fluid as ordered
   b. place client on bed rest in a semi-Fowler's position *to assist in pooling*

| Desired Outcomes | Nursing Actions and ***Selected Purposes/Rationales*** |
|---|---|
| | *or localizing gastrointestinal contents in the pelvis rather than under the diaphragm*<br>c. insert a nasogastric tube if not already present and maintain suction as ordered<br>d. administer antimicrobials if ordered<br>e. administer intravenous fluids and/or blood volume expanders if ordered *to prevent or treat shock (can result from the increased capillary permeability that occurs with inflammation and the subsequent escape of protein, fluid, and electrolytes from the vascular space into the peritoneal cavity)*<br>f. prepare client for surgical intervention (e.g. repair of site of anastomosis, stomal reconstruction) if planned<br>g. provide emotional support to client and significant others. |
| 4.b. The client will maintain adequate stomal circulation and integrity as evidenced by:<br>1. medium pink to red stomal coloring<br>2. expected stomal height<br>3. absence of excessive bleeding and increasing edema of the stoma. | 4.b.1. Assess for and report signs and symptoms of impaired stomal circulation and/or integrity (e.g. pale, dark red, blue-black, or purple color of stoma; increased height of stoma; increased stomal edema or bleeding). Use only clear pouches and a 2-piece pouch system during the immediate postoperative period *to allow easy visibility of stoma.*<br>2. Implement measures *to maintain adequate stomal circulation and integrity:*<br>a. ensure that openings of the adhesive disk, skin barrier, faceplate, and/or pouch are not too small and carefully center stoma in the openings<br>b. apply pouch system securely *to prevent it from slipping and irritating or shearing stoma*<br>c. always cleanse stoma gently using a soft cloth, gauze, or tissue.<br>3. If signs and symptoms of impaired stomal circulation and/or integrity occur:<br>a. perform wound care as ordered<br>b. prepare client for surgical revision of stoma if planned<br>c. provide emotional support to client and significant others. |
| 4.c. The client will not develop stomal obstruction as evidenced by:<br>1. expected amount and consistency of ileostomy output<br>2. no complaints of abdominal cramping, nausea, or increased feeling of fullness<br>3. absence of vomiting. | 4.c.1. Assess for and report signs and symptoms of stomal obstruction:<br>a. less than expected amount of ileostomy output (after return of peristalsis, output may be as high as 2000 ml/day and will gradually decrease to about 400-800 ml/day)<br>b. change in effluent consistency from a thicker consistency to a thin, watery liquid (postoperatively, effluent gradually becomes thicker; a return to thin, watery consistency may indicate blockage of stoma)<br>c. complaints of abdominal cramping, nausea, or increased feeling of fullness<br>d. vomiting.<br>2. Implement measures *to prevent stomal obstruction:*<br>a. if a continent ileostomy was constructed:<br>1. perform actions *to prevent inadvertent removal of stomal catheter* (e.g. secure tubing, instruct client not to pull on catheter)<br>2. perform actions *to maintain patency of stomal catheter* (e.g. avoid kinks in tubing, irrigate as ordered)<br>b. administer oral medications crushed and mixed in water or in liquid or chewable form *(undigested pills can block stoma)*<br>c. when oral intake is allowed, perform actions *to prevent blockage of stoma by food:*<br>1. slowly advance diet as ordered and tolerated<br>2. instruct client to chew food thoroughly<br>3. instruct client to avoid or eat only small amounts of foods that are high in fiber *(fibrous foods absorb water in the intestinal tract)* and/or are hard to digest (e.g. popcorn, coconut, raw vegetables, fruits with seeds, bean sprouts, bamboo shoots, whole kernel corn, potato skins, bran, nuts, fruit skins). |

3. If food blockage occurs, implement measures *to aid in evacuation of effluent:*
   a. perform actions *to stimulate peristalsis* (e.g. drink hot tea)
   b. perform actions *to reduce abdominal muscle tension* (e.g. administer analgesic if indicated, apply warm compresses to abdomen unless contraindicated, encourage participation in relaxing activities such as reading and listening to music)
   c. perform actions *to break up or shift food blockage:*
      1. encourage fluid intake unless contraindicated
      2. instruct and assist client to assume a knee-chest position
      3. gently massage peristomal area unless contraindicated
      4. assist with or gently perform digital dilation of stoma if ordered
   d. irrigate the ileostomy if ordered.
4. If signs and symptoms of stomal obstruction persist:
   a. withhold all food and fluid as ordered
   b. maintain intravenous therapy as ordered *to prevent fluid volume deficit and increased viscosity of effluent*
   c. insert a nasogastric tube and maintain suction as ordered
   d. prepare client for surgical intervention to remove obstruction if indicated
   e. provide emotional support to client and significant others.

## 5. NURSING DIAGNOSIS: Altered sexuality patterns

related to feelings of loss of femininity/masculinity and sexual attractiveness, fear of offensive odor or leakage of effluent from the pouch, fear of rejection by partner, discomfort associated with surgical incision, and depression.

| Desired Outcome | Nursing Actions and ***Selected Purposes/Rationales*** |
|---|---|
| 5. The client will demonstrate beginning adjustment to effects of the ileostomy on sexuality as evidenced by:<br>a. verbalization of a perception of self as sexually acceptable and adequate<br>b. maintenance of relationship with significant other. | 5.a. Assess for signs and symptoms of altered sexuality patterns (e.g. verbalization of sexual concerns, alteration in relationship with significant other).<br>b. Implement measures *to facilitate client's adjustment to effects of changes in appearance and body functioning on his/her sexuality:*<br>1. facilitate communication between client and his/her partner; focus on feelings the couple share and assist them to identify changes which may affect their sexual relationship<br>2. perform actions to facilitate psychological adjustment to the changes that have occurred (see Postoperative Nursing Diagnoses 6, actions d-t; 7, action c; and 8, action b)<br>3. instruct client in ways *to reduce risk for leakage of effluent during sexual activity:*<br>a. empty pouch or drain reservoir before sexual activity<br>b. secure pouch system seal with tape for added security<br>4. if client is concerned about odor, instruct him/her to:<br>a. shower or bathe before sexual activity<br>b. use a pouch deodorizer<br>c. use cologne or perfume if desired<br>d. keep room well ventilated<br>5. if client is concerned about the presence of the stoma and pouch system, discuss the possibility of:<br>a. using opaque or patterned pouches or decorative pouch covers<br>b. wearing underwear with the crotch removed (for females), boxer |

| Desired Outcome | Nursing Actions and ***Selected Purposes/Rationales*** |
|---|---|
| | shorts (for males), or wide elastic wrap or cummerbund around abdomen during sexual activity |
| | 6. if client is concerned that operative site discomfort will interfere with usual sexual activity: |
| | a. assure him/her that discomfort is temporary and will diminish as the incision heals |
| | b. encourage use of positions that decrease pressure on surgical site (e.g. side-lying) until the incision heals |
| | 7. discuss ways to be creative in expressing sexuality (e.g. massage, fantasies, cuddling) |
| | 8. perform actions *to decrease possibility of rejection by partner:* |
| | a. assist the partner to acknowledge feelings about changes in the client |
| | b. if appropriate, involve partner in ostomy care *to facilitate adjustment to the changes in client's appearance and body functioning* |
| | 9. arrange for uninterrupted privacy during hospital stay if desired by the couple |
| | 10. encourage client to obtain written information regarding sexual activity and sexuality from the United Ostomy Association and from manufacturers of ostomy products |
| | 11. include partner in above discussions and encourage his/her continued support of the client. |
| | c. Consult physician if counseling appears indicated. |

## 6. NURSING DIAGNOSIS: Self-concept disturbance*

related to:
a. change in appearance associated with presence of stoma and pouch;
b. embarrassment associated with sound and odor resulting from gas and effluent;
c. dependence (usually temporary) on others for assistance with ostomy management;
d. loss of control over bowel elimination (will be temporary if continent ileostomy was constructed or permanent if client has conventional ileostomy).

*This diagnostic label includes the nursing diagnoses of body image disturbance, self-esteem disturbance, and altered role performance.

| Desired Outcome | Nursing Actions and ***Selected Purposes/Rationales*** |
|---|---|
| 6. The client will demonstrate beginning adaptation to changes in appearance and body functioning as evidenced by: | 6.a. Assess for signs and symptoms of a self-concept disturbance (e.g. verbal or nonverbal cues denoting a negative response to change in body functioning or appearance such as denial of or preoccupation with changes that have occurred, refusal to look at or touch stoma, or withdrawal from significant others). |
| a. verbalization of feelings of self-worth and sexual adequacy | b. Determine the meaning of changes in appearance and body functioning to the client by encouraging him/her to verbalize feelings and by noting nonverbal responses to the changes experienced. |
| b. maintenance of relationships with significant others | c. Implement measures to facilitate the grieving process (see Postoperative Nursing Diagnosis 8, action b). |
| | d. Implement measures *to assist client to increase self-esteem* (e.g. limit negative self-assessment, encourage positive comments about self, assist to |

c. active participation in activities of daily living
d. active interest in personal appearance
e. willingness to pursue usual roles and participate in social activities
f. verbalization of a beginning plan for integrating changes in appearance and bowel elimination into life style.

identify strengths, give positive feedback about accomplishments and behaviors that are indicative of high self-esteem).

e. Reinforce actions to assist client to cope with the effects of the ileostomy (see Postoperative Nursing Diagnosis 7, action c).
f. Implement measures to facilitate client's adjustment to the effects of changes in appearance and body functioning on his/her sexuality (see Postoperative Nursing Diagnosis 5, action b).
g. Instruct client in ways *to reduce gas formation:*
   1. avoid activities that can cause air swallowing (e.g. chewing gum, sucking on hard candy, smoking)
   2. limit intake of carbonated beverages and gas-producing foods (e.g. cabbage, onions, beans, radishes, cucumbers, sauerkraut).
h. Instruct client in and assist with measures *to reduce odor resulting from ileostomy drainage and/or gas:*
   1. use a pouch deodorizer and/or a pouch with a deodorizing flatus filter
   2. empty pouch regularly; rinse inside of pouch and clean off any effluent before closing pouch
   3. drain the reservoir of continent ileostomy as ordered to reduce possibility of leakage
   4. use a disposable pouch and change it regularly or clean reusable pouch thoroughly
   5. empty or change pouch in a well-ventilated area; use room deodorizers if desired
   6. perform actions to achieve an adequate pouch seal (see Postoperative Nursing Diagnosis 3, action b.4.k.3)
   7. limit intake of foods that cause effluent to have a strong odor (e.g. onions, garlic, fish, eggs, cheese, asparagus, broccoli)
   8. increase intake of foods/fluids that control odor (e.g. spinach, parsley, yogurt, buttermilk)
   9. take charcoal tablets or antiflatulents such as bismuth subgallate or bismuth subcarbonate (the bismuth combines with sulfur in intestine to reduce odor)
   10. change bed linens and clothing promptly if they become soiled.
i. Inform client that the pouch and clothing muffle sounds of bowel activity.
j. Assure client that once the stomal edema and surgical discomfort have resolved, he/she will be able to dress as before with minor, if any, modifications.
k. Show client and significant others some of the attractive ostomy products that are available (e.g. opaque or patterned pouches, pouch covers).
l. Assist client with usual grooming and makeup habits if necessary.
m. Promote activities which require client to confront the body changes that have occurred (e.g. active participation in ostomy care). Be aware that integration of the change in body image does not usually occur until 2-6 months after the actual physical change has occurred.
n. Demonstrate acceptance of client using techniques such as touch and frequent visits. Encourage significant others to do the same.
o. Assess for and support behaviors suggesting positive adaptation to changes that have occurred (e.g. willingness to care for ileostomy, compliance with treatment plan, verbalization of feelings of self-worth, maintenance of relationships with significant others).
p. Encourage significant others to allow client to do what he/she is able *so that independence can be reestablished and/or self-esteem redeveloped.*
q. Assist client's and significant others' adjustment by listening, facilitating communication, and providing information.
r. Encourage visits and support from significant others.
s. Encourage client to pursue usual roles and interests and to continue involvement in social activities.
t. Provide information about and encourage utilization of community

| Desired Outcome | Nursing Actions and ***Selected Purposes/Rationales*** |
|---|---|
| | agencies and support groups (e.g. ostomy groups; sexual, family, individual, and/or financial counseling).<br>u. Consult physician about psychological counseling if client desires or if he/she seems unwilling or unable to adapt to changes resulting from the ileostomy. |

## 7. NURSING DIAGNOSIS: Ineffective individual coping

related to fear, anxiety, change in usual method of bowel elimination, difficulty performing ileostomy care or incorporating the care into life style, fear of rejection by others, and inadequate support system.

| Desired Outcome | Nursing Actions and ***Selected Purposes/Rationales*** |
|---|---|
| 7. The client will demonstrate the use of effective coping skills as evidenced by:<br>a. verbalization of ability to cope with the ileostomy<br>b. utilization of appropriate problem-solving techniques<br>c. willingness to participate in treatment plan and meet basic needs<br>d. absence of destructive behavior toward self and others<br>e. appropriate use of defense mechanisms<br>f. recognition and utilization of available support systems. | 7.a. Assess for and report signs and symptoms of ineffective individual coping (e.g. verbalization of inability to cope; inability to ask for help, problem solve, or meet basic needs; reluctance to participate in treatment plan; destructive behavior toward self or others; inappropriate use of defense mechanisms; inability to meet role expectations).<br>b. Assess client's perception of current situation including precipitating factors and effectiveness of coping mechanisms.<br>c. Implement measures *to promote effective coping:*<br>1. allow time for client to adjust to the ileostomy; if frequent diarrhea and cramping had limited client's activities before surgery, stress positive effects ileostomy will have on life style<br>2. assist client to recognize and manage inappropriate denial if it is present<br>3. arrange for a visit from a person of similar age and same sex who has successfully adjusted to an ileostomy<br>4. perform actions to reduce fear and anxiety (see Standardized Postoperative Care Plan, Nursing Diagnosis 20, action b [p. 134])<br>5. encourage verbalization about current situation<br>6. assist client to identify personal strengths and resources that can be utilized to facilitate coping with the current situation<br>7. demonstrate acceptance of client but set limits on inappropriate behavior<br>8. create an atmosphere of trust and support<br>9. maintain consistency of approaches and explanations<br>10. do not overload client with information irrelevant to present stage of ostomy management unless client is questioning or expressing an interest<br>11. encourage participation in ostomy care as soon as possible<br>12. use products that client will be using when discharged<br>13. ensure adequate time for and privacy during ostomy care<br>14. include client in planning of care, encourage maximum participation in ostomy care, and allow choices when possible *to enable him/her to maintain a sense of control*<br>15. instruct client in effective problem-solving techniques (e.g. accurate identification of stressors, determination of various options to solve problem)<br>16. assist client to maintain usual daily routines whenever possible<br>17. assist client through methods such as role playing to prepare for negative reactions from others because of ileostomy |

18. instruct client to have extra ostomy products readily available at all times
19. administer antianxiety and/or antidepressant agents if ordered
20. assist client to identify and use available support systems; provide information about available community resources that can assist client and significant others in coping with effects of the ileostomy (e.g. stress management classes, local ostomy support groups, United Ostomy Association, counseling services)
21. discuss with significant others the fear of rejection client may be experiencing and encourage their continued support
22. encourage client to share with significant others the kind of support that would be most beneficial (e.g. listening, inspiring hope, providing reassurance and accurate information)
23. support behaviors suggesting positive adaptation to changes (e.g. participation in self-care, verbalization of ability to cope, utilization of effective problem-solving strategies).

d. Consult physician about psychological counseling if appropriate. Initiate a referral if necessary.

## 8. NURSING DIAGNOSIS: Grieving*

related to loss of usual manner of bowel elimination and change in appearance associated with presence of stoma.

*This diagnostic label includes anticipatory grieving and grieving following the actual losses.

| Desired Outcome | Nursing Actions and ***Selected Purposes/Rationales*** |
|---|---|
| 8. The client will demonstrate beginning progression through the grieving process as evidenced by:<br>a. verbalization of feelings about the ileostomy<br>b. expression of grief<br>c. participation in treatment plan and self-care activities<br>d. utilization of available support systems<br>e. verbalization of a plan for integrating ostomy care into life style. | 8.a. Assess for signs and symptoms of grieving (e.g. change in eating habits, inability to concentrate, insomnia, anger, noncompliance, withdrawal from significant others, denial of loss). Be aware that client's response to a loss will be affected by factors such as previous experience with loss, age, developmental stage, available support systems, spiritual and cultural background, current health status, and significance of the loss.<br>b. Implement measures *to facilitate the grieving process:*<br>1. assist client to acknowledge losses experienced *so grief work can begin;* assess for factors that may hinder and facilitate acknowledgment<br>2. discuss the grieving process and assist client to accept the phases of grieving as an expected response to actual and/or anticipated losses<br>3. allow time for client to progress through the phases of grieving (phases vary among theorists but progress from shock and alarm to acceptance); be aware that not every phase is expressed by all individuals, that recurrence of phases is common, and that the grieving process may take months to years<br>4. provide an atmosphere of care and concern (e.g. provide privacy, be available and nonjudgmental, display empathy and respect) *so client will feel free to verbalize feelings*<br>5. perform actions *to promote trust* (e.g. answer questions honestly, provide requested information)<br>6. encourage the verbal expression of anger and sadness about the losses experienced; recognize displacement of anger and assist client to see the actual cause of angry feelings and resentment; establish limits on abusive behavior if demonstrated<br>7. encourage client to express his/her feelings in whatever ways are comfortable (e.g. writing, drawing, conversation) |

| Desired Outcome | Nursing Actions and ***Selected Purposes/Rationales*** |
|---|---|
| | 8. perform actions to promote effective coping (see Postoperative Nursing Diagnosis 7, action c)<br>9. support realistic hope about effects of the bowel diversion on his/her life (e.g. increased comfort)<br>10. support behaviors suggesting successful grief work (e.g. verbalizing feelings about ileostomy, focusing on ways to adapt to changes in bowel elimination and presence of stoma, learning ostomy care)<br>11. explain the phases of the grieving process to significant others; encourage their support and understanding<br>12. facilitate communication between the client and significant others; be aware that they may be in different phases of the grieving process<br>13. provide information regarding counseling services and support groups that might assist client in working through grief<br>14. arrange for a visit from clergy if desired by client.<br>c. Consult physician regarding referral for counseling if signs of dysfunctional grieving (e.g. persistent denial of losses, excessive anger or sadness, hysteria, suicidal behaviors) occur. |

## 9. NURSING DIAGNOSIS: Knowledge deficit

regarding follow-up care.

| Desired Outcomes | Nursing Actions and ***Selected Purposes/Rationales*** |
|---|---|
| 9.a. The client will verbalize a basic understanding of the anatomical changes that have occurred as a result of the bowel diversion. | 9.a. Reinforce teaching regarding the anatomical changes that have occurred as a result of the bowel diversion. Use appropriate teaching aids (e.g. pictures, videotapes, anatomical models). |
| 9.b. The client will identify ways to maintain fluid and electrolyte balance. | 9.b. Provide the following instructions on ways to maintain fluid and electrolyte balance:<br>1. instruct client to perform the following actions to prevent excessive ileostomy output:<br>a. avoid excessive intake of foods/liquids that may cause diarrhea (e.g. most raw fruits; extremely hot or cold beverages; highly spiced foods; coffee; fried, greasy foods; rich sauces)<br>b. do not take laxatives or excessive amounts of magnesium-containing antacids<br>c. take antidiarrheal agents as prescribed<br>2. if ileostomy output increases or becomes more watery, instruct client to:<br>a. increase intake of bulk-forming foods (e.g. applesauce, bananas, boiled rice)<br>b. increase intake of foods/liquids such as fruit juices, Gatorade, potatoes, tea, bananas, and bouillon to maintain electrolyte balance<br>c. drink a mixture of baking soda and water (¼-½ teaspoon baking soda and 1 cup of water) if prescribed by physician to maintain acid-base balance. |
| 9.c. The client will verbalize ways to maintain an optimal nutritional status. | 9.c. Provide instructions regarding ways to maintain an optimal nutritional status:<br>1. reinforce ways to prevent excessive ileostomy output (see action b.1 in this diagnosis) |

2. stress the need to chew food thoroughly in order to enhance digestion and subsequent absorption of nutrients
3. stress the importance of taking vitamins and minerals as prescribed.

| | |
|---|---|
| 9.d. The client will identify methods of controlling odor and sound associated with ostomy drainage and gas. | 9.d.1. Reinforce instructions regarding ways to reduce gas formation and odor associated with ileostomy drainage and gas (see Postoperative Nursing Diagnosis 6, actions g and h).<br>2. Inform client that the ostomy pouch and clothing will muffle the sound. |
| 9.e. The client will demonstrate the ability to change the pouch system, maintain integrity of the peristomal and perianal skin, and maintain adequate stomal circulation and integrity. | 9.e.1. Reinforce teaching regarding application of the pouch system, prevention of peristomal and perianal skin irritation and breakdown, and maintenance of adequate stomal circulation and integrity (see Postoperative Nursing Diagnosis 3, actions b.4 and 5 and Collaborative Diagnosis 4, action b.2, for appropriate measures).<br>2. Support client's efforts to decrease odor of effluent and gas but discourage excessive changing and emptying of pouch or pouch system.<br>3. Instruct and assist client to establish a routine time and system for emptying and changing pouch or emptying continent ileostomy in order to reduce risk of leakage of effluent.<br>4. Instruct client to follow special precautions for products used (e.g. inert, moldable skin barriers must be kept in airtight container; skin sealants should be used only on healthy peristomal skin because they can further irritate reddened and excoriated skin).<br>5. Allow time for questions; clarification; practice; and return demonstration of emptying the pouch, changing the pouch system, and performing appropriate stoma and skin care. |
| 9.f. The client will demonstrate proper use and care of ostomy products. | 9.f.1. Instruct client regarding proper use of ostomy products he/she will be using after discharge.<br>2. Discuss recommended methods of storing ostomy products based on manufacturer's recommendations.<br>3. Demonstrate appropriate cleansing techniques. Emphasize importance of:<br>a. rinsing inside of pouch each time it is emptied<br>b. soaking pouch according to manufacturer's instructions and allowing it to dry thoroughly if it is to be reused.<br>4. Instruct client to avoid reusing disposable products and to discard a reusable pouch if it retains an odor after thorough cleansing or if it becomes brittle.<br>5. Provide client with a list of ostomy products he/she is using (include product name, size, and number) and where these supplies can be obtained.<br>6. Allow time for questions, clarification, and return demonstration. |
| 9.g. The client will demonstrate proper techniques for draining and irrigating a continent ileostomy if present. | 9.g.1. Explain the gradual and progressive clamping routine if catheter will be in the stoma of continent ileostomy at time of discharge.<br>2. When the clamping routine is complete, inform client that he/she will be instructed in the correct method of and schedule for stomal catheter insertion (initially the reservoir will need to be drained for 10-15 minutes every 3-4 hours but after about 6 months it may need emptying only 2-3 times/day).<br>3. Demonstrate correct technique for irrigating a continent ileostomy. Caution client to use only the prescribed amount of irrigant (usually 20-30 ml) in order to avoid overdistending and damaging reservoir.<br>4. Allow time for questions, clarification, and return demonstration of clamping and irrigating techniques. |
| 9.h. The client will identify ways to prevent and treat blockage of the stoma. | 9.h.1. Instruct client in ways to prevent food from blocking the stoma:<br>a. chew food thoroughly<br>b. avoid or eat only small amounts of foods that are high in fiber and/or hard to digest (e.g. popcorn, coconut, raw vegetables, bean sprouts, bamboo shoots, whole kernel corn, potato skins, fruit with seeds, nuts, fruit skins). |

| Desired Outcomes | Nursing Actions and ***Selected Purposes/Rationales*** |
|---|---|
| | 2. Instruct client to do the following if stoma is blocked:<br>a. apply warm compresses to abdomen or stoma<br>b. participate in relaxing activities (e.g. warm bath, reading)<br>c. attempt to break-up or shift food blockage (e.g. assume a knee-chest position, gently massage peristomal area, irrigate the stoma or gently perform digital dilation of the stoma if prescribed).<br>3. Demonstrate techniques such as massage of abdomen, irrigation of stoma, and digital dilation of stoma if appropriate.<br>4. Allow time for questions, clarification, and return demonstration. |
| 9.i. The client will state signs and symptoms to report to the health care provider. | 9.i.1. Refer to Standardized Postoperative Care Plan, Nursing Diagnosis 21, action c (p. 135), for signs and symptoms to report to the health care provider.<br>2. Instruct client to also report:<br>a. dark red, blue-black, purple, or pale stoma<br>b. change in color, consistency, or odor of effluent that is not readily identified as a response to food or fluid intake<br>c. absence of or persistent increase in ileostomy output<br>d. change in contour of stoma (use diagrams and descriptive terms so client does not confuse decreasing stoma size due to resolving edema with actual stomal retraction)<br>e. excessive bleeding of stoma or bloody drainage from stoma<br>f. difficulty accomplishing ostomy care<br>g. persistent skin irritation<br>h. skin breakdown<br>i. persistent thirst, dry mucous membranes, or decreased urine output (may indicate fluid volume deficit)<br>j. signs and symptoms of low potassium (e.g. irregular pulse, muscle weakness and cramping, nausea, vomiting)<br>k. signs and symptoms of low sodium (e.g. headache, abdominal cramps, fatigue, irritability)<br>l. thin, watery ileostomy output; absence of ileostomy output; unusual foul odor of gas; abdominal distention; and/or nausea and vomiting that does not resolve within 2 hours of implementing measures to relieve stomal blockage<br>m. difficulty draining continent ileostomy<br>n. persistent leakage of effluent from continent ileostomy<br>o. persistent low-grade fever; pain or cramping in pouch area; pain when draining the pouch; and/or watery, high-volume ileostomy output (these signs and symptoms can indicate inflammation of the pouch [pouchitis], which is a long-term complication that can develop in the client with a continent ileostomy)<br>p. difficulty adjusting to changes in appearance and body functioning. |
| 9.j. The client will identify appropriate community resources that can assist with home management and adjustment to changes resulting from the bowel diversion. | 9.j.1. Provide information about community resources that can assist the client and significant others with home management and adjustment to changes resulting from bowel diversion (e.g. local ostomy support groups; community health agencies; enterostomal therapist; home health agencies; financial, individual, and family counseling services).<br>2. Initiate a referral if appropriate. |
| 9.k. The client will verbalize an understanding of and a plan for adhering to recommended follow-up care including future appointments | 9.k.1. Refer to Standardized Postoperative Care Plan, Nursing Diagnosis 21 (pp. 135-136), for routine postoperative instructions and measures to improve client compliance.<br>2. Reinforce physician's instructions regarding activity limitations:<br>a. avoid lifting objects over 10 pounds for at least 6 weeks<br>b. avoid participating in contact sports.<br>3. Explain the rationale for, side effects of, and importance of taking |

with health care provider, wound care, activity level, and medications prescribed.

medications prescribed (e.g. electrolyte supplements, bismuth subcarbonate).

4. Stress the fact that oral medications should be crushed or in liquid, chewable, uncoated, or sugar-coated form rather than enteric-coated tablets or timed-release spansules so absorption can take place before the medication is excreted.

# Gastrectomy

Gastrectomy is the surgical removal of all or part of the stomach. A partial gastrectomy (gastric resection) is performed to treat peptic ulcer disease that continues to be symptomatic despite conservative management. It is also indicated when complications of peptic ulcer disease (e.g. perforation, gastric outlet obstruction, hemorrhage) develop or if ulcerated lesions are believed to be precancerous.

The distal 40-75% of the stomach is removed in a partial gastrectomy. The area excised includes the antrum (which contains the gastrin-secreting cells) and usually a portion of the body of the stomach, which results in the removal of some parietal cells. Gastrointestinal continuity is reestablished by an anastomosis of the remaining stomach to the duodenum (gastroduodenostomy or Billroth I) or jejunum (gastrojejunostomy or Billroth II). A gastrojejunostomy usually involves the removal of a greater portion of the stomach and, in this procedure, the duodenal stump is left intact to preserve the flow of bile and pancreatic juices into the jejunum. A vagotomy is usually performed with a partial gastrectomy to further reduce gastric acid secretion. Truncal vagotomy (resection of each vagal nerve trunk at the level of the esophageal hiatus) is very effective in reducing gastric secretions but, because the denervation is so extensive, it also greatly suppresses gastric motility and impairs normal functioning of the pancreas, gallbladder, and small intestine. Although a partial vagotomy is not quite as effective in reducing gastric secretions, it is often the type performed with a partial gastrectomy because the other effects of a vagotomy are also reduced. A total gastrectomy may be performed to treat cancer of the stomach, which is usually quite advanced when it is diagnosed, and advanced cases of Zollinger-Ellison syndrome. Gastrointestinal continuity is reestablished by an esophagojejunostomy (anastomosis of the esophagus to the jejunum). A total gastrectomy is performed infrequently because it is so difficult to maintain an adequate nutritional status postoperatively.

**This care plan focuses on the adult client with intractable peptic ulcer disease who is hospitalized for a partial gastrectomy.** Preoperatively, the goals of care are to reduce fear and anxiety and prepare the client for the postoperative period. Postoperative goals of care are to maintain comfort, assist the client to maintain an adequate nutritional status, prevent complications, and educate the client regarding follow-up care.

## DIAGNOSTIC TESTS

**Refer to Care Plan on Peptic Ulcer.**

## DISCHARGE CRITERIA

Prior to discharge, the client will:

- have no signs and symptoms of complications
- tolerate prescribed diet
- identify ways to prevent recurrence of peptic ulcers
- verbalize an understanding of ways to maintain an adequate nutritional status
- identify ways to control postvagotomy diarrhea if it occurs
- identify ways to manage dumping syndrome if it occurs
- state signs and symptoms to report to the health care provider
- verbalize an understanding of and a plan for adhering to recommended follow-up care including future appointments with health care provider, medications prescribed, activity level, and wound care.

**NURSING/ COLLABORATIVE DIAGNOSES**

**Postoperative**

1. Altered nutrition: less than body requirements △ *612*
2. Diarrhea △ *613*
3. Potential complications:
   a. peritonitis
   b. afferent loop syndrome
   c. early dumping syndrome
   d. late dumping syndrome (postprandial hypoglycemia) △ *613*
4. Knowledge deficit△ *616*

**See Care Plan on Peptic Ulcer and the Standardized Preoperative and Postoperative Care Plans for additional diagnoses.**

## PREOPERATIVE

**Refer to the Care Plan on Peptic Ulcer and the Standardized Preoperative Care Plan.**

## POSTOPERATIVE

**Use in conjunction with the Standardized Postoperative Care Plan.**

### 1. NURSING DIAGNOSIS: Altered nutrition: less than body requirements

related to:

a. decreased oral intake associated with prescribed dietary modifications, discomfort, fear of experiencing dumping syndrome (especially with a gastrojejunostomy) or diarrhea (following a truncal vagotomy), and early satiety resulting from reduced stomach size;
b. decreased absorption of nutrients associated with impaired digestion resulting from:
   1. decreased gastric acid secretion (occurs with vagotomy and removal of gastrin-secreting cells and parietal cells)
   2. rapid entry of food into small intestine (a result of reduced stomach size and removal of pylorus)
   3. decreased stimulation and secretion of pancreatic juice and bile associated with:
      a. reduction in hydrochloric acid and gastrin secretion (these gastric secretions stimulate pancreatic enzyme secretion and gallbladder contraction)
      b. absence of food moving through the duodenum following gastrojejunostomy (the presence of food in the duodenum causes the release of secretin and cholecystokinin-pancreozymin, which stimulate gallbladder contraction and pancreatic enzyme secretion);
c. decreased absorption of iron associated with bypassing the duodenum if a gastrojejunostomy was performed;
d. inadequate nutritional replacement therapy;
e. loss of nutrients associated with diarrhea;
f. increased nutritional needs associated with the increased metabolic rate that occurs during wound healing.

| Desired Outcome | Nursing Actions and ***Selected Purposes/Rationales*** |
|---|---|
| 1. The client will maintain an adequate nutritional status (see Standardized Postoperative Care Plan, Nursing Diagnosis 5 [p. 118], for outcome criteria). | 1.a. Refer to Standardized Postoperative Care Plan, Nursing Diagnosis 5 (p. 118), for measures related to assessment and maintenance of nutritional status.<br>b. Implement additional measures *to maintain an adequate nutritional status when oral intake is allowed:*<br>1. provide small, frequent meals *to compensate for early satiety*<br>2. instruct client to chew food thoroughly *(small food particles are more easily and completely digested)*<br>3. perform actions to prevent or control postvagotomy diarrhea (see Postoperative Nursing Diagnosis 2, action b) and dumping syndrome (see Postoperative Collaborative Diagnosis 3, actions c.2 and 3) *in order to reduce the client's fear of precipitating these conditions and to promote increased absorption of nutrients*<br>4. administer prescribed vitamin and iron supplements in liquid or chewable form *to ensure maximum absorption.* |

## 2. NURSING DIAGNOSIS: Diarrhea*

related to rapid passage of foods/fluids through the small intestine possibly associated with loss of nervous system regulation of bowel activity.

*Referred to as "postvagotomy diarrhea" and is more likely to occur if a truncal rather than partial vagotomy was performed.

| Desired Outcome | Nursing Actions and ***Selected Purposes/Rationales*** |
|---|---|
| 2. The client will not experience or will have diminished postvagotomy diarrhea as evidenced by:<br>a. passage of formed stool<br>b. no complaints of urgency or abdominal cramping. | 2.a. Assess for and report signs and symptoms of postvagotomy diarrhea (e.g. watery stools, urgency, and abdominal cramping within 2 hours after eating).<br>b. When oral intake is allowed, implement measures *to prevent or control postvagotomy diarrhea:*<br>1. advance diet gradually<br>2. encourage client to eat small rather than large meals<br>3. instruct client to drink fluids between rather than with meals<br>4. administer antidiarrheals (e.g. kaolin-pectin compounds, loperamide, diphenoxylate hydrochloride) if ordered.<br>c. Consult physician if postvagotomy diarrhea persists. |

## 3. COLLABORATIVE DIAGNOSES: Potential complications:

a. **peritonitis** related to:
   1. wound infection
   2. leakage of upper gastrointestinal (UGI) contents into the peritoneal cavity associated with loss of integrity of the suture line at the duodenal stump (with gastrojejunostomy) or the site of anastomosis;

b. **afferent loop syndrome** related to partial obstruction of the duodenal loop associated with factors such as edema or presence of a kink in the efferent jejunal limb after gastrojejunostomy;

c. **early dumping syndrome** related to rapid emptying of hypertonic food into the jejunum especially after a gastrojejunostomy (the bolus of food pulls fluid from the vascular space; this distends the bowel lumen and increases intestinal peristalsis and motility);

d. **late dumping syndrome (postprandial hypoglycemia)** related to rapid emptying of food/fluid high in carbohydrates into the jejunum especially after a gastrojejunostomy (this results in increased absorption of glucose into the blood causing increased release of insulin and subsequent hypoglycemia).

| Desired Outcomes | Nursing Actions and ***Selected Purposes/Rationales*** |
|---|---|
| 3.a. The client will not develop peritonitis as evidenced by:<br>1. gradual resolution of abdominal pain<br>2. soft, nondistended abdomen<br>3. temperature declining toward normal<br>4. stable vital signs<br>5. absence of nausea and vomiting<br>6. gradual return of normal bowel sounds<br>7. WBC count declining toward normal. | 3.a.1. Assess for and report:<br>a. bile in wound drain *(indicates leakage from suture lines)*<br>b. hiccoughs (can occur as a result of distention of remaining stomach; distention increases pressure on the suture lines)<br>c. signs and symptoms of peritonitis (e.g. increase in severity of abdominal pain; generalized abdominal pain; rebound tenderness; tense, rigid abdomen; increase in temperature; tachycardia; tachypnea; hypotension; nausea; vomiting; continued diminished or absent bowel sounds).<br>2. Monitor WBC counts. Report levels that increase or fail to decline toward normal.<br>3. Implement measures *to prevent peritonitis:*<br>a. perform actions to prevent and treat wound infection (see Standardized Postoperative Care Plan, Nursing Diagnosis 16, actions b.4 and 5 [p. 129])<br>b. perform actions *to maintain patency of wound drain if present:*<br>1. keep tubing free of kinks<br>2. empty collection device as often as necessary<br>3. maintain suction as ordered<br>c. perform actions *to prevent inadvertent removal of wound drain if present:*<br>1. use caution when changing dressings surrounding drain<br>2. provide extension tubing if necessary *to enable client to move without placing tension on the drain*<br>3. instruct client not to pull on drain and drainage tubing<br>d. perform actions *to prevent stress on and subsequent leakage from the suture line at site of anastomosis:*<br>1. do not change position of the nasogastric tube unless ordered *(the tube is positioned during surgery and moving it can traumatize the suture line)*<br>2. implement measures to prevent nausea and vomiting (see Standardized Postoperative Care Plan, Nursing Diagnosis 7.B, action 2 [p. 120])<br>3. implement measures *to prevent distention of the remaining portion of the stomach:*<br>a. perform actions to reduce the accumulation of gastrointestinal gas and fluid (see Standardized Postoperative Care Plan, Nursing Diagnosis 7.A, action 3 [pp. 119-120]),<br>b. when oral intake is allowed, progress diet slowly and instruct client to avoid drinking fluids with meals<br>e. perform actions to treat afferent loop syndrome if it occurs (see action b.2 in this diagnosis) *in order to prevent distention of the duodenal stump and subsequently reduce the risk of disruption of the duodenal stump sutures following gastrojejunostomy.*<br>4. If signs and symptoms of peritonitis occur:<br>a. withhold all food and fluid as ordered<br>b. place client on bed rest in a semi-Fowler's position *to assist in pooling or localizing gastrointestinal contents in the pelvis rather than under the diaphragm* |

c. assist physician with insertion of a nasogastric tube if not already present and maintain suction as ordered
d. administer antimicrobials as ordered
e. administer intravenous fluids and/or blood volume expanders if ordered *to prevent or treat shock (can result from the increased capillary permeability that occurs with inflammation and the subsequent escape of protein, fluid, and electrolytes from the vascular space into the peritoneal cavity)*
f. prepare client for surgical intervention (e.g. repair of anastomosis) if planned
g. provide emotional support to client and significant others.

3.b. The client will have resolution of afferent loop syndrome if it occurs as evidenced by:
1. no complaints of intense nausea or epigastric fullness and pain 20-60 minutes after eating
2. no episodes of vomiting bile 20-60 minutes after eating.

3.b.1. Assess for and report signs and symptoms of afferent loop syndrome (e.g. complaints of intense nausea and/or epigastric fullness and pain 20-60 minutes after eating, forceful vomiting of large amounts of bile 20-60 minutes after eating).
2. If signs and symptoms of afferent loop syndrome occur:
a. maintain food and fluid restrictions as ordered
b. assist physician with insertion of a nasogastric tube if not already present and maintain suction as ordered
c. administer antimicrobials as ordered *(infection can develop as a result of stasis of secretions in the afferent loop)*
d. assist with endoscopy if performed
e. prepare client for surgical intervention if obstruction is caused by kinking of the efferent jejunal limb.

3.c. The client will not experience dumping syndrome after eating as evidenced by:
1. no complaints of abdominal fullness or abdominal cramping
2. normal bowel sounds
3. skin dry and usual color
4. absence of palpitations, weakness, dizziness, diarrhea, and tremors
5. usual mental status.

3.c.1. Assess for signs and symptoms of
a. early dumping syndrome (e.g. complaints of abdominal fullness or abdominal cramping, hyperactive bowel sounds, diaphoresis, flushing, palpitations, weakness, dizziness, and/or diarrhea within 1 hour after meals)
b. late dumping syndrome (e.g. anxiety, palpitations, dizziness, weakness, diaphoresis, inability to concentrate, incoordination, tremors, and/or confusion occurring 2-3 hours after meals).
2. Implement measures *to prevent dumping syndrome:*
a. instruct client to avoid intake of simple carbohydrates (e.g. jelly, cake, pie, pudding, candy) *because they are hypertonic and tend to rapidly draw fluid into the intestine and because they are more rapidly absorbed into the blood leading to increased insulin release and subsequent hypoglycemia*
b. encourage intake of foods containing moderate to high amounts of fat and protein *(these foods leave the stomach more slowly and are less hypertonic)*
c. instruct client in ways *to delay gastric emptying:*
   1. eat small, dry meals
   2. eat meals slowly
   3. drink fluids between rather than with meals; avoid fluids for at least 1 hour before and after meals
   4. eat in a semi-recumbent position, then lie down for at least 30 minutes after each meal unless contraindicated.
3. If signs and symptoms of dumping syndrome occur:
a. provide client with a rapid-acting carbohydrate (e.g. orange juice, hard candy, sugar-containing soft drink) or glucose tablets or gel (e.g. Glucotabs, Monogel) *to treat the hypoglycemia that characterizes late dumping syndrome*
b. review dietary management and revise as necessary (e.g. reduce size of meals, reduce sugar intake)
c. administer anticholinergics (e.g. dicyclomine, probanthine) 30 minutes before meals if ordered *to delay gastric emptying*

| Desired Outcomes | Nursing Actions and ***Selected Purposes/Rationales*** |
|---|---|
| | within 6-12 months (if symptoms are not controlled, surgical revision of the gastric outlet may be necessary *to delay gastric emptying*). |

## 4. NURSING DIAGNOSIS: Knowledge deficit

regarding follow-up care.

| Desired Outcomes | Nursing Actions and ***Selected Purposes/Rationales*** |
|---|---|
| 4.a. The client will identify ways to prevent recurrence of peptic ulcers. | 4.a.1. Instruct the client in ways to prevent peptic ulcer recurrence:<br>a. drink decaffeinated or caffeine-free tea and colas rather than those containing caffeine<br>b. avoid drinking coffee and alcohol or drink these beverages only in small amounts immediately following a meal<br>c. avoid intake of any foods and fluids that cause gastric distress<br>d. eat regularly scheduled meals and snacks (recommended frequency and amount will vary depending on the size of the remaining stomach); do not skip meals<br>e. eat slowly and chew food thoroughly<br>f. maintain a calm, relaxed atmosphere at mealtime and whenever possible<br>g. stop smoking<br>h. maintain a balance of physical activity and rest<br>i. avoid stressful situations<br>j. avoid ingestion of medications such as aspirin, aspirin-containing products, and ibuprofen; if it is necessary to take these or other ulcerogenic medications (e.g. corticosteroids, indomethacin), take them with food whenever possible<br>k. take medications (e.g. antacids, histamine$_2$ receptor antagonists) as prescribed.<br>2. Obtain a dietary consult if client needs assistance in planning meals that incorporate recommended dietary modifications.<br>3. Provide information on community resources that can assist the client in making life-style changes (e.g. stress management classes, smoking cessation programs, counseling services). Initiate a referral if indicated. |
| 4.b. The client will verbalize an understanding of ways to maintain an adequate nutritional status. | 4.b.1. Instruct client regarding ways to maintain an adequate nutritional status:<br>a. eat regularly scheduled meals and snacks (recommended frequency and amount will vary depending on the size of the remaining stomach); do not skip meals<br>b. eat slowly and chew food thoroughly to enhance digestion and absorption of nutrients<br>c. continue with actions to prevent or control postvagotomy diarrhea and dumping syndrome (see actions c.3 and 4 and d.3-5 in this diagnosis); contact health care provider if these conditions are not controlled since they can result in excessive loss of nutrients<br>d. take vitamin and iron supplements as prescribed (usually prescribed in liquid or chewable form to ensure maximum absorption).<br>2. Instruct client to adhere to scheduled follow-up blood studies (e.g. Schilling test) to determine need for vitamin $B_{12}$ injections (pernicious anemia can develop years after the surgery as a result of decreased secretion of the intrinsic factor resulting from loss of the gastrin-secreting and parietal cells). |

| | |
|---|---|
| 4.c. The client will identify ways to control postvagotomy diarrhea if it occurs. | 4.c.1. Inform client that episodes of diarrhea may occur if a vagotomy (especially a truncal vagotomy) was performed.<br>2. Explain that postvagotomy diarrhea can be mild or explosive, usually occurs within 2 hours after eating, is episodic (can occur 2-3 times a week for 1-3 days), and is unpredictable (episodes may last 1-2 months and then not recur for weeks or months). Emphasize that if this condition occurs, it usually resolves within a year.<br>3. Instruct client that eating small rather than large meals and drinking liquids between rather than with meals may help prevent postvagotomy diarrhea.<br>4. Provide teaching regarding antidiarrheal medications recommended or prescribed by physician. |
| 4.d. The client will identify ways to manage dumping syndrome if it occurs. | 4.d.1. Reinforce physician's explanation regarding the factors that cause dumping syndrome. Emphasize that if this condition occurs, it usually resolves within 6-12 months.<br>2. Instruct client to be alert for signs and symptoms of:<br>a. early dumping syndrome (e.g. abdominal fullness, abdominal cramping, weakness, dizziness, and/or diarrhea within an hour after eating)<br>b. late dumping syndrome (e.g. anxiety, palpitations, faintness, weakness, sweating, and/or shakiness 2-3 hours after meals).<br>3. Reinforce teaching regarding ways to prevent dumping syndrome (see Postoperative Collaborative Diagnosis 3, action c.2).<br>4. Provide teaching regarding medications prescribed to prevent dumping syndrome (small doses of an anticholinergic agent may need to be taken 30 minutes before meals if symptoms cannot be prevented with above actions).<br>5. Instruct client to drink fluids with high sugar content (e.g. orange juice, sugar-containing soft drinks) or eat candy that contains sugar if signs and symptoms of late dumping syndrome occur. |
| 4.e. The client will state signs and symptoms to report to the health care provider. | 4.e.1. Refer to Standardized Postoperative Care Plan, Nursing Diagnosis 21, action c (p. 135), for signs and symptoms to report to the health care provider.<br>2. Instruct client to also report:<br>a. persistent nausea and/or vomiting<br>b. persistent or increasing epigastric discomfort or fullness<br>c. bloody, coffee-ground, or green-yellow vomitus<br>d. foul-smelling, greasy bowel movements that float<br>e. black or tarry bowel movements<br>f. persistent diarrhea<br>g. persistent or increasing fatigue and weakness<br>h. weight loss<br>i. signs and symptoms of dumping syndrome (see action d.2 in this diagnosis) that are not controlled using recommended measures. |
| 4.f. The client will verbalize an understanding of and a plan for adhering to recommended follow-up care including future appointments with health care provider, medications prescribed, activity level, and wound care. | 4.f. Refer to Standardized Postoperative Care Plan, Nursing Diagnosis 21 (pp. 135-136), for routine postoperative instructions and measures to improve client compliance. |

# Gastric Reduction

Gastric reduction is a type of bariatric surgery (surgery performed to control obesity) that is accomplished by gastroplasty (e.g. gastric stapling or partitioning) or, less frequently, by gastric bypass. Both of these methods involve reducing the capacity of the stomach to 40-60 ml by partitioning off a small portion of the stomach distal to the gastroesophageal junction and creating a narrow outlet for the pouch so that it does not empty quickly. As a result of the decreased gastric capacity and delayed gastric emptying, the client experiences early satiety and subsequently decreases his/her oral intake and loses weight.

The most frequently performed type of gastroplasty is vertical-banded partitioning. In this approach, the pouch is formed by a vertical staple line on the lesser curvature side of the stomach. The narrow channel created between the pouch and the rest of the stomach is reinforced with mesh or constructed using silicone tubing to reduce the risk of channel widening. Gastric bypass also incorporates gastric partitioning but, in this method of gastric reduction, the stomach is actually transected. The top portion of the stomach forms the pouch and a gastrojejunostomy (Roux-en-Y) is performed. The opening created between the pouch and the jejunal loop is about 1 cm in diameter.

Clients are carefully screened physically and psychologically and must meet certain criteria before undergoing gastric reduction surgery. The criteria usually include massive obesity for at least 5 years, inability to reduce weight using other forms of treatment, weight that is at least 100 pounds or 100% or more over ideal body weight, and obesity that results from a caloric intake greater than the body's needs rather than an underlying metabolic disorder. The client must also be emotionally stable and have access to adequate follow-up medical care.

**This care plan focuses on the adult client hospitalized for gastric reduction surgery.** Preoperative goals of care are to reduce fear and anxiety, prepare the client for the surgery and the postoperative period, and assist him/her to maintain a positive self-concept. Postoperatively, the goals of care are to maintain comfort, prevent complications, assist the client to develop strategies that will help ensure compliance with dietary modifications, and educate him/her regarding follow-up care.

## DISCHARGE CRITERIA

Prior to discharge, the client will:

- have no signs and symptoms of complications
- identify ways to prevent excessive stretching of the gastric pouch and disruption of the staple line (if gastroplasty was performed)
- verbalize an understanding of ways to maintain an adequate nutritional status
- identify ways to reduce the risk of consuming excessive amounts of food, fluid, and calories
- demonstrate the ability to accurately calculate and measure the allotted amounts of food and fluid
- state signs and symptoms to report to the health care provider
- identify community resources that can assist in the adjustment to prescribed dietary modifications and future changes in body image
- verbalize an understanding of and a plan for adhering to recommended follow-up care including future appointments with health care provider, activity level, medications prescribed, and wound care.

## NURSING/COLLABORATIVE DIAGNOSES

**Preoperative**

1. Self-concept disturbance △ *619*

**Postoperative**

1. Ineffective breathing pattern △ *620*
2. Altered nutrition: less than body requirements△ *620*
3. Actual/High risk for impaired skin integrity△ *621*
4. Potential complications:
   a. overdistention of the pouch
   b. peritonitis

c. thromboembolism
d. atelectasis△ *622*
5. Ineffective management of therapeutic regimen△ *625*
6. Knowledge deficit△ *626*

**See Standardized Preoperative and Postoperative Care Plans for additional diagnoses.**

## PREOPERATIVE

**Use in conjunction with the Standardized Preoperative Care Plan.**

### 1. NURSING DIAGNOSIS: Self-concept disturbance*

related to embarrassment associated with obesity and feeling of failure resulting from inability to lose weight by more conventional methods.

*This diagnostic label includes the nursing diagnoses of body image disturbance, self-esteem disturbance, and altered role performance.

| Desired Outcome | Nursing Actions and ***Selected Purposes/Rationales*** |
|---|---|
| 1. The client will demonstrate a positive self-concept as evidenced by:<br>a. verbalization of feelings of self-worth<br>b. positive statements regarding anticipated effects of surgical procedure<br>c. maintenance of relationships with significant others<br>d. active interest in personal appearance<br>e. active participation in preoperative care. | 1.a. Assess for signs and symptoms of a self-concept disturbance (e.g. verbal or nonverbal cues denoting a negative response to self, withdrawal from significant others, refusal to participate in preoperative care or accept responsibility for self-care).<br>b. Determine the meaning of obesity and anticipated effects of the gastric reduction to the client by encouraging him/her to verbalize feelings and by noting nonverbal responses.<br>c. Implement measures *to assist client to increase self-esteem* (e.g. limit negative self-assessment, encourage positive comments about self, assist to identify strengths, give positive feedback about accomplishments, provide positive reinforcement regarding his/her decision to have the surgery and lose weight).<br>d. Implement measures *to reduce client's embarrassment about his/her obesity:*<br>1. before admission, obtain information from physician regarding client's height and weight so that oversized equipment and supplies (e.g. bed, chair, commode, blood pressure cuff, gowns, bathrobe) can be obtained if necessary<br>2. remove unnecessary furniture and equipment from room so client can move around easily<br>3. provide privacy when weighing client<br>4. transfer client to and from operating room in own hospital bed rather than attempting to use a regular-sized stretcher.<br>e. Allow client to wear own clothes rather than hospital gown before and after surgery if desired.<br>f. Assure client that he/she will be assisted with usual grooming and makeup habits after surgery if necessary.<br>g. Demonstrate acceptance of client using techniques such as touch and frequent visits.<br>h. Arrange for a visit from an individual who has achieved weight loss after gastric reduction surgery if client desires.<br>i. If client is expressing concerns about the amount of excess skin he/she will have after the majority of weight loss occurs (usually after 1-1½ |

years), provide information about various clothing styles that may be most flattering (e.g. long-sleeved shirts or blouses) and reconstructive surgery that is available to remove excess skin from abdomen, breasts, upper arms, and thighs.

j. Consult physician if client has unrealistic expectations of postoperative weight loss and dietary management.

## POSTOPERATIVE

**Use in conjunction with the Standardized Postoperative Care Plan.**

### 1. NURSING DIAGNOSIS: Ineffective breathing pattern

related to:

a. depressant effects of anesthesia (effects last longer in the obese client because adipose tissue more readily absorbs and stores anesthetic agents) and some medications (e.g. narcotic analgesics);
b. impaired lung/chest wall expansion associated with:
   1. limited diaphragmatic excursion resulting from large amounts of abdominal adipose tissue, abdominal distention, and reluctance to breathe deeply because of abdominal pain
   2. decreased activity (lung expansion is restricted by the bed surface when client is lying in bed)
   3. increased weight of the chest wall of an obese client (especially in women with pendulous breasts).

| Desired Outcome | Nursing Actions and ***Selected Purposes/Rationales*** |
|---|---|
| 1. The client will maintain an effective breathing pattern (see Standardized Postoperative Care Plan, Nursing Diagnosis 2 [p. 114], for outcome criteria). | 1.a. Refer to Standardized Postoperative Care Plan, Nursing Diagnosis 2 (pp. 114-115), for measures related to assessment and improvement of breathing pattern.<br>b. Implement additional measures *to improve breathing pattern:*<br>1. position client with head of bed elevated at least 30° at all times<br>2. instruct and assist client to use overhead trapeze and turn at least every 2 hours<br>3. add extensions to tubings if necessary *to enable client to turn and move without fear of dislodging tubes*<br>4. assist with ambulation the evening of surgery and at least 4 times/day as ordered. |

### 2. NURSING DIAGNOSIS: Altered nutrition: less than body requirements

related to:

a. decreased oral intake associated with nausea, pain, prescribed dietary modifications, and early satiety resulting from small pouch size;
b. inadequate nutritional replacement therapy;
c. increased nutritional needs associated with the increased metabolic rate that occurs during wound healing.

| Desired Outcome | Nursing Actions and ***Selected Purposes/Rationales*** |
|---|---|
| 2. The client will maintain an adequate nutritional status as evidenced by:<br>a. normal BUN and serum albumin, Hct, Hb, transferrin, and lymphocyte levels<br>b. usual strength and activity tolerance<br>c. healthy oral mucous membrane. | 2.a. Assess for and report signs and symptoms of malnutrition:<br>1. abnormal BUN and low serum albumin, Hct, Hb, transferrin, and lymphocyte levels (decreased Hct and Hb may also result from surgical blood loss)<br>2. weakness and fatigue<br>3. stomatitis.<br>b. Assess for return of bowel function every 2-4 hours. Notify physician when client has normal bowel sounds and is expelling flatus *so that jejunostomy tube feedings and/or oral intake can be started as soon as possible.*<br>c. When oral intake is allowed, monitor client's intake. Report if he/she does not consume prescribed amounts or types of fluids.<br>d. Implement measures *to maintain an adequate nutritional status:*<br>1. maintain jejunostomy tube feeding if ordered<br>2. when oral intake is allowed:<br>a. perform actions to reduce pain (see Standardized Postoperative Care Plan, Nursing Diagnosis 6, action e [p. 119])<br>b. administer antiemetics and/or gastrointestinal stimulants (e.g. metoclopramide) if ordered *to control nausea*<br>c. maintain a clean environment and a relaxed, pleasant atmosphere<br>d. provide oral care before offering fluids<br>e. provide high-protein liquid nourishment as part of fluid allotment as soon as allowed (client is usually allowed to drink dilute liquid protein supplements 4-5 days after surgery)<br>f. reinforce the importance of consuming fluids at scheduled frequency and consuming more nutritious fluids and foods as soon as allowed (client is usually allowed to progress from fluids to solids after 6-8 weeks)<br>3. administer vitamins and minerals if ordered.<br>e. Consult physician if client is unable to tolerate or adhere to prescribed diet. |

## 3. NURSING DIAGNOSIS: Actual/High risk for impaired skin integrity

related to:

a. disruption of skin associated with the surgical procedure;
b. delayed wound healing associated with decreased nutritional status and inadequate blood supply to wound area;
c. irritation of skin associated with contact with wound drainage, pressure from drainage tubes, and use of tape;
d. difficulty keeping deep skin fold areas dry;
e. damage to the skin and/or subcutaneous tissue associated with friction or shearing when moving in bed;
f. ischemia of the skin and subcutaneous tissue associated with pressure on tissues as a result of excessive body weight and decreased activity.

| Desired Outcomes | Nursing Actions and ***Selected Purposes/Rationales*** |
|---|---|
| 3.a. The client will experience normal healing of surgical wounds (see Standardized Postoperative Care Plan, Nursing Diagnosis 9, outcome a [p. 122], for outcome criteria). | 3.a.1. Refer to Standardized Postoperative Care Plan, Nursing Diagnosis 9, action a (pp. 122-123), for measures related to assessment and promotion of wound healing.<br>2. Implement measures to maintain an adequate nutritional status (see Postoperative Nursing Diagnosis 2, action d) *in order to further promote wound healing.* |

| Desired Outcomes | Nursing Actions and ***Selected Purposes/Rationales*** |
|---|---|
| 3.b. The client will maintain skin integrity as evidenced by:<br>1. absence of redness and irritation<br>2. no skin breakdown. | 3.b.1. Inspect the following sites for pallor, redness, and breakdown:<br>a. skin folds of abdomen and groin and under breasts<br>b. skin areas in contact with wound drainage, tape, and drainage tubings<br>c. back, coccyx, and buttocks<br>d. elbows and heels.<br>2. Refer to Standardized Postoperative Care Plan, Nursing Diagnosis 9, action b.2 (p. 123), for measures to prevent skin irritation and breakdown resulting from wound drainage, tape, and drainage tubings.<br>3. Implement additional measures *to reduce the risk for skin breakdown:*<br>a. assist client to turn at least every 2 hours when in bed<br>b. assist client with ambulation as ordered and as frequently as tolerated<br>c. gently massage heels, elbows, and around reddened areas at least every 2 hours<br>d. perform actions *to prevent shearing* (shearing occurs when one tissue layer slides past another) *and skin surface abrasion:*<br>1. apply a thin layer of powder or cornstarch to bottom sheet or skin *to absorb moisture (moist skin is more likely to adhere to sheet) and reduce friction*<br>2. instruct and assist client to use overhead trapeze to lift self off the bed when moving<br>e. instruct or assist client to shift weight every 30 minutes<br>f. if fade time (length of time it takes for reddened area to fade after pressure is removed) is greater than 15 minutes, increase frequency of position change and ambulation<br>g. keep skin lubricated, clean, and dry; assist client to thoroughly cleanse and dry opposing skin surfaces of deep skin folds as often as needed<br>h. apply a thin layer of powder or cornstarch to areas with opposing skin surfaces (e.g. axillae, perineum, beneath breasts) *to absorb moisture and/or reduce friction*<br>i. keep bed linens dry and wrinkle-free<br>j. provide devices to reduce pressure on the skin, decrease shearing, and/or prevent moisture build-up (e.g. alternating pressure mattress or pad, flotation pad, sheepskin) if indicated<br>k. perform actions *to reduce pressure on elbows and heels:*<br>1. encourage client to use overhead trapeze to move self rather than pushing with heels and elbows<br>2. provide elbow and heel protectors if indicated.<br>4. If skin breakdown occurs:<br>a. notify physician<br>b. continue with above measures to prevent further irritation and breakdown<br>c. perform decubitus care as ordered or per standard hospital procedure<br>d. expose opposing skin folds to the air if possible and/or apply protective ointment or cream (e.g. Desitin) as ordered<br>e. assess client closely and report signs and symptoms of infection (e.g. elevated temperature; redness, warmth, and edema around area of breakdown; unusual drainage from site). |

**4. COLLABORATIVE DIAGNOSES:**

**Potential complications:**

a. **overdistention of the pouch** related to:
   1. accumulation of gas and fluid in the pouch associated with decreased peristalsis

2. obstruction of the pouch outlet (the channel between the pouch and distal stomach if gastroplasty performed or the opening between the pouch and jejunal loop if gastric bypass performed) associated with edema and/or ingestion of medications or thick fluids that are not able to pass through pouch outlet
3. excessive oral intake;

b. **peritonitis** related to:
1. wound infection
2. leakage of gastric contents into the peritoneum associated with disruption of the staple line (if gastroplasty performed) or anastomoses (if gastric bypass performed);

c. **thromboembolism** related to:
1. venous stasis associated with decreased activity, fluid volume deficit, and pressure on abdominal vessels from excessive adipose tissue and intestinal distention
2. hypercoagulability associated with increased release of thromboplastin into the blood (occurs as a result of surgical trauma)
3. decreased fibrinolytic activity (occurs in response to surgical trauma)
4. trauma to vein walls during surgery;

d. **atelectasis** related to shallow respirations and stasis of secretions in the alveoli and bronchioles.

| Desired Outcomes | Nursing Actions and ***Selected Purposes/Rationales*** |
|---|---|
| 4.a. The client will not experience overdistention of the pouch as evidenced by:<br>1. decreased complaints of epigastric fullness<br>2. absence of nausea and vomiting. | 4.a.1. Assess for and report signs and symptoms of overdistention of the pouch (e.g. increasing complaints of epigastric fullness, nausea, vomiting).<br>2. Implement measures *to prevent overdistention of the pouch:*<br>a. maintain patency of nasogastric tube *to reduce gas and fluid accumulation during period of decreased peristalsis*<br>b. encourage and assist client with frequent position changes and ambulation as soon as allowed and tolerated *(activity stimulates peristalsis)*<br>c. instruct the client to avoid activities such as chewing gum and smoking *in order to reduce air swallowing*<br>d. do not change position of nasogastric tube unless ordered *(the tube is usually positioned at the pouch outlet to help prevent obstruction of the opening into the distal stomach [if gastroplasty performed] or jejunal loop [if gastric bypass performed])*<br>e. when oral intake is allowed:<br>1. adhere strictly to prescribed oral intake schedule (clients usually begin with hourly liquid feedings of 30 ml and, over at least 6 weeks, progress to 5 or 6 small [1-2 ounce] liquid meals/day with 1-2 ounces of water allowed periodically between meals)<br>2. provide client with allotted amounts of fluids at the proper times; discard skipped "meals" *so client does not ingest feedings too close together*<br>3. instruct client to adhere to the liquid or blenderized diet as ordered *(oral intake that is too thick can block the pouch outlet, which may be narrower in the early postoperative period because of edema)*<br>4. administer oral medication in liquid or chewable form or crushed thoroughly *to prevent blockage of the pouch outlet*<br>f. encourage client to eructate whenever the urge is felt<br>g. encourage use of nonnarcotic analgesics once severe pain has subsided *(narcotic analgesics depress gastrointestinal motility).*<br>3. If signs and symptoms of overdistention occur:<br>a. withhold all oral intake as ordered<br>b. prepare client for upper abdominal x-rays to check placement of nasogastric tube if present |

| Desired Outcomes | Nursing Actions and ***Selected Purposes/Rationales*** |
|---|---|
| | c. assist physician with adjustment or reinsertion of the nasogastric tube if indicated. |
| 4.b. The client will not develop peritonitis as evidenced by:<br>1. gradual resolution of abdominal pain<br>2. soft, nondistended abdomen<br>3. temperature declining toward normal<br>4. stable vital signs<br>5. absence of nausea and vomiting<br>6. gradual return of normal bowel sounds<br>7. WBC count declining toward normal. | 4.b.1. Assess for and report signs and symptoms of peritonitis (e.g. increase in severity of abdominal pain; generalized abdominal pain; rebound tenderness; tense, rigid abdomen; increase in temperature; tachycardia; tachypnea; hypotension; nausea; vomiting; continued diminished or absent bowel sounds).<br>2. Monitor WBC counts. Report levels that increase or fail to decline toward normal.<br>3. Implement measures *to prevent peritonitis:*<br>a. perform actions to prevent and treat wound infection (see Standardized Postoperative Care Plan, Nursing Diagnosis 16, actions b.4 and 5 [p. 129])<br>b. perform actions *to maintain patency of wound drain(s) if present:*<br>1. keep tubing free of kinks<br>2. empty collection device(s) as often as necessary<br>3. maintain suction as ordered<br>c. perform actions *to prevent inadvertent removal of wound drain(s) if present:*<br>1. use caution when changing dressings surrounding drain(s)<br>2. provide extension tubing if necessary *to enable client to move without placing tension on the drain(s)*<br>3. instruct client not to pull on drain(s) and drainage tubing(s)<br>d. perform actions *to prevent stress on the staple line or sites of anastomoses:*<br>1. implement measures to prevent overdistention of pouch (see action a.2 in this diagnosis)<br>2. implement measures to prevent nausea and vomiting (e.g. maintain patency of nasogastric tube, eliminate noxious sights and odors from the environment, instruct client to change positions slowly, administer antiemetics and/or gastrointestinal stimulants as ordered)<br>3. do not adjust position of nasogastric tube unless ordered *(adjustment may cause disruption of staples or perforation at site of proximal anastomosis).*<br>4. If signs and symptoms of peritonitis occur:<br>a. withhold oral intake and jejunostomy tube feeding as ordered<br>b. place client on bed rest in a semi-Fowler's position *to assist in pooling or localizing gastrointestinal contents in the pelvis rather than under the diaphragm*<br>c. assist physician with insertion of a nasogastric tube if not already present and maintain suction as ordered<br>d. administer antimicrobials as ordered<br>e. administer intravenous fluids and/or blood volume expanders if ordered *to prevent or treat shock (can result from the increased capillary permeability that occurs with inflammation and the subsequent escape of protein, fluid, and electrolytes from the vascular space into the peritoneal cavity)*<br>f. prepare client for surgical intervention (e.g. repair of perforation) if planned<br>g. provide emotional support to client and significant others. |
| 4.c. The client will not develop a deep vein thrombus and pulmonary embolism (see Standardized Postoperative Care Plan, Collaborative | 4.c. Refer to Standardized Postoperative Care Plan, Collaborative Diagnosis 19, actions c.1 and 2 (pp. 132-133), for measures related to assessment, prevention, and treatment of a deep vein thrombus and pulmonary embolism. |

| Desired Outcome | Nursing Actions and *Selected Purposes/Rationales* |
|---|---|
| Diagnosis 19, outcomes c.1 and 2 [pp. 132-133], for outcome criteria). | |
| 4.d. The client will not develop atelectasis (see Standardized Postoperative Care Plan, Collaborative Diagnosis 19, outcome b [p. 132], for outcome criteria). | 4.d.1. Refer to Standardized Postoperative Care Plan, Collaborative Diagnosis 19, action b (p. 132), for measures related to assessment, prevention, and treatment of atelectasis.<br>2. Implement additional measures to improve breathing pattern (see Postoperative Nursing Diagnosis 1) *in order to further reduce the risk of development of atelectasis.* |

## 5. NURSING DIAGNOSIS: Ineffective management of therapeutic regimen

related to lack of understanding of the implications of not following the prescribed treatment plan and difficulty integrating prescribed dietary modifications into life style.

| Desired Outcome | Nursing Actions and *Selected Purposes/Rationales* |
|---|---|
| 5. The client will demonstrate the probability of effective management of the therapeutic regimen as evidenced by:<br>a. willingness to learn about and participate in treatments and care<br>b. statements reflecting ways to integrate prescribed dietary plan and exercise program into life style<br>c. statements reflecting an understanding of the implications of not following the prescribed treatment plan. | 5.a. Assess for indications that the client may be unable to effectively manage the therapeutic regimen:<br>1. failure to adhere to treatment plan while in hospital (e.g. not adhering to dietary modifications and fluid restrictions, refusing to increase activity)<br>2. statements reflecting a lack of understanding of dietary modifications and factors that will cause stretching of the gastric pouch or disruption of staple line<br>3. verbalization of an inability to integrate necessary dietary modifications and exercise program into life style<br>4. statements reflecting the belief that the surgical procedure will result in continued weight loss even without adherence to the prescribed dietary modifications or that he/she will return to preoperative weight despite adherence to dietary modifications.<br>b. Implement measures *to promote effective management of the therapeutic regimen:*<br>1. explain the surgical procedure and importance of dietary modifications and a balanced exercise program in terms the client can understand; emphasize that adherence to the treatment program is necessary if he/she is to attain an optimal weight<br>2. inform the client that prescribed food and fluid modifications are not as strict after the surgical area has healed (usually 6-8 weeks)<br>3. stress the positive effects of compliance with dietary modifications and exercise program (e.g. weight loss resulting in change in appearance; decreased risk of development of conditions such as diabetes mellitus, cardiovascular disease, respiratory problems, and arthritis)<br>4. assist client to identify ways he/she can incorporate dietary modifications and exercise program into life style; focus on modifications of life style rather than complete change (e.g. schedule meetings after rather than during lunch, meet friends at a park rather than a restaurant)<br>5. provide a dietary consult to assist client in planning a dietary program based on prescribed modifications and client's likes, dislikes, and daily routines |

| Desired Outcome | Nursing Actions and ***Selected Purposes/Rationales*** |
|---|---|
| | 6. encourage activities other than eating to cope with stress (e.g. exercise)<br>7. initiate and reinforce the discharge teaching outlined in Postoperative Nursing Diagnosis 6 *in order to promote a sense of control and self-reliance*<br>8. encourage questions and allow time for reinforcement and clarification of information provided<br>9. provide written instructions about future appointments with health care provider, dietary modifications, and signs and symptoms to report<br>10. provide information about and encourage utilization of community resources that can assist client to make necessary life-style changes (e.g. weight reduction groups, counseling services, support groups of persons who have had the same or similar surgery, stress management classes)<br>11. reinforce behaviors suggesting future compliance with the therapeutic regimen (e.g. statements reflecting plans for integrating dietary modifications into life style, active participation in planning dietary program, changes in personal habits)<br>12. include significant others in explanations and teaching sessions and encourage their support; reinforce the need for client to assume responsibility for managing as much of care as possible.<br>c. Consult physician regarding referrals to community agencies and/or support groups if continued instruction, support, or supervision is needed. |

## 6. NURSING DIAGNOSIS: Knowledge deficit

regarding follow-up care.

| Desired Outcomes | Nursing Actions and ***Selected Purposes/Rationales*** |
|---|---|
| 6.a. The client will identify ways to prevent excessive stretching of the gastric pouch and disruption of the staple line (if gastroplasty was performed). | 6.a. Instruct client in ways to prevent excessive stretching of the gastric pouch and disruption of the staple line (if gastroplasty was performed):<br>1. decrease risk of blockage of the gastric outlet by:<br>a. limiting oral intake to liquids and blenderized foods for about 6-8 weeks after surgery as prescribed<br>b. taking all prescription and nonprescription medications in liquid or chewable form or crushing them thoroughly<br>c. chewing foods thoroughly<br>2. do not exceed prescribed volume of food/fluid intake<br>3. do not make up for skipped meals while on an hourly drinking/eating schedule<br>4. eat and drink slowly<br>5. avoid intake of carbonated beverages for 6-8 weeks after surgery and limit intake of these beverages after that time<br>6. consume fluids between rather than with meals (recommended intake is usually 50 ounces [1500 ml] of water or low-calorie beverages each day). |
| 6.b. The client will verbalize an understanding of ways to maintain an | 6.b.1. Instruct client regarding ways to maintain an adequate nutritional status:<br>a. do not skip meals<br>b. consume foods/fluids from each food group daily as diet advances<br>c. consume adequate amounts of protein (e.g. blenderized drinks |

adequate nutritional status.

containing peanut butter, pureed meats and fish, creamed cottage cheese) as diet advances
d. take vitamin supplements as prescribed.
2. Obtain dietary consult if indicated to assist client in planning meals.

6.c. The client will identify ways to reduce the risk of consuming excessive amounts of food, fluid, and calories.

6.c. Instruct client in ways to reduce the risk of consuming excessive amounts of food, fluid, and calories:
1. limit food/fluid intake to prescribed volume
2. prepare foods ahead of time, freeze in 1-ounce portions using plastic ice cube trays or plastic bags, and then reheat only allowed amounts at mealtime
3. have jars of prepared strained baby food products rather than high-calorie puddings and snacks on hand
4. have only low-calorie drinks available (other than the required high-protein supplements)
5. decrease the risk of hunger by adhering to a schedule of 5 or 6 meals/day as diet advances (each meal will usually consist of 2-4 tablespoons of food)
6. serve food on a small plate (this provides an illusion that meals are larger than they really are)
7. eat and drink very slowly (use techniques such as putting fork down between bites of food and putting glass down between sips of fluid)
8. if going out to dinner, order an appetizer and have it served with everyone else's entree
9. avoid excessive intake of high-calorie foods/fluids (it is possible to maintain or gain weight if only high-calorie substances are consumed).

6.d. The client will demonstrate the ability to accurately calculate and measure the allotted amounts of food and fluid.

6.d.1. Demonstrate ways to measure foods/fluids accurately using measuring spoons and a cup with 1-ounce markings.
2. Allow time for questions, clarification, and return demonstration.

6.e. The client will state signs and symptoms to report to the health care provider.

6.e.1. Refer to Standardized Postoperative Care Plan, Nursing Diagnosis 21, action c (p. 135), for signs and symptoms to report to the health care provider.
2. Instruct client to also report:
a. nausea and vomiting after consuming prescribed amount of foods/fluids
b. inability to adhere to dietary modifications
c. weight gain
d. inability to lose weight or excessive weight loss (expected weight loss is usually about 10 pounds/month for the 1st year or 30% of preoperative body weight by the end of the 1st year)
e. abdominal cramping, diaphoresis, generalized weakness, and/or dizziness within an hour after eating (indicative of dumping syndrome, which sometimes occurs several weeks after a gastric bypass but is usually self-limiting or easily controlled with dietary modifications).

6.f. The client will identify community resources that can assist in the adjustment to prescribed dietary modifications and future changes in body image.

6.f. 1. Provide information about community resources that can assist the client with adjustment to prescribed dietary modifications and future changes in body image (e.g. weight reduction groups, counseling services, support groups of persons who have had the same or similar surgery).
2. Initiate a referral if indicated.

6.g. The client will verbalize an understanding of and a plan for adhering to

6.g.1. Refer to Standardized Postoperative Care Plan, Nursing Diagnosis 21 (pp. 135-136), for routine postoperative instructions.
2. Reinforce the physician's instructions regarding need to adhere to a schedule of moderate exercise (clients are usually instructed to begin a

| Desired Outcomes | Nursing Actions and ***Selected Purposes/Rationales*** |
|---|---|
| recommended follow-up care including future appointments with health care provider, activity level, medications prescribed, and wound care. | walking program and should be walking 1-2 miles/day by the 4th week after discharge).<br>3. Refer to Postoperative Nursing Diagnosis 5, action b, for measures to promote the client's ability to effectively manage the therapeutic regimen. |

# Inflammatory Bowel Disease: Ulcerative Colitis and Crohn's Disease

Crohn's disease and ulcerative colitis are idiopathic chronic inflammatory bowel diseases, which are often jointly referred to as inflammatory bowel disease (IBD). These disorders have similarities but can usually be differentiated by clinical, radiological, and pathologic findings. Clinical manifestations of inflammatory bowel disease include diarrhea (the most classic symptom), abdominal pain and cramping, bloody stools, and fever. The severity and pattern of signs and symptoms depend on the portion(s) of the bowel affected and depth of bowel wall involvement. Ulcerative colitis involves the mucosa and submucosa of the bowel wall, typically starts in the rectum and sigmoid colon, and progresses in a continuous pattern through the colon. It rarely involves the small intestine. Crohn's disease begins anywhere in the intestinal tract, usually involves the terminal ileum and ascending colon, and has a discontinuous pattern of progression.

Clients with either condition may experience a number of the same complications; however, those with ulcerative colitis have a higher incidence of rectal bleeding, while clients with Crohn's disease have a higher incidence of perianal involvement and fistulas. A small percentage of clients also experience extraintestinal manifestations such as liver and biliary involvement; arthritis; and skin, eye, and oral lesions. Clients with inflammatory bowel disease may require hospitalization during periods of exacerbation if fever and abdominal pain are present and the client is not responding to steroids or if complications are suspected.

**This care plan focuses on the adult client with severe abdominal pain and diarrhea who is hospitalized for medical management of inflammatory bowel disease.** The goals of care are to increase comfort, rest the bowel, maintain adequate nutrition and hydration, prevent complications, and educate the client regarding effective home management of the disease.

## DIAGNOSTIC TESTS

Sigmoidoscopy/proctosigmoidoscopy
Colonoscopy
Barium enema (may be contraindicated during acute illness)
Barium contrast x-ray of upper gastrointestinal tract (small bowel follow-through)
Mucosal biopsies
Stool examination
Complete blood count (CBC)
Erythrocyte sedimentation rate (ESR)
Serum albumin

## DISCHARGE CRITERIA

Prior to discharge, the client will:

- have decreased abdominal pain
- have fewer episodes of diarrhea
- tolerate prescribed diet and have an improved nutritional status
- be free of signs and symptoms of complications

- identify ways to reduce the incidence of disease exacerbation
- verbalize ways to maintain an optimal nutritional status
- state ways to prevent perianal skin breakdown
- verbalize an understanding of medications ordered including rationale, side effects, schedule for taking, and importance of taking as prescribed
- state signs and symptoms to report to the health care provider
- identify resources that can assist in the adjustment to changes resulting from inflammatory bowel disease and its treatment
- share feelings and thoughts about the effects of inflammatory bowel disease on life style and self-concept
- verbalize an understanding of and a plan for adhering to recommended follow-up care including future appointments with health care provider and activity level.

**NURSING/ COLLABORATIVE DIAGNOSES**



## 1. NURSING/ COLLABORATIVE DIAGNOSIS:

### Altered fluid and electrolyte balance:

a. **fluid volume deficit, hypokalemia, hypochloremia, hypomagnesemia, and hypocalcemia** related to:
   1. prolonged inadequate oral intake associated with pain, fatigue, prescribed dietary restrictions, and fear of precipitating an attack of abdominal cramping and diarrhea
   2. impaired absorption of fluid and electrolytes associated with inflammation and ulceration of the intestine
   3. excessive loss of fluid and electrolytes associated with persistent diarrhea;

b. **metabolic acidosis** related to excessive loss of bicarbonate associated with persistent diarrhea.

**Desired Outcome**

1. The client will maintain fluid and electrolyte balance as evidenced by:
   a. normal skin turgor
   b. moist mucous membranes
   c. stable weight
   d. B/P and pulse within normal range for client and stable with position change
   e. small vein filling time less than 3-5 seconds
   f. balanced intake and output
   g. urine specific gravity within normal range
   h. soft, nondistended abdomen with active bowel sounds
   i. usual mental status
   j. absence of cardiac arrhythmias, muscle weakness, paresthesias, twitching, spasms, and dizziness
   k. absence of headache, nausea, and vomiting
   l. negative Chvostek's and Trousseau's signs
   m. serum electrolytes and blood gases within normal range.

**Nursing Actions and *Selected Purposes/Rationales***

1.a. Assess for and report signs and symptoms of:
   1. fluid volume deficit:
      a. decreased skin turgor, dry mucous membranes, thirst
      b. sudden weight loss of 2% or greater
      c. low B/P and/or postural hypotension
      d. weak, rapid pulse
      e. delayed small vein filling time (longer than 3-5 seconds)
      f. decreased urine output with increased specific gravity (reflects an actual rather than potential fluid volume deficit)
      g. significant increase in BUN and Hct above previous levels
   2. hypokalemia (e.g. cardiac arrhythmias, postural hypotension, muscle weakness, paresthesias, nausea and vomiting, abdominal distention, hypoactive or absent bowel sounds)
   3. hypochloremia (e.g. dizziness, irritability, paresthesias, muscle twitching or spasms)
   4. hypomagnesemia and/or hypocalcemia (e.g. anxiousness; irritability; cardiac arrhythmias; positive Chvostek's and Trousseaus's signs; numbness or tingling of fingers, toes, or circumoral area; hyperactive reflexes; tetany; seizures)
   5. metabolic acidosis (e.g. drowsiness; disorientation; stupor; rapid, deep respirations; headache; nausea and vomiting; cardiac arrhythmias).

b. Monitor serum electrolyte and blood gas results. Report abnormal values.

c. Implement measures *to prevent or treat fluid and electrolyte imbalances:*
   1. perform actions to control diarrhea (see Nursing Diagnosis 7, action d)
   2. maintain a fluid intake of at least 2500 ml/day unless contraindicated; if oral intake is inadequate or contraindicated, maintain intravenous therapy as ordered
   3. when oral intake is allowed:
      a. perform actions to improve oral intake (see Nursing Diagnosis 2, action c.4.c)
      b. assist client to select foods/fluids within the prescribed dietary regimen that would replenish electrolytes (be aware that most foods/fluids high in potassium and sodium are contraindicated on a low-residue diet):
         1. foods/fluids high in potassium (e.g. bananas, apricots, potatoes, cantaloupe)
         2. foods/fluids high in sodium (e.g. processed cheese, canned soups and vegetables, bouillon)
         3. foods/fluids high in magnesium (e.g. legumes, seafood)
   4. administer the following if ordered:
      a. electrolyte replacements (e.g. potassium chloride, magnesium sulfate, calcium gluconate, calcium carbonate, sodium chloride, sodium bicarbonate)
      b. vitamin D preparations *to increase intestinal absorption of calcium.*

d. If signs and symptoms of hypomagnesemia or hypocalcemia occur, institute seizure precautions.

e. Consult physician if signs and symptoms of fluid and electrolyte imbalances persist or worsen.

---

**2. NURSING DIAGNOSIS: Altered nutrition: less than body requirements**

related to:

a. decreased oral intake associated with pain, fatigue, prescribed dietary restrictions, and the knowledge that eating often precipitates abdominal cramping and diarrhea;

b. decreased absorption of nutrients associated with inflammation and ulceration of the bowel;
c. loss of nutrients associated with diarrhea;
d. impaired folate absorption associated with treatment with sulfasalazine;
e. increased metabolism of nutrients associated with the increased metabolic rate that may be present during periods of exacerbation.

| Desired Outcome | Nursing Actions and ***Selected Purposes/Rationales*** |
|---|---|
| 2. The client will have an improved nutritional status as evidenced by:<br>a. weight approaching a normal range for client's age, height, and body frame<br>b. improved BUN and serum albumin, Hct, Hb, folate, transferrin, and lymphocyte levels<br>c. increased triceps skinfold thickness<br>d. increased strength and activity tolerance<br>e. healthy oral mucous membrane. | 2 a. Assess for signs and symptoms of malnutrition:<br>1. weight below normal for client's age, height, and body frame<br>2. abnormal BUN and low serum albumin, Hct, Hb, folate, transferrin, and lymphocyte levels<br>3. triceps skinfold thickness less than normal<br>4. weakness and fatigue<br>5. stomatitis.<br>b. When oral intake is allowed, monitor the percentage of meals and snacks client consumes. Report a pattern of inadequate intake.<br>c. Implement measures *to improve nutritional status:*<br>1. administer total parenteral nutrition if ordered<br>2. perform actions to reduce inflammation and hyperactivity of the bowel (see Nursing Diagnosis 7, action d) *in order to reduce episodes of diarrhea and increase absorption of nutrients*<br>3. maintain activity restrictions as ordered (usually bed rest with bedside commode or bathroom privileges) *to reduce caloric requirements*<br>4. when food or fluid is allowed:<br>a. provide elemental formulas (e.g. Vivonex, Criticare HN) if ordered (these formulas are high in calories and nutrients)<br>b. progress diet as tolerated (usual progression is from elemental feedings to a bland, low-residue, high-calorie, high-protein diet)<br>c. perform actions *to improve oral intake:*<br>1. implement measures to reduce pain (see Nursing Diagnosis 3, action e)<br>2. encourage a rest period before meals *to minimize fatigue*<br>3. maintain a clean environment and a relaxed, pleasant atmosphere<br>4. provide oral care before meals<br>5. implement measures *to improve the palatability of elemental formulas* (e.g. offer a variety of flavors, serve chilled)<br>6. obtain a dietary consult if necessary to assist client in selecting bland, low-residue foods/fluids that meet nutritional needs as well as personal and cultural preferences whenever possible<br>7. serve small portions of nutritious foods/fluids that are appealing to client<br>8. allow adequate time for meals; reheat food if necessary<br>5. administer the following if ordered:<br>a. iron preparations (oral iron preparations may not be effective during an acute attack *because they may be poorly absorbed from the inflamed bowel)*<br>b. ascorbic acid *to improve iron absorption and promote healing of ulcerations in the bowel*<br>c. vitamin preparations (e.g. fat-soluble vitamins, cyanocobalamin, folic acid)<br>d. medium-chain triglycerides (MCT) in an oil medium *to provide a source of calories.*<br>d. Perform a 72-hour calorie count if ordered. Report totals to dietitian and physician.<br>e. Consult physician if nutritional status continues to decline. |

## 3. NURSING DIAGNOSIS: Pain:

a. **abdominal pain and cramping** related to:
   1. inflammation and ulceration of the bowel
   2. interference with the flow of intestinal contents associated with narrowing of the intestinal lumen as a result of inflammation and hypertrophy and fibrosis of the bowel wall if present;

b. **joint pain** related to extraintestinal involvement of the joints (arthritis of the large joints, ankylosing spondylitis, and sacroiliitis are the most common);

c. **perianal pain** related to irritation and breakdown of skin in the perianal area associated with persistent diarrhea and/or the presence of an anorectal fistula.

| Desired Outcome | Nursing Actions and ***Selected Purposes/Rationales*** |
|---|---|
| 3. The client will experience diminished pain as evidenced by:<br>a. verbalization of pain relief<br>b. relaxed facial expression and body positioning<br>c. increased participation in activities<br>d. stable vital signs. | 3.a. Determine how the client usually responds to pain.<br>b. Assess client's perception of pain including location, intensity, and type. Use a numerical scale to rate intensity.<br>c. Assess for nonverbal signs of pain (e.g. wrinkled brow, clenched fists, reluctance to move, restlessness, diaphoresis, facial pallor, increased B/P, tachycardia).<br>d. Assess for factors that seem to aggravate and alleviate pain.<br>e. Implement measures *to reduce pain:*<br>1. perform actions *to reduce fear and anxiety about the pain experience* (e.g. assure client that his/her need for pain relief will be met, perform preprocedure teaching)<br>2. medicate prior to painful procedures (e.g. endoscopy) and before pain is severe<br>3. perform actions to reduce inflammation and hyperactivity of the bowel (see Nursing Diagnosis 7, action d) *in order to reduce abdominal pain and cramping*<br>4. perform actions *to reduce joint pain:*<br>a. consult physician regarding:<br>1. application of brace/splint to affected joint<br>2. application of heat to affected joint<br>b. administer anti-inflammatory agents if ordered<br>5. perform actions *to relieve perianal pain:*<br>a. implement measures to control diarrhea (see Nursing Diagnosis 7, action d)<br>b. clean perianal area with medicated wipes such as Tucks after each bowel movement<br>c. apply protective ointment or cream (e.g. BAZA cream, A&D ointment, Desitin, Vaseline) to perianal area after each bowel movement<br>d. consult physician about order for sitz baths<br>e. apply anesthetic preparation (e.g. Nupercainal, Tronolane) to perianal area or into rectum if ordered<br>f. administer corticosteroid foam, suppository, or enema if ordered<br>6. provide or assist with nonpharmacological measures for pain relief (e.g. position change, relaxation techniques, guided imagery, quiet conversation, restful environment, diversional activities)<br>7. administer analgesics if ordered (narcotic analgesics must be administered judiciously *because they slow gastrointestinal motility and can cause toxic megacolon or a bowel obstruction*).<br>f. Consult physician if above measures fail to provide adequate pain relief. |

**4. NURSING DIAGNOSIS: High risk for impaired skin integrity**

related to:

a. damage to the skin and/or subcutaneous tissue associated with prolonged pressure on the tissues, friction, and shearing that can occur when mobility is decreased;
b. frequent contact with irritants associated with persistent diarrhea;
c. increased fragility of skin associated with malnutrition and dryness (may result from fluid volume deficit).

| Desired Outcome | Nursing Actions and ***Selected Purposes/Rationales*** |
|---|---|
| 4. The client will maintain skin integrity as evidenced by:<br>a. absence of redness and irritation<br>b. no skin breakdown. | 4.a. Inspect the skin (especially bony prominences, dependent areas, and perianal area) for pallor, redness, and breakdown.<br>b. Implement measures *to prevent skin breakdown:*<br>1. instruct and/or assist client to turn at least every 2 hours; use all 4 sides (prone, lateral, dorsal) unless contraindicated<br>2. gently massage around reddened areas at least every 2 hours<br>3. perform actions *to prevent shearing* (shearing occurs when one tissue layer slides past another) *and skin surface abrasion:*<br>a. apply a thin layer of powder or cornstarch to bottom sheet or skin *to absorb moisture (moist skin is more likely to adhere to sheet) and reduce friction*<br>b. encourage client to limit length of time he/she is in semi-Fowler's position to 30 minutes *(in this position, client tends to slide down in bed)*<br>4. instruct or assist client to shift weight every 30 minutes<br>5. if fade time (length of time it takes for reddened area to fade after pressure is removed) is greater than 15 minutes, increase frequency of position changes<br>6. keep skin clean and dry<br>7. apply a thin layer of powder or cornstarch to areas with opposing skin surfaces (e.g. axillae, perineum, beneath breasts) if indicated *to absorb moisture and/or reduce friction*<br>8. keep bed linens dry and wrinkle-free<br>9. increase activity as allowed and tolerated<br>10. provide devices to reduce pressure on the skin, decrease shearing, and/or prevent moisture build-up (e.g. alternating pressure mattress or pad, flotation pad)<br>11. perform actions to improve nutritional status (see Nursing Diagnosis 2, action c)<br>12. perform actions *to prevent drying of the skin:*<br>a. encourage a fluid intake of 2500 ml/day unless contraindicated<br>b. provide a mild soap for bathing<br>c. apply moisturizing lotion and/or emollient to skin at least once a day<br>13. perform actions *to prevent skin irritation resulting from diarrhea:*<br>a. implement measures to control diarrhea (see Nursing Diagnosis 7, action d)<br>b. assist client to gently cleanse and dry perianal area with a soft tissue or cloth after each bowel movement; apply a protective ointment or cream (e.g. Desitin, A&D ointment, Vaseline, BAZA cream)<br>c. provide incontinence pads if needed to absorb moisture; do not allow skin to come in contact with plastic portion of the pads. |

| Desired Outcome | Nursing Actions and ***Selected Purposes/Rationales*** |
|---|---|
| | c. If skin breakdown occurs:<br>1. notify physician<br>2. continue with above measures to prevent further irritation and breakdown<br>3. perform decubitus care as ordered or per standard hospital procedure<br>4. assess client closely and report signs and symptoms of infection (e.g. elevated temperature; redness, warmth, and edema around area of breakdown; unusual drainage from site). |

## 5. NURSING DIAGNOSIS: Hyperthermia

related to stimulation of the thermoregulatory center in the hypothalamus by endogenous pyrogens released from neutrophils and macrophages in an inflammatory process.

| Desired Outcome | Nursing Actions and ***Selected Purposes/Rationales*** |
|---|---|
| 5. The client will experience resolution of hyperthermia as evidenced by:<br>a. skin usual temperature and color<br>b. pulse rate between 60-100 beats/minute<br>c. respirations 14-20/minute<br>d. normal body temperature. | 5.a. Assess for signs and symptoms of hyperthermia (e.g. warm, flushed skin; tachycardia; tachypnea; elevated temperature).<br>b. Implement measures *to reduce fever:*<br>1. perform actions to reduce inflammation and hyperactivity of the bowel (see Nursing Diagnosis 7, action d)<br>2. administer antipyretics if ordered.<br>c. Consult physician if temperature remains higher than 38.5° C. |

## 6. NURSING DIAGNOSIS: Activity intolerance

related to:

a. inadequate nutritional status;
b. difficulty resting and sleeping associated with pain, frequent need to defecate, fear, and anxiety;
c. tissue hypoxia associated with anemia resulting from:
   1. blood loss from the ulcerated bowel
   2. decreased oral intake and impaired absorption of iron, vitamin $B_{12}$, and folate;
d. increased energy expenditure associated with the increased metabolic rate that may be present during period of exacerbation.

| Desired Outcome | Nursing Actions and ***Selected Purposes/Rationales*** |
|---|---|
| 6. The client will demonstrate an increased tolerance for activity as evidenced by:<br>a. verbalization of | 6.a. Assess for signs and symptoms of activity intolerance:<br>1. statements of fatigue and weakness<br>2. exertional dyspnea, chest pain, diaphoresis, or dizziness<br>3. abnormal heart rate response to activity (e.g. increase in rate of 20 beats/minute above resting rate, decrease in rate, rate not returning to |

feeling less fatigued and weak
b. ability to perform activities of daily living without exertional dyspnea, chest pain, diaphoresis, dizziness, and a significant change in vital signs.

preactivity level within 3 minutes after stopping activity, change from regular to irregular rate)
4. decreased systolic B/P or a significant increase (10-15 mm Hg) in systolic or diastolic pressure with activity.

b. Implement measures *to improve activity tolerance:*
   1. perform actions *to promote rest and/or conserve energy:*
      a. maintain activity restrictions as ordered
      b. minimize environmental activity and noise
      c. organize nursing care to allow for periods of uninterrupted rest
      d. limit the number of visitors and their length of stay
      e. assist client with self-care activities as needed
      f. keep supplies and personal articles within easy reach
      g. instruct client in energy-saving techniques (e.g. using shower chair when showering, sitting to brush teeth or comb hair)
      h. implement measures to reduce fear and anxiety (see Nursing Diagnosis 11, action b)
      i. implement measures to promote sleep (see Nursing Diagnosis 8, action c)
      j. implement measures to reduce pain (see Nursing Diagnosis 3, action e)
   2. perform actions to reduce inflammation and hyperactivity of the bowel (see Nursing Diagnosis 7, action d) *in order to reduce excess energy demands associated with inflammation, improve absorption of nutrients, reduce pain, and increase client's ability to rest and sleep*
   3. perform actions to improve nutritional status (see Nursing Diagnosis 2, action c)
   4. administer whole blood or packed red cells if ordered
   5. increase client's activity gradually as allowed and tolerated.

c. Instruct client to:
   1. report a decreased tolerance for activity
   2. stop any activity that causes chest pain, shortness of breath, dizziness, or extreme fatigue or weakness.

d. Consult physician if signs and symptoms of activity intolerance persist or worsen.

## 7. NURSING DIAGNOSIS: Diarrhea

related to intestinal hyperactivity and diminished water absorption from the bowel associated with inflammation of the bowel.

| Desired Outcome | Nursing Actions and ***Selected Purposes/Rationales*** |
|---|---|
| 7. The client will have fewer bowel movements and more formed stool. | 7.a. Ascertain client's usual bowel elimination habits.<br>b. Assess for signs and symptoms of diarrhea (e.g. frequent, loose stools; urgency; abdominal pain and cramping).<br>c. Assess bowel sounds regularly. Report an increase in frequency of bowel sounds.<br>d. Implement measures *to reduce inflammation and hyperactivity of the bowel in order to control diarrhea:*<br>1. perform actions *to rest the bowel:*<br>a. maintain food and fluid restrictions as ordered (usually NPO during acute stage)<br>b. maintain activity restrictions as ordered (may initially be limited to bed rest with bedside commode or bathroom privileges) |

| Desired Outcome | Nursing Actions and ***Selected Purposes/Rationales*** |
|---|---|
| | c. implement measures *to reduce stress* (e.g. explain procedures, provide for consistency in staff assigned, perform actions to reduce pain)<br>d. discourage smoking *(nicotine has a stimulant effect on the gastrointestinal tract)*<br>e. when oral intake is allowed:<br>1. progress diet as ordered (diet usually progresses from elemental formulas such as Vivonex or Criticare HN [these formulas are low in fat and residue and are absorbed in the jejunum, which minimizes stimulation of the bowel] to a bland, low-residue diet)<br>2. instruct client to avoid foods/fluids that may be poorly digested or can act as irritants to the inflamed bowel:<br>a. milk and milk products *(clients with Crohn's disease may have an intolerance to lactose-rich foods because of a deficiency of lactase)*<br>b. those high in fat (e.g. butter, cream, whole milk, ice cream, fried foods, gravies)<br>c. those high in fiber or residue (e.g. whole-grain cereals, nuts, raw fruits and vegetables)<br>d. gas producers (e.g. cabbage, onions, beans, cauliflower)<br>e. those high in caffeine (e.g. coffee, tea, colas)<br>f. spicy foods<br>g. extremely hot or cold foods/fluids<br>3. instruct client to add new foods one at a time<br>4. provide small, frequent meals<br>2. administer the following medications if ordered:<br>a. corticosteroids or ACTH *to reduce inflammation of the bowel*<br>b. sulfasalazine or one of its derivatives (e.g. olsalazine, resin-coated mesalamine) *to reduce inflammation of the bowel*<br>c. antidiarrheal agents:<br>1. loperamide hydrochloride *to slow intestinal motility*<br>2. bulk-forming agents (e.g. methylcellulose, psyllium hydrophillic mucilloid, calcium polycarbophil) *to absorb water in the bowel, which results in a more formed stool*<br>d. immunosuppressive agents such as azathioprine or mercaptopurine (used to reduce intestinal symptoms in cases that are persistent and severe; the effectiveness and action of these agents are still undetermined, but it is postulated *that they may decrease the dosage of corticosteroids required).*<br>e. Consult physician if diarrhea persists. |

## 8. NURSING DIAGNOSIS: Sleep pattern disturbance

related to frequent need to defecate, pain, fear, and anxiety.

| Desired Outcome | Nursing Actions and ***Selected Purposes/Rationales*** |
|---|---|
| 8. The client will attain optimal amounts of sleep within the parameters of the treatment regimen as evidenced by:<br>a. statements of feeling well rested | 8.a. Assess for signs and symptoms of a sleep pattern disturbance (e.g. verbal complaints of difficulty falling asleep, sleep interruptions, or not feeling well rested; irritability; lethargy; disorientation; frequent yawning; dark circles under eyes; slight hand tremors).<br>b. Determine the client's usual sleep habits.<br>c. Implement measures *to promote sleep:*<br>1. discourage long periods of sleep during the day unless signs and |

b. usual mental status
c. absence of frequent yawning, dark circles under eyes, and hand tremors.

symptoms of sleep deprivation exist or daytime sleep is usual for client
2. perform actions to reduce fear and anxiety (see Nursing Diagnosis 11, action b)
3. perform actions to reduce pain (see Nursing Diagnosis 3, action e)
4. perform actions to reduce inflammation and hyperactivity of the bowel (see Nursing Diagnosis 7, action d) *in order to reduce abdominal pain and cramping and the frequency of bowel movements*
5. encourage participation in relaxing diversional activities during the evening
6. discourage intake of fluids high in caffeine (e.g. coffee, tea, colas), especially in the evening
7. offer client a high-protein evening snack (e.g. turkey sandwich) if allowed on current diet
8. allow client to continue usual sleep practices (e.g. position, time, bedtime rituals such as reading and meditating) if possible
9. satisfy basic needs such as comfort and warmth before sleep
10. have client empty bladder just before bedtime
11. maintain a quiet, restful atmosphere; have earplugs available for client if needed
12. use relaxation techniques (e.g. progressive relaxation exercises, back massage, meditation, soft music) before sleep
13. ensure good room ventilation
14. administer sedative-hypnotics if ordered
15. perform actions *to reduce interruptions during sleep (80-100 minutes of uninterrupted sleep are usually needed to complete one sleep cycle):*
    a. restrict visitors
    b. group care (e.g. medications, treatments, physical care, assessments) whenever possible.

d. Consult physician if signs and symptoms of sleep deprivation persist or worsen.

## 9. NURSING DIAGNOSIS: High risk for infection

related to:
a. ulcerations in the bowel wall;
b. lowered resistance to infection associated with malnutrition and treatment with corticosteroids and/or immunosuppressives.

| Desired Outcome | Nursing Actions and ***Selected Purposes/Rationales*** |
|---|---|

9. The client will remain free of infection as evidenced by:
a. temperature declining toward normal
b. absence of chills
c. pulse within normal limits
d. normal breath sounds
e. voiding clear urine without complaints of frequency, urgency, and burning
f. no increase in

9.a. Assess for and report signs and symptoms of infection:
1. significant increase in temperature (a temperature may be present due to the bowel inflammation)
2. chills
3. increased pulse
4. abnormal breath sounds
5. cloudy, foul-smelling urine
6. complaints of frequency, urgency, or burning when urinating
7. presence of WBCs, bacteria, and/or nitrites in urine
8. increase in episodes of diarrhea and abdominal cramping and pain
9. heat, pain, redness, swelling, or unusual drainage in any area
10. increase in WBC count above previous levels (WBC count will usually be elevated as a result of bowel inflammation) and/or significant change in differential.

| Desired Outcome | Nursing Actions and ***Selected Purposes/Rationales*** |
|---|---|
| episodes of diarrhea and abdominal cramping and pain<br>g. absence of heat, pain, redness, swelling, and unusual drainage in any area<br>h. no complaints of increased weakness and fatigue<br>i. WBC and differential counts declining toward normal<br>j. negative results of cultured specimens. | b. Obtain specimens (e.g. urine, vaginal, stool, mouth, sputum, blood) for culture as ordered. Report positive results.<br>c. Implement measures *to prevent infection:*<br>1. maintain a fluid intake of at least 2500 ml/day unless contraindicated<br>2. use good handwashing technique and encourage client to do the same<br>3. maintain meticulous aseptic technique during all invasive procedures (e.g. catheterizations, venous and arterial punctures, injections)<br>4. protect client from others with infection and instruct client to continue this after discharge<br>5. change intravenous tubings and solutions and rotate insertion sites according to hospital policy<br>6. perform actions to improve nutritional status (see Nursing Diagnosis 2, action c)<br>7. reinforce importance of good oral care<br>8. perform actions *to reduce stress* (e.g. explain procedures, provide for consistency in staff assigned, perform actions to reduce pain) *in order to prevent excessive secretion of cortisol (cortisol inhibits the immune system)*<br>9. perform actions *to prevent stasis of respiratory secretions* (e.g. instruct client to turn, cough, and deep breathe; increase activity as allowed and tolerated)<br>10. perform actions to prevent skin breakdown (see Nursing Diagnosis 4, action b)<br>11. perform actions to prevent urinary retention (e.g. instruct client to urinate when the urge is first felt, promote relaxation during voiding attempts) *in order to prevent urinary stasis*<br>12. perform actions *to prevent the introduction of microorganisms into the urinary tract* (e.g. assist client with perineal care as needed, instruct and assist female client to wipe from front to back after urinating and defecating, maintain sterile technique during urinary catheterization)<br>13. perform actions to reduce inflammation and hyperactivity of the bowel (see Nursing Diagnosis 7, action d) *in order to prevent further ulceration of the bowel and subsequently reduce the risk for intestinal infection*<br>14. administer antimicrobials if ordered. |

## 10. COLLABORATIVE DIAGNOSES:

**Potential complications:**

a. **renal calculi** related to:
   1. increased serum oxalate (dietary oxalate normally binds with calcium in the intestine and is excreted in the stool; in clients with IBD, calcium is bound with the poorly absorbed fat and oxalate becomes available for absorption)
   2. concentrated urine associated with fluid volume deficit and stasis of urine associated with decreased activity (both contribute to the accumulation and deposition of minerals in the renal pelvis)
   3. treatment with sulfasalazine (this medication may crystallize and precipitate in acidic urine);

b. **perirectal, rectovaginal, enterovesical, and intra-abdominal abscesses, fissures, and fistulas** related to inflammation, ulceration, and localized perforation of the bowel;

c. **toxic megacolon** related to loss of colonic muscle tone associated with the effects of widespread inflammation in the bowel, use of some medications (e.g. opiates, anticholinergics), and hypokalemia;

d. **bowel obstruction** related to narrowing of the intestinal lumen associated with inflammation and scar tissue formation in the bowel;

e. **peritonitis** related to perforation of the bowel or leakage from an abscess or fistula.

| Desired Outcomes | Nursing Actions and ***Selected Purposes/Rationales*** |
|---|---|
| 10.a. The client will not develop renal calculi as evidenced by:<br>1. absence of flank pain, hematuria, urinary frequency and urgency, nausea, and vomiting<br>2. clear urine without calculi. | 10.a.1. Assess for and report signs and symptoms of renal calculi (e.g. dull, aching or severe, colicky flank pain; hematuria; urinary frequency or urgency; nausea; vomiting).<br>2. Obtain a urine specimen for analysis if ordered. Report hyperoxaluria and/or the presence of crystals.<br>3. Implement measures *to prevent renal calculi:*<br>a. perform actions *to prevent urinary stasis:*<br>1. encourage a minimum fluid intake of 2500 ml/day unless contraindicated<br>2. assist client to change positions at least every 2 hours<br>3. progress activity as allowed and tolerated<br>4. implement measures *to facilitate voiding* (e.g. provide privacy, allow client to assume normal voiding position unless contraindicated, pour warm water over perineum)<br>5. instruct client to void whenever the urge is felt<br>6. maintain patency of urinary catheter if present<br>b. if client is taking sulfasalazine:<br>1. monitor pH of urine and report levels below 6 *(sulfasalazine tends to crystallize and precipitate in acidic urine)*<br>2. administer medications that alkalinize the urine (e.g. sodium bicarbonate, citrate preparations) if ordered<br>c. perform actions *to decrease absorption of oxalate from the intestine:*<br>1. encourage client to decrease intake of foods/fluids high in oxalate (e.g. fruit cocktail, tangerines, berries, peanuts, peanut butter, broccoli, chocolate, spinach, rhubarb)<br>2. encourage client to adhere to a low-fat diet *(this reduces the amount of fat available to bind calcium, thereby freeing calcium to bind with oxalate)*<br>d. perform actions to prevent or treat fluid volume deficit (see Nursing Diagnosis 1, actions c.1 and 2)<br>e. administer the following medications if ordered:<br>1. anion-exchange resins (e.g. cholestyramine) *to bind oxalate and decrease its absorption from the bowel*<br>2. calcium preparations (e.g. calcium carbonate, calcium gluconate) *to bind oxalate and decrease its absorption from the bowel*<br>3. citrate preparations *to increase solubility of minerals in the urine.*<br>4. If signs and symptoms of renal calculi occur:<br>a. strain all urine and save any calculi for analysis; report finding to physician<br>b. encourage a minimum fluid intake of 2500 ml/day unless contraindicated<br>c. administer analgesics as ordered<br>d. prepare client for removal of calculi (e.g. extracorporeal shock wave lithotripsy [ESWL], percutaneous ultrasonic or laser lithotripsy) if planned. |
| 10.b. The client will have resolution of any abscesses, fissures, and fistulas that develop as evidenced by:<br>1. temperature declining toward normal<br>2. resolution of abdominal pain<br>3. absence of perianal | 10.b.1. Assess for and report signs and symptoms of abscess and/or fistula formation (e.g. further increase in temperature, increased or more constant abdominal pain, perianal redness and swelling, burning pain in rectum following defecation, fecal drainage from vagina, fecaluria, further increase in WBC count).<br>2. Observe for perianal fissures.<br>3. Implement measures to reduce inflammation and hyperactivity of the bowel (see Nursing Diagnosis 7, action d) *in order to decrease risk of development of abscesses, fissures, and fistulas and promote healing of any that exist.*<br>4. If signs and symptoms of fissures, abscesses, or fistulas occur:<br>a. administer antimicrobials if ordered |

| Desired Outcomes | Nursing Actions and ***Selected Purposes/Rationales*** |
|---|---|
| redness and swelling and burning pain in rectum following defecation<br>4. no unusual vaginal drainage<br>5. clear, yellow urine<br>6. WBC count declining toward normal. | b. perform wound care as ordered<br>c. prepare client for surgical intervention (e.g. incision and drainage of abscess, closure of fistula, colectomy) if planned<br>d. provide emotional support to client and significant others. |
| 10.c. The client will not develop toxic megacolon as evidenced by:<br>1. absence of abdominal distention<br>2. gradual resolution of abdominal pain<br>3. active bowel sounds<br>4. gradual resolution of diarrhea<br>5. temperature and WBC count declining toward normal. | 10.c.1. Assess for and report signs and symptoms of toxic megacolon:<br>a. abdominal distention and increased pain and tenderness<br>b. hypoactive or absent bowel sounds with tympanic percussion note over abdomen<br>c. sudden decrease in episodes of diarrhea<br>d. high fever (usually 40-40.5° C) and tachycardia<br>e. increase in WBC count.<br>2. Monitor abdominal x-ray results. Report findings of colonic dilation.<br>3. Implement measures *to prevent development of toxic megacolon:*<br>a. perform actions to reduce inflammation of the bowel (see Nursing Diagnosis 7, action d)<br>b. administer opiates, opiate-like medications, and anticholinergics judiciously *(all decrease intestinal motility)*<br>c. perform actions to prevent or treat hypokalemia (see Nursing Diagnosis 1, action c).<br>4. If signs and symptoms of toxic megacolon occur:<br>a. withhold all food and fluid as ordered<br>b. consult physician about discontinuing any opiates, opiate-like medications, and anticholinergics ordered<br>c. insert nasogastric or intestinal tube and maintain suction as ordered<br>d. administer the following if ordered:<br>1. intravenous fluids *to maintain adequate vascular volume (third-space fluid shifting occurs as a result of increased capillary permeability associated with increased intraluminal pressure)*<br>2. corticosteroids *to reduce intestinal inflammation*<br>3. antimicrobials *to prevent infection (the risk of perforation is increased when toxic megacolon develops)*<br>e. prepare client for surgical intervention (e.g. colectomy) if planned<br>f. provide emotional support to client and significant others. |
| 10.d. The client will not develop a bowel obstruction as evidenced by:<br>1. absence of vomiting and abdominal distention<br>2. gradual return of normal bowel sounds. | 10.d.1. Assess for and report signs and symptoms of a bowel obstruction:<br>a. vomiting<br>b. abdominal distention<br>c. change in bowel sounds (in mechanical obstruction, bowel sounds are initially high-pitched and hyperactive; in paralytic ileus, bowel sounds are absent).<br>2. Monitor abdominal x-ray results. Report findings of partial or complete bowel obstruction.<br>3. Implement measures to reduce inflammation of the bowel (see Nursing Diagnosis 7, action d) *in order to reduce intestinal narrowing and scar tissue formation.*<br>4. If signs and symptoms of a bowel obstruction occur:<br>a. withhold all food and fluid as ordered<br>b. insert a nasogastric or intestinal tube and maintain suction as ordered<br>c. administer intravenous fluids if ordered *to maintain an adequate vascular volume (dehydration occurs with prolonged vomiting and third-* |

*spacing occurs due to the increased capillary permeability that results from increased intraluminal pressure in a bowel obstruction)*
   d. prepare client for surgical intervention (e.g. colectomy) if planned
   e. provide emotional support to client and significant others.

10.e. The client will not develop peritonitis as evidenced by:
1. temperature declining toward normal
2. soft, nondistended abdomen
3. gradual resolution of abdominal pain
4. gradual return of normal bowel sounds
5. absence of nausea and vomiting
6. stable vital signs
7. WBC count declining toward normal.

10.e.1. Assess for and report signs and symptoms of peritonitis (e.g. further increase in temperature; tense, rigid abdomen; increased abdominal pain; rebound tenderness; diminished or absent bowel sounds; nausea; vomiting; tachycardia; tachypnea; hypotension).
2. Monitor WBC counts. Report levels that increase or fail to decline toward normal.
3. Implement measures to prevent and treat abscesses, fistulas, toxic megacolon, and/or bowel obstruction (see actions b.3 and 4, c.3 and 4, and d.3 and 4 in this diagnosis) *in order to reduce the risk for peritonitis.*
4. If signs and symptoms of peritonitis occur:
   a. withhold all food and fluid as ordered
   b. place client on bed rest in a semi-Fowler's position *to assist in pooling or localizing intestinal contents in the pelvis rather than under the diaphragm*
   c. insert nasogastric tube and maintain suction as ordered
   d. administer antimicrobials as ordered
   e. administer intravenous fluids and/or blood volume expanders if ordered *to prevent or treat shock (can result from the increased capillary permeability that occurs with inflammation and the subsequent escape of protein, fluid, and electrolytes from the vascular space into the peritoneal cavity)*
   f. prepare client for surgical intervention (e.g. repair of perforation, incision and drainage of abscess, colectomy) if planned
   g. provide emotional support to client and significant others.

## 11. NURSING DIAGNOSIS: Anxiety

related to pain; persistent diarrhea with possible social embarrassment; lack of understanding of diagnosis, diagnostic tests, and treatments; unfamiliar environment; uncertain prognosis; and possibility of surgery if current symptoms cannot be controlled.

**Desired Outcome** | **Nursing Actions and *Selected Purposes/Rationales***

11. The client will experience a reduction in anxiety as evidenced by:
   a. verbalization of feeling less anxious and fearful
   b. usual sleep pattern
   c. relaxed facial expression and body movements
   d. stable vital signs
   e. usual perceptual ability and interactions with others.

11.a. Assess client for signs and symptoms of anxiety (e.g. verbalization of fears and concerns, insomnia, tenseness, tremors, irritability, restlessness, diaphoresis, tachypnea, tachycardia, elevated blood pressure, facial pallor or flushing, narrowed perceptual field, withdrawal, noncompliance with treatment plan).
b. Implement measures *to reduce fear and anxiety:*
   1. orient client to hospital environment, equipment, and routines
   2. introduce staff who will be participating in his/her care; if possible, maintain consistency in staff assigned to his/her care *to provide feelings of stability and comfort with the environment*
   3. assure client that staff members are nearby; respond to call signal as soon as possible
   4. maintain a calm, supportive, confident manner when interacting with client
   5. encourage verbalization of fear and anxiety; provide feedback
   6. explain all diagnostic tests
   7. reinforce physician's explanations and clarify misconceptions the

| Desired Outcome | Nursing Actions and ***Selected Purposes/Rationales*** |
|---|---|
| | client has about inflammatory bowel disease, the treatment plan, and prognosis<br>8. perform actions to reduce pain (see Nursing Diagnosis 3, action e)<br>9. perform actions to reduce inflammation and hyperactivity of the bowel (see Nursing Diagnosis 7, action d) *in order to reduce episodes of diarrhea*<br>10. provide a calm, restful environment<br>11. instruct client in relaxation techniques and encourage participation in diversional activities<br>12. assist client to cope with the diagnosis and its implications (see Nursing Diagnosis 13, action c)<br>13. encourage significant others to project a caring, concerned attitude without obvious anxiousness<br>14. if surgical intervention is indicated, begin preoperative teaching<br>15. administer antianxiety agents if ordered.<br>c. Include significant others in orientation and teaching sessions and encourage their continued support of the client.<br>d. Provide information based on current needs of the client and significant others at a level they can understand. Encourage questions and clarification of information provided.<br>e. Consult physician if above actions fail to control fear and anxiety. |

## 12. NURSING DIAGNOSIS: Self-concept disturbance*

related to:
a. dependence on others to meet self-care needs;
b. embarrassment associated with diarrhea;
c. changes in sexual functioning associated with pain, fatigue, and weakness;
d. changes in life style imposed by inflammatory bowel disease and its treatment.

*This diagnostic label includes the nursing diagnoses of body image disturbance, self-esteem disturbance, and altered role performance.

| Desired Outcome | Nursing Actions and ***Selected Purposes/Rationales*** |
|---|---|
| 12. The client will demonstrate beginning adaptation to changes in body functioning, life style, and roles as evidenced by:<br>a. verbalization of feelings of self-worth and sexual adequacy<br>b. maintenance of relationships with significant others<br>c. active participation in activities of daily living<br>d. active interest in personal appearance<br>e. willingness to pursue usual roles | 12.a. Assess for signs and symptoms of a self-concept disturbance (e.g. verbal or nonverbal cues denoting a negative response to the changes that have occurred, withdrawal from significant others).<br>b. Determine the meaning of changes in body functioning and life style/roles to the client by encouraging him/her to verbalize feelings and by noting nonverbal responses to changes experienced.<br>c. Discuss with client improvements in bowel function, comfort, and energy levels that can realistically be expected.<br>d. Implement measures *to assist client to increase self-esteem* (e.g. limit negative self-assessment, encourage positive comments about self, assist to identify strengths, give positive feedback about accomplishments and behaviors that are indicative of high self-esteem).<br>e. Implement measures to assist client to cope with the effects of inflammatory bowel disease (see Nursing Diagnosis 13, action c).<br>f. Implement measures *to reduce embarrassment associated with diarrhea:*<br>1. provide a private room if possible<br>2. keep bedside commode or bedpan within easy reach<br>3. use room deodorizers and empty bedpan or commode as soon as possible after each bowel movement *to reduce odor.* |

| Desired Outcome | Nursing Actions and *Selected Purposes/Rationales* |
|---|---|
| and participate in social activities<br>f. verbalization of a beginning plan for adapting life style to meet restrictions imposed by having inflammatory bowel disease. | g. Encourage client to discuss concerns about sexual functioning. Offer suggestions to assist client to regain optimal level of sexual functioning (e.g. rest before sexual activity).<br>h. Assess for and support behaviors suggesting positive adaptation to changes that have occurred (e.g. compliance with treatment plan, verbalization of feelings of self-worth, maintenance of relationships with significant others).<br>i. Encourage significant others to allow client to do what he/she is able *so that independence can be reestablished and/or self-esteem redeveloped.*<br>j. Assist client's and significant others' adjustment by listening, facilitating communication, and providing information.<br>k. Assist client and significant others to have similar expectations of future life style and to identify ways that personal and family goals can be adjusted rather than abandoned.<br>l. Encourage visits and support from significant others.<br>m. Encourage client to pursue usual roles and interests and to continue involvement in social activities. If previous roles, interests, and hobbies cannot be pursued, encourage development of new ones.<br>n. Provide information about and encourage utilization of community resources (e.g. support groups; sexual, family, and individual counseling).<br>o. Consult physician about psychological counseling if client desires or if he/she seems unwilling or unable to adapt to changes resulting from inflammatory bowel disease. |

## 13. NURSING DIAGNOSIS: Ineffective individual coping

related to:
a. chronicity of condition and effect of disease on life style;
b. pain;
c. fear of eventual need for an ileal diversion;
d. inadequate support system.

| Desired Outcome | Nursing Actions and *Selected Purposes/Rationales* |
|---|---|
| 13. The client will demonstrate the use of effective coping skills as evidenced by:<br>a. verbalization of ability to cope with inflammatory bowel disease and its effects<br>b. utilization of appropriate problem-solving techniques<br>c. willingness to participate in treatment plan and meet basic needs<br>d. absence of destructive behavior | 13.a. Assess for and report signs and symptoms of ineffective individual coping (e.g. verbalization of inability to cope; inability to ask for help, problem solve, or meet basic needs; reluctance to participate in treatment plan; destructive behavior toward self or others; inappropriate use of defense mechanisms; inability to meet role expectations).<br>b. Assess client's perception of current situation including precipitating factors and effectiveness of coping mechanisms.<br>c. Implement measures *to promote effective coping:*<br>1. assist client to recognize and manage inappropriate denial if it is present<br>2. perform actions to reduce fear and anxiety (see Nursing Diagnosis 11, action b)<br>3. perform actions to reduce pain (see Nursing Diagnosis 3, action e)<br>4. encourage verbalization about current situation and ways comparable situations have been handled in the past<br>5. assist client to identify personal strengths and resources that can be used to facilitate coping with the current situation<br>6. demonstrate acceptance of client but set limits on inappropriate behavior |

| Desired Outcome | Nursing Actions and ***Selected Purposes/Rationales*** |
|---|---|
| toward self and others<br>e. appropriate use of defense mechanisms<br>f. recognition and utilization of available support systems. | 7. create an atmosphere of trust and support<br>8. arrange for a visit with another individual who has successfully adjusted to inflammatory bowel disease<br>9. provide consistency in caregivers when possible; inform client if there will be a change in caregivers *so he/she will not interpret the change as rejection*<br>10. include client in planning of care, encourage maximum participation in treatment plan, and allow choices when possible *to enable him/her to maintain a sense of control*<br>11. instruct client in effective problem-solving techniques (e.g. accurate identification of stressors, determination of various options to solve problem)<br>12. assist client to maintain usual daily routines whenever possible<br>13. encourage diversional activities according to client's interests<br>14. assist client as he/she starts to plan for necessary life-style and role changes after discharge; help client to identify priorities and attainable goals<br>15. assist client to prepare for negative reactions from others because of diarrhea and odor of flatus<br>16. assist client to identify and utilize available support systems; provide information regarding available community resources that can assist client and significant others in coping with the disease (e.g. support groups, counseling services)<br>17. administer antianxiety and/or antidepressant agents if ordered<br>18. encourage continued emotional support from significant others; reinforce the importance of maintaining a calm, nonstressful atmosphere during visits<br>19. encourage client to share with significant others the kind of support that would be the most beneficial (e.g. listening, inspiring hope, providing reassurance and accurate information)<br>20. support behaviors suggesting positive adaptation to changes experienced (e.g. increased participation in self-care activities and treatment plan, verbalization of ways to adapt to necessary changes in life style).<br>d. Consult physician about psychological counseling if appropriate. Initiate a referral if necessary. |

## 14. NURSING DIAGNOSIS: Knowledge deficit

regarding follow-up care.

| Desired Outcomes | Nursing Actions and ***Selected Purposes/Rationales*** |
|---|---|
| 14.a. The client will identify ways to reduce the incidence of disease exacerbation. | 14.a.1. Reinforce the importance of adhering to the prescribed treatment regimen in order to reduce the incidence of disease exacerbation.<br>2. Instruct the client regarding ways to reduce bowel irritation:<br>a. avoid foods/fluids likely to be poorly digested or that may irritate the bowel (e.g. raw fruits and vegetables, whole-grain cereals, fried foods, spicy foods, milk products, caffeine-containing beverages, iced drinks)<br>b. avoid use of laxatives<br>c. avoid smoking and alcohol intake.<br>3. Explain that stress can precipitate periods of exacerbation. Provide |

information about stress management classes and counseling services that may assist him/her to manage stress.

| | |
|---|---|
| 14.b. The client will verbalize ways to maintain an optimal nutritional status. | 14.b. Provide instructions regarding ways to maintain an optimal nutritional status:<br>1. reinforce instructions regarding prescribed diet (a low-residue, high-calorie, high-protein diet is often recommended)<br>2. inform client that eating small, frequent meals rather than 3 large meals may help achieve the recommended high-calorie intake<br>3. reinforce the benefits of eating when rested and in a relaxed atmosphere<br>4. stress the importance of taking vitamins and minerals as prescribed. |
| 14.c. The client will state ways to prevent perianal skin breakdown. | 14.c. Provide the following instructions about ways to prevent perianal skin breakdown:<br>1. use soft toilet tissue for wiping after each bowel movement<br>2. cleanse perianal area with a mild soap and warm water after each bowel movement; dry thoroughly<br>3. apply a protective ointment or cream (e.g. BAZA cream, Desitin, Vaseline, A&D ointment) to perianal area after skin has been cleansed. |
| 14.d. The client will verbalize an understanding of medications ordered including rationale, side effects, schedule for taking, and importance of taking as prescribed. | 14.d.1. Explain rationale for, side effects of, and importance of taking medications prescribed.<br>2. If client is discharged on sulfasalazine, instruct to:<br>a. drink at least 10 glasses of liquid/day to reduce risk of kidney stone formation<br>b. expect that urine might be an orange-yellow color<br>c. take medication with food or after meals but do not take with antacids (the absorption time is altered by antacids)<br>d. report a sore throat or mouth, fever, unusual fatigue, continuous headache or aching joint(s), unusual bruising or bleeding, nausea and vomiting, rash, or marked decline in urine output<br>e. notify health care provider if unable to impregnate partner (sulfasalazine may cause a reduction in sperm count)<br>f. keep scheduled appointments for blood and urine studies.<br>3. If client is discharged on a corticosteroid preparation, instruct to:<br>a. take medication exactly as prescribed<br>b. adjust dosage only if prescribed by physician<br>c. notify health care provider if unable to tolerate oral medication<br>d. avoid discontinuing medication suddenly or of own accord<br>e. take with food or antacids to reduce gastric irritation<br>f. eat smaller, more frequent meals if gastric irritation occurs<br>g. weigh self daily and report unusual weight gain<br>h. expect that certain effects such as facial rounding, slight weight gain and swelling, increased appetite, and slight mood changes may occur<br>i. report undesirable effects of corticosteroid therapy such as marked swelling in extremities, significant weight gain, extreme emotional and behavioral changes, extreme weakness, tarry stools, bloody or coffee-ground vomitus, frequent or persistent headaches, insomnia, and lack of menses<br>j. avoid contact with persons who have an infection because corticosteroids lower resistance to infection.<br>4. If client is to administer corticosteroid or mesalamine enemas or suppositories at home, instruct in technique and length of time he/she should retain the solution or suppository. Allow time for questions, clarification, and return demonstration.<br>5. Instruct client to inform physician before taking other prescription and nonprescription medications.<br>6. Instruct client to inform all health care providers of medications being taken. |

| Desired Outcomes | Nursing Actions and ***Selected Purposes/Rationales*** |
|---|---|
| 14.f. The client will state signs and symptoms to report to the health care provider. | 14.f. Instruct client to report the following signs and symptoms:<br>1. recurrent episodes of diarrhea and abdominal pain and cramping<br>2. increasing abdominal distention<br>3. persistent vomiting<br>4. unusual rectal or vaginal drainage<br>5. rectal pain<br>6. yellowing of skin, change in vision, eye pain, or joint pain or swelling (can indicate extraintestinal involvement)<br>7. flank pain. |
| 14.g. The client will identify resources that can assist in the adjustment to changes resulting from inflammatory bowel disease and its treatment. | 14.g.1. Provide information about resources that can assist the client and significant others in adjusting to inflammatory bowel disease and its effects (e.g. local support groups, Crohn's and Colitis Foundation of America, counseling services, stress management classes).<br>2. Initiate a referral if indicated. |
| 14.h. The client will verbalize an understanding of and a plan for adhering to recommended follow-up care including future appointments with health care provider and activity level. | 14.h.1. Reinforce importance of keeping follow-up appointments with health care provider.<br>2. Reinforce importance of frequent rest periods throughout the day.<br>3. Implement measures to improve client compliance:<br>a. include significant others in teaching sessions if possible<br>b. encourage questions and allow time for reinforcement and clarification of information provided<br>c. provide written instructions on future appointments with health care provider, medications prescribed, signs and symptoms to report, and future laboratory studies. |

# Mandibular (Jaw) Fracture with Intermaxillary Fixation

Fracture of the mandible (lower jaw) is one of the most common fractures and is usually the result of blunt trauma to the jaw. The goal of treatment for a mandibular fracture is to correct deformity and restore functional dental occlusion. This is accomplished by closed reduction and 4-6 weeks of intermaxillary fixation (maxillary-mandibular fixation [MMF]) or by open reduction and internal fixation, which is sometimes followed by a shorter period (1-2 weeks) of intermaxillary fixation. Intermaxillary fixation involves attaching wires or arch bars along the upper and lower teeth and connecting these with cross wires or orthodontic elastic bands so that the jaws are held together in correct alignment. The method of reduction and fixation used is determined by the type of fracture and adequacy of the client's teeth. Clients who have a comminuted, compound, or unstable fracture or are edentulous usually require open reduction and internal fixation using transosseous wiring or plates and screws. Those clients with a nondisplaced fracture or a minor degree of displacement and an adequate complement of teeth are more likely to have a closed reduction and intermaxillary fixation.

**This care plan focuses on the adult client with a fracture of the mandible hospitalized for closed reduction and intermaxillary fixation.** Preoperatively, the goals of care are to reduce fear and anxiety, reduce pain, and educate the client regarding ways to prevent postoperative complications. Postoperatively, the goals of care are to maintain a patent airway, jaw immobilization, an adequate nutritional status, and comfort; prevent complications; and educate the client regarding follow-up care.

## DIAGNOSTIC TESTS

X-rays of the mandible
Computed tomography (CT)

## DISCHARGE CRITERIA

Prior to discharge, the client will:

- ❖ have an adequate respiratory status
- ❖ have an adequate oral intake
- ❖ have no signs and symptoms of complications
- ❖ identify ways to maintain a patent airway
- ❖ demonstrate the ability to perform oral hygiene
- ❖ verbalize an understanding of dietary modifications and ways to maintain an adequate nutritional status
- ❖ identify ways to prevent constipation that may result from temporary dietary modifications
- ❖ state signs and symptoms to report to the health care provider
- ❖ share thoughts and feelings regarding temporary alterations in diet, speech, and appearance
- ❖ verbalize an understanding of and a plan for adhering to recommended follow-up care including future appointments with health care provider and medications prescribed.

## NURSING/ COLLABORATIVE DIAGNOSES



**See Standardized Preoperative and Postoperative Care Plans for additional diagnoses.**

## PREOPERATIVE

**Use in conjunction with the Standardized Preoperative Care Plan.**

### 1. NURSING DIAGNOSIS: Anxiety

related to:
a. lack of understanding of planned surgery;
b. anticipated effects of general anesthesia or possibility of discomfort during surgery if local anesthesia is planned;
c. unfamiliar environment and separation from significant others;
d. economic factors associated with hospitalization;

e. anticipated discomfort and effects of surgery and intermaxillary fixation on appearance;
f. anticipated difficulty breathing, swallowing, and talking with jaws wired or banded.

| Desired Outcome | Nursing Actions and ***Selected Purposes/Rationales*** |
|---|---|
| 1. The client will experience a reduction in anxiety (see Standardized Preoperative Care Plan, Nursing Diagnosis 1 [pp. 108-109], for outcome criteria). | 1.a. Refer to Standardized Preoperative Care Plan, Nursing Diagnosis 1 (pp. 108-109), for measures related to assessment and reduction of fear and anxiety.<br>b. Implement additional measures *to reduce fear and anxiety:*<br>1. inform client that the facial edema and ecchymosis that are present following surgery usually diminish after 2-3 days<br>2. discuss alternative methods of communicating after surgery (e.g. magic slate, pad and pencil); stress that client's difficulty communicating verbally will be temporary and that it will improve as facial edema subsides and resolve when intermaxillary fixation device is removed (usually in 4-6 weeks)<br>3. reassure client that he/she will still be able to breathe and swallow when jaws are wired or banded. |

## 2. NURSING DIAGNOSIS: Pain: jaw

related to inflammation and tissue and nerve trauma in the area of the fracture.

| Desired Outcome | Nursing Actions and ***Selected Purposes/Rationales*** |
|---|---|
| 2. The client will experience diminished jaw pain as evidenced by:<br>a. verbalization of a reduction in pain<br>b. relaxed facial expression and body positioning<br>c. stable vital signs. | 2.a. Determine how the client usually responds to pain.<br>b. Assess client's perception of pain including location, intensity, and type. Use a numerical scale to rate intensity.<br>c. Assess for nonverbal signs of pain (e.g. wrinkled brow, clenched fists, rubbing jaw, reluctance to move, restlessness, diaphoresis, facial pallor, increased B/P, tachycardia).<br>d. Assess for factors that seem to aggravate and alleviate pain.<br>e. Implement measures *to reduce pain:*<br>1. perform actions *to reduce fear and anxiety about the pain experience* (e.g. assure client that his/her need for pain relief will be met)<br>2. medicate prior to any painful procedures and before pain is severe<br>3. apply ice packs to jaw if ordered<br>4. provide or assist with nonpharmacological measures for pain relief (e.g. position change, relaxation techniques, quiet conversation, diversional activities)<br>5. administer analgesics if ordered.<br>f. Consult physician if above measures fail to provide adequate pain relief. |

## 3. NURSING DIAGNOSIS: Knowledge deficit

regarding hospital routines associated with surgery, physical preparation for oral surgery, sensations that normally occur following surgery and anesthesia, and postoperative care.

| Desired Outcomes | Nursing Actions and ***Selected Purposes/Rationales*** |
|---|---|
| 3.a. The client will verbalize an understanding of usual preoperative care and postoperative sensations and care. | 3.a.1. Refer to Standardized Preoperative Care Plan, Nursing Diagnosis 4, actions a.1-4 (pp. 111-112), for information to include in preoperative teaching.<br>2. Provide additional information about specific postoperative care following intermaxillary fixation:<br>a. instruct client to avoid trying to open mouth if jaws are wired or banded shut (some surgeons wait until client is fully awake to apply diagonal or vertical wires or bands in order to reduce the risk for aspiration if vomiting occurs)<br>b. inform client that a nasogastric tube may be in place for a short time after surgery to reduce the risk for vomiting<br>c. explain the reason for a liquid or blenderized diet until wires or bands are removed<br>d. instruct client in ways to drink and eat with jaws wired or banded shut:<br>1. sip from a cup or from a spoon<br>2. suck through a straw that has been placed between a gap in teeth or behind last molar between teeth and cheek<br>3. pour liquid or blenderized food into a bulb syringe attached to a tube (e.g. nasogastric tube, rubber catheter) that is placed between a gap in teeth or behind last molar between teeth and cheek<br>e. explain the need for frequent oral hygiene after surgery and instruct client in correct way to rinse mouth and use oral irrigation device (e.g. Water-Pik).<br>3. Allow time for questions, clarification, and return demonstration. |
| 3.b. The client will demonstrate the ability to perform activities designed to prevent postoperative complications. | 3.b.1. Refer to Standardized Preoperative Care Plan, Nursing Diagnosis 4, action b.1 (p. 112), for instructions on ways to prevent postoperative complications.<br>2. Provide additional instructions on ways to prevent postoperative complications following intermaxillary fixation:<br>a. demonstrate use of suction equipment; if possible, have client practice suctioning with teeth clenched (suctioning should be done while leaning forward and suction catheter should be inserted through a gap in the teeth or behind last molar between teeth and cheek)<br>b. instruct client to inform staff if nauseated (treatment of nausea helps prevent vomiting, which decreases the risk for aspiration)<br>c. instruct client regarding appropriate actions if vomiting does occur:<br>1. use call signal to summon help<br>2. turn on side if unable to sit up<br>3. sit up, lean forward, use fingers to pull cheeks away from teeth, and expel as much of vomitus through spaces between teeth as possible<br>4. suction as instructed.<br>3. Allow time for questions, clarification, and return demonstration. |

## POSTOPERATIVE

**Use in conjunction with the Standardized Postoperative Care Plan.**

### 1. NURSING DIAGNOSIS: High risk for aspiration

related to:

a. decreased level of consciousness and absent or diminished gag reflex associated

with the depressant effects of anesthesia (if a general anesthetic was used) and narcotic analgesics;
b. difficulty expelling secretions and/or vomitus associated with intermaxillary fixation;
c. difficulty chewing and swallowing associated with restricted jaw movement.

| Desired Outcome | Nursing Actions and ***Selected Purposes/Rationales*** |
|---|---|
| 1. The client will not aspirate secretions, vomitus, or foods/fluids (see Standardized Postoperative Care Plan, Nursing Diagnosis 18 [p. 131], for outcome criteria). | 1.a. Refer to Standardized Postoperative Care Plan, Nursing Diagnosis 18 (p. 131), for measures related to assessment and prevention of aspiration.<br>b. Implement additional measures *to prevent aspiration:*<br>1. position client on side with head of bed slightly elevated until he/she is fully awake and able to swallow; then keep head of bed elevated at least 45° *to facilitate swallowing and ability to clear airway*<br>2. perform actions to prevent nausea and vomiting (see Postoperative Nursing Diagnosis 4)<br>3. if vomiting does occur:<br>a. position client on his/her side or assist him/her to sit up and lean forward<br>b. instruct and/or assist client to retract cheeks by holding them out and back with fingers *so vomitus does not pool between cheeks and gingivae*<br>c. instruct client to expel vomitus through spaces between teeth<br>d. perform and/or assist client with oral and nasopharyngeal suctioning if necessary<br>e. perform good oral hygiene following vomiting episode *to remove vomitus from mouth*<br>4. administer narcotic analgesics judiciously *to prevent depression of the gag reflex*<br>5. instruct client to avoid intake of carbonated beverages *(the fizzing in the back of the throat can cause choking)*<br>6. stress to client the importance of adhering to a liquid or blenderized diet *(restricted jaw movement makes it difficult to effectively chew and safely swallow solid food).* |

## 2. NURSING DIAGNOSIS: Altered nutrition: less than body requirements

related to:
a. decreased oral intake associated with nausea, mouth and jaw pain, fear of choking, and dislike of the prescribed diet;
b. inadequate nutritional replacement therapy;
c. loss of nutrients associated with vomiting;
d. increased nutritional needs associated with the increased metabolic rate that occurs during wound healing.

| Desired Outcome | Nursing Actions and ***Selected Purposes/Rationales*** |
|---|---|
| 2. The client will maintain an adequate nutritional status (see Standardized Postoperative Care Plan, Nursing Diagnosis 5 [p. 118], for outcome criteria). | 2.a. Refer to Standardized Postoperative Care Plan, Nursing Diagnosis 5 (p. 118), for measures related to assessment and maintenance of an adequate nutritional status.<br>b. Implement additional measures *to maintain an adequate nutritional status:*<br>1. perform actions *to increase oral intake:*<br>a. implement measures to reduce mouth and jaw pain (see Postoperative Nursing Diagnosis 3) |

b. implement measures to prevent nausea and vomiting (see Postoperative Nursing Diagnosis 4)
c. allow client to use the technique he/she is most comfortable with when feeding self (e.g. syringe, spoon, straw, cup) *in order to decrease fear of choking*

2. advance diet from clear liquids to blenderized foods with high-protein dietary supplements when allowed and tolerated.

## 3. NURSING DIAGNOSIS: Pain: mouth and jaw

related to tissue trauma associated with the fracture, closed reduction, application of the intermaxillary fixation device, and presence of protruding wire ends in the mouth postoperatively.

| Desired Outcome | Nursing Actions and ***Selected Purposes/Rationales*** |
|---|---|
| 3. The client will experience diminished mouth and jaw pain (see Standardized Postoperative Care Plan, Nursing Diagnosis 6 [p. 119], for outcome criteria). | 3.a. Refer to Standardized Postoperative Care Plan, Nursing Diagnosis 6 (p. 119), for measures related to assessment and reduction of pain.<br>b. Implement additional measures *to reduce mouth and jaw pain:*<br>1. apply ice packs to jaw for 24-48 hours after surgery if ordered<br>2. instruct client to avoid intake of hot or cold foods/fluids *(the mouth and teeth are very sensitive for a few days after surgery)*<br>3. apply topical anesthetics to painful areas in mouth if ordered<br>4. apply dental or paraffin wax to ends of protruding wires<br>5. administer corticosteroids (e.g. dexamethasone) if ordered *to reduce edema in the operative area.* |

## 4. NURSING DIAGNOSIS: Altered comfort: nausea and vomiting

related to stimulation of the vomiting center associated with:
a. stimulation of the afferent vagal and/or sympathetic pathways resulting from irritation of the gastric mucosa by swallowed blood;
b. cortical stimulation resulting from pain, stress, and the taste of blood.

| Desired Outcome | Nursing Actions and ***Selected Purposes/Rationales*** |
|---|---|
| 4. The client will experience relief of nausea and vomiting (see Standardized Postoperative Care Plan, Nursing Diagnosis 7.B [p. 120], for outcome criteria). | 4.a. Refer to Standardized Postoperative Care Plan, Nursing Diagnosis 7.B (p. 120), for measures related to assessment and prevention of nausea and vomiting.<br>b. Implement additional measures *to prevent nausea and vomiting:*<br>1. keep container of suctioned secretions out of client's sight by covering it or placing it at head of the bed *(noxious stimuli cause cortical stimulation of the vomiting center)*<br>2. instruct and assist client to remove blood and saliva from mouth by suctioning and/or pushing it out through spaces between teeth rather than swallowing it<br>3. maintain patency of nasogastric tube if present<br>4. remind client to report nausea so that antiemetics can be given as soon as needed. |

## 5. NURSING DIAGNOSIS: Impaired verbal communication

related to restricted jaw movement associated with pain, edema, and presence of intermaxillary fixation device.

| Desired Outcome | Nursing Actions and ***Selected Purposes/Rationales*** |
|---|---|
| 5. The client will successfully communicate needs and desires. | 5.a. Assess client for impaired verbal communication (e.g. inability to speak, difficulty forming words or sentences).<br>b. Implement measures *to facilitate communication:*<br>1. answer call signal in person rather than using the intercommunication system<br>2. ask questions that require short answers, eye blinks, or nod of head if client is having difficulty speaking and/or is frustrated or fatigued<br>3. perform actions to reduce mouth and jaw pain (see Postoperative Nursing Diagnosis 3)<br>4. maintain a patient, calm approach; listen attentively and allow ample time for communication<br>5. maintain a quiet environment *so that client does not have to raise voice to be heard*<br>6. provide materials such as magic slate, pad and pencil, or chalk and chalkboard if appropriate; try to ensure that placement of intravenous line does not interfere with use of these aids.<br>c. Inform significant others and health care personnel of techniques being used to facilitate client's ability to communicate. |

## 6. NURSING DIAGNOSIS: Altered oral mucous membrane:

a. **dry, sore lips** related to stretching of the lips during surgery and inability to moisten lips with tongue associated with jaws being banded or wired shut;
b. **irritation and breakdown of oral mucosa** related to:
1. application of intermaxillary fixation device and presence of protruding wires
2. colonization of bacteria associated with trapping of food particles and bacteria in the intermaxillary fixation device and inadequate oral hygiene.

| Desired Outcome | Nursing Actions and ***Selected Purposes/Rationales*** |
|---|---|
| 6. The client will experience improved health of the oral mucous membrane as evidenced by:<br>a. moist lips<br>b. decreased mucosal inflammation<br>c. absence of ulcerations<br>d. decreasing complaints of oral pain. | 6.a. Assess oral mucous membranes frequently (use flashlight and tongue depressor to retract cheeks) being aware that inflammation will be present because of surgical trauma.<br>b. Report any increase in mucosal inflammation, presence of ulcerations, or increased oral pain.<br>c. Implement measures *to maintain or regain integrity of the oral mucous membrane:*<br>1. instruct and assist client with prescribed oral hygiene (e.g. rinsing mouth with warm saline, diluted hydrogen peroxide, or alkaline mouthwash; brushing teeth with a small, soft-bristle toothbrush; using oral irrigation device); avoid products such as lemon-glycerin swabs and commercial mouthwashes containing alcohol *(these products have a drying or irritating effect on the oral mucous membrane)* |

2. avoid using sponge-tipped applicators and cotton swabs to clean teeth *(the sponge or cotton may catch in the intermaxillary fixation device)*
3. stress the importance of performing oral hygiene gently and thoroughly
4. lubricate client's lips frequently with K-Y jelly, ChapStick, Blistex, or mineral oil
5. encourage client to breathe through nose rather than his/her mouth *in order to reduce mouth dryness*
6. encourage a fluid intake of 2500 ml/day unless contraindicated
7. perform actions to maintain an adequate nutritional status (see Postoperative Nursing Diagnosis 2)
8. instruct client to avoid substances that might further irritate the oral mucosa (e.g. extremely hot, spicy, or acidic foods/fluids)
9. encourage client not to smoke *(smoking dries and irritates the mucosa)*
10. if protruding wires are irritating the oral mucosa, apply or assist client to apply paraffin or dental wax to the ends of the wires (wax should be removed before eating and brushing teeth).

d. Consult physician about readjustment of wires and/or alternative methods of oral hygiene if irritation and inflammation of oral mucous membrane persist or worsen.

---

## 7. NURSING DIAGNOSIS: High risk for infection: oral cavity

related to:

a. invasion of pathogens associated with breaks in the oral mucous membrane resulting from intermaxillary fixation;
b. colonization of bacteria in mouth associated with:
   1. difficulty expelling oral secretions and blood resulting from jaws being wired or banded shut
   2. trapping of food particles in intermaxillary fixation device
   3. difficulty performing good oral hygiene;
c. decreased resistance to infection associated with inadequate nutritional status.

| Desired Outcome | Nursing Actions and ***Selected Purposes/Rationales*** |
|---|---|
| 7. The client will remain free of infection in the oral cavity as evidenced by:<br>a. absence of chills and fever<br>b. decreased inflammation and pain in mouth<br>c. absence of ulcerations and white patches in mouth<br>d. absence of foul odor from mouth<br>e. WBC and differential counts returning toward or within normal range<br>f. negative cultures of oral lesions. | 7.a. Assess for and report signs and symptoms of oral cavity infection (e.g. chills, fever, increased inflammation of oral mucous membrane, complaints of increased mouth pain, presence of ulcerations or white patches in mouth, halitosis).<br>b. Monitor for and report persistent elevation of WBC count and significant change in differential.<br>c. Obtain cultures from oral lesions as ordered. Report positive results.<br>d. Implement measures *to prevent infection in the oral cavity:*<br>1. perform actions to maintain or regain integrity of the oral mucous membrane (see Postoperative Nursing Diagnosis 6, action c)<br>2. instruct client to avoid unnecessary handling of wires or bands<br>3. suction oral cavity as needed *to remove secretions, blood, and food particles*<br>4. perform oral hygiene frequently (usual order is every 2 hours and following meals and snacks)<br>5. wash hands thoroughly before performing oral hygiene or suctioning client and instruct client to do the same<br>6. administer the following if ordered:<br>a. antibacterial oral rinse solutions (e.g. Peridex)<br>b. antimicrobial agents. |

## 8. COLLABORATIVE DIAGNOSIS: Potential complication: airway obstruction

related to inability to clear airway effectively associated with:
a. decreased level of consciousness and depressed gag reflex in the early post-operative period;
b. difficulty expelling secretions and/or vomitus as a result of jaws being wired or banded shut.

| Desired Outcome | Nursing Actions and ***Selected Purposes/Rationales*** |
|---|---|
| 8. The client will not experience airway obstruction as evidenced by:<br>a. unlabored respirations at 14-20/minute<br>b. absence of stridor and sternocleidomastoid muscle retraction<br>c. usual mental status<br>d. usual skin color<br>e. blood gases within normal range. | 8.a. Assess for and immediately report:<br>1. signs and symptoms of airway obstruction (e.g. rapid and/or labored respirations, stridor, sternocleidomastoid muscle retraction, restlessness, agitation, cyanosis)<br>2. abnormal blood gases<br>3. significant change in oximetry results.<br>b. Obtain an order from physician regarding the circumstances that warrant cutting the wires or bands and specific instructions as to which wires or bands can be cut. Document these orders on the client's nursing care plan.<br>c. Have wire cutters or scissors and suction equipment at bedside and tracheostomy tray and oxygen equipment readily available.<br>d. Implement measures to prevent aspiration (see Postoperative Nursing Diagnosis 1) *in order to reduce the risk for airway obstruction.*<br>e. If signs and symptoms of airway obstruction occur:<br>1. place client in a high Fowler's position<br>2. administer oxygen as ordered<br>3. perform oral and nasopharyngeal suctioning as indicated<br>4. use wire cutters or scissors to cut wires or bands if absolutely necessary (specific orders regarding the circumstances in which the wires/bands should be cut and which ones to cut should be strictly adhered to)<br>5. prepare client for emergency tracheotomy if indicated<br>6. provide emotional support to client and significant others. |

## 9. NURSING DIAGNOSIS: Body image disturbance

related to impaired verbal communication, difficulty eating, and change in appearance associated with facial edema and presence of intermaxillary fixation device.

| Desired Outcome | Nursing Actions and ***Selected Purposes/Rationales*** |
|---|---|
| 9. The client will demonstrate beginning adaptation to the temporary changes in appearance and ability to eat and communicate verbally as evidenced by:<br>a. communication of feelings of self-worth<br>b. maintenance of | 9.a. Assess for signs and symptoms of a body image disturbance (e.g. verbal or nonverbal cues denoting a negative response to change in appearance such as refusal to look in mirror, reluctance to participate in oral care, or withdrawal from significant others).<br>b. Determine the meaning of change in appearance and difficulty eating and communicating verbally to the client by encouraging him/her to communicate feelings and by noting nonverbal responses to these changes.<br>c. Inform client that facial edema and ecchymosis should start to decrease in 2-3 days and that he/she will be able to speak more clearly once edema |

| | |
|---|---|
| relationships with significant others<br>c. active participation in activities of daily living<br>d. active interest in personal appearance<br>e. willingness to participate in social activities. | resolves. Stress the temporary nature of jaw immobilization (usually 4-6 weeks).<br>d. Implement measures *to assist client to increase self-esteem* (e.g. limit negative self-assessment, encourage positive comments about self).<br>e. Assist the client to identify and utilize coping techniques that have been helpful in the past.<br>f. Provide privacy during oral care and suctioning. Encourage client to suction self or expectorate frequently *to decrease drooling*.<br>g. Provide privacy at mealtime if client is embarrassed (client may need to use syringe to feed self and/or may drool while eating).<br>h. Assist client with usual grooming and makeup habits if necessary.<br>i. Assess for and support behaviors suggesting positive adaptation to changes experienced (e.g. willingness to suction and feed self, attempts at verbal communication).<br>j. Encourage visits and support from significant others. |

## 10. NURSING DIAGNOSIS: Knowledge deficit

regarding follow-up care.

| Desired Outcomes | Nursing Actions and ***Selected Purposes/Rationales*** |
|---|---|
| 10.a. The client will identify ways to maintain a patent airway. | 10.a.1. Instruct client regarding ways to maintain a patent airway during period of jaw immobilization:<br>a. avoid any situation that might lead to nausea and vomiting (e.g. ingestion of foods/fluids that client has not been able to tolerate in the past, noxious sights and odors)<br>b. reduce the risk of choking by:<br>1. sitting up in a chair and leaning forward slightly when eating and drinking<br>2. preparing food as recommended (e.g. blenderized)<br>3. taking all oral medications in liquid form<br>4. avoiding intake of carbonated beverages (the fizzing at the back of the throat can cause choking)<br>5. avoiding alcohol intake (alcohol may cause vomiting and/or depress the gag reflex)<br>c. if vomiting does occur:<br>1. sit up, lean forward, and expel vomitus through spaces between teeth<br>2. use fingers to hold cheeks away from teeth to facilitate removal of vomitus<br>3. use suction equipment if indicated (a soft, small bulb syringe is usually all that is needed after discharge)<br>d. perform good oral hygiene after any episode of emesis and after meals to decrease possibility of aspiration<br>e. avoid swimming and other water activities (increases the risk for aspiration)<br>f. have wire cutters (if wires present) or scissors (if bands present) readily available at all times and cut the wires or bands per physician's instructions.<br>2. Provide instructions to significant others regarding circumstances which require cutting the wires or bands and which wires or bands to cut. |

| Desired Outcomes | Nursing Actions and ***Selected Purposes/Rationales*** |
|---|---|
| 10.b. The client will demonstrate the ability to perform oral hygiene. | 10.b.1. Stress the importance of performing oral hygiene as prescribed.<br>2. Instruct client in proper oral hygiene techniques (e.g. rinsing mouth with saline or diluted hydrogen peroxide, gentle brushing, using oral irrigation device such as Water-Pik).<br>3. Reinforce the proper method of applying paraffin or dental wax to the protruding wires and removing the wax before meals and oral care.<br>4. Instruct client to use a lip moisturizer if lips are dry.<br>5. Allow time for questions, clarification, and return demonstration. |
| 10.c. The client will verbalize an understanding of dietary modifications and ways to maintain an adequate nutritional status. | 10.c. 1. Reinforce prescribed dietary modifications (client usually progresses rapidly from clear liquids to blenderized foods).<br>2. Instruct client in ways to maintain an adequate nutritional status:<br>a. plan well-balanced meals that meet caloric needs<br>b. stimulate appetite by looking at and smelling food before it is blenderized<br>c. drink protein supplements between meals<br>d. experiment with spices that may make diet more appetizing and enhance taste sensation<br>e. take vitamin supplements as ordered.<br>3. Consult dietitian regarding menu planning and food preparation if indicated. |
| 10.d. The client will identify ways to prevent constipation that may result from temporary dietary modifications. | 10.d.1. Inform client of the effect that a decrease in dietary fiber will have on bowel habits.<br>2. Instruct client in ways to prevent constipation:<br>a. drink at least 10 glasses of liquid/day<br>b. continue with measures previously used to stimulate bowel activity (e.g. drink warm tea in the morning, drink prune juice)<br>c. take liquid stool softeners and laxatives as prescribed<br>d. use suppositories or enemas if needed. |
| 10.e. The client will state signs and symptoms to report to the health care provider. | 10.e. 1. Refer to Standardized Postoperative Care Plan, Nursing Diagnosis 21, action c (p. 135), for signs and symptoms to report to health care provider.<br>2. Instruct client to also report:<br>a. difficulty breathing<br>b. jaw pain or oral pain unrelieved by prescribed medications<br>c. constipation not controlled by usual methods, stool softeners, laxatives, suppositories, or enemas<br>d. persistent irritation or breakdown of oral mucosa<br>e. facial swelling that persists or increases<br>f. weight loss of 15 pounds or more during the first 6 weeks after surgery<br>g. inability to adhere to prescribed diet<br>h. unusual mouth odor, drainage, or taste<br>i. discoloration of elastic bands (could indicate bands have stretched) and/or loosening of wires or bands. |
| 10.f. The client will verbalize an understanding of and a plan for adhering to recommended follow-up care including future appointments with health care provider and medications prescribed. | 10.f. 1. Refer to Standardized Postoperative Care Plan, Nursing Diagnosis 21 (pp. 135-136), for routine postoperative instructions and measures to improve client compliance.<br>2. Explain the rationale for, side effects of, and importance of taking medications prescribed (e.g. laxatives, stool softeners, analgesics, antimicrobials, vitamins, corticosteroids).<br>3. Instruct client to keep teeth clenched and contact physician immediately if wires or bands become loose or disconnected or if it was necessary to cut them. |

# Peptic Ulcer

A peptic ulcer is a break in the continuity of the gastrointestinal mucosa that is exposed to acidic digestive secretions. The areas most often involved are the stomach and duodenum. Erosion of these areas of the gastrointestinal mucosa can result from direct damage to the mucosal barrier by irritants such as excessive amounts of hydrochloric acid, refluxed bile and pancreatic secretions, alcohol, certain spices, caffeine, and some drugs (e.g. aspirin). Erosion can also result from a decrease in the blood supply to the mucosa and/or an increase in mucosal permeability which impair mucosal resistance and allow for the back diffusion of hydrogen ions.

Peptic ulcers are usually classified by location (e.g. gastric, duodenal) and by the extensiveness of erosion (e.g. acute [superficial erosion with minimal inflammation], chronic [erosion of mucosa and submucosa with scar tissue formation]). Causative factors and the relationship between eating and occurrence of pain vary depending on the location of the ulcer. The characteristic symptom of a peptic ulcer is chronic, intermittent epigastric pain that is described as burning, aching, gnawing, or cramping. Remissions and exacerbations are typical of peptic ulcer disease.

Medical treatment of a peptic ulcer focuses on removing ulcerogenic factors and increasing the gastroduodenal pH. Surgical intervention (e.g. vagotomy, partial gastrectomy) may be indicated if symptoms cannot be medically controlled after repeated attempts to do so; if ulcers recur frequently; or if complications such as hemorrhage, perforation, or obstruction occur in the ulcerated area(s).

**This care plan focuses on the adult client hospitalized for evaluation and medical treatment of a peptic ulcer that has become increasingly symptomatic.** The goals of care are to relieve pain, maintain an adequate nutritional status, prevent complications, and educate the client regarding follow-up care.

## DIAGNOSTIC TESTS

Endoscopy of the upper gastrointestinal (UGI) tract
Barium radiological studies of the UGI tract
Serum gastrin level
Gastric analysis
Complete blood count (CBC)
Stool analysis for occult blood

## DISCHARGE CRITERIA

Prior to discharge, the client will:

- have pain controlled
- have no signs and symptoms of complications
- identify ways to promote healing of the existing ulcer and prevent recurrence of peptic ulcer
- verbalize an understanding of medications ordered including rationale, side effects, schedule for taking, and importance of taking as prescribed
- state signs and symptoms to report to the health care provider
- identify community resources that can assist with making life-style changes necessary to promote healing and prevent recurrence of peptic ulcer
- verbalize an understanding of and a plan for adhering to recommended follow-up care including future appointments with health care provider.

## NURSING/COLLABORATIVE DIAGNOSES

## 1. NURSING DIAGNOSIS: Altered nutrition: less than body requirements

related to:
a. decreased oral intake associated with pain (especially with a gastric ulcer because pain often increases after eating);
b. failure to eat a well-balanced diet associated with prescribed or self-imposed dietary modifications.

| Desired Outcome | Nursing Actions and ***Selected Purposes/Rationales*** |
|---|---|
| 1. The client will maintain an adequate nutritional status as evidenced by:<br>a. weight within normal range for client's age, height, and body frame<br>b. normal BUN and serum albumin, Hct, Hb, transferrin, and lymphocyte levels<br>c. triceps skinfold thickness within normal range<br>d. usual strength and activity tolerance<br>e. healthy oral mucous membrane. | 1.a. Assess for and report signs and symptoms of malnutrition:<br>1. weight below normal for client's age, height, and body frame<br>2. abnormal BUN and low serum albumin, Hct, Hb, transferrin, and lymphocyte levels (Hct and Hb may also be decreased because of bleeding of the ulcerated area)<br>3. triceps skinfold thickness less than normal<br>4. weakness and fatigue<br>5. stomatitis.<br>b. Monitor percentage of meals and snacks client consumes. Report a pattern of inadequate intake.<br>c. Implement measures *to maintain an adequate nutritional status:*<br>1. when food or fluid is allowed, perform actions *to improve oral intake:*<br>a. implement measures to reduce epigastric pain (see Nursing Diagnosis 2, actions e.1.c-g, 2, and 3)<br>b. obtain a dietary consult if necessary to assist client in selecting foods/fluids that meet nutritional needs and dietary modifications as well as personal and cultural preferences whenever possible<br>c. maintain a clean environment and a relaxed, pleasant atmosphere<br>d. provide oral care before meals<br>e. serve small portions of nutritious foods/fluids that are appealing to the client<br>f. allow adequate time for meals; reheat food if necessary<br>2. ensure that meals are well balanced and high in essential nutrients; offer dietary supplements between meals if indicated<br>3. administer vitamins and minerals if ordered.<br>d. Perform a 72-hour calorie count if ordered. Report totals to dietitian and physician.<br>e. Consult physician regarding the need for parenteral nutrition if client does not consume enough food or fluids to meet nutritional needs. |

## 2. NURSING DIAGNOSIS: Pain: epigastric

related to:
a. inflammation of the ulcerated area;
b. stimulation of exposed nerve endings and reflex muscle spasm (occurs when gastric or duodenal secretions or other irritants come in contact with the ulcer).

**Desired Outcome**

2. The client will experience diminished pain as evidenced by:
   a. verbalization of pain relief
   b. relaxed facial expression and body positioning
   c. increased participation in activities.

**Nursing Actions and *Selected Purposes/Rationales***

2.a. Determine how the client usually responds to pain.
  b. Assess client's perception of pain including location, intensity, and type. Utilize a numerical scale to rate intensity.
  c. Assess for nonverbal signs of pain (e.g. wrinkled brow, rubbing epigastric area, clenched fists, reluctance to move, restlessness).
  d. Assess for factors that seem to aggravate and alleviate pain.
  e. Implement measures *to reduce epigastric pain:*
    1. perform actions *to prevent further tissue irritation and/or promote healing of the ulcer:*
      a. withhold foods/fluids as ordered *to reduce stimulation of gastric acid secretion*
      b. insert a nasogastric tube and maintain suction as ordered *to remove gastric secretions*
      c. administer the following medications if ordered:
        1. histamine$_2$ receptor antagonists (e.g. cimetidine, famotidine, ranitidine, nizatidine), anticholinergics (e.g. clidinium, glycopyrrolate), and/or proton-pump inhibitors (e.g. omeprazole) *to inhibit gastric acid secretion*
        2. antacids *to neutralize gastric secretions*
        3. cytoprotective agents (e.g. sucralfate) *to protect the ulcerated area*
        4. synthetic prostaglandins (e.g. misoprostol) *to inhibit gastric acid secretion and protect the ulcerated area*
      d. implement measures to reduce fear and anxiety (see Nursing Diagnosis 4, action b) *in order to reduce stimulation of the vagus nerve and subsequent increase in basal acid output*
      e. when foods/fluids are allowed:
        1. instruct client to:
          a. avoid intake of coffee; caffeine-containing tea and colas; spices such as black pepper, chili powder, and nutmeg; and extremely hot foods/fluids
          b. chew food thoroughly and eat slowly *(a large bolus of food causes an increased output of hydrochloric acid and pepsin)*
          c. limit intake of milk and milk products and drink milk with rather than between meals *(protein and calcium are potent stimulators of gastrin secretion which causes increased output of gastric acid)*
          d. avoid intake of foods/fluids that produce pain (this is often referred to as a "free-choice" diet)
        2. provide regularly scheduled meals and snacks as ordered *to neutralize gastric acid* (3 moderate-sized meals are usually recommended; eating frequent, small meals to buffer gastric acid is not often prescribed *because it is more effective to actually reduce gastric acid secretion with medication therapy*)
      f. encourage client to stop smoking
      g. if client needs to take ulcerogenic medications (e.g. corticosteroids, aspirin, indomethacin), administer them with meals or snacks *to decrease gastric irritation*
      h. prepare client for a vagotomy if indicated *to reduce gastric acid production*
    2. provide or assist with nonpharmacological measures for pain relief (e.g. relaxation techniques, quiet conversation, restful environment, diversional activities)
    3. administer analgesics if ordered.
  f. Consult physician if above measures fail to provide adequate pain relief.

## 3. COLLABORATIVE DIAGNOSES:

**Potential complications:**

a. **hypovolemic shock** related to upper gastrointestinal (UGI) bleeding associated with:
   1. erosion of numerous small blood vessels (the gastric and duodenal mucosa have a rich blood supply)
   2. erosion of a major blood vessel (can occur if the ulcer is deep);

b. **peritonitis** related to leakage of gastrointestinal contents into the peritoneal cavity associated with perforation of the wall of the stomach or duodenum (can occur if the ulcer is deep);

c. **gastric outlet obstruction** related to narrowing of the pylorus associated with inflammation, spasm, and/or scar tissue formation (can occur if the ulcer is at or near the gastric outlet).

| Desired Outcomes | Nursing Actions and ***Selected Purposes/Rationales*** |
|---|---|
| 3.a. The client will not develop hypovolemic shock as evidenced by:<br>1. usual mental status<br>2. stable vital signs<br>3. skin warm, dry, and usual color<br>4. palpable peripheral pulses<br>5. urine output at least 30 ml/hour. | 3.a.1. Assess for and report signs and symptoms of UGI bleeding (e.g. hematemesis, bright red or coffee-ground drainage from nasogastric tube, increased epigastric pain, complaints of epigastric fullness, decreased B/P, increased pulse rate).<br>2. Monitor RBC, Hct, and Hb levels. Report declining values.<br>3. Assess for and report signs and symptoms of hypovolemic shock:<br>a. restlessness, agitation, confusion<br>b. significant decrease in B/P<br>c. postural hypotension<br>d. rapid, thready pulse<br>e. rapid respirations<br>f. cool, moist skin<br>g. pallor, cyanosis<br>h. diminished or absent peripheral pulses<br>i. urine output less than 30 ml/hour.<br>4. Implement measures to prevent further tissue irritation and/or promote healing of the ulcer (see Nursing Diagnosis 2, action e.1) *in order to prevent UGI bleeding*.<br>5. If signs and symptoms of UGI bleeding occur:<br>a. insert nasogastric tube if not already present and maintain suction as ordered<br>b. assist with measures to control bleeding (e.g. gastric lavage, endoscopic electrocoagulation, selective arterial embolization, intravenous or intra-arterial administration of vasopressin) if ordered<br>c. administer blood products and/or volume expanders if ordered<br>d. prepare client for surgical intervention (e.g. ligation of bleeding vessels, partial gastrectomy) if planned.<br>6. If signs and symptoms of hypovolemic shock occur:<br>a. continue with above measures to control bleeding<br>b. place client flat in bed with legs elevated unless contraindicated<br>c. monitor vital signs frequently<br>d. administer oxygen as ordered<br>e. administer blood products and/or volume expanders as ordered<br>f. prepare client for insertion of hemodynamic monitoring devices (e.g. central venous catheter, intra-arterial catheter) if planned<br>g. provide emotional support to client and significant others. |
| 3.b. The client will not develop peritonitis as evidenced by:<br>1. no complaints of increased | 3.b.1. Assess for and report:<br>a. signs and symptoms of perforation of the gastric or duodenal wall (e.g. sudden, sharp, severe upper abdominal pain; extreme abdominal tenderness; abdominal x-ray showing free air in peritoneal cavity) |

abdominal pain and tenderness
2. soft, nondistended abdomen
3. afebrile status
4. stable vital signs
5. absence of nausea and vomiting
6. normal bowel sounds
7. WBC count within normal range.

b. signs and symptoms of peritonitis (e.g. increase in severity of abdominal pain; rebound tenderness; tense, rigid abdomen; elevated temperature; tachycardia; tachypnea; hypotension; nausea; vomiting; diminished or absent bowel sounds)
c. increase in WBC count.

2. Implement measures to prevent further tissue irritation and/or promote healing of the ulcer (see Nursing Diagnosis 2, action e.1) *in order to prevent perforation.*
3. If signs and symptoms of peritonitis occur:
   a. withhold all food and fluid as ordered
   b. place client on bed rest in a semi-Fowler's position *to assist in pooling or localizing gastrointestinal contents in the pelvis rather than under the diaphragm*
   c. insert a nasogastric tube if not already present and maintain suction as ordered
   d. administer antimicrobials as ordered
   e. administer intravenous fluids and/or blood volume expanders if ordered *to prevent or treat shock (can result from the increased capillary permeability that occurs with inflammation and the subsequent escape of protein, fluid, and electrolytes from the vascular space into the peritoneal cavity)*
   f. prepare client for surgical repair of the perforation if indicated
   g. provide emotional support to client and significant others.

3.c. The client will not experience gastric outlet obstruction as evidenced by:
1. soft, nondistended epigastric area
2. no complaints of epigastric fullness or bloating
3. absence of anorexia, nausea, and vomiting.

3.c. 1. Assess for and report signs and symptoms of gastric outlet obstruction (e.g. epigastric distention, complaints of epigastric fullness or bloating, anorexia, nausea, vomiting, foul-smelling vomitus containing particles of food ingested many hours earlier).
2. Implement measures to prevent further tissue irritation and/or promote healing of the ulcer (see Nursing Diagnosis 2, action e.1) *in order to reduce the risk of narrowing the lumen of the gastric outlet if the ulcer is at or near the pylorus.*
3. If signs and symptoms of gastric outlet obstruction occur:
   a. withhold all food and fluid as ordered
   b. insert a nasogastric tube if not already present and maintain suction as ordered
   c. administer intravenous fluid and electrolyte replacements as ordered
   d. prepare client for surgical intervention (e.g. partial gastrectomy, pyloroplasty) if planned
   e. provide emotional support to client and significant others.

## 4. NURSING DIAGNOSIS: Anxiety

related to pain; lack of understanding of the diagnosis, diagnostic tests, and treatment plan; unfamiliar environment; financial concerns; and probable need to change life style in order to control symptoms and prevent ulcer recurrence.

| Desired Outcome | Nursing Actions and ***Selected Purposes/Rationales*** |
|---|---|
| 4. The client will experience a reduction in anxiety as evidenced by:<br>a. verbalization of feeling less anxious and fearful<br>b. usual sleep pattern | 4.a. Assess client for signs and symptoms of anxiety (e.g. verbalization of fears and concerns, insomnia, tenseness, tremors, irritability, restlessness, tachypnea, tachycardia, elevated blood pressure, narrowed perceptual field, withdrawal, noncompliance with treatment plan).<br>b. Implement measures *to reduce fear and anxiety:*<br>1. orient client to hospital environment, equipment, and routines<br>2. introduce staff who will be participating in his/her care; if possible, |

| Desired Outcome | Nursing Actions and ***Selected Purposes/Rationales*** |
|---|---|
| c. relaxed facial expression and body movements<br>d. stable vital signs<br>e. usual perceptual ability and interactions with others. | maintain consistency in staff assigned to his/her care *to provide feelings of stability and comfort with the environment*<br>3. assure client that staff members are nearby; respond to call signal as soon as possible<br>4. maintain a calm, supportive, confident manner when interacting with client<br>5. encourage verbalization of fear and anxiety; provide feedback<br>6. reinforce physician's explanations and clarify misconceptions client has about the peptic ulcer, the treatment plan, and the prognosis<br>7. explain all diagnostic tests<br>8. perform actions to reduce epigastric pain (see Nursing Diagnosis 2, action e)<br>9. provide a calm, restful environment<br>10. instruct client in relaxation techniques and encourage participation in diversional activities<br>11. assist client to identify specific stressors and ways to cope with them<br>12. encourage significant others to project a caring, concerned attitude without obvious anxiousness<br>13. initiate financial and/or social service referrals if indicated<br>14. administer antianxiety agents if ordered.<br>c. Include significant others in orientation and teaching sessions and encourage their continued support of the client.<br>d. Provide information based on current needs of client and significant others at a level they can understand. Encourage questions and clarification of information provided.<br>e. Consult physician if above actions fail to control fear and anxiety. |

## 5. NURSING DIAGNOSIS: Ineffective management of therapeutic regimen

related to:
a. lack of understanding of the implications of not following the prescribed treatment plan;
b. difficulty modifying personal habits.

| Desired Outcome | Nursing Actions and ***Selected Purposes/Rationales*** |
|---|---|
| 5. The client will demonstrate the probability of effective management of the therapeutic regimen as evidenced by:<br>a. willingness to learn about and participate in the treatment plan<br>b. statements reflecting ways to modify personal habits and integrate treatments into life style<br>c. statements reflecting an understanding of the implications of | 5.a. Assess for indications that the client may be unable to effectively manage the therapeutic regimen:<br>1. statements reflecting that he/she was unable to adhere to treatment plan at home<br>2. failure to adhere to treatment plan while in hospital (e.g. refusing medications, not adhering to dietary modifications)<br>3. statements reflecting a lack of understanding of factors that aggravate or cause peptic ulcers<br>4. statements reflecting an unwillingness or inability to modify personal habits and integrate necessary treatments into life style<br>5. statements reflecting view that the peptic ulcer will resolve without any treatment, that an absence of epigastric pain indicates that the ulcer is cured, or that recurrence and complications are inevitable and efforts to comply with treatments are useless.<br>b. Implement measures *to promote effective management of the therapeutic regimen:*<br>1. explain peptic ulcer disease in terms the client can understand; stress |

| | |
|---|---|
| not following the prescribed treatment plan. | the fact that complications can occur and/or ulcer will recur if treatment plan is not followed<br>2. inform client that prescribed dietary modifications and medication therapy will not be as extensive after the existing ulcer has healed (usually 6-8 weeks)<br>3. initiate and reinforce the discharge teaching outlined in Nursing Diagnosis 6 *in order to promote a sense of control over disease progression*<br>4. encourage questions and clarify misconceptions the client has about the peptic ulcer and its effects<br>5. discuss the importance of developing and utilizing stress reduction techniques (stress can increase basal acid output and is often a factor contributing to some of the behaviors such as cigarette smoking, aspirin ingestion, alcohol and/or caffeinated beverage intake, and irregular eating habits that increase the risk for peptic ulcer formation)<br>6. assist client to identify ways he/she can incorporate treatments into life style; focus on modifications of life style rather than complete change (e.g. drinking decaffeinated rather than caffeine-containing tea and colas)<br>7. provide a dietary consult to assist client in planning a dietary program that incorporates the prescribed modifications and his/her likes, dislikes, and daily routines<br>8. provide information about various antacids available if appropriate; instruct client to alternate types of antacids in order to minimize side effects such as diarrhea and constipation<br>9. assist client in setting up a medication schedule that he/she can incorporate into daily activities<br>10. encourage questions and allow time for reinforcement and clarification of information provided<br>11. provide written instructions about future appointments with health care provider, dietary modifications, medications, and signs and symptoms to report<br>12. if client has concerns regarding the cost of medications, obtain a social service consult to assist him/her with financial planning and to obtain financial aid if indicated<br>13. provide information about and encourage utilization of community resources that can assist client to make necessary life-style changes (e.g. smoking cessation programs, stress management classes, counseling services)<br>14. reinforce behaviors suggesting future compliance with the therapeutic regimen (e.g. participation in the treatment plan, statements reflecting ways to modify personal habits).<br>c. Include significant others in explanations and teaching sessions and encourage their support. |

## 6. NURSING DIAGNOSIS: Knowledge deficit

regarding follow-up care.

| Desired Outcomes | Nursing Actions and ***Selected Purposes/Rationales*** |
|---|---|
| 6.a. The client will identify ways to promote healing of the existing ulcer and prevent | 6.a. 1. Instruct client in ways to promote healing of the existing ulcer and prevent recurrence of peptic ulcer:<br>a. drink decaffeinated or caffeine-free tea and colas rather than those containing caffeine |

| Desired Outcomes | Nursing Actions and ***Selected Purposes/Rationales*** |
|---|---|
| recurrence of peptic ulcer. | b. avoid drinking coffee and alcohol or drink these beverages only in small amounts during or immediately following a meal<br>c. avoid ingestion of foods that are known to irritate gastric mucosa directly or increase gastric acid production (e.g. whole grains, chocolate, rich pastries, spicy foods, meat extracts, extremely hot foods)<br>d. avoid intake of any foods and fluids that cause gastric distress<br>e. eat 3 regularly scheduled meals; do not skip meals<br>f. eat slowly and chew food thoroughly<br>g. maintain a calm, pleasant atmosphere at mealtime and whenever possible<br>h. stop smoking<br>i. maintain a balance of physical activity and rest<br>j. avoid stressful situations<br>k. avoid ingestion of over-the-counter medications such as aspirin and ibuprofen; if it is necessary to take these or other ulcerogenic medications (e.g. corticosteroids, indomethacin), take them with antacids or food whenever possible<br>l. take medications prescribed for ulcer treatment as prescribed.<br>2. Obtain a dietary consult if client needs assistance in planning meals that incorporate dietary modifications with his/her likes, dislikes, and daily routines.<br>3. Assist client to identify ways he/she can make necessary life-style changes. |
| 6.b. The client will verbalize an understanding of medications ordered including rationale, side effects, schedule for taking, and importance of taking as prescribed. | 6.b.1. Explain the rationale for, side effects of, schedule for taking, and importance of taking medications prescribed.<br>2. If client is discharged on antacid therapy, instruct to:<br>a. take as prescribed (usually 7 times/day [1 hour and 3 hours after each meal and at bedtime] or 4 times/day [1 hour after each meal and at bedtime] for 4-6 weeks)<br>b. take antacid suspensions rather than tablets, especially those tablets that are swallowed rather than chewed, whenever possible *(suspensions neutralize gastric acid more effectively)*<br>c. thoroughly chew tablets that are labelled as "chewable"<br>d. shake antacid suspensions vigorously before taking dose<br>e. check the sodium content of antacids and avoid use of those high in sodium (e.g. Amphojel, Basaljel, Di-Gel, Delcid) if hypertensive or on a sodium-restricted diet<br>f. alternate aluminum-containing antacids (e.g. Amphojel, ALternaGel) and magnesium-containing antacids (e.g. Milk of Magnesia, Mag-Ox) periodically or take aluminum and magnesium hydroxide combination antacids (e.g. Maalox, Di-Gel, Gaviscon, Mylanta II) if constipation or diarrhea develops<br>g. avoid excessive use of antacids high in calcium (e.g. Titralac, Tums) and sodium bicarbonate (e.g. baking soda, Alka-Seltzer, Bromo-Seltzer)<br>h. expect that stool may be speckled or whitish<br>i. observe for and report:<br>1. thirst, dry mouth, weakness, lethargy *(may indicate hypernatremia resulting from excessive amounts of antacids containing sodium)* and/or swelling of extremities and weight gain *(can occur with the subsequent water retention)*<br>2. constipation not resolved by increased fluid intake, laxatives, stool softeners, and switching to an antacid containing magnesium<br>3. diarrhea not controlled by antidiarrheal medication and switching to an antacid containing aluminum.<br>3. If client is discharged on sucralfate (Carafate), instruct to:<br>a. take it an hour before meals and at bedtime |

b. avoid taking antacids for at least 30 minutes before and after taking the medication
c. monitor for and report persistent constipation, nausea, or indigestion.

4. If client is discharged on a histamine$_2$ receptor antagonist (e.g. cimetidine, nizatidine, famotidine, ranitidine), instruct to:
   a. avoid taking antacids within an hour before or after taking the drug
   b. avoid taking sucralfate within 2 hours before or after taking cimetidine
   c. monitor for and report persistent constipation, diarrhea, or headache; dizziness; or rash
   d. monitor for and report breast enlargement (in males) or milk production (in females) if taking cimetidine.
5. If client is discharged on misoprostol (e.g. Cytotec), instruct to:
   a. avoid taking it with food or antacids
   b. monitor for and report:
      1. persistent diarrhea, nausea, headache, or fatigue
      2. menstrual irregularities (e.g. spotting, cramps, excessive bleeding)
   c. notify physician if pregnancy is suspected (misoprostol may induce miscarriage).
6. If client is discharged on omeprazole (e.g. Losec, Prilosec), instruct to monitor for and report persistent diarrhea, headache, constipation, or nausea; dizziness; or rash.
7. Caution client to consult physician before stopping any medications prescribed for peptic ulcer treatment.
8. Instruct client to inform health care providers of medications being taken for the treatment of peptic ulcer (many of the drugs prescribed can alter the absorption of other medications).

6.c. The client will state signs and symptoms to report to the health care provider.

6.c. Instruct client to report:
1. black or tarry stools
2. bloody or coffee-ground vomitus
3. abdominal distention
4. persistent epigastric fullness or bloating, nausea, and/or vomiting
5. weight loss
6. persistent or increased epigastric or abdominal pain
7. weakness and fatigue
8. undesirable side effects of medications prescribed (see actions b.2.i, 3.c, 4.c and d, 5.b, and 6 in this diagnosis)
9. persistent high stress levels
10. difficulty taking medications as prescribed.

6.d. The client will identify community resources that can assist with making life-style changes necessary to promote healing and prevent recurrence of peptic ulcer.

6.d.
1. Provide information about community resources that can assist client to make life-style changes necessary to promote healing and prevent recurrence of peptic ulcer (e.g. smoking cessation programs, stress management classes, counseling services).
2. Initiate a referral if indicated.

6.e. The client will verbalize an understanding of and a plan for adhering to recommended follow-up care including future appointments with health care provider.

6.e.
1. Reinforce the importance of follow-up appointments with health care provider.
2. Refer to Nursing Diagnosis 5, action b, for measures to promote the client's ability to effectively manage the therapeutic regimen.

UNIT
# XV

# *Nursing Care of the Client with Disturbances of the Liver, Biliary Tract, and Pancreas*

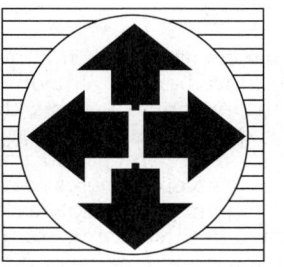

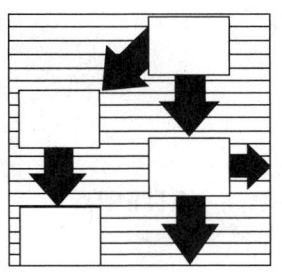

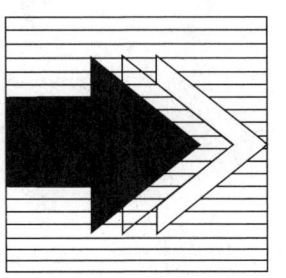

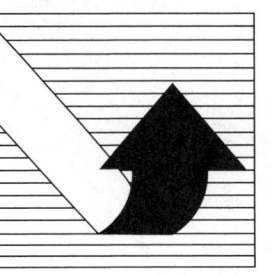

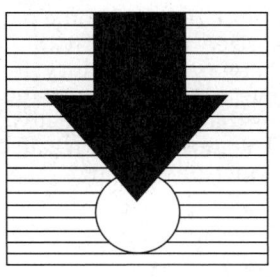

# Acute Pancreatitis

Acute pancreatitis is an inflammation of the pancreas that occurs when the enzymes it produces become activated in the pancreas rather than in the duodenum. The subsequent autodigestion causes pathologic changes that range from mild pancreatic inflammation and edema to severe pancreatic damage, which is characterized by hemorrhage and extensive tissue necrosis. In addition, life-threatening complications can develop as the activated enzymes escape into the systemic circulation. Following an episode of acute pancreatitis, the structure and function of the pancreas is usually restored. If the damage has been extensive, irreversible changes can occur and chronic pancreatitis can develop.

It is theorized that pancreatic duct obstruction, pancreatic ischemia, direct injury to the acinar cells, and reflux of bile into the pancreatic duct are among the mechanisms that trigger the activation of enzymes in the pancreas. The most common causes of acute pancreatitis are biliary tract disease and heavy alcohol intake. Additional causes include external trauma to the abdomen, trauma to the pancreas during abdominal surgery, viral infections, drugs (e.g. tetracycline, estrogen, hydrochlorothiazide, furosemide), and metabolic disorders such as hyperparathyroidism and hyperlipidemia.

The focus of medical treatment is to prevent further autodigestion of the pancreas by decreasing stimulation of the pancreatic enzymes until normal outflow resumes. If the cause of the pancreatitis is biliary tract disease, surgery (e.g. removal of gallstones that may be blocking the pancreatic duct) is usually performed after pancreatic inflammation has subsided and the client is in stable condition.

**This care plan focuses on the adult client hospitalized with probable acute pancreatitis.** The goals of care are to control pain, maintain an adequate nutritional status, prevent complications, and educate the client regarding follow-up care.

## DIAGNOSTIC TESTS

Serum and urine amylase
Pancreatic isoamylase
Serum lipase
Amylase/creatinine clearance ratio
Ultrasonography
Computed tomography (CT)

## DISCHARGE CRITERIA

Prior to discharge, the client will:

- have no signs and symptoms of complications
- have relief of severe pain
- have an adequate nutritional intake
- identify ways to prevent overstimulation of and further trauma to the pancreas
- verbalize an understanding of recommended dietary modifications
- state signs and symptoms to report to the health care provider
- verbalize an understanding of and a plan for adhering to recommended follow-up care including future appointments with health care provider and medications prescribed.

## NURSING/ COLLABORATIVE DIAGNOSES

1. Ineffective breathing pattern△ *669*
2. Altered fluid and electrolyte balance:
   a. fluid volume deficit, hypokalemia, and hypochloremia
   b. hypocalcemia
   c. metabolic alkalosis
   d. third-spacing△ *670*
3. Altered nutrition: less than body requirements△ *671*
4. Pain: epigastric or abdominal with radiation to the back△ *672*

## 1. NURSING DIAGNOSIS: Ineffective breathing pattern

related to:
a. reluctance to breathe deeply associated with severe abdominal pain;
b. depressant effects of some medications (e.g. narcotic analgesics);
c. impaired lung/chest expansion associated with:
   1. decreased activity
   2. positioning (client often positions self on his/her side with knees and trunk flexed to reduce pain)
   3. pleural effusion if it occurs
   4. pressure on the diaphragm resulting from ascites if present and accumulation of gastrointestinal gas and fluid.

| Desired Outcome | Nursing Actions and ***Selected Purposes/Rationales*** |
|---|---|
| 1. The client will maintain an effective breathing pattern as evidenced by:<br>a. normal rate and depth of respirations<br>b. absence of dyspnea<br>c. blood gases within normal range. | 1.a. Assess for signs and symptoms of an ineffective breathing pattern (e.g. shallow respirations, dyspnea).<br>b. Monitor for and report the following:<br>1. abnormal blood gases<br>2. significant changes in oximetry results.<br>c. Implement measures *to improve breathing pattern:*<br>1. perform actions to reduce pain (see Nursing Diagnosis 4, action e)<br>2. perform actions *to reduce pressure on the diaphragm:*<br>a. implement measures to reduce the accumulation of gastrointestinal gas and fluid (see Nursing Diagnosis 5.B, action 3)<br>b. administer salt-poor albumin if ordered *to reduce ascites*<br>3. perform actions to prevent and treat pleural effusion (see Collaborative Diagnosis 7, actions e.3 and 4)<br>4. when severe pain has subsided, place client in a semi- to high Fowler's position unless contraindicated<br>5. assist client to turn from side to side at least every 2 hours while in bed<br>6. instruct client to deep breathe or use incentive spirometer at least every 2 hours<br>7. increase activity as allowed and tolerated<br>8. administer central nervous system depressants judiciously; hold medication and consult physician if respiratory rate is less than 12/minute.<br>d. Consult physician if:<br>1. ineffective breathing pattern continues<br>2. signs and symptoms of atelectasis (e.g. diminished or absent breath |

| Desired Outcome | Nursing Actions and ***Selected Purposes/Rationales*** |
|---|---|
| | sounds, dull percussion note over affected area, increased respiratory rate, dyspnea, tachycardia, elevated temperature) develop<br>3. signs and symptoms of impaired gas exchange (e.g. restlessness, irritability, confusion, decreased $PaO_2$ and increased $PaCO_2$ levels) are present. |

## 2. NURSING/COLLABORATIVE DIAGNOSIS:

**Altered fluid and electrolyte balance:**

a. **fluid volume deficit, hypokalemia, and hypochloremia** related to decreased oral intake and excessive loss of fluid and electrolytes associated with vomiting and nasogastric tube drainage;

b. **hypocalcemia** related to:
   1. binding of calcium to the undigested fats in the intestine (lipase and phospholipase A are not released into the intestinal tract to digest fats so calcium binds with the free fats and is excreted in the stool)
   2. loss of albumin into peritoneal cavity associated with increased vascular permeability (albumin transports nonionized calcium in the blood)
   3. binding of calcium to free fatty acids in areas of tissue necrosis (lipolysis of pancreatic, peripancreatic, and fatty tissue occurs as lipases are activated in the pancreas and released into the surrounding area and systemic circulation);

c. **metabolic alkalosis** related to hypokalemia, hypochloremia, and excessive loss of hydrochloric acid associated with vomiting and nasogastric tube drainage;

d. **third-spacing** related to increased vascular permeability associated with the inflammatory response and activation of bradykinin and kallidin by kallikrein (the plasma peptide kallikrein is activated by the pancreatic enzyme trypsin, which enters the systemic circulation during acute pancreatitis).

| Desired Outcomes | Nursing Actions and ***Selected Purposes/Rationales*** |
|---|---|
| 2.a. The client will maintain fluid and electrolyte balance as evidenced by:<br>1. normal skin turgor<br>2. moist mucous membranes<br>3. stable weight<br>4. B/P and pulse within normal range for client and stable with position change<br>5. small vein filling time less than 3-5 seconds<br>6. balanced intake and output<br>7. urine specific gravity within normal range<br>8. soft, nondistended abdomen with | 2.a.1. Assess for and report signs and symptoms of:<br>a. fluid volume deficit:<br>1. decreased skin turgor, dry mucous membranes, thirst<br>2. sudden weight loss of 2% or greater<br>3. low B/P and/or postural hypotension<br>4. weak, rapid pulse<br>5. delayed small vein filling time (longer than 3-5 seconds)<br>6. decreased urine output with increased specific gravity (reflects an actual rather than potential fluid volume deficit)<br>7. increased BUN and Hct<br>b. hypokalemia (e.g. cardiac arrhythmias, postural hypotension, muscle weakness, paresthesias, nausea and vomiting, abdominal distention, hypoactive or absent bowel sounds)<br>c. hypochloremia and metabolic alkalosis (e.g. dizziness, irritability, paresthesias, muscle twitching or spasms, hypoventilation)<br>d. hypocalcemia (e.g. anxiousness; irritability; cardiac arrhythmias; numbness or tingling of fingers, toes, or circumoral area; positive Chvostek's and Trousseau's signs; hyperactive reflexes; tetany; seizures).<br>2. Monitor serum electrolyte and blood gas results. Report abnormal values.<br>3. Implement measures *to prevent or treat fluid and electrolyte imbalances:*<br>a. perform actions to reduce nausea and vomiting (see Nursing Diagnosis 5.A, action 2) |

normal bowel sounds
9. absence of cardiac arrhythmias, muscle weakness, paresthesias, twitching, spasms, dizziness, tetany, and seizure activity
10. usual mental status
11. negative Chvostek's and Trousseau's signs
12. BUN, Hct, serum electrolyte, and blood gases within normal range.

b. if irrigation of nasogastric tube is indicated, use normal saline rather than water
c. administer fluid and electrolyte replacements if ordered
d. maintain a fluid intake of at least 2500 ml/day unless contraindicated
e. when oral intake is allowed:
   1. assist client to select the following foods/fluids:
      a. those high in potassium (e.g. bananas, potatoes, cantaloupe, raisins, figs, apricots, dates)
      b. those high in sodium (e.g. bouillon, canned soups, dill pickles, processed cheese, cured meats, catsup, canned vegetables)
      c. those high in calcium such as milk and milk products (if client is on a low-fat diet, items such as ice cream, whole milk, butter, and cream will not be allowed)
   2. administer pancreatic enzymes (e.g. pancreatin, pancrelipase) if ordered *to promote fat digestion so that there is less fat available for calcium to bind to*
f. perform actions to prevent or treat fat necrosis (see Collaborative Diagnosis 7, actions g.2 and 3) *in order to reduce sequestration of calcium in those areas.*

4. Consult physician if signs and symptoms of fluid and electrolyte imbalances persist or worsen.

2.b. The client will not experience third-spacing as evidenced by:
1. absence of ascites
2. absence of dyspnea
3. audible breath sounds
4. B/P and pulse within normal range for client and stable with position change
5. balanced intake and output.

2.b.1. Assess for and report signs and symptoms of third-spacing:
   a. ascites
   b. dyspnea and diminished or absent breath sounds
   c. evidence of vascular depletion (e.g. postural hypotension; weak, rapid pulse; decreased urine output).
2. Monitor chest x-ray results. Report findings of pleural effusion.
3. Monitor serum albumin levels. Report below-normal levels *(albumin maintains plasma colloid osmotic pressure).*
4. Implement measures *to prevent third-spacing and/or promote mobilization of fluid back into vascular space:*
   a. encourage client to rest periodically in a recumbent position if tolerated *(lying flat promotes venous return and results in lower venous hydrostatic pressure and subsequent reshifting of fluid back into vascular space)*
   b. administer salt-poor albumin if ordered *to increase colloid osmotic pressure*
   c. perform actions to decrease pancreatic stimulation (see Nursing Diagnosis 4, action e.3) *in order to decrease inflammation and activation of kallikrein and subsequently decrease vascular permeability.*
5. Consult physician if signs and symptoms of third-spacing persist or worsen.

**3. NURSING DIAGNOSIS: Altered nutrition: less than body requirements**

related to:
a. decreased oral intake associated with nausea, pain, prescribed dietary restrictions, and early satiety resulting from abdominal distention;
b. loss of nutrients associated with vomiting;
c. decreased utilization of nutrients associated with impaired digestion of fats, proteins, and carbohydrates resulting from obstructed outflow of pancreatic enzymes.

| Desired Outcome | Nursing Actions and ***Selected Purposes/Rationales*** |
|---|---|
| 3. The client will maintain an adequate nutritional status as evidenced by:<br>a. weight within normal range for client's age, height, and body frame<br>b. normal BUN and serum albumin, Hct, Hb, transferrin, and lymphocyte levels<br>c. triceps skinfold thickness within normal range<br>d. usual strength and activity tolerance<br>e. healthy oral mucous membrane. | 3.a. Assess for and report signs and symptoms of malnutrition:<br>1. weight below normal for client's age, height, and body frame<br>2. abnormal BUN and low serum albumin, Hct, Hb, transferrin, and lymphocyte levels (albumin levels can also be low because of increased vascular permeability)<br>3. triceps skinfold thickness less than normal<br>4. weakness and fatigue<br>5. stomatitis.<br>b. When oral intake is allowed, monitor percentage of meals and snacks client consumes. Report a pattern of inadequate intake.<br>c. Implement measures *to maintain an adequate nutritional status:*<br>1. administer total parenteral nutrition if ordered<br>2. when food or fluid is allowed:<br>a. perform actions *to improve oral intake:*<br>1. implement measures to reduce pain and abdominal distention (see Nursing Diagnoses 4, action e and 5.B, action 3)<br>2. implement measures to reduce nausea and vomiting (see Nursing Diagnosis 5.A, action 2)<br>3. increase activity as allowed and tolerated *(activity stimulates appetite)*<br>4. obtain a dietary consult if necessary to assist client in selecting foods/fluids that meet nutritional needs and dietary modifications as well as personal and cultural preferences whenever possible<br>5. maintain a clean environment and a relaxed, pleasant atmosphere<br>6. provide oral hygiene before meals<br>7. serve small portions of nutritious foods/fluids that are appealing to client<br>8. allow adequate time for meals; reheat food if necessary<br>9. limit fluid intake (unless it has a high nutritional value) with meals *to reduce early satiety and subsequent decreased food intake*<br>b. ensure that meals are well balanced and high in essential nutrients; offer dietary supplements between meals if indicated<br>c. administer the following if ordered:<br>1. vitamins and minerals<br>2. pancreatic enzymes (e.g. pancreatin, pancrelipase) *to facilitate the digestion of proteins, fats, and carbohydrates.*<br>d. Perform a 72-hour calorie count if ordered. Report totals to dietitian and physician.<br>e. Reassess nutritional status on a regular basis and report decline. |

## 4. NURSING DIAGNOSIS: Pain: epigastric or abdominal with radiation to the back

related to:
a. distention of the pancreas associated with inflammation and obstruction of pancreatic ducts;
b. peritoneal irritation associated with escape of activated pancreatic enzymes into the peritoneum.

| Desired Outcome | Nursing Actions and ***Selected Purposes/Rationales*** |
|---|---|
| 4. The client will experience diminished pain as evidenced by: | 4.a. Determine how the client usually responds to pain.<br>b. Assess client's perception of pain including location, intensity, and type. Use a numerical scale to rate intensity. |

a. verbalization of pain relief
b. relaxed facial expression and body positioning
c. increased participation in activities
d. stable vital signs.

c. Assess for nonverbal signs of pain (e.g. wrinkled brow; clenched fists; guarding of abdomen; rubbing back; reluctance to move; restlessness; diaphoresis; rapid, shallow respirations; facial pallor; increased B/P; tachycardia).
d. Assess for factors that seem to aggravate and alleviate pain.
e. Implement measures *to reduce pain:*
   1. perform actions *to reduce fear and anxiety about the pain experience* (e.g. assure client that his/her need for pain relief will be met)
   2. medicate prior to any painful procedure and before pain is severe
   3. perform actions *to reduce pancreatic stimulation:*
      a. withhold all food and fluid as ordered *(food and fluid [especially those with a high protein or fat content] entering the duodenum cause the release of cholecystokinin, which stimulates the secretion of pancreatic enzymes)*
      b. insert nasogastric tube and maintain suction as ordered *to reduce the amount of acid that enters the duodenum (hydrochloric acid stimulates secretin, which then stimulates the output of pancreatic enzymes)*
      c. administer the following medications if ordered *to reduce the amount of acid that enters the duodenum:*
         1. antacids *to neutralize gastric acid*
         2. histamine$_2$ receptor antagonists (e.g. cimetidine, famotidine, ranitidine) *to reduce gastric output of hydrochloric acid*
      d. minimize client's exposure to odor and sight of food until oral intake is allowed *in order to prevent the stimulation of gastrin and subsequent pancreatic enzyme secretion*
   4. allow client to sit or lie with knees flexed and trunk slightly flexed *(this position relieves pressure on the inflamed pancreas)*
   5. provide or assist with additional nonpharmacological measures for pain relief (e.g. back rub, relaxation techniques, quiet conversation, restful environment, diversional activities)
   6. administer analgesics as ordered or encourage client to use patient-controlled analgesia (PCA) device as instructed (meperidine is usually the analgesic prescribed *because morphine sulfate often intensifies pain by increasing spasms of the sphincter of Oddi)*
   7. when oral intake is allowed, perform actions *to maintain reduced pancreatic activity:*
      a. continue to administer antacids and histamine$_2$ receptor antagonists as ordered
      b. advance diet slowly
      c. provide small, frequent meals rather than 3 large ones
      d. maintain dietary restrictions of fat intake as ordered.
f. Consult physician if above measures fail to provide adequate pain relief.

---

**5.A. NURSING DIAGNOSIS:**

**Altered comfort: nausea and vomiting**

related to stimulation of the vomiting center associated with:
1. stimulation of the afferent vagal and/or sympathetic pathways resulting from visceral irritation associated with abdominal distention and inflammation of the pancreas;
2. cortical stimulation resulting from pain and stress.

| Desired Outcome | Nursing Actions and ***Selected Purposes/Rationales*** |
|---|---|
| 5.A. The client will experience relief of | 5.A.1. Assess client for nausea and vomiting.<br>2. Implement measures *to reduce nausea and vomiting:* |

| Desired Outcome | Nursing Actions and ***Selected Purposes/Rationales*** |
|---|---|
| nausea and vomiting as evidenced by:<br>1. verbalization of relief of nausea<br>2. absence of vomiting. | a. perform actions to reduce fear and anxiety (see Nursing Diagnosis 8, action b)<br>b. perform actions to reduce pain (see Nursing Diagnosis 4, action e)<br>c. perform actions to reduce the accumulation of gastrointestinal gas and fluid (see Nursing Diagnosis 5.B, action 3) *in order to prevent abdominal distention and the subsequent visceral irritation*<br>d. maintain food and fluid restrictions as ordered<br>e. maintain patency of nasogastric tube (e.g. keep tubing free of kinks, irrigate and maintain suction as ordered) if present<br>f. eliminate noxious sights and odors from the environment *(noxious stimuli cause cortical stimulation of the vomiting center)*<br>g. encourage client to take deep, slow breaths when nauseated<br>h. instruct client to change positions slowly *(rapid movement stimulates the afferent vestibulocerebellar pathway with resultant stimulation of the chemoreceptor trigger zone)*<br>i. provide oral hygiene every 2 hours and after each emesis<br>j. when oral intake is allowed:<br>1. avoid serving foods with an overpowering aroma; remove lids from hot foods before entering room<br>2. provide small, frequent meals; instruct client to ingest foods and fluids slowly<br>3. instruct client to eat dry foods (e.g. toast, crackers) and avoid drinking liquids with meals if nauseated<br>4. instruct client to avoid foods/fluids that irritate the gastric mucosa (e.g. spicy foods; caffeine-containing beverages such as tea, coffee, and colas)<br>5. instruct client to avoid foods/fluids high in fat (e.g. butter, cream, whole milk, ice cream, fried foods, gravies, nuts) *in order to reduce nausea associated with impaired fat digestion*<br>6. instruct the client to rest after eating with head of bed elevated<br>k. administer antiemetics if ordered.<br>3. Consult physician if above measures fail to control nausea and vomiting. |

## 5.B. NURSING DIAGNOSIS: Altered comfort: abdominal distention and gas pain

related to accumulation of gastrointestinal gas or fluid associated with:
1. an inability to digest fats properly resulting from obstruction of the flow of lipase;
2. decreased gastrointestinal motility resulting from some medications (e.g. narcotic analgesics) and decreased activity.

| Desired Outcome | Nursing Actions and ***Selected Purposes/Rationales*** |
|---|---|
| 5.B. The client will experience diminished abdominal distention and gas pain as evidenced by:<br>1. verbalization of same<br>2. relaxed facial | 5.B.1. Assess for verbal complaints of abdominal fullness or gas pain.<br>2. Assess for nonverbal signs of abdominal distention or gas pain (e.g. grimacing, clutching or guarding of abdomen, restlessness, reluctance to move, increasing abdominal girth).<br>3. Implement measures *to reduce the accumulation of gastrointestinal gas and fluid in order to decrease abdominal distention and gas pain:*<br>a. encourage and assist client with frequent position changes and ambulation as allowed and tolerated *(activity stimulates peristalsis and expulsion of flatus)* |

expression and body positioning
3. decrease in abdominal girth.

b. instruct the client to avoid activities such as gum chewing and smoking *in order to reduce air swallowing*
c. maintain food and fluid restrictions as ordered
d. maintain patency of nasogastric tube if present
e. when oral intake is allowed, instruct client to avoid the following:
   1. carbonated beverages and gas-producing foods (e.g. cabbage, onions, baked beans)
   2. foods/fluids high in fat (e.g. butter, cream, whole milk, ice cream, fried foods, gravies, nuts)
f. encourage client to eructate and expel flatus whenever the urge is felt
g. administer the following medications if ordered:
   1. antiflatulents (e.g. simethicone) *to reduce gas accumulation*
   2. pancreatic enzymes (e.g. pancreatin, pancrelipase) *to improve fat digestion*
h. encourage the use of nonnarcotic analgesics once the period of severe pain has subsided *(narcotic analgesics depress gastrointestinal motility).*

4. Consult physician if signs and symptoms of abdominal distention and gas pain persist or worsen.

## 6. NURSING DIAGNOSIS: Altered oral mucous membrane: dryness

related to:
a. fluid volume deficit associated with fluid loss and fluid restrictions;
b. decreased salivation associated with fluid volume deficit, restricted oral intake, and some medications (e.g. narcotic analgesics);
c. mouth breathing when nasogastric tube is in place.

| Desired Outcome | Nursing Actions and ***Selected Purposes/Rationales*** |
|---|---|
| 6. The client will maintain a moist, intact oral mucous membrane. | 6.a. Assess client for dryness of the oral mucosa. |

b. Implement measures *to decrease dryness of the oral mucous membrane:*
   1. instruct and assist client to perform good oral hygiene as often as needed
   2. encourage client to rinse mouth frequently with water or dilute mouthwash
   3. instruct client to avoid products such as lemon-glycerin swabs and commercial mouthwashes containing alcohol *(these products have a drying or irritating effect on the oral mucous membrane)*
   4. lubricate client's lips frequently with K-Y jelly, ChapStick, Blistex, or mineral oil
   5. encourage client to breathe through nose rather than his/her mouth
   6. encourage client not to smoke *(smoking irritates and dries the mucosa)*
   7. maintain intravenous fluid therapy as ordered; when oral intake is allowed, encourage a fluid intake of at least 2500 ml/day unless contraindicated
   8. advance diet as allowed and tolerated *to stimulate salivation.*

c. If oral mucosa is irritated or cracked, implement measures *to relieve discomfort and promote healing:*
   1. assist client to select soft, bland foods
   2. instruct client to avoid foods/fluids that are extremely hot
   3. use a soft-bristle brush, sponge-tipped applicator, or low-pressure power spray for oral hygiene

| Desired Outcome | Nursing Actions and ***Selected Purposes/Rationales*** |
|---|---|
| | 4. administer topical anesthetics, oral protective pastes or coating agents, and topical and systemic analgesics if ordered.<br>d. Consult physician if dryness, irritation, and/or discomfort persist. |

## 7. COLLABORATIVE DIAGNOSES:

**Potential complications:**

a. **hypovolemic shock** related to:
   1. fluid volume deficit associated with fluid loss and fluid restrictions
   2. peripheral vasodilation and increased vascular permeability with subsequent third-spacing associated with activation of bradykinin and kallidin (trypsin activates the peptide kallikrein, which then activates these vasoactive substances)
   3. hemorrhage associated with destruction of elastic fibers of the blood vessels by the proteolytic enzyme elastase (elastase is activated in the pancreas by trypsin and causes localized vessel damage in addition to the vessel wall destruction that occurs when it enters the systemic circulation);

b. **pancreatic pseudocyst or abscess formation** related to inflammation and necrosis of the pancreatic and surrounding tissue associated with destruction of the tissue by the activated proteolytic enzymes;

c. **peritonitis** related to:
   1. presence of activated pancreatic enzymes in the peritoneum
   2. leakage of necrotic substances into the peritoneum associated with rupture of a pancreatic pseudocyst or abscess;

d. **hyperglycemia** related to increased release of glucagon and decreased release of insulin associated with injury to the alpha and beta cells;

e. **pleural effusion** related to:
   1. increased capillary permeability associated with damage to pleural vessels resulting from the escape of activated pancreatic enzymes into the systemic circulation
   2. passage of exudate from the peritoneal cavity to the pleural cavity through the diaphragmatic lymph channels;

f. **adult respiratory distress syndrome (ARDS)** related to disruption of the alveolar-capillary membrane associated with the release of activated pancreatic enzymes into the systemic circulation;

g. **fat necrosis** related to destruction of fatty tissue by activated pancreatic enzymes such as lipase and phospholipase A that escape from the pancreas into the systemic circulation and tissues.

| Desired Outcomes | Nursing Actions and ***Selected Purposes/Rationales*** |
|---|---|
| 7.a. The client will not develop hypovolemic shock as evidenced by:<br>1. usual mental status<br>2. stable vital signs<br>3. skin warm, dry, and usual color<br>4. palpable peripheral pulses<br>5. urine output at least 30 ml/hour. | 7.a.1. Assess for and report signs and symptoms of:<br>a. fluid volume deficit and third-spacing (see Nursing Diagnosis 2, actions a.1.a and b.1 for signs and symptoms)<br>b. bleeding (e.g. gray-blue discoloration around umbilicus [Cullen's sign], green-blue or purple-blue discoloration of flanks [Grey Turner's sign], increased abdominal or back pain, increased abdominal girth, declining B/P and increased pulse rate, decreased Hct and Hb levels)<br>c. hypovolemic shock:<br>1. restlessness, agitation, confusion<br>2. significant decrease in B/P<br>3. postural hypotension<br>4. rapid, thready pulse<br>5. rapid respirations<br>6. cool, moist skin<br>7. pallor, cyanosis |

8. diminished or absent peripheral pulses
9. urine output less than 30 ml/hour.

2. Implement measures *to prevent hypovolemic shock:*
   a. perform actions to prevent or treat fluid and electrolyte imbalances (see Nursing Diagnosis 2, actions a.3 and b.4)
   b. perform actions to reduce pancreatic stimulation (see Nursing Diagnosis 4, action e.3) *in order to decrease the amount of elastase that is activated and released into the tissue and systemic circulation and thereby reduce the risk for bleeding.*
3. If signs and symptoms of hypovolemic shock occur:
   a. continue with above actions
   b. place client flat in bed with legs elevated unless contraindicated
   c. monitor vital signs frequently
   d. administer oxygen as ordered
   e. administer blood products and/or volume expanders as ordered
   f. prepare client for insertion of hemodynamic monitoring devices (e.g. central venous catheter, intra-arterial catheter) if indicated
   g. provide emotional support to client and significant others.

7.b. The client will have resolution of a pancreatic pseudocyst or abscess if it develops as evidenced by:
1. decrease in abdominal pain
2. temperature declining toward normal
3. WBC count declining toward normal.

7.b.1. Assess for and report signs and symptoms of a pancreatic pseudocyst or abscess formation (e.g. increased or more constant abdominal pain, persistent or recurrent increase in temperature, further increase in WBC count).
2. If signs and symptoms of a pancreatic pseudocyst or abscess occur:
   a. prepare client for diagnostic studies (e.g. computed tomography, ultrasonography)
   b. administer antimicrobials if ordered
   c. prepare client for drainage of the pseudocyst or abscess if planned.

7.c. The client will have resolution of peritonitis if it occurs as evidenced by:
1. gradual resolution of abdominal pain
2. soft, nondistended abdomen
3. temperature declining toward normal
4. stable vital signs
5. decreased nausea and vomiting
6. gradual return of normal bowel sounds
7. WBC count declining toward normal.

7.c.1. Assess for and report signs and symptoms of peritonitis (e.g. increase in severity of abdominal pain; generalized abdominal pain; rebound tenderness; tense, rigid abdomen; further increase in temperature; tachycardia; tachypnea; hypotension; increased nausea and vomiting; diminished or absent bowel sounds).
2. Monitor WBC counts. Report levels that increase or fail to decline toward normal.
3. If signs and symptoms of peritonitis occur:
   a. withhold all food and fluid as ordered
   b. place client on bed rest in a semi-Fowler's position *to assist in pooling or localizing gastrointestinal contents in the pelvis rather than under the diaphragm*
   c. insert a nasogastric tube if not already present and maintain suction as ordered
   d. administer antimicrobials as ordered
   e. administer intravenous fluids and/or blood volume expanders if ordered *to prevent or treat shock (can result from the increased capillary permeability that occurs with inflammation and the subsequent escape of protein, fluid, and electrolytes from the vascular space into the peritoneal cavity)*
   f. prepare client for and assist with peritoneal lavage if performed *to remove toxins from the peritoneal cavity*
   g. provide emotional support to client and significant others.

7.d. The client will maintain a safe blood glucose level as evidenced by:

7.d.1. Assess for and report signs and symptoms of hyperglycemia (e.g. polydipsia; polyuria; polyphagia; change in mental status).
2. Monitor blood glucose levels. Report blood glucose values above 200 mg/dl or values as otherwise specified by physician.

| Desired Outcomes | Nursing Actions and ***Selected Purposes/Rationales*** |
|---|---|
| 1. absence of polydipsia, polyuria, and polyphagia<br>2. usual mental status<br>3. serum glucose between 60-200 mg/dl. | 3. Implement measures *to prevent hyperglycemia:*<br>a. perform actions to reduce pancreatic stimulation (see Nursing Diagnosis 4, action e.3) *in order to prevent further damage to the alpha and beta cells*<br>b. perform actions to reduce fear and anxiety and pain (see Nursing Diagnoses 8, action b and 4, action e) *in order to reduce emotional and physiological stress (stress causes an increased output of epinephrine, norepinephrine, glucagon, and cortisol, which results in a further increase in blood glucose).*<br>4. If signs and symptoms of hyperglycemia occur:<br>a. administer insulin or oral hypoglycemic agents if ordered<br>b. assess for and report signs and symptoms of ketoacidosis (e.g. hypotension; warm, flushed skin; thirst; weakness; lethargy; increased abdominal pain; fruity odor on breath; Kussmaul respirations; blood glucose above 300 mg/dl; ketones in blood and urine; low serum pH and $CO_2$ content)<br>c. if client does not have a history of diabetes or chronic pancreatitis, assure him/her that the hyperglycemia is expected to resolve as the pancreatitis does. |
| 7.e. The client will not experience pleural effusion as evidenced by:<br>1. unlabored respirations at 14-20/minute<br>2. usual chest excursion<br>3. resonant percussion note throughout lung fields<br>4. normal breath sounds. | 7.e.1. Assess for and report signs and symptoms of pleural effusion (e.g. dyspnea; decreased chest excursion, dull percussion note, and diminished or absent breath sounds over the affected area).<br>2. Monitor chest x-ray results. Report findings of pleural effusion.<br>3. Implement measures to reduce pancreatic stimulation (see Nursing Diagnosis 4, action e.3) *in order to reduce the release of activated pancreatic enzymes into the systemic circulation and diaphragmatic lymph channels.*<br>4. If signs and symptoms of pleural effusion occur, prepare client for thoracentesis if planned. |
| 7.f. The client will not experience ARDS as evidenced by:<br>1. unlabored respirations at 14-20/minute<br>2. usual skin color<br>3. usual mental status<br>4. blood gases within normal range. | 7.f.1. Assess for and report signs and symptoms of ARDS (e.g. rapid, shallow respirations; sternocleidomastoid muscle retraction; dusky or cyanotic skin color; drowsiness; confusion).<br>2. Monitor for and report:<br>a. abnormal blood gas values (progressive arterial hypoxemia even when receiving oxygen is indicative of ARDS)<br>b. significant changes in oximetry results<br>c. findings of atelectasis or pulmonary edema on chest x-ray.<br>3. Implement measures to reduce pancreatic stimulation (see Nursing Diagnosis 4, action e.3) *in order to reduce the amount of pancreatic enzymes in the systemic circulation and the subsequent increased risk for disruption of the alveolar-capillary membranes.*<br>4. If signs and symptoms of ARDS occur:<br>a. administer diuretics if ordered *to reduce pulmonary edema*<br>b. maintain oxygen therapy as ordered<br>c. assist with intubation, mechanical ventilation, and transfer to intensive care unit if indicated<br>d. provide emotional support to client and significant others. |
| 7.g. The client will not experience signs and symptoms of fat necrosis as evidenced by:<br>1. absence of | 7.g.1. Assess for and report signs and symptoms of fat necrosis (e.g. reddened, tender nodules in affected areas [usually on the lower extremities]; further increase in temperature and WBC count).<br>2. Implement measures to reduce pancreatic stimulation (see Nursing Diagnosis 4, action e.3) *in order to reduce the amount of pancreatic enzymes that escape from the pancreas into the systemic circulation and tissues.* |

| | |
|---|---|
| reddened, tender nodules in affected areas<br>2. WBC count within normal range. | 3. If signs and symptoms of fat necrosis occur:<br>a. administer antimicrobials if ordered *to prevent or treat infection in areas of fat necrosis*<br>b. prepare client for incision and drainage or removal of the necrotic areas. |

## 8. NURSING DIAGNOSIS: Anxiety

related to severe pain; unknown diagnosis; unfamiliar environment; and lack of understanding of diagnostic tests, treatment plan, and prognosis.

| Desired Outcome | Nursing Actions and ***Selected Purposes/Rationales*** |
|---|---|
| 8. The client will experience a reduction in anxiety as evidenced by:<br>a. verbalization of feeling less anxious and fearful<br>b. usual sleep pattern<br>c. relaxed facial expression and body movements<br>d. stable vital signs<br>e. usual perceptual ability and interactions with others. | 8.a. Assess client for signs and symptoms of anxiety (e.g. verbalization of fears and concerns, insomnia, tenseness, tremors, irritability, restlessness, diaphoresis, tachypnea, tachycardia, elevated blood pressure, facial pallor or flushing, narrowed perceptual field, withdrawal, noncompliance with treatment plan). Validate perceptions carefully, remembering that some behavior may be a physiological response to pain.<br>b. Implement measures *to reduce fear and anxiety:*<br>1. perform actions to reduce pain (see Nursing Diagnosis 4, action e)<br>2. orient client to hospital environment, equipment, and routines<br>3. introduce staff who will be participating in his/her care; if possible, maintain consistency in staff assigned to his/her care *to provide feelings of stability and comfort with the environment*<br>4. assure client that staff members are nearby; respond to call signal as soon as possible<br>5. maintain a calm, supportive, confident manner when interacting with client<br>6. encourage verbalization of fear and anxiety; provide feedback<br>7. explain all diagnostic tests<br>8. reinforce physician's explanations and clarify misconceptions the client has about pancreatitis, the treatment plan, and prognosis<br>9. provide a calm, restful environment<br>10. instruct client in relaxation techniques and encourage participation in diversional activities once severe pain has subsided<br>11. assist client to identify specific stressors and ways to cope with them<br>12. encourage significant others to project a caring, concerned attitude without obvious anxiousness<br>13. administer antianxiety agents if ordered.<br>c. Include significant others in orientation and teaching sessions and encourage their continued support of the client.<br>d. Provide information based on current needs of client and significant others at a level they can understand. Encourage questions and clarification of information provided.<br>e. Consult physician if above measures fail to control fear and anxiety. |

## 9. NURSING DIAGNOSIS: Knowledge deficit

regarding follow-up care.

| Desired Outcomes | Nursing Actions and ***Selected Purposes/Rationales*** |
|---|---|
| 9.a. The client will identify ways to prevent overstimulation of and further trauma to the pancreas. | 9.a.1. Instruct client in importance of avoiding overstimulation of the pancreas for the length of time specified by the physician (may be for a few months or for his/her lifetime depending on the cause of the pancreatitis and if permanent pancreatic damage has occurred).<br>2. Instruct client in ways to prevent overstimulation of and further trauma to the pancreas:<br>a. maintain a balanced program of rest and exercise<br>b. avoid stressful situations<br>c. avoid drinking alcohol<br>d. adhere to recommended dietary modifications (see action b.1 in this diagnosis)<br>e. maintain a relaxed atmosphere during and after meals.<br>3. Assist client to identify ways he/she can make necessary changes in personal habits and life style. |
| 9.b. The client will verbalize an understanding of recommended dietary modifications. | 9.b.1. Instruct client regarding dietary modifications necessary to prevent overstimulation of the pancreas during the recovery period:<br>a. eat small, frequent meals rather than 3 large ones<br>b. avoid foods/fluids high in fat (e.g. butter, cream, whole milk, ice cream, fried foods, gravies, nuts)<br>c. avoid caffeine-containing beverages (e.g. coffee, tea, colas).<br>2. Obtain a dietary consult if client needs assistance in planning meals that incorporate dietary modifications. |
| 9.c. The client will state signs and symptoms to report to the health care provider. | 9.c. Instruct client to report:<br>1. bowel movements that float and are grayish, greasy, and foul-smelling (indicates stool with a very high fat content resulting from impaired flow of the pancreatic enzyme lipase into the intestinal tract)<br>2. severe abdominal, epigastric, or back pain<br>3. persistent nausea or vomiting<br>4. abdominal distention or increasing feeling of fullness<br>5. excessive thirst or excessive urination<br>6. irritability or confusion<br>7. continued or unexplained weight loss<br>8. bluish areas on the back or abdomen<br>9. elevated temperature that lasts more than 2 days<br>10. tremors or seizures<br>11. difficulty breathing<br>12. reddened, tender nodules on skin. |
| 9.d. The client will verbalize an understanding of and a plan for adhering to recommended follow-up care including future appointments with health care provider and medications prescribed. | 9.d.1. Reinforce the importance of keeping follow-up appointments with health care provider.<br>2. Explain the rationale for, side effects of, and importance of taking medications prescribed (e.g. vitamins, antacids, histamine$_2$ receptor antagonists, pancreatic enzymes, antimicrobials).<br>3. Implement measures to improve client compliance:<br>a. include significant others in teaching sessions if possible<br>b. encourage questions and allow time for reinforcement and clarification of information provided<br>c. provide written instructions on scheduled appointments with health care provider, medications prescribed, and signs and symptoms to report. |

# Cholecystectomy

A cholecystectomy is the surgical removal of the gallbladder. It is commonly performed to treat symptomatic cholecystitis and/or cholelithiasis. A cholecystectomy can be done via a laparoscopy or through a right subcostal incision. A laparoscopic cholecystectomy involves a small umbilical incision for insertion of a laparoscope and 3 other small incisions in the abdomen for insertion of instruments. The procedure is considered to be minor surgery and the client is usually discharged the day of or the day following surgery. Acute cholecystitis with tissue distortion and/or the presence of large stones in the biliary duct system usually require the more traditional approach via a right subcostal incision. If stones are present in the common bile duct, a choledocholithotomy is performed and a T tube is usually placed in the common bile duct to maintain adequate flow or drainage of bile until ductal edema subsides.

**This care plan focuses on the adult client hospitalized for a cholecystectomy with common bile duct exploration.** Preoperatively, the goals of care are to maintain comfort, reduce fear and anxiety, and prepare the client for the postoperative period. Postoperative goals of care are to maintain comfort, maintain skin integrity, prevent complications, and educate the client regarding follow-up care.

## DIAGNOSTIC TESTS

**Refer to Care Plan on Cholelithiasis/Cholecystitis.**

## DISCHARGE CRITERIA

Prior to discharge, the client will:

- have pain controlled
- tolerate prescribed diet
- have no signs and symptoms of complications
- demonstrate the ability to appropriately care for T tube and surrounding skin if T tube is present
- verbalize an understanding of the rationale for and components of a low- to moderate-fat diet if prescribed
- state signs and symptoms to report to the health care provider
- verbalize an understanding of and a plan for adhering to recommended follow-up care including future appointments with health care provider, wound care, medications prescribed, and activity level.

## NURSING/COLLABORATIVE DIAGNOSES

**Postoperative**

1. Ineffective breathing pattern△ *682*
2. Altered nutrition: less than body requirements△ *682*
3. Actual/High risk for impaired skin integrity△ *683*
4. Potential complications:
   a. abscess formation
   b. fistula formation
   c. peritonitis
   d. continued obstruction of bile flow△ *683*
5. Knowledge deficit△ *685*

**See Care Plan on Cholelithiasis/Cholecystitis and the Standardized Preoperative and Postoperative Care Plans for additional diagnoses.**

## PREOPERATIVE

**Refer to the Care Plan on Cholelithiasis/Cholecystitis and the Standardized Preoperative Care Plan.**

## POSTOPERATIVE

**Use in conjunction with the Standardized Postoperative Care Plan.**

### 1. NURSING DIAGNOSIS: Ineffective breathing pattern

related to:
a. reluctance to breathe deeply associated with incisional pain;
b. depressant effects of anesthesia and some medications (e.g. narcotic analgesics);
c. impaired lung/chest wall expansion associated with positioning, weakness, fatigue, and abdominal distention if present;
d. fear and anxiety.

| Desired Outcome | Nursing Actions and ***Selected Purposes/Rationales*** |
|---|---|
| 1. The client will maintain an effective breathing pattern (see Standardized Postoperative Care Plan, Nursing Diagnosis 2 [p. 114], for outcome criteria). | 1.a. Refer to Standardized Postoperative Care Plan, Nursing Diagnosis 2 (pp. 114-115), for measures related to assessment and management of an ineffective breathing pattern.<br>b. Implement additional measures *to improve breathing pattern:*<br>1. instruct client to bend knees while coughing and deep breathing *in order to relieve tension on abdominal muscles and incision*<br>2. instruct and assist client to splint incision with hands or pillow when coughing and deep breathing. |

### 2. NURSING DIAGNOSIS: Altered nutrition: less body requirements

related to:
a. loss of nutrients associated with vomiting and nasogastric tube drainage;
b. decreased oral intake associated with prescribed dietary modifications, pain, fatigue, nausea, and dislike of prescribed diet;
c. inadequate nutritional replacement therapy;
d. increased nutritional needs associated with the increased metabolic rate that occurs during healing;
e. decreased absorption of fats and fat-soluble vitamins associated with excessive loss or obstructed flow of bile.

| Desired Outcome | Nursing Actions and ***Selected Purposes/Rationales*** |
|---|---|
| 2. The client will maintain an adequate nutritional status (see Standardized Postoperative Care Plan, Nursing Diagnosis 5 [p. 118], for outcome criteria). | 2.a. Refer to Standardized Postoperative Care Plan, Nursing Diagnosis 5 (p. 118), for measures related to assessment and maintenance of an adequate nutritional status.<br>b. Clamp T tube before, during, and after meals if ordered and as tolerated (it is usually clamped 1-2 hours before meals and then unclamped 1-2 hours after meals if tolerated) *to allow bile to drain into the duodenum and aid digestion and the absorption of fat-soluble vitamins.* |

**3. NURSING DIAGNOSIS: Actual/High risk for impaired skin integrity**

related to:
a. disruption of skin associated with the surgical procedure;
b. delayed wound healing associated with decreased nutritional status and inadequate blood supply to wound area;
c. irritation of skin associated with pressure from drainage tubes, use of tape, and contact with wound drainage (bile is extremely irritating to the skin).

| Desired Outcomes | Nursing Actions and ***Selected Purposes/Rationales*** |
|---|---|
| 3.a. The client will experience normal healing of surgical wounds (see Standardized Postoperative Care Plan, Nursing Diagnosis 9, outcome a [p. 122], for outcome criteria). | 3.a. Refer to Standardized Postoperative Care Plan, Nursing Diagnosis 9, action a (pp. 122-123), for measures related to assessment and promotion of wound healing. |
| 3.b. The client will maintain skin integrity (see Standardized Postoperative Care Plan, Nursing Diagnosis 9, outcome b [p. 123], for outcome criteria). | 3.b. Refer to Standardized Postoperative Care Plan, Nursing Diagnosis 9, action b (p. 123), for measures related to assessment and prevention of skin irritation and breakdown. |

**4. COLLABORATIVE DIAGNOSES: Potential complications:**

a. **abscess formation** related to accumulation of drainage in the surgical area and subsequent invasion of the area by microorganisms and neutrophils;
b. **fistula formation** related to perforation of biliary duct associated with surgical trauma and/or increased ductal pressure;
c. **peritonitis** related to escape of bile into the peritoneal cavity associated with surgical trauma to the gallbladder and biliary duct;
d. **continued obstruction of bile flow** related to residual stones in the biliary duct system or persistent inflammation and/or strictures of the common bile duct associated with surgical trauma.

| Desired Outcomes | Nursing Actions and ***Selected Purposes/Rationales*** |
|---|---|
| 4.a. The client will not develop an abscess or fistula as evidenced by:<br>1. gradual resolution of abdominal pain<br>2. temperature | 4.a.1. Assess for and report signs and symptoms of abscess and/or fistula formation (e.g. increased or more constant abdominal pain, increase in temperature and pulse rate, further increase in WBC count).<br>2. Implement measures *to prevent accumulation of drainage in the surgical area in order to reduce risk of abscess and fistula formation:*<br>a. perform actions *to maintain patency of wound drain and/or T tube if present:* |

| Desired Outcomes | Nursing Actions and ***Selected Purposes/Rationales*** |
|---|---|
| declining toward normal<br>3. WBC count declining toward normal. | 1. implement measures *to prevent stasis and reflux of drainage:*<br>a. keep drainage tubing free of dependent loops and kinks (prevent kinking by placing a gauze roll under the drain tube and anchoring it to the skin with tape)<br>b. keep collection device(s) below drain insertion site(s)<br>c. empty collection device(s) as often as necessary and at least every shift<br>2. implement measures *to prevent inadvertent removal of wound drain and/or T tube:*<br>a. instruct client not to pull on drain(s) and drainage tubing<br>b. use caution when changing dressings surrounding drain(s)<br>c. attach collection device(s) securely to abdominal dressing<br>b. maintain client in a semi-Fowler's position as much as possible when in bed.<br>3. If signs and symptoms of an abscess or fistula occur:<br>a. prepare client for diagnostic tests (e.g. ultrasonography, computed tomography)<br>b. administer antimicrobials if ordered<br>c. prepare client for surgical intervention (e.g. incision and drainage of abscess, closure of fistula) if planned<br>d. provide emotional support to client and significant others. |
| 4.b. The client will not develop peritonitis as evidenced by:<br>1. gradual resolution of abdominal pain<br>2. soft, nondistended abdomen<br>3. temperature declining toward normal<br>4. stable vital signs<br>5. absence of nausea and vomiting<br>6. gradual return of normal bowel sounds<br>7. WBC count declining toward normal. | 4.b.1. Assess for and report signs and symptoms of peritonitis (e.g. increase in severity of abdominal pain; generalized abdominal pain; rebound tenderness; tense, rigid abdomen; increase in temperature; tachycardia; tachypnea; hypotension; nausea; vomiting; continued diminished or absent bowel sounds).<br>2. Monitor WBC counts. Report levels that increase or fail to decline toward normal.<br>3. Implement measures to maintain patency and prevent inadvertent removal of T tube if present (see actions a.2.a in this diagnosis) *in order to prevent bile from leaking into the peritoneum.*<br>4. If signs and symptoms of peritonitis occur:<br>a. withhold all food and fluid as ordered<br>b. place client on bed rest in a semi-Fowler's position *to assist in pooling or localizing gastrointestinal contents in the pelvis rather than under the diaphragm*<br>c. insert a nasogastric tube (if not already present) or intestinal tube and maintain suction as ordered<br>d. administer antimicrobials as ordered<br>e. administer intravenous fluids and/or blood volume expanders if ordered *to prevent or treat shock (can result from the increased capillary permeability that occurs with inflammation and the subsequent escape of protein, fluid, and electrolytes from the vascular space into the peritoneal cavity)*<br>f. prepare client for surgical intervention (e.g. repair of leakage site) if planned<br>g. provide emotional support to client and significant others. |
| 4.c. The client will experience normal bile flow within 7-10 days after surgery as evidenced by:<br>1. decline in output of bile in T tube to less than 400 ml/day<br>2. absence of pain, nausea, and feeling | 4.c.1. Assess for and report signs and symptoms of continued bile flow obstruction (e.g. T tube draining more than 1000 ml in 24 hours; a marked increase in T tube drainage after it has started to decline; persistent pain, nausea, or feeling of fullness when T tube is clamped; jaundice; clay-colored stools; dark amber urine).<br>2. If signs and symptoms of bile flow obstruction occur:<br>a. leave T tube unclamped<br>b. perform actions to maintain patency of T tube (see action a.2.a in this diagnosis)<br>c. prepare client for T tube cholangiogram if planned |

| Desired Outcomes | Nursing Actions and *Selected Purposes/Rationales* |
|---|---|
| of fullness when T tube is clamped<br>3. absence of jaundice, clay-colored stools, and dark amber urine. | d. assist with or perform irrigation of T tube if ordered<br>e. prepare client for endoscopic sphincterotomy and/or basket removal of stones or surgery if planned<br>f. provide emotional support to client and significant others. |

## 5. NURSING DIAGNOSIS: Knowledge deficit

regarding follow-up care.

| Desired Outcomes | Nursing Actions and ***Selected Purposes/Rationales*** |
|---|---|
| 5.a. The client will demonstrate the ability to appropriately care for T tube and surrounding skin if T tube is present. | 5.a.1. If the client is to be discharged with a T tube in place, instruct regarding care of the T tube and surrounding skin:<br>a. cleanse the skin around the T tube insertion site daily and cover the site with a dry sterile dressing<br>b. always keep the T tube drainage collection device below the insertion site<br>c. keep the tubing pinned to the dressing and avoid any strain or pull on the tubing<br>d. empty the drainage collection device at least twice daily or more often if needed; keep a record of the amount of drainage<br>e. when emptying the drainage collection device, check to see that the tube has not become dislodged (this can be easily monitored if the tube is marked at the skin line before discharge)<br>f. clamp T tube only as instructed.<br>2. Allow time for questions, clarification, and return demonstration of care of T tube and surrounding skin. |
| 5.b. The client will verbalize an understanding of the rationale for and components of a low- to moderate-fat diet if prescribed. | 5.b.1. Explain the rationale for avoiding excessive fat intake for the first 4-6 weeks after surgery (some physicians instruct client to avoid only those foods that cause epigastric discomfort).<br>2. Instruct client to increase fat intake gradually and introduce foods/fluids high in fat (e.g. butter, cream, whole milk, ice cream, fried foods, gravies, nuts) one at a time. |
| 5.c. The client will state signs and symptoms to report to the health care provider. | 5.c.1 Refer to Standardized Postoperative Care Plan, Nursing Diagnosis 21, action c (p. 135), for signs and symptoms to report to health care provider.<br>2. Instruct client to report these additional signs and symptoms:<br>a. development of increased itchiness or yellowing of skin<br>b. clay-colored stools or dark amber urine<br>c. green-brown drainage around T tube or from wound site<br>d. a significant increase in or more than 500 ml/day of drainage from T tube<br>e. persistent heartburn or feeling of bloating<br>f. loose stools that continue for longer than 2-3 months. |
| 5.d. The client will verbalize an understanding of and a plan for adhering to recommended follow-up care | 5.d.1. Refer to Standardized Postoperative Care Plan, Nursing Diagnosis 21 (pp. 135-136), for routine postoperative instructions and measures to improve client compliance.<br>2. Instruct client to avoid lifting objects weighing over 10 pounds for 4-6 weeks after surgery. |

| Desired Outcomes | Nursing Actions and ***Selected Purposes/Rationales*** |
|---|---|
| including future appointments with health care provider, wound care, medications prescribed, and activity level. | |

# Cholelithiasis/Cholecystitis

Cholelithiasis refers to the presence of gallstones in the gallbladder. The two major types of gallstones are cholesterol stones and pigment stones. Cholesterol stones, the most prevalent type, form when bile becomes supersaturated with cholesterol, which then precipitates and starts to form stones. Stones either remain in the gallbladder or migrate into the duct system where they may cause partial or complete obstruction. The severity of the client's symptoms depends on the degree of bile flow obstruction.

Cholecystitis is inflammation of the gallbladder wall. It can be acute or chronic and in the majority of cases is associated with cholelithiasis. Cholecystitis results when stones lodge in the neck of the gallbladder or in the biliary duct system causing obstruction of bile flow. The bile trapped in the gallbladder acts as a chemical irritant causing inflammation and edema of the gallbladder wall. The inflammation and distention of the gallbladder cause venous congestion and subsequent impairment of blood flow to the gallbladder. If necrosis occurs, there is a high risk for bacterial invasion. Scarring of the gallbladder can occur following an acute attack, which can result in loss of normal gallbladder function.

In most cases, the treatment of choice for symptomatic cholelithiasis and cholecystitis is cholecystectomy and choledocholithotomy if stones have migrated into the biliary duct system. A cholecystostomy may be done to relieve symptoms if the client has severe symptoms and is a poor surgical risk. Nonsurgical treatment modalities for cholelithiasis such as dissolution of stones using oral bile acids (e.g. ursodeoxycholic acid [ursodiol, Actigall]), percutaneous instillation of a dissolution agent such as methyl tertiary butyl ether (MTBE) into the gallbladder, and extracorporeal shock-wave lithotripsy are currently being tried on some clients.

**This care plan focuses on the adult client hospitalized with probable cholelithiasis and/or cholecystitis.** The goals of treatment are to relieve discomfort, restore or maintain fluid and electrolyte balance, prevent complications, and educate the client regarding follow-up care.

## DIAGNOSTIC TESTS

Abdominal x-ray
Ultrasonography
Cholecystography
Percutaneous transhepatic cholangiography
Endoscopic retrograde cholangiopancreatography (ERCP)
Radionuclide imaging (e.g. HIDA or DISIDA scan)
Computed tomography (CT)
White blood cell (WBC) count and differential
Serum bilirubin and amylase
Serum enzymes (e.g. AST [SGOT], LDH, alkaline phosphatase)
Prothrombin time

## DISCHARGE CRITERIA

Prior to discharge, the client will:

- have relief of severe pain

- tolerate prescribed diet
- be free of signs and symptoms of complications
- verbalize an understanding of ways to reduce the risk for recurrent gallbladder attacks
- state signs and symptoms to report to the health care provider
- verbalize an understanding of and a plan for adhering to recommended follow-up care including future appointments with health care provider and medications prescribed.

**NURSING/ COLLABORATIVE DIAGNOSES**



**1. NURSING/ COLLABORATIVE DIAGNOSIS:**

**Altered fluid and electrolyte balance: fluid volume deficit, hypokalemia, hypochloremia, and metabolic alkalosis**

related to decreased oral intake and excessive loss of fluid and electrolytes associated with vomiting and nasogastric tube drainage.

| Desired Outcome | Nursing Actions and ***Selected Purposes/Rationales*** |
|---|---|
| 1. The client will maintain fluid and electrolyte balance as evidenced by:<br>a. normal skin turgor<br>b. moist mucous membranes<br>c. stable weight<br>d. B/P and pulse within normal range for client and stable with position change<br>e. small vein filling time less than 3-5 seconds<br>f. balanced intake and output | 1.a. Assess for and report signs and symptoms of:<br>1. fluid volume deficit:<br>a. decreased skin turgor, dry mucous membranes, thirst<br>b. sudden weight loss of 2% or greater<br>c. low B/P and/or postural hypotension<br>d. weak, rapid pulse<br>e. delayed small vein filling time (longer than 3-5 seconds)<br>f. decreased urine output with increased specific gravity (reflects an actual rather than potential fluid volume deficit)<br>g. increased BUN and Hct<br>2. hypokalemia (e.g. cardiac arrhythmias, postural hypotension, muscle weakness, paresthesias, nausea and vomiting, abdominal distention, hypoactive or absent bowel sounds)<br>3. hypochloremia and metabolic alkalosis (e.g. dizziness, irritability, paresthesias, muscle twitching or spasms, hypoventilation). |

| Desired Outcome | Nursing Actions and ***Selected Purposes/Rationales*** |
|---|---|
| g. urine specific gravity within normal range<br>h. soft, nondistended abdomen with normal bowel sounds<br>i. absence of cardiac arrhythmias, muscle weakness, paresthesias, twitching, spasms, and dizziness<br>j. BUN, Hct, serum electrolytes, and blood gases within normal range. | b. Monitor serum electrolyte and blood gas results. Report abnormal values.<br>c. Implement measures *to prevent or treat fluid and electrolyte imbalances:*<br>1. perform actions to reduce nausea and vomiting (see Nursing Diagnosis 4.B, action 2)<br>2. if irrigation of nasogastric tube is indicated, use normal saline rather than water<br>3. administer fluid and electrolyte replacements if ordered<br>4. maintain a fluid intake of at least 2500 ml/day unless contraindicated<br>5. when oral intake is allowed, assist client to select foods/fluids high in potassium (e.g. bananas, potatoes, raisins, figs, apricots, dates, orange juice, cantaloupe) and sodium (e.g. bouillon, canned soups, processed cheese, canned vegetables).<br>d. Consult physician if signs and symptoms of fluid and electrolyte imbalances persist or worsen. |

## 2. NURSING DIAGNOSIS: Altered nutrition: less than body requirements

related to:

a. decreased oral intake associated with nausea, dyspepsia, pain, and self-imposed or prescribed dietary restrictions;
b. loss of nutrients associated with vomiting;
c. decreased absorption of fats and fat-soluble vitamins associated with bile flow obstruction.

| Desired Outcome | Nursing Actions and ***Selected Purposes/Rationales*** |
|---|---|
| 2. The client will maintain an adequate nutritional status as evidenced by:<br>a. weight within normal range for client's age, height, and body frame<br>b. normal BUN and serum albumin, Hct, Hb, transferrin, and lymphocyte levels<br>c. triceps skinfold thickness within normal range<br>d. usual strength and activity tolerance<br>e. healthy oral mucous membrane. | 2.a. Assess for and report signs and symptoms of malnutrition:<br>1. weight below normal for client's age, height, and body frame<br>2. abnormal BUN and low serum albumin, Hct, Hb, transferrin, and lymphocyte levels<br>3. triceps skinfold thickness less than normal<br>4. weakness and fatigue<br>5. stomatitis.<br>b. Monitor percentage of meals and snacks client consumes. Report a pattern of inadequate intake.<br>c. Implement measures *to maintain an adequate nutritional status:*<br>1. when food or fluid is allowed, perform actions *to improve oral intake:*<br>a. implement measures to reduce nausea, vomiting, and dyspepsia (see Nursing Diagnoses 4.B, action 2 and 4.C, action 3)<br>b. implement measures to reduce pain (see Nursing Diagnosis 3, action e)<br>c. obtain a dietary consult if necessary to assist client in selecting foods/fluids that meet dietary restrictions and nutritional needs as well as personal and cultural preferences whenever possible<br>d. provide oral care before meals<br>e. serve small portions of nutritious foods/fluids that are appealing to the client<br>f. maintain a clean environment and a relaxed, pleasant atmosphere<br>g. allow adequate time for meals; reheat food if necessary<br>2. ensure that meals are well balanced and high in essential nutrients (diet may be advanced from powdered protein and carbohydrate |

supplements in skim milk to a low- to moderate-fat diet); offer dietary supplements between meals if indicated
3. administer fat-soluble vitamins if ordered.

d. Perform a 72-hour calorie count if ordered. Report totals to dietitian and physician.
e. Consult physician regarding alternative methods of providing nutrition (e.g. parenteral nutrition) if client does not consume enough food or fluids to meet nutritional needs.

## 3. NURSING DIAGNOSIS: **Pain: epigastric area or right upper quadrant of abdomen with radiation to interscapular area or right scapula or shoulder**

related to:
a. inflammation and distention of the gallbladder;
b. ductal spasms associated with blockage of bile flow if gallstones are present in the duct system.

| Desired Outcome | Nursing Actions and ***Selected Purposes/Rationales*** |
|---|---|
| 3. The client will experience diminished pain as evidenced by:<br>a. verbalization of pain relief<br>b. relaxed facial expression and body positioning<br>c. increased participation in activities<br>d. stable vital signs. | 3.a. Determine how the client usually responds to pain.<br>b. Assess client's perception of pain including location, severity, and type of pain (increased pain with transient inspiratory arrest upon deep palpation of the right upper quadrant [Murphy's sign] is indicative of cholecystitis). Use a numerical scale to rate intensity of pain.<br>c. Assess for nonverbal signs of pain (e.g. wrinkled brow; clenched fists; guarding of abdomen; rubbing right shoulder; reluctance to move; facial pallor; rapid, shallow respirations; increased B/P; tachycardia).<br>d. Assess for factors that seem to aggravate and alleviate pain.<br>e. Implement measures *to reduce pain:*<br>1. perform actions *to reduce fear and anxiety about the pain experience* (e.g. assure client that his/her need for pain relief will be met, perform preprocedure teaching)<br>2. medicate prior to any painful procedure and before pain is severe<br>3. perform actions *to reduce stimulation of gallbladder contractions:*<br>a. maintain NPO status as ordered<br>b. insert nasogastric tube and maintain suction as ordered<br>c. when oral intake is allowed, maintain dietary restrictions of fat as ordered (avoid foods/fluids high in fat such as butter, cream, whole milk, ice cream, fried foods, gravies, and nuts)<br>4. provide or assist with nonpharmacological measures for pain relief (e.g. back rub, position change, relaxation techniques, quiet conversation, restful environment, diversional activities)<br>5. administer the following if ordered:<br>a. analgesics (meperidine is often the medication of choice *because morphine sulfate increases spasms of the sphincter of Oddi)*<br>b. antimicrobials *to prevent or treat infection and subsequently reduce inflammation of the gallbladder wall*<br>6. consult physician about order for patient-controlled analgesia (PCA) if adequate relief cannot be achieved with usual pain control methods<br>7. prepare client for surgery, endoscopic ductal stone removal, percutaneous infusion of cholesterol stone solvent into gallbladder, or extracorporeal shock-wave lithotripsy if planned.<br>f. Consult physician if above measures fail to provide adequate pain relief. |

## 4.A. NURSING DIAGNOSIS:

**Altered comfort: pruritus**

related to irritation of the skin by bile salts, which deposit in the skin as a result of bile flow obstruction.

| Desired Outcome | Nursing Actions and ***Selected Purposes/Rationales*** |
|---|---|
| 4.A. The client will experience relief of pruritus as evidenced by:<br>1. verbalization of same<br>2. no scratching or rubbing of skin. | 4.A.1. Assess client's pruritus including onset, characteristics, location, and factors that aggravate and alleviate it.<br>2. Instruct client in and/or implement measures *to relieve pruritus:*<br>a. perform actions *to promote capillary constriction:*<br>1. apply cool, moist compresses to pruritic areas<br>2. maintain a cool environment<br>b. apply emollient creams or ointments frequently *to prevent dryness*<br>c. add emollients, cornstarch, baking soda, or oatmeal preparations to bath water<br>d. use tepid water and mild soaps for bathing<br>e. pat skin dry, making sure to dry thoroughly<br>f. encourage participation in diversional activity<br>g. utilize cutaneous stimulation techniques (e.g. massage, pressure, vibration, stroking with soft brush) at the sites of itching or acupressure points<br>h. encourage client to wear loose cotton garments<br>i. utilize relaxation techniques<br>j. administer the following medications if ordered:<br>1. antihistamines<br>2. cholestyramine *to bind bile salts and reduce their accumulation in the skin.*<br>3. Consult physician if above measures fail to alleviate pruritus or if the skin becomes excoriated. |

## 4.B. NURSING DIAGNOSIS:

**Altered comfort: nausea and vomiting**

related to stimulation of the vomiting center associated with:

1. stimulation of the afferent vagal and/or sympathetic pathways as a result of visceral irritation that occurs with gallbladder and bile duct inflammation;
2. cortical stimulation resulting from pain and stress.

| Desired Outcome | Nursing Actions and ***Selected Purposes/Rationales*** |
|---|---|
| 4.B. The client will experience relief of nausea and vomiting as evidenced by:<br>1. verbalization of relief of nausea<br>2. absence of vomiting. | 4.B.1. Assess client for nausea and vomiting.<br>2. Implement measures *to reduce nausea and vomiting:*<br>a. maintain patency of nasogastric tube (e.g. keep tubing free of kinks, irrigate and maintain suction as ordered) if present<br>b. eliminate noxious sights and odors from the environment *(noxious stimuli cause cortical stimulation of the vomiting center)*<br>c. instruct client to change positions slowly *(rapid movement stimulates the afferent vestibulocerebellar pathway with resultant stimulation of the chemoreceptor trigger zone)*<br>d. provide oral hygiene every 2 hours and after each emesis<br>e. perform actions to reduce fear and anxiety (see Nursing Diagnosis 7, action b) |

f. perform actions to reduce pain (see Nursing Diagnosis 3, action e)
g. encourage client to take deep, slow breaths when nauseated
h. maintain food and fluid restrictions as ordered
i. when oral intake is allowed:
    1. advance diet as tolerated
    2. avoid serving foods with an overpowering aroma; remove lids from hot foods before entering room
    3. provide small, frequent meals; instruct client to ingest foods and fluids slowly
    4. instruct client to eat dry foods (e.g. toast, crackers) and avoid drinking liquids with meals if nauseated
    5. instruct client to avoid the following:
        a. foods/fluids high in fat (e.g. butter, cream, whole milk, ice cream, fried foods, gravies, nuts)
        b. foods/fluids that irritate the gastric mucosa (e.g. spicy foods; caffeine-containing beverages such as tea, coffee, and colas)
    6. instruct client to rest after eating with head of bed elevated
j. administer antiemetics if ordered (phenothiazines should be used cautiously *because of their potential cholestatic effect).*

3. Consult physician if above measures fail to control nausea and vomiting.

---

**4.C. NURSING DIAGNOSIS:** **Altered comfort: dyspepsia**
related to impaired fat digestion associated with bile flow obstruction.

| Desired Outcome | Nursing Actions and ***Selected Purposes/Rationales*** |
|---|---|
| 4.C. The client will verbalize relief of dyspepsia. | 4.C.1. Assess client for verbal complaints of dyspepsia (e.g. epigastric discomfort, feeling of fullness or bloating, nausea).<br>2. Determine if particular foods/fluids contribute to dyspepsia (client usually reports an intolerance of fatty foods).<br>3. Implement measures *to reduce dyspepsia:*<br>a. perform actions to reduce nausea once oral intake is allowed (see Nursing Diagnosis 4.B, action 2.i)<br>b. perform actions *to reduce the accumulation of gas in the gastrointestinal tract:*<br>1. encourage and assist client with frequent position changes and ambulation as allowed and tolerated *(activity stimulates peristalsis and expulsion of flatus)*<br>2. instruct client to avoid activities such as chewing gum and smoking *in order to reduce air swallowing*<br>3. encourage client to eructate and expel flatus whenever the urge is felt<br>4. administer antiflatulents (e.g. simethicone) if ordered.<br>4. Consult physician if above measures fail to control dyspepsia. |

---

**5. NURSING DIAGNOSIS:** **Altered oral mucous membrane: dryness**
related to:
a. fluid volume deficit associated with fluid loss and fluid restrictions;

b. decreased salivation associated with fluid volume deficit, restricted oral intake, and treatment with some medications (e.g. narcotic analgesics);
c. mouth breathing when nasogastric tube is in place.

| Desired Outcome | Nursing Actions and ***Selected Purposes/Rationales*** |
|---|---|
| 5. The client will maintain a moist, intact oral mucous membrane. | 5.a. Assess client for dryness of the oral mucosa.<br>b. Implement measures *to relieve dryness of the oral mucous membrane:*<br>1. instruct and assist client to perform good oral hygiene as often as needed; avoid products such as lemon-glycerin swabs and commercial mouthwashes containing alcohol *(these products have a drying or irritating effect on oral mucous membrane)*<br>2. encourage client to rinse mouth frequently with water or dilute mouthwash<br>3. lubricate client's lips frequently with K-Y jelly, ChapStick, Blistex, or mineral oil<br>4. encourage client to breathe through nose rather than his/her mouth<br>5. encourage client not to smoke *(smoking irritates and dries the mucosa)*<br>6. maintain intravenous fluid administration as ordered *to improve hydration*<br>7. provide sips of water frequently if allowed<br>8. advance diet as allowed and tolerated *to stimulate salivation.*<br>c. If oral mucosa is irritated or cracked, implement measures *to relieve discomfort and promote healing:*<br>1. assist client to select soft, bland foods<br>2. instruct client to avoid foods/fluids that are extremely hot<br>3. use a soft-bristle brush, sponge-tipped applicator, or low-pressure power spray for oral hygiene<br>4. administer topical anesthetics, oral protective pastes or coating agents, and topical and systemic analgesics if ordered.<br>d. Consult physician if dryness, irritation, and/or discomfort persist. |

## 6. COLLABORATIVE DIAGNOSES:

**Potential complications:**

a. **abscess or fistula formation** related to presence of increased cholecystic and ductal pressure (can cause perforation of the gallbladder into localized, contained area [abscess] or wall of an adjacent organ [fistula]);
b. **peritonitis** related to escape of bile into the peritoneal cavity associated with perforation of the gallbladder;
c. **pancreatitis** related to obstruction of the flow of pancreatic secretions as a result of a stone or inflammation in the common bile duct;
d. **cholangitis** related to:
   1. irritation of the bile ducts associated with presence of ductal stones
   2. possible bacterial invasion of biliary system associated with stasis of bile.

| Desired Outcomes | Nursing Actions and ***Selected Purposes/Rationales*** |
|---|---|
| 6.a. The client will experience resolution of any abscess or fistula that develops as evidenced by:<br>1. decrease in abdominal pain | 6.a.1. Assess for and report signs and symptoms of abscess and/or fistula formation (e.g. increased or more constant abdominal pain, further increase in temperature and pulse rate, further increase in WBC count).<br>2. If signs and symptoms of an abscess or fistula occur:<br>a. prepare client for diagnostic studies (e.g. ultrasonography, computed tomography)<br>b. administer antimicrobials if ordered |

2. temperature and pulse declining toward normal
3. WBC count declining toward normal.

c. prepare client for surgical intervention (e.g. cholecystectomy or cholecystostomy with incision and drainage of abscess or closure of fistula) if planned
d. provide emotional support to client and significant others.

6.b. The client will have resolution of peritonitis if it occurs as evidenced by:
1. gradual resolution of abdominal pain
2. soft, nondistended abdomen
3. temperature declining toward normal
4. stable vital signs
5. decreased nausea and vomiting
6. gradual return of normal bowel sounds
7. WBC count declining toward normal.

6.b.1. Assess for and report signs and symptoms of peritonitis (e.g. transient pain relief; diffuse abdominal pain; rebound tenderness; tense, rigid abdomen; further increase in temperature; tachycardia; tachypnea; hypotension; increased nausea and vomiting; diminished or absent bowel sounds).
2. Monitor WBC counts. Report levels that increase or fail to decline toward normal.
3. If signs and symptoms of peritonitis occur:
a. withhold all food and fluid as ordered
b. place client on bed rest in a semi-Fowler's position *to assist in pooling or localizing gastrointestinal contents in the pelvis rather than under the diaphragm*
c. insert a nasogastric tube (if not already present) or intestinal tube and maintain suction as ordered
d. administer antimicrobials as ordered
e. administer intravenous fluids and/or blood volume expanders if ordered *to prevent or treat shock (can result from the increased capillary permeability that occurs with inflammation and the subsequent escape of protein, fluid, and electrolytes from the vascular space into the peritoneal cavity)*
f. prepare client for surgery (e.g. cholecystectomy or cholecystostomy with peritoneal lavage) if planned
g. provide emotional support to client and significant others.

6.c. The client will experience resolution of pancreatitis if it occurs as evidenced by:
1. gradual resolution of abdominal pain
2. temperature declining toward normal
3. stable B/P and pulse
4. serum amylase and lipase levels declining toward normal
5. renal amylase/creatinine clearance ratio returning toward normal
6. WBC count declining toward normal.

6.c.1. Assess for and report signs and symptoms of pancreatitis (e.g. extension of pain to left upper quadrant or back, further increase in temperature, tachycardia, hypotension, elevated serum amylase and lipase levels).
2. Collect a timed (usually 2-hour) urine specimen if ordered. Report an elevated renal amylase/creatinine clearance ratio.
3. Monitor WBC counts. Report levels that increase or fail to decline toward normal.
4. If signs and symptoms of pancreatitis occur:
a. assist client to assume position of greatest comfort (e.g. side-lying, sitting with trunk and knees flexed, sitting and leaning forward)
b. maintain food and fluid restrictions as ordered
c. insert nasogastric tube if not already present and maintain suction as ordered *(removal of gastric secretions reduces pancreatic stimulation)*
d. administer the following if ordered:
1. analgesics
2. antacids and histamine$_2$ receptor antagonists (e.g. cimetidine, ranitidine, famotidine) *to decrease the acidity of gastric contents and thereby reduce stimulation of the pancreas (when acidic gastric contents enter the duodenum and jejunum, secretin is released; secretin stimulates pancreatic secretion)*
e. prepare client for endoscopic sphincterotomy or stone extraction or surgery to relieve ductal obstruction if planned
f. refer to Care Plan on Pancreatitis for additional care measures.

6.d. The client will experience resolution of cholangitis if it occurs as evidenced by:
1. gradual resolution of abdominal pain

6.d.1. Assess for signs and symptoms of cholangitis (e.g. increased abdominal pain, jaundice, chills, increase in temperature, further increase in WBC count). Be aware that lethargy, confusion, and hypotension may indicate septic shock, which can develop with suppurative cholangitis.
2. Monitor serum bilirubin and enzymes (e.g. alkaline phosphatase, ALT [SGPT], AST [SGOT]). Report increased levels.
3. Obtain blood cultures as ordered. Report positive results.

| Desired Outcomes | Nursing Actions and ***Selected Purposes/Rationales*** |
|---|---|
| 2. absence of jaundice and chills<br>3. temperature declining toward normal<br>4. WBC count declining toward normal. | 4. If signs and symptoms of cholangitis occur:<br>a. administer antimicrobials if ordered<br>b. prepare client for endoscopic sphincterotomy, insertion of a percutaneous transhepatic catheter (to decompress duct), or surgical removal of ductal stone if planned<br>c. provide emotional support to client and significant others. |

## 7. NURSING DIAGNOSIS: Anxiety

related to discomfort, unknown diagnosis, unfamiliar environment, lack of understanding of diagnostic tests and treatments, and possibility of surgery.

| Desired Outcome | Nursing Actions and ***Selected Purposes/Rationales*** |
|---|---|
| 7. The client will experience a reduction in anxiety as evidenced by:<br>a. verbalization of feeling less anxious and fearful<br>b. usual sleep pattern<br>c. relaxed facial expression and body movements<br>d. stable vital signs<br>e. usual perceptual ability and interactions with others. | 7.a. Assess client for signs and symptoms of anxiety (e.g. verbalization of fears and concerns, insomnia, tenseness, tremors, irritability, restlessness, diaphoresis, tachypnea, tachycardia, elevated blood pressure, facial pallor or flushing, narrowed perceptual field, withdrawal, noncompliance with treatment plan). Validate perceptions carefully, remembering that some behavior may result from pain.<br>b. Implement measures *to reduce fear and anxiety:*<br>1. orient client to hospital environment, equipment, and routines<br>2. introduce staff who will be participating in his/her care; if possible, maintain consistency in staff assigned to his/her care *to provide feelings of stability and comfort with the environment*<br>3. assure client that staff members are nearby; respond to call signal as soon as possible<br>4. maintain a calm, supportive, confident manner when interacting with client<br>5. encourage verbalization of fear and anxiety; provide feedback<br>6. explain all diagnostic tests<br>7. reinforce physician's explanations and clarify misconceptions client has about cholelithiasis and/or cholecystitis and the treatment plan<br>8. perform actions to reduce discomfort (see Nursing Diagnoses 3, action e; 4.A, action 2; 4.B, action 2; and 4.C, action 3)<br>9. provide a calm, restful environment<br>10. instruct client in relaxation techniques and encourage participation in diversional activities once severe pain has subsided<br>11. assist client to identify specific stressors and ways to cope with them<br>12. encourage significant others to project a caring, concerned attitude without obvious anxiousness<br>13. if surgical intervention is indicated, begin preoperative teaching<br>14. administer antianxiety agents if ordered.<br>c. Include significant others in orientation and teaching sessions and encourage their continued support of the client.<br>d. Provide information based on current needs of the client and significant others at a level they can understand. Encourage questions and clarification of information provided.<br>e. Consult physician if above actions fail to control fear and anxiety. |

## 8. NURSING DIAGNOSIS: Knowledge deficit

regarding follow-up care.

| Desired Outcomes | Nursing Actions and ***Selected Purposes/Rationales*** |
|---|---|
| 8.a. The client will verbalize an understanding of ways to reduce the risk for recurrent gallbladder attacks. | 8.a. Instruct client regarding ways to reduce the risk for recurrent gallbladder attacks:<br>1. adhere to a low- to moderate-fat diet (avoid foods/fluids high in fat such as butter, cream, whole milk, ice cream, fried foods, gravies, and nuts)<br>2. lose weight if obese but avoid rapid weight loss (*rapid weight loss has been shown to increase biliary cholesterol saturation*)<br>3. exercise regularly<br>4. consult physician prior to or regarding continued use of estrogen preparations/oral contraceptives (*estrogen preparations increase biliary cholesterol levels and subsequently increase the risk for gallstones*). |
| 8.b. The client will state signs and symptoms to report to the health care provider. | 8.b. Instruct client to report the following signs and symptoms:<br>1. persistent indigestion, flatulence, and loose stools<br>2. nausea and vomiting<br>3. recurrent episodes of abdominal pain<br>4. development of or persistent itching, yellow coloring of skin or eyes, dark color of urine, or clay-colored stools (*indicative of bile flow obstruction*)<br>5. persistent or recurrent temperature elevation. |
| 8.c. The client will verbalize an understanding of and a plan for adhering to recommended follow-up care including future appointments with health care provider and medications prescribed. | 8.c.1. Reinforce importance of keeping follow-up appointments with health care provider.<br>2. Explain the rationale for, side effects of, and importance of taking prescribed medications (e.g. fat-soluble vitamins, cholestyramine, ursodiol, antimicrobials).<br>3. Implement measures to improve client compliance:<br>a. include significant others in teaching sessions if possible<br>b. encourage questions and allow time for reinforcement and clarification of information provided<br>c. provide written instructions on future appointments with health care provider, medications prescribed, and signs and symptoms to report. |

# Cirrhosis

Cirrhosis is a chronic progressive liver disease which occurs because of extensive destruction of the parenchymal cells in the liver. These cells are eventually replaced by fibrous scar tissue with subsequent change in the structure and functioning of the liver. The structural changes impair portal blood flow which results in venous congestion in other organs and systems such as the spleen and gastrointestinal tract. The four major types of cirrhosis are alcoholic (e.g. Laennec's portal, nutritional), postnecrotic, biliary, and cardiac. Alcoholic cirrhosis is the most common type seen in North America. Malnutrition is not a cause of any type of cirrhosis but is thought to possibly potentiate the harmful effects of alcohol on the liver and augment the development of cirrhosis.

All types of cirrhosis have similar signs and symptoms which are manifestations of impaired liver function and the venous congestion that occurs with portal hypertension. Alcohol-related cirrhosis may have additional manifestations such as cerebral degeneration and demyelinating neuropathies that are thought to be a direct result of the toxic effects of alcohol. Treatment of cirrhosis includes removing the causative factor if possible, providing a diet that prevents further malnutrition and promotes liver regeneration, and encouraging rest to reduce the metabolic demands on the liver. Liver transplantation is often indicated for treatment of end-stage liver disease. There has been little enthusiasm for using transplants for treating alcoholic cirrhosis, however, particularly if another alcohol-related disease is present. Abstinence from alcohol (usually for a minimum of 6 months) is currently a criterion used for evaluation and selection of the alcoholic client for liver transplantation.

**This care plan focuses on the adult client with alcoholic (Laennec's) cirrhosis hospitalized for management of increasing ascites and peripheral edema.** The goals of care are to maintain comfort, improve nutritional status and fluid balance, prevent complications, and educate the client regarding follow-up care.

## DIAGNOSTIC TESTS

Serum enzymes (e.g. AST [SGOT], ALT [SGPT], LDH, alkaline phosphatase)
Serum proteins and protein electrophoresis
Serum bilirubin
Serum ammonia
Serum cholesterol and electrolytes
Complete blood count (CBC)
Urine bilirubin and urobilinogen
Prothrombin time (PT)
Ultrasonography
Computed tomography (CT)
Liver biopsy
Percutaneous transhepatic portography
Esophagoscopy and/or barium contrast x-ray of upper gastrointestinal (UGI) tract (may be performed to determine the presence of esophageal varices)

## DISCHARGE CRITERIA

Prior to discharge, the client will:

- ❖ have an adequate nutritional intake
- ❖ perform activities of daily living without extreme fatigue or dyspnea
- ❖ have a reduction in or resolution of ascites and edema
- ❖ have no evidence of life-threatening complications
- ❖ identify ways to prevent further liver damage
- ❖ verbalize an understanding of the rationale for and components of the recommended diet
- ❖ identify ways to reduce stress on esophageal vessels
- ❖ identify ways to prevent bleeding
- ❖ identify ways to reduce the risk of infection
- ❖ identify ways to relieve pruritus
- ❖ state signs and symptoms to report to the health care provider

- identify community resources that can assist with home management and adjustment to life-style changes necessary for effective management of cirrhosis
- share concerns and feelings about the diagnosis of cirrhosis; prognosis; and effects of the disease process and its treatment on self-concept, life style, and roles
- verbalize an understanding of and a plan for adhering to recommended follow-up care including future appointments with health care provider, medications prescribed, and activity level.

**Use in conjunction with the Care Plan on Immobility.**

**NURSING/ COLLABORATIVE DIAGNOSES**



**See Care Plan on Immobility for additional diagnoses.**

## 1. NURSING DIAGNOSIS: Ineffective breathing pattern

related to impaired lung/chest wall expansion associated with:
a. weakness;
b. positioning (client often remains on back in a semi-Fowler's position because of ascites);
c. pressure on the diaphragm as a result of peritoneal fluid accumulation;
d. pleural effusion (can occur as a result of fluid volume excess and passage of

ascitic fluid into the pleural space through a probable pressure-related defect in the diaphragm).

| Desired Outcome | Nursing Actions and ***Selected Purposes/Rationales*** |
|---|---|
| 1. The client will have an improved breathing pattern as evidenced by:<br>a. normal rate and depth of respirations<br>b. decreased dyspnea<br>c. blood gases within normal range. | 1.a. Assess for signs and symptoms of an ineffective breathing pattern (e.g. shallow respirations, dyspnea, use of accessory muscles when breathing).<br>b. Monitor for and report the following:<br>1. abnormal blood gases<br>2. significant changes in oximetry results.<br>c. Implement measures *to improve breathing pattern:*<br>1. perform actions to increase strength and activity tolerance (see Nursing Diagnosis 7)<br>2. perform actions to restore fluid balance (see Nursing Diagnosis 2, action a.4) *in order to reduce fluid accumulation in the peritoneal cavity and the risk for pleural effusion*<br>3. assist client to turn from side to side at least every 2 hours while in bed<br>4. place client in a semi-Fowler's position (a high Fowler's position is uncomfortable if ascites is severe); position with pillows *to prevent slumping*<br>5. instruct client to deep breathe or use incentive spirometer at least every 2 hours<br>6. instruct client to avoid intake of gas-forming foods (e.g. beans, cauliflower, cabbage, onions), carbonated beverages, and large meals *in order to prevent gastric distention and additional pressure on the diaphragm*<br>7. assist with IPPB treatments if ordered<br>8. increase activity as allowed and tolerated<br>9. administer central nervous system depressants judiciously; hold medication and consult physician if respiratory rate is less then 12/minute<br>10. assist with thoracentesis and/or paracentesis if performed *to remove pleural and/or peritoneal fluid in order to allow increased lung expansion.*<br>d. Consult physician if:<br>1. ineffective breathing pattern continues<br>2. signs and symptoms of impaired gas exchange (e.g. restlessness, irritability, confusion, decreased $Pa{O_2}$ and increased $Pa{CO_2}$ levels) are present. |

**2. NURSING/COLLABORATIVE DIAGNOSIS:**

**Altered fluid and electrolyte balance:**

a. **fluid volume excess** related to:
   1. sodium and water retention associated with an increased aldosterone level resulting from:
      a. inability of the liver to metabolize aldosterone
      b. activation of the renin-angiotensin-aldosterone mechanism as a result of decreased renal blood flow (occurs because of a decrease in the effective intravascular volume that results from third-spacing and sequestration of fluid in the splanchnic system)
   2. decreased water excretion associated with increased antidiuretic hormone (ADH) output (a compensatory response to a decrease in the effective intravascular volume that results from third-spacing and sequestration of fluid in the splanchnic system);

b. **third-spacing** related to:
   1. low plasma colloid osmotic pressure associated with decreased plasma proteins (primarily a result of decreased hepatic synthesis of plasma proteins)
   2. increased pressure in the portal system and hepatic lymph system associated with blood flow backup resulting from structural changes in the liver
   3. generalized increase in hydrostatic pressure associated with fluid volume excess;

c. **hypokalemia** related to excessive potassium loss associated with an increased aldosterone level (aldosterone causes potassium excretion) and diuretic therapy;

d. **hyponatremia** related to dietary restriction of sodium, hemodilution associated with fluid volume excess, and sodium loss associated with diuretic therapy.

| Desired Outcomes | Nursing Actions and ***Selected Purposes/Rationales*** |
|---|---|

**Desired Outcomes**

2.a. The client will experience resolution of fluid imbalance as evidenced by:
   1. decline in weight toward client's normal
   2. B/P and pulse within normal range for client and stable with position change
   3. absence or resolution of $S_3$ heart sound
   4. balanced intake and output
   5. usual mental status
   6. serum sodium returning toward normal range
   7. small vein emptying time less than 3-5 seconds
   8. decreased dyspnea, peripheral edema, and neck vein distention
   9. improved breath sounds
   10. resolution of ascites.

**Nursing Actions and *Selected Purposes/Rationales***

2.a.1. Assess for signs and symptoms of the following:
   a. fluid volume excess:
      1. weight gain
      2. elevated B/P (B/P may not be elevated if fluid has shifted out of the vascular space)
      3. development or worsening of $S_3$ heart sound
      4. intake greater than output
      5. change in mental status (may also reflect impending hepatic encephalopathy)
      6. low serum sodium (may also result from diuretic therapy and a low sodium diet)
      7. delayed small vein emptying time (longer than 3-5 seconds)
      8. dyspnea, orthopnea
      9. peripheral edema
      10. distended neck veins
      11. crackles (rales), diminished or absent breath sounds
   b. third-spacing:
      1. ascites as evidenced by:
         a. increase in abdominal girth (abdominal girth should be measured daily at the same time and in the same location on the abdomen with client in same position)
         b. dull percussion note over abdomen with finding of shifting dullness
         c. presence of abdominal fluid wave
         d. protruding umbilicus and bulging flanks
      2. dyspnea and diminished or absent breath sounds
      3. evidence of vascular depletion (e.g. postural hypotension; weak, rapid pulse; decreased urine output).

2. Monitor chest x-ray results. Report findings of pulmonary vascular congestion, pleural effusion, or pulmonary edema.

3. Monitor serum albumin levels. Report below-normal levels *(albumin maintains plasma colloid osmotic pressure).*

4. Implement measures *to restore fluid balance:*
   a. perform actions *to reduce fluid volume excess:*
      1. maintain fluid restrictions as ordered
      2. restrict sodium intake as ordered
      3. implement measures to promote mobilization of fluid back into the vascular space (see action a.4.b. in this diagnosis) *in order to improve renal blood flow and reduce ADH output*
      4. administer diuretics if ordered (aldosterone antagonists [e.g. spironolactone] are often used initially)
   b. perform actions *to prevent further third-spacing and promote mobilization of fluid back into the vascular space:*

Desired Outcomes | Nursing Actions and ***Selected Purposes/Rationales***

1. implement measures to reduce fluid volume excess (see action a.4.a in this diagnosis)
2. encourage client to rest periodically in a recumbent position if tolerated *(lying flat promotes reshifting of fluid into vascular space)*
3. administer salt-poor albumin if ordered *to increase colloid osmotic pressure*
4. prepare client for surgical insertion of a peritoneovenous shunt (e.g. Denver shunt, LeVeen shunt) if planned.

5. Consult physician if signs and symptoms of fluid imbalance persist or worsen.

2.b. The client will maintain a safe serum potassium level as evidenced by:
1. regular pulse at 60-100 beats/minute
2. B/P within normal range for client and stable with position change
3. usual muscle tone and strength
4. absence of paresthesias, nausea, and vomiting
5. soft, nondistended abdomen with normal bowel sounds
6. normal ECG reading
7. serum potassium within normal range.

2.b.1. Assess for and report signs and symptoms of hypokalemia (e.g. cardiac arrhythmias; postural hypotension; muscle weakness; paresthesias; nausea and vomiting; abdominal distention; hypoactive or absent bowel sounds; ECG reading showing ST segment depression, T wave inversion or flattening, and presence of U waves; low serum potassium level).

2. Implement measures *to prevent or treat hypokalemia:*
   a. administer intravenous and oral potassium replacements as ordered (monitor serum potassium and urine output closely when giving supplemental potassium; consult physician if potassium level increases above normal and/or urine output is less than 30 ml/hour)
   b. if client is taking a potassium-depleting diuretic or if signs and symptoms of hypokalemia are present, encourage intake of foods/fluids high in potassium (e.g. bananas, potatoes, raisins, figs, apricots, dates, cantaloupe, white beans).

3. Consult physician if signs and symptoms of hypokalemia persist or worsen.

2.c. The client will maintain a safe serum sodium level as evidenced by:
1. absence of nausea and abdominal cramps
2. usual mental status
3. usual muscle strength
4. absence of tremors and seizure activity
5. serum sodium within normal range.

2.c.1. Assess for and report signs and symptoms of hyponatremia (e.g. nausea, abdominal cramps, lethargy, confusion, weakness, tremors, seizures, low serum sodium level).

2. Implement measures *to prevent or treat hyponatremia:*
   a. maintain fluid restrictions as ordered
   b. administer loop diuretics (e.g. furosemide) if ordered *(loop diuretics induce a fairly isotonic diuresis so that water loss can occur without further hyponatremia)*
   c. administer hypertonic saline solutions if ordered (not commonly given until hyponatremia is severe *because of the risk of intravascular volume overload).*

3. Consult physician if signs and symptoms of hyponatremia persist or worsen.

**3. NURSING DIAGNOSIS: Altered nutrition: less than body requirements**

related to:

a. poor eating habits prior to admission;
b. decreased oral intake associated with abdominal pain, dyspepsia, fatigue, dyspnea, dislike of the prescribed diet, and early satiety (a result of increased intra-abdominal pressure that occurs with ascites);
c. reduced metabolism and storage of nutrients by the liver associated with a reduction of functional liver tissue;
d. malabsorption of fats and fat-soluble vitamins associated with impaired bile production and flow.

| Desired Outcome | Nursing Actions and ***Selected Purposes/Rationales*** |
|---|---|
| 3. The client will have an improved nutritional status as evidenced by:<br>a. dry weight approaching normal range for client's age, height, and body frame (dry weight is achieved after fluid volume excess has been resolved)<br>b. improved serum albumin, Hct, Hb, $B_{12}$, folate, transferrin, and lymphocyte levels<br>c. triceps skinfold thickness approaching normal range<br>d. improved strength and activity tolerance<br>e. healthy oral mucous membrane. | 3.a. Assess for and report signs and symptoms of malnutrition:<br>1. dry weight below normal for client's age, height, and body frame<br>2. decreased serum albumin, Hct, Hb, $B_{12}$, folate, transferrin, and lymphocyte levels<br>3. triceps skinfold thickness less than normal<br>4. weakness and fatigue<br>5. stomatitis.<br>b. Monitor percentage of meals and snacks client consumes. Report a pattern of inadequate intake.<br>c. Implement measures *to improve nutritional status:*<br>1. perform actions *to improve oral intake:*<br>a. implement measures to relieve abdominal pain and dyspepsia (see Nursing Diagnoses 4, action e and 5.B, action 3)<br>b. obtain a dietary consult if necessary to assist the client in selecting foods/fluids that meet dietary modifications and nutritional needs as well as personal and cultural preferences whenever possible<br>c. encourage a rest period before meals *to minimize fatigue*<br>d. maintain a clean environment and a relaxed, pleasant atmosphere<br>e. provide oral care before meals<br>f. serve small portions of nutritious foods/fluids that are appealing to the client<br>g. elevate head of bed as tolerated for meals *to help relieve dyspnea and feeling of fullness* (a high Fowler's position may be too uncomfortable if ascites is severe)<br>h. instruct client to use herbs, spices, and salt substitutes (if approved by physician) *in order to make low-sodium diet more palatable*<br>i. allow adequate time for meals; reheat food if necessary<br>j. increase activity as allowed and tolerated *(activity stimulates appetite)*<br>k. limit fluid intake (unless it has a high nutritional value) with meals *to reduce early satiety and subsequent decreased food intake*<br>2. assist and instruct client to adhere to the following dietary recommendations:<br>a. avoid skipping meals<br>b. consume a diet high in calories (2000-3000 calories/day) and carbohydrates; suck on hard candy and drink fruit juices if unable to tolerate solid foods<br>c. maintain a moderate to high protein intake (generally at least 1 gm of protein/kg of body weight is recommended unless the serum ammonia level is high or clinical evidence of encephalopathy is present) *in order to promote liver cell regeneration*<br>d. consume meals that are well balanced and high in essential nutrients; supplement meals with snacks if having difficulty consuming adequate calories |

| Desired Outcome | Nursing Actions and ***Selected Purposes/Rationales*** |
|---|---|
| | 3. administer the following if ordered:<br>a. trace elements (e.g. zinc, magnesium, selenium)<br>b. vitamin preparations (e.g. fat-soluble vitamins, B-complex vitamins, folic acid).<br>d. Perform a 72-hour calorie count if ordered. Report totals to dietitian and physician.<br>e. Consult physician about alternative methods of providing nutrition (e.g. parenteral nutrition, tube feedings) if client does not consume enough food or fluids to meet nutritional needs. |

## 4. NURSING DIAGNOSIS: Pain: abdominal

related to swelling and distention of the liver capsule and distention of the peritoneum associated with excessive fluid accumulation.

| Desired Outcome | Nursing Actions and ***Selected Purposes/Rationales*** |
|---|---|
| 4. The client will experience diminished abdominal pain as evidenced by:<br>a. verbalization of pain relief<br>b. relaxed facial expression and body positioning<br>c. increased participation in activities. | 4.a. Determine how the client usually responds to pain.<br>b. Assess client's perception of pain including location, intensity, and type. Use a numerical scale to rate intensity.<br>c. Assess for nonverbal signs of pain (e.g. wrinkled brow, clenched fists, guarding of abdomen, reluctance to move, restlessness).<br>d. Assess for factors that seem to aggravate and alleviate pain.<br>e. Implement measures *to reduce pain:*<br>1. perform actions to restore fluid balance (see Nursing Diagnosis 2, action a.4) *in order to reduce peritoneal fluid accumulation*<br>2. provide or assist with nonpharmacological measures for pain relief (e.g. position change, relaxation techniques, quiet conversation, restful environment, diversional activities)<br>3. administer analgesics if ordered; be aware of the following:<br>a. lower doses of narcotics are usually ordered *because the liver cannot detoxify narcotics at a normal rate*<br>b. narcotic analgesics may cause biliary spasm (particularly morphine sulfate) and the physician should be notified if they fail to relieve or actually intensify pain<br>c. acetaminophen may be ordered (despite its potential hepatotoxic effect) rather than acetylsalicylic acid *because of the increased risk for gastric irritation and bleeding with acetylsalicylic acid.*<br>f. Consult physician if above measures fail to provide adequate pain relief. |

## 5.A. NURSING DIAGNOSIS: Altered comfort: pruritus

related to irritation of the skin by bile salts, which deposit in the skin as a result of bile flow obstruction.

| Desired Outcome | Nursing Actions and ***Selected Purposes/Rationales*** |
|---|---|
| 5.A. The client will experience relief of pruritus as evidenced by:<br>1. verbalization of same<br>2. no scratching or rubbing of skin. | 5.A.1. Assess client's pruritus including onset, characteristics, location, and factors that aggravate and alleviate it.<br>2. Instruct client in and/or implement measures *to relieve pruritus:*<br>a. apply cool, moist compresses to pruritic areas<br>b. apply emollient creams or ointments frequently *to prevent dryness*<br>c. add emollients, cornstarch, baking soda, or oatmeal preparations to bath water<br>d. use tepid water and mild soaps for bathing<br>e. pat skin dry, making sure to dry thoroughly<br>f. maintain a cool environment<br>g. encourage participation in diversional activity<br>h. utilize relaxation techniques<br>i. utilize cutaneous stimulation techniques (e.g. massage, pressure, vibration, stroking with soft brush) at sites of itching or acupressure points<br>j. encourage client to wear loose cotton garments; launder clothing in mild soap<br>k. administer the following medications if ordered:<br>1. antihistamines<br>2. cholestyramine *to bind bile salts and reduce their accumulation in the skin.*<br>3. Consult physician if above measures fail to alleviate pruritus or if the skin becomes excoriated. |

**5.B. NURSING DIAGNOSIS:**

**Altered comfort: dyspepsia**

related to:

1. impaired fat digestion associated with bile flow obstruction;
2. reflux of gastric contents associated with increased intra-abdominal pressure resulting from ascites;
3. impaired gastrointestinal functioning associated with venous congestion in the gastrointestinal tract as a result of portal hypertension.

| Desired Outcome | Nursing Actions and ***Selected Purposes/Rationales*** |
|---|---|
| 5.B. The client will verbalize relief of dyspepsia. | 5.B.1. Assess client for verbal complaints of dyspepsia (e.g. epigastric discomfort, feeling of fullness or bloating, nausea).<br>2. Determine if particular foods/fluids contribute to dyspepsia.<br>3. Implement measures *to reduce dyspepsia:*<br>a. perform actions *to reduce gastroesophageal reflux:*<br>1. keep head of bed elevated for 2-3 hours after meals<br>2. provide small, frequent meals rather than 3 large ones<br>3. implement measures to restore fluid balance (see Nursing Diagnosis 2, action a.4) *in order to reduce ascites*<br>b. instruct client to ingest foods and fluids slowly<br>c. instruct client to avoid foods/fluids that may cause gastric irritation (e.g. spicy foods; caffeine-containing beverages such as coffee, tea, and colas; decaffeinated coffee)<br>d. instruct client to eat dry foods (e.g. toast, crackers) and avoid drinking liquids with meals if nauseated<br>e. encourage client not to smoke<br>f. instruct client to avoid foods high in fat *in order to prevent a delay in gastric emptying and reduce nausea associated with impaired fat digestion* |

| Desired Outcome | Nursing Actions and ***Selected Purposes/Rationales*** |
|---|---|
| | g. administer antacids and histamine$_2$ receptor antagonists (e.g. famotidine, ranitidine) if ordered *to reduce acidity of gastric contents and thereby reduce esophageal irritation if reflux occurs.*<br>4. Consult physician if above measures fail to control dyspepsia. |

## 6. NURSING DIAGNOSIS: High risk for impaired skin integrity

related to:

a. ischemia of the skin and subcutaneous tissue associated with prolonged pressure on the tissues as a result of decreased mobility;
b. damage to the skin and/or subcutaneous tissue associated with friction or shearing;
c. increased fragility of the skin associated with edema and malnutrition;
d. excessive scratching associated with pruritus.

| Desired Outcome | Nursing Actions and ***Selected Purposes/Rationales*** |
|---|---|
| 6. The client will maintain skin integrity as evidenced by:<br>a. absence of redness and irritation<br>b. no skin breakdown. | 6.a. Inspect the skin (especially bony prominences and dependent, edematous, and pruritic areas) for pallor, redness, and breakdown.<br>b. Refer to Care Plan on Immobility, Nursing Diagnosis 4, action b (pp. 141-142), for measures to prevent skin breakdown.<br>c. Implement additional measures *to prevent skin breakdown:*<br>1. perform actions *to prevent skin irritation resulting from scratching:*<br>a. implement measures to relieve pruritus (see Nursing Diagnosis 5.A, action 2)<br>b. keep nails trimmed and/or apply mittens if necessary<br>c. instruct client to apply firm pressure to pruritic areas rather than scratching<br>2. perform actions to improve nutritional status (see Nursing Diagnosis 3, action c)<br>3. perform actions to reduce fluid volume excess (see Nursing Diagnosis 2, action a.4.a.) *in order to reduce edema.*<br>d. If skin breakdown occurs:<br>1. notify physician<br>2. continue with above measures to prevent further irritation and breakdown<br>3. perform decubitus care as ordered or per standard hospital procedure<br>4. assess client closely and report signs and symptoms of infection (e.g. elevated temperature; redness, warmth, and edema around area of breakdown; unusual drainage from site). |

## 7. NURSING DIAGNOSIS: Activity intolerance

related to:

a. tissue hypoxia associated with anemia resulting from:
   1. decreased production of RBCs resulting from a decreased oral intake of vitamins and minerals (particularly vitamin $B_{12}$ and folic acid), an inability of the liver to store vitamins and minerals, and the toxic effect of alcohol on the bone marrow
   2. excessive RBC destruction resulting from hypersplenism (if venous conges-

tion has resulted in splenomegaly, the spleen will destroy RBCs faster than usual)
3. blood loss if bleeding has occurred;

b. loss of muscle mass, tone, and strength associated with malnutrition and disuse if mobility has been limited for an extended period;
c. decrease in available energy associated with inability of the liver to metabolize glucose and fats properly;
d. difficulty resting and sleeping associated with dyspnea, discomfort, frequent assessments and treatments, fear, anxiety, and unfamiliar environment.

| Desired Outcome | Nursing Actions and ***Selected Purposes/Rationales*** |
|---|---|
| 7. The client will demonstrate an increased tolerance for activity (see Care Plan on Immobility, Nursing Diagnosis 5 [p. 143], for outcome criteria). | 7.a. Refer to Care Plan on Immobility, Nursing Diagnosis 5 (p. 143), for measures related to assessment and improvement of activity tolerance.<br>b. Implement additional measures *to improve activity tolerance:*<br>1. perform additional actions *to promote rest:*<br>a. implement measures to reduce fear and anxiety (see Nursing Diagnosis 15)<br>b. implement measures to promote sleep (see Nursing Diagnosis 10)<br>c. implement measures to reduce discomfort (see Nursing Diagnoses 4, action e; 5.A, action 2; and 5.B, action 3)<br>d. implement measures to improve breathing pattern (see Nursing Diagnosis 1, action c) *in order to decrease dyspnea*<br>2. maintain oxygen therapy as ordered<br>3. perform actions to improve nutritional status (see Nursing Diagnosis 3, action c)<br>4. administer packed red cells if ordered. |

## 8. NURSING DIAGNOSIS: Self-care deficit

related to:
a. weakness, fatigue, and dyspnea;
b. altered thought processes.

| Desired Outcome | Nursing Actions and ***Selected Purposes/Rationales*** |
|---|---|
| 8. The client will demonstrate increased participation in self-care activities within physical and mental limitations and prescribed activity restrictions. | 8.a. Refer to Care Plan on Immobility, Nursing Diagnosis 7 (pp. 144-145), for measures related to planning for and meeting the client's self-care needs.<br>b. Implement measures *to further facilitate the client's ability to perform self-care activities:*<br>1. perform actions to increase strength and activity tolerance (see Nursing Diagnosis 7)<br>2. perform actions to maintain optimal thought processes (see Nursing Diagnosis 9, action c)<br>3. perform actions to improve breathing pattern (see Nursing Diagnosis 1, action c) *in order to decrease dyspnea.* |

## 9. NURSING DIAGNOSIS: Altered thought processes

related to disturbances in central nervous system functioning associated with accumulation of toxic substances (e.g. ammonia) in the brain, toxic effects of long term alcohol use, deficiencies of certain vitamins (e.g. thiamine, vitamin $B_{12}$), and hypoxia if anemia is moderate to severe.

| Desired Outcome | Nursing Actions and ***Selected Purposes/Rationales*** |
|---|---|
| 9. The client will demonstrate improvement in thought processes as evidenced by:<br>a. improved verbal response time<br>b. improved memory<br>c. longer attention span<br>d. absence or resolution of personality changes and confusion. | 9.a. Assess client for altered thought processes (e.g. slowed verbal responses, impaired memory, shortened attention span, personality changes, confusion).<br>b. Ascertain from significant others client's usual level of intellectual and emotional functioning and whether personality changes have occurred.<br>c. Implement measures *to maintain optimal thought processes:*<br>1. perform actions to improve nutritional status (see Nursing Diagnosis 3, action c) *in order to provide vitamins that are essential for normal neurological functioning and treatment of anemia*<br>2. perform actions to prevent or manage hepatic coma (see Collaborative Diagnosis 13, actions d.3-5) *and subsequently reduce levels of cerebral toxins*<br>3. administer central nervous system depressants such as narcotics, sedative-hypnotics, and antianxiety agents with extreme caution *(many of these agents are metabolized in the liver);* question any order for a normal adult dose of these medications<br>4. administer vitamin $B_{12}$ (e.g. cyanocobalamin) or thiamine if ordered *to prevent further neurological manifestations.*<br>d. If client shows evidence of altered thought processes:<br>1. reorient client to person, place, and time as necessary<br>2. address client by name<br>3. place familiar objects, clock, and calendar within client's view<br>4. approach client in a slow, calm manner; allow adequate time for communication<br>5. repeat instructions as necessary using clear, simple language and short sentences<br>6. maintain a consistent and fairly structured routine and write out a schedule of activities for client to refer to if desired<br>7. have client perform only one activity at a time and allow adequate time for performance of activities<br>8. encourage client to make lists of planned activities, questions, and concerns<br>9. assist client to problem solve if necessary<br>10. maintain realistic expectations of client's ability to learn, comprehend, and remember information provided; provide client with a written copy of instructions<br>11. encourage significant others to be supportive of client; instruct them in methods of dealing with client's altered thought processes<br>12. inform client and significant others that intellectual and emotional functioning are likely to improve with treatment<br>13. consult physician if altered thought processes worsen. |

## 10. NURSING DIAGNOSIS: Sleep pattern disturbance

related to unfamiliar environment, frequent assessments and treatments, decreased physical activity, discomfort, fear, anxiety, and inability to assume usual sleep position as a result of orthopnea.

| Desired Outcome | Nursing Actions and ***Selected Purposes/Rationales*** |
|---|---|
| 10. The client will attain optimal amounts of sleep within the parameters of the treatment regimen (see Care Plan on Immobility, Nursing Diagnosis 10 [p. 147], for outcome criteria). | 10.a. Refer to Care Plan on Immobility, Nursing Diagnosis 10 (p. 147), for measures related to assessment and promotion of sleep.<br>b. Implement additional measures *to promote sleep:*<br>1. if client has orthopnea, assist him/her to assume a position *that facilitates breathing* (e.g. head of bed elevated with arms supported on pillows, sitting in a chair)<br>2. maintain oxygen therapy during sleep if indicated<br>3. perform actions to reduce discomfort (see Nursing Diagnoses 4, action e; 5.A, action 2; and 5.B, action 3)<br>4. administer sedative-hypnotics if ordered remembering that these agents must be used cautiously *because many are metabolized by the liver* (diphenhydramine is often preferred if a sleep aid is necessary). |

## 11. NURSING DIAGNOSIS: High risk for infection

related to:
a. lowered resistance to infection associated with:
   1. diminished function of the Kupffer cells in the liver (these cells normally phagocytize bacteria)
   2. malnutrition
   3. leukopenia resulting from the toxic effect of alcohol on the bone marrow and hypersplenism (if venous congestion has resulted in splenomegaly, the spleen will destroy leukocytes faster than usual);
b. stasis of secretions in the lungs and urinary stasis if mobility is decreased.

| Desired Outcome | Nursing Actions and ***Selected Purposes/Rationales*** |
|---|---|
| 11. The client will remain free of infection as evidenced by:<br>a. absence of fever and chills<br>b. pulse within normal limits<br>c. normal breath sounds<br>d. voiding clear urine without complaints of frequency, urgency, and burning<br>e. absence of heat, pain, redness, swelling, and unusual drainage in any area<br>f. no complaints of increased weakness and fatigue<br>g. WBC and differential counts within normal range<br>h. negative results of cultured specimens. | 11.a. Assess for and report signs and symptoms of infection:<br>1. elevated temperature<br>2. chills<br>3. increased pulse<br>4. abnormal breath sounds<br>5. cloudy, foul-smelling urine<br>6. complaints of frequency, urgency, or burning when urinating<br>7. presence of WBCs, bacteria, and/or nitrites in urine<br>8. heat, pain, redness, swelling, or unusual drainage in any area<br>9. complaints of increased weakness or fatigue<br>10. elevated WBC count and/or significant change in differential.<br>b. Obtain specimens (e.g. urine, vaginal, mouth, sputum, blood) for culture as ordered. Report positive results.<br>c. Implement measures *to prevent infection:*<br>1. perform actions to prevent skin breakdown (see Nursing Diagnosis 6, actions b and c)<br>2. maintain the maximum fluid intake allowed<br>3. use good handwashing technique and encourage client to do the same<br>4. maintain meticulous aseptic technique during all invasive procedures (e.g. catheterization, venous and arterial punctures, injections)<br>5. change intravenous tubings and solutions and rotate insertion sites according to hospital policy<br>6. protect client from others with infection<br>7. perform actions to improve nutritional status (see Nursing Diagnosis 3, action c)<br>8. provide or assist with good oral hygiene |

| Desired Outcome | Nursing Actions and ***Selected Purposes/Rationales*** |
|---|---|
| | 9. perform actions to reduce stress (e.g. relieve discomfort; explain procedures and treatments; provide a quiet, restful environment) *in order to prevent excessive secretion of cortisol (cortisol inhibits the immune response)*<br>10. perform actions *to prevent stasis of respiratory secretions* (e.g. assist client to turn, cough, and deep breathe; increase activity as allowed and tolerated)<br>11. perform actions to prevent urinary retention (e.g. instruct client to urinate when the urge is first felt, promote relaxation during voiding attempts) *in order to prevent urinary stasis*<br>12. perform actions *to prevent the introduction of microorganisms into the urinary tract* (e.g. assist client with perineal care as needed, instruct and assist female client to wipe from front to back after urinating and defecating, maintain sterile technique during urinary catheterization). |

## 12. NURSING DIAGNOSIS: High risk for trauma

related to:

a. falls associated with:
   1. weakness
   2. dizziness (can result from anemia and the postural hypotension that occurs with third-spacing)
   3. balance and gait disturbances that can occur with deficiencies of thiamine and/or vitamin $B_{12}$
   4. altered thought processes;

b. burns and cuts associated with:
   1. altered thought processes
   2. paresthesias that can occur with deficiencies of thiamine and vitamin $B_{12}$
   3. delirium tremens ("DTs") if present.

| Desired Outcome | Nursing Actions and ***Selected Purposes/Rationales*** |
|---|---|
| 12. The client will not experience falls, burns, or cuts. | 12.a. Implement measures *to reduce the risk for trauma:*<br>1. perform actions *to prevent falls:*<br>a. keep bed in low position with side rails up when client is in bed<br>b. keep needed items within easy reach<br>c. encourage client to request assistance whenever needed; have call signal within easy reach<br>d. instruct and assist client to get out of bed slowly *in order to reduce dizziness associated with postural hypotension*<br>e. use lap belt when client is in chair if indicated<br>f. instruct client to wear well-fitting slippers/shoes with nonslip soles and low heels when ambulating<br>g. keep floor free of clutter and wipe up spills promptly<br>h. accompany client during ambulation using a transfer safety belt if he/she is weak or dizzy<br>i. provide ambulatory aids (e.g. walker, cane) if the client is weak or unsteady on feet<br>j. instruct client to ambulate in well-lit areas and to use handrails if needed<br>k. do not rush client; allow adequate time for ambulation to the bathroom and in hallway<br>l. perform actions to increase strength and activity tolerance (see Nursing Diagnosis 7) |

m. reinforce instructions from physical therapist on correct transfer and ambulation techniques if client has gait disturbances
n. make sure that bathtub and shower have nonslip bottom surfaces and that shower chair, secure bath mat, call light, hand grips, and adequate lighting are present

2. perform actions *to prevent burns:*
   a. let hot foods and fluids cool slightly before serving
   b. supervise client while smoking if indicated
   c. assess temperature of bath water before and during use
3. assist client with tasks that require fine motor skills (e.g. shaving) *in order to prevent cuts*
4. if client is confused or irrational:
   a. reorient frequently to surroundings and necessity of adhering to safety precautions
   b. provide constant supervision (e.g. staff member, significant other) if indicated
   c. consult physician about the temporary use of jacket or wrist restraints if necessary
   d. administer antianxiety and antipsychotic medications if ordered
5. administer central nervous system depressants with extreme caution *(many of these agents are metabolized in the liver);* question any order for a normal adult dose of these medications.

b. Include client and significant others in planning and implementing measures to prevent trauma.
c. If injury does occur, initiate appropriate first aid and notify physician.

## 13. COLLABORATIVE DIAGNOSES:

**Potential complications:**

a. **bleeding** related to:
   1. decreased production of clotting factors associated with impaired liver function and impaired vitamin K absorption (normal bile flow is necessary for absorption of vitamin K)
   2. thrombocytopenia associated with toxic effects of alcohol on the bone marrow and hypersplenism (if venous congestion has resulted in splenomegaly, the spleen will destroy platelets faster than usual);
b. **hepatorenal syndrome** possibly related to decreased renal blood flow associated with:
   1. a decrease in the effective intravascular volume resulting from third-spacing and sequestration of fluid in the portal system
   2. intrarenal vasoconstriction resulting from altered prostaglandin levels and an increase in renin output and sympathetic nervous system activity that occur in response to the decreased effective intravascular volume;
c. **bleeding esophageal varices** (varices are a result of the development of collateral circulation in the low-pressure vessels of the esophagus as a result of portal hypertension) related to:
   1. large increases in portal pressure associated with volume overload and sudden increases in intra-abdominal pressure
   2. increased bleeding tendency;
d. **hepatic (portal-systemic) encephalopathy (hepatic coma)** related to altered brain function associated with the effect of toxic substances (e.g. ammonia, mercaptans) on the brain and increased brain sensitivity to certain substances and conditions.

| Desired Outcomes | Nursing Actions and ***Selected Purposes/Rationales*** |
|---|---|
| 13.a. The client will not experience unusual | 13.a.1. Assess client for and report signs and symptoms of unusual bleeding:<br>a. petechiae, purpura, ecchymoses |

| Desired Outcomes | Nursing Actions and ***Selected Purposes/Rationales*** |
|---|---|
| bleeding as evidenced by:<br>1. skin and mucous membranes free of petechiae, purpura, ecchymoses, and active bleeding<br>2. absence of unusual joint pain<br>3. no further increase in abdominal girth<br>4. absence of frank and occult blood in stool, urine, and vomitus<br>5. usual menstrual flow<br>6. vital signs within normal range for client<br>7. stable or improved Hct and Hb. | b. gingival bleeding<br>c. prolonged bleeding from puncture sites<br>d. epistaxis, hemoptysis<br>e. unusual joint pain<br>f. further increase in abdominal girth<br>g. frank or occult blood in the stool, urine, or vomitus<br>h. menorrhagia<br>i. restlessness, confusion<br>j. declining B/P and increased pulse rate<br>k. decline in Hct and Hb levels.<br>2. Monitor platelet count and coagulation test results (e.g. prothrombin time, activated partial thromboplastin time, bleeding time). Report abnormal values.<br>3. If platelet count is low, coagulation test results are abnormal, or Hct and Hb levels decline, test all stools, urine, and vomitus for occult blood. Report positive results.<br>4. Implement measures *to prevent bleeding:*<br>a. perform actions to reduce risk of bleeding from esophageal varices (see action c.3 in this diagnosis)<br>b. use smallest gauge needle possible when giving injections and performing venous and arterial punctures<br>c. apply gentle, prolonged pressure to puncture sites after injections, venous and arterial punctures, and procedures such as paracentesis<br>d. take B/P only when necessary and avoid overinflating the cuff<br>e. caution client to avoid activities that increase the risk for trauma (e.g. shaving with a straight-edge razor, using stiff-bristle toothbrush or dental floss)<br>f. gently perform procedures that can cause injury to the rectal mucosa (e.g. taking temperature rectally, inserting a rectal suppository, administering an enema)<br>g. pad side rails if client is confused or restless<br>h. perform actions to prevent falls (see Nursing Diagnosis 12, action a.1)<br>i. instruct client to avoid blowing nose forcefully or straining to have a bowel movement; consult physician about an order for a decongestant, stool softener, and/or laxative if indicated<br>j. administer the following if ordered *to improve clotting ability:*<br>1. vitamin K (e.g. phytonadione) injections<br>2. platelets<br>3. fresh blood or plasma *(the liver cannot detoxify the preservative in stored blood).*<br>5. If bleeding occurs and does not subside spontaneously:<br>a. apply firm, prolonged pressure to bleeding area(s) if possible<br>b. if epistaxis occurs, place client in a high Fowler's position and apply pressure and ice pack to nasal area<br>c. maintain oxygen therapy as ordered<br>d. implement measures identified in action c.4 in this diagnosis if gastric or esophageal bleeding occurs<br>e. administer vitamin K (e.g. phytonadione) injections and blood products (e.g. fresh frozen plasma or whole blood, platelets) as ordered<br>f. assess for and report signs and symptoms of hypovolemic shock (e.g. restlessness; confusion; significant decrease in B/P; rapid, thready pulse; rapid respirations; cool, pale skin; urine output less than 30 ml/hour)<br>g. prepare client for surgical repair of bleeding vessels if planned<br>h. provide emotional support to client and significant others. |

13.b. The client will maintain adequate renal function as evidenced by:
1. BUN and serum creatinine levels within normal range
2. normal urine sodium
3. urine output at least 30 ml/hour.

13.b.1. Assess for and report signs and symptoms of the hepatorenal syndrome (e.g. increased BUN and serum creatinine, low urine sodium, urine output less than 30 ml/hour).
2. Implement measures *to reduce the risk for hepatorenal syndrome:*
   a. perform actions *to maintain adequate renal blood flow:*
      1. maintain an adequate fluid intake; if client is on a fluid restriction, maintain the maximum fluid intake allowed
      2. administer the following if ordered *to increase the effective intravascular volume:*
         a. salt-poor albumin
         b. volume expanders
   b. consult with physician regarding discontinuation of prescribed medications that may precipitate the hepatorenal syndrome (e.g. indomethacin, ibuprofen, naproxen).
3. If signs and symptoms of the hepatorenal syndrome occur:
   a. continue with above actions
   b. consult physician regarding discontinuation of nephrotoxic agents (e.g. neomycin) if any have been ordered
   c. prepare client for dialysis if indicated
   d. refer to Care Plan on Renal Failure for additional care measures.

13.c. The client will not experience bleeding of esophageal varices as evidenced by:
1. absence of hematemesis, hematochezia, and melena
2. B/P and pulse within normal range for client
3. stable or improved RBC, Hct, and Hb levels.

13.c.1. Assess for and report signs and symptoms of bleeding esophageal varices (e.g. hematemesis, hematochezia, melena, decreased B/P, increased pulse).
2. Monitor RBC, Hct, and Hb levels. Report declining values.
3. Implement measures *to reduce risk of bleeding from esophageal varices:*
   a. perform actions to reduce fluid volume excess (see Nursing Diagnosis 2, action a.4.a) *in order to reduce portal hypertension and pressure in esophageal vessels*
   b. instruct client to avoid activities such as straining to have a bowel movement, coughing, sneezing, and bending at the waist *in order to prevent an increase in intra-abdominal pressure;* consult physician about an order for stool softener, laxative, antitussive, and/or decongestant if indicated
   c. administer vitamin K and blood products if ordered *to improve clotting ability.*
4. If signs and symptoms of bleeding esophageal varices occur:
   a. place client on his/her side *to reduce risk of aspiration*
   b. maintain oxygen therapy as ordered
   c. assist with insertion of a gastroesophageal balloon tube (e.g. Sengstaken-Blakemore tube, Minnesota tube); maintain balloon pressure and suction and perform saline lavage as ordered
   d. assist with administration of vasopressin if ordered *to constrict splanchnic vessels and reduce blood flow to the portal vein* (nitroglycerin may be given concurrently *to reduce drug side effects)*
   e. assist with endoscopic sclerotherapy if performed
   f. administer vitamin K (e.g. phytonadione) injections and blood products (e.g. fresh frozen plasma or whole blood, platelets) as ordered
   g. assess for and immediately report signs and symptoms of hypovolemic shock (e.g. restlessness; confusion; further decline in B/P and increase in pulse; rapid respirations; cool, pale skin; urine output less than 30 ml/hour)
   h. prepare client for surgery (e.g. ligation of bleeding vessels, portal-systemic shunt) if planned
   i. provide emotional support to client and significant others.

13.d. The client will not develop hepatic encephalopathy as evidenced by:

13.d.1. Assess for and report signs and symptoms of hepatic encephalopathy (e.g. change in handwriting, inability to draw simple figures or numbers, slow or slurred speech, inability to concentrate, emotional lability, disordered sleep, agitation, belligerence, disorientation,

| Desired Outcomes | Nursing Actions and ***Selected Purposes/Rationales*** |
|---|---|
| 1. usual speech and handwriting<br>2. usual mental status<br>3. absence of asterixis and fetor hepaticus<br>4. serum ammonia level within normal range. | lethargy, asterixis, fetor hepaticus [musty, sweet odor on breath], unresponsiveness).<br>2. Monitor serum ammonia results. Report elevated values.<br>3. Implement measures *to reduce the risk of hepatic coma:*<br>a. perform actions *to eliminate or control the following factors that increase levels of ammonia and other nitrogenous substances:*<br>1. constipation *(results in increased formation and absorption of ammonia and mercaptans from the gut)*<br>2. gastrointestinal hemorrhage *(intestinal bacteria convert the protein in blood to ammonia and other nitrogenous substances)*<br>3. hypokalemia and/or metabolic alkalosis *(hypokalemia contributes to alkalosis and increases renal production of ammonia; alkalosis increases the dissociation of $NH_4$ to $NH_3$, which more readily crosses the blood brain barrier)*<br>4. renal failure *(results in decreased excretion of ammonia)*<br>5. excessive protein intake *(intestinal bacteria convert protein to ammonia and other nitrogenous substances)*<br>6. infection *(increases tissue breakdown, which increases the level of nitrogenous substances)*<br>7. dehydration/hypovolemia *(reduced blood flow to the liver results in decreased detoxification of ammonia and other toxins)*<br>b. consult physician about discontinuation of prescribed medications that are known or potential hepatotoxins (e.g. isoniazid, methyldopa, phenytoin) *in order to prevent further liver damage.*<br>4. Administer central nervous system depressants such as narcotics, sedative-hypnotics, and antianxiety agents with extreme caution *(many of these agents are metabolized in the liver and may precipitate nonnitrogenous coma).*<br>5. If signs and symptoms of hepatic encephalopathy occur:<br>a. maintain client on strict bed rest *to reduce metabolic demands on the liver*<br>b. maintain dietary protein restrictions as ordered (usually 0-40 gm/day)<br>c. ensure a high carbohydrate intake or administer intravenous glucose or tube feedings as ordered *to provide a rapid energy source and decrease metabolism of endogenous proteins*<br>d. administer enemas and/or cathartics as ordered *to hasten expulsion of intestinal contents so that bacteria have less time to convert proteins to ammonia and other nitrogenous substances*<br>e. administer the following medications if ordered:<br>1. neomycin *to destroy intestinal bacteria and subsequently decrease protein breakdown*<br>2. lactulose *to stimulate catharsis and create an acidic medium in the intestine (the acidity reduces bacterial growth and the resultant formation of nitrogenous substances and also traps ammonia in the colon by promoting the conversion of $NH_3$ to the poorly absorbed $NH_4$)*<br>f. institute general safety precautions<br>g. provide emotional support to client and significant others. |

## 14. NURSING DIAGNOSIS: Sexual dysfunction

related to:

a. impotence associated with:
   1. testicular atrophy that can occur as a result of high levels of estrogen (results

from impaired hepatic clearance) and a possible toxic effect of alcohol on the testes
2. psychogenic factors;
b. decreased libido associated with hormonal imbalances, weakness, fatigue, and an altered self-concept.

| Desired Outcome | Nursing Actions and ***Selected Purposes/Rationales*** |
|---|---|
| 14. The client will demonstrate beginning acceptance of changes in sexual functioning as evidenced by:<br>a. verbalization of a perception of self as sexually acceptable and adequate<br>b. statements reflecting beginning adjustment to effects of cirrhosis on sexual functioning<br>c. maintenance of relationship with significant other. | 14.a. Assess for signs and symptoms of sexual dysfunction (e.g. verbalization of sexual concerns or inability to achieve sexual satisfaction, alteration in relationship with significant other).<br>b. Provide accurate information about the possible effects of cirrhosis and alcohol intake on sexual functioning. Encourage questions and clarify misconceptions.<br>c. Implement measures *to promote optimal sexual functioning:*<br>1. facilitate communication between client and his/her partner; focus on feelings the couple share and assist them to identify changes which may affect their sexual relationship<br>2. discuss ways to be creative in expressing sexuality (e.g. massage, fantasies, cuddling)<br>3. arrange for uninterrupted privacy during hospital stay if desired by the couple<br>4. perform actions to improve client's self-concept (see Nursing Diagnosis 16)<br>5. if impotence is a problem:<br>a. encourage client to discuss impotence and various treatment options (e.g. penile prothesis) with physician<br>b. suggest alternative methods of sexual gratification if appropriate<br>6. encourage client to rest before sexual activity.<br>d. Include partner in above discussions and encourage his/her continued support of the client.<br>e. Consult physician if counseling appears indicated. |

## 15. NURSING DIAGNOSIS: Anxiety

related to difficulty breathing; discomfort; lack of understanding of diagnosis, diagnostic tests, and treatments; uncertainty of prognosis; financial concerns; unfamiliar environment; and possibility of changes in life style and roles.

| Desired Outcome | Nursing Actions and ***Selected Purposes/Rationales*** |
|---|---|
| 15. The client will experience a reduction in anxiety (see Care Plan on Immobility, Nursing Diagnosis 13 [p. 153], for outcome criteria). | 15.a. Refer to Care Plan on Immobility, Nursing Diagnosis 13 (p. 153), for measures related to assessment and reduction of fear and anxiety.<br>b. Implement additional measures *to reduce fear and anxiety:*<br>1. perform actions to improve breathing pattern (see Nursing Diagnosis 1, action c) *in order to decrease dyspnea*<br>2. perform actions to reduce pain and dyspepsia (see Nursing Diagnoses 4, action e and 5.B, action 3). |

## 16. NURSING DIAGNOSIS: Self-concept disturbance*

related to:

a. changes in appearance (e.g. edema, ascites, jaundice, spider angiomas, palmar erythema, gynecomastia);
b. alterations in sexual functioning;
c. infertility associated with hypogonadism if present;
d. dependence on others to meet self-care needs;
e. altered thought processes;
f. stigma of having a chronic illness;
g. possible changes in life style and roles.

*This diagnostic label includes the nursing diagnoses of body image disturbance, self-esteem disturbance, and altered role performance.

| Desired Outcome | Nursing Actions and ***Selected Purposes/Rationales*** |
|---|---|
| 16. The client will demonstrate beginning adaptation to changes in appearance, level of independence, body functioning, life style, and roles (see Care Plan on Immobility, Nursing Diagnosis 14 [pp. 153-154], for outcome criteria). | 16.a. Refer to Care Plan on Immobility, Nursing Diagnosis 14 (pp. 153-154), for measures related to assessment and promotion of a positive self-concept.<br>b. Implement additional measures *to assist client to adapt to changes in appearance, level of independence, body functioning, life style, and roles:*<br>1. encourage client to discuss concerns about fertility with physician; discuss alternative methods of parenting (e.g. adoption, artificial insemination)<br>2. inform client that many of changes in appearance may be lessened by adherence to treatment regimen<br>3. perform actions to promote optimal sexual functioning (see Nursing Diagnosis 14, action c)<br>4. discuss techniques the client can use *to adapt to altered thought processes:*<br>a. encourage client to make lists and jot down messages and refer to these notes rather than relying on memory<br>b. instruct client to place self in a calm environment when making decisions<br>c. encourage client to validate decisions, clarify information, and seek assistance to problem solve<br>5. assist client *to attain and maintain optimal independence:*<br>a. perform actions to increase client's strength and activity tolerance (see Nursing Diagnosis 7)<br>b. consult social services and occupational therapist about a home evaluation before discharge to identify ways that client's home environment can be modified so that he/she can function more independently<br>c. reinforce benefits of using portable oxygen if it has been prescribed<br>6. encourage maximum participation in self-care within the prescribed activity restrictions and encourage significant others to allow client to do what he/she is able *so that independence can be reestablished and self-esteem redeveloped.* |

## 17. NURSING DIAGNOSIS: Ineffective management of therapeutic regimen

related to:

a. lack of understanding of the implications of not following the prescribed treatment plan;
b. difficulty modifying personal habits (e.g. dietary habits, alcohol intake);
c. insufficient financial resources.

| Desired Outcome | Nursing Actions and ***Selected Purposes/Rationales*** |
|---|---|
| 17. The client will demonstrate the probability of effective management of the therapeutic regimen as evidenced by:<br>a. willingness to learn about and participate in treatment plan and care<br>b. statements reflecting ways to modify personal habits and integrate treatments into life style<br>c. statements reflecting an understanding of the implications of not following the prescribed treatment plan. | 17.a. Assess for indications that the client may be unable to effectively manage the therapeutic regimen:<br>1. statements reflecting that he/she was unable to manage care at home<br>2. failure to adhere to treatment plan while in hospital (e.g. not adhering to dietary modifications and fluid restrictions, refusing medications)<br>3. statements reflecting a lack of understanding of the factors that will cause further progression of liver failure<br>4. statements reflecting an unwillingness or inability to modify personal habits and integrate necessary treatments into life style<br>5. statements reflecting the view that cirrhosis has resolved once he/she is feeling better or that there is no way to control the disease and efforts to comply with treatments are useless.<br>b. Implement measures *to promote effective management of the therapeutic regimen:*<br>1. explain cirrhosis in terms the client can understand; stress the fact that cirrhosis is a chronic disease and adherence to the treatment plan is necessary in order to delay and/or prevent complications<br>2. encourage questions and clarify misconceptions client has about cirrhosis and its effects<br>3. encourage client to participate in the treatment plan<br>4. initiate and reinforce the discharge teaching outlined in Nursing Diagnosis 18 *in order to promote a sense of control and self-reliance*<br>5. provide instructions on weighing self and calculating dietary sodium and protein content; allow time for return demonstration; determine areas of difficulty and misunderstanding and reinforce teaching as necessary<br>6. provide client with written instructions about scheduled appointments with health care provider, medications, signs and symptoms to report, weighing self, and dietary modifications<br>7. assist client to identify ways he/she can incorporate treatments into life style; focus on modifications of life style rather than complete change<br>8. encourage client to discuss his/her concerns about the cost of hospitalization, medications, and lifelong follow-up care; obtain a social service consult to assist with financial planning and to obtain financial aid if indicated<br>9. provide information about and encourage utilization of community resources that can assist client to make necessary life-style changes (e.g. drug and alcohol rehabilitation programs)<br>10. reinforce behaviors suggesting future compliance with the therapeutic regimen (e.g. statements reflecting plans for integrating treatments into life style, participation in diet planning, statements reflecting an understanding of the importance of eliminating alcohol intake)<br>11. include significant others in explanations and teaching sessions and encourage their support; reinforce the need for client to assume responsibility for managing as much of care as possible.<br>c. Consult physician about referrals to community health agencies if continued instruction, support, or supervision is needed. |

## 18. NURSING DIAGNOSIS: Knowledge deficit

regarding follow-up care.

| Desired Outcomes | Nursing Actions and ***Selected Purposes/Rationales*** |
|---|---|
| 18.a. The client will identify ways to prevent further liver damage. | 18.a. Provide the following instructions regarding ways to prevent further liver damage:<br>1. avoid the following hepatotoxic agents:<br>a. alcohol<br>b. cleaning agents containing carbon tetrachloride (these are toxic even when inhaled)<br>2. take acetaminophen (e.g. Tylenol) only when necessary and do not exceed the recommended dose because of its potential toxic effect on the liver<br>3. adhere to the following precautions to prevent hepatitis:<br>a. wash hands thoroughly after using the bathroom<br>b. eat only in restaurants that have been inspected and approved by health authorities<br>c. if blood transfusions are necessary, receive autologous blood or blood from donor known not to have hepatitis<br>d. avoid sharing food or eating utensils and handling toiletry items of others<br>e. avoid intimate contact with known carrier of hepatitis<br>f. avoid oral-anal sex since it is one way that hepatitis A can be transmitted. |
| 18.b. The client will verbalize an understanding of the rationale for and components of the recommended diet. | 18.b.1. Explain to client that adherence to the recommended diet will promote healing of the liver and reduce the risk of further liver damage.<br>2. Reinforce the dietary instructions outlined in Nursing Diagnosis 3, action c.2.<br>3. Explain the rationale for a diet low in sodium and provide information about decreasing sodium intake:<br>a. be aware that the terms salt and sodium are often used interchangeably but are not synonymous; there is 40% sodium in table salt<br>b. read food labels and calculate sodium content of items (often expressed in milligrams [2 gm is 2000 mg])<br>c. do not add salt when cooking foods or to prepared foods; use low sodium herbs and spices if desired<br>d. avoid canned soups and vegetables<br>e. avoid processed convenience foods and commercial sauces<br>f. avoid cured and smoked foods<br>g. avoid salty snack foods.<br>4. Obtain a dietary consult to assist client in planning meals that will meet prescribed dietary modifications. |
| 18.c. The client will identify ways to reduce stress on esophageal vessels. | 18.c. Provide the following instructions about ways to reduce stress on esophageal vessels:<br>1. adhere to prescribed measures to reduce fluid retention (e.g. fluid restriction, low-sodium diet, diuretics)<br>2. avoid activities that increase intra-abdominal pressure (e.g. straining to have a bowel movement, coughing, sneezing, lifting heavy objects). |
| 18.d. The client will identify ways to prevent bleeding. | 18.d.1. Instruct client about ways to minimize risk of bleeding:<br>a. avoid taking aspirin, aspirin-containing products, and ibuprofen on a regular basis<br>b. use an electric rather than a straight-edge razor<br>c. floss and brush teeth gently<br>d. cut nails carefully<br>e. avoid situations that could result in injury (e.g. contact sports)<br>f. avoid blowing nose forcefully<br>g. avoid straining to have a bowel movement<br>h. avoid putting sharp objects (e.g. toothpicks) in mouth<br>i. do not walk barefoot.<br>2. Instruct client to control any bleeding by applying firm, prolonged pressure to the area if possible. |

| | |
|---|---|
| 18.e. The client will identify ways to reduce the risk of infection. | 18.e. Instruct client in ways to reduce risk of infection:<br>1. continue with coughing and deep breathing or use of incentive spirometer every 2 hours while awake as long as activity is limited<br>2. increase activity as tolerated<br>3. avoid contact with persons who have an infection<br>4. avoid crowds, especially during flu and cold seasons<br>5. decrease or stop smoking<br>6. drink at least 10 glasses of liquid/day unless on a fluid restriction<br>7. adhere to recommended diet<br>8. take supplemental vitamins and minerals as prescribed<br>9. maintain good personal hygiene. |
| 18.f. The client will identify ways to relieve pruritus. | 18.f.1. Reinforce instructions in Nursing Diagnosis 5.A, action 2, regarding ways to relieve itching.<br>2. Instruct client to take cholestyramine or an antihistamine as prescribed. |
| 18.g. The client will state signs and symptoms to report to the health care provider. | 18.g. Stress the importance of reporting the following signs and symptoms:<br>1. rapid weight gain or loss<br>2. increasing size of abdomen<br>3. increased swelling of lower extremities<br>4. increasing shortness of breath<br>5. increased itchiness or yellowing of skin<br>6. temperature elevation that lasts more than 2 days<br>7. blood in stools, urine, or vomitus; persistent bleeding from nose, mouth, or skin; prolonged or excessive menses; excessive bruising; severe headache; or sudden abdominal or back pain<br>8. persistent impotence or decrease in libido<br>9. tremors or changes in behavior, speech, or handwriting. |
| 18.h. The client will identify community resources that can assist with home management and adjustment to life-style changes necessary for effective management of cirrhosis. | 18.h.1. Provide information regarding community resources that can assist client and significant others with home management and adjustment to changes necessary for effective management of cirrhosis (e.g. Meals on Wheels, home health agencies, transportation services, drug and alcohol rehabilitation programs, counseling services).<br>2. Initiate a referral if indicated. |
| 18.i. The client will verbalize an understanding of and a plan for adhering to recommended follow-up care including future appointments with health care provider, medications prescribed, and activity level. | 18.i. 1. Reinforce the importance of keeping follow-up appointments with health care provider.<br>2. Explain the rationale for, side effects of, and importance of taking medications prescribed.<br>3. Reinforce physician's instructions regarding activity level. Stress the importance of rest in relation to the liver's ability to heal.<br>4. Implement measures outlined in Nursing Diagnosis 17, action b, to promote the client's ability to effectively manage the therapeutic regimen. |

# Hepatitis

Hepatitis is widespread inflammation of the liver that results in focal degeneration and necrosis of liver cells with subsequent organized regeneration of the cells in the majority of cases. It can be caused by bacteria, hepatotoxic agents (e.g. drugs, industrial chemicals) or, most commonly, a virus.

The five agents that have been identified as causes of acute viral hepatitis are the hepatitis A virus (HAV), hepatitis B virus (HBV), hepatitis C virus (HCV), hepatitis E virus (HEV), and the delta virus or hepatitis D virus (HDV). Hepatitis A is often referred to as infectious hepatitis and is transmitted almost exclusively by the fecal-oral route. Hepatitis B is transmitted parenterally, sexually, and perinatally. Parenteral transmission occurs primarily in intravenous drug users and in health care workers who have accidental exposure to infected blood. Screening of blood donors has minimized the incidence of transfusion-related cases of hepatitis B. Hepatitis C was formerly referred to as post-transfusion non-A, non-B hepatitis. Approximately 90% of the cases of post-transfusion hepatitis are caused by the hepatitis C virus; however, only a small percentage of the cases of hepatitis C are transfusion related. The majority of cases are associated with parenteral drug use and unknown factors. Hepatitis D appears to require the presence of the hepatitis B virus for its replication and is seen only in HBV-infected persons. Hepatitis E (formerly called enterically-transmitted non-A, non-B hepatitis) is similar in many respects to hepatitis A. It is transmitted by the fecal-oral route, usually by sewage-contaminated water, and seen predominantly in underdeveloped countries or in persons who have traveled to those countries.

The clinical manifestations and course of the disease are similar in all types of viral hepatitis. The majority of signs and symptoms are associated with alterations in the structure and function of the liver. The extrahepatic manifestations result from activation of the complement system by the antigen-antibody immune complexes. There are 3 stages or phases of viral hepatitis. The earliest is the preicteric or prodromal stage in which the client experiences a variety of flu-like symptoms. The disease is communicable during this stage and, in many cases, does not progress further. The next stage is the icteric stage. It is characterized by jaundice, dark-colored urine, and light-colored stools, which are manifestations of the cholestasis that is often present during this period. The third stage (posticteric or convalescent stage) lasts several weeks to months. During this time, symptoms subside and liver function tests return to normal.

Acute viral hepatitis is a major public health problem because it is highly communicable, is transmissible prior to the onset of symptoms, and, as yet, has no effective drug treatment. The majority of cases are self-limited and resolve completely without complications. The treatment is primarily supportive and directed toward reducing metabolic demands on the liver and promoting cell regeneration. Hospitalization is usually not required; however, it is indicated for clients with persistent nausea and vomiting, extreme elevation of liver function tests, a prolonged prothrombin time, or evidence of progressive deterioration, especially encephalopathy. A certain percentage of cases of acute viral hepatitis (approximately 20% of hepatitis B and 50% of hepatitis C) progress to a chronic state. Interferon alfa-2b has shown promise and been approved for treatment of chronic hepatitis B and C.

**This care plan focuses on the adult client in the icteric stage of acute viral hepatitis hospitalized to treat persistent nausea and vomiting and determine the type of hepatitis and extent of liver damage.** The goals of care are to ensure adequate rest, maintain an optimal nutritional status, reduce discomfort, prevent complications, and educate the client regarding follow-up care. It is the responsibility of each health care provider to maintain appropriate precautions for the type of hepatitis diagnosed in order to prevent the spread of infection to others.

## DIAGNOSTIC TESTS

Serum enzymes (e.g. ALT [SGPT], AST [SGOT], alkaline phosphatase)
Serum and urine bilirubin
Serum albumin and globulin
Antigen and antibody tests (e.g. $HB_sAg$, $HB_eAg$, IgM anti-$HB_c$, IgM anti-HAV, IgM anti-HDV, anti-HCV)
Complete blood count (CBC) and differential
Prothrombin time (PT)

## DISCHARGE CRITERIA

Prior to discharge, the client will:

- have resolution of nausea and vomiting
- have no evidence of bleeding or progressive liver degeneration

- have an adequate nutritional intake
- perform activities of daily living without fatigue
- identify ways to prevent the spread of hepatitis to others
- identify ways to prevent further liver damage
- verbalize an understanding of the rationale for and components of the recommended diet
- state signs and symptoms to report to the health care provider
- verbalize an understanding of and a plan for adhering to recommended follow-up care including future appointments with health care provider and for laboratory studies and activity level.

**NURSING/ COLLABORATIVE DIAGNOSES**



**1. NURSING/ COLLABORATIVE DIAGNOSIS:**

## Altered fluid and electrolyte balance:

a. **fluid volume deficit, hypokalemia, and hypochloremia** related to:
   1. excessive loss of fluid and electrolytes associated with persistent vomiting
   2. decreased oral intake associated with anorexia and nausea;

b. **metabolic alkalosis** related to excessive loss of potassium, chloride, and hydrochloric acid associated with persistent vomiting.

| Desired Outcome | Nursing Actions and ***Selected Purposes/Rationales*** |
|---|---|
| 1. The client will maintain fluid and electrolyte balance as evidenced by:<br>a. normal skin turgor<br>b. moist mucous membranes<br>c. stable weight<br>d. B/P and pulse within normal range for client and stable with position change | 1.a. Assess for and report signs and symptoms of:<br>1. fluid volume deficit:<br>a. decreased skin turgor, dry mucous membranes, thirst<br>b. sudden weight loss of 2% or greater<br>c. low B/P and/or postural hypotension<br>d. weak, rapid pulse<br>e. delayed small vein filling time (longer than 3-5 seconds)<br>f. decreased urine output with increased specific gravity (reflects an actual rather than potential fluid volume deficit)<br>g. increased BUN and Hct<br>2. hypokalemia (e.g. cardiac arrhythmias, postural hypotension, muscle |

| Desired Outcome | Nursing Actions and ***Selected Purposes/Rationales*** |
|---|---|
| e. small vein filling time less than 3-5 seconds<br>f. balanced intake and output<br>g. urine specific gravity within normal range<br>h. soft, nondistended abdomen with normal bowel sounds<br>i. absence of cardiac arrhythmias, muscle weakness, paresthesias, twitching, spasms, and dizziness<br>j. BUN, Hct, serum electrolytes, and blood gases within normal range. | weakness, paresthesias, nausea and vomiting, abdominal distention, hypoactive or absent bowel sounds)<br>3. hypochloremia and metabolic alkalosis (e.g. dizziness, irritability, paresthesias, muscle twitching or spasms, hypoventilation).<br>b. Monitor serum electrolyte and blood gas results. Report abnormal values.<br>c. Implement measures *to prevent or treat fluid and electrolyte imbalances:*<br>1. perform actions to reduce nausea and vomiting (see Nursing Diagnosis 4.B, action 2)<br>2. administer fluid and electrolyte replacements if ordered<br>3. maintain a fluid intake of at least 2500 ml/day unless contraindicated<br>4. perform actions to improve oral intake (see Nursing Diagnosis 2, action c.1)<br>5. when nausea and vomiting subside, assist client to select foods/fluids high in potassium (e.g. bananas, raisins, figs, apricots, potatoes, dates, cantaloupe, white beans, orange juice) and sodium (e.g. processed cheese, canned soups and vegetables, bouillon).<br>d. Consult physician if signs and symptoms of fluid and electrolyte imbalances persist or worsen. |

## 2. NURSING DIAGNOSIS: Altered nutrition: less than body requirements

related to:
a. decreased oral intake associated with anorexia and nausea;
b. loss of nutrients associated with persistent vomiting;
c. reduced metabolism and storage of nutrients by the liver associated with an alteration in normal liver function as a result of inflammation;
d. malabsorption of fats and fat-soluble vitamins associated with impaired bile flow resulting from inflammation of the liver;
e. increased utilization of nutrients associated with the increased metabolic rate that is present with infection.

| Desired Outcome | Nursing Actions and ***Selected Purposes/Rationales*** |
|---|---|
| 2. The client will maintain an adequate nutritional status as evidenced by:<br>a. weight within normal range for client's age, height, and body frame<br>b. normal BUN and serum albumin, Hct, Hb, $B_{12}$, folate, and transferrin levels<br>c. triceps skinfold thickness within normal range<br>d. improved strength and activity tolerance<br>e. healthy oral mucous membrane. | 2.a. Assess for and report signs and symptoms of malnutrition:<br>1. weight below normal for client's age, height, and body frame<br>2. abnormal BUN and low serum albumin, Hct, Hb, $B_{12}$, folate, and transferrin levels (some of these values also reflect impaired liver function)<br>3. triceps skinfold thickness less than normal<br>4. weakness and fatigue<br>5. stomatitis.<br>b. Monitor percentage of meals and snacks client consumes. Report a pattern of inadequate intake.<br>c. Implement measures *to maintain an adequate nutritional status:*<br>1. perform actions *to improve oral intake:*<br>a. implement measures to reduce nausea and vomiting (see Nursing Diagnosis 4.B, action 2)<br>b. obtain a dietary consult if necessary to assist client in selecting foods/fluids that meet nutritional needs as well as personal and cultural preferences whenever possible<br>c. encourage a rest period before meals *to minimize fatigue*<br>d. maintain a clean environment and a relaxed, pleasant atmosphere<br>e. provide oral care before meals |

f. serve small portions of nutritious foods/fluids that are appealing to client
g. offer larger meals in the morning *since nausea and anorexia are often not as severe early in the day*
h. allow adequate time for meals; reheat food if necessary
i. limit fluid intake (unless it has a high nutritional value) with meals *to reduce early satiety and subsequent decreased food intake*
j. increase activity as allowed and tolerated *(activity stimulates appetite)*

2. encourage client to consume meals that are well balanced and high in essential nutrients; supplement meals with snacks if client's caloric intake is inadequate
3. assist and instruct client to adhere to the following dietary recommendations:
   a. avoid skipping meals
   b. consume a diet high in calories (2000-3000 calories/day) and carbohydrates; if unable to tolerate food, suck on hard candy and drink fruit juices and regular soft drinks
   c. maintain a moderate to high protein intake (unless the serum ammonia level is high or clinical evidence of encephalopathy is present) *in order to promote healing of the liver*
4. administer vitamin preparations (e.g. vitamin K, B-complex vitamins, vitamin C) if ordered.

d. Perform a 72-hour calorie count if ordered. Report totals to dietitian and physician.
e. Consult physician about alternative methods of providing nutrition (e.g. parenteral nutrition, tube feeding) if client does not consume enough food or fluids to meet nutritional needs.

**3. NURSING DIAGNOSIS: Pain:**

a. **upper abdominal pain** related to inflammation of the liver;
b. **joint pain (arthralgia)** related to immune complex-mediated tissue injury associated with a viral infection.

| Desired Outcome | Nursing Actions and ***Selected Purposes/Rationales*** |
|---|---|
| 3. The client will experience diminished pain as evidenced by:<br>a. verbalization of pain relief<br>b. relaxed facial expression and body positioning<br>c. increased participation in activities. | 3.a. Determine how the client usually responds to pain.<br>b. Assess client's perception of pain including location, intensity, and type. Use a numerical scale to rate intensity.<br>c. Assess for nonverbal signs of pain (e.g. wrinkled brow, guarding of abdomen, rubbing joints, reluctance to move, restlessness).<br>d. Assess for factors that seem to aggravate and alleviate pain.<br>e. Implement measures *to reduce pain:*<br>1. consult physician about application of heat to painful joints<br>2. provide or assist with nonpharmacological measures for pain relief (e.g. back rub, position change, relaxation techniques, quiet conversation, restful environment, diversional activities)<br>3. administer analgesics if ordered; be aware of the following:<br>a. lower doses of narcotics are usually ordered *because the liver cannot detoxify narcotics at a normal rate*<br>b. acetaminophen may be ordered (despite its potential hepatotoxic effect) rather than acetylsalicylic acid *because of the increased risk of bleeding with acetylsalicylic acid.*<br>f. Consult physician if above measures fail to provide adequate pain relief. |

## 4.A. NURSING DIAGNOSIS: Altered comfort: pruritus

related to:
1. irritation of the skin by bile salts, which deposit in the skin as a result of the bile flow obstruction;
2. rash (sometimes occurs as a result of activation of the complement system by the immune complexes formed in response to a viral infection).

| Desired Outcome | Nursing Actions and ***Selected Purposes/Rationales*** |
|---|---|
| 4.A. The client will experience relief of pruritus as evidenced by:<br>1. verbalization of same<br>2. no scratching or rubbing of skin. | 4.A.1. Assess client's pruritus including onset, characteristics, location, and factors that aggravate and alleviate it.<br>2. Instruct client in and/or implement measures *to relieve pruritus:*<br>a. apply cool, moist compresses to pruritic areas<br>b. apply emollient cream or ointment frequently *to prevent dryness*<br>c. add emollients, cornstarch, baking soda, or oatmeal preparations to bath water<br>d. use tepid water and mild soaps for bathing<br>e. pat skin dry, making sure to dry thoroughly<br>f. maintain a cool environment<br>g. encourage participation in diversional activity<br>h. utilize relaxation techniques<br>i. utilize cutaneous stimulation techniques (e.g. massage, pressure, vibration, stroking with a soft brush) at the sites of itching or acupressure points<br>j. encourage client to wear loose cotton garments<br>k. administer the following medications if ordered:<br>1. antihistamines<br>2. cholestyramine *to bind bile salts and reduce their accumulation in the skin.*<br>3. Consult physician if above measures fail to alleviate pruritus or if the skin becomes excoriated. |

## 4.B. NURSING DIAGNOSIS: Altered comfort: nausea and vomiting

related to stimulation of the vomiting center associated with stimulation of the afferent vagal and/or sympathetic pathways as a result of visceral irritation that occurs with:
1. inflammation of the gastrointestinal tract resulting from the viral infection and subsequent immune complex-mediated tissue damage;
2. gaseous distention resulting from impaired fat digestion (a result of bile flow obstruction);
3. venous congestion in the gastrointestinal tract if portal hypertension has developed.

| Desired Outcome | Nursing Actions and ***Selected Purposes/Rationales*** |
|---|---|
| 4.B. The client will experience relief of nausea and vomiting as evidenced by: | 4.B.1. Assess client for nausea and vomiting.<br>2. Implement measures *to reduce nausea and vomiting:*<br>a. eliminate noxious sights and odors from the environment *(noxious stimuli cause cortical stimulation of the vomiting center)* |

1. verbalization of relief of nausea
2. absence of vomiting.

b. instruct client to change positions slowly *(rapid movement stimulates the afferent vestibulocerebellar pathway with resultant stimulation of the chemoreceptor trigger zone)*
c. provide oral hygiene after each emesis and before meals
d. encourage client to take deep, slow breaths when nauseated
e. encourage client to avoid intake of foods/fluids high in fat (e.g. butter, cream, whole milk, ice cream, fried foods, gravies, nuts) *to prevent a delay in gastric emptying and reduce nausea associated with impaired fat digestion*
f. avoid serving foods with an overpowering aroma; remove lids from hot foods before entering room
g. instruct client to eat dry foods (e.g. toast, crackers) and avoid drinking liquids with meals if nauseated
h. provide small, frequent meals; instruct client to ingest foods and fluids slowly
i. instruct client to avoid foods/fluids that irritate the gastric mucosa (e.g. spicy foods; caffeine-containing beverages such as tea, coffee, and colas)
j. instruct client to rest after eating with head of bed elevated
k. administer antiemetics if ordered (phenothiazines are contraindicated *because of their potential cholestatic effects).*

3. If above measures fail to control nausea and vomiting:
   a. consult physician
   b. be prepared to insert nasogastric tube and maintain suction as ordered.

## 5. NURSING DIAGNOSIS: Activity intolerance

related to:
a. inadequate nutritional status;
b. increased energy utilization associated with the increased metabolic rate present in infectious processes;
c. difficulty resting and sleeping associated with frequent assessments and treatments, discomfort, and unfamiliar environment.

| Desired Outcome | Nursing Actions and ***Selected Purposes/Rationales*** |
|---|---|

5. The client will demonstrate an increased tolerance for activity as evidenced by:
   a. verbalization of feeling less fatigued and weak
   b. ability to perform activities of daily living without exertional dyspnea, chest pain, diaphoresis, dizziness, and a significant change in vital signs.

5.a. Assess for signs and symptoms of activity intolerance:
   1. statements of fatigue and weakness
   2. exertional dyspnea, chest pain, diaphoresis, or dizziness
   3. abnormal heart rate response to activity (e.g. increase in rate of 20 beats/minute above resting rate, decrease in rate, rate not returning to preactivity level within 3 minutes after stopping activity, change from regular to irregular rate)
   4. decreased systolic B/P or a significant increase (10-15 mm Hg) in systolic or diastolic pressure with activity.

b. Implement measures *to improve activity tolerance:*
   1. perform actions *to promote rest and/or conserve energy:*
      a. maintain activity restrictions as ordered
      b. minimize environmental activity and noise
      c. organize nursing care to allow for periods of uninterrupted rest
      d. limit the number of visitors and their length of stay
      e. assist client with self-care activities as needed
      f. keep supplies and personal articles within easy reach

| Desired Outcome | Nursing Actions and ***Selected Purposes/Rationales*** |
|---|---|
| | g. instruct client in energy-saving techniques (e.g. using shower chair when showering, sitting to brush teeth or comb hair)<br>h. implement measures to reduce discomfort (see Nursing Diagnoses 3, action e; 4.A, action 2; and 4.B, action 2)<br>2. perform actions to maintain an adequate nutritional status (see Nursing Diagnosis 2, action c)<br>3. increase client's activity gradually as allowed and tolerated.<br>c. Instruct client to:<br>1. report a decreased tolerance for activity<br>2. stop any activity that causes chest pain, shortness of breath, dizziness, or extreme fatigue or weakness.<br>d. Consult physician if signs and symptoms of activity intolerance persist or worsen. |

## 6. COLLABORATIVE DIAGNOSES:

**Potential complications:**

a. **bleeding** related to:
  1. decreased production of clotting factors associated with impaired liver function and impaired vitamin K absorption (normal bile flow is necessary for absorption of vitamin K)
  2. thrombocytopenia associated with hypersplenism (if venous congestion has resulted in splenomegaly, the spleen will destroy platelets faster than usual);

b. **progressive liver degeneration** related to extensive necrosis of liver cells (a rare complication that may develop in persons with hepatitis C or hepatitis B).

| Desired Outcomes | Nursing Actions and ***Selected Purposes/Rationales*** |
|---|---|
| 6.a. The client will not experience unusual bleeding as evidenced by:<br>1. skin and mucous membranes free of petechiae, purpura, ecchymoses, and active bleeding<br>2. absence of unusual joint pain<br>3. no increase in abdominal girth<br>4. absence of frank and occult blood in stool, urine, and vomitus<br>5. usual menstrual flow<br>6. vital signs within normal range for client | 6.a.1. Assess client for and report signs and symptoms of unusual bleeding:<br>a. petechiae, purpura, ecchymoses<br>b. gingival bleeding<br>c. prolonged bleeding from puncture sites<br>d. epistaxis, hemoptysis<br>e. unusual joint pain<br>f. increase in abdominal girth<br>g. frank or occult blood in stool, urine, or vomitus<br>h. menorrhagia<br>i. restlessness, confusion<br>j. declining B/P and an increased pulse rate<br>k. decline in Hct and Hb levels.<br>2. Monitor platelet count and coagulation test results (e.g. prothrombin time, activated partial thromboplastin time, bleeding time). Report abnormal values.<br>3. If platelet count is low, coagulation test results are abnormal, or Hct and Hb levels decline, test all stools, urine, and vomitus for occult blood. Report positive results.<br>4. Implement measures *to prevent bleeding:*<br>a. use the smallest gauge needle possible when giving injections and performing venous and arterial punctures<br>b. apply gentle, prolonged pressure to puncture sites after injections and venous and arterial punctures |

7. stable or improved Hct and Hb.

c. take B/P only when necessary and avoid overinflating cuff
d. caution client to avoid activities that increase the risk for trauma (e.g. shaving with a straight-edge razor, using stiff-bristle toothbrush or dental floss)
e. pad side rails if client is confused or restless
f. gently perform procedures that can cause injury to the rectal mucosa (e.g. inserting a rectal suppository or tube, administering an enema)
g. perform actions *to reduce the risk for falls* (e.g. avoid unnecessary clutter in room, instruct client to wear shoes/slippers with nonslip soles when ambulating)
h. instruct client to avoid blowing nose forcefully or straining to have a bowel movement; consult physician about an order for a decongestant, stool softener, and/or laxative if indicated
i. administer the following if ordered *to improve clotting ability:*
   1. vitamin K (e.g. phytonadione) injections
   2. platelets
   3. fresh blood or plasma *(the liver may be unable to detoxify the preservative in stored blood).*

5. If bleeding occurs and does not subside spontaneously:
   a. apply firm, prolonged pressure to bleeding area(s) if possible
   b. if epistaxis occurs, place client in a high Fowler's position and apply pressure and ice pack to nasal area
   c. maintain oxygen therapy as ordered
   d. if gastric or esophageal bleeding occurs:
      1. position client on his/her side *to reduce the risk for aspiration*
      2. assist with insertion of a gastroesophageal balloon tube (e.g. Sengstaken-Blakemore tube, Minnesota tube); maintain balloon pressure, suction client, and perform saline lavage if ordered
      3. assist with administration of vasopressin if ordered *to constrict splanchnic vessels and reduce blood flow to the portal vein*
      4. assist with endoscopic sclerotherapy if performed
   e. administer vitamin K (e.g. phytonadione) injections and blood products (e.g. fresh frozen plasma or whole blood, platelets) as ordered
   f. assess for and report signs and symptoms of hypovolemic shock (e.g. restlessness; confusion; significant decrease in B/P; rapid, thready pulse; rapid respirations; cool, pale skin; urine output less than 30 ml/hour)
   g. prepare client for surgical repair of bleeding vessels if planned
   h. provide emotional support to client and significant others.

6.b. The client will not experience progressive liver degeneration as evidenced by:
1. resolution of signs and symptoms of hepatitis
2. absence of edema, ascites, and bleeding
3. usual mental status
4. coagulation test results and serum AST (SGOT), ALT (SGPT), alkaline phosphatase, and bilirubin levels returning toward normal.

6.b.1. Assess for signs and symptoms of progressive liver degeneration:
   a. worsening of signs and symptoms of hepatitis (e.g. increased jaundice, weakness, anorexia, nausea, and vomiting)
   b. edema, ascites
   c. bleeding (see action a.1 in this diagnosis)
   d. encephalopathy (e.g. change in handwriting, slow or slurred speech, emotional lability, agitation, disorientation, lethargy)
   e. further elevation of coagulation and liver function test results.

2. Implement measures identified in this care plan to promote healing of the liver.
3. Consult physician if signs and symptoms of progressive liver degeneration occur.

## 7. NURSING DIAGNOSIS: Social isolation

related to:
a. temporary restrictions of some usual activities (e.g. vigorous exercise, contact sports, sexual activity, alcohol consumption);
b. limited contact with others associated with fear of transmitting hepatitis and others' fear of contracting hepatitis.

| Desired Outcome | Nursing Actions and ***Selected Purposes/Rationales*** |
|---|---|
| 7. The client will experience a decreased sense of isolation as evidenced by:<br>a. maintenance of relationships with significant others<br>b. verbalization of decreasing feelings of aloneness and rejection. | 7.a. Ascertain client's usual degree of social interaction.<br>b. Assess for indications of social isolation (e.g. absence of supportive significant others; uncommunicative and withdrawn; expression of feelings of rejection, being different from others, or aloneness imposed by others; hostility; sad, dull affect).<br>c. Implement measures *to decrease social isolation:*<br>1. assist client to identify reasons for feeling isolated and alone; aid him/her in developing a plan of action to reduce these feelings<br>2. convey acceptance of client<br>3. encourage significant others to visit<br>4. encourage client to maintain telephone contact with others<br>5. educate client and significant others about mode of disease transmission and ways to prevent spread of infection (see Nursing Diagnosis 8, action a.1) *in order to reduce fear of disease transmission.* |

## 8. NURSING DIAGNOSIS: Knowledge deficit

regarding follow-up care.

| Desired Outcomes | Nursing Actions and ***Selected Purposes/Rationales*** |
|---|---|
| 8.a. The client will identify ways to prevent the spread of hepatitis to others. | 8.a.1. Provide the following instructions on ways to prevent the spread of hepatitis to others:<br>a. if client has hepatitis A, instruct him/her to adhere to the following precautions for 1-2 weeks after the onset of jaundice:<br>1. wash hands thoroughly after defecating and before meals<br>2. use separate toilet facilities if possible; if separate toilet facilities are not available, clean toilet seat with a chlorine solution after use<br>3. wash bedding, towels, and underwear separately from other articles in hot, soapy water<br>4. do not donate blood or work in food services until approved by physician<br>b. if client has hepatitis B, C, or D, instruct him/her to adhere to the following precautions until certain antigen/antibody tests (e.g. $HB_sAg$, $HB_eAg$, anti-HCV) are negative:<br>1. wash hands thoroughly after urinating and defecating<br>2. do not share personal articles (e.g. toothbrush, straight-edge razor, thermometer, washcloth)<br>3. use disposable eating utensils or wash utensils separately in hot, soapy water<br>4. do not share food or eating utensils<br>5. if any injections (e.g. insulin, vitamin $B_{12}$) are given at home, use |

disposable equipment and dispose of it properly to reduce the risk of others coming in contact with contaminated needles
6. avoid intimate sexual contact; once sexual activity is resumed, avoid intercourse during menstruation and intermenstrual bleeding and make sure that a condom is used during intercourse
7. do not donate blood.

2. Instruct client to inform household and sexual contacts to see health care provider for appropriate immunization and testing for early detection of hepatitis.

| | |
|---|---|
| 8.b. The client will identify ways to prevent further liver damage. | 8.b. Provide the following instructions regarding ways to prevent further liver damage:<br>1. avoid alcohol intake for a minimum of 6 months (many sources recommend a year)<br>2. avoid contact with industrial toxins (e.g. paint solvents, cleaning agents containing carbon tetrachloride)<br>3. take acetaminophen (e.g. Tylenol) only when necessary and do not exceed the recommended dose because of its potential toxic effect on the liver<br>4. take precautions to prevent recurrent hepatitis (client is immune only to the viral type he/she has had):<br>a. if client has hepatitis A, instruct in ways to reduce the risk for hepatitis B, C, and D:<br>1. receive autologous blood or blood from donor known not to have hepatitis if transfusions are necessary<br>2. avoid intimate sexual contact with known carriers of hepatitis<br>3. avoid sharing food and eating utensils and handling toiletry items of others<br>4. avoid contact with contaminated needles<br>b. if client has hepatitis B or D:<br>1. instruct in ways to prevent occurrence of hepatitis A:<br>a. wash hands thoroughly after defecating and before meals<br>b. eat only in restaurants that have been inspected and approved by health authorities<br>c. avoid oral-anal sex<br>2. instruct in ways to reduce the risk for hepatitis C (see action 4.a above)<br>c. if client has hepatitis C, instruct in ways to prevent hepatitis B, D, and A (see actions 4.a and b.1. above). |
| 8.c. The client will verbalize an understanding of the rationale for and components of the recommended diet. | 8.c.1. Explain to client that adherence to the recommended diet will promote healing of the liver and reduce the risk of further liver damage.<br>2. Reinforce the dietary instructions outlined in Nursing Diagnosis 2, action c.3.<br>3. Instruct client to avoid intake of foods high in fat (e.g. butter, cream, ice cream, pork, fried foods, gravy) until gastrointestinal symptoms such as nausea and indigestion subside. |
| 8.d. The client will state signs and symptoms to report to the health care provider. | 8.d. Stress the importance of reporting the following signs and symptoms:<br>1. persistent or recurrent loss of appetite, nausea and vomiting, or weight loss<br>2. persistent fatigue<br>3. increased itchiness or yellowing of skin<br>4. blood in stools, urine, or vomitus; prolonged or excessive bleeding from nose, mouth, or skin; prolonged or excessive menses; excessive bruising; severe headache; or sudden abdominal or back pain<br>5. changes in behavior, speech, or handwriting. |
| 8.e. The client will verbalize an understanding of and plan for adhering to recommended follow- | 8.e.1. Reinforce the importance of keeping follow-up appointments with health care provider and for laboratory studies (liver enzyme levels and serological markers provide information about immunity, presence of a carrier state, and chronicity, which helps determine the need for additional treatment [e.g. interferon alfa-2B] and teaching). |

| Desired Outcomes | Nursing Actions and ***Selected Purposes/Rationales*** |
|---|---|
| up care including future appointments with health care provider and for laboratory studies and activity level. | 2. Reinforce physician's instructions regarding activity level. Stress the importance of rest during convalescent phase (from 6 weeks to 6 months).<br>3. Provide client with information about and encourage participation in drug and alcohol rehabilitation programs if indicated.<br>4. Implement measures to improve client compliance:<br>a. include significant others in teaching sessions if possible<br>b. encourage questions and allow time for reinforcement and clarification of information provided<br>c. provide written instructions regarding scheduled appointments with health care provider and for laboratory studies, activity restrictions, and signs and symptoms to report. |

UNIT

XVI

# *Nursing Care of the Client with Disturbances of Metabolic Function*

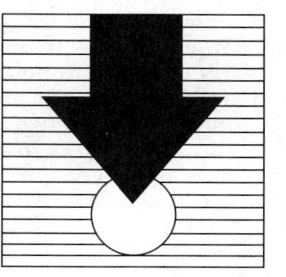

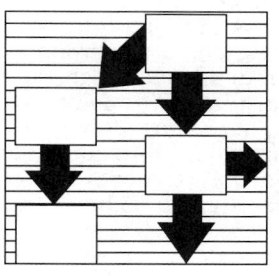

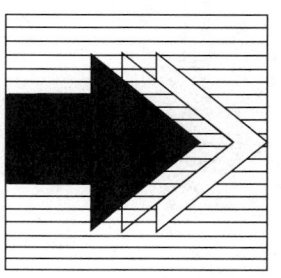

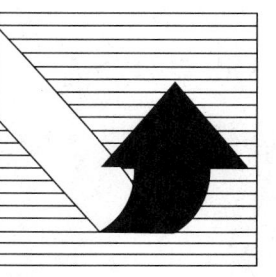

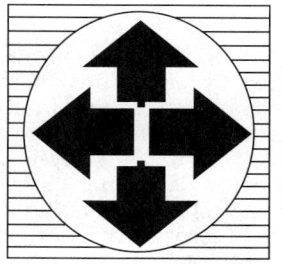

# Diabetes Mellitus

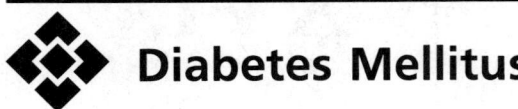

Diabetes mellitus is a chronic systemic syndrome characterized by alterations in carbohydrate, fat, and protein metabolism resulting from an inadequate supply of insulin and/or a defective cellular response to insulin. The hallmark of this metabolic disorder is hyperglycemia. Diabetes* is further characterized by structural and functional abnormalities in the blood vessels and nerves. The atherosclerotic and arteriosclerotic changes that occur in the large vessels (macroangiopathy) affect the cardiac, cerebral, and peripheral circulation. Thickening of the basement membrane of the capillaries (microangiopathy) also occurs and involves vessels of the eyes and kidneys. Neurological manifestations are thought to be due in part to an insufficient blood supply to the nerves but appear to be primarily a result of a metabolic defect in the polyol pathway leading to an accumulation of byproducts (e.g. sorbitol) in nerve tissue. These byproducts act as toxins and cause demyelination and decreased nerve conduction.

The two major classifications of diabetes are insulin-dependent diabetes mellitus (IDDM), also referred to as type I, and noninsulin-dependent diabetes mellitus (NIDDM), often called type II. Insulin-dependent diabetics have an absolute insulin deficiency and are dependent on insulin therapy to prevent ketosis. The insulin deficiency is a result of pancreatic beta cell destruction that is thought to be related to genetic, immunologic, and/or environmental (e.g. virus) factors. Noninsulin-dependent diabetics have a relative deficiency of insulin due to faulty insulin secretion (often a delayed and prolonged output), decreased tissue responsiveness to insulin, and/or accelerated hepatic glucose production. Genetics is a major factor in the development of type II diabetes. Additional classifications of diabetes are related to stage of development or etiology and include impaired glucose tolerance diabetes, gestational diabetes, and diabetes associated with other conditions such as pancreatic disease and endocrine disorders (e.g. Cushing's syndrome, acromegaly) or use of medications such as glucocorticoids, estrogens, and thiazides.

A sequence of pathophysiological events occur in diabetes. When an insulin deficiency exists, glucose cannot be transported into the cells for energy metabolism. As a result, glucose accumulates in the blood and starts to spill into the urine once the level exceeds the renal threshold (180 mg/dl or greater). The high blood glucose acts as an osmotic diuretic, which leads to excessive diuresis and subsequent fluid volume deficit. Because the glucose cannot be utilized as an energy source by many cells, protein and fat stores are broken down to provide a source of energy for the starving cells. The free fatty acids that are mobilized from adipose tissue are converted by the liver to ketones (acetoacetate, acetone, β-hydroxybutyrate) to be used as an energy source. The ketones are strong acids and eventually deplete the body's buffer system and respiratory compensatory ability, leading to a state of acidosis. Continuation of these metabolic derangements leads to life-threatening imbalances.

**This care plan focuses on the adult client who has had diabetes for many years and is being hospitalized because of difficulty stabilizing blood glucose levels.** Many of the long-term vascular and neurological complications have been included in this care plan and should be individualized based on the client's current status. The goals of care are to maintain glucose levels within a safe range, prevent further complications, and educate the client regarding follow-up care. This care plan should be used in conjunction with the care plans on Heart Failure, Myocardial Infarction, Cerebrovascular Accident, Hypertension, and/or Chronic Renal Failure if the client is also being treated for one of these vascular complications of diabetes.

*Diabetes mellitus will be referred to as diabetes throughout this care plan.

## DIAGNOSTIC TESTS

Fasting plasma glucose (fasting blood sugar [FBS])
Postprandial blood sugar (PPBS)
Capillary blood glucose (CBG)
Glycosylated hemoglobin (Hgb $A_1$, Hgb $A_{1c}$)
Urine ketones and protein
Serum cholesterol, triglycerides, and lipoprotein profile

## DISCHARGE CRITERIA

Prior to discharge, the client will:

- have blood glucose stabilized within a desired range

- ❖ verbalize a basic understanding of diabetes mellitus
- ❖ verbalize an understanding of medications ordered including rationale, side effects, schedule for taking, and importance of taking as prescribed
- ❖ demonstrate the ability to correctly draw up and administer insulin if prescribed
- ❖ verbalize an understanding of the principles of dietary management and be able to calculate and plan meals within the prescribed caloric distribution
- ❖ demonstrate the ability to correctly perform blood glucose and urine tests and accurately interpret results
- ❖ verbalize an understanding of the role of exercise in the management of diabetes
- ❖ identify health care and hygiene practices that should be integrated into life style
- ❖ identify appropriate safety measures to follow because of the diagnosis of diabetes
- ❖ state signs and symptoms of hypoglycemia and ketoacidosis and appropriate actions for prevention and treatment
- ❖ state signs and symptoms to report to the health care provider
- ❖ share feelings and concerns about diabetes and its effect on life style
- ❖ identify resources that can assist in the adjustment to and management of diabetes
- ❖ verbalize an understanding of and a plan for adhering to recommended follow-up care including future appointments with health care provider and for laboratory studies.

**NURSING/ COLLABORATIVE DIAGNOSES**

## 1. NURSING DIAGNOSIS: Altered tissue perfusion

related to:
a. vascular abnormalities (arteriosclerosis, atherosclerosis, microangiopathies) that develop with diabetes;
b. postural hypotension associated with neuropathy of the autonomic nervous system.

### Desired Outcome

1. The client will maintain adequate tissue perfusion as evidenced by:
   a. B/P and pulse within normal range for client
   b. usual mental status
   c. extremities warm with absence of pallor and cyanosis
   d. palpable peripheral pulses
   e. capillary refill time less than 3 seconds
   f. absence of exercise-induced pain
   g. balanced intake and output.

### Nursing Actions and ***Selected Purposes/Rationales***

1.a. Assess for signs and symptoms of autonomic neuropathy involving the cardiovascular system:
   1. lightheadedness upon standing
   2. resting pulse rate greater than 100 beats/minute
   3. decline in systolic B/P of 30 mm Hg or more when client changes from a lying to sitting or standing position.

b. Assess for and report signs and symptoms of diminished tissue perfusion (e.g. significant decrease in B/P, restlessness, confusion, cool extremities, pallor or cyanosis of extremities, diminished or absent peripheral pulses, slow capillary refill, claudication, angina, oliguria).

c. Monitor serum cholesterol, triglycerides, and lipoprotein profile. Report abnormalities. *(Elevated lipid levels may contribute to atherosclerosis.)*

d. Implement measures *to maintain adequate tissue perfusion:*
   1. perform actions *to promote adequate circulation in lower extremities:*
      a. increase activity as allowed; instruct client with intermittent claudication to walk slowly and alternate activity with periods of rest
      b. discourage positions that compromise blood flow in lower extremities (e.g. crossing legs, pillows under knees, use of knee gatch, prolonged sitting or standing)
      c. instruct client in and assist with active foot and leg exercises every 1-2 hours
   2. perform actions *to reduce postural hypotension:*
      a. instruct client to change from a horizontal to a vertical position slowly *in order to allow time for autoregulatory mechanisms to adjust to upright position*
      b. keep head of bed elevated at least 30°
      c. apply elastic stockings as ordered; remove for 30-60 minutes at least twice daily
      d. administer fludrocortisone acetate if ordered
   3. instruct client to avoid foods high in saturated fat and cholesterol (e.g. butter, cheese, ice cream, eggs, red meat) *in order to reduce progression of atherogenesis*
   4. perform actions to maintain blood glucose at a near-normal level (see Nursing Diagnosis 3, action d); *maintaining blood glucose at a near-normal level may prevent or delay development of some of the vascular complications*
   5. perform actions to prevent fluid volume deficit (see Nursing Diagnosis 2, action b)
   6. perform actions *to prevent vasoconstriction:*
      a. implement measures *to reduce stress* (e.g. explain procedures, maintain a calm environment, reduce discomfort)
      b. discourage smoking
      c. implement measures *to keep client from getting cold* (e.g. maintain a comfortable room temperature, provide adequate clothing and blankets)
   7. administer the following medications if ordered:

a. antilipemic agents (e.g. lovastatin, gemfibrizol) *to prevent further atherogenesis*
b. pentoxifylline (Trental) *to improve blood flow (increases erythrocyte flexibility, reduces blood viscosity, and has a mild vasodilator effect).*

e. Consult physician if signs and symptoms of diminished tissue perfusion persist or worsen.

**2. NURSING DIAGNOSIS:**

**High risk for fluid volume deficit**

related to excessive loss of fluid associated with the osmotic diuresis that can result from hyperglycemia.

| Desired Outcome | Nursing Actions and ***Selected Purposes/Rationales*** |
|---|---|
| 2. The client will not experience a fluid volume deficit as evidenced by:<br>a. normal skin temperature and turgor<br>b. moist mucous membranes<br>c. stable weight<br>d. B/P and pulse within normal range for client and stable with position change<br>e. small vein filling time less than 3-5 seconds<br>f. balanced intake and output<br>g. urine specific gravity within normal range<br>h. Hct within normal range. | 2.a. Assess for and report signs and symptoms of fluid volume deficit:<br>1. warm, flushed skin<br>2. decreased skin turgor<br>3. dry mucous membranes, thirst<br>4. sudden weight loss of 2% or greater (many clients with diabetes are on weight reduction diets, so some weight loss is expected)<br>5. low B/P and/or postural hypotension<br>6. weak, rapid pulse<br>7. delayed small vein filling time (longer than 3-5 seconds)<br>8. decreased urine output with increased specific gravity (reflects an actual rather than potential fluid deficit; if client has diabetic nephropathy, specific gravity may not be a useful indicator of hydration status)<br>9. elevated Hct.<br>b. Implement measures *to prevent fluid volume deficit:*<br>1. perform actions *to prevent or treat hyperglycemia in order to prevent osmotic diuresis:*<br>a. encourage client to adhere to the diabetic diet prescribed (commonly the American Diabetic Association [ADA] diet)<br>b. administer insulin as ordered and in an area where maximum absorption will occur *(there is decreased absorption of insulin if it is administered in an area where tissue is hypertrophied);* if client has an insulin pump, maintain prescribed basal infusion rate and ensure that client receives preprandial boluses as ordered<br>c. administer prescribed oral hypoglycemic agent 30-60 minutes before meals<br>d. minimize client's exposure to emotional and physiological stress *(stress causes an increased output of epinephrine, glucagon, and cortisol, all of which increase blood sugar)*<br>2. maintain a fluid intake of at least 2500 ml/day unless contraindicated; if oral intake is inadequate or contraindicated, maintain intravenous therapy as ordered. |

**3. NURSING DIAGNOSIS:**

**Altered nutrition***

related to:
a. inability to metabolize carbohydrates, fats, and proteins properly associated with insulin deficiency;
b. noncompliance with prescribed dietary regimen.

*This diagnostic label includes altered nutrition: less than and more than body requirements.

| Desired Outcome | Nursing Actions and ***Selected Purposes/Rationales*** |
|---|---|
| 3. The client will maintain an adequate nutritional status as evidenced by:<br>a. maintenance of or return toward normal weight<br>b. serum albumin, Hct, Hb, transferrin, and lymphocyte levels within normal range<br>c. triceps skinfold thickness within or approaching normal range<br>d. usual strength and activity tolerance. | 3.a. Assess for signs and symptoms of an altered nutritional status:<br>1. abnormal weight for client's age, height, and body frame (many clients with type II diabetes are overweight)<br>2. low serum albumin, Hct, Hb, transferrin, and lymphocyte levels<br>3. triceps skinfold thickness less than or greater than normal<br>4. weakness and fatigue.<br>b. Monitor blood glucose levels regularly. Report values below 60 mg/dl or above 200 mg/dl or outside of the parameters specified by physician.<br>c. Monitor percentage of meals and snacks client consumes. Report a pattern of inadequate or excessive intake.<br>d. Implement measures *to maintain blood glucose at a near-normal level, achieve ideal weight, and provide necessary nutrients in order to maintain an adequate nutritional status:*<br>1. obtain a dietary consult to reinforce teaching about the diet prescribed and ways to adapt it to personal and cultural preferences and specific needs (dietary restrictions will vary but are most often prescribed as specific percentages of carbohydrate, fat, and protein within an optimal calorie level; it is recommended that 50-60% of calories be derived from carbohydrate [the majority of which should be complex carbohydrates], 20-30% from fat [primarily polyunsaturated], and 15-20% from protein)<br>2. assist client to calculate and select appropriate foods utilizing an exchange list<br>3. provide meals and snacks on time and at evenly spaced intervals *to maintain desired balance between insulin and glucose*<br>4. administer insulin and/or oral hypoglycemic agent as ordered *to enhance cellular utilization of glucose and promote normal metabolism of fats and proteins*<br>5. perform actions to prevent or treat hypoglycemia (see Collaborative Diagnosis 12, actions b.3 and 4)<br>6. perform actions to treat gastroparesis and relieve gastric discomfort if present (see Nursing Diagnosis 4.B, action 3) *in order to promote even absorption of nutrients and an adequate oral intake*<br>7. reinforce importance of weight loss if client is obese *(studies have shown that weight loss significantly reduces symptoms of diabetes in grossly overweight clients).*<br>e. Perform a 72-hour calorie count if ordered. Report totals to dietitian and physician. |

## 4.A. NURSING DIAGNOSIS:

**Altered comfort: burning, aching, cramping, numbness, and/or tingling (particularly in lower extremities)**
related to peripheral neuropathies and peripheral vascular insufficiency.

| Desired Outcome | Nursing Actions and ***Selected Purposes/Rationales*** |
|---|---|
| 4.A. The client will experience diminished discomfort as evidenced by:<br>1. verbalization of a reduction of burning, aching, cramping, | 4.A.1. Determine how client usually responds to discomfort.<br>2. Assess for signs and symptoms of peripheral neuropathies and peripheral vascular insufficiency (can occur anywhere but most often occur in the lower extremities):<br>a. persistent burning or aching sensation that often becomes worse at night<br>b. numbness or tingling<br>c. diminished or absent reflexes |

numbness, and tingling in involved areas
2. relaxed facial expression and body positioning
3. increased participation in activities
4. stable vital signs.

d. cramps, especially in calf muscles, during ambulation *(indicative of intermittent claudication).*
3. Assess for nonverbal signs of discomfort (e.g. wrinkled brow, clenched fists, guarding of affected area, reluctance to move, restlessness, diaphoresis, facial pallor, increased B/P, tachycardia).
4. Assess for factors that seem to aggravate and alleviate discomfort.
5. Implement measures *to reduce discomfort:*
   a. perform actions *to reduce fear and anxiety about discomfort* (e.g. assure client that his/her discomfort is recognized and attempts will be made to relieve it)
   b. medicate before pain is severe
   c. provide a bed cradle *to keep bedding off affected extremities*
   d. assist client with ambulation if walking relieves discomfort (walking usually relieves lower extremity discomfort associated with neuropathies of the lower extremities); if client is experiencing intermittent claudication, encourage short, more frequent walks *since longer walks exacerbate pain associated with vascular insufficiency*
   e. provide or assist with additional nonpharmacological measures for relief of discomfort (e.g. position change, relaxation techniques, guided imagery, quiet conversation, restful environment, diversional activities)
   f. plan methods for controlling discomfort with client *to enable him/her to maintain a sense of control over the discomfort*
   g. administer the following medications if ordered *to control discomfort:*
      1. analgesics (narcotic analgesics are avoided as long as possible *because the pain may be chronic;* some painful neuropathies may, however, subside after a few months)
      2. tricyclic antidepressants (e.g. amitriptyline)
      3. carbamazepine (has been useful in treatment of some sharp or stabbing neuralgia pain)
      4. capsaicin cream (e.g. Zostrix)
      5. pentoxifylline (Trental) *to improve blood flow and reduce discomfort associated with intermittent claudication.*
6. Consult physician if above measures fail to provide adequate relief of discomfort.

## 4.B. NURSING DIAGNOSIS: Altered comfort: gastric fullness, pyrosis, and/or nausea

related to accumulation of gas and fluid in the stomach associated with gastroparesis resulting from autonomic neuropathy.

| Desired Outcome | Nursing Actions and ***Selected Purposes/Rationales*** |
|---|---|
| 4.B. The client will experience a reduction in gastric discomfort as evidenced by:<br>1. verbalization of same<br>2. relaxed facial expression and body positioning. | 4.B.1. Assess client for verbal complaints of gastric fullness or bloating, heartburn, or nausea.<br>2. Assess for nonverbal signs of gastric discomfort (e.g. grimacing, clutching or guarding of stomach, restlessness, reluctance to move).<br>3. Implement measures *to reduce gastric discomfort:*<br>a. perform actions *to reduce the accumulation of gas and fluid in the stomach:*<br>1. encourage and assist client with frequent position change and ambulation as tolerated *(activity stimulates gastric motility)*<br>2. have client sit up during meals and for 1-2 hours after meals *(gravity promotes passage of food and fluid through the gastrointestinal tract)* |

| Desired Outcome | Nursing Actions and ***Selected Purposes/Rationales*** |
|---|---|
| | 3. provide small, frequent meals rather than 3 large ones; instruct client to ingest foods and fluids slowly<br>4. encourage client to drink warm liquids *in order to initiate the gastrocolic and duodenocolic reflexes and stimulate peristalsis*<br>5. instruct client to avoid activities such as gum chewing and smoking *in order to reduce air swallowing*<br>6. instruct client to avoid carbonated beverages and gas-producing foods (e.g. cabbage, onions, beans)<br>7. encourage client to eructate whenever the urge is felt<br>8. administer gastrointestinal stimulants (e.g. metoclopramide) and antiflatulents (e.g. simethicone) if ordered<br>b. perform actions *to reduce nausea if present:*<br>1. encourage client to take deep, slow breaths when nauseated<br>2. avoid foods/fluids that irritate the gastric mucosa (e.g. spicy foods; caffeine-containing beverages such as coffee, tea, and colas)<br>3. eliminate noxious sights and odors from the environment *(noxious stimuli cause cortical stimulation of the vomiting center)*<br>4. instruct client to change positions slowly *(rapid movement stimulates the afferent vestibulocerebellar pathway with resultant stimulation of the chemoreceptor trigger zone)*<br>5. avoid serving foods with an overpowering aroma; remove lids from hot foods before entering room<br>6. administer antiemetics if ordered<br>c. administer antacids and histamine$_2$ receptor antagonists (e.g. cimetidine, ranitidine, famotidine) if ordered *to reduce gastric acidity.*<br>4. Consult physician if gastric discomfort persists or worsens. |

## 5. NURSING DIAGNOSIS: Sensory/perceptual alteration: visual

related to:
a. osmotic swelling of the lens associated with hyperglycemia and the subsequent accumulation of sorbitol in the lens;
b. changes in the retinal vessels (retinopathy);
c. presence of cataracts and/or glaucoma (there is a higher incidence of these conditions in clients with diabetes).

| Desired Outcome | Nursing Actions and ***Selected Purposes/Rationales*** |
|---|---|
| 5. The client will not experience further progression of visual disturbances and will demonstrate adaptation to existing ones. | 5.a. Assess for visual disturbances (e.g. complaints of blurred vision [usually associated with a high blood sugar, which results in accumulation of sugar and fluid in the lens]; statements of partial or total loss of vision or the presence of "floaters," halos, or flashing lights).<br>b. Examine the fundus of the eye or review the report of the physician's examination to determine if signs and symptoms of retinopathy (e.g. small retinal hemorrhages, dilated veins, cotton-wool spots) are present.<br>c. Implement measures *to prevent further visual disturbances:*<br>1. perform actions identified in Nursing Diagnosis 2, action b.1, to control hyperglycemia *(maintenance of blood sugar at a stable, near-normal level may reduce small vessel disease)*<br>2. prepare client for laser photocoagulation or vitrectomy if planned.<br>d. If vision is impaired:<br>1. implement measures to reduce the risk for trauma (see Nursing Diagnosis 11, action a)<br>2. avoid startling client (e.g. speak client's name and identify yourself |

when entering room and before any physical contact, describe activities and reasons for various noises in the room)
3. assist client with personal hygiene he/she is unable to perform independently
4. identify where items are placed on his/her plate and tray, cut food, open packages, and feed client if necessary
5. assist with activities such as filling out menus and reading mail and legal documents as needed
6. instruct client in use of appropriate self-help devices (e.g. magnifier for insulin syringe, insulin pen that delivers fixed amount of insulin, needle guide for insulin vial, glucometer that displays blood glucose values in bold numbers); monitor client's accuracy in testing blood glucose and administering insulin
7. provide auditory rather than visual diversionary activities
8. inform client of resources available if he/she desires additional information about visual aids (e.g. publications such as Aids for the Blind; American Federation for the Blind).

e. Reassess visual status regularly and consult physician if visual status worsens.

## 6. NURSING DIAGNOSIS: High risk for impaired skin integrity

related to:

a. increased fragility of the skin associated with inadequate tissue perfusion and dryness (can occur because of sweat gland dysfunction that sometimes results from autonomic neuropathy);
b. damage to the skin and/or subcutaneous tissue associated with prolonged pressure on the tissues, friction, or shearing if mobility is decreased;
c. abnormal pressure distribution on plantar aspect of feet (results from muscle weakness in feet associated with peripheral neuropathy) and undetected foot injuries associated with diminished sensation (results from vascular insufficiency and neuropathy);
d. frequent contact with irritants if diarrhea occurs;
e. development of ulcerative skin lesions (diabetic dermopathy, necrobiosis lipoidica diabeticorum).

**Desired Outcome** / **Nursing Actions and *Selected Purposes/Rationales***

6. The client will maintain skin integrity as evidenced by:
   a. absence of redness and irritation
   b. no skin breakdown.

6.a. Inspect skin for areas of pallor, redness, and breakdown with particular attention to:
1. skinfolds of abdomen and groin and under breasts
2. spaces between toes
3. feet and lower legs
4. dependent areas
5. bony prominences
6. perianal area
7. areas where sensation is diminished *(client may be unaware of development of blisters and ulcerations).*

b. Implement measures *to prevent skin breakdown:*
1. assist client to turn every 2 hours if activity is limited
2. gently massage around reddened areas at least every 2 hours
3. perform actions *to prevent shearing* (shearing occurs when one tissue layer slides past another) *and skin surface abrasion:*
   a. apply a thin layer of powder or cornstarch to bottom sheet or skin *to absorb moisture (moist skin is more likely to adhere to sheet) and reduce friction*

| Desired Outcome | Nursing Actions and ***Selected Purposes/Rationales*** |
|---|---|

b. limit length of time client is in semi-Fowler's position to 30 minutes *(in this position, client tends to slide down in bed)*

4. instruct or assist client to shift weight every 30 minutes
5. if fade time (length of time it takes for reddened area to fade after pressure is removed) is greater than 15 minutes, increase frequency of position changes
6. keep skin clean and dry
7. apply a thin layer of powder or cornstarch to areas with opposing skin surfaces (e.g. axillae, perineum, beneath breasts) if indicated *to absorb moisture and/or reduce friction*
8. keep bed linens dry and wrinkle-free
9. increase activity as allowed and tolerated
10. provide devices to reduce pressure on the skin, decrease shearing, and/or prevent moisture build-up (e.g. alternating pressure mattress or pad, flotation pad, sheepskin)
11. perform actions to maintain an adequate nutritional status (see Nursing Diagnosis 3, action d)
12. perform actions *to prevent drying of the skin:*
    a. encourage a fluid intake of 2500 ml/day unless contraindicated
    b. provide a mild soap for bathing
    c. apply moisturizing lotion and/or emollient to skin at least once a day
13. perform actions *to prevent skin irritation resulting from diarrhea if present:*
    a. implement measures to control diarrhea (see Nursing Diagnosis 9, action d)
    b. assist client to thoroughly cleanse and dry perineal area with soft tissue or cloth after each bowel movement; apply a protective ointment or cream (e.g. Desitin, A&D ointment, Vaseline)
14. perform actions to maintain adequate tissue perfusion (see Nursing Diagnosis 1, action d)
15. perform meticulous foot care:
    a. wash feet daily with warm water and a mild soap
    b. dry feet thoroughly using a soft towel or cloth, paying particular attention to interdigital spaces
    c. apply lanolin or other lubricating lotion to feet (except between toes) daily
16. perform actions *to prevent trauma to feet:*
    a. caution client to always wear socks and shoes or sturdy slippers when ambulating
    b. do not place heating pad on feet
    c. check the temperature of bath water before client immerses feet.

c. If skin breakdown occurs:

1. notify physician
2. continue with above measures to prevent further irritation and breakdown
3. perform wound care as ordered or per hospital procedure
4. implement additional measures *to promote wound healing:*
    a. perform actions *to maintain adequate circulation to the wound area:*
        1. implement measures to maintain adequate tissue perfusion (see Nursing Diagnosis 1, action d)
        2. do not apply dressings tightly *(excessive pressure impairs circulation to the area)*
    b. perform actions to prevent infection in wound (see Nursing Diagnosis 10, action c.10)
5. assess for and report signs and symptoms of impaired wound healing (e.g. increasing redness and swelling at wound site, pale or necrotic tissue in wound, separation of wound edges).

## 7. NURSING DIAGNOSIS: Urinary retention

related to loss of bladder sensation and diminished contractility of the detrusor muscle associated with neuropathy of the pelvic nerves.

| Desired Outcome | Nursing Actions and ***Selected Purposes/Rationales*** |
|---|---|
| 7. The client will not experience urinary retention as evidenced by:<br>a. voiding at normal intervals<br>b. no complaints of bladder fullness or suprapubic discomfort<br>c. absence of bladder distention and dribbling of urine<br>d. balanced intake and output. | 7.a. Determine client's usual urinary elimination pattern.<br>b. Assess for signs and symptoms of urinary retention:<br>1. frequent voiding of small amounts (25-60 ml) of urine<br>2. complaints of bladder fullness or suprapubic discomfort<br>3. bladder distention<br>4. dribbling of urine<br>5. output less than intake.<br>c. Assist with urodynamic studies (e.g. cystometrogram) if ordered.<br>d. Implement measures *to prevent urinary retention:*<br>1. offer bedpan or urinal or assist client to bedside commode or bathroom every 2-3 hours if indicated<br>2. instruct client to urinate when the urge is first felt<br>3. perform actions *to provide sensory stimulation that may help trigger the micturition reflex* (e.g. run water, place client's hands in warm water, pour warm water over perineum)<br>4. allow client to assume a normal position for voiding unless contraindicated<br>5. instruct client to lean his/her upper body forward and/or gently press downward on lower abdomen during voiding attempts unless contraindicated *in order to put pressure on the bladder area (pressure helps trigger the micturition reflex and promotes more complete bladder emptying)*<br>6. instruct client to perform the Valsalva maneuver during urination unless contraindicated<br>7. administer cholinergic drugs (e.g. bethanechol) if ordered *to stimulate bladder contraction.*<br>e. Consult physician about intermittent catheterization or insertion of an indwelling catheter if above actions fail to alleviate urinary retention. |

## 8. NURSING DIAGNOSIS: Constipation

related to colonic atony or dilatation associated with autonomic neuropathy of the large bowel.

| Desired Outcome | Nursing Actions and ***Selected Purposes/Rationales*** |
|---|---|
| 8. The client will not experience constipation as evidenced by:<br>a. usual frequency of bowel movements<br>b. passage of soft, formed stool<br>c. absence of headache, anorexia, abdominal | 8.a. Ascertain client's usual bowel elimination habits.<br>b. Assess for signs and symptoms of constipation (e.g. decrease in frequency of stools; passage of hard, formed stools; headache; anorexia; abdominal distention and pain; feeling of fullness or pressure in rectum; straining at stool).<br>c. Assess bowel sounds. Report a pattern of decreasing bowel sounds.<br>d. Implement measures *to prevent constipation:*<br>1. encourage client to defecate whenever the urge is felt<br>2. assist client to toilet or bedside commode or place in a high Fowler's |

| Desired Outcome | Nursing Actions and ***Selected Purposes/Rationales*** |
|---|---|
| distention and pain, rectal pressure, and straining at stool. | position on bedpan for bowel movements unless contraindicated; provide privacy and adequate ventilation<br>3. instruct client to increase intake of foods high in fiber (e.g. bran, whole-grain breads and cereals, raw fruits and vegetables) unless contraindicated; obtain a dietary consult if indicated to assist client with ways to incorporate high-fiber foods into prescribed diabetic diet<br>4. instruct client to maintain a minimum fluid intake of 2500 ml/day unless contraindicated<br>5. encourage client to drink warm liquids upon arising in the morning *in order to initiate the gastrocolic and duodenocolic reflexes and stimulate peristalsis*<br>6. increase activity as allowed and tolerated<br>7. encourage client to perform isometric abdominal strengthening exercises unless contraindicated<br>8. administer laxatives, stool softeners, and/or enemas if ordered.<br>e. Consult physician if signs and symptoms of constipation persist. |

## 9. NURSING DIAGNOSIS: Diarrhea

related to autonomic neuropathy involving the small intestine.

| Desired Outcome | Nursing Actions and ***Selected Purposes/Rationales*** |
|---|---|
| 9. The client will have fewer bowel movements and more formed stool if diarrhea occurs. | 9.a. Ascertain client's usual bowel elimination habits.<br>b. Assess for and report signs and symptoms of diarrhea (e.g. frequent, loose stools; urgency; abdominal pain and cramping). Be aware that the diarrhea that these clients have often occurs at night.<br>c. Assess bowel sounds regularly. Report an increase in frequency of bowel sounds.<br>d. Administer the following medications if ordered *to control diarrhea* (the diarrhea caused by diabetic neuropathy is typically controlled by medications rather than dietary modifications):<br>1. opiate or opiate-like substances (e.g. loperamide, diphenoxylate hydrochloride) *to decrease gastrointestinal motility*<br>2. bulk-forming agents (e.g. methylcellulose, psyllium hydrophilic mucilloid, calcium polycarbophil) *to absorb water in the bowel, which results in a more formed stool*<br>3. antimicrobial agents *(it is thought by some practitioners that diarrhea may be partly due to bacterial overgrowth in the small intestine).*<br>e. Consult physician if diarrhea persists. |

## 10. NURSING DIAGNOSIS: High risk for infection

related to:

a. high glucose levels that create a good medium for growth of pathogens;

b. impaired leukocyte function (appears to be directly related to control of blood glucose levels);
c. delayed healing of any break in skin integrity associated with decreased tissue perfusion and altered nutritional status;
d. increased bacterial growth in urinary tract associated with urinary stasis (can result from retention and decreased mobility if present);
e. stasis of respiratory secretions if mobility is decreased.

| Desired Outcome | Nursing Actions and ***Selected Purposes/Rationales*** |
|---|---|
| 10. The client will remain free of infection as evidenced by:<br>a. absence of fever and chills<br>b. pulse within normal limits<br>c. normal breath sounds<br>d. absence of any unusual vaginal discharge<br>e. voiding clear urine without complaints of frequency, urgency, and burning<br>f. absence of heat, pain, redness, swelling, and unusual drainage in any area<br>g. WBC and differential counts within normal range<br>h. negative results of cultured specimens. | 10.a. Assess for and report signs and symptoms of infection:<br>1. elevated temperature<br>2. chills<br>3. increased pulse<br>4. abnormal breath sounds<br>5. unusual vaginal discharge and pruritus in vulvovaginal area<br>6. cloudy, foul-smelling urine<br>7. complaints of frequency, urgency, or burning when urinating<br>8. presence of WBCs, bacteria, and/or nitrites in urine<br>9. heat, pain, redness, swelling, or unusual drainage in any area<br>10. elevated WBC count and/or significant change in differential.<br>b. Obtain specimens (e.g. urine, vaginal, mouth, sputum, blood) for culture as ordered. Report positive results.<br>c. Implement measures *to prevent infection:*<br>1. maintain a fluid intake of at least 2500 ml/day unless contraindicated<br>2. perform actions to maintain an adequate nutritional status and a near-normal blood glucose level (see Nursing Diagnosis 3, action d)<br>3. instruct and assist client with good oral hygiene<br>4. use good handwashing technique and encourage client to do the same<br>5. maintain meticulous aseptic technique during all invasive procedures (e.g. catheterizations, venous and arterial punctures, injections)<br>6. change equipment and solutions used for procedures such as irrigations and wound care according to hospital policy<br>7. change intravenous tubings and solutions and rotate insertion sites according to hospital policy<br>8. protect client from others with infection<br>9. perform actions to prevent skin breakdown (see Nursing Diagnosis 6, action b)<br>10. perform actions *to prevent infection in any existing wound:*<br>a. instruct client to avoid touching dressings or open wounds<br>b. maintain meticulous aseptic technique during all dressing changes and wound care<br>c. administer antimicrobials if ordered prophylactically<br>11. perform actions *to prevent stasis of respiratory secretions* (e.g. assist client to turn, cough, and deep breathe; increase activity as allowed and tolerated)<br>12. perform actions to prevent urinary retention (see Nursing Diagnosis 7, action d) *in order to prevent urinary stasis*<br>13. perform actions *to prevent the introduction of microorganisms into the urinary tract* (e.g. assist client with perineal care as needed, instruct and assist female client to wipe from front to back after urinating and defecating, maintain sterile technique during urinary catheterization)<br>14. assist female client to maintain meticulous perineal care *in order to reduce risk of vaginal infection.* |

## 11. NURSING DIAGNOSIS: High risk for trauma

related to:

a. falls associated with:
   1. gait abnormalities, decreased ability to perceive position or movement of a body part, diminished or absent reflexes, and/or muscle weakness resulting from motor and sensory neuropathies
   2. dizziness and syncope resulting from postural hypotension (can occur with neuropathy of the autonomic nervous system)
   3. visual disturbances;

b. burns associated with paresthesias that can occur with sensory neuropathy;

c. cuts associated with visual disturbances and decreased ability to perceive position or movement of a body part (results from neuropathy of proprioceptive fibers).

| Desired Outcome | Nursing Actions and ***Selected Purposes/Rationales*** |
|---|---|
| 11. The client will not experience falls, burns, or cuts. | 11.a. Implement measures *to reduce the risk for trauma:*<br>1. perform actions *to prevent falls:*<br>a. keep bed in low position with side rails up when client is in bed<br>b. keep needed items within easy reach<br>c. encourage client to request assistance whenever needed; have call signal within easy reach<br>d. instruct and assist client to get out of bed slowly *in order to reduce dizziness and syncope associated with postural hypotension*<br>e. use lap belt when client is in chair if indicated<br>f. instruct client to wear well-fitting slippers/shoes with nonslip soles and low heels when ambulating<br>g. if vision is impaired, orient client to surroundings, room, and arrangement of furniture and identify obstacles during ambulation<br>h. keep floor free of clutter and wipe up spills promptly<br>i. accompany client during ambulation using a transfer safety belt if he/she is weak or dizzy<br>j. provide ambulatory aids (e.g. walker, cane) if client is weak or unsteady on feet<br>k. instruct client to ambulate in well-lit areas and to use handrails if needed<br>l. do not rush client; allow adequate time for ambulation to the bathroom and in hallway<br>m. make sure that bathtub and shower have nonslip bottom surfaces and that shower chair, secure bath mat, call light, hand grips, and adequate lighting are present<br>2. perform actions *to prevent burns:*<br>a. let hot foods and fluids cool slightly before serving<br>b. supervise client while smoking if indicated<br>c. assess temperature of bath water and heating pad before and during use<br>3. assist client with tasks that require fine motor skills (e.g. shaving) *in order to prevent cuts*<br>4. administer central nervous system depressants judiciously.<br>b. Include client and significant others in planning and implementing measures to prevent trauma.<br>c. If injury does occur, initiate appropriate first aid measures and notify physician. |

**12. COLLABORATIVE DIAGNOSES:**

**Potential acute complications:**

a. **diabetic ketoacidosis (DKA)** related to hyperglycemia and accelerated ketogenesis associated with insulin deficiency and glucagon excess (DKA may be precipitated by administration of inadequate amounts of insulin; excessive food intake; and/or the presence of stressors such as illness, trauma, or infection);
b. **hypoglycemia** related to administration of too much insulin or oral hypoglycemic agent, inadequate food intake, erratic insulin absorption, and/or decreased excretion of insulin if renal function is impaired;
c. **hyperosmolar nonketotic coma** related to severe dehydration associated with sustained osmotic diuresis resulting from uncontrolled hyperglycemia.

| Desired Outcomes | Nursing Actions and ***Selected Purposes/Rationales*** |
|---|---|
| 12.a. The client will not experience ketoacidosis as evidenced by:<br>1. stable vital signs<br>2. usual skin temperature and color<br>3. absence of unusual weakness, lethargy, nausea, vomiting, abdominal pain, and fruity odor on breath<br>4. unlabored respirations at 14-20/minute<br>5. blood glucose less than 300 mg/dl<br>6. absence of ketones in blood and urine<br>7. blood pH and bicarbonate level within normal range. | 12.a.1. Assess for and report signs and symptoms of ketoacidosis (clients at greatest risk are insulin-dependent diabetics):<br>a. evidence of fluid volume deficit (e.g. hypotension; weak, rapid pulse; warm, flushed skin; thirst)<br>b. weakness, lethargy<br>c. nausea, vomiting, abdominal pain<br>d. acetone (fruity) odor on breath<br>e. Kussmaul respirations<br>f. blood glucose above 300 mg/dl<br>g. ketones in blood and urine<br>h. low pH and bicarbonate ($CO_2$ content) level.<br>2. Implement measures to prevent or treat hyperglycemia (see Nursing Diagnosis 2, action b.1) *in order to prevent ketoacidosis.*<br>3. If signs and symptoms of ketoacidosis occur:<br>a. maintain client on bed rest<br>b. administer the following if ordered:<br>1. insulin (usually a continuous intravenous infusion of regular insulin)<br>2. intravenous fluid and electrolyte replacements:<br>a. isotonic or half-strength normal saline (usually rapidly infused until B/P is stabilized and urine output is adequate)<br>b. combination saline and glucose solutions once blood sugar falls to 250-300 mg/dl *(prevents hypoglycemia which could result from the rapid drop in blood sugar)*<br>c. potassium chloride or potassium phosphate *(hypokalemia and hypophosphatemia result from osmotic diuresis and a shift of potassium and phosphorus into the cells during insulin therapy)*<br>d. sodium bicarbonate if the serum pH drops below 7.0-7.1; if bicarbonate is administered, it should be discontinued when the pH reaches 7.2-7.3 *because reversing acidosis too quickly has harmful physiological effects.* |
| 12.b. The client will not experience hypoglycemia as evidenced by:<br>1. pulse rate between 60-100 beats/minute<br>2. absence of palpitations<br>3. warm, dry skin | 12.b.1. Assess for and report signs and symptoms of hypoglycemia (at greatest risk are clients taking insulin or long-acting sulfonureas, those having adjustments in insulin dosages or having difficulty maintaining an adequate oral intake, and clients with liver disease or end-stage renal failure):<br>a. mild hypoglycemia—tachycardia; palpitations; cool, pale skin; diaphoresis; weakness; nervousness; tremors *(these signs and symptoms reflect increased sympathetic nervous system activity)*; be aware that early sympathetic warning symptoms may not be present in some clients *because of a decreased epinephrine output that may occur* |

**Desired Outcomes** | **Nursing Actions and *Selected Purposes/Rationales***

4. usual mental status
5. absence of slurred speech, gait abnormalities, mood swings, and seizures
6. blood glucose above 50 mg/dl.

*with type I diabetes* and that early warning symptoms may also be diminished if client is taking a beta-adrenergic blocking agent

b. moderate hypoglycemia—headache, inability to concentrate, somnolence, slurred speech, staggering gait, mood swings, irrational behavior, double or blurred vision, and confusion *(these signs and symptoms reflect that the brain is being deprived of glucose)*
c. severe hypoglycemia—disorientation, seizures, coma *(these signs and symptoms reflect that the brain cells are starving)*
d. blood glucose below 50 mg/dl.

2. Determine from client whether he/she has nightsweats, nightmares, or an early-morning headache *(these symptoms are indicative of hypoglycemia occurring during sleep).*
3. Implement measures *to prevent hypoglycemia:*
   a. administer insulin as ordered being careful to inject it into an area that has adequate subcutaneous tissue
   b. perform actions *to ensure that client has adequate caloric intake:*
      1. provide meal within 1 hour after administering a rapid-acting insulin (especially routine morning dose)
      2. provide protein snacks in midafternoon and at bedtime if client is receiving an intermediate or long-acting insulin
      3. consult dietitian about appropriate supplements if client does not eat all of the meals and snacks provided
   c. consult physician about altering prescribed insulin dose and/or providing alternative forms of intake (e.g. intravenous therapy) if client is to receive nothing by mouth in preparation for a diagnostic test or surgery or is unable to maintain an adequate oral intake.
4. If signs and symptoms of hypoglycemia occur, administer the following depending on the severity of hypoglycemia:
   a. mild hypoglycemia—10-15 gm of a rapid-acting carbohydrate (e.g. 4-6 oz of juice or regular soft drink, 6-10 Lifesavers, 2 packets of sugar, 2-3 commercial glucose tablets, or glucose gel [e.g. Monogel]); repeat in 10-15 minutes if symptoms have not resolved
   b. moderate hypoglycemia—15-30 gm of a rapid-acting carbohydrate followed in 10-15 minutes by a snack of longer-acting carbohydrate (e.g. glass of low-fat or skim milk, crackers, cheese)
   c. severe hypoglycemia—glucagon or intravenous 50% dextrose solution followed by a simple sugar until nausea subsides, then a small snack or meal.

12.c. The client will not experience hyperosmolar nonketotic coma as evidenced by:
1. stable vital signs
2. usual skin temperature and color
3. absence of motor and sensory deficits and seizure activity
4. blood glucose less than 600 mg/dl.

12.c.1. Assess for and report signs and symptoms of hyperosmolar nonketotic coma (clients at greatest risk are persons over 60 years of age; noninsulin-dependent diabetics; clients with inadequate fluid intake or excessive fluid loss; those who are experiencing unusual emotional or physical stress [e.g. acute illness, infection, surgery]; and clients receiving corticosteroids, diuretics, phenytoin, hyperalimentation, or dialysis treatments):
   a. evidence of fluid volume deficit (e.g. hypotension; weak, rapid pulse; warm, flushed skin; decreased skin turgor; thirst)
   b. extremely high serum osmolality (usually above 350 mOsm/liter)
   c. neurological signs such as hemiparesis, aphasia, lethargy, disorientation, and seizures
   d. blood glucose above 600 mg/dl with absent or only slight elevation of ketones in urine and serum.

2. Implement measures *to prevent hyperosmolar nonketotic coma:*
   a. perform actions *to prevent or treat hyperglycemia* (see Nursing Diagnosis 2, action b.1) *in order to prevent hyperosmolarity and the subsequent osmotic diuresis*
   b. notify physician if client is unable to take in an adequate amount of

oral fluids or if he/she is experiencing diarrhea or unusual emotional stress.

3. If signs and symptoms of hyperosmolar nonketotic coma occur, administer the following if ordered:
   a. fluid replacement (isotonic or half-strength saline is infused rapidly until B/P is stabilized and urine output is adequate; once blood sugar falls to 250-300 mg/dl, 5% glucose is added to prevent hypoglycemia, which could result from the rapid drop in blood sugar)
   b. insulin (usually a continuous intravenous infusion of regular insulin)
   c. intravenous potassium chloride or potassium phosphate *(hypokalemia and hypophosphatemia result from osmotic diuresis and a shift of potassium and phosphorus into the cells during insulin therapy).*

## 13. NURSING DIAGNOSIS: Sexual dysfunction

related to:

a. impotence associated with autonomic neuropathy involving nerves that control erection, decreased penile blood flow resulting from angiopathy, and/or psychogenic factors;
b. decreased libido associated with depression, stress, and discomfort.

| Desired Outcome | Nursing Actions and ***Selected Purposes/Rationales*** |
|---|---|
| 13. The client will perceive self as sexually adequate and acceptable as evidenced by:<br>a. verbalization of same<br>b. maintenance of relationship with significant other. | 13.a. Assess for signs and symptoms of sexual dysfunction (e.g. verbalization of sexual concerns or inability to achieve sexual satisfaction, alteration in relationship with significant other).<br>b. Provide accurate information about the effects of diabetes on sexual functioning. Encourage questions and clarify misconceptions.<br>c. Implement measures *to promote optimal sexual functioning:*<br>1. facilitate communication between client and his/her partner; focus on the feelings the couple share and assist them to identify changes which may affect their sexual relationship<br>2. discuss ways to be creative in expressing sexuality (e.g. massage, fantasies, cuddling)<br>3. arrange for uninterrupted privacy during hospital stay if desired by couple<br>4. if impotence is a problem:<br>a. encourage client to discuss impotence and various treatment options (e.g. penile prosthesis, external vacuum device, papaverine and phentolamine injections) with physician<br>b. suggest alternative methods of sexual gratification if appropriate<br>c. discuss alternative methods of parenting (e.g. adoption, artificial insemination) if of concern to client<br>5. perform actions to reduce feelings of powerlessness and promote effective coping (see Nursing Diagnoses 14, actions c-m and 15, action c) *in order to reduce depression.*<br>d. Include partner in above discussions and encourage his/her continued support of the client.<br>e. Consult physician if counseling appears indicated. |

## 14. NURSING DIAGNOSIS: Powerlessness

related to:
a. disease progression despite efforts to comply with treatment regimen;
b. dependence on others for assistance with care;
c. need to modify life style as a result of having diabetes.

| Desired Outcome | Nursing Actions and ***Selected Purposes/Rationales*** |
|---|---|
| 14. The client will demonstrate increased feelings of control over his/her situation as evidenced by:<br>a. verbalization of same<br>b. active participation in planning of care<br>c. participation in self-care and treatment plan. | 14.a. Assess for behaviors that may indicate feelings of powerlessness (e.g. verbalization of lack of control over self-care or current situation, anger, apathy, hostility, excessive dependency, lack of participation in care planning or self-care).<br>b. Obtain information from client and significant others regarding client's usual response to situations in which he/she has had limited control (e.g. loss of job, financial stress).<br>c. Evaluate with client his/her perceptions of current situation, strengths, weaknesses, expectations, and parts of current situation which are under his/her control. Correct misinformation and inaccurate perceptions and encourage discussion of feelings about areas in which he/she perceives a lack of control.<br>d. Assist client to establish realistic short- and long-term goals.<br>e. Reinforce physician's explanations about diabetes and the importance of adhering to the treatment plan as a way to prevent and/or delay the development of complications. Clarify misconceptions.<br>f. Implement measures to promote effective coping (see Nursing Diagnosis 15, action c) *in order to promote an increased sense of control over his/her situation.*<br>g. Support realistic hope about his/her ability to control the disease process and prevent or delay the development of complications.<br>h. Remind client of his/her right to ask questions about diabetes and the prescribed treatment plan.<br>i. Support client's efforts to increase knowledge of and control over condition. Provide relevant pamphlets and audiovisual materials.<br>j. Include client in the planning of care, encourage maximum participation in the treatment plan, and allow choices whenever possible *to promote a sense of control.*<br>k. Inform client of scheduled procedures and tests *so that unpredictability is eliminated as much as possible and a feeling of control is promoted.*<br>l. Encourage significant others to allow client to do as much as he/she is able *so that a feeling of independence can be maintained.*<br>m. Encourage client's participation in self-help groups if indicated. |

## 15. NURSING DIAGNOSIS: Ineffective individual coping

related to fear of complications and inability to manage them; discomfort; need to alter life style; feeling of powerlessness; knowledge that condition is chronic and will require lifelong medical supervision, dietary regulation, and medication therapy; and an inadequate support system.

| Desired Outcome | Nursing Actions and ***Selected Purposes/Rationales*** |
|---|---|
| 15. The client will demonstrate the use of effective coping skills as evidenced by:<br>a. verbalization of ability to cope with diabetes and its management<br>b. utilization of appropriate problem-solving techniques<br>c. willingness to participate in treatment plan and meet basic needs<br>d. appropriate use of defense mechanisms<br>e. recognition and utilization of available support systems. | 15.a. Assess for and report signs and symptoms of ineffective individual coping (e.g. verbalization of inability to cope; inability to problem solve, ask for help, or meet basic needs; reluctance to participate in treatment plan; inappropriate use of defense mechanisms; inability to meet role expectations).<br>b. Assess client's perception of current situation including precipitating factors and effectiveness of coping mechanisms.<br>c. Implement measures *to promote effective coping:*<br>1. assist client to recognize and manage inappropriate denial if it is present<br>2. encourage verbalization about current situation and ways comparable situations have been handled in the past<br>3. perform actions to reduce feelings of powerlessness (see Nursing Diagnosis 14, actions c-m)<br>4. assist client to identify personal strengths and resources that can be utilized to facilitate coping with the current situation<br>5. create an atmosphere of trust and support<br>6. assist client to maintain usual daily routines whenever possible<br>7. perform actions to reduce discomfort (see Nursing Diagnoses 4.A, action 5 and 4.B, action 3)<br>8. instruct client in effective problem-solving techniques (e.g. identification of stressors, determination of various options to solve problems)<br>9. provide diversional activities according to client's interests and abilities<br>10. assist client as he/she starts to plan for necessary changes in life style<br>11. assist client to identify and utilize available support systems; provide information regarding available community resources that can assist client and significant others in coping with effects of diabetes (e.g. counseling services, diabetic education classes, diabetes support groups)<br>12. encourage client to share with significant others the kind of support that would be most beneficial (e.g. listening, inspiring hope, providing reassurance and accurate information)<br>13. encourage continued emotional support from significant others<br>14. support behaviors suggesting positive adaptation to changes experienced (e.g. active participation in the treatment plan, verbalization of plans for altering life style, verbalization of ability to cope).<br>d. Consult physician about psychological counseling if appropriate. Initiate a referral if necessary. |

## 16. NURSING DIAGNOSIS: Ineffective management of therapeutic regimen

related to:

a. lack of understanding of the implications of not following the prescribed treatment plan;
b. feeling of lack of control over disease progression despite efforts to follow prescribed treatment plan;
c. difficulty modifying personal habits and integrating necessary treatments and dietary regimen into life style;
d. insufficient financial resources.

| Desired Outcome | Nursing Actions and ***Selected Purposes/Rationales*** |
|---|---|
| 16. The client will demonstrate the probability of effective management of the therapeutic regimen as evidenced by:<br>a. willingness to learn about and participate in treatments and care<br>b. statements reflecting ways to modify personal habits and integrate treatments into life style<br>c. statements reflecting an understanding of the implications of not following the prescribed treatment plan. | 16.a. Assess for indications that client may be unable to effectively manage the therapeutic regimen:<br>1. statements reflecting that he/she was unable to manage care at home<br>2. failure to adhere to treatment plan while in hospital (e.g. refusing medications, not adhering to dietary restrictions)<br>3. statements reflecting a lack of understanding of factors that contribute to acute and chronic complications<br>4. statements reflecting an unwillingness or inability to modify personal habits and integrate necessary treatments into life style<br>5. statements reflecting the view that diabetes is curable or that the situation is hopeless and that efforts to comply with treatments are useless.<br>b. Implement measures *to promote effective management of the therapeutic regimen:*<br>1. determine client's understanding of diabetes; clarify misconceptions and stress the fact that diabetes is a chronic condition and adherence to the treatment plan may delay and/or prevent complications; caution client that some complications may occur despite strict adherence to treatment plan<br>2. encourage client to participate in assessments and treatments (e.g. blood glucose monitoring, selection of diet, insulin administration)<br>3. review with client his/her technique for drawing up and administering insulin, testing blood glucose, and menu selection; determine areas of difficulty and misunderstanding and reinforce teaching as necessary<br>4. provide client with written instructions about future appointments with health care provider, diet, medications, exercise, and signs and symptoms to report<br>5. discuss with client difficulties he/she has had incorporating treatments into life style; assist client to identify ways to modify life style rather than completely change it<br>6. encourage client to discuss his/her concerns about the cost of medications, food, and supplies; obtain a social service consult to assist with financial planning and obtain financial aid if indicated<br>7. perform actions to reduce feeling of powerlessness and promote effective coping (see Nursing Diagnoses 14, actions c-m and 15, action c)<br>8. initiate and reinforce the discharge teaching outlined in Nursing Diagnosis 17 *in order to promote a sense of control and self-reliance*<br>9. encourage client to attend follow-up diabetic education classes<br>10. provide information about and encourage utilization of resources that can assist client to make necessary life-style changes (e.g. diabetes support groups, counseling services, American Diabetes Association, diabetic cookbooks, publications such as Diabetes Forecast)<br>11. reinforce behaviors suggesting future compliance with the therapeutic regimen (e.g participation in the treatment plan, statements reflecting plans for integrating treatments into life style)<br>12. include significant others in explanations and teaching sessions and encourage their support; reinforce the need for client to assume responsibility for managing as much of care as possible.<br>c. Consult physician about referrals to community health agencies if continued instruction or supervision is needed. |

## 17. NURSING DIAGNOSIS: Knowledge deficit

regarding follow-up care.

| Desired Outcomes | Nursing Actions and ***Selected Purposes/Rationales*** |
|---|---|
| 17.a. The client will verbalize a basic understanding of diabetes mellitus. | 17.a. Determine from client his/her understanding of diabetes mellitus. Clarify misconceptions and reinforce teaching as necessary. Utilize available teaching aids (e.g. pamphlets, videotapes). |
| 17.b. The client will verbalize an understanding of medications ordered including rationale, side effects, schedule for taking, and importance of taking as prescribed. | 17.b.1. Explain the rationale for, side effects of, and importance of taking medications prescribed.<br>2. Provide the following instructions if client is to administer own insulin injections after discharge:<br>a. store the bottle(s) of insulin currently being used at room temperature unless the room temperature is above 86° F (insulin is stable for up to 1 month at room temperature)<br>b. store unopened bottle(s) of insulin in refrigerator<br>c. periodically check expiration date and discard outdated bottle(s) of insulin<br>d. do not use insulin that has changed color or contains granules or clumped particles<br>e. let refrigerated insulin return to room temperature before use if possible<br>f. do not change type or strength of insulin unless directed by physician<br>g. rotate injection sites using the following guidelines:<br>1. no site should be used more than once a month<br>2. there should be at least 2.5 cm (1 inch) between sites<br>3. avoid giving injections right at the waistline or within 2.5 cm (1 inch) of the umbilicus<br>4. avoid using an area that will be heavily exercised that day (insulin will be more rapidly absorbed from that area)<br>5. do not give injections into areas where the skin appears raised, thickened, or "wasted"<br>h. clean insulin delivery devices per manufacturer's instructions<br>i. plan meals and snacks keeping the onset, peak action, and length of action of the insulin(s) prescribed in mind<br>j. adjust insulin dosage based on blood sugar results and parameters established by physician<br>k. consult health care provider immediately if unable to tolerate food or fluid for 4 hours<br>l. if local reaction such as itching, redness, or tenderness occurs after injections and persists for more than 4 weeks, consult health care provider<br>m. always have a rapid-acting carbohydrate readily available (e.g. glucose tablets, hard candy, sugar cubes or packets, small tube of cake icing [e.g. Cakemate gel]) and take when initial symptoms of hypoglycemia occur; if symptoms do not subside after taking a rapid-acting carbohydrate every 10-15 minutes within a 30-minute period, contact health care provider immediately<br>n. consult health care provider if repeated episodes of sweating, nervousness, weakness, hunger, shakiness, slurred speech, blurred or double vision, and difficulty concentrating occur (may indicate need to reduce insulin dose)<br>o. consult health care provider if experiencing unusual emotional or physical stress (e.g. acute illness, physical trauma, pregnancy) so that insulin dose can be increased to provide adequate coverage.<br>3. If client is discharged with a button infuser or an insulin pump device, provide instructions regarding its management (e.g. changing the needle and tubing or device every 1-3 days, filling syringes, changing batteries in pump). Allow time for practice and return demonstration. |

| Desired Outcomes | Nursing Actions and ***Selected Purposes/Rationales*** |
|---|---|
| | 4. If client is discharged on an oral hypoglycemic agent, instruct to:<br>a. take medication exactly as prescribed<br>b. notify health care provider if unable to tolerate food and fluid<br>c. limit alcohol intake to small amounts and be aware that a hypersensitivity to alcohol as evidenced by nausea, vomiting, shortness of breath, sweating, weakness, flushing of face, or pounding heartbeat sometimes develops when taking an oral hypoglycemic agent (most frequently occurs with chlorpropamide)<br>d. adhere strictly to the prescribed diet (oral hypoglycemics are not a substitute for good dietary management)<br>e. consult health care provider if experiencing unusual emotional or physical stress (e.g. acute illness, physical injury) so that dosage may be adjusted to provide adequate coverage.<br>5. Instruct client to consult health care provider before taking other prescription and nonprescription medications.<br>6. Instruct client to inform all health care providers of medications being taken. |
| 17.c. The client will demonstrate the ability to correctly draw up and administer insulin if prescribed. | 17.c. If client is to be discharged on insulin, reinforce the following instructions regarding preparation and administration:<br>1. mix insulin before use by gently rotating or rolling bottle between palms or palm and thigh; do not vigorously shake the bottle<br>2. read the label carefully, making sure the syringe and insulin concentrations match and that it is the correct type of insulin (e.g. regular, NPH)<br>3. clean the top of the bottle(s) with alcohol<br>4. withdraw the correct amount of insulin making sure to remove air bubbles<br>5. if mixing two insulins, withdraw in the same order every time (usually recommended that the rapid-acting insulin be drawn up first in order to reduce the risk of contaminating the vial of rapid-acting insulin with a longer-acting insulin)<br>6. insert needle into subcutaneous tissue and inject insulin (the recommended technique for insulin administration may vary among institutions and should be reviewed before client teaching)<br>7. following insulin injection, apply gentle pressure to site rather than rubbing it. |
| 17.d. The client will verbalize an understanding of the principles of dietary management and be able to calculate and plan meals within the prescribed caloric distribution. | 17.d.1. Reinforce dietary instructions regarding the prescribed diabetic diet and methods of calculating the foods/fluids allowed (e.g. ADA exchange list).<br>2. Have client plan sample menus before discharge to ensure that he/she is able to calculate the diet correctly.<br>3. Explain the purpose of weight reduction if client has been placed on a reducing diet. Reinforce need to avoid fasting and fad diets.<br>4. Instruct client on appropriate dietary adjustments that should be made if meal schedule or activity level has been significantly altered.<br>5. Reinforce the following principles of good dietary management:<br>a. eat 3 or more regularly spaced meals each day and do not skip meals<br>b. weigh or measure foods rather than estimating serving sizes<br>c. avoid intake of concentrated sweets (e.g. sugar, candy, syrups, jams, jellies, cakes, pies, pastries, fruits packed in heavy syrup) and foods high in saturated fat and cholesterol (e.g. butter, cheese, eggs, ice cream, red meat)<br>d. read processed food/fluid labels and avoid those foods/fluids that contain significant amounts of sugar, honey, and alternative forms of sugar such as xylitol, sorbitol, and fructose<br>e. incorporate any alcoholic beverages consumed into diabetic diet by substituting for fat exchanges. |

17.e. The client will demonstrate the ability to correctly perform blood glucose and urine tests and accurately interpret results.

17.e.1. Review with client how to perform a capillary blood glucose (CBG) measurement and test urine for ketones.
2. Have client demonstrate blood and urine tests. Reinforce teaching as necessary.
3. Instruct client to keep a record of test results.
4. Provide instructions on actions client should take when test results are abnormal (some clients are instructed to adjust insulin dose and dietary intake; others are instructed to notify appropriate health care provider).

17.f. The client will verbalize an understanding of the role of exercise in the management of diabetes.

17.f.1. Explain how exercise affects blood sugar levels.
2. Provide the following instructions about exercise:
   a. maintain a regular exercise program
   b. wait 1-1½ hours after meals to engage in exercise
   c. avoid exercising during insulin peak action time
   d. adjust dietary intake if there are significant changes in activity level (insulin-dependent diabetics should eat a 10-15 gm carbohydrate snack before planned increases in activity)
   e. perform blood glucose tests more frequently during periods of significant variation in activity level
   f. avoid exercise if blood sugar is greater than 250 mg/dl and ketones are present in urine
   g. carry a rapid-acting carbohydrate source (e.g. hard candy, glucose tablets) during exercise (especially if insulin dependent and if exercise is expected to be prolonged or vigorous)
   h. stop any activity that causes extreme weakness, trembling, incoordination, or nausea.

17.g. The client will identify health care and hygiene practices that should be integrated into life style.

17.g.1. Reinforce the importance of adhering to the following health care practices:
   a. daily oral hygiene including brushing and flossing teeth
   b. regular dental appointments
   c. regular eye examinations
   d. not smoking (smoking contributes to the risk of cardiovascular complications)
   e. meticulous care of cuts, burns, and scratches.
2. Provide instructions about foot care:
   a. inspect feet daily for cuts, redness, cracks, blisters, corns, and calluses; use a mirror to check bottoms of feet if necessary
   b. wash feet daily with a mild soap and warm water and dry gently but thoroughly
   c. apply lanolin or other lubricating lotion to feet (except between toes) daily
   d. keep feet dry by:
      1. applying a mild powder
      2. wearing cotton socks
      3. avoiding shoes with rubber or plastic soles (cause feet to sweat)
   e. soak feet before cutting nails, cut nails straight across, and smooth them with an emery board after cutting
   f. see a podiatrist rather than using home remedies to treat corns, calluses, and ingrown nails
   g. avoid wearing socks, stockings, or garters that are tight (may further compromise peripheral blood flow)
   h. buy shoes that fit well and break them in gradually
   i. wear shoes or slippers when walking to protect feet from injury
   j. do not use a heating pad or hot water bottle on feet (if paresthesias are present, burns may occur)
   k. protect feet from extreme cold to prevent vasoconstriction and possible frostbite.

17.h. The client will identify appropriate safety measures to

17.h. Teach client the following safety precautions:
1. always carry an identification card and wear a Medic-Alert tag
2. always carry a rapid-acting carbohydrate such as Lifesavers, sugar

| Desired Outcomes | Nursing Actions and ***Selected Purposes/Rationales*** |
|---|---|
| follow because of the diagnosis of diabetes. | cubes or packets, or glucose tablets<br>3. if insulin-dependent, always have insulin readily available (carry in purse or briefcase)<br>4. consult physician about plans for pregnancy and maintain close prenatal supervision<br>5. keep a glucagon kit readily available and know how and when to use it; make sure significant other is also trained in how to use it<br>6. if ill but able to tolerate some foods/fluids:<br>a. take usual dose of insulin or oral hypoglycemic agent<br>b. consume soft foods or liquids from bread/starch, milk, fruit, and vegetable exchange list if unable to tolerate usual diet or drink at least 4 ounces of a sugar-containing liquid every hour<br>c. test blood glucose and urine ketones every 4 hours<br>d. do not exercise<br>7. notify physician if oral intake is inadequate for longer than 24 hours, vomiting or severe diarrhea persists for more than 4 hours, and/or blood glucose is significantly higher than usual and ketones are present in urine<br>8. inform all health care providers of diabetic condition. |
| 17.i. The client will state signs and symptoms of hypoglycemia and ketoacidosis and appropriate actions for prevention and treatment. | 17.i.1. Reinforce the following information about hypoglycemia:<br>a. factors that precipitate hypoglycemia (e.g. too much insulin or oral hypoglycemic agent, insufficient oral intake, excessive exercise, excessive alcohol intake)<br>b. signs and symptoms of hypoglycemia (e.g. shakiness, nervousness, weakness, hunger, sweating, nightmares, early-morning headache, incoordination, blood sugar less than 50)<br>c. actions to take if signs and symptoms of hypoglycemia occur:<br>1. immediately take a rapid-acting carbohydrate (e.g. half a glass of orange or grapefruit juice or regular soft drink, 2 teaspoons of honey or syrup, 2 packets or cubes of sugar, 6-10 Lifesavers, glucose tablets)<br>2. if symptoms persist, take the same amount of carbohydrate again every 10-15 minutes; consult health care provider if symptoms persist for more than 30 minutes<br>3. after the hypoglycemic episode, consume a longer-acting carbohydrate snack (e.g. crackers, glass of low-fat or skim milk).<br>2. Teach significant others how to prepare and administer glucagon in case client loses consciousness.<br>3. Reinforce the following information about ketoacidosis:<br>a. factors that precipitate ketoacidosis (e.g. emotional stress, infection, failure to take insulin or oral hypoglycemic agent, dietary excess)<br>b. signs and symptoms of impending or actual ketoacidosis (e.g. unusual thirst; excessive urination; weakness; warm, flushed skin; blood sugar higher than 300; ketones in urine; abdominal pain; nausea and vomiting)<br>c. immediate actions to take if signs and symptoms of ketoacidosis occur:<br>1. drink a cup or more of broth or tea if able to tolerate it<br>2. administer insulin (if previously instructed in insulin coverage based on blood glucose results)<br>3. consult health care provider. |
| 17.j. The client will state signs and symptoms to report to the health care provider. | 17.j. Instruct client to report the following:<br>1. unexplained episodes of hypoglycemia and ketoacidosis (see actions i.1.b and 3.b in this diagnosis for signs and symptoms)<br>2. unusual variations in blood glucose results<br>3. a cut, scratch, or burn that becomes red, swollen, tender, or does not start to heal within 24 hours |

4. nausea and vomiting or severe diarrhea that lasts more than 4 hours
5. temperature elevation that lasts more than 2 days
6. change in vision
7. development or worsening of symptoms that are indicative of long-term complications (e.g. burning or aching pain in extremity, decreased sensation in extremity, persistent gastric discomfort, frequent urination of small amounts, impotence, gait disturbances, chest pain, extreme fatigue, persistent dizziness or lightheadedness).

17.k. The client will identify resources that can assist in the adjustment to and management of diabetes.

17.k.1. Provide information about resources that can assist client and significant others in adjustment to and management of diabetes (e.g. American Diabetes Association, diabetic education classes, weight loss programs, diabetes support groups, counseling services, publications such as Diabetes Forecast).
2. Initiate a referral if indicated.

17.l. The client will verbalize an understanding of and a plan for adhering to recommended follow-up care including future appointments with health care provider and for laboratory studies.

17.l. 1. Reinforce the importance of keeping follow-up appointments with health care provider and for laboratory studies.
2. Refer to Nursing Diagnosis 16, action b, for measures to promote the client's ability to effectively manage the therapeutic regimen.

# Thyroidectomy

Thyroidectomy is the surgical removal of the thyroid gland. It may be performed to treat thyroid carcinoma, unusually large goiters, or hyperthyroidism that has been refractory to conservative treatment. A subtotal thyroidectomy (removal of up to 90% of the thyroid gland) is the preferred procedure unless the surgery is being done to treat a malignancy, in which case a total thyroidectomy will usually be performed. Following a subtotal thyroidectomy, the remaining gland tissue usually hypertrophies enough to supply adequate amounts of thyroid hormone.

The client is usually given antithyroid agents for 4-6 weeks prior to hospitalization for a thyroidectomy in order to achieve a euthyroid state and minimize the risk of thyroid crisis. Iodine preparations are also administered for 7-10 days prior to surgery to reduce vascularity of the thyroid gland and the risk for hemorrhage in the intraoperative and postoperative period. During this prehospitalization period, it is also important for an optimal nutritional state and cardiovascular status to be attained.

**This care plan focuses on the adult client with hyperthyroidism whose condition has been medically stabilized and who is being hospitalized for a subtotal thyroidectomy.** Preoperative goals of care are to reduce fear and anxiety and educate the client regarding postoperative care. Postoperatively, the goals of care are to maintain comfort, prevent complications, and educate the client regarding follow-up care.

## DISCHARGE CRITERIA

Prior to discharge, the client will:

- have no signs and symptoms of complications
- verbalize an understanding of range of motion exercises of the neck
- state signs and symptoms to report to the health care provider
- verbalize an understanding of and a plan for adhering to recommended follow-

up care including future appointments with health care provider, medications prescribed, activity level, and wound care.

**NURSING/ COLLABORATIVE DIAGNOSES**



**See Standardized Preoperative and Postoperative Care Plans for additional diagnoses.**

## PREOPERATIVE

**Use in conjunction with the Standardized Preoperative Care Plan.**

### 1. NURSING DIAGNOSIS: Knowledge deficit

regarding hospital routines associated with surgery, physical preparation for a thyroidectomy, sensations that normally occur following surgery and anesthesia, and postoperative care.

| Desired Outcomes | Nursing Actions and ***Selected Purposes/Rationales*** |
|---|---|
| 1.a. The client will verbalize an understanding of usual preoperative care and postoperative sensations and care. | 1.a.1. Refer to Standardized Preoperative Care Plan, Nursing Diagnosis 4, actions a.1-4 (pp. 111-112), for information to include in preoperative teaching.<br>2. Inform client that he/she will be assessed for voice changes routinely after surgery. Explain that hoarseness is expected for a few days and unnecessary talking should be avoided during that time.<br>3. Allow time for questions and clarification of information provided. |
| 1.b. The client will demonstrate the ability to perform activities designed to prevent postoperative complications. | 1.b.1. Refer to Standardized Preoperative Care Plan, Nursing Diagnosis 4, action b.1 (p. 112), for instructions on ways to prevent postoperative complications.<br>2. Provide additional instructions on ways to prevent complications after a thyroidectomy:<br>a. instruct client on ways to minimize stress on the suture line:<br>1. support head and neck with hands when turning head, coughing, and moving in bed for first few days after surgery<br>2. avoid turning head abruptly and hyperextending neck<br>b. inform client that he/she will need to do neck range of motion exercises beginning 2-4 days after surgery; demonstrate flexion, extension, rotation, and lateral movement of head and neck.<br>3. Allow time for questions, clarification, and return demonstration. |

## POSTOPERATIVE

**Use in conjunction with the Standardized Postoperative Care Plan.**

### 1. NURSING DIAGNOSIS: Ineffective airway clearance

related to:
a. blockage of pharynx by base of tongue associated with muscular flaccidity resulting from effects of anesthesia and some medications (e.g. narcotic analgesics);
b. stasis of secretions associated with:
   1. decreased activity
   2. poor cough effort resulting from the effects of anesthesia and some medications (e.g. narcotic analgesics), pain, weakness, and fear of disrupting incision;
c. increased secretions associated with irritation of the respiratory tract (can result from inhalation anesthetics and endotracheal intubation);
d. tracheal compression associated with edema or bleeding in the surgical area.

| Desired Outcome | Nursing Actions and ***Selected Purposes/Rationales*** |
|---|---|
| 1. The client will maintain clear, open airways (see Standardized Postoperative Care Plan, Nursing Diagnosis 3 [p. 115], for outcome criteria). | 1.a. Refer to Standardized Postoperative Care Plan, Nursing Diagnosis 3 (pp. 115-116) for measures related to assessment and promotion of effective airway clearance.<br>b. Implement additional measures *to promote effective airway clearance:*<br>1. perform actions *to minimize edema in the surgical area and subsequently reduce pressure on the trachea:*<br>a. keep head of bed elevated at least 30°<br>b. apply ice packs to neck as ordered *to reduce inflammation*<br>2. perform actions to reduce stress on the incision (see Postoperative Nursing Diagnosis 2, action b) *in order to reduce the risk of bleeding and a subsequent increase in pressure on the trachea.* |

### 2. NURSING DIAGNOSIS: Impaired skin integrity

related to:
a. disruption of skin associated with the surgical procedure;
b. delayed wound healing associated with decreased nutritional status and unusual stress on incision (can result from excessive movement of head and neck, persistent or vigorous coughing, vomiting, and edema or hematoma formation at the surgical site).

| Desired Outcome | Nursing Actions and ***Selected Purposes/Rationales*** |
|---|---|
| 2. The client will experience normal healing of surgical wound (see Standardized Postoperative Care Plan, Nursing Diagnosis 9, outcome a [p. 122], for outcome criteria). | 2.a. Refer to Standardized Postoperative Care Plan, Nursing Diagnosis 9, action a (pp. 122-123), for measures related to assessment and promotion of wound healing.<br>b. Implement additional measures *to reduce stress on the incision:*<br>1. place client in a semi-Fowler's position with small pillow under head<br>2. maintain client's head and neck in proper alignment using pillows or sandbags<br>3. support client's head and neck during position change until client is able to do so independently |

| Desired Outcome | Nursing Actions and ***Selected Purposes/Rationales*** |
|---|---|
| | 4. reinforce preoperative instructions about supporting head and neck and remind client to avoid turning head abruptly and hyperextending neck<br>5. perform actions to prevent nausea and vomiting (see Standardized Postoperative Care Plan, Nursing Diagnosis 7.B, action 2 [p. 120])<br>6. place personal articles and call signal within easy reach *so client does not have to turn head and neck or strain to reach them*<br>7. focus on deep breathing and use of incentive spirometer rather than vigorous coughing to promote an effective breathing pattern and airway clearance (some physicians prefer that client not cough *because it increases stress on suture line)*<br>8. stress importance of doing neck range of motion exercises gently (exercises are usually started 2-4 days postoperatively). |

## 3. COLLABORATIVE DIAGNOSES:

**Potential complications:**

a. **hemorrhage** related to surgery in a highly vascular area;
b. **respiratory distress** related to airway obstruction associated with:
   1. tracheal compression resulting from edema or bleeding in the surgical area
   2. closure of the glottis resulting from paralysis of the vocal cords (can occur with injury to the bilateral recurrent laryngeal nerves)
   3. laryngeal spasm resulting from calcium deficiency;
c. **hypocalcemia** related to damage to or inadvertent removal of the parathyroid gland(s) during surgery;
d. **thyroid storm (thyrotoxic crisis)**—a rare complication that is possibly related to an altered peripheral response to thyroid hormone and sympathetic nervous system stimulation associated with surgical trauma;
e. **recurrent laryngeal nerve damage** related to surgical trauma or compression of the nerve(s) associated with edema or bleeding in the surgical area.

| Desired Outcomes | Nursing Actions and ***Selected Purposes/Rationales*** |
|---|---|
| 3.a. The client will not have excessive bleeding in the surgical area as evidenced by:<br>1. absence of feeling of tightness of neck dressing and sensation of pressure or fullness at incision site<br>2. expected amount of drainage on dressing<br>3. absence of excessive swallowing, choking sensation, and respiratory distress<br>4. stable vital signs. | 3.a.1. Assess for and report signs and symptoms of hemorrhage (e.g. increased tightness of neck dressing; complaints of fullness or pressure in neck; excessive bloody drainage on dressing, pillow, or back of neck; statements of excessive swallowing or a choking sensation; difficulty breathing; tachycardia; decline in B/P).<br>2. Implement measures *to reduce the risk of hemorrhage:*<br>a. maintain pressure dressing over incision site as ordered<br>b. perform actions to reduce stress on the incision (see Postoperative Nursing Diagnosis 2, action b)<br>c. perform actions *to decrease venous pressure in the surgical area:*<br>1. keep head of bed elevated at least 30°<br>2. discourage vigorous coughing<br>d. apply ice packs to neck as ordered.<br>3. If signs and symptoms of bleeding occur:<br>a. loosen dressing *to promote drainage of blood and reduce the risk of respiratory distress*<br>b. notify physician<br>c. assist with suture/clip removal and drainage of hematoma if indicated<br>d. assist with emergency tracheostomy if respiratory distress develops<br>e. prepare client for surgical intervention (e.g. ligation of bleeding vessels) if planned<br>f. provide emotional support to client and significant others. |

3.b. The client will not experience respiratory distress as evidenced by:
1. unlabored respirations at 14-20/minute
2. absence of stridor and sternocleidomastoid muscle retraction
3. usual mental status
4. usual skin color
5. blood gases within normal range.

3.b.1. Assess for and immediately report:
a. increased edema or expanding hematoma in surgical area
b. deviation of trachea from midline
c. persistent or increased difficulty swallowing or choking sensation
d. signs and symptoms of respiratory distress (e.g. rapid and/or labored respirations, stridor, sternocleidomastoid muscle retraction, restlessness, agitation, cyanosis)
e. abnormal blood gases
f. significant changes in oximetry results.

2. Have oxygen and skin clip or suture removal, tracheostomy, and suction equipment readily available.
3. Implement measures *to prevent respiratory distress:*
a. perform actions to minimize edema in the surgical area (see Postoperative Nursing Diagnosis 1, action b.1)
b. perform actions to reduce the risk of hemorrhage or treat bleeding if it occurs (see actions a.2 and 3 in this diagnosis)
c. assess for and immediately report signs and symptoms of hypocalcemia (see action c.1 in this diagnosis) *so that treatment can be initiated and risk of laryngeal spasm reduced.*
4. If signs and symptoms of respiratory distress occur:
a. place client in a high Fowler's position unless he/she is hypotensive
b. loosen dressing on neck *to prevent further compression of trachea*
c. maintain oxygen therapy as ordered
d. suction client if indicated
e. assist with emergency tracheostomy if performed
f. provide emotional support to client and significant others.

3.c. The client will experience resolution of hypocalcemia if it occurs as evidenced by:
1. usual mental status
2. absence of numbness and tingling in fingers, toes, and circumoral area
3. negative Chvostek's and Trousseau's signs
4. regular pulse at 60-100 beats/minute
5. absence of muscle twitching and spasms and seizure activity
6. serum calcium level within normal range.

3.c.1. Assess for and report signs and symptoms of hypocalcemia (e.g. anxiousness; irritability; numbness or tingling of fingers, toes, or circumoral area; positive Chvostek's and Trousseau's signs; cardiac arrhythmias; muscle twitching or spasms; seizures; low serum calcium).
2. If signs and symptoms of hypocalcemia occur:
a. institute seizure precautions
b. perform actions to treat respiratory distress if it occurs (see action b.4 in this diagnosis)
c. administer oral calcium preparations or intravenous calcium gluconate or calcium chloride if ordered
d. provide emotional support to client and significant others.

3.d. The client will not develop thyroid storm as evidenced by:
1. stable vital signs
2. usual mental status
3. absence of tremors, nausea, vomiting, and diarrhea.

3.d.1. Assess for and report signs and symptoms of thyroid storm:
a. significant temperature elevation (usually above 39° C), profuse diaphoresis
b. marked increase in client's usual pulse rate and B/P
c. increasing restlessness
d. agitation, irritability, tremors
e. nausea, vomiting, diarrhea
f. delirium, coma.
2. If signs and symptoms of thyroid storm occur:

| Desired Outcomes | Nursing Actions and ***Selected Purposes/Rationales*** |
|---|---|
| | a. utilize hypothermia techniques (e.g. cooling blanket, tepid sponge bath) *to reduce fever*<br>b. maintain intravenous fluid and electrolyte therapy as ordered<br>c. maintain oxygen therapy as ordered<br>d. institute appropriate safety measures if client is irrational, delirious, or comatose<br>e. administer the following medications if ordered:<br>1. antipyretics *to reduce fever* (avoid aspirin *because it increases free thyroid hormone levels*)<br>2. antithyroid agents (e.g. propylthiouracil, methimazole) and iodine preparations (e.g. sodium iodide) *to suppress production and release of thyroid hormone from the remaining thyroid tissue; propylthiouracil also blocks the peripheral conversion of $T_4$ to the more potent $T_3$*<br>3. glucocorticoids (e.g. dexamethasone, hydrocortisone) *to aid the body in handling stress, replenish endogenous glucocorticoids that have probably been depleted by the increased metabolism, and block the peripheral conversion of $T_4$ to $T_3$*<br>4. adrenergic inhibiting agents (e.g. propranolol) *to reduce the severity of many of the clinical manifestations*<br>5. vitamin supplements *to replace vitamins used during increased metabolism*<br>f. provide emotional support to client and significant others. |
| 3.e. The client will experience resolution of recurrent laryngeal nerve damage if it occurs as evidenced by:<br>1. improved voice tone and quality<br>2. gradual resolution of hoarseness<br>3. absence of respiratory distress. | 3.e.1. Assess for the following indications of recurrent laryngeal nerve damage:<br>a. voice changes (e.g. hoarseness; weak, whispery voice; inability to speak)<br>b. respiratory distress (see action b.1.d in this diagnosis for signs and symptoms).<br>2. Implement measures *to reduce the risk of recurrent laryngeal nerve damage:*<br>a. perform actions to reduce edema in the surgical area (see Postoperative Nursing Diagnosis 1, action b.1)<br>b. perform actions to reduce the risk of hemorrhage or treat bleeding if it occurs (see actions a.2 and 3 in this diagnosis).<br>3. If signs and symptoms of recurrent laryngeal nerve damage occur:<br>a. encourage client to avoid unnecessary talking in order to rest the vocal cords<br>b. implement measures *to facilitate communication* (e.g. ask questions that require a short answer or nod of head, provide materials such as magic slate or pad and pencil, answer call signal in person rather than using intercommunication system)<br>c. notify physician immediately if signs and symptoms of respiratory distress occur, client is unable to speak, or hoarseness or voice changes worsen. |

## 4. NURSING DIAGNOSIS: Knowledge deficit

regarding follow-up care.

| Desired Outcomes | Nursing Actions and ***Selected Purposes/Rationales*** |
|---|---|
| 4.a. The client will verbalize an | 4.a.1. Reinforce preoperative teaching about range of motion exercises of the neck. Instruct client to do the exercises as prescribed by physician |

understanding of range of motion exercises of the neck. (exercises are usually begun 2-4 days after surgery and are done 3-4 times/day for a few weeks).

2. Allow time for questions and clarification.

4.b. The client will state signs and symptoms to report to the health care provider.

4.b.1. Refer to Standardized Postoperative Care Plan, Nursing Diagnosis 21, action c (p. 135), for signs and symptoms to report to the health care provider.

2. Instruct client to also report signs and symptoms of:
   a. recurrent hyperthyroidism (e.g. insomnia, heat intolerance, diarrhea, restlessness, unexplained weight loss)
   b. hypothyroidism (e.g. unexplained weight gain, persistent fatigue and weakness, drowsiness, cold intolerance, constipation)
   c. hypoparathyroidism (e.g. numbness or tingling of toes or fingers or around mouth, muscle twitching or spasms).

4.c. The client will verbalize an understanding of and a plan for adhering to recommended follow-up care including future appointments with health care provider, medications prescribed, activity level, and wound care.

4.c.1. Refer to Standardized Postoperative Care Plan, Nursing Diagnosis 21 (pp. 135-136), for routine postoperative instructions and measures to improve client compliance.

2. Teach client the rationale for, side effects of, schedule for taking, and importance of taking medications prescribed (e.g. thyroid hormone, calcium supplements).

UNIT

# XVII

# *Nursing Care of the Client with Disturbances of Musculoskeletal Function*

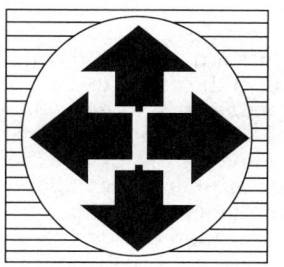

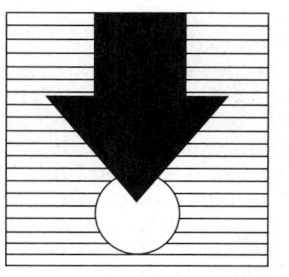

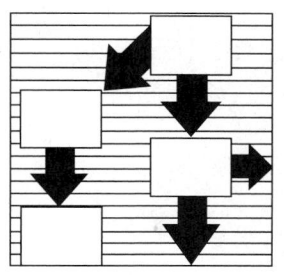

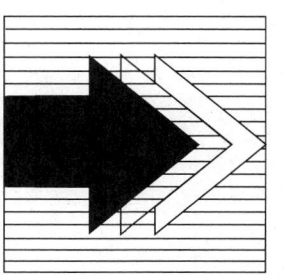

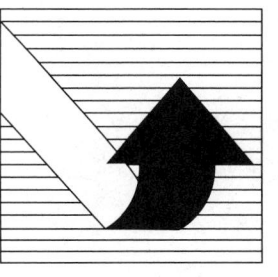

# Amputation

An amputation is the removal of all or part of a limb. Amputation of the upper extremities is usually the result of trauma and tends to occur in younger people. The majority of amputations, however, are surgically performed and involve the lower extremities of persons with inadequate peripheral circulation resulting from atherosclerosis or diabetes mellitus. In these instances, amputation is considered to be a reconstructive surgery performed to improve quality of life by relieving severe, persistent discomfort. Amputation may also be indicated in the treatment of clients who have experienced severe tissue destruction as a result of mechanical or thermal trauma, cancer, uncontrollable infection, gangrene, or congenital anomalies.

The two types of surgical amputations are open and closed. The open or guillotine type is used for the client with an infected limb. The wound is left open, treated until infection resolves, and then closed during a second surgical procedure. A closed amputation, which consists of soft tissue flaps sutured over the bone, is performed on the client with no evidence of infection. The point of amputation is determined by the adequacy of circulation in the involved extremity and by prosthetic requirements. A disarticulation is a closed amputation of a limb through a joint.

The three basic techniques for postoperative residual limb management are the use of a soft compression dressing with delayed prosthetic fitting, casting with early prosthetic fitting (usually in 10-30 days), and casting with immediate prosthetic fitting. The technique selected depends on the underlying pathological condition, physiological and psychological status of the client, and his/her age.

**This care plan focuses on the adult client hospitalized for a planned below the knee, closed amputation.** Preoperatively, goals of care are to reduce fear and anxiety and educate the client regarding postoperative care and expectations. Goals of postoperative care are to maintain comfort, prevent complications, assist the client to adjust to the change in body image and effects of the amputation on mobility, assist with rehabilitative efforts, and educate the client regarding follow-up care. If an above the knee amputation is planned, refer to medical-surgical nursing texts for additional nursing diagnoses and related actions that might be appropriate.

## DIAGNOSTIC TESTS

Arteriography
Doppler ultrasonography
Laser doppler measurements
Skin fluorescent studies
Xenon$^{133}$ ($^{133}$Xe) skin clearance
Plethysmography
Transcutaneous oxygen tension
Skin perfusion pressure measurements

## DISCHARGE CRITERIA

Prior to discharge, the client will:

- have no signs and symptoms of complications
- demonstrate appropriate ways to prevent contractures, increase strength, and improve mobility
- demonstrate the ability to transfer self safely
- identify ways to assess and maintain health of the remaining extremities
- demonstrate the ability to appropriately care for the residual limb
- verbalize how to appropriately care for the prosthesis
- identify ways to manage phantom limb pain if it occurs
- state signs and symptoms to report to the health care provider
- share feelings and thoughts about the change in body image and effects of the amputation on life style and roles
- identify community resources that can assist with home management and adjustment to changes resulting from the amputation
- verbalize an understanding of and a plan for adhering to recommended follow-up care including future appointments with health care provider, prosthetist, and physical therapist; medications prescribed; and activity level.

**NURSING/ COLLABORATIVE DIAGNOSES**

**Preoperative**



**Postoperative**



**See Standardized Preoperative and Postoperative Care lans for additional diagnoses.**

## PREOPERATIVE

**Use in conjunction with the Standardized Preoperative Care Plan.**

### 1. NURSING DIAGNOSIS: Anxiety

related to:
a. impending mutilating surgery;
b. lack of understanding of diagnostic tests and reason for amputation;
c. anticipated loss of control, effects of anesthesia, and postoperative pain;
d. unfamiliar environment and separation from significant others;
e. economic factors associated with hospitalization;
f. changes in usual life style and roles as a result of the amputation.

| Desired Outcome | Nursing Actions and ***Selected Purposes/Rationales*** |
|---|---|
| 1. The client will experience a reduction in anxiety (see Standardized Preoperative Care Plan, Nursing Diagnosis 1 [pp. 108-109], for outcome criteria). | 1.a. Refer to Standardized Preoperative Care Plan, Nursing Diagnosis 1 (pp. 108-109), for measures related to assessment and reduction of fear and anxiety.<br>b. Implement additional measures *to reduce fear and anxiety:*<br>1. reinforce physician's explanation about the level of amputation planned including that final determination of the level will be made during the surgical procedure once adequacy of circulation in the operative limb is confirmed<br>2. if desired by client, arrange for a visit with an amputee who has successfully adjusted to the loss of a lower limb. |

## 2. NURSING DIAGNOSIS: Knowledge deficit

regarding:
a. hospital routines associated with surgery;
b. physical preparation for the amputation;
c. sensations that normally occur following surgery and anesthesia including phantom limb phenomena;
d. postoperative care and management of the residual limb;
e. postoperative activity and exercise schedule.

| Desired Outcomes | Nursing Actions and ***Selected Purposes/Rationales*** |
|---|---|
| 2.a. The client will verbalize an understanding of usual preoperative care and postoperative sensations and care. | 2.a.1. Refer to Standardized Preoperative Care Plan, Nursing Diagnosis 4, actions a.1-4 (pp. 111-112), for information to include in preoperative teaching.<br>2. Explain the phantom limb sensation that is experienced by all clients after an amputation. Emphasize that the sensation is typically strongest in the immediate postoperative period and tends to diminish over time.<br>3. Reinforce the physician's explanation about the phantom limb pain that may also be experienced postoperatively. Explanation may include that:<br>a. it does not occur in all clients<br>b. it may begin immediately after surgery but usually starts several weeks postoperatively and disappears gradually over several months to years<br>c. the type of pain experienced varies from client to client and can be very similar to pain experienced before the amputation (e.g. burning, squeezing, cramping, electric shock-like or tingling sensations)<br>d. it may be triggered by pressure on other body areas.<br>4. Explain that limited ambulation will be encouraged within 48 hours postoperatively if a temporary prosthesis is in place.<br>5. Allow time for questions and clarification of information provided. |
| 2.b. The client will demonstrate the ability to perform recommended activities to prevent postoperative complications. | 2.b.1. Refer to Standardized Preoperative Care Plan, Nursing Diagnosis 4, action b.1 (p. 112), for instructions on ways to prevent postoperative complications.<br>2. Provide additional instructions on ways to prevent complications following a below the knee amputation:<br>a. inform client that the following precautions will need to be adhered to postoperatively in order to prevent flexion, abduction, and/or external rotation of the hip and contractures of the knee (if residual limb is not casted):<br>1. avoid sitting for long periods<br>2. avoid placing pillows under residual limb<br>3. maintain residual limb in proper alignment<br>4. lie prone for several periods during the day unless contraindicated to promote hip extension<br>b. instruct in range of motion exercises that will help prevent hip and knee contractures.<br>3. Allow time for questions and clarification of information provided and practice and return demonstration of recommended exercises. |
| 2.c. The client will demonstrate ways to improve strength and facilitate mobility postoperatively. | 2.c.1. Instruct client in the following exercises performed to improve strength and facilitate mobility postoperatively:<br>a. knee flexion and extension, hip extension and abduction, straight leg raising, and quadriceps-setting<br>b. range of motion and strengthening exercises for the upper extremities, chest, and abdominal muscles to facilitate crutch walking and transfer activities. |

2. Provide instructions related to:
   a. use of overhead trapeze
   b. transfer techniques
   c. use of mobility aids (e.g. crutches, walker)
   d. weight-bearing modifications for the affected side; emphasize that full weight-bearing will not be done until the permanent prosthesis is in place.
3. Allow time for practice and return demonstration of exercises and transfer techniques.

| | |
|---|---|
| 2.d. The client will verbalize an understanding of the prosthesis and dressings planned. | 2.d.1. Reinforce the physician's explanation about the type of prosthesis and dressings planned.<br>2. If an immediate or early prosthetic fitting is planned:<br>a. show client what the prosthesis will look like and how it will be held in place<br>b. inform client that:<br>1. the residual limb will be wrapped with a soft material or "sock" and casted or encased in an air splint<br>2. the purpose of applying the air splint or casting the residual limb is to facilitate shaping, provide controlled pressure in order to reduce edema and support tissue, minimize pain on movement, and allow attachment of a temporary prosthetic extension (pylon) and/or artificial foot/ankle assembly<br>3. the cast will be changed as the residual limb shrinks (the first cast is usually replaced about 7-10 days after surgery).<br>3. If prosthesis fitting is delayed or not planned:<br>a. explain that a cast or compression dressing will be applied to support tissue, reduce edema, and promote residual limb maturation<br>b. inform client of the type and frequency of wound care.<br>4. Allow time for questions and clarification of information provided. |

## POSTOPERATIVE

**Use in conjunction with the Standardized Postoperative Care Plan.**

### 1. NURSING DIAGNOSIS: Pain:

a. **incisional pain** related to tissue trauma and reflex muscle spasms associated with the amputation;
b. **phantom limb pain** possibly related to an interruption of the neural reflex pathways or psychological factors.

| Desired Outcome | Nursing Actions and ***Selected Purposes/Rationales*** |
|---|---|
| 1. The client will experience diminished pain (see Standardized Postoperative Care Plan, Nursing Diagnosis 6 [p. 119], for outcome criteria). | 1.a. Refer to Standardized Postoperative Care Plan, Nursing Diagnosis 6 (p. 119), for measures related to assessment and management of pain.<br>b. Encourage client to report phantom limb pain.<br>c. Implement measures *to reduce phantom limb pain if it occurs:*<br>1. instruct client to apply pressure on residual limb by walking on pylon or pressing limb against a firm surface<br>2. consult physician about use of transcutaneous electrical nerve stimulation (TENS) or application of heat to residual limb<br>3. instruct client to mentally put absent limb through range of motion exercises<br>4. administer tricyclic antidepressants (e.g. amitriptyline) if ordered. |

## 2. NURSING DIAGNOSIS: Actual/High risk for impaired skin integrity

related to:
a. disruption of skin associated with the amputation;
b. delayed wound healing associated with:
  1. inadequate nutritional status
  2. decreased blood supply to wound area resulting from the underlying disease process, edema of the residual limb, and/or excessive pressure on operative site (may occur as a result of noncompliance with weight-bearing limitations; improper residual limb wrapping; and/or slippage of the cast, air splint, or compression dressing);
c. irritation of skin associated with contact with wound drainage, pressure from drainage tube, and use of tape;
d. damage to the skin and/or subcutaneous tissue associated with prolonged pressure on tissues, friction, and shearing while mobility is decreased.

| Desired Outcomes | Nursing Actions and ***Selected Purposes/Rationales*** |
|---|---|
| 2.a. The client will experience normal healing of surgical wound (see Standardized Postoperative Care Plan, Nursing Diagnosis 9, outcome a [p. 122], for outcome criteria). | 2.a.1. Refer to Standardized Postoperative Care Plan, Nursing Diagnosis 9, actions a.1 and 2 (pp. 122-123), for measures related to assessment and promotion of wound healing.<br>2. Implement additional measures *to promote wound healing:*<br>a. perform actions to prevent excessive edema in residual limb (see Postoperative Collaborative Diagnosis 5, action b.2)<br>b. assess for and report slippage of cast, air splint, or compression dressing *(can act as a tourniquet and impede circulation);* assist with reapplication if indicated<br>c. caution client to comply with weight-bearing limitations *in order to prevent excessive pressure on wound site.* |
| 2.b. The client will maintain skin integrity (see Standardized Postoperative Care Plan, Nursing Diagnosis 9, outcome b [p. 123], for outcome criteria). | 2.b.1. Inspect the following sites for pallor, redness, and breakdown:<br>a. skin areas in contact with wound drainage, tape, and drainage tubing<br>b. back, coccyx, and buttocks<br>c. elbows and remaining heel.<br>2. Refer to Standardized Postoperative Care Plan, Nursing Diagnosis 9, action b (p. 123), for measures related to assessment and prevention of skin irritation or breakdown resulting from contact with wound drainage, drainage tubings, and/or tape.<br>3. Implement additional measures *to prevent skin breakdown:*<br>a. assist client to turn at least every 2 hours; use all 4 sides (prone, lateral, dorsal) unless contraindicated<br>b. gently massage around reddened areas at least every 2 hours<br>c. perform actions *to prevent shearing* (shearing occurs when one tissue layer slides past another) *and skin surface abrasion:*<br>1. apply a thin layer of powder or cornstarch to bottom sheet or skin *to absorb moisture (moist skin is more likely to adhere to sheet) and reduce friction*<br>2. lift and move client carefully using a turn sheet and adequate assistance<br>3. limit length of time client is in semi-Fowler's position to 30 minutes *(in this position, client tends to slide down in bed)*<br>d. instruct or assist client to shift weight every 30 minutes<br>e. if fade time (length of time it takes for reddened area to fade after pressure is removed) is greater than 15 minutes, increase frequency of position changes and/or provide more effective method of cushioning, padding, and positioning<br>f. keep skin lubricated, clean, and dry |

g. keep bed linens dry and wrinkle-free
h. provide devices to reduce pressure on the skin, decrease shearing, and/or prevent moisture build-up (e.g. alternating pressure mattress or pad, flotation pad, sheepskin)
i. increase activity as allowed and tolerated.

4. If skin breakdown occurs:
   a. notify physician
   b. continue with above measures to prevent further irritation and breakdown
   c. perform wound and decubitus care as ordered or per standard hospital procedure
   d. assess client closely and report signs and symptoms of infection (e.g. elevated temperature; redness, warmth, and edema around area of breakdown; unusual drainage from site).

## 3. NURSING DIAGNOSIS: Impaired physical mobility

related to:
a. pain, weakness, and fatigue;
b. depressant effects of anesthesia and some medications (e.g. narcotic analgesics);
c. balance difficulties associated with change in the body's center of gravity as a result of loss of a lower limb;
d. inability to control prosthesis;
e. activity restrictions imposed by the treatment plan;
f. fear of falling and compromising surgical wound.

| Desired Outcome | Nursing Actions and ***Selected Purposes/Rationales*** |
|---|---|
| 3. The client will achieve maximum physical mobility within limitations imposed by the amputation and prescribed activity restrictions. | 3.a. Refer to Standardized Postoperative Care Plan, Nursing Diagnosis 11 (p. 125), for measures to increase client's mobility.<br>b. Implement additional measures *to increase mobility:*<br>1. perform actions to reduce pain (see Postoperative Nursing Diagnosis 1)<br>2. reinforce physical therapist's instructions on ways to adapt to the body's new center of gravity (e.g. change position slowly)<br>3. reinforce preoperative instructions and assist client with exercises, transfer activities, and ambulation techniques (ambulation with crutches is typically begun the 2nd postoperative day)<br>4. assure client that pylon or air splint will provide adequate support during ambulation<br>5. reinforce prosthetist's instructions about control and use of prosthesis and correct gait technique<br>6. if application of a prosthesis is delayed or not planned, assist client with exercises to:<br>a. develop standing balance and strength (e.g. knee bends, standing on toes, hopping on the remaining foot while holding on to a chair, balancing on the unoperative leg without support, quadriceps- and gluteal-setting exercises)<br>b. increase strength of arm extensor and shoulder depressor muscles (e.g. pushups, use of trapeze to lift body off bed, flexion and extension of arms holding traction weights or a weighted wand, arm pulley exercises) *to facilitate crutch walking.* |

## 4. NURSING DIAGNOSIS: High risk for trauma

related to falls associated with:
a. weakness and fatigue;
b. postural hypotension resulting from peripheral pooling of blood and blood loss during surgery;
c. central nervous system depressant effects of some medications (e.g. narcotic analgesics);
d. difficulty with balance, prosthesis control, and transfer and ambulation techniques.

| Desired Outcome | Nursing Actions and ***Selected Purposes/Rationales*** |
|---|---|
| 4. The client will not experience falls. | 4.a. Refer to Standardized Postoperative Care Plan, Nursing Diagnosis 17 (p. 130), for measures to prevent falls.<br>b. Implement additional measures *to prevent falls:*<br>1. perform actions to increase client's mobility and stability (see Postoperative Nursing Diagnosis 3)<br>2. encourage client to ask for assistance when he/she wishes to ambulate; accompany client until control of the prosthesis and transfer and ambulation techniques are mastered. |

## 5. COLLABORATIVE DIAGNOSES: Potential complications:

a. **hematoma formation** related to inadequate hemostasis during or following surgical procedure and/or impaired drainage from operative area;
b. **residual limb edema** related to slippage of the cast, air splint, or compression dressing; inadequate residual limb bandaging; and/or prolonged dependent positioning;
c. **necrosis of skin flap** related to impaired wound healing and infection;
d. **knee flexion and hip contractures on the operative side** (particularly with delayed prosthesis fitting) related to poor positioning and failure to perform prescribed exercises.

| Desired Outcomes | Nursing Actions and ***Selected Purposes/Rationales*** |
|---|---|
| 5.a. The client will not develop a hematoma at the operative site as evidenced by:<br>1. expected amount of drainage<br>2. no unusual increase in swelling and pain in operative area<br>3. no increase in skin | 5.a.1. Assess for and report signs and symptoms of hematoma formation (e.g. less than expected amount of drainage from wound drain; oozing of blood from suture line; increased swelling, pain, and/or discoloration in surgical area).<br>2. Implement measures *to prevent hematoma formation:*<br>a. maintain patency of drain (e.g. keep tubing free of kinks, empty collection device as often as necessary, maintain suction if ordered) if present<br>b. wrap residual limb properly if it is not casted or in an air splint *so that adequate pressure is maintained to site*<br>c. protect the residual limb from trauma. |

| | |
|---|---|
| discoloration at surgical site. | 3. If a hematoma develops, prepare client for aspiration of blood and reapplication of a pressure dressing if planned. |
| 5.b. The client will experience limited residual limb edema. | 5.b.1. Assess for and report increasing edema of residual limb.<br>2. Implement measures *to prevent excessive edema in residual limb:*<br>a. use proper residual limb wrapping technique<br>b. maintain elevation of foot of bed if ordered<br>c. caution client to avoid placing residual limb in a dependent position (e.g. over side of bed) for long periods; instruct client to maintain residual limb in an extended position when sitting in a chair (e.g. use additional chair to support residual limb)<br>d. securely attach cast suspension straps to waist belt when client is transferring or ambulating *to prevent cast from slipping*<br>e. if cast or air splint slippage occurs, immediately wrap residual limb firmly with elastic bandages and notify physician.<br>3. If residual limb edema becomes excessive, prepare client for and assist with recasting or reapplication of a soft compression dressing if indicated. |
| 5.c. The client will not experience necrosis of the skin flap as evidenced by:<br>1. skin warm and usual color<br>2. no skin breakdown<br>3. absence of a foul odor. | 5.c.1. Assess for and report signs and symptoms of necrosis of skin flap (e.g. pale, cool, darkened skin; skin breakdown; foul odor).<br>2. Implement measures *to prevent necrosis of the skin flap:*<br>a. perform actions to promote wound healing (see Postoperative Nursing Diagnosis 2, action a)<br>b. perform actions to prevent and treat wound infection (see Standardized Postoperative Care Plan, Nursing Diagnosis 16, actions b.4 and 5 [p. 129]).<br>3. If necrosis occurs:<br>a. prepare client for surgical revision of the residual limb<br>b. provide emotional support to client and significant others. |
| 5.d. The client will not develop knee flexion and hip contractures on the operative side as evidenced by the ability to move joints through their full range of motion. | 5.d.1. Assess client frequently for beginning development of knee flexion and hip contractures (e.g. inability to fully extend knee and/or extend, adduct, or internally rotate residual limb).<br>2. Implement measures *to prevent knee flexion and/or hip contractures:*<br>a. if residual limb elevation is ordered postoperatively, place bed in Trendelenburg position rather than placing limb on pillows (elevation of residual limb may be ordered for the first 24 hours postoperatively)<br>b. turn client to prone position at least once the 1st postoperative day then several times daily unless contraindicated *in order to promote hip extension;* place a pillow under abdomen and residual limb *to maintain hip extension and stretch flexor muscles*<br>c. position legs close to one another in good alignment *to prevent hip abduction*<br>d. caution client not to raise head of the bed or sit for extended periods<br>e. place trochanter roll or sandbags along outer aspect of thigh when client is supine *to prevent external rotation of hip*<br>f. encourage client to keep knee straight when lying or sitting<br>g. assist client with range of motion and prescribed exercise program at least 3-4 times/day<br>h. encourage crutch walking as soon as allowed and tolerated<br>i. perform actions to reduce pain (see Postoperative Nursing Diagnosis 1) *in order to reduce the risk of client flexing residual limb in response to pain.*<br>3. If contractures develop:<br>a. assist with rehabilitative efforts to improve range of motion of knee and hip<br>b. provide emotional support to client and significant others. |

## 6. NURSING DIAGNOSIS: Self-concept disturbance*

related to:
a. change in appearance and mobility associated with loss of a limb;
b. inability to participate in usual life style and roles associated with physical limitations imposed by loss of a limb;
c. dependence on others to meet self-care needs.

*This diagnostic label includes the nursing diagnoses of body image disturbance, self-esteem disturbance, and altered role performance.

### Desired Outcome

6. The client will demonstrate beginning adaptation to the loss of a lower limb and resulting changes in body functioning, life style, and roles as evidenced by:
   a. verbalization of feelings of self-worth
   b. maintenance of relationships with significant others
   c. active participation in activities of daily living
   d. active interest in personal appearance
   e. willingness to pursue usual roles and participate in social activities
   f. verbalization of a beginning plan for adapting life style to meet restrictions imposed by the loss of a lower limb.

### Nursing Actions and ***Selected Purposes/Rationales***

6.a. Assess for signs and symptoms of a self-concept disturbance (e.g. verbal or nonverbal cues denoting a negative response to changes in body functioning and appearance such as denial of or preoccupation with changes that have occurred, refusal to look at or touch residual limb, or withdrawal from significant others).

b. Determine the meaning of changes in body image and functioning, life style, and roles to the client by encouraging him/her to verbalize feelings and by noting nonverbal responses to changes experienced.

c. Implement measures to facilitate the grieving process (see Postoperative Nursing Diagnosis 7, action b).

d. Stay with the client during first dressing change *to provide support as he/she views the residual limb for the first time.*

e. Discuss with client the availability of a natural-looking prosthesis.

f. Implement measures *to assist client to increase self-esteem* (e.g. limit negative self-assessment, encourage positive comments about self, assist to identify strengths, give positive feedback about accomplishments and behaviors that are indicative of high self-esteem).

g. Assist client to identify and utilize coping techniques that have been helpful in the past.

h. Clarify misconceptions about future limitations on physical activity. Emphasize that a high level of mobility can be achieved with a prosthesis in place and/or use of crutches.

i. Assist client with usual grooming and makeup habits if necessary.

j. Promote activities which require client to confront the body changes that have occurred (e.g. exercise, bathing, wrapping residual limb). Be aware that integration of the change in body image does not usually occur until 2-6 months after the actual physical change has occurred.

k. Demonstrate acceptance of client using techniques such as touch and frequent visits. Encourage significant others to do the same.

l. Assess for and support behaviors suggesting positive adaptation to loss of lower limb (e.g. willingness to care for residual limb, compliance with treatment plan, verbalization of feelings of self-worth, maintenance of relationships with significant others).

m. Encourage significant others to allow client to do what he/she is able *so that independence can be reestablished and/or self-esteem redeveloped.*

n. Encourage client contact with others *so that he/she can test and establish a new self-image.*

o. Assist client's and significant others' adjustment by listening, facilitating communication, and providing information.

p. Provide opportunity for client to discuss life-style changes he/she feels might be necessary as a result of the amputation. Assist him/her to explore available options.

q. Assist client and significant others to have similar expectations and understanding of future life style and to identify ways that personal and family goals can be adjusted rather than abandoned.

r. Teach client the rationale for treatments and encourage maximum participation in treatment regimen *to enable him/her to maintain a sense of control over life.*

s. Encourage visits and support from significant others.

t. Encourage client to continue involvement in social activities and to pursue usual roles and interests. If previous roles, interests, and hobbies cannot be pursued, encourage development of new ones.

u. Arrange for a visit with an amputee who has successfully adjusted to loss of a limb.

v. Provide information about and encourage utilization of community agencies and support groups (e.g. National Amputation Foundation; vocational rehabilitation; family, individual, and/or financial counseling).

w. Consult physician about psychological counseling if client desires or if he/she seems unwilling or unable to adapt to changes that have occurred as a result of the amputation.

## 7. NURSING DIAGNOSIS: Grieving*

related to the loss of a limb and resulting changes in body image and usual life style and roles.

*This diagnostic label includes anticipatory grieving and grieving following the actual losses.

| Desired Outcome | Nursing Actions and ***Selected Purposes/Rationales*** |
|---|---|
| 7. The client will demonstrate beginning progression through the grieving process as evidenced by:<br>a. verbalization of feelings about the loss of his/her leg<br>b. expression of grief<br>c. participation in treatment plan and self-care activities<br>d. utilization of available support systems<br>e. verbalization of a plan for integrating prescribed follow-up care into life style. | 7.a. Assess for signs and symptoms of grieving (e.g. change in eating habits, inability to concentrate, insomnia, anger, noncompliance, withdrawal from significant others, denial of loss). Be aware that client's response to a loss will be affected by factors such as previous experience with loss, age, developmental stage, available support systems, spiritual and cultural background, current health status, and significance of the loss.<br>b. Implement measures *to facilitate the grieving process:*<br>1. assist client to acknowledge the losses experienced *so grief work can begin;* assess for factors that may hinder and facilitate acknowledgment<br>2. discuss the grieving process and assist client to accept the phases of grieving as an expected response to the loss of his/her limb and anticipated life-style changes<br>3. allow time for client to progress through the phases of grieving (phases vary among theorists but progress from shock and alarm to acceptance); be aware that not every phase is expressed by all individuals, that recurrence of phases is common, and that the grieving process may take months to years<br>4. provide an atmosphere of care and concern (e.g. provide privacy, be available and nonjudgmental, display empathy and respect) *so client will feel free to verbalize feelings*<br>5. perform actions *to promote trust* (e.g. answer questions honestly, provide requested information)<br>6. encourage the verbal expression of anger and sadness about the losses experienced; recognize displacement of anger and assist client to see the actual cause of angry feelings and resentment; establish limits on abusive behavior if demonstrated<br>7. encourage client to express his/her feelings in whatever ways are comfortable (e.g. writing, drawing, conversation) |

| Desired Outcome | Nursing Actions and ***Selected Purposes/Rationales*** |
|---|---|
| | 8. assist client to identify personal strengths that have helped him/her to cope in previous situations of loss<br>9. support realistic hope about his/her ability to be successfully rehabilitated<br>10. support behaviors suggesting successful resolution of grief work (e.g. verbalizing feelings about loss of the leg, focusing on ways to adapt to losses, learning needed skills, developing or renewing relationships)<br>11. explain the phases of the grieving process to significant others; encourage their support and understanding<br>12. facilitate communication between the client and significant others; be aware that they may be in different phases of the grieving process<br>13. provide information regarding counseling services and support groups that might assist client in working through grief<br>14. arrange for visit from clergy if desired by client.<br>c. Consult physician regarding referral for counseling if signs of dysfunctional grieving (e.g. persistent denial of loss, excessive anger or sadness, hysteria, suicidal behaviors) occur. |

## 8. NURSING DIAGNOSIS: Knowledge deficit

regarding follow-up care.

| Desired Outcomes | Nursing Actions and ***Selected Purposes/Rationales*** |
|---|---|
| 8.a. The client will demonstrate appropriate ways to prevent contractures, increase strength, and improve mobility. | 8.a.1. Instruct client in the following ways to prevent contractures, increase strength, and improve mobility:<br>a. performing range of motion exercises of residual limb and unaffected extremities<br>b. lying prone several times a day with pillow under abdomen and residual limb (maintains hip extension and stretches flexor muscles)<br>c. performing knee bends, standing on toes, hopping on remaining foot while holding on to a chair, balancing on the unoperative leg without support, and performing quadriceps- and gluteal-setting exercises<br>d. performing pushups, flexion and extension of arms holding weights, and arm pulley exercises (facilitates crutch walking).<br>2. Allow time for questions, clarification, and return demonstration. |
| 8.b. The client will demonstrate the ability to transfer self safely. | 8.b.1. Reinforce instructions from physical therapist on ways to transfer self safely.<br>2. Allow time for questions, clarification, practice, and return demonstration of techniques. |
| 8.c. The client will identify ways to assess and maintain health of the remaining extremities. | 8.c.1. Instruct client in ways to maintain health of the remaining extremities:<br>a. wear a well-fitting shoe to protect remaining foot from pressure and trauma<br>b. perform foot and nail care using appropriate technique<br>c. avoid breaks in the skin to reduce risk of infection<br>d. stop smoking<br>e. adhere to regular follow-up care if diabetes or peripheral vascular disease was a factor leading to the need for amputation.<br>2. Instruct client to report signs and symptoms of altered circulation in extremities (e.g. tingling, color changes, numbness, swelling, pallor, absent peripheral pulses).<br>3. Demonstrate how to check peripheral pulses if appropriate.<br>4. Allow time for questions, clarification, and return demonstration. |

8.d. The client will demonstrate the ability to appropriately care for the residual limb.

8.d.1. Reinforce preoperative teaching about the purpose of bandaging the residual limb.
2. Instruct client in ways to care for the residual limb:
   a. inspect all aspects of residual limb daily using a hand mirror if necessary to check for redness, skin irritation, breakdown, and drainage
   b. massage residual limb daily toward suture line to mobilize scar and prevent adhesions
   c. if the residual limb is bandaged:
      1. instruct client and significant others in appropriate wrapping technique; stress importance of using the proper width and length of elastic wraps (below the knee amputee usually needs 4-inch double length bandages)
      2. instruct client to use clean bandages each day and rewrap the residual limb at least 4 times/day (wrap should be worn 24 hours/day until prosthetic fitting is completed and/or residual limb size has stabilized)
   d. if the residual limb is casted:
      1. instruct client in cast care and importance of wearing cast suspension belt when ambulating and/or transferring in order to maintain proper position of cast
      2. inform client that a shrinker device (elastic sock or bandages, removable cast) will be used when wound is healed and cast is removed (usually 3-5 weeks) to prepare residual limb for a permanent prosthesis
   e. if client has a prosthesis, instruct to:
      1. wash residual limb daily using a mild soap, rinse thoroughly, and pat dry; allow the limb to air dry for at least an hour before applying prosthesis
      2. avoid use of emollients and powders on residual limb
      3. toughen residual limb once healing has taken place by massaging it, pushing it against a firm surface, pulling on it with a hand-held towel, and/or applying alcohol to scar (a toughened limb is more resistent to irritation and breakdown from the constant pressure exerted by the prosthesis)
      4. wear a residual limb sock next to skin to reduce friction between residual limb and socket
      5. use only residual limb socks recommended by the prosthetist; socks should be changed daily, laundered gently in cool water with a mild soap, and laid flat to dry
      6. replace worn or damaged residual limb socks; never mend them
      7. emphasize the need to monitor fit of the socket; inform client that the residual limb will continue to shrink for up to 2 years and adjustments of socket will need to be done by prosthetist as this occurs; caution client not to make even minor adjustments on his/her own
      8. caution client to follow weight-bearing limitations until healing is complete
      9. if skin breakdown occurs, avoid use of prosthesis until area has been checked by physician and/or prosthetist
      10. apply prosthesis on arising and wear for prescribed length of time to prevent residual limb edema
      11. apply shrinker device whenever prosthesis is removed to prevent edema of the residual limb and subsequent difficulty in reapplication of the prosthesis.
3. Allow time for questions, clarification, and return demonstration.

8.e. The client will verbalize how to

8.e. Instruct client in ways to care for the prosthesis:
   1. cleanse socket daily with a damp cloth; dry thoroughly
   2. do not allow leather or metal components of prosthesis to get wet

| Desired Outcomes | Nursing Actions and ***Selected Purposes/Rationales*** |
|---|---|
| appropriately care for the prosthesis. | 3. have prosthesis examined by a prosthetist on a regular basis<br>4. have prosthesis readjusted if a weight loss or gain of 10 pounds occurs<br>5. make sure that shoes worn with prosthesis are in good repair to avoid damage to prosthesis and gait alteration. |
| 8.f. The client will identify ways to manage phantom limb pain if it occurs. | 8.f.1. Instruct client in ways to manage phantom limb pain if it occurs:<br>a. apply intermittent pressure to residual limb by walking on pylon or pressing the limb against a firm surface<br>b. mentally put absent limb through range of motion exercises<br>c. apply moist or dry heat to residual limb<br>d. participate in diversional activities.<br>2. Reassure client that phantom limb pain should gradually disappear. |
| 8.g. The client will state signs and symptoms to report to the health care provider. | 8.g.1. Refer to Standardized Postoperative Care Plan, Nursing Diagnosis 21, action c (p. 135), for signs and symptoms to report to the health care provider.<br>2. Instruct client to report these additional signs and symptoms:<br>a. occurrence of and/or persistent phantom limb pain<br>b. persistent or increased residual limb swelling<br>c. difficulty with full extension of residual limb<br>d. inability to maintain balance<br>e. difficulty controlling prosthesis<br>f. numbness, tingling, color changes, or swelling of residual limb and/or remaining extremities<br>g. absent peripheral pulses. |
| 8.h. The client will identify community resources that can assist with home management and adjustment to changes resulting from the amputation. | 8.h.1. Provide information about community resources that can assist the client and significant others with home management and adjustment to changes resulting from the amputation (e.g. home health agency; social services; individual, family, and occupational counseling; amputee support groups; National Amputation Foundation).<br>2. Initiate a referral if indicated. |
| 8.i. The client will verbalize an understanding of and a plan for adhering to recommended follow-up care including future appointments with health care provider, prosthetist, and physical therapist; medications prescribed; and activity level. | 8.i. 1. Refer to Standardized Postoperative Care Plan, Nursing Diagnosis 21 (pp. 135-136), for routine postoperative instructions and measures to improve client compliance.<br>2. Emphasize the importance of adhering to recommended progression of weight-bearing on residual limb. |

# Fractured Hip with Internal Fixation or Prosthesis Insertion

A fractured hip is the term used to describe a fracture of the proximal end of the femur which includes the head, neck, and trochanteric area of the femur. A fractured hip is classified according to the specific location of the fracture. An intracapsular fracture occurs in the femoral neck and may be specifically identified as a subcapital or transcervical fracture. An extracapsular fracture occurs distal to the hip joint and may be classified as intertrochanteric or subtrochanteric.

A fractured hip is one of the most common orthopedic injuries in the elderly because of the increased incidence of osteoporosis and falls in the elderly population. Although a fractured hip can be treated by traction for 8-12 weeks, the preferred treatment is surgery because it allows earlier mobility. Surgery involves internal fixation of the fracture or insertion of a femoral head prosthesis. If the fracture occurred in the intracapsular region, the femoral head and neck may be replaced with a prosthetic device (e.g. Austin Moore or bipolar prosthesis), although internal fixation with preservation of the femoral head is again becoming a popular method of treating femoral neck fractures. If the fracture occurred in the extracapsular region, internal fixation of the fracture with pins, nails, a nail and plate device, or a compression screw device will be performed. Ideally, surgery is performed within 12-24 hours after the injury, especially if the client has a displaced femoral neck. During the preoperative period, traction is usually applied to stabilize and reduce the fracture and reduce muscle spasms and pain.

**This care plan focuses on the elderly adult client who is hospitalized for surgical repair of a hip fracture.** The goals of preoperative care are to reduce fear and anxiety, maintain comfort, and prevent neurovascular dysfunction. Postoperatively, the goals of care are to maintain comfort, prevent complications, assist the client to regain maximum mobility and independence, and educate the client regarding follow-up care.

## DIAGNOSTIC TESTS

X-rays of the hip

## DISCHARGE CRITERIA

Prior to discharge, the client will:

- ❖ demonstrate evidence of fracture reduction and healing
- ❖ have hip pain controlled
- ❖ have no signs and symptoms of complications
- ❖ verbalize an understanding of activity and position restrictions necessary to prevent dislocation of the prosthesis or internal fixation device
- ❖ demonstrate correct transfer and ambulation techniques and proper use of ambulatory aids
- ❖ demonstrate the ability to correctly perform the prescribed exercises
- ❖ identify ways to reduce the risk of falls in the home environment
- ❖ share thoughts and feelings about the need to transfer to an extended care facility if planned
- ❖ state signs and symptoms to report to the health care provider
- ❖ identify community resources that can assist with home management and provide transportation
- ❖ verbalize an understanding of and a plan for adhering to recommended follow-up care including future appointments with health care provider and physical therapist, medications prescribed, activity level, and wound care.

**NURSING/ COLLABORATIVE DIAGNOSES**



**See Standardized Preoperative and Postoperative Care Plans for additional diagnoses.**

## PREOPERATIVE

**Use in conjunction with the Standardized Preoperative Care Plan.**

### 1. NURSING DIAGNOSIS: Anxiety

related to:
a. severe pain;
b. lack of understanding of traction device and planned surgical procedure;
c. unfamiliar environment and separation from significant others;
d. anticipated effects of anesthesia and postoperative discomfort;
e. economic factors associated with hospitalization;
f. possibility of changes in usual life style, permanent disability, or death.

| Desired Outcome | Nursing Actions and ***Selected Purposes/Rationales*** |
|---|---|
| 1. The client will experience a reduction in anxiety (see Standardized Preoperative Care Plan, Nursing Diagnosis 1 [pp. 108-109], for outcome criteria). | 1.a. Refer to Standardized Preoperative Care Plan, Nursing Diagnosis 1 (pp. 108-109), for measures related to assessment and reduction of fear and anxiety.<br>b. Implement additional measures *to reduce fear and anxiety:*<br>1. perform actions to reduce pain (see Preoperative Nursing Diagnosis 2, action e)<br>2. explain the purpose of traction and how it works<br>3. assure client that staff are knowledgeable about traction equipment<br>4. reassure client that modern treatment methods for a fractured hip have significantly reduced permanent disability and death rates; inform client that he/she will probably begin ambulation by the 2nd postoperative day. |

**2. NURSING DIAGNOSIS: Pain: hip**

related to fracture of the bone, soft tissue injury, and muscle spasms.

| Desired Outcome | Nursing Actions and ***Selected Purposes/Rationales*** |
|---|---|
| 2. The client will experience diminished hip pain as evidenced by:<br>a. verbalization of a reduction of pain<br>b. relaxed facial expression and body positioning<br>c. stable vital signs. | 2.a. Determine how the client usually responds to pain.<br>b. Assess client's perception of pain including location, intensity, and type. Utilize a numerical scale to rate intensity.<br>c. Assess for nonverbal signs of pain (e.g. wrinkled brow, clenched fists, reluctance to move, clutching hip or thigh, restlessness, diaphoresis, facial pallor, increased B/P, tachycardia).<br>d. Assess for factors that seem to aggravate and alleviate pain.<br>e. Implement measures *to reduce pain:*<br>1. perform actions *to reduce fear and anxiety about the pain experience* (e.g. assure client that his/her need for pain relief will be met)<br>2. medicate prior to any painful treatments or procedures (e.g. application of traction) and before pain is severe<br>3. perform actions *to maintain effective traction on the injured extremity* (client is usually placed in Buck's traction with 5 pounds of weight preoperatively *to stabilize and reduce the fracture and reduce muscle spasms and pain):*<br>a. ensure that weights are hanging freely<br>b. do not allow footplate or ropes to rest on end of bed<br>c. keep affected heel off bed<br>d. keep knots away from pulley device<br>e. do not remove traction unless specifically ordered<br>f. do not lift the weights in order to facilitate lifting and other care *(this reduces traction pull and can cause severe muscle spasm)*<br>g. limit head of bed elevation to 20-25° except for meals and toileting *in order to maintain the prescribed traction force*<br>4. avoid bumping the traction device<br>5. place a trochanter roll or sandbag firmly against the lateral aspect of injured hip and upper thigh (should extend from iliac crest to midthigh) *in order to maintain leg in proper alignment*<br>6. consult physician if extremity appears out of alignment; do not attempt to realign extremity *(an attempt to realign the extremity may cause further tissue injury)*<br>7. move client carefully, keeping injured extremity well supported<br>8. if turning is allowed, place pillow between legs before turning *in order to prevent adduction and further strain on the fracture site*<br>9. provide or assist with additional nonpharmacological measures for pain relief (e.g. relaxation techniques, quiet conversation, diversional activities)<br>10. administer analgesics and muscle relaxants if ordered.<br>f. Consult physician if above measures fail to provide adequate pain relief. |

**3. NURSING DIAGNOSIS: High risk for peripheral neurovascular dysfunction: fractured extremity**

related to trauma to the nerves or blood vessels as a result of the injury; displaced bone fragments; and improper wrapping, alignment, or traction of the injured extremity.

| Desired Outcome | Nursing Actions and ***Selected Purposes/Rationales*** |
|---|---|
| 3. The client will maintain normal neurovascular function in the injured extremity as evidenced by:<br>a. palpable pedal pulses<br>b. capillary refill time in toes less than 3 seconds<br>c. extremity warm and usual color<br>d. ability to flex and extend foot and toes<br>e. absence of numbness and tingling in leg and foot<br>f. absence of foot pain during passive movement of toes and foot<br>g. no increase in pain in extremity. | 3.a. Assess for and report signs and symptoms of neurovascular dysfunction in the injured extremity:<br>1. diminished or absent pedal pulses<br>2. capillary refill time in toes greater than 3 seconds<br>3. pallor, blanching, cyanosis, or coolness of the extremity<br>4. inability to flex or extend foot or toes<br>5. numbness or tingling in leg or foot<br>6. pain in foot during passive motion of toes or foot<br>7. increased pain in extremity.<br>b. Implement measures *to prevent neurovascular dysfunction in injured extremity:*<br>1. maintain traction as ordered<br>2. place a trochanter roll or sandbag firmly against lateral aspect of injured hip and upper thigh (should extend from the iliac crest to midthigh) *in order to help maintain proper alignment*<br>3. do not attempt to realign injured leg unless specifically ordered *(an attempt to align extremity may cause further trauma to the nerves)*<br>4. make sure elastic wraps are applied properly (if necessary to reapply elastic wraps, obtain assistance *so that one person can maintain traction on the leg during the reapplication process*)<br>5. make sure that excessive or prolonged pressure is not exerted on Achilles tendon and medial and lateral aspects of knee and ankle<br>6. do not turn client on injured side unless specifically ordered *(may cause further displacement of fracture and decrease blood flow to area).*<br>c. If signs and symptoms of neurovascular dysfunction occur:<br>1. assess for and correct improper positioning of the injured extremity and traction device and external causes of uneven or excessive pressure<br>2. notify physician if the signs and symptoms persist or worsen<br>3. prepare client for surgical intervention (e.g. internal fixation, insertion of hip prosthesis) if planned. |

## POSTOPERATIVE

**Use in conjunction with the Standardized Postoperative Care Plan.**

### 1. NURSING DIAGNOSIS: High risk for peripheral neurovascular dysfunction: operative extremity

related to trauma to the nerves or blood vessels as a result of surgery and the initial injury, blood accumulation and edema in the surgical area, improper alignment of operative extremity, improper stabilization of abductor device, or dislocation of prosthesis or internal fixation device postoperatively.

| Desired Outcome | Nursing Actions and ***Selected Purposes/Rationales*** |
|---|---|
| 1. The client will maintain normal neurovascular function in the operative extremity (see Preoperative Nursing Diagnosis 3, for outcome criteria). | 1.a. Assess for signs and symptoms of neurovascular dysfunction in the operative extremity (see Preoperative Nursing Diagnosis 3, action a, for signs and symptoms).<br>b. Implement measures *to prevent neurovascular dysfunction in the operative extremity:*<br>1. maintain extremity in proper alignment<br>2. perform actions to prevent dislocation of prosthesis or internal fixation device (see Postoperative Collaborative Diagnosis 6, action a.2)<br>3. make sure that straps on abductor device are not too tight and are not |

exerting pressure on the popliteal space, lateral calf immediately below the knee, and lateral malleolus
4. consult physician about application of ice to surgical site if edema develops.

c. If signs and symptoms of neurovascular dysfunction occur:
1. assess for and correct improper positioning of operative extremity; do not attempt realignment if extreme rotation has occurred
2. notify physician if the signs and symptoms persist or worsen
3. prepare client for closed reduction or return to surgery if planned.

## 2. NURSING DIAGNOSIS: Pain: hip

related to tissue trauma and reflex muscle spasms associated with the surgery and the initial injury.

| Desired Outcome | Nursing Actions and ***Selected Purposes/Rationales*** |
|---|---|
| 2. The client will experience diminished hip pain (see Standardized Postoperative Care Plan, Nursing Diagnosis 6 [p. 119], for outcome criteria). | 2.a. Refer to Standardized Postoperative Care Plan, Nursing Diagnosis 6 (p. 119), for measures related to assessment and reduction of pain.<br>b. Implement additional measures *to reduce pain in operative extremity:*<br>1. maintain extremity in proper alignment<br>2. keep pillows between legs when turning and while in a side-lying position *in order to prevent adduction and the resultant strain on surgical site*<br>3. move the operative extremity gently. |

## 3. NURSING DIAGNOSIS: Impaired physical mobility

related to:

a. pain and weakness in weight-bearing extremity associated with the fracture and subsequent surgical repair;
b. prescribed activity and weight-bearing restrictions following internal fixation or prosthesis insertion;
c. generalized weakness associated with surgery;
d. depressant effects of some medications (e.g. narcotic analgesics, central-acting muscle relaxants);
e. fear of falling, moving operative hip improperly, and compromising surgical wound.

| Desired Outcome | Nursing Actions and ***Selected Purposes/Rationales*** |
|---|---|
| 3. The client will achieve maximum physical mobility within prescribed activity and weight-bearing restrictions. | 3.a. Refer to Standardized Postoperative Care Plan, Nursing Diagnosis 11 (p. 125), for measures to increase client's mobility.<br>b. Implement additional measures *to increase client's mobility:*<br>1. perform actions to reduce pain (see Postoperative Nursing Diagnosis 2)<br>2. instruct client in and assist with isometric quadriceps- and gluteal-setting exercises *to strengthen muscles needed for ambulation*<br>3. encourage client to use overhead trapeze to move self *in order to strengthen arm and shoulder muscles needed for proper use of ambulatory aids*<br>4. reinforce physical therapist's instructions regarding muscle |

| Desired Outcome | Nursing Actions and ***Selected Purposes/Rationales*** |
|---|---|
| | strengthening exercises, transfer and ambulation techniques, and use of ambulatory aids<br>5. perform actions to prevent falls (see Postoperative Nursing Diagnosis 5, actions a and b) *in order to decrease client's fear of injury*<br>6. assist client with ambulation as soon as allowed (usually by the 2nd postoperative day).<br>c. Consult physician if client is unable to achieve expected level of mobility. |

## 4. NURSING DIAGNOSIS: High risk for infection

related to:

a. stasis of pulmonary secretions and high risk for aspiration (in immediate post-operative period);
b. wound contamination (risk is increased because of close proximity of wound to perineal area);
c. decreased resistance to infection associated with an inadequate nutritional status and decreased effectiveness of immune system if client is elderly;
d. colonization of bacteria in the urine associated with urinary stasis if mobility is decreased and introduction of pathogens if indwelling catheter is present.

| Desired Outcome | Nursing Actions and ***Selected Purposes/Rationales*** |
|---|---|
| 4. The client will remain free of infection as evidenced by:<br>a. absence of fever and chills<br>b. pulse within normal limits<br>c. normal breath sounds<br>d. voiding clear urine without complaints of frequency, urgency, and burning<br>e. absence of redness, heat, and swelling around wound<br>f. usual drainage from wound<br>g. no new or increased discomfort in hip<br>h. sedimentation rate and WBC and differential counts returning toward normal range<br>i. negative results of cultured specimens. | 4.a. Refer to Standardized Postoperative Care Plan, Nursing Diagnosis 16 (pp. 128-129), for measures related to assessment and prevention of infection.<br>b. Assess for and report additional signs and symptoms that may be indicative of wound infection or osteomyelitis:<br>1. elevated sedimentation rate<br>2. complaints of increased hip discomfort.<br>c. Maintain patency of wound drainage system (e.g. prevent kinking of tubing, keep collection device below surgical wound, keep suction device compressed) *to prevent the accumulation of drainage and subsequent colonization of pathogens in the surgical area.*<br>d. If signs and symptoms of wound infection or osteomyelitis occur:<br>1. prepare client for surgical debridement of wound and/or wound irrigation if planned<br>2. administer antimicrobials as ordered. |

## 5. NURSING DIAGNOSIS: High risk for trauma

related to falls associated with:

a. weakness, fatigue, and postural hypotension resulting from the effects of major surgery and physiological changes that may have occurred if client is elderly;
b. central nervous system depressant effects of some medications (e.g. narcotic analgesics, central-acting muscle relaxants);
c. weakness and pain in weight-bearing extremity as a result of the surgery and initial injury;
d. improper transfer and ambulation techniques.

| Desired Outcome | Nursing Actions and ***Selected Purposes/Rationales*** |
|---|---|
| 5. The client will not experience falls. | 5.a. Refer to Standardized Postoperative Care Plan, Nursing Diagnosis 17, action a (p. 130), for measures to prevent falls.<br>b. Implement additional measures *to reduce the risk for falls:*<br>1. perform actions *to assist client to increase muscle strength:*<br>a. instruct and encourage client to perform isometric quadriceps- and gluteal-setting exercises<br>b. encourage client to use the overhead trapeze to lift self *(strengthens arm and shoulder muscles which will facilitate use of crutches or walker)*<br>2. reinforce physical therapist's instructions regarding correct transfer and ambulation techniques and proper use of ambulatory aids (e.g. walker)<br>3. administer prescribed analgesics before exercise and ambulation sessions *in order to reduce hip pain and subsequently maximize client's ability to utilize proper transfer and ambulation techniques.*<br>c. Include client and significant others in planning and implementing measures to prevent falls.<br>d. If client falls, initiate first aid measures if appropriate and notify physician. |

## 6. COLLABORATIVE DIAGNOSES: Potential complications:

a. **dislocation of prosthesis or internal fixation device** related to improper positioning of operative extremity, early weight-bearing, delayed healing of the fracture, or infection of the bone or surrounding tissue;
b. **thromboembolism** related to:
   1. venous stasis associated with positioning during and following surgery, fluid volume deficit, decreased activity, and pressure exerted on blood vessels by abductor device
   2. hypercoagulability associated with increased release of tissue thromboplastin into the blood (occurs as a result of surgical trauma)
   3. decreased fibrinolytic activity (occurs in response to surgical trauma)
   4. trauma to vein walls during surgery;
c. **avascular necrosis** related to an inadequate blood supply to the bone (occurs primarily following intracapsular fractures);
d. **delayed healing of the fractured bone** (with eventual nonunion) related to inadequate reduction and internal fixation of fracture, diminished blood supply to fracture site, thin or absent periosteum in neck of femur (decreases the healing potential), inadequate nutritional status, preexisting osteoporosis if present, or development of infection in the fractured bone and/or surrounding tissue.

| Desired Outcomes | Nursing Actions and ***Selected Purposes/Rationales*** |
|---|---|
| 6.a. The client will not experience dislocation of the prosthesis or internal fixation device as evidenced by:<br>1. continued resolution of hip pain<br>2. ability to maintain operative leg in proper alignment<br>3. length of operative extremity equal to unoperative extremity<br>4. ability to adhere to exercise and ambulation regimen<br>5. normal neurovascular status in operative leg. | 6.a.1. Assess for and report signs and symptoms of dislocation of the hip prosthesis or internal fixation device:<br>a. sudden, severe pain in operative hip<br>b. significant (greater than 10°) external or internal rotation of the operative leg<br>c. operative extremity more than 2.5 cm (1 inch) shorter than unoperative extremity<br>d. sudden inability to participate in usual exercise and ambulation regimen<br>e. decline in neurovascular status in operative leg.<br>2. Implement measures *to reduce the risk for dislocation of the prosthesis or internal fixation device:*<br>a. perform actions to promote healing of the fracture (see action c.2 in this diagnosis)<br>b. perform actions *to prevent adduction of the operative extremity:*<br>1. keep 2-3 pillows or abductor device between legs at all times<br>2. remind client not to cross legs<br>3. do not move operative extremity past midline<br>c. maintain the operative extremity in proper alignment (be particularly alert to preventing internal rotation)<br>d. maintain restrictions on head of bed elevation if ordered (some physicians order a 45-60° maximum elevation for the first few days after surgery) *to reduce hip flexion*<br>e. perform actions *to prevent extreme (beyond 90°) hip flexion:*<br>1. instruct client not to lean forward to reach objects on end of bed or on floor or to put on slippers, socks, or shoes<br>2. raise the entire bed to client's midthigh level before he/she gets in or out of bed *in order to reduce the degree of hip flexion that occurs when client sits on edge of bed*<br>3. provide a high, firm chair (or elevate sitting surface with pillows) and raised toilet seat for client's use *in order to reduce degree of hip flexion when client sits down*<br>4. do not elevate operative leg when sitting in chair<br>f. maintain restrictions on turning (usually allowed to turn on unoperative side only) and always turn client with pillows between legs<br>g. reinforce weight-bearing limitations ordered (partial weight-bearing is usually allowed as soon as ambulation is started following prosthesis insertion; weight-bearing restrictions vary following internal fixation but often progress from no weight-bearing initially to partial weight-bearing before discharge)<br>h. perform actions to prevent and treat wound infection and osteomyelitis (see Standardized Postoperative Care Plan, Nursing Diagnosis 16, actions b.4 and 5 [p. 129] and Postoperative Nursing Diagnosis 4, actions c and d).<br>3. If signs and symptoms of dislocation of prosthesis or internal fixation device occur:<br>a. maintain client on bed rest<br>b. prepare client for x-rays of surgical area<br>c. prepare client for closed reduction or surgical repair of the dislocation if planned<br>d. provide emotional support to client and significant others. |
| 6.b. The client will not develop a deep vein thrombus or pulmonary embolism (see Standardized | 6.b.1. Refer to Standardized Postoperative Care Plan, Collaborative Diagnosis 19, actions c.1 and 2 (pp. 132-133), for measures related to assessment, prevention, and treatment of a deep vein thrombus and pulmonary embolism.<br>2. Implement additional measures *to prevent thrombus formation:* |

| Desired Outcome | Nursing Actions and *Selected Purposes/Rationales* |
|---|---|
| Postoperative Care Plan, Collaborative Diagnosis 19, outcomes c.1 and 2 [pp. 132-133], for outcome criteria). | a. make sure that straps on abductor device do not exert uneven or excessive pressure on any area<br>b. encourage client to perform active foot exercises every 1-2 hours while awake; provide adequate analgesia *to promote client compliance*<br>c. administer anticoagulants (e.g. low-dose warfarin or heparin) or antiplatelet agents (e.g. low-dose aspirin) if ordered<br>d. assist client with ambulation as soon as allowed. |
| 6.c. The client will not experience avascular necrosis or delayed healing of the fracture as evidenced by:<br>1. resolution of hip pain<br>2. proper alignment of operative extremity<br>3. expected progression in prescribed physical therapy program<br>4. x-rays showing evidence of normal stages of bone healing. | 6.c.1. Assess for and report signs and symptoms of avascular necrosis and/or delayed healing of the fracture:<br>a. persistent hip pain<br>b. inability to maintain operative leg in proper alignment<br>c. inability to make expected progress in physical therapy program<br>d. x-rays showing delayed healing of fracture.<br>2. Implement measures *to promote healing of the fracture:*<br>a. maintain operative leg in proper alignment<br>b. maintain restrictions on weight-bearing as ordered<br>c. maintain an adequate nutritional status (see Standardized Postoperative Care Plan, Nursing Diagnosis 5, action d [p. 118])<br>d. encourage client to consume foods/fluids high in calcium and vitamin D (e.g. fortified dairy products)<br>e. perform actions to prevent and treat wound infection and osteomyelitis (see Standardized Postoperative Care Plan, Nursing Diagnosis 16, actions b.4 and 5 [p. 129] and Postoperative Nursing Diagnosis 4, actions c and d)<br>f. discourage smoking *(evidence strongly suggests that smoking decreases tissue perfusion and may delay bone union)*<br>g. administer the following medications if ordered:<br>1. calcium preparations (e.g. calcium carbonate)<br>2. vitamin D (e.g. calcitriol, calcifediol)<br>3. estrogen preparations *to inhibit further bone resorption.*<br>3. If signs and symptoms of avascular necrosis or delayed healing of the fracture occur:<br>a. continue with above measures to promote healing<br>b. prepare client for surgical intervention (e.g. bone grafting, prosthesis insertion) if planned<br>c. provide emotional support to client and significant others. |

## 7. NURSING DIAGNOSIS: Powerlessness

related to temporary physical limitations, dependence on others to meet basic needs, and possible change in roles and future living situation.

| Desired Outcome | Nursing Actions and *Selected Purposes/Rationales* |
|---|---|
| 7. The client will demonstrate increased feelings of control over his/her situation as evidenced by:<br>a. verbalization of same<br>b. active participation in planning of care and decision-making regarding future living situation | 7.a. Assess for behaviors that may indicate feelings of powerlessness (e.g. verbalization of lack of control over self-care or current situation, anger, apathy, hostility, excessive dependence, lack of participation in self-care or discharge planning).<br>b. Obtain information from client and significant others regarding client's usual response to situations in which he/she has had limited control (e.g. loss of job, financial stress).<br>c. Encourage client to verbalize feelings about current situation and possible changes in roles and living situation (e.g. transfer to an extended care facility, need for a live-in attendant, move to another person's home). Focus on the positive aspects of the planned living arrangement changes. |

| Desired Outcome | Nursing Actions and ***Selected Purposes/Rationales*** |
|---|---|
| c. participation in self-care activities within physical limitations. | d. Reinforce physician's explanations about the hip surgery and rehabilitation plan. Clarify misconceptions.<br>e. Support realistic hope about effects of rehabilitation and probability of future independence.<br>f. Assist client to establish realistic short- and long-term goals.<br>g. Remind client of his/her right to ask questions about condition and plan of care.<br>h. Include client in planning of care, encourage maximum participation in the treatment plan, and allow choices whenever possible *to promote a sense of control.*<br>i. Encourage significant others to allow client to do as much as he/she is able *so that a feeling of independence can be maintained.*<br>j. Inform client of schedule (e.g. planned care, physical therapy schedule) *so that unpredictability is eliminated as much as possible and feeling of control is promoted.*<br>k. Consult occupational therapist if indicated about assistive devices and environmental modifications that would allow client more independence in performing activities of daily living.<br>l. Encourage client to be as active as possible in making decisions about his/her living situation. |

## 8. NURSING DIAGNOSIS: Knowledge deficit

regarding follow-up care.

| Desired Outcomes | Nursing Actions and ***Selected Purposes/Rationales*** |
|---|---|
| 8.a. The client will verbalize an understanding of activity and position restrictions necessary to prevent dislocation of the prosthesis or internal fixation device. | 8.a. Instruct client to adhere to the following activity and position restrictions for at least 2 months (time may vary depending on physician preference) in order to prevent dislocation of prosthesis or internal fixation device:<br>1. turn only as directed by physician (many physicians allow turning to unoperative side only and instruct client to keep pillows between legs when turning and while on side)<br>2. never cross legs<br>3. do not sit on low chairs, stools, or toilets; place a cushion on low chairs, rent or purchase a raised toilet seat for home use, and use the high toilets designed for the handicapped when in public facilities<br>4. do not elevate operative leg higher than hip when sitting<br>5. sit in chairs with arms and use the arms to raise self off chair<br>6. support weight on unoperative leg when raising self from a sitting position<br>7. do not bend down to reach objects on the floor or in low cupboards or drawers<br>8. do not reach to end of bed to pull covers up<br>9. do not put on shoes or socks without using an assistive device (e.g. long-handled shoehorn)<br>10. keep operative leg in proper alignment and avoid extreme internal and external rotation of leg<br>11. when riding in a car:<br>a. sit on a firm pillow or cushion to prevent hip flexion of more than 90°<br>b. keep operative leg extended (a sudden impact of the knee against the dashboard can dislodge the prosthesis) |

12. do not resume sexual activity until approved by physician
13. when sexual activity is resumed, avoid positions that involve turning knee and hip inward, flexing hip beyond 90°, and moving operative leg past the midline
14. avoid lifting heavy objects, excessive twisting and turning of body, and activities that place excessive strain on hip (e.g. jogging).

8.b. The client will demonstrate correct transfer and ambulation techniques and proper use of ambulatory aids.

8.b.1. Reinforce instructions about correct transfer and ambulation techniques, amount of weight-bearing allowed, and proper use of ambulatory aids (a walker is preferable for most of these clients because it provides the greatest stability).
2. Allow time for questions, clarification, and practice of transfer and ambulation techniques.

8.c. The client will demonstrate the ability to correctly perform the prescribed exercises.

8.c.1. Reinforce instructions on muscle strengthening and range of motion exercises.
2. Explain importance of continuing muscle strengthening and range of motion exercises 3-4 times/day.
3. Allow time for questions, clarification, and return demonstration of prescribed exercises.

8.d. The client will identify ways to reduce the risk of falls in the home environment.

8.d. If client is to return home, provide the following instructions on how to reduce risk for falls at home:
1. keep electrical cords out of pathways
2. remove unnecessary furniture and provide wide pathways for ambulation
3. remove scatter rugs
4. provide adequate lighting at all times
5. do not climb stairs until permission is given by physician.

8.e. The client will state signs and symptoms to report to the health care provider.

8.e.1. Refer to Standardized Postoperative Care Plan, Nursing Diagnosis 21, action c (p. 135), for signs and symptoms to report to the health care provider.
2. Instruct client to report these additional signs and symptoms:
a. persistent or increased pain or spasms in operative extremity
b. loss of sensation or movement in operative extremity
c. inability to maintain operative extremity in a neutral position
d. inability to bear weight on operative extremity once weight-bearing is allowed
e. shortening of operative extremity (will probably be noticed as a limp once full weight-bearing is resumed).

8.f. The client will identify community resources that can assist with home management and provide transportation.

8.f.1. Provide information about community resources that can assist the client and significant others with home management and provide transportation (e.g. home health agencies, Meals on Wheels, church groups, transportation services).
2. Initiate a referral if indicated.

8.g. The client will verbalize an understanding of and a plan for adhering to recommended follow-up care including future appointments with health care provider and physical therapist, medications prescribed, activity level, and wound care.

8.g.1. Refer to Standardized Postoperative Care Plan, Nursing Diagnosis 21 (pp. 135-136), for routine postoperative instructions and measures to improve client compliance.
2. Reinforce the importance of keeping appointments with physical therapist.

# Laminectomy/Diskectomy with or without Fusion

A laminectomy is the surgical removal of the lamina of a vertebra. It may be performed to allow for the removal of a neoplasm or bone fragments that are putting pressure on spinal nerve roots or the spinal cord or to enable a rhizotomy or cordotomy to be performed to treat intractable pain. Most commonly, a laminectomy or a laminotomy (the surgical division of the lamina of a vertebra) is performed to gain access to a herniated nucleus pulposus ("ruptured disk") so that a diskectomy (removal of the herniated portion of the disk) can be accomplished.

Disk herniation is usually the result of trauma (e.g. falls, vehicular accidents, penetrating wounds) or strain caused by factors such as improper lifting of heavy objects, continued poor posture, awkward movement, sneezing, or coughing. Degenerative changes in the disks, supporting ligaments, and vertebrae are known to begin about age 30 and make the disks more prone to rupture. The most common sites of disk herniation are C5-6, C6-7, L4-5, and L5-S1. These areas of the spine are the most flexible and therefore are subjected to a greater amount of movement and strain. Signs and symptoms of lumbar disk herniation can include low back pain which radiates down the buttock, thigh, calf, and ankle on affected side; muscle spasms in lower back; muscle weakness, numbness, or tingling in affected lower extremity; constipation; and/or urinary retention. Clinical manifestations of cervical disk herniation can include neck pain which radiates to the shoulder, arm, and fingers on affected side; muscle weakness, numbness, or tingling in affected arm and fingers; and/or muscle spasms in the neck.

A diskectomy is usually indicated if conservative measures such as bed rest and anti-inflammatory medications fail to control pain or neurological impairments persist or worsen. Disk removal can be accomplished by a percutaneous lateral diskectomy, microdiskectomy, or most commonly, a laminectomy. A laminectomy can be performed using an anterior or posterior approach depending on the location of the protruding disk and physician preference. A spinal fusion (immobilization of the vertebrae using bone from client's iliac crest or from a bone bank and/or using a fixation device such as wire and/or rods) may be performed with the laminectomy if the vertebral column in the surgical area is unstable.

**This care plan focuses on the adult client hospitalized for a laminectomy* that is being performed to remove a herniated nucleus pulposus that has not responded to conservative management.** Preoperatively, goals of care are to reduce fear and anxiety and educate the client regarding postoperative management. Postoperative goals of care are to maintain comfort, prevent complications, and educate the client regarding follow-up care.

---

*The care of a client hospitalized for a laminectomy with spinal fusion is also discussed. If a fusion is performed and activity is limited for longer than 72 hours, refer to the Care Plan on Immobility.

## DIAGNOSTIC TESTS

Spinal x-rays
Computed tomography (CT) of the spine
Magnetic resonance imaging (MRI)
Myelography
Diskography
Electromyography
Nerve conduction studies

## DISCHARGE CRITERIA

Prior to discharge, the client will:

- have pain controlled
- have no signs and symptoms of complications
- identify ways to prevent recurrent disk herniation
- demonstrate the ability to correctly apply and remove stabilization device if one is required
- verbalize an understanding of ways to maintain skin integrity when wearing a stabilization device
- state signs and symptoms to report to the health care provider
- verbalize an understanding of and a plan for adhering to recommended follow-up care including future appointments with health care provider, medications prescribed, activity level, and wound care.

**NURSING/ COLLABORATIVE DIAGNOSES**



**See Standardized Preoperative and Postoperative Care Plans for additional diagnoses.**

## PREOPERATIVE

**Use in conjunction with the Standardized Preoperative Care Plan.**

### 1. NURSING DIAGNOSIS: Knowledge deficit

regarding hospital routines associated with surgery, physical preparation for laminectomy and spinal fusion (if planned), sensations that normally occur following surgery and anesthesia, and postoperative care.

| Desired Outcomes | Nursing Actions and ***Selected Purposes/Rationales*** |
|---|---|
| 1.a. The client will verbalize an understanding of usual preoperative care and postoperative sensations and care. | 1.a.1. Refer to Standardized Preoperative Care Plan, Nursing Diagnosis 4, actions a.1-4 (pp. 111-112), for information to include in preoperative teaching.<br>2. Provide additional information regarding postoperative care:<br>a. explain that client may begin progressive activity the evening of or morning after a laminectomy<br>b. if client is to wear a stabilization device such as a soft cervical collar or back brace while the surgical area heals, explain that the device is to be worn during activity (some physicians order a stabilization device for 4-6 weeks following a laminectomy if the surgery is fairly extensive and/or the client has a tendency to be too active)<br>c. if a spinal fusion is also planned:<br>1. explain that progressive activity usually begins 1-3 days after surgery depending on physician preference and extensiveness of the surgery<br>2. reinforce physician's explanation about the type of stabilization device client will need to wear while the surgical area heals (usually a rigid cervical collar or halo device following a cervical fusion and a lumbar brace or body jacket following a lumbar fusion)<br>d. if client has muscle weakness or numbness or tingling in the affected extremity, explain that it may take weeks to months to resolve after surgery due to surgical trauma and the time it takes the peripheral nerves to heal<br>e. explain to client that the pain he/she is experiencing preoperatively |

| Desired Outcomes | Nursing Actions and ***Selected Purposes/Rationales*** |
|---|---|
| | may still be present postoperatively due to nerve irritation and edema resulting from the surgery; assure him/her that the presence of pain does not indicate that the surgery was unsuccessful.<br>3. Allow time for questions and clarification of information provided. |
| 1.b. The client will demonstrate the ability to perform activities designed to prevent postoperative complications. | 1.b.1. Refer to Standardized Preoperative Care Plan, Nursing Diagnosis 4, action b.1 (p. 112), for instructions on ways to prevent postoperative complications.<br>2. Provide additional instructions about ways to prevent postoperative complications:<br>a. instruct client how to logroll and stress the importance of turning in this manner after surgery (the length of time logrolling is necessary increases if a fusion was performed)<br>b. instruct client to avoid extreme flexion, hyperextension, and twisting of the cervical or lumbar spine postoperatively<br>c. demonstrate the correct way to change from a lying to standing position (e.g. keeping spine in proper alignment, utilizing arm and leg muscles)<br>d. reinforce physician's or physical therapist's instructions about exercises to strengthen arm, leg, and abdominal muscles (increased strength of these muscles decreases strain on the spine)<br>e. demonstrate proper posture and good body mechanics and stress the importance of lifelong adherence to these principles.<br>3. Allow time for questions, clarification, and return demonstration. |

## POSTOPERATIVE

**Use in conjunction with the Standardized Postoperative Care Plan.**

### 1. NURSING DIAGNOSIS: High risk for peripheral neurovascular dysfunction

related to:
a. trauma to the nerves or blood vessels associated with surgery;
b. blood accumulation and inflammation in the surgical area;
c. dislocation of the bone graft and/or fixation device (if a fusion was performed);
d. excessive pressure exerted by stabilization device (client may need to wear one temporarily following surgery).

| Desired Outcome | Nursing Actions and ***Selected Purposes/Rationales*** |
|---|---|
| 1. The client will maintain normal peripheral neurovascular function as evidenced by:<br>a. palpable peripheral pulses<br>b. capillary refill time less than 3 seconds<br>c. extremities warm and usual color<br>d. ability to flex and extend feet and toes | 1.a. Assess for and report signs and symptoms of peripheral neurovascular dysfunction (check upper extremities after surgery on the cervical area and lower extremities after surgery on the lumbar area):<br>1. diminished or absent peripheral pulses<br>2. capillary refill time greater than 3 seconds<br>3. pallor, blanching, cyanosis, or coolness of extremities<br>4. inability to flex or extend foot or toes or hands or fingers<br>5. decreased tone or strength in biceps or quadriceps<br>6. development of or increase in numbness or tingling in extremities<br>7. increase in pain in extremities.<br>b. Implement measures *to reduce the risk for peripheral neurovascular dysfunction:*<br>1. perform actions to reduce strain on surgical area (see Postoperative |

and hands and fingers
e. usual tone and strength in biceps and quadriceps
f. expected resolution of numbness and tingling in extremities
g. no increase in pain in extremities.

Nursing Diagnosis 2, action b.1) *in order to prevent bleeding and subsequent hematoma formation in the surgical area and to reduce the risk for dislocation of the bone graft and/or fixation device (if fusion was performed)*
2. maintain wound suction and patency of wound drain *to reduce the accumulation of blood in the surgical area and subsequently prevent increased pressure on nerves and blood vessels*
3. apply stabilization device properly; notify orthotist if it appears to create excessive pressure on any area
4. administer corticosteroids (e.g. dexamethasone) if ordered *to reduce inflammation in the surgical area.*

c. If signs and symptoms of peripheral neurovascular dysfunction occur:
1. assess for and correct improper body alignment and external causes of excessive pressure (e.g. tight or improperly applied stabilization device)
2. notify physician if signs and symptoms persist
3. prepare client for surgical intervention (e.g. evacuation of hematoma, repositioning of dislocated bone graft and/or fixation device) if planned.

## 2. NURSING DIAGNOSIS: Pain

related to:
a. tissue trauma and reflex muscle spasms associated with the surgery;
b. removal of bone (client's own bone [usually taken from the iliac crest] may be used to achieve spinal fusion);
c. stretching and compression of sensory nerves associated with blood accumulation and inflammation in the surgical area;
d. irritation from drainage tube (wound drain may be present, especially following a spinal fusion);
e. stress on surgical area associated with movement;
f. release of pressure on compressed spinal nerve root following removal of the herniated nucleus pulposus (improved sensory nerve function can cause a temporary increase in pain in area[s] of previously diminished sensation).

| Desired Outcome | Nursing Actions and ***Selected Purposes/Rationales*** |
|---|---|
| 2. The client will experience diminished pain (see Standardized Postoperative Care Plan, Nursing Diagnosis 6 [p. 119], for outcome criteria). | 2.a. Refer to Standardized Postoperative Care Plan, Nursing Diagnosis 6 (p. 119), for measures related to assessment and management of pain.<br>b. Implement additional measures *to reduce pain:*<br>1. perform actions *to reduce strain on the surgical area:*<br>a. logroll client for first 48 hours postoperatively and then instruct him/her to continue to logroll when turning self<br>b. ensure that client is always positioned with spine in proper alignment<br>c. apply stabilization device if ordered *to provide additional support to surgical area*<br>d. reinforce preoperative instructions to avoid hyperextension, extreme flexion, and twisting of spine<br>e. if lumbar laminectomy was performed, assist client to maintain a position that results in flattening of the lumbosacral spine (e.g. slight knee flexion when supine, knees flexed while in side-lying position, feet elevated on footstool when sitting in chair) *in order to reduce stretching of the nerves and muscles in the lower back*<br>f. instruct client to avoid sitting for longer than 30 minutes (some physicians allow clients to sit only for meals for first few postoperative days) |

| Desired Outcome | Nursing Actions and ***Selected Purposes/Rationales*** |
|---|---|
| | g. instruct client to avoid straining to have a bowel movement (especially after lumbar laminectomy) and vigorous coughing; consult physician about an order for a laxative, stool softener, and antitussive if indicated<br>2. if appropriate, perform actions *to reduce pressure on bone graft donor site* (e.g. position client so he/she is not lying on site, protect the site with padding if stabilization device is worn over it)<br>3. administer corticosteroids (e.g. dexamethasone) if ordered *to reduce inflammation in the surgical area.* |

## 3. NURSING DIAGNOSIS: Actual/High risk for impaired skin integrity

related to:
a. disruption of skin associated with the surgical procedure;
b. irritation of skin associated with contact with wound drainage, use of tape, and pressure from drainage tube and/or stabilization device if present.

| Desired Outcomes | Nursing Actions and ***Selected Purposes/Rationales*** |
|---|---|
| 3.a. The client will experience normal healing of the surgical wound (see Standardized Postoperative Care Plan, Nursing Diagnosis 9, outcome a [p. 122], for outcome criteria). | 3.a. Refer to Standardized Postoperative Care Plan, Nursing Diagnosis 9, action a (pp. 122-123), for measures related to assessment and promotion of wound healing. |
| 3.b. The client will maintain skin integrity as evidenced by:<br>1. absence of redness and irritation<br>2. no skin breakdown. | 3.b.1. Inspect the following skin areas for signs and symptoms of irritation and breakdown:<br>a. areas in contact with wound drainage, tape, and drainage tubing<br>b. area under stabilization device.<br>2. Refer to Standardized Postoperative Care Plan, Nursing Diagnosis 9, action b.2 (p. 123), for measures related to prevention of skin irritation and breakdown resulting from contact with wound drainage, drainage tubing, and tape.<br>3. Implement measures *to prevent skin irritation and breakdown under stabilization device:*<br>a. apply device securely enough to keep it from rubbing and irritating the skin but not too tightly<br>b. position client so that the device is not causing excessive pressure on any area<br>c. assist client to put a cotton T-shirt on under the brace or body jacket and ensure that the shirt is dry and wrinkle-free<br>d. apply cornstarch to skin under stabilization device *in order to keep skin dry and reduce friction and subsequent skin irritation*<br>e. pad areas over bony prominences before applying stabilization device<br>f. keep stabilization device clean and dry<br>g. instruct client to refrain from poking anything under the stabilization device<br>h. consult physician, physical therapist, or orthotist if stabilization device is putting excessive pressure on the skin. |

4. If skin breakdown occurs:
   a. notify physician
   b. continue with above measures to prevent further irritation and breakdown
   c. perform wound or decubitus care as ordered or per standard hospital procedure
   d. assess client closely and report signs and symptoms of infection (e.g. elevated temperature; redness, warmth, and edema around incision or area of breakdown; unusual drainage from site).

## 4. NURSING DIAGNOSIS: Urinary retention

related to:

a. pooling of urine in kidney and bladder associated with horizontal positioning;
b. inability to urinate associated with:
   1. indirect sympathetic nervous system stimulation of bladder and urinary sphincters resulting from pain, fear, and anxiety
   2. direct stimulation of the sympathetic fibers that innervate the bladder (may occur with a lumbar laminectomy);
c. decreased bladder muscle tone and perception of bladder fullness associated with depressant effects of some medications (e.g. anesthetic agents, narcotic analgesics, central-acting muscle relaxants).

| Desired Outcome | Nursing Actions and ***Selected Purposes/Rationales*** |
|---|---|
| 4. The client will not experience urinary retention (see Standardized Postoperative Care Plan, Nursing Diagnosis 13 [p. 126], for outcome criteria). | 4. Refer to Standardized Postoperative Care Plan, Nursing Diagnosis 13 (p. 126), for measures related to assessment and management of urinary retention. |

## 5. COLLABORATIVE DIAGNOSES: Potential complications:

a. **respiratory distress** related to:
   1. damage to the phrenic nerve during surgery or compression of the nerve associated with inflammation (this is a possibility in clients who have had a cervical laminectomy because the phrenic nerve arises at the C3-5 level)
   2. tracheal compression associated with inflammation or accumulation of blood in the surgical area following a cervical laminectomy (particularly if the anterior approach was used)
   3. closure of the glottis associated with paralysis of the vocal cords as a result of injury to the bilateral recurrent laryngeal nerves during an anterior cervical laminectomy;
b. **cerebrospinal fistula** related to inadvertent damage to and/or incomplete closure of the dura (care is taken during surgery to keep the dura intact; however, it is sometimes necessary to incise dura that extends along the involved nerve root);
c. **recurrent laryngeal nerve damage** related to surgical trauma or pressure on the nerve(s) associated with inflammation or accumulation of blood in the surgical area (can occur with an anterior cervical laminectomy);

d. **paralytic ileus** related to:
   1. impaired innervation of the intestinal tract following a lumbar laminectomy associated with stimulation of sympathetic nerves and/or loss of parasympathetic nerve function in the operative area
   2. depressant effects of anesthesia and some medications (e.g. central-acting muscle relaxants, narcotic analgesics).

| Desired Outcomes | Nursing Actions and ***Selected Purposes/Rationales*** |
|---|---|
| 5.a. The client will not experience respiratory distress as evidenced by:<br>1. unlabored respirations at 14-20/minute<br>2. absence of stridor and sternocleidomastoid muscle retraction<br>3. usual mental status<br>4. usual skin color<br>5. blood gases within normal range. | 5.a.1. Following a cervical laminectomy, assess for and report:<br>a. increased edema or an expanding hematoma in surgical area<br>b. deviation of trachea from midline<br>c. statements of difficulty swallowing or choking sensation<br>d. signs and symptoms of respiratory distress (e.g. rapid and/or labored respirations, stridor, sternocleidomastoid muscle retraction, restlessness, agitation, cyanosis)<br>e. abnormal blood gases<br>f. significant change in oximetry results.<br>2. Have tracheostomy equipment readily available following a cervical laminectomy.<br>3. Implement measures *to prevent respiratory distress following a cervical laminectomy:*<br>a. perform actions *to reduce inflammation and/or prevent bleeding and subsequent hematoma formation in the surgical area:*<br>1. implement measures to reduce strain on the surgical area (see Postoperative Nursing Diagnosis 2, action b.1)<br>2. elevate head of bed 30-45° unless contraindicated<br>3. apply ice pack to incisional area as ordered<br>4. administer corticosteroids (e.g. dexamethasone) if ordered<br>b. maintain wound suction and patency of wound drain *to prevent the accumulation of blood in the surgical area.*<br>4. If signs and symptoms of respiratory distress occur:<br>a. place client in a high Fowler's position unless contraindicated<br>b. loosen neck dressing or cervical brace or collar if it appears tight<br>c. administer oxygen as ordered<br>d. assist with intubation or emergency tracheostomy if indicated<br>e. prepare client for surgical evacuation of hematoma or repair of the bleeding vessel(s) if indicated<br>f. provide emotional support to client and significant others. |
| 5.b. The client will not develop a cerebrospinal fistula as evidenced by:<br>1. absence of cerebrospinal fluid drainage from lower back or neck incision<br>2. no complaints of headache. | 5.b.1. Assess for and report signs and symptoms of a cerebrospinal fluid leak *(indicates a tear in the dura):*<br>a. presence of glucose in wound drainage as shown by positive results on a glucose reagent strip (e.g. Tes-Tape, Dextrostix); be aware that any drainage containing blood will also test positive for glucose<br>b. clear halo or watery, yellowish ring around bloody or serosanguineous drainage on lower back or neck dressing, sheet, or pillowcase<br>c. complaints of a headache.<br>2. Implement measures to reduce strain on surgical area (see Postoperative Nursing Diagnosis 2, action b.1) *in order to promote healing of the dura and prevent subsequent development of cerebrospinal fistula.*<br>3. If signs and symptoms of cerebrospinal fistula occur:<br>a. maintain activity restrictions as ordered *to reduce stress on the dural tear*<br>b. maintain meticulous sterile technique when changing dressings<br>c. change dressings as soon as they become damp<br>d. administer antimicrobials if ordered<br>e. assess for and report signs and symptoms of meningitis (e.g. fever, |

chills, increasing or persistent headache, nuchal rigidity, photophobia, positive Kernig's and Brudzinski's signs)
f. prepare client for surgical repair of the torn dura if it does not heal spontaneously
g. provide emotional support to the client and significant others.

5.c. The client will experience resolution of recurrent laryngeal nerve damage if it occurs as evidenced by:
1. improved voice tone and quality
2. gradual resolution of hoarseness
3. absence of respiratory distress.

5.c.1. Assess for the following indications of recurrent laryngeal nerve damage:
a. voice changes (e.g. hoarseness; weak, whispery voice; inability to speak)
b. respiratory distress (see action a.1.d in this diagnosis).
2. Implement measures to reduce inflammation and/or prevent bleeding and subsequent hematoma formation in the surgical area (see action a.3 in this diagnosis) *in order to reduce pressure on the recurrent laryngeal nerves.*
3. If signs and symptoms of recurrent laryngeal nerve damage occur:
a. encourage client to limit verbal communication *in order to rest the vocal cords*
b. implement measures to facilitate communication (e.g. provide pad and pencil, flash cards, or magic slate; maintain quiet environment *so client does not have to raise voice to be heard*)
c. reinforce physician's explanation regarding the permanence of voice changes (voice tone and quality usually return to normal as inflammation subsides)
d. notify physician immediately if signs and symptoms of respiratory distress occur, client is unable to speak, or hoarseness or voice changes worsen.

5.d. The client will not develop a paralytic ileus (see Standardized Postoperative Care Plan, Collaborative Diagnosis 19, outcome d [p. 133], for outcome criteria).

5.d. Refer to Standardized Postoperative Care Plan, Collaborative Diagnosis 19, action d (p. 133), for measures related to assessment and management of a paralytic ileus.

## 6. NURSING DIAGNOSIS: Knowledge deficit

regarding follow-up care.

| Desired Outcomes | Nursing Actions and ***Selected Purposes/Rationales*** |
|---|---|
| 6.a. The client will identify ways to prevent recurrent disk herniation. | 6.a.1. Provide instructions regarding ways to reduce back and/or neck strain and reduce risk of recurrent disk herniation:<br>a. maintain an optimal weight<br>b. provide adequate support for spine (e.g. sleep on a firm mattress; sit on firm, straight-backed or contoured chairs; wear stabilization device as prescribed)<br>c. always use proper body mechanics (e.g. bend at the knees rather than waist, push rather than pull objects, carry items close to body)<br>d. always maintain good posture<br>e. begin prescribed, progressive exercise program to strengthen back, neck, arms, legs, and abdominal muscles when allowed.<br>2. Provide a dietary consult regarding a weight reduction program if indicated. |

| Desired Outcomes | Nursing Actions and ***Selected Purposes/Rationales*** |
|---|---|
| | 3. Allow time for client to practice good posture when sitting, standing, and walking; proper positioning when resting; and any exercises allowed in immediate postoperative period. Encourage client to think about and plan movements before doing them.<br>4. Allow time for questions, clarification, and return demonstration of proper body mechanics, positioning, and exercises allowed. |
| 6.b. The client will demonstrate the ability to correctly apply and remove stabilization device if one is required. | 6.b.1. Reinforce instructions on the correct way to apply and remove stabilization device if client needs to wear one after discharge.<br>2. Allow time for questions, clarification, and return demonstration. |
| 6.c. The client will verbalize an understanding of ways to maintain skin integrity when wearing a stabilization device. | 6.c.1. If client is to be discharged with a stabilization device, instruct him/her to examine skin daily when device is off during personal hygiene (if device should not be removed, demonstrate how to examine underneath it using a mirror and flashlight).<br>2. Instruct client in ways to maintain skin integrity if he/she needs to wear a stabilization device:<br>a. apply device properly and maintain spine in good alignment to avoid undue pressure in any area<br>b. wear a cotton T-shirt under brace or body jacket and keep shirt dry and wrinkle-free<br>c. apply cornstarch to skin under stabilization device to keep skin dry and reduce irritation caused by friction<br>d. avoid poking anything under the device<br>e. pad areas between stabilization device and bony prominences. |
| 6.d. The client will state signs and symptoms to report to the health care provider. | 6.d.1. Refer to Standardized Postoperative Care Plan, Nursing Diagnosis 21, action c (p. 135), for signs and symptoms to report to the health care provider.<br>2. Instruct client to report these additional signs and symptoms:<br>a. decreased movement or sensation in extremities<br>b. coolness or bluish color of extremities<br>c. increasing or recurrent numbness, tingling, or pain in surgical area or extremity<br>d. difficulty standing up straight (after lumbar surgery) or keeping neck straight (after cervical surgery)<br>e. persistent and/or severe headache<br>f. drainage of clear or bloody fluid from incision<br>g. persistent hoarseness (following anterior cervical laminectomy)<br>h. reddened or irritated area on skin underneath stabilization device<br>i. loosening of stabilization device. |
| 6.e. The client will verbalize an understanding of and a plan for adhering to recommended follow-up care including future appointments with health care provider, medications prescribed, activity level, and wound care. | 6.e.1. Refer to Standardized Postoperative Care Plan, Nursing Diagnosis 21 (pp. 135-136), for routine postoperative instructions and measures to improve client compliance.<br>2. Reinforce physician's instructions regarding activity (the restrictions will vary depending on extensiveness of surgery, client condition, and physician preference):<br>a. avoid lifting heavy objects<br>b. progress through exercise program at the rate prescribed<br>c. avoid sitting or standing for longer than 30 minutes at a time (especially after surgery on lumbar area)<br>d. schedule adequate rest periods<br>e. avoid driving a car (causes increased flexion of the spine) and taking long car rides (the vibrations can jar the spine and long periods without significant changes in position can increase stiffness and discomfort) until allowed. |

# Total Hip Replacement

A total hip replacement (arthroplasty) is a surgical procedure in which the ball and socket components of the hip joint are replaced with prosthetic devices. There are a variety of prosthetic devices available. The prostheses are either cemented in place using an agent called methylmethacrylate or are uncemented (cementless). Uncemented prostheses have porous surfaces that permit bone ingrowth to occur and provide biological fixation. A total hip replacement is performed to relieve joint pain that has been resistant to conservative management and/or improve joint mobility in persons with severe degenerative or rheumatoid arthritis, avascular necrosis of the femoral head, or congenital hip deformity. It may also be performed following failure of previous reconstructive hip surgery.

**This care plan focuses on the adult client hospitalized for a total hip replacement.** Preoperative goals of care are to reduce fear and anxiety and educate the client regarding ways to prevent postoperative complications and facilitate rehabilitation. Postoperatively, the goals of care are to maintain comfort, prevent complications, assist the client to regain maximum mobility, and educate the client regarding follow-up care. Prevention of infection is of major importance in caring for the client who has had a total hip replacement since infection of the operative hip usually necessitates surgical debridement and/or removal of the prostheses.

## DIAGNOSTIC TESTS

X-rays of the hip and femoral shaft

## DISCHARGE CRITERIA

Prior to discharge, the client will:

- have reduced hip pain
- have expected degree of mobility of hip joint
- have no signs and symptoms of complications
- verbalize an understanding of activity and position restrictions necessary to prevent dislocation of the hip prostheses
- demonstrate correct transfer and ambulation techniques and proper use of ambulatory aids
- demonstrate the ability to correctly perform the prescribed exercises
- identify ways to reduce the risk of falls in the home environment
- state signs and symptoms to report to the health care provider
- identify community resources that can assist with home management and provide transportation
- verbalize an understanding of and a plan for adhering to recommended follow-up care including future appointments with health care provider and physical therapist, medications prescribed, activity level, and wound care.

## NURSING/COLLABORATIVE DIAGNOSES

**6.** High risk for trauma△ *801*
**7.** Potential complications:
  **a.** hemorrhage and/or hematoma formation
  **b.** dislocation of hip prosthesis(es)
  **c.** thromboembolism△ *802*
**8.** Knowledge deficit△ *804*

**See Standardized Preoperative and Postoperative Care Plans for additional diagnoses.**

## PREOPERATIVE

**Use in conjunction with the Standardized Preoperative Care Plan.**

### 1. NURSING DIAGNOSIS: Knowledge deficit

regarding hospital routines associated with surgery, physical preparation for the total hip replacement, sensations that normally occur following surgery and anesthesia, and postoperative care.

| Desired Outcomes | Nursing Actions and ***Selected Purposes/Rationales*** |
|---|---|
| 1.a. The client will verbalize an understanding of usual preoperative care and postoperative sensations and care. | 1.a.1. Refer to Standardized Preoperative Care Plan, Nursing Diagnosis 4, actions a.1-4 (pp. 111-112), for information to include in preoperative teaching.<br>2. Provide additional information on specific preoperative care for clients having a total hip replacement:<br>a. explain that the following measures will be performed to reduce risk of a postoperative hip infection:<br>1. the operative hip and thigh will be scrubbed with an antiseptic solution (e.g. povidone-iodine) before surgery<br>2. injections will not be given in the operative extremity<br>3. existing infections will be treated before surgery; instruct client to report any symptoms of infection (e.g. cough, runny nose, burning on urination)<br>4. antimicrobials will probably be administered prophylactically before and after surgery<br>b. explain that anticoagulants (e.g. heparin, warfarin) and/or antiplatelet agents (e.g. low-molecular-weight dextran, low-dose aspirin) may be administered before surgery to reduce risk of postoperative thrombus formation; inform client that coagulation studies are usually done before starting these medications, especially if he/she has been taking aspirin, aspirin-containing compounds, or ibuprofen.<br>3. Allow time for questions and clarification of information provided. |
| 1.b. The client will demonstrate the ability to perform activities designed to prevent postoperative complications. | 1.b.1. Refer to Standardized Preoperative Care Plan, Nursing Diagnosis 4, action b.1 (p. 112), for instructions on ways to prevent postoperative complications.<br>2. Provide additional instructions about ways to prevent complications following total hip replacement:<br>a. reinforce physician's or physical therapist's instructions on:<br>1. transfer techniques that can be performed without flexing hip beyond the prescribed limit |

2. exercises (e.g. quadriceps- and gluteal-setting, upper extremity strengthening, active heel slides, straight leg raising)
3. ambulation techniques and proper use of ambulatory aids (weight-bearing limitations are determined by the physician and vary depending on the type of prostheses used; weight-bearing is allowed earlier with cemented prostheses)

b. instruct client in the correct way to use overhead trapeze and unoperative extremity to move self
c. explain the following activity and positioning limitations that need to be adhered to postoperatively to prevent dislocation of the prosthesis(es):
1. operative extremity will be maintained in an abducted position by a balanced suspension device, abduction wedge, or 2-3 pillows for first few days after surgery
2. operative leg should not be brought toward the midline, crossed, or rotated inwardly
3. if turning is allowed, it should be done only with assistance of trained personnel
4. hip flexion of 45-60° will be permitted initially and then should not exceed 90° during the rehabilitation phase.

3. Allow time for questions, clarification, and return demonstration.

## POSTOPERATIVE

**Use in conjunction with the Standardized Postoperative Care Plan.**

### 1. NURSING DIAGNOSIS: High risk for peripheral neurovascular dysfunction: operative extremity

related to trauma to the nerves or blood vessels associated with surgery, blood accumulation and edema in the surgical area, improper alignment of operative extremity, excessive pressure exerted by balanced suspension device or abductor wedge, and dislocation of the prosthesis(es).

| Desired Outcome | Nursing Actions and ***Selected Purposes/Rationales*** |
|---|---|
| 1. The client will maintain normal neurovascular function in the operative extremity as evidenced by:<br>a. palpable pedal pulses<br>b. capillary refill time in toes less than 3 seconds<br>c. extremity warm and usual color<br>d. ability to flex and extend foot and toes<br>e. absence of numbness and tingling in foot and toes<br>f. absence of foot pain | 1.a. Assess for and report signs and symptoms of neurovascular dysfunction in the operative extremity:<br>1. diminished or absent peripheral pulses<br>2. capillary refill time in toes greater than 3 seconds<br>3. pallor, blanching, cyanosis, or coolness of the extremity<br>4. inability to flex or extend foot or toes<br>5. numbness or tingling in foot or toes<br>6. pain in foot during passive motion of the toes or foot<br>7. increased pain in the extremity.<br>b. Implement measures *to prevent neurovascular dysfunction in the operative extremity:*<br>1. perform actions to prevent hematoma formation (see Postoperative Collaborative Diagnosis 7, action a.2)<br>2. make sure that elastic wraps, trochanter roll, balanced suspension device, and abductor wedge are not exerting pressure on the popliteal space, Achilles tendon, and lateral and medial aspects of the knee and ankle |

| Desired Outcome | Nursing Actions and ***Selected Purposes/Rationales*** |
|---|---|
| during passive movement of foot and toes<br>g. no increase in pain in extremity. | 3. perform actions to prevent dislocation of the prostheses (see Postoperative Collaborative Diagnosis 7, action b.2).<br>c. If signs and symptoms of neurovascular dysfunction occur:<br>1. assess for and correct causes of uneven pressure (e.g. tight elastic wraps, improper positioning of abductor wedge)<br>2. notify physician if the signs and symptoms persist<br>3. prepare client for closed reduction (e.g. traction) or surgical intervention (e.g. relocation of prosthesis, hematoma evacuation) if planned. |

## 2. NURSING DIAGNOSIS: Pain: hip

related to tissue trauma and reflex muscle spasms associated with the surgery, blood accumulation and edema in surgical area, and improper positioning of the operative extremity.

| Desired Outcome | Nursing Actions and ***Selected Purposes/Rationales*** |
|---|---|
| 2. The client will experience diminished hip pain (see Standardized Postoperative Care Plan, Nursing Diagnosis 6 [p. 119], for outcome criteria). | 2.a. Refer to Standardized Postoperative Care Plan, Nursing Diagnosis 6 (p. 119), for measures related to assessment and reduction of pain.<br>b. Implement additional measures *to reduce pain:*<br>1. keep operative extremity in an abducted position (some physicians ensure this position by placing the extremity in balanced suspension for 24 hours after surgery; others order placement of an abduction wedge or 2-3 pillows between legs at all times)<br>2. maintain restrictions on the degree of hip flexion as ordered (usually a 45-60° maximum is allowed for first 2-3 days with a maximum of 90° during rehabilitation period)<br>3. place trochanter or hip roll against the operative site for first 24-48 hours after surgery *(pressure on the operative area helps maintain alignment and prevent hematoma formation)*<br>4. maintain patency of wound drainage system (e.g. prevent kinking of tubing, empty collection device as needed, keep collection device below surgical wound, maintain suction as ordered) *to reduce accumulation of fluid in surgical area*<br>5. move operative extremity gently<br>6. if turning is allowed, keep pillows between legs when turning and while in side-lying position *to prevent adduction and resultant strain on surgical site*<br>7. administer prescribed analgesics before exercise and ambulation sessions. |

## 3. NURSING DIAGNOSIS: Actual/High risk for impaired skin integrity

related to:

a. disruption of skin associated with the surgical procedure;
b. delayed wound healing associated with decreased nutritional status and inadequate blood supply to wound area;
c. irritation of skin associated with contact with wound drainage, pressure from drainage tubes, and use of tape;

d. excessive or prolonged pressure on tissues from balanced suspension device, abductor wedge, and elastic wraps or stockings;
e. damage to the skin and/or subcutaneous tissue associated with prolonged pressure on tissues, friction, and shearing while mobility is decreased.

| Desired Outcomes | Nursing Actions and ***Selected Purposes/Rationales*** |
|---|---|
| 3.a. The client will experience normal healing of the surgical wound (see Standardized Postoperative Care Plan, Nursing Diagnosis 9, outcome a [p. 122], for outcome criteria). | 3.a. Refer to Standardized Postoperative Care Plan, Nursing Diagnosis 9, action a (pp. 122-123), for measures related to assessment and promotion of wound healing. |
| 3.b. The client will maintain skin integrity as evidenced by:<br>1. absence of redness and irritation<br>2. no skin breakdown. | 3.b.1. Inspect the following sites for pallor, redness, and breakdown:<br>a. skin in contact with wound drainage, tape, and drainage tubing<br>b. back, coccyx, and buttocks<br>c. elbows and heels<br>d. pressure points on operative extremity in contact with balanced suspension device<br>e. areas in contact with abductor wedge<br>f. areas under elastic wraps or stockings.<br>2. Refer to Standardized Postoperative Care Plan, Nursing Diagnosis 9, action b.2 (p. 123), for measures related to prevention of skin irritation and breakdown resulting from contact with wound drainage, drainage tubings, and tape.<br>3. Implement measures *to prevent skin breakdown associated with decreased mobility:*<br>a. instruct client to use overhead trapeze to lift self and shift weight every 30 minutes<br>b. gently massage around reddened areas at least every 2 hours<br>c. perform actions *to prevent shearing* (shearing occurs when one tissue layer slides past another) *and skin surface abrasion:*<br>1. apply a thin layer of powder or cornstarch to bottom sheet or skin *to absorb moisture (moist skin is more likely to adhere to sheet) and reduce friction*<br>2. lift and move client carefully using a turn sheet and adequate assistance<br>3. limit length of time client is in semi-Fowler's position to 30 minutes *(in this position, client tends to slide down in bed)*<br>d. turn client every 2 hours if allowed (may be allowed to turn on unoperative side)<br>e. if fade time (length of time it takes for reddened area to fade after pressure is removed) is greater than 15 minutes, increase the frequency of position changes and massages<br>f. keep skin lubricated, clean, and dry<br>g. keep bed linens dry and wrinkle-free<br>h. provide devices to reduce pressure on the skin, decrease shearing, and/or prevent moisture build-up (e.g. alternating pressure mattress or pad, flotation pad, sheepskin)<br>i. increase activity as allowed and tolerated.<br>4. Implement measures *to prevent skin breakdown associated with excessive or uneven pressure caused by balanced suspension device or abductor wedge:*<br>a. make sure metal parts on suspension device are not resting on any area of extremity |

| Desired Outcomes | Nursing Actions and ***Selected Purposes/Rationales*** |
|---|---|
| | b. maintain proper alignment of extremity in suspension device<br>c. make sure that straps holding abductor wedge in place are not too tight.<br>5. Implement measures *to prevent irritation and breakdown on elbows and heels:*<br>a. massage elbows and heels with lotion frequently<br>b. encourage client to use overhead trapeze to move self rather than pushing up with heel and elbows<br>c. provide elbow and heel protectors if indicated.<br>6. Implement measures *to prevent skin breakdown under elastic wraps or stockings:*<br>a. remove elastic wraps or stockings at least twice daily, bathe and thoroughly dry skin, and reapply smoothly<br>b. check wraps or stockings frequently and reapply if they have slipped or become wrinkled<br>c. if areas of redness develop under wraps or stockings, consult physician before reapplying.<br>7. If skin breakdown occurs:<br>a. notify physician<br>b. continue with above measures to prevent further irritation and breakdown<br>c. perform wound and decubitus care as ordered or per standard hospital procedure<br>d. assess client closely and report signs and symptoms of infection (e.g. elevated temperature; redness, warmth, and edema around area of breakdown; unusual drainage from site). |

## 4. NURSING DIAGNOSIS: Impaired physical mobility

related to:
a. pain and weakness in weight-bearing extremity associated with surgery on the hip;
b. prescribed activity and weight-bearing restrictions following total hip replacement;
c. generalized weakness associated with surgery;
d. depressant effects of some medications (e.g. narcotic analgesics, central-acting muscle relaxants);
e. fear of falling, dislodging drainage tube, dislocating prostheses, and compromising surgical wound.

| Desired Outcome | Nursing Actions and ***Selected Purposes/Rationales*** |
|---|---|
| 4. The client will maintain maximum physical mobility within prescribed activity and weight-bearing restrictions. | 4.a. Refer to Standardized Postoperative Care Plan, Nursing Diagnosis 11 (p. 125), for measures to increase client's mobility.<br>b. Implement additional measures *to increase client's mobility:*<br>1. perform actions to reduce pain (see Postoperative Nursing Diagnosis 2)<br>2. instruct client in and assist with quadriceps- and gluteal-setting exercises *to strengthen muscles needed for ambulation*<br>3. encourage client to use overhead trapeze to move self *in order to strengthen arm and shoulder muscles needed for proper use of ambulatory aids*<br>4. reinforce physical therapist's instructions regarding additional muscle strengthening exercises, transfer and ambulation techniques, and use of ambulatory aids<br>5. perform actions to prevent falls (see Postoperative Nursing Diagnosis 6, actions a and b) *to decrease client's fear of injury* |

6. assist client with ambulation as soon as allowed (usually by the 2nd postoperative day).

c. Consult physician if client is unable to achieve expected level of mobility.

## 5. NURSING DIAGNOSIS: High risk for infection: operative hip

related to:
a. introduction of pathogens into the wound during or after surgery;
b. hematoma formation (increases the likelihood of infection by providing a good medium for bacterial growth and compromising blood flow to the area);
c. increased susceptibility to infection associated with decreased effectiveness of immune system if client is elderly and immunosuppression if client has been taking corticosteroids to treat the joint disorder necessitating the surgery (e.g. rheumatoid arthritis).

| Desired Outcome | Nursing Actions and ***Selected Purposes/Rationales*** |
|---|---|
| 5. The client will remain free of infection in the operative hip (see Standardized Postoperative Care Plan, Nursing Diagnosis 16, outcome b [p. 129], for outcome criteria). | 5.a. Assess for and report the following:<br>1. continuous drainage of fluid from incision *(may be indicative of a sinus tract)*<br>2. sloughing or necrosis of skin in the operative area<br>3. signs and symptoms of wound infection (e.g. chills; fever; redness, warmth, and swelling of wound area; unusual wound drainage; foul odor from wound area; persistent or increased pain in operative hip; elevated sedimentation rate).<br>b. Refer to Standardized Postoperative Care Plan, Nursing Diagnosis 16, actions b.4 and 5 (p. 129), for measures related to prevention and treatment of wound infection.<br>c. Implement additional measures *to reduce risk for infection in the operative hip:*<br>1. use strict aseptic technique when performing wound care and emptying wound drainage device (some physicians do not allow other health care personnel to empty drainage device *because of risk of contamination)*<br>2. maintain patency of wound drainage device *in order to reduce risk of hematoma formation*<br>3. do not administer injections in operative extremity<br>4. avoid urinary catheterization but if it becomes necessary, take precautions to prevent urinary tract infection (e.g. use strict aseptic technique during catheter insertion, remove catheter as soon as possible); *the increased possibility of urinary tract infection associated with the presence of a urinary catheter increases the risk for lymphatic or hematogenous seeding of the hip wound*<br>5. administer prophylactic antimicrobials if ordered (they are usually started before surgery and continued for 2-5 days after surgery)<br>6. prepare client for drainage of hematoma or grafting of any area of skin sloughing or necrosis if planned.<br>d. If signs and symptoms of wound infection occur, prepare client for wound irrigation, surgical debridement, and/or removal of prostheses if planned. |

## 6. NURSING DIAGNOSIS: High risk for trauma

related to falls associated with:
a. weakness, fatigue, and postural hypotension resulting from effects of major

surgery (there is often significant blood loss and subsequent anemia because the hip is a very vascular area);
b. central nervous system depressant effects of some medications (e.g. narcotic analgesics, central-acting muscle relaxants);
c. weakness and pain in weight-bearing extremity as a result of the surgery;
d. improper transfer and ambulation techniques.

| Desired Outcome | Nursing Actions and ***Selected Purposes/Rationales*** |
|---|---|
| 6. The client will not experience falls. | 6.a. Refer to Standardized Postoperative Care Plan, Nursing Diagnosis 17, action a (p. 130), for measures to prevent falls.<br>b. Implement additional measures *to reduce risk of falls:*<br>1. reinforce preoperative instructions about and assist client with exercises to improve muscle strength, transfer and ambulation techniques, and use of ambulatory aids<br>2. administer prescribed analgesics before exercise and ambulation sessions *in order to reduce hip pain and subsequently maximize client's ability to utilize proper transfer and ambulation techniques*<br>3. administer blood products if ordered *to reduce weakness associated with anemia.*<br>c. Include client and significant others in planning and implementing measures to prevent falls.<br>d. If falls occur, initiate first aid measures if appropriate and notify physician. |

## 7. COLLABORATIVE DIAGNOSES:

**Potential complications:**

a. **hemorrhage and/or hematoma formation** related to surgical trauma to blood vessels (the hip is a very vascular area) and use of anticoagulants or antiplatelet agents before and after surgery;
b. **dislocation of hip prosthesis(es)** related to weakness of the hip muscles, improper positioning of the operative extremity, and/or noncompliance with weight-bearing limitations;
c. **thromboembolism** related to:
   1. trauma to vein walls during surgery
   2. venous stasis associated with decreased mobility, fluid volume deficit, and pressure exerted by balanced suspension device or abductor wedge
   3. hypercoagulability associated with increased release of tissue thromboplastin into the blood (occurs as a result of surgical trauma)
   4. decreased fibrinolytic activity (occurs in response to surgical trauma).

| Desired Outcomes | Nursing Actions and ***Selected Purposes/Rationales*** |
|---|---|
| 7.a. The client will not experience hemorrhage or hematoma formation as evidenced by:<br>1. expected amount of wound drainage<br>2. no further decline in RBC, Hct, and Hb<br>3. no significant increase in hip pain | 7.a.1. Assess for and report the following:<br>a. excessive wound drainage (expected loss is 200-500 ml in the first 24 hours, diminishing to 30 ml/shift by 48 hours after surgery)<br>b. significant decline in RBC, Hct, and Hb levels<br>c. signs and symptoms of hematoma formation (e.g. increased pain and tense swelling in buttock and/or thigh).<br>2. Implement measures *to reduce operative site bleeding and/or prevent hematoma formation:*<br>a. maintain pressure dressing over operative site as ordered<br>b. keep trochanter roll or sandbag placed firmly against operative site for the first 24-48 hours after surgery *to provide additional pressure on surgical site* |

4. absence of tense swelling at surgical site.

c. apply ice pack to operative hip if ordered
d. maintain patency of wound drainage system if present.

3. If signs and symptoms of excessive bleeding or hematoma formation occur, prepare client for return to surgery to ligate bleeding vessels and/or drain hematoma if planned.

7.b. The client will not experience dislocation of the hip prosthesis(es) as evidenced by:
1. continued resolution of hip pain
2. ability to maintain operative leg in proper alignment
3. ability to adhere to expected exercise and ambulation regimen
4. usual length of operative extremity
5. normal neurovascular status in operative leg.

7.b.1. Assess for and report signs and symptoms of dislocation of hip prosthesis(es):
a. sudden, severe hip pain followed by continued pain and muscle spasms during hip movement
b. abnormal rotation of operative leg
c. inability to move or bear weight on operative leg
d. shortening of operative leg
e. decline in neurovascular status in operative leg.

2. Implement measures *to prevent dislocation of the prosthesis(es):*
a. maintain bed rest as ordered (may be on bed rest for first 24 hours after surgery)
b. perform actions *to prevent adduction of the operative extremity:*
1. maintain extremity in abducted position using balanced suspension device or an abduction wedge or 2-3 pillows between legs
2. remind client to avoid crossing legs
3. do not move operative extremity past midline
4. turn client only as ordered and always with pillows between legs
c. maintain operative extremity in proper alignment (be particularly alert to preventing internal rotation)
d. instruct client to avoid extreme internal and external rotation of operative leg
e. maintain restrictions on head of bed elevation if ordered (some physicians order a 45-60° maximum for first 2-3 days after surgery) *to reduce hip flexion*
f. perform actions *to prevent extreme (beyond 90°) hip flexion:*
1. instruct client not to lean forward to reach objects on end of bed or on floor or to put on slippers, socks, or shoes
2. raise the entire bed to client's midthigh level before he/she gets in or out of bed *in order to reduce the degree of hip flexion that occurs when client sits on edge of bed*
3. provide a high, firm chair (or elevate sitting surface with pillows) and a raised toilet seat for client's use *in order to reduce degree of hip flexion when client sits down*
4. do not elevate operative leg when client is sitting in chair
g. reinforce importance of adhering to recommended weight-bearing restrictions (the amount of weight-bearing allowed is based on the type of prostheses inserted; with cemented prostheses, partial weight-bearing is usually allowed as soon as ambulation is started)
h. instruct and assist client to pivot and bear weight on the unoperative leg when transferring from bed to chair and raising self out of chair.

3. If signs and symptoms of dislocation of the prosthesis(es) occur:
a. maintain client on bed rest
b. prepare client for x-rays of the surgical area
c. prepare client for closed reduction (e.g. traction) or surgical relocation of the prosthesis(es) if planned
d. provide emotional support to client and significant others.

7.c. The client will not develop a deep vein thrombus or pulmonary embolism

7.c.1. Refer to Standardized Postoperative Care Plan, Collaborative Diagnosis 19, actions c.1 and 2 (pp. 132-133), for measures related to assessment, prevention, and treatment of a deep vein thrombus and pulmonary embolism.

| Desired Outcomes | Nursing Actions and ***Selected Purposes/Rationales*** |
|---|---|
| (see Standardized Postoperative Care Plan, Collaborative Diagnosis 19, outcomes c.1 and 2 [pp. 132-133], for outcome criteria). | 2. Implement additional measures *to prevent thrombus formation:*<br>a. assist client with exercises and ambulation as allowed<br>b. promote active foot and leg exercises by having client rock in a rocking chair once activity is progressed<br>c. perform actions *to reduce risk of compromising venous return:*<br>1. make sure elastic wraps or stockings are not too tight<br>2. make sure that sling on balanced suspension device and elastic wraps or stockings are not exerting pressure on popliteal space<br>3. avoid use of knee gatch or pillows under knees<br>4. discourage prolonged sitting or standing<br>5. make sure that straps on abductor wedge do not exert uneven or excessive pressure on any area<br>d. administer anticoagulants (e.g. low-dose warfarin or heparin) or antiplatelet agents (e.g. low-molecular-weight dextran, low-dose aspirin) as ordered. |

## 8. NURSING DIAGNOSIS: Knowledge deficit

regarding follow-up care.

| Desired Outcomes | Nursing Actions and ***Selected Purposes/Rationales*** |
|---|---|
| 8.a. The client will verbalize an understanding of activity and position restrictions necessary to prevent dislocation of the hip prostheses. | 8.a. Instruct client to adhere to the following activity and position restrictions in order to prevent dislocation of the hip prostheses (length of time the restrictions are necessary varies but ranges from 2-6 months):<br>1. turn only as directed by physician (many physicians allow turning to unoperative side only and instruct client to keep pillow between legs when turning and while on side)<br>2. never cross legs<br>3. do not sit on low chairs, stools, or toilets; place a cushion on low chairs, rent or purchase a raised toilet seat for home use, and use the high toilets designated for the handicapped when in public facilities<br>4. do not elevate operative leg higher than hip when sitting<br>5. sit in chairs with arms and use the arms to raise self off chair<br>6. support weight on unoperative leg when raising self from a sitting position<br>7. do not bend down to reach objects on the floor or in low cupboards or drawers<br>8. do not reach to the end of bed to pull covers up<br>9. do not put on shoes or socks without using an assistive device<br>10. keep operative leg in proper alignment and avoid extreme internal and external rotation of leg<br>11. when riding in a car:<br>a. sit on a firm pillow or cushion to prevent hip flexion of more than 90°<br>b. keep operative leg extended (a sudden impact of the knee against the dashboard can dislodge the prostheses)<br>12. do not resume sexual activity until approved by physician (usually about 6 weeks postoperatively)<br>13. when sexual activity is resumed, avoid positions that involve turning leg inward, flexing hip beyond 90°, and moving operative leg past the midline |

| | |
|---|---|
| | 14. avoid lifting heavy objects, excessive twisting and turning of body, and activities that place excessive strain on hip (e.g. jogging, jumping). |
| 8.b. The client will demonstrate correct transfer and ambulation techniques and proper use of ambulatory aids. | 8.b.1. Reinforce instructions about correct transfer and ambulation techniques and proper use of walker, quad cane, or crutches.<br>2. Reinforce physician's instructions about amount of weight-bearing on operative extremity.<br>3. Allow time for questions, clarification, and practice of transfer and ambulation techniques. |
| 8.c. The client will demonstrate the ability to correctly perform the prescribed exercises. | 8.c.1. Reinforce the physical therapist's instructions on prescribed exercises and the importance of continuing the exercises for at least a year after surgery.<br>2. Inform client that walking and swimming are good aerobic exercises but that hiking, running, tennis, skiing, and stair climbing should be avoided.<br>3. Allow time for questions, clarification, and return demonstration of prescribed exercises. |
| 8.d. The client will identify ways to reduce the risk of falls in the home environment. | 8.d. Provide the following instructions on ways to reduce risk of falls at home:<br>1. keep electrical cords out of pathways<br>2. remove unnecessary furniture and provide wide pathways for ambulation<br>3. remove scatter rugs<br>4. provide adequate lighting at all times<br>5. avoid unnecessary stair climbing. |
| 8.e. The client will state signs and symptoms to report to the health care provider. | 8.e.1. Refer to Standardized Postoperative Care Plan, Nursing Diagnosis 21, action c (p. 135), for signs and symptoms to report to the health care provider.<br>2. Instruct client to report these additional signs and symptoms:<br>a. persistent or increased pain or spasms in operative extremity<br>b. loss of sensation or movement in operative extremity<br>c. inability to bear weight on operative extremity<br>d. inability to maintain operative extremity in a neutral position<br>e. shortening of operative extremity (will probably be noticed as a limp). |
| 8.f. The client will identify community resources that can assist with home management and provide transportation. | 8.f.1. Provide information about community resources that can assist the client and significant others with home management and provide transportation (e.g. home health agencies, Meals on Wheels, church groups, transportation services).<br>2. Initiate a referral if indicated. |
| 8.g. The client will verbalize an understanding of and a plan for adhering to recommended follow-up care including future appointments with health care provider and physical therapist, medications prescribed, activity level, and wound care. | 8.g.1. Refer to Standardized Postoperative Care Plan, Nursing Diagnosis 21 (pp. 135-136), for routine postoperative instructions and measures to improve client compliance.<br>2. Reinforce importance of keeping appointments with physical therapist.<br>3. Instruct client to inform other health care providers of history of total hip replacement so prophylactic antimicrobials may be started before any dental work, invasive diagnostic procedures, or surgery is performed. |

# Total Knee Replacement

A total knee replacement (arthroplasty) is a surgical procedure in which the articular surfaces of the tibia and femur and sometimes the patella are replaced with prosthetic devices. It is performed to relieve joint pain that has not been controlled by conservative management and/or improve joint mobility in persons with severe degenerative, rheumatoid, or traumatic arthritis; congenital knee deformity; hemophilic arthropathy; or severe intra-articular injury.

There are a variety of prostheses available. Most prostheses have a metal femoral component, a metal-backed polyethylene tibial component, and a polyethylene patellar component (the patella is not always replaced). Prostheses may be fully constrained (hinge prosthesis), semi-constrained, or unconstrained (unlinked). The hinge prosthesis is a one-piece prosthesis. With this type of prosthesis, the greatest portion of the load (weight supported) is placed on the prosthesis itself which contributes to a high rate of loosening. For this reason, the hinge prosthesis is being used less frequently. Unconstrained prostheses have separate femoral, tibial, and patellar components with a greater portion of the load absorbed by the surrounding capsule and ligaments as occurs in a normal knee. Fixation of the prostheses is accomplished by using a cement-like agent called methylmethacrylate or, if left uncemented, by bone ingrowth into the porous outer surface on the prostheses.

**This care plan focuses on the adult client hospitalized for a total knee replacement.** Preoperative goals of care are to reduce fear and anxiety and educate the client regarding ways to prevent postoperative complications and facilitate rehabilitation. Postoperatively, the goals of care are to maintain comfort, prevent complications, assist the client to regain maximum mobility, and educate the client regarding follow-up care. Prevention of infection is of major importance in caring for the client who has had a total knee replacement since infection of the operative knee usually necessitates surgical debridement and/or removal of the prosthesis(es).

## DIAGNOSTIC TESTS

X-rays of the knee
Arthrography
Computed tomography (CT)
Magnetic resonance imaging (MRI)

## DISCHARGE CRITERIA

Prior to discharge, the client will:

- have reduced knee pain
- have expected degree of mobility of knee joint
- have no signs and symptoms of complications
- demonstrate correct transfer and ambulation techniques and proper use of ambulatory aids
- demonstrate the ability to correctly perform the prescribed exercises
- identify ways to reduce the risk of loosening of the prosthesis(es)
- identify ways to reduce the risk of falls in the home environment
- state signs and symptoms to report to the health care provider
- identify community resources that can assist with home management and provide transportation
- verbalize an understanding of and a plan for adhering to recommended follow-up care including future appointments with health care provider and physical therapist, medications prescribed, activity level, and wound care.

**NURSING/ COLLABORATIVE DIAGNOSES**



**See Standardized Preoperative and Postoperative Care Plans for additional diagnoses.**

## PREOPERATIVE

**Use in conjunction with the Standardized Preoperative Care Plan.**

### 1. NURSING DIAGNOSIS: Knowledge deficit

regarding hospital routines associated with surgery, physical preparation for total knee replacement, sensations that normally occur following surgery and anesthesia, and postoperative care.

| Desired Outcomes | Nursing Actions and ***Selected Purposes/Rationales*** |
|---|---|
| 1.a. The client will verbalize an understanding of usual preoperative care and postoperative sensations and care. | 1.a.1. Refer to Standardized Preoperative Care Plan, Nursing Diagnosis 4, actions a.1-4 (pp. 111-112), for information to include in preoperative teaching.<br>2. Provide additional information about specific preoperative care for clients having a total knee replacement:<br>a. explain that the following measures will be performed to reduce risk of a postoperative knee infection:<br>1. the operative leg will be scrubbed with an antiseptic solution (e.g. povidone-iodine) before surgery<br>2. existing infections will be treated before surgery; instruct client to report any symptoms of infection (e.g. cough, runny nose, burning on urination)<br>3. antimicrobials will probably be administered prophylactically before and after surgery<br>b. explain that anticoagulants (e.g. heparin, warfarin) and/or antiplatelet agents (e.g. low-molecular-weight dextran, low-dose aspirin) may be administered before surgery to reduce risk of postoperative thrombus formation; inform client that coagulation studies are usually done before starting these medications, especially if he/she has been taking aspirin, aspirin-containing compounds, or ibuprofen<br>c. explain that a physical therapist will fit crutches or walker and provide instructions on postoperative physical therapy regimen. |

| Desired Outcomes | Nursing Actions and ***Selected Purposes/Rationales*** |
|---|---|
| | 3. Allow time for questions and clarification of information provided. |
| 1.b. The client will demonstrate the ability to perform activities designed to prevent postoperative complications. | 1.b.1. Refer to Standardized Preoperative Care Plan, Nursing Diagnosis 4, action b.1 (p. 112), for instructions on ways to prevent postoperative complications.<br>2. Provide additional instructions about ways to prevent complications following total knee replacement:<br>a. reinforce physician's or physical therapist's instructions on:<br>1. exercises to improve strength and facilitate mobility:<br>a. quadriceps- and gluteal-setting<br>b. upper extremity strengthening<br>c. knee flexion<br>d. sling-assisted and independent straight leg raising<br>2. transfer and ambulation techniques and proper use of ambulatory aids (weight-bearing limitations are determined by the physician and vary depending on the type of prostheses inserted (usually partial weight-bearing is allowed initially with progressive weight-bearing as tolerated)<br>b. instruct client in the correct way to use overhead trapeze and unoperative extremity to move self<br>c. inform client that he/she will need to avoid extreme flexion of the knee for first few weeks after surgery in order to prevent displacement of the prosthesis(es)<br>d. explain the need to leave operative extremity in the continuous passive motion (CPM) machine if ordered<br>e. describe or show client knee immobilizer and explain purpose for wearing immobilizer.<br>3. Allow time for questions, clarification, and return demonstration. |

## POSTOPERATIVE

**Use in conjunction with the Standardized Postoperative Care Plan.**

### 1. NURSING DIAGNOSIS: High risk for peripheral neurovascular dysfunction: operative extremity

related to trauma to the nerves or blood vessels associated with surgery, blood accumulation and edema in the surgical area, improper alignment of operative extremity, excessive pressure exerted by immobilizing device or CPM machine, or dislocation of the prosthesis(es).

| Desired Outcome | Nursing Actions and ***Selected Purposes/Rationales*** |
|---|---|
| 1. The client will maintain normal neurovascular function in operative extremity as evidenced by:<br>a. palpable peripheral pulses<br>b. capillary refill time in toes less than 3 seconds | 1.a. Assess for and report signs and symptoms of neurovascular dysfunction in the operative extremity:<br>1. diminished or absent peripheral pulses<br>2. capillary refill time in toes greater than 3 seconds<br>3. pallor, blanching, cyanosis, or coolness of the extremity<br>4. inability to flex or extend foot or toes<br>5. numbness or tingling in foot or toes<br>6. pain in foot during passive motion of toes or foot<br>7. increased pain in extremity.<br>b. Implement measures *to prevent neurovascular dysfunction in the operative extremity:* |

| Desired Outcome | Nursing Actions and *Selected Purposes/Rationales* |
|---|---|
| c. extremity warm and usual color<br>d. ability to flex and extend foot and toes<br>e. absence of numbness and tingling in foot and toes<br>f. absence of foot pain during passive movement of toes and foot<br>g. no increase in pain in extremity. | 1. apply ice packs to operative knee for the first 24-48 hours after surgery if ordered *to reduce bleeding and edema in surgical area*<br>2. maintain patency of wound drainage system (e.g. prevent kinking of tubing, empty collection device as needed, keep collection device below wound level, maintain suction as ordered) *to reduce accumulation of fluid in the surgical area*<br>3. maintain extremity in proper alignment<br>4. position leg so that immobilizing device and CPM machine are not causing uneven or excessive pressure on any area<br>5. loosen straps of knee immobilizer if it appears to be too tight<br>6. notify physician if dressing appears to be too tight<br>7. perform actions to prevent dislocation of the prosthesis(es) and stress fracture of the tibia and femur (see Postoperative Collaborative Diagnosis 7, action a.2).<br>c. If signs and symptoms of neurovascular dysfunction occur:<br>1. assess for and correct causes of uneven or excessive pressure<br>2. notify physician if the signs and symptoms persist<br>3. prepare client for closed reduction or surgical intervention (e.g. realignment of the prosthesis) if planned. |

## 2. NURSING DIAGNOSIS: Pain: knee

related to tissue trauma and reflex muscle spasms associated with the surgery, blood accumulation and edema in the surgical area, and improper positioning of the operative extremity.

| Desired Outcome | Nursing Actions and *Selected Purposes/Rationales* |
|---|---|
| 2. The client will experience diminished knee pain (see Standardized Postoperative Care Plan, Nursing Diagnosis 6 [p. 119], for outcome criteria). | 2.a. Refer to Standardized Postoperative Care Plan, Nursing Diagnosis 6 (p. 119), for measures related to assessment and reduction of pain.<br>b. Implement additional measures *to reduce pain:*<br>1. maintain operative extremity in proper alignment<br>2. move the operative extremity carefully<br>3. apply ice packs to the operative knee for first 24-48 hours after surgery if ordered *to reduce bleeding and edema in the surgical area*<br>4. maintain patency of the wound drainage system if present *to prevent accumulation of fluid in the surgical area*<br>5. remind client to avoid flexing operative knee beyond prescribed limits<br>6. maintain proper placement and function of transcutaneous electrical nerve stimulator (TENS) if ordered<br>7. administer prescribed analgesics before exercise and ambulation sessions<br>8. apply ice packs to operative knee for 20-30 minutes before and after exercise and ambulation sessions as ordered. |

## 3. NURSING DIAGNOSIS: Actual/High risk for impaired skin integrity

related to:

a. disruption of skin associated with the surgical procedure;
b. delayed wound healing associated with decreased nutritional status and inadequate blood supply to wound area;

c. irritation of skin associated with contact with wound drainage, pressure from drainage tubes, and use of tape;
d. excessive or prolonged pressure on tissues from immobilizing device (e.g. compression dressing, knee immobilizer) or CPM machine;
e. damage to the skin and/or subcutaneous tissue associated with prolonged pressure on tissues, friction, and shearing while mobility is decreased.

| Desired Outcomes | Nursing Actions and ***Selected Purposes/Rationales*** |
|---|---|
| 3.a. The client will experience normal healing of the surgical wound (see Standardized Postoperative Care Plan, Nursing Diagnosis 9, outcome a [p. 122], for outcome criteria). | 3.a. Refer to Standardized Postoperative Care Plan, Nursing Diagnosis 9, action a (pp. 122-123), for measures related to assessment and promotion of wound healing. |
| 3.b. The client will maintain skin integrity as evidenced by:<br>1. absence of redness and irritation<br>2. no skin breakdown. | 3.b.1. Inspect the following areas for pallor, redness, and breakdown:<br>a. skin in contact with wound drainage, tape, and drainage tubings<br>b. back, coccyx, and buttocks<br>c. elbows and heels<br>d. edges of compression dressing or knee immobilizer<br>e. areas in contact with CPM machine.<br>2. Refer to Standardized Postoperative Care Plan, Nursing Diagnosis 9, action b.2 (p. 123), for measures related to prevention of skin irritation and breakdown resulting from contact with wound drainage, drainage tubings, and tape.<br>3. Implement measures *to prevent skin breakdown associated with decreased mobility:*<br>a. instruct client to use overhead trapeze to lift self and shift weight every 30 minutes<br>b. gently massage around reddened areas at least every 2 hours<br>c. perform actions *to prevent shearing* (shearing occurs when one tissue layer slides past another) *and skin surface abrasion:*<br>1. apply a thin layer of powder or cornstarch to bottom sheet or skin *to absorb moisture (moist skin is more likely to adhere to sheet) and reduce friction*<br>2. lift and move client carefully using a turn sheet and adequate assistance<br>3. limit length of time client is in semi-Fowler's position to 30 minutes *(in this position, client tends to slide down in bed)*<br>d. if turning is allowed (some physicians may not allow turning for first 48 hours), turn client every 2 hours keeping pillows between legs and operative knee extended<br>e. if fade time (length of time it takes for reddened area to fade after pressure is removed) is greater than 15 minutes, increase the frequency of position changes and massages<br>f. keep skin lubricated, clean, and dry<br>g. keep bed linens dry and wrinkle-free<br>h. provide devices to reduce pressure on the skin, decrease shearing, and/or prevent moisture build-up (e.g. alternating pressure mattress or pad, flotation pad, sheepskin)<br>i. increase activity as allowed and tolerated.<br>4. Implement measures *to prevent irritation and breakdown on elbows and heels:*<br>a. massage elbows and heels with lotion frequently |

b. encourage client to use overhead trapeze to move self rather than pushing up with heel and elbows
c. provide elbow and heel protectors if indicated.

5. Implement measures *to prevent skin breakdown in areas in contact with the immobilizing device or CPM machine:*
   a. assess for and report tightness of the dressing or burning sensation under the immobilizing device
   b. loosen straps on knee immobilizer if it appears to be too tight
   c. apply cornstarch to skin under immobilizer *in order to keep skin dry and reduce friction and subsequent skin irritation*
   d. keep dressing dry
   e. position the operative extremity so that the immobilizing device and CPM machine are not causing uneven or excessive pressure on any area
   f. make sure CPM machine is padded adequately
   g. instruct client to refrain from poking anything inside the immobilizing device.
6. If skin breakdown occurs:
   a. notify physician
   b. continue with above measures to prevent further irritation and breakdown
   c. perform wound and decubitus care as ordered or per standard hospital procedure
   d. assess client closely and report signs and symptoms of infection (e.g. elevated temperature; redness, warmth, and edema around area of breakdown; unusual drainage from site; foul odor from dressing).

## 4. NURSING DIAGNOSIS: Impaired physical mobility

related to:
a. pain and weakness in weight-bearing extremity associated with surgery on the knee;
b. prescribed activity and weight-bearing restrictions following total knee replacement;
c. generalized weakness associated with surgery;
d. depressant effects of some medications (e.g. narcotic analgesics, central-acting muscle relaxants);
e. fear of falling, dislocating prostheses, and compromising surgical wound.

| Desired Outcome | Nursing Actions and ***Selected Purposes/Rationales*** |
|---|---|
| 4. The client will maintain maximum physical mobility within prescribed activity and weight-bearing restrictions. | 4.a. Refer to Standardized Postoperative Care Plan, Nursing Diagnosis 11 (p. 125), for measures to increase client's mobility.<br>b. Implement additional measures *to increase client's mobility:*<br>1. perform actions to reduce pain (see Postoperative Nursing Diagnosis 2)<br>2. encourage client to keep operative leg in CPM machine for the prescribed time *in order to improve range of motion and prevent stiffening of the knee*<br>3. encourage client to perform quadriceps- and gluteal-setting, straight leg raising, and knee flexion-extension exercises as soon as allowed (usually started 2-4 days postoperatively)<br>4. encourage client to use overhead trapeze to move self *in order to strengthen arm and shoulder muscles needed for proper use of ambulatory aids*<br>5. reinforce physical therapist's instructions regarding transfer and |

| Desired Outcome | Nursing Actions and ***Selected Purposes/Rationales*** |
|---|---|
| | ambulation techniques and use of ambulatory aids (e.g. crutches, walker)<br>6. perform actions to prevent falls (see Postoperative Nursing Diagnosis 6, actions a and b) *in order to decrease client's fear of injury*<br>7. assist client with ambulation as soon as allowed (usually by the 2nd postoperative day).<br>c. Consult physician if client is unable to make expected progress with knee flexion or if any other joint motion becomes restricted. |

## 5. NURSING DIAGNOSIS: High risk for infection: operative knee

related to:

a. introduction of pathogens into the wound during or following surgery;

b. increased susceptibility to infection associated with decreased effectiveness of immune system if client is elderly and immunosuppression if client has been taking corticosteroids to treat the joint disorder necessitating the surgery (e.g. rheumatoid arthritis).

| Desired Outcome | Nursing Actions and ***Selected Purposes/Rationales*** |
|---|---|
| 5. The client will remain free of infection in the operative knee (see Standardized Postoperative Care Plan, Nursing Diagnosis 16, outcome b [p. 129], for outcome criteria). | 5.a. Assess for and report the following:<br>1. continuous drainage of fluid from incision *(may indicate a sinus tract)*<br>2. sloughing or necrosis of skin in operative area<br>3. signs and symptoms of wound infection (e.g. chills; fever; redness, warmth, and swelling of wound area; unusual wound drainage; foul odor from wound area; persistent or increased pain in knee; elevated sedimentation rate).<br>b. Refer to Standardized Postoperative Care Plan, Nursing Diagnosis 16, actions b.4 and 5 (p. 129), for measures related to prevention and treatment of wound infection.<br>c. Implement additional measures *to reduce risk for infection in the operative knee:*<br>1. use strict aseptic technique when performing wound care and emptying wound drainage device (some physicians do not want other health care personnel to empty drainage device *because of risk of contamination)*<br>2. maintain patency of the wound drainage device *in order to prevent accumulation of drainage in surgical area*<br>3. keep CPM machine off the floor when not in use<br>4. avoid urinary catheterization but if it becomes necessary, take precautions to prevent urinary tract infection (e.g. use strict aseptic technique during catheter insertion, remove catheter as soon as possible); *the increased possibility of urinary tract infection associated with the presence of a urinary catheter increases the risk for lymphatic or hematogenous seeding of the knee wound*<br>5. administer prophylactic antimicrobials if ordered (they are usually started before surgery and continued for 2-5 days after surgery).<br>d. If signs and symptoms of wound infection occur, prepare client for wound irrigation, surgical debridement, and/or removal of prostheses if planned. |

## 6. NURSING DIAGNOSIS: High risk for trauma

related to falls associated with:
a. weakness, fatigue, and postural hypotension resulting from the effects of major surgery;
b. central nervous system depressant effects of some medications (e.g. narcotic analgesics, central-acting muscle relaxants);
c. weakness and pain in weight-bearing extremity as a result of the surgery;
d. improper transfer and ambulation techniques.

| Desired Outcome | Nursing Actions and ***Selected Purposes/Rationales*** |
|---|---|
| 6. The client will not experience falls. | 6.a. Refer to Standardized Postoperative Care Plan, Nursing Diagnosis 17, action a (p. 130), for measures to prevent falls.<br>b. Implement additional measures *to reduce the risk for falls:*<br>1. reinforce preoperative instructions about and assist client with transfer and ambulation techniques, use of ambulatory aids, and exercises to improve muscle strength<br>2. administer prescribed analgesics and/or apply ice packs to operative knee before exercise and ambulation sessions *in order to reduce knee pain and subsequently maximize the client's ability to use proper transfer and ambulation techniques*<br>3. ensure that client has knee immobilizer on for ambulation sessions *to provide additional support of operative leg.*<br>c. Include client and significant others in planning and implementing measures to prevent falls.<br>d. If falls occur, initiate first aid measures if appropriate and notify physician. |

## 7. COLLABORATIVE DIAGNOSES: Potential complications:

a. **dislocation of knee prosthesis(es) or stress fracture of tibia or femur** related to rotation of or excessive pressure on the knee;
b. **thromboembolism** related to:
   1. trauma to vein walls during surgery
   2. venous stasis associated with use of a tourniquet on operative leg during surgery, pressure created by the immobilizing device or CPM machine, decreased mobility, and fluid volume deficit
   3. hypercoagulability associated with increased release of tissue thromboplastin into the blood (occurs as a result of surgical trauma)
   4. decreased fibrinolytic activity (occurs in response to surgical trauma).

| Desired Outcomes | Nursing Actions and ***Selected Purposes/Rationales*** |
|---|---|
| 7.a. The client will not experience dislocation of the knee prosthesis(es) or stress fracture of tibia or femur as evidenced by:<br>1. continued resolution of knee pain<br>2. ability to maintain operative leg in | 7.a.1. Assess for and report signs and symptoms of dislocation of the knee prosthesis(es) and/or stress fracture of tibia or femur:<br>a. sudden, severe knee pain followed by continued pain and muscle spasms during knee movement<br>b. abnormal rotation of the lower portion of operative leg<br>c. inability to move or bear weight on operative leg<br>d. decline in neurovascular status in operative leg.<br>2. Implement measures *to prevent dislocation of the prosthesis(es) and stress fracture of the tibia and femur:*<br>a. instruct client to avoid hyperextension, rotation, and acute flexion of knee |

| Desired Outcomes | Nursing Actions and Selected Purposes/Rationales |
|---|---|
| proper alignment<br>3. ability to adhere to planned exercise and ambulation regimen<br>4. normal neurovascular status in operative leg. | b. reinforce physician's instructions regarding the amount of weight-bearing allowed (usual order is partial weight-bearing initially with progressive weight-bearing as tolerated)<br>c. reinforce instructions and assist client with gait training and proper use of ambulatory aids<br>d. reinforce the importance of wearing knee immobilizer when ambulating.<br>3. If signs and symptoms of prosthesis(es) dislocation or stress fracture occur:<br>a. maintain client on bed rest<br>b. prepare client for x-rays of operative leg<br>c. prepare client for closed reduction or surgical intervention if planned<br>d. provide emotional support to client and significant others. |
| 7.b. The client will not develop a deep vein thrombus or pulmonary embolism (see Standardized Postoperative Care Plan, Collaborative Diagnosis 19, outcomes c.1 and 2 [pp. 132-133], for outcome criteria). | 7.b.1. Refer to Standardized Postoperative Care Plan, Collaborative Diagnosis 19, actions c.1 and 2 (pp. 132-133), for measures related to assessment, prevention, and treatment of a deep vein thrombus and pulmonary embolism.<br>2. Implement additional measures *to prevent thrombus formation:*<br>a. perform actions *to improve venous return:*<br>1. maintain continuous passive motion of extremity if ordered<br>2. assist client to perform leg exercises and ambulate as soon as allowed<br>3. implement measures *to reduce risk of compromising venous return:*<br>a. consult physician if dressing appears to be too tight<br>b. loosen knee immobilizer if it appears to be too tight<br>c. make sure exercise sling is not exerting pressure on the popliteal space<br>d. avoid use of the knee gatch or pillows under knees<br>e. discourage prolonged sitting or standing<br>b. administer anticoagulants (e.g. low-dose warfarin or heparin) or antiplatelet agents (e.g. low-dose aspirin) as ordered. |

## 8. NURSING DIAGNOSIS: Knowledge deficit
regarding follow-up care.

| Desired Outcomes | Nursing Actions and ***Selected Purposes/Rationales*** |
|---|---|
| 8.a. The client will demonstrate correct transfer and ambulation techniques and proper use of ambulatory aids. | 8.a.1. Reinforce instructions about correct transfer and ambulation techniques and proper use of crutches, cane, or walker.<br>2. Reinforce the importance of adhering to weight-bearing restrictions if prescribed.<br>3. Allow time for questions, clarification, and practice of transfer and ambulation techniques. |
| 8.b. The client will demonstrate the ability to correctly perform the prescribed exercises. | 8.b.1. Reinforce the physical therapist's instructions about prescribed exercises.<br>2. Reinforce the importance of continuing prescribed exercises for at least a year after surgery.<br>3. Allow time for questions, clarification, and return demonstration of prescribed exercises. |
| 8.c. The client will identify ways to reduce the risk of loosening of the prosthesis(es). | 8.c.1. Inform client of the possibility of loosening of the prosthesis (usually does not occur until 2-3 years after surgery).<br>2. Instruct client to report increasing pain or instability of operative knee (may indicate loosening of the prosthesis). |

| | |
|---|---|
| | 3. Instruct client regarding ways to minimize risk of loosening of the prosthesis(es):<br>a. adhere to weight-bearing restrictions if prescribed<br>b. avoid unusual twisting of knee<br>c. avoid contact sports<br>d. do not force knee beyond comfortable degree of flexion and avoid kneeling<br>e. avoid placing undue stress on knees (e.g. do not lift and carry heavy objects, maintain ideal body weight, avoid activities such as jogging). |
| 8.d. The client will identify ways to reduce the risk of falls in the home environment. | 8.d. Provide the following instructions on ways to reduce risk of falls at home:<br>1. keep electrical cords out of pathways<br>2. remove unnecessary furniture and provide wide pathways for ambulation<br>3. remove scatter rugs<br>4. provide adequate lighting at all times<br>5. avoid unnecessary stair climbing. |
| 8.e. The client will state signs and symptoms to report to the health care provider. | 8.e.1. Refer to Standardized Postoperative Care Plan, Nursing Diagnosis 21, action c (p. 135), for signs and symptoms to report to the health care provider.<br>2. Instruct client to report these additional signs and symptoms:<br>a. persistent or increased pain or spasms in operative extremity<br>b. loss of sensation or movement in operative extremity<br>c. inability to bear expected amount of weight on operative extremity<br>d. inability to maintain operative extremity in a neutral position<br>e. instability of operative extremity (feeling of knee "giving out"). |
| 8.f. The client will identify community resources that can assist with home management and provide transportation. | 8.f.1. Provide information about community resources that can assist client and significant others with home management and provide transportation (e.g. home health agencies, Meals on Wheels, church groups, transportation services).<br>2. Initiate a referral if indicated. |
| 8.g. The client will verbalize an understanding of and a plan for adhering to recommended follow-up care including future appointments with health care provider and physical therapist, medications prescribed, activity level, and wound care. | 8.g.1. Refer to Standardized Postoperative Care Plan, Nursing Diagnosis 21 (pp. 135-136), for routine postoperative instructions and measures to improve client compliance.<br>2. Reinforce the importance of keeping appointments with physical therapist.<br>3. Instruct client to inform other health care providers of history of total knee replacement so prophylactic antimicrobials may be started before any dental work, invasive diagnostic procedures, or surgery is performed. |

UNIT

# XVIII

# *Nursing Care of the Client with Disturbances of the Breast and Reproductive System*

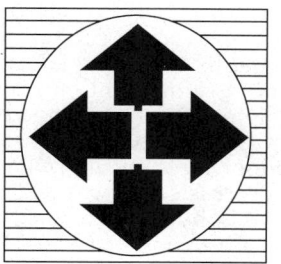

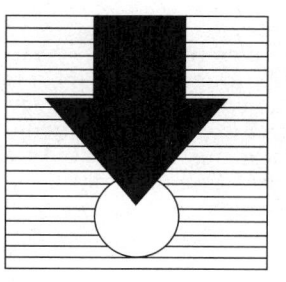

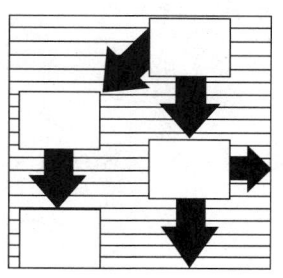

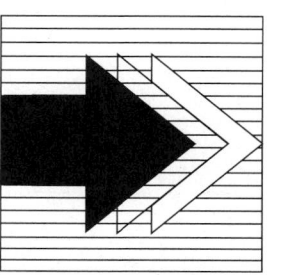

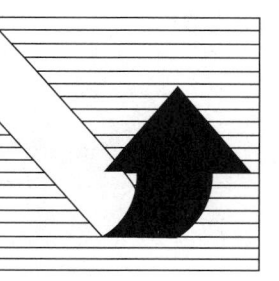

# Colporrhaphy (Anterior and Posterior Repair)

Colporrhaphy is the surgical tightening of the vagina and repair of incompetent muscles and ligaments of the pelvic floor. An anterior colporrhaphy is performed to correct a cystocele, which is a protrusion or displacement of the bladder through the pubocervical fascia into the vagina and occasionally beyond the introitus. A posterior colporrhaphy is performed to repair a rectocele, which is a protrusion of part of the anterior rectal wall upward into the vagina. Cystoceles and rectoceles are caused by relaxation of the pelvic musculature and ligaments usually associated with aging and tissue damage during childbirth. They can occur alone or in conjunction with prolapse of the uterus.

Signs and symptoms of a cystocele include back pain, stress incontinence, urinary urgency and frequency, and/or vaginal pressure. A rectocele is manifested by difficult or incomplete emptying of the rectum, constipation, backache, hemorrhoids, and/or a feeling of pelvic pressure. Colporrhaphy is indicated when conservative management (e.g. perineal exercises, insertion of a pessary) no longer controls signs and symptoms.

Repair of a cystocele is accomplished with a U-shaped incision in the anterior vaginal wall. Repair of a rectocele typically involves an incision in the posterior vaginal wall and the perineum. Reconstruction of the posterior fourchette to repair a lax vaginal introitus is almost always performed simultaneously with a posterior colporrhaphy because perineal body laxity usually accompanies a rectocele. Bladder suspension surgery (e.g. Gittes, Stamey, Raz) may be performed at the same time to restore the bladder neck and proximal urethra to a high retropubic position if the client is also experiencing severe stress incontinence.

**This care plan focuses on the adult female client hospitalized for an elective anterior and posterior colporrhaphy.** Preoperatively, the goals of care are to reduce fear and anxiety and prepare the client for the surgical experience. The goals of postoperative care are to maintain comfort, prevent complications, and educate the client regarding follow-up care.

## DIAGNOSTIC TESTS

Cystoscopy
Proctoscopy

## DISCHARGE CRITERIA

Prior to discharge, the client will:

- have surgical pain controlled
- have no signs and symptoms of complications
- identify ways to decrease the risk of reherniation of the bladder and rectum into the vagina
- identify ways to relieve surgical site discomfort
- state signs and symptoms to report to the health care provider
- verbalize an understanding of and a plan for adhering to recommended follow-up care including future appointments with health care provider, medications prescribed, and limitations on sexual activity.

## NURSING/COLLABORATIVE DIAGNOSES

**Postoperative**

1. Pain△ *819*
2. Urinary retention△ *819*
3. Constipation△ *820*
4. High risk for infection:
   a. wound infection
   b. urinary tract infection△ *820*
5. Potential complication: reherniation of bladder and rectum△ *821*
6. Knowledge deficit△ *821*

**See Standardized Preoperative and Postoperative Care Plans for additional diagnoses.**

**PREOPERATIVE** **Refer to the Standardized Preoperative Care Plan.**

**POSTOPERATIVE** **Use in conjunction with the Standardized Postoperative Care Plan.**

## 1. NURSING DIAGNOSIS: Pain

related to tissue trauma and reflex muscle spasms associated with the surgical procedure.

| Desired Outcome | Nursing Actions and ***Selected Purposes/Rationales*** |
| --- | --- |
| 1. The client will experience diminished pain as evidenced by:<br>a. verbalization of pain relief<br>b. relaxed facial expression and body positioning<br>c. ability to sit and walk more comfortably<br>d. increased participation in activities<br>e. stable vital signs. | 1.a. Refer to Standardized Postoperative Care Plan, Nursing Diagnosis 6 (p. 119), for measures related to assessment and management of postoperative pain.<br>b. Implement additional measures *to reduce pain:*<br>1. apply ice packs to the perineal area for the first 24 hours postoperatively if ordered<br>2. instruct client in and assist with sitz baths as ordered<br>3. encourage client to lie flat or in semi-Fowler's position when in bed *in order to minimize pressure on surgical site*<br>4. administer the following if ordered:<br>a. topical anesthetics if perineal incision is present<br>b. genitourinary smooth muscle relaxants (e.g. oxybutynin, flavoxate) *to reduce discomfort associated with bladder spasms if present.* |

## 2. NURSING DIAGNOSIS: Urinary retention

related to:

a. edema of the bladder neck and urethra associated with surgical trauma and irritation of tissue by the urethral catheter;
b. decreased bladder muscle tone and perception of bladder fullness associated with pelvic edema, nerve trauma that can result from surgery, and depressant effects of some medications (e.g. anesthetic agents, narcotic analgesics);
c. inability to urinate associated with sympathetic nervous system stimulation of bladder and urinary sphincters resulting from pain, fear, and anxiety.

| Desired Outcome | Nursing Actions and ***Selected Purposes/Rationales*** |
| --- | --- |
| 2. The client will not experience urinary retention (see Standardized Postoperative Care Plan, Nursing Diagnosis 13 [p. 126], for outcome criteria). | 2. Refer to Standardized Postoperative Care Plan, Nursing Diagnosis 13 (p. 126), for measures related to assessment, prevention, and treatment of urinary retention (client will usually have an indwelling catheter for several days postoperatively until bladder neck and urethral edema subside). |

## 3. NURSING DIAGNOSIS: Constipation

related to:
a. decreased gastrointestinal motility associated with anesthesia, narcotic analgesics, and decreased activity;
b. reluctance to defecate associated with fear of pain and reherniation of rectum;
c. decreased intake of fluids and foods high in fiber.

| Desired Outcome | Nursing Actions and ***Selected Purposes/Rationales*** |
|---|---|
| 3. The client will not experience constipation (see Standardized Postoperative Care Plan, Nursing Diagnosis 14 [p. 127], for outcome criteria). | 3.a. Refer to Standardized Postoperative Care Plan, Nursing Diagnosis 14 (p. 127), for measures related to assessment and prevention of constipation.<br>b. Instruct client to request an analgesic prior to attempting to defecate *in order to ease the surgical site pain associated with the increased intra-abdominal and perineal pressure that occur with defecation.* |

## 4. NURSING DIAGNOSIS: High risk for infection:

a. **wound infection** related to break in the vaginal mucosa and close proximity of the incision to the rectum (particularly with rectocele repair);
b. **urinary tract infection** related to:
   1. increased bacterial growth associated with urinary stasis
   2. introduction of pathogens associated with an indwelling catheter and presence of vaginal drainage.

| Desired Outcomes | Nursing Actions and ***Selected Purposes/Rationales*** |
|---|---|
| 4.a. The client will remain free of wound infection (see Standardized Postoperative Care Plan, Nursing Diagnosis 16, outcome b [p. 129], for outcome criteria). | 4.a.1. Refer to Standardized Postoperative Care Plan, Nursing Diagnosis 16, action b (p. 129), for measures related to assessment, prevention, and management of postoperative wound infection.<br>2. Implement additional measures *to reduce risk of wound infection:*<br>a. instruct client to wipe from front to back following defecation<br>b. administer perineal care 2-3 times/day and after defecation<br>c. if urinary catheter is present, perform catheter care each shift and as necessary<br>d. if douches are ordered, use sterile equipment and solution. |
| 4.b. The client will remain free of urinary tract infection (see Standardized Postoperative Care Plan, Nursing Diagnosis 16, outcome c [p. 129], for outcome criteria). | 4.b. Refer to Standardized Postoperative Care Plan, Nursing Diagnosis 16, action c (p. 129), for measures related to the assessment, prevention, and management of urinary tract infection. |

**5. COLLABORATIVE DIAGNOSIS:** **Potential complication: reherniation of bladder and rectum**

related to stress on suture lines in vagina associated with increased intra-abdominal, bladder, rectal, or vaginal pressure.

| Desired Outcome | Nursing Actions and ***Selected Purposes/Rationales*** |
|---|---|
| 5. The client will not experience reherniation of the bladder and rectum into the vagina as evidenced by:<br>a. absence of stress incontinence<br>b. no difficulty with evacuation of stool<br>c. absence of urinary frequency and urgency<br>d. gradual resolution of back pain and pelvic and vaginal pressure. | 5.a. Assess for signs and symptoms of reherniation of the bladder or rectum into the vagina (e.g. stress incontinence, difficulty evacuating stool, urinary frequency and urgency, voiding small amounts, back pain, pelvic and vaginal pressure).<br>b. Implement measures *to prevent stress on the vaginal suture lines and subsequent reherniation of the bladder and rectum into the vagina:*<br>1. perform actions to prevent urinary retention (see Standardized Postoperative Care Plan, Nursing Diagnosis 13 [p. 126]) *in order to prevent accumulation of urine in the bladder*<br>2. perform actions to prevent constipation (e.g. increase intake of oral fluids and foods high in fiber as allowed and tolerated, administer laxatives and stool softeners as prescribed) *in order to prevent distention of the rectum*<br>3. perform actions *to prevent increased intra-abdominal pressure:*<br>a. instruct client to lie flat or in a semi-Fowler's position while in bed<br>b. instruct client to avoid any activities that may create a Valsalva response (e.g. straining to have a bowel movement, lifting or carrying a heavy object, holding breath while moving, coughing)<br>c. administer a stool softener, laxative, antiemetic, and antitussive if ordered *to prevent straining to have a bowel movement and control nausea, vomiting, and persistent cough*<br>4. caution client to avoid prolonged standing and sitting<br>5. if douches are ordered, insert nozzle carefully, slowly instill small amounts of solution, and rotate nozzle gently.<br>c. If reherniation occurs:<br>1. maintain client on bed rest<br>2. prepare client for surgical repair of the vaginal wall<br>3. provide emotional support to client and significant others. |

**6. NURSING DIAGNOSIS:** **Knowledge deficit**

regarding follow-up care.

| Desired Outcomes | Nursing Actions and ***Selected Purposes/Rationales*** |
|---|---|
| 6.a. The client will identify ways to decrease the risk of reherniation of the bladder and rectum into the vagina. | 6.a.1. Provide the following instructions on ways to minimize pressure on the suture lines and decrease the risk of reherniation of the bladder and/or rectum:<br>a. reinforce instructions about avoiding prolonged sitting and standing and any activity that may create a Valsalva response (e.g. straining to have a bowel movement, lifting or carrying heavy objects, holding breath while moving, coughing) for at least 6 weeks<br>b. instruct client to urinate whenever she feels the urge or at least every 4 hours |

| Desired Outcomes | Nursing Actions and ***Selected Purposes/Rationales*** |
|---|---|
| | c. if douches are ordered, instruct client to carefully insert nozzle, slowly instill small amounts of solution, and rotate nozzle gently<br>d. reinforce instructions about how to prevent constipation (e.g. drink at least 8 glasses of water daily, increase intake of foods high in fiber, take stool softeners and laxatives as prescribed).<br>2. Encourage client to do perineal exercises (e.g. stopping and starting urinary stream, alternately contracting and relaxing the gluteal muscles) when healing is complete (usually 6 weeks) in order to improve vaginal tone and further decrease the risk of reherniation of the bladder and rectum. |
| 6.b. The client will identify ways to relieve surgical site discomfort. | 6.b. Provide the following instructions regarding ways to relieve discomfort in the surgical area:<br>1. take a sitz bath 2-3 times/day<br>2. apply a topical anesthetic (e.g. dibucaine, benzocaine) to perineum as needed<br>3. douche if permitted by physician<br>4. avoid prolonged sitting and standing<br>5. sit on a foam pad or pillow<br>6. take analgesics as prescribed. |
| 6.c. The client will state signs and symptoms to report to the health care provider. | 6.c. 1. Refer to Standardized Postoperative Care Plan, Nursing Diagnosis 21, action c (p. 135), for signs and symptoms to report to the health care provider.<br>2. Instruct the client to report these additional signs and symptoms:<br>a. foul-smelling vaginal discharge<br>b. heavy vaginal bleeding<br>c. stress incontinence<br>d. vaginal leakage of urine or stool<br>e. excessive perineal edema or pain. |
| 6.d. The client will verbalize an understanding of and a plan for adhering to recommended follow-up care including future appointments with health care provider, medications prescribed, and limitations on sexual activity. | 6.d.1. Refer to Standardized Postoperative Care Plan, Nursing Diagnosis 21 (pp. 135-136), for routine postoperative instructions and measures to improve client compliance.<br>2. Instruct client not to have sexual intercourse until permitted by physician (usually 6 weeks).<br>3. Inform client that loss of vaginal sensation is usually temporary but may persist for several months. |

# Hysterectomy with Salpingectomy and Oophorectomy

Hysterectomy is the surgical removal of the uterus. It is performed to treat conditions of the uterus such as benign or malignant tumors, endometriosis, dysfunctional bleeding, and prolapse. A vaginal approach may be used if only the uterus is to be removed, repairs to the vaginal wall or pelvic floor are necessary, or if the client is obese. An abdominal approach is commonly used if the uterus is enlarged and/or if oophorectomy (removal of the ovaries) and salpingectomy (removal of the fallopian tubes) are performed at the same time.

**This care plan focuses on the adult female client hospitalized for a hysterectomy with salpingectomy and oophorectomy.** Preoperatively, the goals of care are to reduce fear and anxiety and prepare the client for the surgical experience. Postoperative goals are to maintain comfort, prevent complications, assist the client to adjust to changes in body image, and educate her regarding follow-up care.

## DISCHARGE CRITERIA

Prior to discharge, the client will:

- ❖ have surgical pain controlled
- ❖ tolerate expected level of activity
- ❖ have no signs and symptoms of complications
- ❖ verbalize an understanding of the effects of surgical menopause
- ❖ identify ways to achieve optimal sexual satisfaction
- ❖ verbalize an understanding of medications ordered including rationale, side effects, schedule for taking, and importance of taking as prescribed
- ❖ state signs and symptoms to report to the health care provider
- ❖ share feelings about the loss of reproductive ability
- ❖ verbalize an understanding of and a plan for adhering to recommended follow-up care including future appointments with health care provider, activity limitations, and wound care.

## NURSING/COLLABORATIVE DIAGNOSES



**See Standardized Preoperative and Postoperative Care Plans for additional diagnoses.**

## PREOPERATIVE

**Use in conjunction with the Standardized Preoperative Care Plan.**

## 1. NURSING DIAGNOSIS: Anxiety

related to:
a. anticipated loss of control, effects of anesthesia, and postoperative discomfort;
b. anticipated effects of surgery on feelings of femininity and reproductive ability;
c. fear of rejection by partner;
d. unfamiliar environment;
e. potential embarrassment or loss of dignity associated with exposure of genitals during preoperative care, surgery, and postoperative care.

| Desired Outcome | Nursing Actions and ***Selected Purposes/Rationales*** |
|---|---|
| 1. The client will experience a reduction in anxiety (see Standardized Preoperative Care Plan, Nursing Diagnosis 1 [pp. 108-109], for outcome criteria). | 1.a. Refer to Standardized Preoperative Care Plan, Nursing Diagnosis 1 (pp. 108-109), for measures related to assessment and reduction of fear and anxiety.<br>b. Implement additional measures *to reduce fear and anxiety:*<br>1. encourage client to verbalize concerns and feelings about loss of ovarian function and reproductive ability; provide feedback<br>2. discuss alternative methods of parenting (e.g. adoption) if of concern to client<br>3. assure client she will not suffer needless body exposure during preoperative care, surgery, and postoperative care. |

## POSTOPERATIVE

**Use in conjunction with the Standardized Postoperative Care Plan.**

## 1. NURSING DIAGNOSIS: Urinary retention

related to:
a. decreased bladder muscle tone and perception of bladder fullness associated with pelvic edema, nerve trauma that can result from surgery, and the depressant effects of some medications (e.g. anesthetic agents, narcotic analgesics);
b. inability to urinate associated with sympathetic nervous system stimulation of the bladder and urinary sphincters resulting from pain, fear, and anxiety.

| Desired Outcome | Nursing Actions and ***Selected Purposes/Rationales*** |
|---|---|
| 1. The client will not experience urinary retention (see Standardized Postoperative Care Plan, Nursing Diagnosis 13 [p. 126], for outcome criteria). | 1. Refer to Standardized Postoperative Care Plan, Nursing Diagnosis 13 (p. 126), for measures related to assessment, prevention, and treatment of urinary retention (client will usually have an indwelling urinary catheter for first 24-48 hours after surgery). |

**2. COLLABORATIVE DIAGNOSES:**

**Potential complications:**

a. **bladder or ureteral injury** related to accidental tear or ligation during the surgical procedure;
b. **thromboembolism** related to:
   1. pressure on the vessels in lower extremities during surgery if the client was in lithotomy position
   2. trauma to the large pelvic veins associated with manipulation during surgery
   3. venous stasis associated with decreased activity, fluid volume deficit, and abdominal distention (the distended intestine may put pressure on the abdominal vessels)
   4. hypercoagulability associated with increased release of tissue thromboplastin into the blood (occurs as a result of surgical trauma)
   5. decreased fibrinolytic activity (occurs in response to surgical trauma).

| Desired Outcomes | Nursing Actions and ***Selected Purposes/Rationales*** |
|---|---|
| 2.a. The client will experience resolution of bladder or ureteral injury if it occurs as evidenced by:<br>1. gradual resolution of hematuria and backache<br>2. output greater than 200 ml within 6-8 hours after surgery. | 2.a.1. Assess for and report signs and symptoms of bladder or ureteral injury (e.g. hematuria, backache, output less than 200 ml in first 6-8 hours after surgery).<br>2. If signs and symptoms of bladder or ureteral injury are present:<br>a. continue to monitor output carefully<br>b. prepare client for surgical repair of the bladder or ureter if planned<br>c. provide emotional support to client and significant others. |
| 2.b. The client will not develop a deep vein thrombus or pulmonary embolism (see Standardized Postoperative Care Plan, Collaborative Diagnosis 19, outcomes c.1 and 2 [pp. 132-133], for outcome criteria). | 2.b. Refer to Standardized Postoperative Care Plan, Collaborative Diagnosis 19, actions c.1 and 2 (pp. 132-133), for measures related to assessment, prevention, and treatment of a deep vein thrombus and pulmonary embolism. |

**3. NURSING DIAGNOSIS:**

**Body image disturbance**

related to:
a. loss of reproductive organs with subsequent inability to bear children;
b. feeling of loss of femininity and sexual attractiveness.

| Desired Outcome | Nursing Actions and ***Selected Purposes/Rationales*** |
|---|---|
| 3. The client will demonstrate beginning adaptation to changes in | 3.a. Assess for signs and symptoms of a body image disturbance (e.g. verbal or nonverbal cues denoting a negative response to changes in body functioning such as denial of or preoccupation with changes that have occurred or withdrawal from significant others). |

| Desired Outcome | Nursing Actions and ***Selected Purposes/Rationales*** |
|---|---|
| body functioning as evidenced by:<br>a. verbalization of feelings of self-worth and sexual adequacy<br>b. maintenance of relationships with significant others<br>c. active participation in activities of daily living<br>d. active interest in personal appearance. | b. Determine the meaning of the loss of reproductive organs to the client by encouraging her to verbalize feelings and by noting nonverbal responses to the changes experienced.<br>c. Implement measures to facilitate the grieving process (see Postoperative Nursing Diagnosis 4, action b).<br>d. Implement measures *to assist client to increase self-esteem* (e.g. limit negative self-assessment, encourage positive comments about self, assist to identify strengths, give positive feedback about accomplishments and behaviors that are indicative of high self-esteem).<br>e. Implement measures *to facilitate client's adjustment to the effects of the loss of her reproductive organs on her sexuality:*<br>1. encourage questions and clarify misconceptions the client has about the effect of loss of the uterus, ovaries, and fallopian tubes on sexual functioning; encourage questions and clarify misconceptions<br>2. facilitate communication between client and her partner; focus on feelings the couple share and assist them to identify changes which may affect their sexual relationship<br>3. arrange for uninterrupted privacy during hospital stay if desired by couple<br>4. discuss ways to be creative in expressing sexuality (e.g. massage, cuddling).<br>f. Assist client to identify and utilize coping techniques that have been helpful in the past.<br>g. Assist client with usual grooming and makeup habits if necessary.<br>h. Assess for and support behaviors suggesting positive adaptation to loss of reproductive organs (e.g. active interest in personal appearance, verbalization of feelings of self-worth, maintenance of relationships with significant others).<br>i. Assist client's and significant others' adjustment by listening, facilitating communication, and providing information.<br>j. Encourage visits and support from significant others.<br>k. If client expresses an interest in the adoption of children, provide names of appropriate community agencies.<br>l. Consult physician about psychological counseling if client desires or if she seems unwilling or unable to adapt to changes resulting from the surgery. |

## 4. NURSING DIAGNOSIS: Grieving*

related to loss of reproductive organs and its effect on body image and functioning (e.g. surgical menopause, inability to reproduce).

*This diagnostic label includes anticipatory grieving and grieving following the actual losses.

| Desired Outcome | Nursing Actions and ***Selected Purposes/Rationales*** |
|---|---|
| 4. The client will demonstrate beginning progression through the grieving process as evidenced by:<br>a. verbalization of feelings about the loss of reproductive organs | 4.a. Assess for signs and symptoms of grieving (e.g. change in eating habits, inability to concentrate, insomnia, anger, noncompliance, withdrawal from significant others, denial of loss). Be aware that client's response to a loss will be affected by factors such as previous experience with loss, age, developmental stage, available support systems, spiritual and cultural background, current health status, and significance of the loss.<br>b. Implement measures *to facilitate the grieving process:*<br>1. assist client to acknowledge the losses experienced *so grief work can begin;* assess for factors that may hinder and facilitate acknowledgment |

b. expression of grief
c. participation in treatment plan and self-care activities
d. utilization of available support systems.

2. discuss the grieving process and assist client to accept the phases of grieving as an expected response to loss of her reproductive organs and usual body functioning
3. allow time for client to progress through the phases of grieving (phases vary among theorists but progress from shock and alarm to acceptance); be aware that not every phase is expressed by all individuals, that recurrence of phases is common, and that the grieving process may take months to years
4. provide an atmosphere of care and concern (e.g. provide privacy, be available and nonjudgmental, display empathy and respect) *so that client will feel free to verbalize feelings*
5. perform actions *to promote trust* (e.g. answer questions honestly, provide requested information)
6. encourage the verbal expression of anger and sadness about the losses experienced; recognize displacement of anger and assist client to see the actual cause of angry feelings and resentment
7. encourage client to express her feelings in whatever ways are comfortable (e.g. writing, drawing, conversation)
8. assist client to identify personal strengths that have helped her to cope in previous situations of loss
9. support behaviors suggesting successful grief work (e.g. verbalizing feelings about changes in physical functioning, expressing sorrow, focusing on ways to adapt to loss of reproductive function)
10. explain the phases of the grieving process to significant others; encourage their support and understanding
11. facilitate communication between client and significant others; be aware that they may be in different phases of the grieving process
12. provide information about counseling services and support groups that might assist client in working through grief
13. arrange for visit from clergy if desired by client.

c. Consult physician about referral for counseling if signs of dysfunctional grieving (e.g. persistent denial of losses, excessive anger or sadness, hysteria, suicidal behaviors) occur.

## 5. NURSING DIAGNOSIS: Knowledge deficit

regarding follow-up care.

| Desired Outcomes | Nursing Actions and ***Selected Purposes/Rationales*** |
|---|---|
| 5.a. The client will verbalize an understanding of the effects of surgical menopause. | 5.a. Reinforce the physician's explanation of surgical menopause and its possible effects (e.g. hot flashes, facial hair growth, decrease in vaginal lubrication, insomnia, nervousness, palpitations, depression). |
| 5.b. The client will identify ways to achieve optimal sexual satisfaction. | 5.b.1. Explain the effects of the surgery on sexual functioning (e.g. painful intercourse because of vaginal dryness).<br>2. Instruct client in ways to improve sexual satisfaction:<br>a. use a water-soluble lubricant in the vagina to prevent pain during intercourse (the amount of vaginal lubrication decreases as a result of the effects of surgically-induced menopause)<br>b. take hormone replacements (e.g. estrogen) as prescribed.<br>3. Reinforce physician's instructions regarding when client can resume sexual intercourse (usually 4-6 weeks). |

| Desired Outcomes | Nursing Actions and ***Selected Purposes/Rationales*** |
|---|---|
| 5.c. The client will verbalize an understanding of medications ordered including rationale, side effects, schedule for taking, and importance of taking as prescribed. | 5.c.1. Explain the rationale for, side effects of, schedule for taking, and importance of taking medications prescribed.<br>2. If client is discharged on estrogen replacement therapy, instruct her to:<br>a. apply patch as prescribed; take oral medication with food or at bedtime to prevent nausea<br>b. be aware that depression, headache, weight gain, acne, increased skin pigmentation, nausea, and tender breasts are potential side effects of estrogen therapy<br>c. wear a supportive bra if breasts are tender<br>d. stop smoking (smoking may increase the incidence of some side effects of estrogen)<br>e. report the following to the health care provider:<br>1. side effects that are not controlled or tolerable<br>2. visual blurring or acuity changes or contact lens intolerance<br>3. numbness, swelling, pain, or redness of an extremity<br>f. keep scheduled follow-up appointments with health care provider while on estrogen replacement therapy. |
| 5.d. The client will state signs and symptoms to report to the health care provider. | 5.d.1. Refer to Standardized Postoperative Care Plan, Nursing Diagnosis 21, action c (p. 135), for signs and symptoms to report to the health care provider.<br>2. Instruct the client to report these additional signs and symptoms:<br>a. foul-smelling vaginal discharge<br>b. heavy vaginal bleeding (it is normal for a slight discharge to occur about 2 weeks postoperatively when internal sutures are absorbed)<br>c. excessive depression or difficulty dealing with changes in body image<br>d. excessive discomfort associated with effects of surgical menopause. |
| 5.e. The client will verbalize an understanding of and a plan for adhering to recommended follow-up care including future appointments with health care provider, activity limitations, and wound care. | 5.e.1. Refer to Standardized Postoperative Care Plan, Nursing Diagnosis 21 (pp. 135-136), for routine postoperative instructions and measures to promote client compliance.<br>2. Reinforce the physician's instructions regarding:<br>a. the need to avoid lifting objects over 10 pounds, sitting for long periods, stair climbing, and strenuous physical activity (e.g. aerobics) for 6-8 weeks postoperatively<br>b. resumption of douching and tub bathing (usually 4-6 weeks postoperatively) and driving a car (usually 2 weeks postoperatively). |

# Mammoplasty

A mammoplasty is the surgical reconstruction of the breast(s) that is performed to augment or reduce breast size or to shape and build a new breast mound following a mastectomy. It may be performed immediately following the mastectomy or delayed 3-12 months depending on physician preference, extensiveness of the tumor, lymph node status, planned treatment program, and age and desire of the client.

The technique used for reconstruction following a mastectomy will depend on when it is performed in relation to the mastectomy; amount, condition, and laxness of the skin on the chest wall; thickness of the skin flaps; and presence of pectoralis major muscle. In some women, a subpectoral prosthetic implant is all that is necessary. In others who have extensive skin, tissue, and muscle loss or radiation-induced skin damage, reconstruction may involve the use of autologous tissue such as the gluteus maximus, latissimus dorsi, or rectus abdominis muscle or rarely, the omentum. An additional prosthetic implant may not be necessary when this type of grafting is done, and the procedure will generally result in a softer, more natural-appearing breast mound. If the client has very taut skin on the chest wall or if the reconstruction is initiated at the time of the mastectomy, the use of a tissue expander may be necessary to facilitate stretching of the skin. With this procedure, an inflatable device is placed beneath the pectoral muscle and then gradually filled with saline over a period of several weeks to months. When the skin has stretched sufficiently to allow for inflation of the expander to 25% beyond the desired cosmetic size, it is replaced with a permanent prosthesis. There are tissue expanders available that can serve as the permanent implant. With this type, only the filling port is removed when adequate expansion has been achieved. The construction of a nipple-areola complex may be performed concurrently but is usually delayed until satisfactory breast symmetry has been achieved and placement can be more accurately determined. The areola is constructed by utilizing a graft from the pigmented upper, inner aspect of the thigh; postauricular area; labia minora; or the contralateral breast if the areola is of sufficient size. Intradermal tattooing can also be done to simulate an areola or to achieve a more appropriate color in grafted tissue. The nipple prominence is created by partitioning the nipple on the remaining breast, by utilizing a small portion of the earlobe or scar tissue, or by using skin and fat at the site of the new nipple (Skate flap). The majority of women who undergo breast reconstruction following a mastectomy will also have surgery (e.g. reduction, augmentation, mastopexy) on the contralateral breast in order to achieve symmetry.

**This care plan focuses on the adult female client hospitalized for breast reconstruction following a mastectomy.** Preoperatively, the goals of care are to reduce fear and anxiety and educate the client regarding postoperative expectations and management. Postoperative goals of care are to prevent complications, assist the client to adjust to her new body image, and educate her regarding follow-up care.

## DISCHARGE CRITERIA

Prior to discharge, the client will:

- be able to perform activities of daily living
- have no signs and symptoms of complications
- verbalize an understanding of the importance of doing a routine breast self-examination (BSE)
- demonstrate the ability to correctly perform a BSE
- demonstrate the appropriate technique to prevent capsule formation around breast implant(s)
- demonstrate the ability to care for wound drain insertion site(s), empty collection device, measure wound drainage, and reestablish negative pressure in collection device
- state signs and symptoms to report to the health care provider
- share feelings and thoughts about the change in body image
- verbalize an understanding of and a plan for adhering to recommended follow-up care including future appointments with health care provider, medications prescribed, activity restrictions, and wound care.

## NURSING/ COLLABORATIVE DIAGNOSES



**See Standardized Preoperative and Postoperative Care Plans for additional diagnoses.**

## PREOPERATIVE

**Use in conjunction with the Standardized Preoperative Care Plan.**

### 1. NURSING DIAGNOSIS: Knowledge deficit

regarding:
a. hospital routines associated with surgery;
b. physical preparation for the mammoplasty;
c. sensations that normally occur following surgery and anesthesia;
d. postoperative care;
e. appearance of the breast(s) following reconstruction.

| Desired Outcomes | Nursing Actions and ***Selected Purposes/Rationales*** |
|---|---|
| 1.a. The client will verbalize an understanding of usual preoperative care and postoperative sensations and care. | 1.a.1. Refer to Standardized Preoperative Care Plan, Nursing Diagnosis 4, actions a.1-4 (pp. 111-112), for information to include in preoperative teaching.<br>2. Provide information about expected sensations associated with breast reconstruction:<br>a. if the use of a tissue expander is planned, explain that a feeling of tightness and pressure in the chest will be present<br>b. if a latissimus dorsi flap will be used, explain that a feeling of back stiffness or tightness may be present as a result of muscle loss<br>c. explain that a loss of sensitivity in grafted nipples and skin around the suture lines is a common occurrence.<br>3. Allow time for questions and clarification. Provide feedback. |
| 1.b. The client will demonstrate the ability to perform activities designed to prevent postoperative complications. | 1.b.1. Refer to Standardized Preoperative Care Plan, Nursing Diagnosis 4, action b.1 (p. 112), for instructions on ways to prevent postoperative complications.<br>2. Provide additional instructions regarding ways to prevent complications following a mammoplasty:<br>a. if client is to have subpectoral implant(s), inform her that a bra should not be worn for several weeks following surgery to allow prosthesis(es) to settle into pocket(s) created in chest wall and to decrease the risk of capsule formation around implant(s)<br>b. inform client that she will need to keep upper arm on operative side(s) close to her body for a week after surgery (length of time may vary according to physician preference) in order to prevent tension on the suture lines and subsequent hematoma and seroma formation.<br>3. Allow time for questions and clarification of information provided. |
| 1.c. The client will verbalize an awareness of expected appearance of the breast(s) after reconstruction. | 1.c.1. Provide the following information on expected appearance of the breast(s) after reconstruction:<br>a. reinforce physician's explanation that the goal of reconstructive surgery after a mastectomy is to achieve a normal appearance in clothing; emphasize that it is impossible to duplicate the size, shape, and contour of a natural breast<br>b. explain that the breast(s) will be swollen and discolored in the immediate postoperative period and will appear unusually high on the chest wall if a subpectoral implant has been done; assure client and significant other that this is temporary<br>c. inform client that when one breast is reconstructed, symmetry does not usually occur until the tissue surrounding the implant has stretched.<br>2. Allow time for questions and clarification of information provided.<br>3. Consult physician if client has unrealistic expectations about the postoperative appearance of the breast(s). |

## POSTOPERATIVE

**Use in conjunction with the Standardized Postoperative Care Plan.**

### 1. NURSING DIAGNOSIS: Self-care deficit

related to impaired physical mobility associated with pain, depressant effects of some medications (e.g. narcotic analgesics), fear of injury to surgical site, and prescribed arm movement restrictions on operative side(s).

| Desired Outcome | Nursing Actions and ***Selected Purposes/Rationales*** |
|---|---|
| 1. The client will perform self-care activities within physical limitations and postoperative activity restrictions. | 1.a. Refer to Standardized Postoperative Care Plan, Nursing Diagnosis 12 (p. 125), for measures related to planning for and meeting client's self-care needs.<br>b. Assist client with personal hygiene tasks that require extension and abduction of the arm on the operative side (e.g. bathing, combing and washing hair). |

### 2. COLLABORATIVE DIAGNOSES: Potential complications:

a. **hematoma formation** related to inadequate hemostasis during surgical procedure, stress on vessels in operative area, and impaired drainage from the operative area;
b. **seroma formation** related to delayed or impaired flap adherence associated with irregular shape of chest wall, impaired wound drainage, and movement of operative site with arm and shoulder use;
c. **extrusion of prosthesis(es) or tissue expander** related to inadequate pocket size for implant(s), necrosis of skin flap(s), or trauma to surgical site;
d. **necrosis of skin flap(s) and/or grafted nipple(s)** related to:
   1. inadequate blood supply associated with stretching or rotation of blood vessels in grafted tissue during operative procedure and hematoma or seroma formation
   2. presence of infection;
e. **tissue expander failure** related to accidental puncture during operative procedure, defect in device, or excessive pressure on chest wall.

| Desired Outcomes | Nursing Actions and ***Selected Purposes/Rationales*** |
|---|---|
| 2.a. The client will not develop a hematoma at the surgical site as evidenced by:<br>1. no unusual increase in pain, edema, and skin discoloration in operative area<br>2. expected amount of wound drainage in collection device. | 2.a.1. Assess for and report signs and symptoms of hematoma formation (e.g. increased pain, edema, and skin discoloration in operative area; less than expected amount of wound drainage in collection device).<br>2. Implement measures *to prevent hematoma formation:*<br>a. caution client to keep elbows at sides for 7 days after surgery *in order to prevent strain on the surgical site and reduce the risk of subsequent bleeding*<br>b. maintain patency of wound drains (e.g. keep tubing free of kinks)<br>c. maintain wound drain suction as ordered.<br>3. If signs and symptoms of hematoma formation occur, prepare client for evacuation of hematoma and repair of bleeding vessels if planned. |
| 2.b. The client will not develop a seroma at | 2.b.1. Assess for and report signs and symptoms of seroma formation (e.g. continued drainage from incision, less than expected amount of wound |

| Desired Outcomes | Nursing Actions and ***Selected Purposes/Rationales*** |
|---|---|
| the surgical site as evidenced by:<br>1. absence of continued drainage from incision<br>2. expected amount of wound drainage in collection device. | drainage in collection device).<br>2. Implement measures *to prevent seroma formation:*<br>a. maintain patency of wound drains (e.g. keep tubing free of kinks)<br>b. maintain wound drain suction as ordered<br>c. place needed items within easy reach *to prevent unnecessary arm and shoulder movement*<br>d. reinforce importance of adhering to prescribed arm and shoulder movement restrictions.<br>3. If seroma formation occurs:<br>a. prepare client for needle aspiration of excessive fluid if planned<br>b. assist with application of compression dressing if planned<br>c. administer antimicrobials if ordered. |
| 2.c. The client will not experience extrusion of the breast prosthesis(es) or tissue expander as evidenced by maintenance of implant(s) or tissue expander under skin flap(s). | 2.c.1. Assess for and report:<br>a. conditions such as trauma to operative site, separation of suture line, or necrosis of skin flap that may place client at risk for extrusion of prosthesis(es) or tissue expander<br>b. extrusion of the prosthesis(es) or tissue expander.<br>2. Implement measures *to prevent extrusion of prosthesis(es) or tissue expander:*<br>a. perform actions to prevent skin flap necrosis (see action d.2 in this diagnosis)<br>b. caution client to avoid placing undue pressure on reconstructed area(s) until healing has occurred.<br>3. If extrusion of prosthesis(es) or tissue expander occurs:<br>a. prepare client for surgical replacement or removal of the implant(s) or tissue expander<br>b. provide emotional support to client and significant others. |
| 2.d. The client will not experience necrosis of the skin flap(s) or grafted nipple(s) as evidenced by:<br>1. skin flap(s) and nipple(s) warm and expected color<br>2. approximated wound edges<br>3. absence of foul odor from flap area and grafted nipple(s). | 2.d.1. Assess for and report signs and symptoms of:<br>a. impaired blood flow in skin flap and/or nipple (e.g. decreased warmth of skin flap and/or nipple; blue, white, or red appearing skin flap; capillary refill time greater than 3 seconds)<br>b. skin flap or grafted nipple necrosis (e.g. pale, cool, darkened tissue; separation of wound edges; foul odor).<br>2. Implement measures *to prevent necrosis of skin flap(s) and grafted nipple(s):*<br>a. perform actions *to maintain adequate circulation to wound area:*<br>1. implement measures to prevent hematoma and seroma formation (see actions a.2 and b.2 in this diagnosis)<br>2. ascertain that dressings and clothing are not too tight<br>3. keep client warm *to prevent generalized vasoconstriction*<br>4. position client on unoperative side or back *to prevent pressure on the surgical area*<br>5. encourage client not to smoke *(smoking causes vasoconstriction)*<br>b. administer oxygen if ordered *to increase oxygen availability to grafted nipple(s) and skin flap(s)*<br>c. perform actions to promote healing of surgical incision and prevent and treat wound infection (see Standardized Postoperative Care Plan, Nursing Diagnoses 9, action a.2 [pp. 122-123] and 16, actions b.4 and 5 [p. 129])<br>d. use caution when changing dressings, being careful not to disturb graft site(s).<br>3. If signs and symptoms of necrosis of skin flap(s) or grafted nipple(s) occur:<br>a. prepare client for surgical revision of reconstructed area<br>b. provide emotional support to client and significant others. |
| 2.e. The client will maintain a functional and intact tissue expander as evidenced by: | 2.e.1. Assess for and report signs and symptoms of tissue expander failure (e.g. deflation of breast mound, sudden reduction in sensations of tightness or pressure in reconstructed breast in early postoperative period). |

| Desired Outcomes | Nursing Actions and *Selected Purposes/Rationales* |
|---|---|
| 1. maintenance of inflation of breast mound<br>2. statements of feeling of skin and chest tightness and pressure in reconstructed breast in early postoperative period. | 2. Implement measures *to prevent excessive pressure on reconstructed area in order to reduce the risk for tissue expander failure:*<br>a. notify physician if dressings appear to be too tight<br>b. make sure that clothing worn over area is loose<br>c. instruct client to lie on unoperative side or back.<br>3. If signs and symptoms of tissue expander failure occur:<br>a. prepare client for surgical replacement or removal of expander if planned<br>b. provide emotional support to client and significant others. |

## 3. NURSING DIAGNOSIS: Knowledge deficit

regarding follow-up care.

| Desired Outcomes | Nursing Actions and ***Selected Purposes/Rationales*** |
|---|---|
| 3.a. The client will verbalize an understanding of the importance of doing a routine breast self-examination (BSE). | 3.a.1. Explain the reasons for a monthly BSE.<br>2. Discuss with client the importance of being familiar with what is "normal" for her breasts as a result of surgery.<br>3. Explore with client ways to remember to carry out BSE. The examination should be done one week after conclusion of menses or on a specific date if postmenopausal. |
| 3.b. The client will demonstrate the ability to correctly perform a BSE. | 3.b.1. Demonstrate the technique for performing BSE using a model, film, or chart.<br>2. Allow time for questions, clarification, and return demonstration. |
| 3.c. The client will demonstrate the appropriate technique to prevent capsule formation around breast implant(s). | 3.c.1. Instruct client on massage technique that is used to maintain mobility of the implant(s) and prevent capsule formation.<br>2. Emphasize the necessity of massaging and moving the implant(s) at least 4-6 times/day as soon as permitted by physician (massage should be continued for several months postoperatively).<br>3. Allow time for questions and clarification. |
| 3.d. The client will demonstrate the ability to care for wound drain insertion site(s), empty collection device, measure wound drainage, and reestablish negative pressure in collection device. | 3.d.1. Instruct client in care of wound drain insertion site(s) and wound drainage system. Demonstrate the following:<br>a. cleaning of drain insertion site(s)<br>b. emptying collection device<br>c. measuring and recording the amount of wound drainage<br>d. establishing negative pressure in collection device.<br>2. Allow time for questions, clarification, and return demonstration. |
| 3.e. The client will state signs and symptoms to report to the health care provider. | 3.e.1. Refer to Standardized Postoperative Care Plan, Nursing Diagnosis 21, action c (p. 135), for signs and symptoms to report to the health care provider.<br>2. Instruct client to report these additional signs and symptoms:<br>a. thinning, change of color, or breakdown of skin over implant or flap site<br>b. increasing redness of or drainage from donor site if grafting was done<br>c. sudden change in position of implants. |

| Desired Outcomes | Nursing Actions and ***Selected Purposes/Rationales*** |
|---|---|
| 3.f. The client will verbalize an understanding of and a plan for adhering to recommended follow-up care including future appointments with health care provider, medications prescribed, activity restrictions, and wound care. | 3.f.1. Refer to Standardized Postoperative Care Plan, Nursing Diagnosis 21 (pp. 135-136), for routine postoperative instructions and measures to improve client compliance.<br>2. If client has subpectoral implant(s), reinforce that a bra should not be worn for several weeks following surgery (this allows the prosthesis[es] to settle and decreases the risk of capsule formation).<br>3. If client had a tissue expander inserted:<br>a. emphasize importance of keeping appointments every 7-14 days to enlarge expander (in some cases, the client will eventually be taught to do the instillation at home); explain that a sterile solution will be added until a slight feeling of tightness is felt around the expander<br>b. instruct her to report pain, change in color of tissue over expander, redness of area, and/or separation of incision edges<br>c. provide suggestions for clothing styles to minimize the appearance of breast asymmetry.<br>4. Caution client to limit arm movement as prescribed.<br>5. Caution client to avoid pressure on chest wall during sexual activity and to avoid sleeping in prone position until healing is complete.<br>6. Instruct client to avoid lifting or pushing objects over 5 pounds for at least a month in order to prevent strain on pectoral muscles. |

# Mastectomy

A mastectomy is the surgical removal of all or part of the breast and is usually performed to treat breast cancer. The three major types of mastectomies performed today are the total mastectomy with axillary node dissection (modified radical), wide excision of the primary tumor (e.g. lumpectomy, tylectomy, segmental resection), and a subcutaneous mastectomy. The total mastectomy with axillary node dissection includes removal of the breast, some or all of the axillary nodes, and possibly the pectoralis minor muscle. The pectoralis major muscle is preserved with this procedure which allows the client to retain the shape of her chest and facilitates reconstructive surgery. Reconstruction may be performed at the time of the mastectomy or may be delayed for several months depending on physician and client preference and additional treatment planned. Breast-conserving surgery (wide-excision) followed by irradiation of the breast is an option today for women with grade I and II breast cancer in lieu of a total mastectomy. It involves the excision of the tumor with a surrounding margin of normal tissue and an axillary node dissection. Variables such as the location and size of the tumor, breast size, client preference, and the presence of collagen vascular disease will determine whether breast-conserving surgery is an option. A subcutaneous mastectomy may be performed for premalignant conditions or in situations in which the woman is at high risk for developing cancer of the breast. In this procedure, the subcutaneous breast tissue is removed, leaving the skin and nipple-areola complex intact.

**This care plan focuses on the adult female client hospitalized for a total mastectomy with axillary node dissection.** Goals of preoperative care are to reduce fear and anxiety and prepare the client for the postoperative period. Postoperatively, the goals of care are to maintain comfort, prevent complications, assist the client to adjust to the change in body image, and educate her regarding follow-up care. This care plan should be used in conjunction with the Care Plan on Mammoplasty if appropriate.

## DIAGNOSTIC TESTS

Mammography
Breast biopsy

## DISCHARGE CRITERIA

Prior to discharge, the client will:

- have surgical pain controlled
- be able to perform activities of daily living
- identify ways to reduce the risk of trauma to and infection in the arm on the operative side
- identify ways to prevent and treat lymphedema of the arm on the operative side
- demonstrate the ability to perform appropriate hand, arm, and shoulder exercises
- verbalize an understanding of the importance of doing a routine breast self-examination (BSE) on the remaining breast and operative site
- demonstrate the ability to correctly perform a BSE
- state the factors to consider in selecting a breast prosthesis
- state signs and symptoms to report to the health care provider
- share thoughts and feelings about the change in body image
- identify community resources that can assist with home management and adjustment to the diagnosis of cancer and the loss of a breast
- verbalize an understanding of and a plan for adhering to recommended follow-up care including future appointments with health care provider, medications prescribed, activity level, and wound care.

## NURSING/COLLABORATIVE DIAGNOSES



**See Standardized Preoperative and Postoperative Care Plans for additional diagnoses.**

## PREOPERATIVE

**Use in conjunction with the Standardized Preoperative Care Plan.**

### 1. NURSING DIAGNOSIS: Anxiety

related to:

a. diagnosis of cancer, treatment plan, and prognosis;
b. anticipated loss of control, effects of anesthesia, and surgical findings;
c. anticipated loss of femininity, physical attractiveness, and possible change in

relationship with significant other associated with the disfiguring effects of the mastectomy;
d. unfamiliar environment and separation from significant others;
e. anticipated postoperative discomfort and limitations.

| Desired Outcome | Nursing Actions and ***Selected Purposes/Rationales*** |
|---|---|
| 1. The client will experience a reduction in anxiety (see Standardized Preoperative Care Plan, Nursing Diagnosis 1 [pp. 108-109], for outcome criteria). | 1.a. Refer to Standardized Preoperative Care Plan, Nursing Diagnosis 1 (pp. 108-109), for measures related to assessment and reduction of preoperative fear and anxiety.<br>b. Implement additional measures *to reduce fear and anxiety:*<br>1. arrange for a Reach to Recovery volunteer to visit client if appropriate<br>2. if immediate reconstruction is not planned, reinforce information from physician about the possibility of future breast reconstruction if desired by client<br>3. reinforce physician's explanation about the positive effects of the mastectomy on her prognosis. |

## 2. NURSING DIAGNOSIS: Knowledge deficit

regarding hospital routines associated with surgery, physical preparation for a mastectomy, sensations that normally occur following surgery and anesthesia, and postoperative care.

| Desired Outcomes | Nursing Actions and ***Selected Purposes/Rationales*** |
|---|---|
| 2.a. The client will verbalize an understanding of usual preoperative care and postoperative sensations and care. | 2.a.1. Refer to Standardized Preoperative Care Plan, Nursing Diagnosis 4, actions a.1-4 (pp. 111-112), for information to include in preoperative teaching.<br>2. Provide the following information on phantom sensations that may occur after a mastectomy:<br>a. explain to client that it is common to experience sensations of itching, coldness, heaviness, pain, numbness, nipple twinges, and/or "pins and needles" in the absent breast (most clients will notice it within the first week after surgery)<br>b. assure client that women experience the sensation of both breasts being present most of the time; explain that a physical awareness of the loss may occur when leaning on a solid object (e.g. table) or crossing her arms<br>c. explain to client that she may feel unbalanced at first, particularly if breasts are large.<br>3. Allow time for questions and clarification of information provided. |
| 2.b. The client will demonstrate the ability to perform activities designed to prevent postoperative complications. | 2.b.1. Refer to Standardized Preoperative Care Plan, Nursing Diagnosis 4, action b.1 (p. 112), for instructions on ways to prevent postoperative complications.<br>2. Provide additional instructions regarding ways to prevent complications following a mastectomy:<br>a. inform the client that she must keep upper arm on operative side close to her body for about a week after surgery (length of time will vary according to physician preference) in order to prevent tension on the suture lines and subsequent hematoma and seroma formation<br>b. explain that exercise of the hand, arm, and shoulder on the operative |

side is essential in order to facilitate and improve lymphatic and blood circulation, maintain muscle tone, and prevent contractures
   c. demonstrate recommended postmastectomy exercises (e.g. flexion and extension of the fingers and wrist, wall climbing, pulley motion, rope turning)
   d. instruct client on ways to minimize or prevent lymphedema of the arm on operative side:
      1. keep arm on operative side elevated on pillows with elbow at heart level and hand higher than elbow in the early postoperative period
      2. perform recommended postmastectomy exercises as soon as allowed (hand and wrist exercises are usually begun the day of surgery and gradually progress to full range of motion of shoulder on operative side when sutures are removed)
      3. inform client that no venipunctures, injections, or B/P measurements should be performed on that arm (these procedures increase risk of infection or trauma and subsequent lymphedema).
3. Allow time for questions, clarification, practice, and return demonstration of exercises.

## POSTOPERATIVE

**Use in conjunction with the Standardized Postoperative Care Plan.**

---

### 1. NURSING DIAGNOSIS: Self-care deficit

related to impaired physical mobility associated with pain, depressant effects of some medications (e.g. narcotic analgesics), fear of injury to surgical site, and prescribed arm movement restrictions on the operative side.

| Desired Outcome | Nursing Actions and ***Selected Purposes/Rationales*** |
|---|---|
| 1. The client will perform self-care activities within physical limitations and postoperative activity restrictions. | 1.a. Refer to Standardized Postoperative Care Plan, Nursing Diagnosis 12 (p. 125), for measures related to planning for and meeting client's self care needs.<br>b. Instruct and assist client with postmastectomy exercises as soon as allowed *in order to strengthen extremity on operative side and increase client's ability to perform self-care.*<br>c. Assist client with personal hygiene tasks that require extension and abduction of arm on operative side (e.g. combing and washing hair, bathing). |

---

### 2. COLLABORATIVE DIAGNOSES: Potential complications:

a. **lymphedema of arm on operative side** related to interruption in usual lymph flow associated with extensive removal of axillary nodes and infection of or trauma to operative arm;
b. **motor and sensory impairment of the arm and/or shoulder on the operative side** related to:
   1. transection of or trauma to the nerves during surgical procedure
   2. pressure on nerves associated with lymphedema if it occurs
   3. noncompliance with prescribed exercise program;

c. **seroma formation** related to:
   1. large potential dead space beneath flap
   2. delayed or impaired flap adherence associated with irregular shape of chest wall, impaired wound drainage, and movement of operative area with arm and shoulder use;

d. **hematoma formation** related to inadequate hemostasis during surgical procedure, stress on vessels in operative area, and impaired drainage from the operative area;

e. **necrosis of skin flap** related to inadequate blood supply in flap or infection of surgical wound.

| Desired Outcomes | Nursing Actions and ***Selected Purposes/Rationales*** |
|---|---|
| 2.a. The client will not develop lymphedema of the arm on the operative side as evidenced by:<br>1. normal motor and sensory function of the arm<br>2. absence of pain and edema in the arm. | 2.a.1. Assess for and report signs and symptoms of lymphedema of the arm on the operative side:<br>a. sensory or motor deficits<br>b. pain, sensation of heaviness<br>c. edema (measure arm on operative side at points 4 inches above and below elbow).<br>2. Implement measures *to prevent lymphedema of arm on operative side:*<br>a. place client in a semi-Fowler's position during the immediate postoperative period; elevate arm on the operative side on pillows, keeping elbow at heart level and hand higher than elbow<br>b. avoid prolonged adduction of arm *to prevent pressure on axilla (pressure can impede lymphatic flow)*<br>c. place a sign above bed to remind personnel not to use arm on operative side for venipunctures, injections, and B/P measurement *in order to decrease risk of infection or trauma and subsequent lymphedema*<br>d. perform actions to prevent and treat wound infection (see Standardized Postoperative Care Plan, Nursing Diagnosis 16, actions b.4 and 5 [p. 129])<br>e. instruct and assist client to perform postmastectomy exercises as soon as allowed *in order to promote adequate lymphatic drainage.*<br>3. If signs and symptoms of lymphedema occur:<br>a. continue with above measures<br>b. administer the following medications if ordered:<br>1. antimicrobials *to prevent or treat cellulitis and lymphangitis*<br>2. diuretics *to reduce fluid accumulation in tissues*<br>c. apply an elastic bandage or elastic pressure gradient sleeve to the affected arm if ordered *to reduce edema*<br>d. assist and instruct client in use of an intermittent pneumatic compression sleeve on affected arm if ordered<br>e. restrict sodium intake if ordered<br>f. provide emotional support to client and significant others. |
| 2.b. The client will maintain normal motor and sensory function of the arm and shoulder on the operative side as evidenced by:<br>1. ability to put arm and shoulder through expected range of motion<br>2. absence of numbness, tingling, and muscle weakness. | 2.b.1. Assess for and report signs and symptoms of motor and/or sensory impairment of the arm and shoulder on operative side (e.g. inability to move joints through expected range of motion, numbness, tingling, muscle weakness).<br>2. Implement measures *to prevent arm and shoulder dysfunction:*<br>a. perform actions to prevent lymphedema (see action a.2 in this diagnosis)<br>b. initiate postmastectomy exercises (e.g. wall climbing) as soon as allowed<br>c. encourage use of arm on operative side to perform activities of daily living as soon as allowed.<br>3. If signs and symptoms of impaired arm or shoulder function occur:<br>a. continue with above measures<br>b. assist with prescribed physical therapy<br>c. provide emotional support to client and significant others. |

2.c. The client will not develop a seroma at the surgical site as evidenced by:
1. absence of continued drainage from incision
2. expected amount of wound drainage in collection device.

2.c.1. Assess for and report signs and symptoms of seroma formation (e.g. continued drainage from incision, less than expected amount of wound drainage in collection device).
2. Implement measures *to prevent seroma formation:*
   a. maintain patency of wound drain (e.g. keep tubing free of kinks)
   b. maintain wound drain suction as ordered
   c. place needed items within easy reach *to prevent unnecessary arm and shoulder movement*
   d. reinforce importance of adhering to arm and shoulder movement restrictions.
3. If seroma formation occurs:
   a. prepare client for needle aspiration of excessive fluid if planned
   b. assist with application of compression dressing if planned
   c. administer antimicrobials if ordered.

2.d. The client will not develop a hematoma at the surgical site as evidenced by:
1. no unusual increase in pain, edema, and skin discoloration in operative area
2. expected amount of wound drainage in collection device.

2.d.1. Assess for and report signs and symptoms of hematoma formation (e.g. increased pain, edema, and discoloration of operative site; less than expected amount of wound drainage in collection device).
2. Implement measures *to prevent hematoma formation:*
   a. caution client to adhere to arm and shoulder movement restrictions *in order to prevent strain on the surgical site and subsequent bleeding*
   b. maintain patency of wound drain (e.g. keep tubing free of kinks)
   c. maintain wound drain suction as ordered.
3. If signs and symptoms of hematoma formation occur, prepare client for evacuation of hematoma and repair of bleeding vessels if planned.

2.e. The client will not experience necrosis of the skin flap as evidenced by:
1. skin flap warm and expected color
2. approximated wound edges
3. absence of foul odor from flap area.

2.e.1. Assess for and report signs and symptoms of:
   a. impaired blood flow in skin flap (e.g. decreased warmth of skin flap; blue, white, or red appearing skin flap; capillary refill time greater than 3 seconds)
   b. skin flap necrosis (e.g. pale, cool, darkened tissue; separation of wound edges; foul odor).
2. Implement measures *to prevent skin flap necrosis:*
   a. perform actions *to maintain adequate circulation to wound area:*
      1. implement measures to prevent seroma and hematoma formation (see actions c.2 and d.2 in this diagnosis)
      2. consult physician regarding loosening of dressing if client complains of increased tightness of dressing or if dressing appears too restrictive
      3. position client on unoperative side or back
      4. encourage client not to smoke *(smoking causes vasoconstriction)*
   b. perform actions to promote healing of surgical incision and prevent and treat wound infection (see Standardized Postoperative Care Plan, Nursing Diagnoses 9, action a.2 [pp. 122-123] and 16, actions b.4 and 5 [p. 129]).
3. If signs and symptoms of skin flap necrosis occur:
   a. prepare client for surgical revision of flap
   b. provide emotional support to client and significant others.

## 3. NURSING DIAGNOSIS: Self-concept disturbance*

related to:
a. loss of a breast;
b. dependence on others for assistance with self-care associated with restricted arm movement;

*This diagnostic label includes the nursing diagnoses of body image disturbance, self-esteem disturbance, and altered role function.

c. possible altered sexuality patterns associated with decreased libido, perceived loss of femininity, and fear of rejection by partner.

| Desired Outcome | Nursing Actions and ***Selected Purposes/Rationales*** |
|---|---|
| 3. The client will demonstrate beginning adaptation to the loss of her breast and integration of the change in body image as evidenced by:<br>a. verbalization of feelings of self-worth and sexual adequacy<br>b. maintenance of relationships with significant others<br>c. active participation in activities of daily living<br>d. active interest in personal appearance<br>e. willingness to look at surgical site<br>f. willingness to pursue usual roles and participate in social activities. | 3.a. Assess for signs and symptoms of a self-concept disturbance (e.g. verbal or nonverbal cues denoting a negative response to the loss of a breast such as denial of or preoccupation with the loss, refusal to look at or touch mastectomy site, or withdrawal from significant others).<br>b. Determine the meaning of the loss of a breast to the client by encouraging her to verbalize feelings and by noting nonverbal responses to the loss experienced.<br>c. Implement measures to facilitate the grieving process (see Postoperative Nursing Diagnosis 5, action b).<br>d. Implement measures to assist client to cope with the effects of the mastectomy (see Postoperative Nursing Diagnosis 4, action c).<br>e. Implement measures *to assist client to increase self-esteem* (e.g. limit negative self-assessment, encourage positive comments about self, assist to identify strengths, give positive feedback about accomplishments and behaviors that are indicative of high self-esteem).<br>f. Implement measures *to facilitate client's adjustment to the effects of the loss of her breast on her sexuality:*<br>1. facilitate communication between client and her partner; focus on the feelings the couple share and assist them to identify factors which may affect their sexual relationship<br>2. arrange for uninterrupted privacy during hospital stay if desired by the couple.<br>g. If appropriate, involve partner in care of the client's wound *to facilitate partner's adjustment to the change in client's body image and subsequently decrease the possibility of partner's rejection of client.*<br>h. Assist client with usual grooming and makeup habits if necessary.<br>i. Demonstrate acceptance of client using techniques such as touch and frequent visits. Encourage significant others to do the same.<br>j. Stay with client during first dressing change and encourage her to express her feelings about appearance of incision and change in her body. Be aware that the integration of the change in body image does not occur until 2-6 months after the actual physical change has occurred.<br>k. If the client is unwilling to look at the surgical site, provide support and encouragement to do so before discharge.<br>l. If a mammoplasty has not been performed:<br>1. encourage client to discuss possibilities for future reconstruction of her breast with the physician if desired<br>2. discuss the variety of prostheses available and ways to obtain one.<br>m. Assist client's and significant others' adjustment by listening, facilitating communication, and providing information.<br>n. Assess for and support behaviors suggesting positive adaptation to loss of the breast (e.g. willingness to look at and care for wound, compliance with exercise program, maintenance of relationships with significant others).<br>o. Encourage significant others to allow client to do what she is able *so that independence can be reestablished and/or self-esteem redeveloped.*<br>p. Encourage client contact with others *so that she can test and establish a new self-image.*<br>q. Encourage visits and support from significant others.<br>r. Encourage client to pursue usual roles and interests and to continue involvement in social activities.<br>s. Provide information about and encourage utilization of community |

agencies and support groups (e.g. Reach to Recovery; sexual, family, and individual counseling services; American Cancer Society).

t. Consult physician about psychological counseling if client desires or if she seems unwilling or unable to adapt to the loss of her breast.

## 4. NURSING DIAGNOSIS: Ineffective individual coping

related to:

a. perceived loss of femininity and embarrassment associated with loss of a breast;
b. fear of rejection by significant others;
c. fear, anxiety, and feelings of loss of control associated with the diagnosis of cancer, adjuvant therapy (e.g. chemotherapy, radiation therapy) if planned, and possibility of disease recurrence;
d. inadequate support system.

| Desired Outcome | Nursing Actions and ***Selected Purposes/Rationales*** |
|---|---|
| 4. The client will demonstrate the use of effective coping skills as evidenced by:<br>a. verbalization of ability to cope with the loss of a breast<br>b. utilization of appropriate problem-solving techniques<br>c. willingness to participate in treatment plan and meet basic needs<br>d. absence of destructive behavior toward self and others<br>e. appropriate use of defense mechanisms<br>f. recognition and utilization of available support systems. | 4.a. Assess for and report signs and symptoms of ineffective individual coping (e.g. verbalization of inability to cope; inability to ask for help, problem solve, or meet basic needs; reluctance to participate in the treatment plan; destructive behavior toward self or others; inappropriate use of defense mechanisms; inability to meet role expectations).<br>b. Assess client's perception of current situation including effectiveness of coping mechanisms.<br>c. Implement measures *to promote effective coping:*<br>1. allow time for client to adjust psychologically to the mastectomy; inform client that a peak period of emotional distress may occur several weeks postoperatively<br>2. assist client to recognize and manage inappropriate denial if it is present<br>3. arrange for a Reach to Recovery volunteer to visit client<br>4. perform actions to improve self-concept (see Postoperative Nursing Diagnosis 3, actions e-s)<br>5. perform actions to reduce fear and anxiety (see Standardized Postoperative Care Plan, Nursing Diagnosis 20, action b [p. 134])<br>6. encourage verbalization about current situation<br>7. assist client to identify personal strengths and resources that can be utilized to facilitate coping with the current situation<br>8. demonstrate acceptance of client but set limits on inappropriate behavior<br>9. create an atmosphere of trust and support<br>10. include client in planning of care, encourage maximum participation in treatment plan, and allow choices when possible *to enable her to maintain a sense of control*<br>11. instruct client in effective problem-solving techniques (e.g. accurate identification of stressors, determination of various options to solve problem)<br>12. assist client to maintain usual daily routines whenever possible<br>13. assist client through methods such as role playing to prepare for negative reactions from others because of the loss of her breast and the diagnosis of cancer<br>14. administer antianxiety and/or antidepressant agents if ordered<br>15. assist client to identify and utilize available support systems; provide information about available community resources that can assist client |

| Desired Outcome | Nursing Actions and ***Selected Purposes/Rationales*** |
|---|---|
| | and significant others in coping with the mastectomy (e.g. American Cancer Society, counselors, mastectomy support groups)<br>16. encourage the client to share with significant others the kind of support that would be most beneficial (e.g. listening, inspiring hope, providing reassurance and accurate information).<br>d. Consult physician about psychological counseling if appropriate. Initiate a referral if necessary. |

## 5. NURSING DIAGNOSIS: Grieving*

related to:
a. loss of a breast and subsequent change in body image;
b. potential for premature death associated with the diagnosis of cancer.

*This diagnostic label includes anticipatory grieving and grieving following the actual loss.

| Desired Outcome | Nursing Actions and ***Selected Purposes/Rationales*** |
|---|---|
| 5. The client will demonstrate beginning progression through the grieving process as evidenced by:<br>a. verbalization of feelings about the loss of a breast and diagnosis of cancer<br>b. expression of grief<br>c. participation in treatment plan and self-care activities<br>d. utilization of available support systems. | 5.a. Assess for signs and symptoms of grieving (e.g. change in eating habits, inability to concentrate, insomnia, anger, noncompliance, withdrawal from significant others, denial of loss and diagnosis). Be aware that client's response to the diagnosis of cancer and loss experienced will be affected by factors such as previous experience with loss, age, developmental stage, available support systems, spiritual and cultural background, current health status, and significance of the diagnosis and loss.<br>b. Implement measures *to facilitate the grieving process:*<br>1. assist client to acknowledge the changes resulting from loss of her breast and diagnosis of cancer *so grief work can begin;* assess for factors that may hinder and facilitate acknowledgment<br>2. discuss the grieving process and assist client to accept the phases of grieving as an expected response to loss of a breast and diagnosis of cancer<br>3. allow time for client to progress through the phases of grieving (phases vary among theorists but progress from shock and alarm to acceptance); be aware that not every phase is expressed by all individuals, that recurrence of phases is common, and that the grieving process may take months to years<br>4. provide an atmosphere of care and concern (e.g. provide privacy, be available and nonjudgmental, display empathy and respect) *so client will feel free to verbalize feelings*<br>5. perform actions *to promote trust* (e.g. answer questions honestly, provide requested information)<br>6. encourage the verbal expression of anger and sadness about the diagnosis of cancer and the loss of her breast; recognize displacement of anger and assist client to see the actual cause of angry feelings and resentment<br>7. encourage client to express her feelings in whatever ways are comfortable (e.g. writing, drawing, conversation)<br>8. perform actions to promote effective coping (see Postoperative Nursing Diagnosis 4, action c)<br>9. support realistic hope about the effect of surgery on the disease process and the possibility of breast reconstruction if it has not been done |

10. support behaviors suggesting successful grief work (e.g. verbalizing feelings about loss of a breast, expressing sorrow)
11. explain the phases of the grieving process to significant others; encourage their support and understanding
12. facilitate communication between the client and significant others; be aware that they may be in different phases of the grieving process
13. provide information regarding counseling services and support groups that might assist client in working through grief
14. arrange for visit from clergy if desired by client.

c. Consult physician regarding referral for counseling if signs of dysfunctional grieving (e.g. persistent denial of loss, excessive anger or sadness, hysteria, suicidal behaviors) occur.

## 6. NURSING DIAGNOSIS: Knowledge deficit

regarding follow-up care.

| Desired Outcomes | Nursing Actions and ***Selected Purposes/Rationales*** |
|---|---|
| 6.a. The client will identify ways to reduce the risk of trauma to and infection in the arm on the operative side. | 6.a.1. Provide the following instructions regarding ways to reduce the risk of trauma to and infection in the arm on operative side (these recommendations are based on the American Cancer Society's guidelines):<br>a. push cuticles back instead of cutting them<br>b. use heavy work gloves when gardening and rubber gloves when in contact with steel wool or water for prolonged periods<br>c. use insulated gloves when reaching into a hot oven<br>d. use a thimble when sewing in order to avoid pinpricks<br>e. avoid wearing tight jewelry or constrictive clothing on the affected arm to prevent unnecessary pressure<br>f. carry heavy objects such as purse or packages with the unaffected arm<br>g. offer only the unaffected arm for blood pressure readings, injections, and blood testing<br>h. wash any break in the skin on the affected arm with soap and water and cover the area with a protective dressing<br>i. use an electric rather than a straight-edge razor when shaving underarm area<br>j. apply a lanolin hand cream several times/day to prevent drying and cracking of the skin<br>k. avoid prolonged exposure to the sun in order to prevent burns.<br>2. Instruct client to contact physician immediately should any injury to the arm on the operative side occur. |
| 6.b. The client will identify ways to prevent and treat lymphedema of the arm on the operative side. | 6.b.1. Instruct client in ways to prevent lymphedema of the arm on operative side:<br>a. elevate the affected arm for 30 minutes every 2 hours for the first 2 weeks postoperatively and then for 30 minutes 3 times a day for the next 6 weeks<br>b. sleep on unaffected side or back with affected arm elevated (forearm should be higher than the elbow and elbow level with or higher than the heart) for 8 weeks postoperatively<br>c. adhere to recommended measures for reducing the risk of trauma to and preventing infection in the arm on the operative side (see action a.1 in this diagnosis). |

| Desired Outcomes | Nursing Actions and ***Selected Purposes/Rationales*** |
|---|---|
| | 2. Reinforce physician's instructions regarding ways to treat lymphedema if present:<br>a. adhere to a diet low in sodium<br>b. take diuretics and antimicrobials as prescribed<br>c. use elastic bandage or pressure gradient sleeve as recommended. |
| 6.c. The client will demonstrate the ability to perform appropriate hand, arm, and shoulder exercises. | 6.c.1. Reinforce teaching about postmastectomy exercises.<br>2. Emphasize the need to exercise hand, arm, and shoulder on operative side daily as prescribed.<br>3. Allow time for questions, clarification, and return demonstration. |
| 6.d. The client will verbalize an understanding of the importance of doing a routine breast self-examination (BSE) on the remaining breast and operative site. | 6.d.1. Explain the reasons for monthly BSE of the remaining breast and operative site.<br>2. Explore with client ways to remember to carry out BSE. The examination should be done a week after conclusion of menses or on a specific date if postmenopausal. |
| 6.e. The client will demonstrate the ability to correctly perform a BSE. | 6.e.1. Demonstrate, using a model, film, or chart, how to do a BSE.<br>2. Allow time for questions, clarification, and return demonstration. |
| 6.f. The client will state the factors to consider in selecting a breast prosthesis. | 6.f.1. Invite a Reach to Recovery volunteer or prosthetist to share information about the various prostheses available.<br>2. Suggest a soft, temporary prosthesis until complete healing of the incision has occurred.<br>3. Encourage the client to take significant other or a close friend with her for the initial fitting in order to provide emotional support.<br>4. Emphasize that it is important to select or make a prosthesis that will balance the chest in order to avoid difficulties with posture and subsequent back, shoulder, and neck discomfort.<br>5. Discuss ways to improvise breast forms (e.g. fill bra cup with soft material) and maintain symmetry when using a light, temporary prosthesis (e.g. anchor bra to other undergarments, place drapery weights in bra cup on affected side to achieve balance, wear long-line bra). |
| 6.g. The client will state signs and symptoms to report to the health care provider. | 6.g.1. Refer to Standardized Postoperative Care Plan, Nursing Diagnosis 21, action c (p. 135), for signs and symptoms to report to the health care provider.<br>2. Instruct client to report these additional signs and symptoms:<br>a. tingling, stiffness, or increased numbness in hand, arm, or shoulder on operative side (explain that a residual numbness may persist in the chest wall and arm)<br>b. increasing weakness of the affected arm<br>c. warmth or redness of the affected arm<br>d. increase in size of arm on affected side (client may be instructed to measure arm circumference weekly at points 4 inches above and below elbow and compare with unaffected arm); inform client that transient edema may occur as she increases her use of affected arm and that this should subside as collateral lymphatic circulation develops<br>e. decreased ability to move shoulder or arm on operative side through their full range of motion (full range of motion should be regained within 3-6 months). |
| 6.h. The client will identify community resources that can assist with | 6.h.1. Provide information about community resources that can assist the client and significant others with home management and adjustment to the diagnosis of cancer and the mastectomy (e.g. American Cancer Society, |

home management and adjustment to the diagnosis of cancer and the loss of a breast.

Reach to Recovery, mastectomy support groups, social services, home health agencies, individual and family counselors).

2. Initiate a referral if appropriate.

6.i. The client will verbalize an understanding of and a plan for adhering to recommended follow-up care including future appointments with health care provider, medications prescribed, activity level, and wound care.

6.i.1. Refer to Standardized Postoperative Care Plan, Nursing Diagnosis 21 (pp. 135-136), for routine postoperative instructions and measures to improve client compliance.

2. Reinforce physician's explanations and instructions regarding future treatment (e.g. chemotherapy, radiation therapy, breast reconstruction) if planned.

# Radical Prostatectomy

A radical prostatectomy involves removal of the prostate gland, prostatic capsule, seminal vesicles, part of the vas deferens, and cuff of the bladder neck. It is accomplished via a retropubic or perineal approach depending on the size and position of the prostate and physician preference. A pelvic lymphadenectomy may be done concurrently. Radical prostatectomy is a curative treatment for cancer of the prostate if the cancer is basically confined to the prostate gland. Surgery may be followed by a course of external radiation therapy (teletherapy) if there is evidence of metastasis to the lymph nodes.

**This care plan focuses on the adult male client with cancer of the prostate who is admitted for a radical prostatectomy.** The goals of preoperative care are to reduce fear and anxiety and provide emotional support. Postoperatively, goals of care are to maintain comfort, prevent complications, facilitate the client's adjustment to the effects of the diagnosis and its treatment, and educate him regarding follow-up care.

## DIAGNOSTIC TESTS*

Blood studies (e.g. prostatic acid phosphatase, prostate-specific antigen [PSA])
Biopsy of the prostate
Transrectal ultrasonography
Computed tomography (CT) of pelvis and lower abdomen
Bone scan
Magnetic resonance imaging (MRI)
Lymphangiography
Excretory urography (intravenous pyelography)

*May be performed to confirm the diagnosis and stage the disease.

## DISCHARGE CRITERIA

Prior to discharge, the client will:

- have surgical pain controlled
- have no signs and symptoms of complications
- demonstrate the ability to perform care related to the urinary catheter and drainage system

- identify ways to manage urinary incontinence if it occurs following catheter removal
- identify ways to manage bowel incontinence if present
- share feelings and concerns about the diagnosis of cancer, the prognosis, and changes in body functioning that may occur as a result of a radical prostatectomy
- state signs and symptoms to report to the health care provider
- verbalize an understanding of and a plan for adhering to recommended follow-up care including future appointments with health care provider, medications prescribed, activity level, wound care, and plans for subsequent treatment.

**NURSING/ COLLABORATIVE DIAGNOSES**



**See Standardized Preoperative and Postoperative Care Plans for additional diagnoses.**

## PREOPERATIVE

**Use in conjunction with the Standardized Preoperative Care Plan.**

### 1. NURSING DIAGNOSIS: Anxiety

related to:
a. diagnosis of cancer, treatment plan, and prognosis;
b. potential embarrassment or loss of dignity associated with exposure of genitals during preoperative care, surgery, and postoperative assessments and treatments;
c. anticipated loss of control, effects of anesthesia, postoperative discomfort, and effects of radical prostatectomy on body functioning;
d. risk of contracting disease if blood transfusions are necessary;
e. unfamiliar environment and separation from significant others;
f. ability to independently perform urinary catheter care following discharge;
g. economic factors associated with hospitalization.

| Desired Outcome | Nursing Actions and ***Selected Purposes/Rationales*** |
|---|---|
| 1. The client will experience a reduction in anxiety (see Standardized Preoperative Care Plan, Nursing Diagnosis 1, [pp. 108-109], for outcome criteria). | 1.a. Refer to Standardized Preoperative Care Plan, Nursing Diagnosis 1, (pp. 108-109), for measures related to assessment and reduction of fear and anxiety.<br>b. Implement additional measures *to reduce fear and anxiety:*<br>1. allow time for verbalization of concerns regarding the effects of the radical prostatectomy on body functioning (e.g. sterility, possible impotence, possible urinary and/or bowel incontinence); if appropriate, reinforce physician's explanation about the success of nerve-sparing surgical techniques which have greatly reduced the incidence of impotence<br>2. instruct client to expect the following postoperatively *so that he is not overly concerned when they occur:*<br>a. presence of a urinary catheter (the catheter will be removed about 2-3 weeks after surgery)<br>b. frequent dressing changes and/or presence of wound drainage collection device for the first 2-4 days after surgery<br>c. possible need for bladder irrigations to keep catheter patent<br>d. presence of some blood in urine (can occur occasionally during the first 1-3 days after surgery)<br>3. reinforce physician's explanation about the positive effects of surgery (when diagnosed and treated in early stages, prostatic cancer is a highly curable disease)<br>4. assure client that privacy will be maintained during preoperative care and postoperative assessments and treatments<br>5. assure client that he will receive thorough instructions about management of the urinary catheter prior to discharge. |

## POSTOPERATIVE

**Use in conjunction with the Standardized Postoperative Care Plan.**

### 1. NURSING DIAGNOSIS: Pain

related to tissue trauma and reflex muscle spasms associated with the surgery; irritation from drainage tubes; and stress on surgical area associated with movement, sitting (especially following a perineal approach), and straining to have a bowel movement.

| Desired Outcome | Nursing Actions and ***Selected Purposes/Rationales*** |
|---|---|
| 1. The client will experience diminished pain (see Standardized Postoperative Care Plan, Nursing Diagnosis 6 [p. 119], for outcome criteria). | 1.a. Refer to Standardized Postoperative Care Plan, Nursing Diagnosis 6 (p. 119), for measures related to assessment and management of pain.<br>b. Implement additional measures *to reduce pain:*<br>1. instruct client to avoid straining to have a bowel movement *in order to prevent increased pressure on operative site;* consult physician about an order for a stool softener and/or laxative if indicated<br>2. if client has a perineal incision:<br>a. provide a pillow or foam pad for him to sit on if desired<br>b. assist with sitz baths if ordered following removal of perineal wound drains (some physicians will not order sitz baths until the urinary catheter is also removed). |

## 2. NURSING DIAGNOSIS: Urinary retention

related to obstruction of the urinary catheter.

| Desired Outcome | Nursing Actions and ***Selected Purposes/Rationales*** |
|---|---|
| 2. The client will not experience urinary retention as evidenced by:<br>a. no complaints of bladder fullness or suprapubic discomfort<br>b. absence of bladder distention<br>c. balanced intake and output within 48 hours after surgery. | 2.a. Assess for and report signs and symptoms of urinary retention (e.g. complaints of bladder fullness or suprapubic discomfort, bladder distention, absence of urine in drainage tubing, output that continues to be less than intake 48 hours after surgery).<br>b. Implement measures *to maintain patency of urinary catheter in order to prevent urinary retention:*<br>1. keep drainage tubing free of kinks<br>2. keep collection container below level of bladder<br>3. tape catheter securely to abdomen or thigh *in order to prevent inadvertent removal*<br>4. perform bladder irrigations as ordered *to flush out blood clots if present (the clots could obstruct the catheter).*<br>c. Consult physician if signs and symptoms of urinary retention persist. |

## 3. NURSING DIAGNOSIS: Bowel incontinence

related to:

a. unavoidable or inadvertent damage to the anal sphincter or to the pudendal nerve during surgery (this nerve controls the anal sphincter);
b. compression of the pudendal nerve associated with postoperative edema in the surgical area;
c. loss of perineal muscle tone associated with surgical incision if a perineal approach was used.

| Desired Outcome | Nursing Actions and ***Selected Purposes/Rationales*** |
|---|---|
| 3. The client will maintain optimal bowel control as evidenced by absence of or decreased episodes of incontinence. | 3.a. Monitor for episodes of bowel incontinence.<br>b. Implement measures *to reduce the risk of bowel incontinence:*<br>1. instruct client to perform perineal exercises (e.g. stopping and starting stream during voiding; squeezing buttocks together, then relaxing the muscles) when allowed *in order to increase anal sphincter tone and strengthen pelvic floor muscles, which will help maintain the normal anorectal angle*<br>2. have bedside commode or bedpan readily available to client and provide easy access to bathroom *in order to reduce delays in toileting.*<br>c. If bowel incontinence occurs, consult physician about initiating a bowel care program *so that client is able to routinely evacuate contents of lower colon and reduce the risk of incontinence.* |

## 4. NURSING DIAGNOSIS: High risk for infection:

a. **wound infection** related to wound contamination (especially with a perineal approach because incision is close to the anus);

b. **urinary tract infection** related to:
   1. introduction of pathogens associated with presence of indwelling urinary catheter
   2. colonization of bacteria in the urine associated with urinary stasis resulting from decreased activity or urinary retention (can occur if the catheter becomes obstructed).

| Desired Outcomes | Nursing Actions and ***Selected Purposes/Rationales*** |
|---|---|
| 4.a. The client will remain free of wound infection (see Standardized Postoperative Care Plan, Nursing Diagnosis 16, outcome b [p. 129], for outcome criteria). | 4.a.1. Refer to Standardized Postoperative Care Plan, Nursing Diagnosis 16, action b (p. 129), for measures related to assessment, prevention, and treatment of wound infection.<br>2. If a perineal approach was used, implement additional measures *to prevent wound infection:*<br>a. instruct and assist client to perform good perineal care immediately after bowel movements<br>b. use a double-tailed T-binder, scrotal support, or jockey shorts to secure perineal dressings *(movement of loose dressings can cause skin irritation and subsequent breakdown)*<br>c. assist with sitz baths if ordered *to cleanse the wound and promote healing* (sitz baths are often ordered following removal of the perineal wound drains although some physicians wait until the catheter is also removed). |
| 4.b. The client will remain free of urinary tract infection as evidenced by:<br>1. clear urine<br>2. no unusual odor to urine<br>3. absence of chills and fever<br>4. absence of nitrites, bacteria, and WBCs in urine<br>5. negative urine culture. | 4.b.1. Assess for and report signs and symptoms of urinary tract infection (e.g. cloudy, foul-smelling urine; chills; elevated temperature).<br>2. Monitor urinalysis and report presence of nitrites, bacteria, and/or WBCs.<br>3. Obtain a urine specimen for culture and sensitivity if ordered. Report abnormal results.<br>4. Implement measures *to prevent urinary tract infection:*<br>a. perform actions to prevent urinary retention (see Postoperative Nursing Diagnosis 2, action b)<br>b. maintain a fluid intake of at least 2500 ml/day unless contraindicated<br>c. maintain sterile technique during bladder irrigations if performed<br>d. perform catheter care as often as needed *to prevent accumulation of mucus and blood around the meatus*<br>e. keep urine collection container below bladder level at all times *to prevent reflux or stasis of urine*<br>f. if frequent bladder irrigations are necessary, consult physician about initiation of continuous, closed system irrigation *(frequent intermittent irrigations increase the risk of introduction of pathogens)*<br>g. increase activity as allowed and tolerated *to decrease urinary stasis*<br>h. administer antimicrobials if ordered.<br>5. If signs and symptoms of urinary tract infection are present, continue with above actions. |

## 5. COLLABORATIVE DIAGNOSES:

**Potential complications:**

a. **hypovolemic shock** related to:
   1. fluid volume deficit associated with excessive fluid loss and inadequate fluid replacement
   2. hemorrhage associated with:
      a. high vascularity of prostate gland
      b. transection of the dorsal vein complex (occurs with a retropubic approach)

c. increased fibrinolytic activity (the prostate gland is a source of plasminogen which, when activated, increases lysis of blood clots; secretion and activation of plasminogen appear to also increase with cancer of the prostate);

b. **thromboembolism** related to:
1. trauma to large pelvic veins during surgery
2. venous stasis associated with:
   a. pressure on the pelvic and calf vessels during surgery if client was in lithotomy position (this position is used during a perineal approach)
   b. decreased activity
   c. fluid volume deficit
   d. abdominal distention (if the intestine is distended it can place pressure on the abdominal vessels)
3. hypercoagulability associated with increased release of tissue thromboplastin into the blood (occurs as a result of surgical trauma);

c. **continued extravasation of urine** related to loss of integrity of sutures at the site of anastomosis of the bladder and urethra.

| Desired Outcomes | Nursing Actions and ***Selected Purposes/Rationales*** |
|---|---|
| 5.a. The client will not develop hypovolemic shock (see Standardized Postoperative Care Plan, Collaborative Diagnosis 19, outcome a [pp. 131-132], for outcome criteria). | 5.a.1. Assess for and report the following:<br>a. excessive operative site bleeding:<br>1. excessive bloody drainage on dressings or from drains<br>2. increased swelling and/or blue-black discoloration in surgical area<br>3. persistent redness of or blood clots in urine<br>4. significant decline in RBC, Hct, and Hb levels<br>b. persistent vomiting<br>c. difficulty maintaining intravenous or oral fluid intake<br>d. signs and symptoms of hypovolemic shock (see Standardized Postoperative Care Plan, Collaborative Diagnosis 19, action a.3 [p. 132]).<br>2. Refer to Standardized Postoperative Care Plan, Collaborative Diagnosis 19, actions a.4 and 5 (p. 132), for measures to prevent and treat hypovolemic shock.<br>3. Implement measures *to minimize pressure on the operative area in order to prevent hemorrhage and subsequently reduce the risk of hypovolemic shock:*<br>a. perform actions to prevent urinary retention (see Postoperative Nursing Diagnosis 2, action b) *in order to avoid distention of the bladder which could create strain on the newly coagulated blood vessels and suture lines*<br>b. instruct client to avoid sitting for long periods<br>c. instruct client to avoid straining to have a bowel movement; consult physician regarding an order for a stool softener and laxative if indicated<br>d. instruct client to return to bed and limit activity for a few hours if urine becomes red when ambulating or sitting in chair. |
| 5.b. The client will not develop a deep vein thrombus or pulmonary embolism (see Standardized Postoperative Care Plan, Collaborative Diagnosis 19, outcomes c.1 and 2 [pp. 132-133], for outcome criteria). | 5.b. Refer to Standardized Postoperative Care Plan, Collaborative Diagnosis 19, actions c.1 and 2 (pp. 132-133), for measures related to assessment, prevention, and treatment of a deep vein thrombus and pulmonary embolism. Be aware that prophylactic anticoagulant and antiplatelet medications are usually contraindicated *because of the high risk of hemorrhage during and following surgery on the prostate gland.* |
| 5.c. The client will experience resolution | 5.c.1. Assess for and report signs and symptoms of continued extravasation of urine (e.g. presence of urine in drainage from wound drains or incision |

of urine extravasation as evidenced by:
1. absence of urine in drainage from wound drains and incision
2. no statements of new or increased pressure or fullness in rectal or perineal area.

beyond expected time, statements of new or increased pressure or fullness in the rectal or perineal area).
2. Implement measures *to promote healing of the site of anastomosis of the bladder and urethra in order to prevent continued extravasation of urine:*
   a. perform actions to prevent urinary retention (see Postoperative Nursing Diagnosis 2, action b) *in order to prevent bladder distention and subsequent stress on the suture lines*
   b. anchor urinary catheter securely to abdomen or thigh *in order to prevent excessive movement of the catheter and subsequent tissue trauma at the site of anastomosis.*
3. If signs and symptoms of extravasation of urine persist:
   a. continue with above actions
   b. assist with insertion of a suprapubic catheter and possible removal of urethral catheter if indicated
   c. prepare client for surgical revision of the site of anastomosis if planned
   d. provide emotional support to client and significant others.

## 6. NURSING DIAGNOSIS: Sexual dysfunction

related to:
a. decreased libido associated with fear of bowel incontinence, fear of urinary incontinence following catheter removal, surgical site discomfort, anxiety, and depression;
b. impotence associated with psychological factors and damage to the pudendal nerve and/or neurovascular supply to the corpora cavernosa during surgery if physician was unable to use a nerve-sparing technique (the possibility of impotence is higher with the perineal approach);
c. absence of ejaculation associated with removal of seminal vesicles and transection of the vas deferens.

**Desired Outcome**

6. The client will demonstrate beginning acceptance of changes in sexual functioning as evidenced by:
   a. verbalization of a perception of self as sexually acceptable and adequate
   b. statements reflecting beginning adjustment to effects of radical prostatectomy on sexual functioning
   c. maintenance of relationship with significant other.

**Nursing Actions and *Selected Purposes/Rationales***

6.a. Assess for signs and symptoms of sexual dysfunction (e.g. verbalization of sexual concerns, alteration in relationship with significant other, limitations imposed by effects of radical prostatectomy).
  b. Provide accurate information about the effects of the radical prostatectomy on sexual functioning. Encourage questions and clarify misconceptions.
  c. Implement measures *to promote optimal sexual functioning:*
    1. facilitate communication between client and his partner; focus on the feelings the couple share and assist them to identify changes which may affect their sexual relationship
    2. discuss ways to be creative in expressing sexuality (e.g. massage, fantasies, cuddling)
    3. arrange for uninterrupted privacy during hospital stay if desired by the couple
    4. perform actions to facilitate client's psychological adjustment to the diagnosis and effects of the surgery (see Postoperative Nursing Diagnoses 7, actions e-p, and 8 action b)
    5. if impotence is a problem:
       a. encourage client to discuss it and various treatment options (e.g. penile prosthesis) with physician
       b. suggest alternative methods of sexual gratification if appropriate
    6. if bowel incontinence is a problem and/or urinary incontinence is

| Desired Outcome | Nursing Actions and ***Selected Purposes/Rationales*** |
|---|---|
| | anticipated following catheter removal, encourage client to defecate and/or urinate just before intercourse and other sexual activity<br>7. if client is concerned that operative site discomfort will interfere with usual sexual activity:<br>a. assure him that the discomfort is temporary and will diminish as incision heals<br>b. encourage alternatives to intercourse and, when intercourse is allowed, use of positions that decrease pressure on the surgical site (e.g. side-lying).<br>d. Include partner in above discussions and encourage his/her continued support.<br>e. Consult physician if counseling appears indicated. |

## 7. NURSING DIAGNOSIS: Self-concept disturbance*

related to:

a. presence of urinary catheter (the catheter is usually not removed until 2-3 weeks after surgery);
b. bowel incontinence if present and possible urinary incontinence following removal of the catheter;
c. sterility associated with removal of the prostate gland, vas deferens, and seminal vesicles;
d. alteration in sexual functioning.

*This diagnostic label includes the nursing diagnoses of body image disturbance, self-esteem disturbance, and altered role performance.

| Desired Outcome | Nursing Actions and ***Selected Purposes/Rationales*** |
|---|---|
| 7. The client will demonstrate beginning adaptation to changes in body functioning as evidenced by:<br>a. verbalization of feelings of self-worth and sexual adequacy<br>b. maintenance of relationships with significant others<br>c. active participation in activities of daily living<br>d. active interest in personal appearance<br>e. willingness to pursue usual roles and participate in social activities. | 7.a. Assess for signs and symptoms of a self-concept disturbance (e.g. verbal or nonverbal cues denoting a negative response to changes in body functioning such as denial of or preoccupation with changes that have occurred, refusal to look at or touch genitals, or withdrawal from significant others).<br>b. Determine the meaning of changes in body functioning to the client by encouraging him to verbalize feelings and by noting nonverbal responses to the changes experienced.<br>c. Implement measures to promote optimal sexual functioning (see Postoperative Nursing Diagnosis 6, action c).<br>d. Implement measures to facilitate the grieving process (see Postoperative Nursing Diagnosis 8, action b).<br>e. Discuss with client improvements in bowel, bladder, and sexual function that can realistically be expected.<br>f. Implement measures *to assist client to increase self-esteem* (e.g. limit negative self-assessment, encourage positive comments about self, assist to identify strengths, give positive feedback about accomplishments and behaviors that are indicative of high self-esteem.<br>g. Assist client to identify and utilize coping techniques that have been helpful in the past.<br>h. Assist client with usual grooming if necessary.<br>i. Inform client that when he is discharged, he will be able to connect his urinary catheter to a leg bag and that this bag will not be visible to others when he is dressed. |

j. If client is incontinent of stool and/or if incontinence of urine is an anticipated problem following catheter removal:
   1. reinforce the importance of doing perineal exercises when allowed *in order to improve bowel and bladder control*
   2. assist him to establish a routine bowel care program *to reduce the risk of bowel incontinence*
   3. instruct in ways to minimize incontinence *so that social interaction is possible* (e.g. placing disposable liners in underwear, wearing absorbent undergarments such as Attends).

k. Because sterility is expected and impotence may occur, discuss alternative methods of becoming a parent (e.g. adoption) if of concern to client.

l. Assess for and support behaviors suggesting positive adaptation to changes that have occurred (e.g. verbalization of feelings of self-worth, compliance with treatment plan, maintenance of relationships with significant others).

m. Assist client's and significant others' adjustment by listening, facilitating communication, and providing information.

n. Encourage visits and support from significant others.

o. Encourage client to pursue usual roles and interests and to continue involvement in social activities.

p. Provide information about and encourage utilization of community agencies and support groups (e.g. sexual, family, or individual counseling; Help for Incontinent People [HIP]; Impotence Anonymous).

q. Consult physician about psychological counseling if client desires or if he seems unwilling or unable to adapt to changes resulting from the radical prostatectomy.

## 8. NURSING DIAGNOSIS: Grieving*

related to impotence and loss of bowel control (if they occur), possible loss of bladder control following removal of the urinary catheter, diagnosis of cancer, and possibility of premature death.

*This diagnostic label includes anticipatory grieving and grieving following the actual losses.

| Desired Outcome | Nursing Actions and ***Selected Purposes/Rationales*** |
|---|---|
| 8. The client will demonstrate beginning progression through the grieving process as evidenced by:<br>a. verbalization of feelings about changes in body functioning and diagnosis of cancer<br>b. expression of grief<br>c. participation in treatment plan and self-care activities<br>d. utilization of available support systems. | 8.a. Assess for signs and symptoms of grieving (e.g. change in eating habits, inability to concentrate, insomnia, anger, noncompliance, withdrawal from significant others, denial of losses). Be aware that client's response to a loss will be affected by factors such as previous experience with loss, age, developmental stage, available support systems, spiritual and cultural background, current health status, and significance of the loss.<br>b. Implement measures *to facilitate the grieving process:*<br>1. assist client to acknowledge the losses experienced *so grief work can begin;* assess for factors that may hinder and facilitate acknowledgment<br>2. discuss the grieving process and assist client to accept the phases of grieving as an expected response to actual and/or anticipated losses<br>3. allow time for client to progress through the phases of grieving (phases vary among theorists but progress from shock and alarm to acceptance); be aware that not every phase is expressed by all individuals, that recurrence of phases is common, and that the grieving process may take months to years<br>4. provide an atmosphere of care and concern (e.g. provide privacy, be |

| Desired Outcome | Nursing Actions and ***Selected Purposes/Rationales*** |
|---|---|
| | available and nonjudgmental, display empathy and respect) *so client will feel free to verbalize feelings*<br>5. perform actions *to promote trust* (e.g. answer questions honestly, provide requested information)<br>6. encourage the verbal expression of anger and sadness about the losses experienced; recognize displacement of anger and assist client to see the actual cause of angry feelings and resentment<br>7. encourage client to express his feelings in whatever ways are comfortable (e.g. writing, drawing, conversation)<br>8. assist client to identify personal strengths that have helped him to cope in previous situations of loss<br>9. if appropriate, support realistic hope that bowel and/or bladder control will improve if he continues to do perineal exercises<br>10. support behaviors suggesting successful grief work (e.g. verbalizing feelings about losses, focusing on ways to adapt to losses, learning needed skills, developing or renewing relationships)<br>11. explain the phases of the grieving process to significant others; encourage their support and understanding<br>12. facilitate communication between the client and significant others; be aware that they may be in different phases of the grieving process<br>13. provide information about counseling services and support groups that might assist client in working through grief<br>14. arrange for visit from clergy if desired by client.<br>c. Consult physician regarding referral for counseling if signs of dysfunctional grieving (e.g. persistent denial of losses, excessive anger or sadness, hysteria, suicidal behaviors) occur. |

## 9. NURSING DIAGNOSIS: Knowledge deficit

regarding follow-up care.

| Desired Outcomes | Nursing Actions and ***Selected Purposes/Rationales*** |
|---|---|
| 9.a. The client will demonstrate the ability to perform care related to the urinary catheter and drainage system. | 9.a.1. Instruct client in care related to the urinary catheter and drainage system including:<br>a. cleansing the urinary meatus with soap and water at least twice a day<br>b. anchoring the catheter tubing securely to abdomen or thigh<br>c. keeping catheter and urine collection bag tubing free of kinks<br>d. keeping urine collection bag below the level of the bladder<br>e. changing from the leg bag to bedside collection bag when lying down for more than a few hours<br>f. emptying the leg bag and the bedside collection bag<br>g. measuring and recording the amount of urine output if necessary.<br>2. Allow time for questions, clarification, practice, and return demonstration. |
| 9.b. The client will identify ways to manage urinary incontinence if it occurs following catheter removal. | 9.b.1. Provide information about ways to reduce the risk of urinary incontinence following removal of the urinary catheter (incontinence can occur as a result of trauma to urinary sphincters during surgery and/or irritation from the urinary catheter, damage to pelvic nerves during surgery, and/or a temporary decrease in bladder capacity because of the continued decompression of the bladder while the catheter was in place): |

a. try to urinate every 2-3 hours and when the urge is felt
b. urinate in a standing or sitting position to facilitate complete bladder emptying
c. avoid drinking large quantities of liquid (especially alcohol) over a short period
d. avoid drinking caffeine-containing beverages (e.g. coffee, tea, colas)
e. stop drinking liquids a few hours before bedtime (reduces risk of nighttime incontinence)
f. avoid activities that make it difficult to empty bladder as soon as the urge is felt (e.g. long car rides, lengthy meetings).

2. Reinforce the importance of performing perineal exercises (e.g. stopping and starting stream during voiding; squeezing buttocks together, then relaxing the muscles) when allowed in order to improve urinary control if possible. Assist client to set up a schedule that will remind him to do the exercises (e.g. before and after each meal, during television commercials, when talking on telephone).
3. Inform client that if urinary incontinence occurs following catheter removal, he should:
   a. wash and dry perineal area after each episode of incontinence
   b. wear disposable underwear liners or absorbent undergarments such as Attends if needed
   c. consult physician about use of devices such as an external catheter if indicated.

9.c. The client will identify ways to manage bowel incontinence if present.

9.c. If client is experiencing bowel incontinence, instruct him to:
1. adhere to a routine bowel care program
2. perform perineal exercises (e.g. stopping and starting stream during voiding; squeezing buttocks together, then relaxing the muscles) when allowed in order to improve bowel control if possible
3. wash and dry perineal area after each episode of incontinence
4. wear disposable underwear liners or absorbent undergarments such as Attends if needed.

9.d. The client will state signs and symptoms to report to the health care provider.

9.d.1. Refer to Standardized Postoperative Care Plan, Nursing Diagnosis 21, action c (p. 135), for signs and symptoms to report to the health care provider.
2. Instruct client to also report if he experiences unexpected loss of bladder or bowel control or impotence.

9.e. The client will verbalize an understanding of and a plan for adhering to recommended follow-up care including future appointments with health care provider, medications prescribed, activity level, wound care, and plans for subsequent treatment.

9.e.1. Refer to Standardized Postoperative Care Plan, Nursing Diagnosis 21 (pp. 135-136), for routine postoperative instructions and measures to improve client compliance.
2. Reinforce physician's explanations and instructions regarding adjuvant therapy (e.g. radiation therapy) if planned.

# Transurethral Resection of the Prostate (TURP)

Transurethral resection of the prostate (TURP) is the surgical removal of a prostatic adenoma through the urethra, while leaving the true prostate and its fibrous capsule intact. It may be performed to remove a small cancerous prostatic tumor but most frequently is done to remove a benign prostatic neoplasm that has enlarged enough to block the bladder outlet or urethra. The most common cause of a benign neoplasm is benign prostatic hyperplasia (BPH).

BPH is common in men over 50 years of age and results from age-associated changes in levels of testosterone and estrogen. Hyperplasia usually occurs gradually and involves the medial portion of the prostate gland which surrounds the urethra. Treatment is indicated when signs and symptoms of prostatism (e.g. urgency, frequency, hesitancy, decreased force of urinary stream, nocturia, incontinence) become problematic or when complications such as recurrent urinary tract infection, urinary retention, hematuria, renal calculi, or hydronephrosis occur. TURP is the most common method of treatment of BPH. If the prostate gland is quite large, an open prostatectomy using a suprapubic, retropubic, or perineal approach may be necessary. Measures other than prostatectomy that may be used to relieve the urinary obstruction caused by BPH include pharmacological therapy (e.g. antiandrogens, sympathetic alpha-adrenergic inhibitors), prostatic massage, sitz baths, prostatic balloon dilatation (transcystoscopic urethroplasty), and/or transurethral incision of the bladder neck.

**This care plan focuses on the adult male client with BPH who is hospitalized for a transurethral resection of the prostate.** Preoperative goals of care are to reduce fear and anxiety, promote adequate urinary elimination, and educate the client regarding postoperative management. Postoperatively, goals of care are to maintain comfort, prevent complications, and educate the client regarding follow-up care.

## DIAGNOSTIC TESTS

Catheterization for residual urine
Urodynamic studies (e.g. cystometrogram)
Cystourethroscopy
Transrectal and suprapubic ultrasonography

## DISCHARGE CRITERIA

Prior to discharge, the client will:

- void 100-200 ml with minimal discomfort every 2-4 hours
- have no signs and symptoms of complications
- identify ways to prevent bleeding in the surgical area
- identify ways to regain or maintain control of bladder emptying
- state signs and symptoms to report to the health care provider
- verbalize an understanding of and a plan for adhering to recommended follow-up care including future appointments with health care provider, medications prescribed, and activity level.

## NURSING/ COLLABORATIVE DIAGNOSES

**Preoperative**

1. Urinary retention△ *857*
2. Knowledge deficit△ *857*

**Postoperative**

1. Altered fluid balance: fluid volume excess or water intoxication ("TUR syndrome")△ *859*
2. Altered comfort: bladder spasms△ *859*
3. Altered urinary elimination:
   a. retention
   b. incontinence following catheter removal△ *860*
4. High risk for infection: urinary tract△ *862*

**5.** Potential complications:
  **a.** hypovolemic shock
  **b.** thromboembolism△ *862*
**6.** Knowledge deficit△ *863*

**See Standardized Preoperative and Postoperative Care Plans for additional diagnoses.**

## PREOPERATIVE

**Use in conjunction with the Standardized Preoperative Care Plan.**

### 1. NURSING DIAGNOSIS: Urinary retention

related to:
a. obstruction of the urethra and/or bladder neck by the enlarged prostate;
b. loss of bladder muscle tone associated with hypertrophy of the bladder wall (as BPH develops, the detrusor muscle hypertrophies in an attempt to increase its ability to push urine past the bladder neck or urethral obstruction; this hypertrophied muscle has poor contractility).

| Desired Outcome | Nursing Actions and ***Selected Purposes/Rationales*** |
|---|---|
| 1. The client will experience resolution of urinary retention if it occurs as evidenced by:<br>a. no complaints of bladder fullness and suprapubic discomfort<br>b. absence of bladder distention and dribbling of urine<br>c. balanced intake and output. | 1.a. Determine client's usual urinary elimination pattern.<br>b. Assess for signs and symptoms of urinary retention:<br>1. frequent voiding of small amounts (25-60 ml) of urine<br>2. complaints of bladder fullness or suprapubic discomfort<br>3. bladder distention<br>4. dribbling of urine<br>5. output less than intake.<br>c. Implement measures *to treat urinary retention if present:*<br>1. insert or assist with insertion of a urethral catheter as ordered (if insertion is difficult because of obstruction of the prostatic urethra or bladder neck, it may be necessary to use a stylet or a firm, specially angled catheter)<br>2. assist with insertion of a suprapubic catheter if unable to insert a urethral catheter because of obstruction.<br>d. If a urinary catheter is present, implement measures *to maintain patency of the catheter in order to prevent urinary retention:*<br>1. keep drainage tubing free of kinks<br>2. keep collection container below level of bladder<br>3. tape catheter securely to abdomen or thigh *in order to prevent inadvertent removal.*<br>e. Consult physician if signs and symptoms of urinary retention persist despite implementation of above actions. |

### 2. NURSING DIAGNOSIS: Knowledge deficit

regarding hospital routines associated with surgery, physical preparation for the TURP, sensations that normally occur following surgery and anesthesia, and post-operative care.

| Desired Outcomes | Nursing Actions and ***Selected Purposes/Rationales*** |
|---|---|
| 2.a. The client will verbalize an understanding of usual preoperative care and postoperative sensations and care. | 2.a. 1. Refer to Standardized Preoperative Care Plan, Nursing Diagnosis 4, actions a.1-4 (pp. 111-112), for information to include in preoperative teaching.<br>2. Provide additional information regarding care following a TURP:<br>a. explain that bed rest is usually ordered for 6-18 hours after surgery; activity is then increased gradually (the level of activity allowed depends on physician preference, extensiveness of the resection, and the amount of postoperative bleeding client experiences)<br>b. explain that a urinary catheter will be in place for 24-72 hours after surgery (a urethral catheter with 3 lumens [e.g. 3-way Foley catheter] is usually inserted to allow drainage of bladder and simultaneous infusion of irrigation solution if needed)<br>c. describe the procedure and rationale for intermittent and continuous bladder irrigations<br>d. explain that traction may be applied to the catheter for 4-6 hours postoperatively and again as needed to put pressure on the surgical site in order to control bleeding (traction is accomplished by pulling down on the urethral catheter and anchoring it securely to the client's leg so that tension is maintained)<br>e. explain that the following can be expected:<br>1. red urine that gradually lightens in color (urine color usually goes from bright red to pink within 24-36 hours and to light pink or dark amber within 72 hours) but often temporarily becomes more red when activity increases<br>2. some blood clots in urine<br>3. some bloody drainage from urethra<br>f. describe signs and symptoms that can be indicative of bladder spasms (e.g. leakage of urine around catheter, feeling of an urgent need to urinate or defecate, pressure in bladder); stress that these signs and symptoms should be reported to the nurse so that catheter patency can be checked and medication can be given as needed to reduce discomfort<br>g. explain that after the catheter is removed:<br>1. a mild to moderate burning sensation may be experienced when urinating and that this is expected to decrease with each voiding and resolve within 1-2 days<br>2. urinary symptoms experienced preoperatively (e.g. urgency, frequency, hesitancy, dribbling) may still be present or may even increase temporarily postoperatively due to poor bladder muscle tone and/or tissue trauma from the surgery and catheter.<br>3. Reinforce physician's explanation regarding effects of TURP on sexual functioning (after surgery, the client usually experiences retrograde ejaculation as a result of direct trauma to the internal urinary sphincter and/or widening of the bladder neck; normal ejaculatory function usually returns within weeks or months).<br>4. Allow time for questions and clarification of information provided. |
| 2.b. The client will demonstrate the ability to perform activities designed to prevent postoperative complications. | 2.b. 1. Refer to Standardized Preoperative Care Plan, Nursing Diagnosis 4, action b.1 (p. 112), for instructions on ways to prevent postoperative complications.<br>2. Provide additional instructions about ways to prevent complications following TURP:<br>a. when oral fluid intake is allowed after surgery, drink one glass of fluid each hour while awake to keep urine dilute (helps keep catheter patent and reduces the risk for urinary tract infection)<br>b. avoid activities that will put excessive pressure on the surgical area (e.g. straining to have a bowel movement, attempting to urinate around catheter, excessive coughing, pulling on catheter, walking or sitting for too long).<br>3. Allow time for questions, clarification, and return demonstration. |

## POSTOPERATIVE

**Use in conjunction with the Standardized Postoperative Care Plan.**

### 1. NURSING DIAGNOSIS: Altered fluid balance: fluid volume excess or water intoxication ("TUR syndrome")

related to:
a. vigorous fluid therapy during and immediately after surgery;
b. increased secretion of antidiuretic hormone (output of ADH is stimulated by trauma, pain, anesthetic agents, and narcotic analgesics);
c. excessive absorption of irrigation solution via the prostatic veins during and following surgery.

| Desired Outcome | Nursing Actions and ***Selected Purposes/Rationales*** |
|---|---|
| 1. The client will not experience fluid volume excess or water intoxication (see Standardized Postoperative Care Plan, Nursing Diagnosis 4, outcome b [p. 117], for outcome criteria). | 1.a. Refer to Standardized Postoperative Care Plan, Nursing Diagnosis 4, action b (p. 117), for measures related to assessment, prevention, and treatment of fluid volume excess and water intoxication.<br>b. Implement measures *to reduce absorption of fluid via the prostatic veins in order to further reduce the risk for fluid volume excess and/or water intoxication:*<br>1. use normal saline rather than hypotonic solutions for bladder irrigations<br>2. do not increase frequency of bladder irrigations or speed up continuous irrigation unless indicated. |

### 2. NURSING DIAGNOSIS: Altered comfort: bladder spasms

related to:
a. irritation of the bladder wall associated with tissue trauma during surgery, presence of urinary catheter, rapid infusion of irrigation solution, and distention of the bladder (can occur if urine flow becomes obstructed);
b. increased pressure on the bladder neck and prostatic fossa if traction is applied to the urethral catheter (traction may be applied to pull the catheter balloon into the prostatic fossa in order to put pressure on bleeding vessels).

| Desired Outcome | Nursing Actions and ***Selected Purposes/Rationales*** |
|---|---|
| 2. The client will experience relief of bladder spasms as evidenced by:<br>a. verbalization of relief of suprapubic discomfort<br>b. no complaints of an urgent need to urinate or defecate<br>c. no leakage of urine around the urinary catheter. | 2.a. Assess for signs and symptoms of bladder spasms:<br>1. complaints of suprapubic discomfort<br>2. statements of an urgent need to urinate or defecate<br>3. leakage of urine around the urinary catheter.<br>b. Implement measures *to decrease the risk of bladder spasms:*<br>1. maintain patency of catheter (e.g. irrigate as needed, keep tubing free of kinks) *to prevent distention of bladder*<br>2. perform actions *to keep urinary catheter from irritating the bladder mucosa:*<br>a. tape catheter securely to client's abdomen or thigh<br>b. instruct client to avoid pulling on and twisting the catheter<br>3. release traction on the catheter as soon as ordered *to reduce pressure on the bladder neck and prostatic fossa*<br>4. do not increase frequency of bladder irrigations or speed up continuous irrigation unless bleeding or blood clots are present *because irrigation solution can irritate the bladder mucosa*<br>5. instruct client to avoid attempting to urinate around the catheter and |

| Desired Outcome | Nursing Actions and ***Selected Purposes/Rationales*** |
|---|---|
| | straining to urinate after catheter is removed *(attempts to forcefully contract bladder can stimulate bladder spasms)*<br>6. perform actions to prevent urinary retention following removal of catheter (see Postoperative Nursing Diagnosis 3, action a.3) *in order to prevent distention of the bladder.*<br>c. If bladder spasms occur:<br>1. encourage client to take short, frequent walks unless contraindicated *(walking seems to reduce spasms)*<br>2. decrease the rate of continuous bladder irrigation if urine is not red and blood clots are not present<br>3. administer the following medications if ordered:<br>a. belladonna and opium (B&O) rectal suppositories (this combination of an antimuscarinic and narcotic analgesic *reduces spasm of the bladder muscle and the client's perception of discomfort;* it is usually only prescribed when the urinary catheter is present *because it can cause urinary retention)*<br>b. other genitourinary smooth muscle relaxants (e.g. oxybutynin, flavoxate).<br>d. Consult physician if above measures fail to control bladder spasms. |

## 3. NURSING DIAGNOSIS: Altered urinary elimination:

a. **retention** related to:
   1. obstruction of the urinary catheter
   2. difficulty urinating following removal of the catheter associated with:
      a. loss of bladder muscle tone resulting from hypertrophy of the detrusor muscle as BPH developed and overdistention of the bladder preoperatively
      b. sympathetic nervous system stimulation of the bladder and urinary sphincters resulting from surgical site discomfort, fear, and anxiety
      c. obstruction of the urethra and bladder neck by blood clots and/or edema resulting from surgical trauma and irritation of the tissues by the urinary catheter, particularly if traction had been applied to the catheter to control bleeding;

b. **incontinence following catheter removal** related to:
   1. trauma to the urinary sphincter(s) associated with surgical instrumentation and presence of urethral catheter
   2. decreased bladder capacity associated with continued decompression of the bladder while the catheter was in place.

| Desired Outcomes | Nursing Actions and ***Selected Purposes/Rationales*** |
|---|---|
| 3.a. The client will not experience urinary retention as evidenced by:<br>1. no complaints of bladder fullness and suprapubic | 3.a.1. Assess for and report signs and symptoms of the following:<br>a. urinary retention when catheter is present (e.g. complaints of bladder fullness or suprapubic discomfort, bladder distention, absence of fluid in urinary drainage tubing, output that continues to be less than intake 48 hours after surgery)<br>b. progressive narrowing of the urethra or bladder neck after catheter removal (e.g. complaints of decreasing size of urinary stream, |

discomfort
2. absence of bladder distention
3. balanced intake and output within 48 hours after surgery
4. voiding adequate amounts at expected intervals after removal of catheter.

increasing need to strain to empty bladder, and increasing urgency)
c. urinary retention following removal of catheter (e.g. complaints of bladder fullness or suprapubic discomfort, frequent voiding of small amounts [25-60 ml] of urine, bladder distention, output that continues to be less than intake 48 hours after surgery).

2. Implement measures *to maintain patency of the urinary catheter in order to prevent urinary retention:*
   a. keep drainage tubing free of kinks
   b. keep collection container below level of bladder
   c. tape catheter securely to abdomen or thigh *in order to prevent inadvertent removal.*
3. Following removal of the catheter, implement the following measures *to prevent urinary retention:*
   a. offer urinal or assist client to bathroom every 2-3 hours if indicated
   b. instruct client to urinate when the urge is first felt *(bladder is still hypotonic and can easily become distended)*
   c. perform actions *to promote relaxation during voiding attempts* (e.g. provide privacy, play soft music, encourage client to read)
   d. perform actions to relieve discomfort (see Postoperative Nursing Diagnosis 2, actions b and c)
   e. perform actions *to provide sensory stimulation that may help trigger the micturition reflex and promote voluntary relaxation of the perineal muscles and external urinary sphincter* (e.g. run water, place client's hands in warm water, encourage client to urinate when in shower)
   f. allow client to assume a normal position for voiding unless contraindicated.
4. If signs and symptoms of urinary retention occur after removal of the catheter, consult physician about intermittent catheterization or reinsertion of an indwelling catheter.

3.b. The client will experience urinary continence.

3.b.1. Assess for urinary incontinence after removal of the urinary catheter (catheter is usually removed 1-3 days after surgery).

2. Implement measures *to maintain urinary continence:*
   a. perform actions *to prevent trauma to the urinary sphincter(s) while the catheter is in place in order to reduce the risk of urinary incontinence following removal of the catheter:*
      1. if urethral catheter traction is ordered to control bleeding, release it as soon as allowed (traction should not be maintained for longer than 4-6 hours without being released) *in order to reduce pressure on and possible damage to the internal urinary sphincter*
      2. tape catheter securely to client's abdomen or thigh *in order to prevent excessive movement of the catheter*
   b. following removal of the catheter:
      1. keep urinal within client's reach and provide easy access to bathroom *in order to reduce delays in toileting*
      2. allow client to assume a normal position for voiding unless contraindicated *in order to promote complete bladder emptying*
      3. instruct client to perform perineal exercises (e.g. stopping and starting stream during voiding; squeezing buttocks together, then relaxing the muscles) *in order to strengthen pelvic floor muscles*
      4. limit oral fluid intake in the evening *to decrease the possibility of nighttime incontinence*
      5. instruct client to avoid drinking beverages containing caffeine *(caffeine is a mild diuretic and may make urinary control more difficult)*
      6. instruct client to space fluids evenly throughout the day rather than drinking a large quantity at one time *(rapid filling of bladder can result in incontinence if client has decreased urinary sphincter tone).*
3. If urinary incontinence persists, consult physician regarding intermittent catheterization, reinsertion of an indwelling catheter, or use of external catheter.

## 4. NURSING DIAGNOSIS: High risk for infection: urinary tract

related to:

a. introduction of pathogens associated with instrumentation of urinary tract during surgery, presence of indwelling catheter, and frequent bladder irrigations;

b. increased bacterial growth associated with urinary stasis resulting from decreased activity and urinary retention if it occurs.

| Desired Outcome | Nursing Actions and ***Selected Purposes/Rationales*** |
|---|---|
| 4. The client will remain free of urinary tract infection (see Standardized Postoperative Care Plan, Nursing Diagnosis 16, outcome c [p. 129], for outcome criteria). | 4.a. Refer to Standardized Postoperative Care Plan, Nursing Diagnosis 16, action c (p. 129), for measures related to assessment, prevention, and treatment of urinary tract infection.<br>b. Implement additional measures *to prevent urinary tract infection:*<br>1. perform actions to prevent urinary retention (see Postoperative Nursing Diagnosis 3, actions a.2 and 3)<br>2. consult physician about removal of the catheter as soon as the urine is clear and free of blood clots *(risk of urinary tract infection increases the longer the catheter is in place).* |

## 5. COLLABORATIVE DIAGNOSES: Potential complications:

a. **hypovolemic shock** related to hemorrhage (the prostate gland is very vascular) and inadequate fluid replacement;

b. **thromboembolism** related to venous stasis associated with:
   1. pressure on the pelvic and calf vessels during surgery (the client is usually in lithotomy position)
   2. decreased activity.

| Desired Outcomes | Nursing Actions and ***Selected Purposes/Rationales*** |
|---|---|
| 5.a. The client will not develop hypovolemic shock (see Standardized Postoperative Care Plan, Collaborative Diagnosis 19, outcome a [pp. 131-132], for outcome criteria). | 5.a.1. Assess for and report the following:<br>a. excessive operative site bleeding:<br>1. bright red, viscous drainage (could indicate arterial bleeding) or persistent darker drainage (venous bleeding) in urinary catheter<br>2. persistent redness of and blood clots in serial urines after removal of the catheter<br>3. significant decline in RBC, Hct, and Hb levels<br>b. signs and symptoms of hypovolemic shock (see Standardized Postoperative Care Plan, Collaborative Diagnosis 19, action a.3 [p. 132]).<br>2. Refer to Standardized Postoperative Care Plan, Collaborative Diagnosis 19, actions a.4 and 5 (p. 132), for measures to prevent and treat hypovolemic shock.<br>3. Implement additional measures *to prevent or control hemorrhage in order to prevent hypovolemic shock:*<br>a. maintain traction on the urethral catheter as ordered<br>b. perform actions *to prevent trauma to and/or unnecessary pressure on the prostatic area:*<br>1. tape catheter tubing securely to client's abdomen or thigh *in order to minimize movement of catheter* |

2. caution client to avoid pulling on the catheter
3. instruct client to take short rather than long walks and to avoid sitting for long periods
4. instruct client to avoid excessive coughing, sneezing, and straining to have a bowel movement; consult physician regarding an order for an antitussive, decongestant, stool softener, and/or laxative if indicated
5. implement measures to prevent urinary retention (see Postoperative Nursing Diagnosis 3, actions a.2 and 3) *in order to prevent distention of the bladder and subsequent stretching of the newly coagulated blood vessels in the operative area*

c. instruct client to return to bed and limit activity for a few hours if urine becomes more red when ambulating or sitting in chair.

| | |
|---|---|
| 5.b. The client will not develop a deep vein thrombus or pulmonary embolism (see Standardized Postoperative Care Plan, Collaborative Diagnosis 19, outcomes c.1 and 2 [pp. 132-133], for outcome criteria). | 5.b. Refer to Standardized Postoperative Care Plan, Collaborative Diagnosis 19, actions c.1 and 2 (pp. 132-133), for measures related to assessment, prevention, and treatment of a deep vein thrombus and pulmonary embolism. Be aware that prophylactic anticoagulant and antiplatelet medications are usually contraindicated *because of the risk of hemorrhage during and following surgery on the highly vascular prostate gland.* |

## 6. NURSING DIAGNOSIS: Knowledge deficit

regarding follow-up care.

| Desired Outcomes | Nursing Actions and ***Selected Purposes/Rationales*** |
|---|---|
| 6.a. The client will identify ways to prevent bleeding in the surgical area. | 6.a. Instruct client in ways to prevent pressure on the surgical area in order to prevent bleeding:<br>1. avoid straining during bowel movements (provide instructions about increasing fluid intake and intake of foods high in fiber if client tends to be constipated)<br>2. avoid long walks, prolonged sitting, long car rides, running, climbing stairs quickly, strenuous exercise, sexual intercourse, and lifting objects over 5-10 pounds for as long as recommended by physician (usually for 3-6 weeks after discharge). |
| 6.b. The client will identify ways to regain or maintain control of bladder emptying. | 6.b.1. Instruct client in ways to regain or maintain control of bladder emptying:<br>a. try to urinate every 2-3 hours and whenever the urge is felt<br>b. urinate in a standing or sitting position to facilitate bladder emptying<br>c. avoid drinking large quantities of liquids (especially alcohol) over a short period<br>d. avoid drinking caffeine-containing beverages (e.g. coffee, tea, colas)<br>e. stop drinking liquids a few hours before bedtime (reduces risk of urine retention and nighttime incontinence)<br>f. avoid activities that make it difficult to empty bladder as soon as the urge is felt (e.g. long car rides, lengthy meetings) in order to prevent retention and the subsequent risk for incontinence<br>g. perform perineal exercises (e.g. stopping and starting stream during voiding; squeezing buttocks together, then relaxing the muscles) 10- |

| Desired Outcomes | Nursing Actions and ***Selected Purposes/Rationales*** |
|---|---|
| | 20 times/hour while awake until urinary control is regained; assist client to set up a schedule that will remind him to do the exercises (e.g. before and after each meal, during television commercials, when talking on telephone).<br>2. If client is experiencing urinary incontinence, instruct him to:<br>a. wear disposable underwear liners or absorbent undergarments such as Attends if necessary<br>b. consult physician if urinary incontinence persists, worsens, or interferes with daily life so that various options (e.g. external urinary catheter, insertion of artificial urinary sphincter) can be discussed. |
| 6.c. The client will state signs and symptoms to report to the health care provider. | 6.c. 1. Refer to Standardized Postoperative Care Plan, Nursing Diagnosis 21, action c (p. 135), for signs and symptoms to report to the health care provider.<br>2. Instruct client to report these additional signs and symptoms:<br>a. persistent bright red urine (inform client that some blood is expected intermittently for 2-3 weeks after surgery but that urine should become pink to amber after he rests and increases fluid intake for a couple of hours)<br>b. presence of large blood clots or continued passage of smaller clots<br>c. increase in frequency, burning, or pain when urinating<br>d. decrease in urine output or force and caliber of urinary stream<br>e. bladder distention<br>f. unexpected loss of bladder control<br>g. persistent or increased bladder spasms. |
| 6.d. The client will verbalize an understanding of and a plan for adhering to recommended follow-up care including future appointments with health care provider, medications prescribed, and activity level. | 6.d.1. Refer to Standardized Postoperative Care Plan, Nursing Diagnosis 21 (pp. 135-136), for routine postoperative instructions and measures to improve client compliance.<br>2. Reinforce the physician's instructions regarding the importance of lying down and increasing fluid intake for a few hours if amount of blood or number of blood clots in the urine increases.<br>3. Explain the importance of having a digital rectal examination and a blood test for prostatic-specific antigen (PSA) done each year (cancer of the prostate and recurrent BPH can develop since the entire prostate gland is not removed during a TURP). |

UNIT

# XIX

# *Nursing Care of the Client with Disturbances of the Head and Neck*

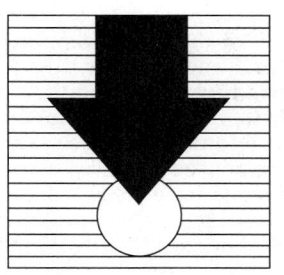

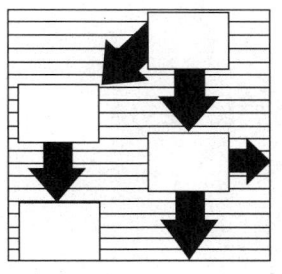

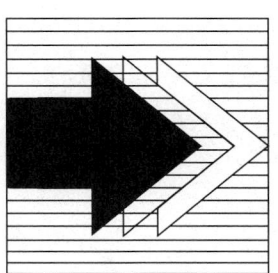

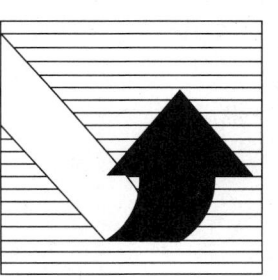

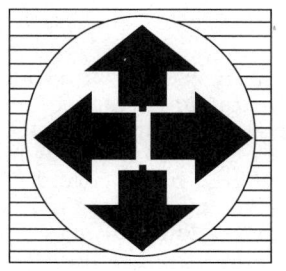

# Total Laryngectomy with Radical Neck Dissection

A total laryngectomy with radical neck dissection is the usual treatment for cancer of the larynx with metastasis to regional lymph nodes and/or adjacent neck structures. A total laryngectomy includes removal of the larynx, the hyoid bone, cricoid cartilage, pre-epiglottic space, and 2-3 tracheal rings. The extent of metastasis dictates which additional neck structures are removed during the concurrent radical neck dissection. A comprehensive radical neck dissection includes the removal of all lymph node regions of one side of the neck from the inferior border of the mandible to the clavicle and from the lateral border of the strap muscles to the anterior border of the trapezius muscle. The current trend is to perform a modified or functional neck dissection if possible to reduce the morbidity associated with the surgery. With this procedure, the spinal accessory nerve, the sternocleidomastoid muscle, and/or the internal jugular vein are spared. Myocutaneous flaps using the pectoralis major, latissimus dorsi, or the lateral trapezius muscle or free flaps are commonly used in reconstruction of the neck and oral cavity if remaining tissue is not sufficient.

A tracheoesophageal puncture (TEP) may also be performed at the time of the surgery to create a fistula for the insertion of a voice prosthesis (e.g. Blom-Singer) early in the postoperative period. The prosthesis allows for diversion of exhaled air into the pharynx by occlusion of the stoma. Sound is produced by the vibration of the mucosa above the expired air stream and is converted to speech by the client's intact articulatory structures—the tongue, lips, teeth, and palate.

**This care plan focuses on the adult client with cancer of the larynx hospitalized for a laryngectomy with radical neck dissection.** Preoperatively, the goals of care are to reduce fear and anxiety and prepare the client for the postoperative period. The goals of postoperative care are to prevent complications, assist the client to cope with the change in body image and functioning, facilitate rehabilitative efforts, and educate the client regarding follow-up care. The care plan will need to be individualized according to the extensiveness of the dissection, the amount and type of grafting necessary, and the physiological and psychological status of the client. If the client has received a preoperative course of radiation therapy, refer to the Care Plan on External Radiation Therapy for specific nursing care measures related to side effects the client may still be experiencing.

## DIAGNOSTIC TESTS

Endoscopy of larynx, lungs, and/or esophagus
Biopsy of larynx
X-rays of the chest and larynx
Laryngography
Computed tomography (CT) of neck
Magnetic resonance imaging (MRI) of larynx and neck structures
Barium swallow

## DISCHARGE CRITERIA

Prior to discharge, the client will:

- have an adequate respiratory status
- be able to communicate effectively
- have an adequate nutritional status
- have no signs and symptoms of complications
- demonstrate appropriate stomal care, suctioning, tracheostomy tube care, oral hygiene, and tube feeding techniques
- demonstrate the ability to effectively use and care for an artificial larynx
- demonstrate the ability to care for the tracheoesophageal puncture (TEP) and voice prosthesis if in place
- identify appropriate safety precautions related to the presence of a tracheostomy and nerve damage resulting from surgery
- identify signs and symptoms to report to the health care provider
- share feelings and thoughts about the effects of radical neck surgery on body image and usual life style and roles

- identify community resources that can assist with home management and adjustment to the effects of surgery
- communicate an understanding of and a plan for adhering to recommended follow-up care including future appointments with health care provider and speech pathologist, medications prescribed, exercises, pain control measures, activity level, and wound care.

**NURSING/ COLLABORATIVE DIAGNOSES**



**See Standardized Preoperative and Postoperative Care Plans for additional diagnoses.**

## PREOPERATIVE

**Use in conjunction with the Standardized Preoperative Care Plan.**

### 1. NURSING DIAGNOSIS: Anxiety

related to:

a. impending disfiguring surgery that will result in loss of normal speech and a marked change in physical appearance and functioning;
b. lack of understanding of diagnostic tests, surgical procedure, and care required for the airway diversion and speech prosthesis (if planned);
c. anticipated loss of control, effects of anesthesia, and postoperative discomfort;
d. economic factors associated with hospitalization;
e. unfamiliar environment and separation from significant others;
f. possible rejection by significant others;
g. ability to independently care for self following discharge and anticipated changes in usual life style and roles;
h. diagnosis of cancer with uncertain prognosis.

| Desired Outcome | Nursing Actions and ***Selected Purposes/Rationales*** |
|---|---|
| 1. The client will experience a reduction in anxiety (see Standardized Preoperative Care Plan, Nursing Diagnosis 1 [pp. 108-109], for outcome criteria). | 1.a. Refer to Standardized Preoperative Care Plan, Nursing Diagnosis 1 (pp. 108-109), for measures related to assessment and reduction of fear and anxiety.<br>b. Implement additional measures *to reduce fear and anxiety:*<br>1. support client's decision to accept and endure aggressive treatment for his/her disease<br>2. discuss and plan with client and speech pathologist a method of communicating during the postoperative period (e.g. artificial larynx, paper and pencil, picture or word board, magic slate, flash cards)<br>3. arrange for a visit with a volunteer from the Lost Chord or New Voice Club or International Association of Laryngectomees who has successfully adjusted to a laryngectomy.<br>c. Discuss with significant others the effects of their positive outlook and reactions on the client's anxiety level and mental status. |

## 2. NURSING DIAGNOSIS: Knowledge deficit

regarding hospital routines associated with surgery, physical preparation for the laryngectomy and radical neck dissection, sensations that normally occur following surgery and anesthesia, and postoperative care and expectations.

| Desired Outcomes | Nursing Actions and ***Selected Purposes/Rationales*** |
|---|---|
| 2.a. The client will verbalize an understanding of usual preoperative care and postoperative sensations and care. | 2.a.1. Refer to Standardized Preoperative Care Plan, Nursing Diagnosis 4, actions a.1-4 (pp. 111-112), for information to include in preoperative teaching.<br>2. Explain purpose of each part of a tracheostomy tube and how it works. Allow client to handle a tube or use a chart or model to show where the tube will be inserted if one is to be used (some physicians prefer not to use a tracheostomy tube because the stoma will be a permanent one which is sutured open and there is less tissue reaction and better stoma formation when a tube is not used).<br>3. Provide additional information regarding specific expectations and care after laryngectomy and radical neck dissection:<br>a. length of time the tracheostomy tube will be in place (usually 2-3 weeks but depends on physician preference and length of healing time)<br>b. purpose, frequency, and procedure for tracheostomy care<br>c. suctioning procedure and purpose and sensations (e.g. pain, choking, pressure) that client may experience during the procedure<br>d. techniques that will be used to provide moisture to inspired air (e.g. nebulizer, moist bib, humidifier)<br>e. temporary need for tube feedings to minimize contamination of internal suture lines and to prevent fluid from leaking through the suture line into the trachea until healing has occurred; assure client that oral feedings will be initiated as soon as suture line has healed (usually 8-10 days after surgery, but a longer healing time [12-14 days] may be necessary if client has had radiation therapy to the operative area)<br>f. presence and purpose of closed wound drainage system<br>g. involvement in wound care, suctioning, and tube feeding very early in the postoperative period<br>h. appearance of neck if a TEP is planned during the surgical procedure (will return from surgery with a stent protruding from stoma and |

taped to neck; stent is removed and prosthesis is inserted about the 5th postoperative day)
i. different methods of speech production that can be learned postoperatively if a TEP is not performed or is planned as a subsequent surgery.
4. Allow time for questions and clarification. Provide feedback.

2.b. The client will demonstrate the ability to perform activities designed to prevent postoperative complications.

2.b.1. Refer to Standardized Preoperative Care Plan, Nursing Diagnosis 4, action b.1 (p. 112), for teaching related to prevention of postoperative complications.
2. Provide additional instructions on ways to prevent complications associated with a laryngectomy and radical neck dissection:
a. demonstrate oral hygiene techniques that will be used postoperatively (e.g. low-pressure power spray, irrigations with saline or hydrogen peroxide and water)
b. demonstrate exercises (e.g. shoulder flexion, abduction, and external rotation; wall climbing with fingers; pulley exercises) that may be ordered to prevent shoulder and neck dysfunction on the affected side
c. emphasize the need to stop smoking in order to help prevent respiratory infection and irritation of oral mucosa.
3. Allow time for questions, clarification, practice, and return demonstration of exercises and oral hygiene techniques.

## POSTOPERATIVE

**Use in conjunction with the Standardized Postoperative Care Plan.**

### 1. NURSING DIAGNOSIS: Ineffective airway clearance

related to:
a. obstruction or dislodgment of tracheostomy tube;
b. stasis of secretions associated with decreased activity and poor cough effort resulting from depressant effects of anesthesia and some medications (e.g. narcotic analgesics), pain, weakness, fatigue, and inability to raise intrathoracic pressure as a result of removal of the larynx;
c. tenacious secretions associated with fluid loss; decreased fluid intake; and inhalation of cool, dry air because of rerouting of normal air passages (the nose and mouth normally humidify and warm inspired air);
d. increased secretions associated with irritation of the respiratory tract resulting from inhalation anesthetics, endotracheal intubation, and presence of tube in trachea;
e. tracheal compression associated with edema, bleeding, and positioning of the neck (especially if large compression dressing is in place).

| Desired Outcome | Nursing Actions and ***Selected Purposes/Rationales*** |
|---|---|
| 1. The client will maintain clear, open airways (see Standardized Postoperative Care Plan, Nursing Diagnosis 3 [p. 115], for outcome criteria). | 1.a. Refer to Standardized Postoperative Care Plan, Nursing Diagnosis 3 (pp. 115-116), for measures related to assessment and promotion of effective airway clearance.<br>b. Implement additional measures *to promote effective airway clearance:*<br>1. perform actions *to decrease risk of dislodgment of tracheostomy tube:*<br>a. obtain adequate assistance when changing tube ties<br>b. fasten tube ties securely; check them frequently to be sure that they have not become loose |

| Desired Outcome | Nursing Actions and ***Selected Purposes/Rationales*** |
|---|---|
| | c. minimize movement of outer cannula when removing or replacing inner cannula *(movement can irritate the trachea and stimulate coughing)*<br>d. cover stomal area with a nonraveling material *to prevent lint from entering tube and stimulating coughing*<br>e. discourage vigorous coughing<br>f. consult physician about an order for an antitussive if client is coughing excessively<br>2. if tracheostomy tube does become dislodged, perform or assist with immediate replacement according to hospital procedure (proper size tracheostomy tube should be kept at the bedside)<br>3. cleanse tracheostomy tube as necessary *in order to remove excessive secretions*<br>4. perform additional measures *to liquefy and facilitate removal of tenacious pulmonary secretions:*<br>a. instill small amounts (usually 2-5 ml) of sterile normal saline into tracheostomy tube before suctioning<br>b. maintain humidification of inspired air:<br>1. place a moist, thin 4 x 4 gauze pad over stomal opening<br>2. place humidifier in room<br>3. provide oxygen mist by nebulizer as ordered<br>5. perform actions *to decrease risk or degree of tracheal compression:*<br>a. keep head of bed elevated at least 30° *to decrease edema in surgical area*<br>b. implement measures to reduce stress on the surgical site (see Postoperative Nursing Diagnosis 5, actions a.2.c.2-6) *in order to prevent bleeding and hematoma formation.* |

## 2. NURSING DIAGNOSIS: Altered nutrition: less than body requirements

related to:

a. decreased oral intake associated with:
   1. prescribed dietary modifications
   2. anorexia resulting from factors such as discomfort, fatigue, depression, and an impaired sense of taste and smell (olfactory stimulation does not occur because of altered nasal airflow)
   3. dysphagia resulting from edema, nerve damage, and removal of some muscles and structures necessary for swallowing;

b. inadequate nutritional replacement therapy;

c. increased nutritional needs associated with the increased metabolic rate that occurs during wound healing.

| Desired Outcome | Nursing Actions and ***Selected Purposes/Rationales*** |
|---|---|
| 2. The client will maintain an adequate nutritional status (see Standardized Postoperative Care Plan, Nursing Diagnosis 5 [p. 118], for outcome criteria). | 2.a. Refer to Standardized Postoperative Care Plan, Nursing Diagnosis 5 (p. 118), for measures related to assessment and maintenance of nutritional status.<br>b. Implement additional measures *to maintain an adequate nutritional status:*<br>1. administer tube feedings as ordered (usually progress from water to a commercial formula)<br>2. perform actions *to improve oral intake when allowed* (oral feedings are usually initiated 8-14 days after surgery):<br>a. implement measures to improve client's ability to swallow (see Postoperative Nursing Diagnosis 3, action b)<br>b. implement measures *to compensate for impaired taste and smell* (assure client that both senses usually return to some degree):<br>1. serve foods warm *to stimulate the sense of smell* |

2. provide extra sweeteners for foods/fluids
3. encourage client to experiment with spices and other seasonings (e.g. lemon, garlic, onion, mint) *to enhance taste sensation*

c. assist client with oral hygiene before meals *to eliminate unpleasant tastes*
d. implement measures to facilitate client's psychological adjustment to the effects of the surgery (see Postoperative Nursing Diagnoses 10, actions f-x; 11, action c; and 13, action b) *in order to reduce depression and improve appetite*
e. support client during self-feeding attempts by staying with him/her and offering encouragement
f. provide privacy for client during early self-feeding attempts *in order to reduce the embarrassment associated with eating difficulties.*

---

## 3. NURSING DIAGNOSIS: Impaired swallowing

related to:
a. edema of surgical area;
b. impaired tongue movement associated with damage to the hypoglossal nerve;
c. mouth and neck pain;
d. structural changes in the pharynx (results in difficulty moving food bolus from pharynx into esophagus);
e. xerostomia if client had radiation therapy preoperatively.

| Desired Outcome | Nursing Actions and ***Selected Purposes/Rationales*** |
|---|---|
| 3. The client will experience an improvement in swallowing as evidenced by:<br>a. communication of same<br>b. absence of food in oral cavity after swallowing<br>c. absence of coughing and choking when eating and drinking. | 3.a. Assess for signs and symptoms of impaired swallowing (e.g. communication of difficulty swallowing, stasis of food in oral cavity, coughing or choking when eating or drinking).<br>b. Implement measures *to improve ability to swallow:*<br>1. place client in high Fowler's position for meals and snacks; head and neck should be tilted forward slightly *to facilitate posterior movement of the tongue*<br>2. perform actions *to reduce discomfort associated with swallowing* (e.g. medicate before meals)<br>3. when oral intake is first allowed, provide thick fluids or thicken thin fluids with substances such as "Thick-it," gelatin, or baby cereal as ordered<br>4. assist client to select foods that have a distinct texture and are easy to swallow (e.g. custard, cottage cheese, pureed meat, mashed potatoes)<br>5. instruct client to avoid mixing foods of different texture in his/her mouth at same time<br>6. avoid serving foods that are sticky (e.g. peanut butter, soft bread, bananas)<br>7. moisten dry foods with gravy or sauces (e.g. catsup, sour cream, salad dressings)<br>8. utilize assistive devices (e.g. long-handled spoon) to place food in back of mouth if tongue movement is impaired<br>9. perform actions *to improve impaired swallowing due to xerostomia:*<br>a. implement measures *to stimulate salivation:*<br>1. provide oral care before meals<br>2. provide a piece of sour, hard candy for client to suck on just before meals unless contraindicated<br>3. serve foods that are visually pleasing<br>4. place a piece of lemon or sour pickle on client's plate |

| Desired Outcome | Nursing Actions and ***Selected Purposes/Rationales*** |
|---|---|
| | b. encourage a fluid intake of 2500 ml/day unless contraindicated<br>c. encourage client to use artificial saliva<br>10. encourage client to avoid milk and milk products (unless boiled) and chocolate *(when combined with saliva, these produce very thick secretions)*<br>11. instruct client to avoid putting too much food/fluid in mouth at one time<br>12. encourage client to concentrate on the act of swallowing<br>13. if client is retaining food/fluid in mouth, instruct him/her to tilt head to unaffected side when eating and drinking<br>14. if client has decreased lip control, instruct him/her to close lips with hand prior to swallowing<br>15. consult speech pathologist about methods for dealing with impaired swallowing; reinforce recommended exercises and techniques.<br>c. Consult physician if swallowing difficulties persist or worsen. |

## 4. NURSING DIAGNOSIS: Impaired verbal communication

related to the surgical removal of the larynx.

| Desired Outcome | Nursing Actions and ***Selected Purposes/Rationales*** |
|---|---|
| 4. The client will successfully communicate needs and desires. | 4.a. Implement measures *to facilitate communication:*<br>1. maintain a patient, calm approach; listen attentively and allow ample time for communication<br>2. answer call signal in person rather than using the intercommunication system<br>3. if client is frustrated or fatigued, try to anticipate needs *in order to minimize the necessity of communication attempts*<br>4. ask questions that require short answers, eye blinks, or nod of head if client is having difficulty communicating and is frustrated or fatigued<br>5. provide materials such as magic slate, pad and pencil, word cards, and/or picture board; try to ensure that placement of intravenous line does not interfere with use of these communication aids<br>6. reinforce communication techniques prescribed by speech pathologist<br>7. if a TEP has been performed and voice prosthesis is in place (usually 5th postoperative day), reinforce instructions from speech pathologist about its use<br>8. assist client to operate artificial larynx if indicated.<br>b. Post a sign on the door, intercommunication system, and above bed to remind health care personnel that the client is nonverbal.<br>c. Inform significant others and health care personnel of techniques being used to facilitate client's ability to communicate. Stress the importance of consistent use of these techniques.<br>d. Encourage client to communicate with the physician about the possibility of future surgical reconstruction of the larynx (possible in a limited number of cases) or a TEP with voice prosthesis *in order to allow him/her to regain the ability to speak in a more normal fashion.* |

## 5. NURSING DIAGNOSIS: Actual/High risk for impaired skin integrity

related to:
a. disruption of skin associated with the surgical procedure and grafting (if performed);
b. delayed wound healing associated with:
   1. compromised circulation to area resulting from preoperative radiation to tumor site and/or excessive pressure or stress on wound area
   2. air or fluid accumulation under skin flaps (extensive skin flaps are created with a radical neck dissection)
   3. inadequate nutritional status;
c. irritation of skin associated with contact with wound drainage, pressure from drainage tubes, and use of tape.

| Desired Outcomes | Nursing Actions and ***Selected Purposes/Rationales*** |
|---|---|
| 5.a. The client will experience normal healing of surgical wounds (see Standardized Postoperative Care Plan, Nursing Diagnosis 9, outcome a [p. 122], for outcome criteria). | 5.a.1. Refer to Standardized Postoperative Care Plan, Nursing Diagnosis 9, action a (pp. 122-123), for measures related to assessment and promotion of wound healing.<br>2. Implement additional measures *to promote wound healing:*<br>a. cleanse peristomal area gently with normal saline or half-strength hydrogen peroxide *to promote healing of tracheal stoma*<br>b. use a bed cradle if indicated *to protect donor site from pressure of linens*<br>c. perform actions *to reduce stress on and trauma to graft site, suture lines, and/or surrounding tissue:*<br>1. position client as ordered (e.g. head elevated at least 30° and supported with pillows) *to maintain head alignment and promote venous and lymphatic drainage*<br>2. instruct client to avoid manipulation of nasogastric tube<br>3. support client's head and neck during position change until client is able to do so<br>4. instruct client to support head and neck with hands when moving in bed and to avoid turning head abruptly and hyperextending neck<br>5. place personal articles and call signal within easy reach *so client does not have to turn or strain to reach them*<br>6. maintain patency of wound drainage system *in order to prevent fluid accumulation under the skin flaps*<br>7. make sure that gown and tracheostomy tube ties are not too tight<br>8. use an isolation mask rather than tape to secure dressings<br>9. soak adherent dressings with sterile normal saline before removal<br>10. implement measures to improve airway clearance (see Postoperative Nursing Diagnosis 1) *in order to prevent strenuous respiratory efforts and resultant use of accessory muscles in the operative area*<br>11. instruct client to focus on deep breathing rather than vigorous coughing to promote effective airway clearance (some physicians prefer that their clients not cough *because it increases stress on the suture line)*<br>d. perform actions to maintain an adequate nutritional status (see Postoperative Nursing Diagnosis 2)<br>e. perform actions to prevent and treat wound infection (see Postoperative Nursing Diagnosis 7). |
| 5.b. The client will maintain skin integrity (see Standardized Postoperative Care | 5.b.1. Refer to Standardized Postoperative Care Plan, Nursing Diagnosis 9, actions b.1 and 2 (p. 123), for measures related to assessment and prevention of skin irritation and breakdown resulting from contact with wound drainage, drainage tubings, and tape. |

| Desired Outcomes | Nursing Actions and ***Selected Purposes/Rationales*** |
|---|---|
| Plan, Nursing Diagnosis 9, outcome b [p. 123], for outcome criteria). | 2. Implement additional measures *to prevent skin irritation and breakdown:*<br>a. secure neck dressings with an isolation mask rather than tape<br>b. soak adherent dressings with sterile normal saline before removal<br>c. change dressings as needed *to prevent maceration of tissue.*<br>3. If skin irritation or breakdown occurs:<br>a. notify physician<br>b. continue with above measures to prevent further irritation and breakdown<br>c. perform wound care as ordered or per standard hospital procedure<br>d. assess client closely and report signs and symptoms of infection (e.g. elevated temperature; redness, warmth, and edema around incision or area of breakdown; unusual drainage from site). |

## 6. NURSING DIAGNOSIS: Constipation

related to:
a. decreased gastrointestinal motility associated with anesthesia, narcotic analgesics, and decreased activity;
b. decreased fluid intake;
c. decreased intake of foods high in fiber associated with dietary restrictions and difficulty swallowing;
d. inability to bear down or strain to have a bowel movement (client is not able to perform a Valsalva maneuver as a result of removal of the larynx).

| Desired Outcome | Nursing Actions and ***Selected Purposes/Rationales*** |
|---|---|
| 6. The client will not experience constipation as evidenced by:<br>a. usual frequency of bowel movements when usual oral intake is resumed<br>b. passage of soft, formed stool<br>c. absence of headache, anorexia, abdominal distention and pain, and rectal pressure. | 6.a. Refer to Standardized Postoperative Care Plan, Nursing Diagnosis 14 (p. 127), for measures related to assessment, prevention, and management of constipation.<br>b. Establish a routine time for defecation based on client's usual bowel elimination pattern.<br>c. Implement measures to improve oral intake when allowed (see Postoperative Nursing Diagnosis 2, action b.2). |

## 7. NURSING DIAGNOSIS: High risk for infection: wound

related to:
a. wound contamination and continuous exposure of suture lines to saliva (there is an increased concentration of bacteria in saliva);
b. increased colonization of pathogens associated with accumulation of drainage around tracheostomy and beneath flaps (can result from a large dead space and/or obstruction of the wound drainage system);
c. decreased resistance to infection associated with inadequate nutritional status and diminished tissue perfusion to operative site.

| Desired Outcome | Nursing Actions and ***Selected Purposes/Rationales*** |
|---|---|
| 7. The client will remain free of wound infection (see Standardized Postoperative Care Plan, Nursing Diagnosis 16, outcome b [p. 129], for outcome criteria). | 7.a. Refer to Standardized Postoperative Care Plan, Nursing Diagnosis 16, action b (p. 129), for measures related to assessment, prevention, and management of wound infection.<br>b. Implement additional actions *to prevent wound infection:*<br>1. perform actions to promote wound healing (see Postoperative Nursing Diagnosis 5, action a.)<br>2. apply an antimicrobial ointment to tracheal stoma and suture lines if ordered<br>3. perform tracheostomy care as needed *to prevent the accumulation of secretions.* |

**8. COLLABORATIVE DIAGNOSES:**

**Potential complications:**

a. **hypovolemic shock** related to:
   1. hemorrhage associated with carotid artery erosion and subsequent rupture resulting from:
      a. prolonged exposure of vessel to atmospheric air during surgery (causes drying and subsequent destruction of the vessel wall)
      b. wound infection, tissue necrosis, and/or fistula formation
      c. weakening of the vessel wall as a result of preoperative radiation to tumor site
   2. fluid volume deficit associated with excessive fluid loss and inadequate fluid replacement;

b. **necrosis of the skin flaps** related to inadequate blood supply to flaps associated with:
   1. excessive tension on wound margins, preoperative radiation in excess of 4500 cGy to wound area, mechanical obstruction of blood flow within the flap, and vascular congestion (can result from pressure differences in blood flow to and from flap)
   2. elevation of flaps resulting from wound infection, hematoma or seroma formation, and/or development of a fistula;

c. **salivary fistula** related to dehiscence or necrosis of mucosal suture line in pharynx associated with wound infection, inadequate nutritional status, excessive tension on suture lines resulting from removal of a large amount of tissue, and impaired vascularity of the wound;

d. **thoracic duct (chylous) fistula** related to injury to the thoracic duct or one of its tributaries (if the neck dissection is on the left side) or to the lymphatic channel (if the neck dissection is on the right side) during the surgical procedure;

e. **shoulder and neck dysfunction** related to denervation of the trapezius muscle associated with removal of or damage to the spinal accessory nerve during surgery (current trend is to spare the spinal accessory nerve if possible).

| Desired Outcomes | Nursing Actions and ***Selected Purposes/Rationales*** |
|---|---|
| 8.a. The client will not develop hypovolemic shock (see Standardized Postoperative Care Plan, Collaborative Diagnosis 19, outcome a [pp. 131-132], for outcome criteria). | 8.a.1. Assess for and report:<br>a. signs and symptoms of conditions that could lead to carotid artery rupture:<br>1. impaired circulation to wound and surrounding skin (e.g. change in skin color from red to pale or black, coolness, increased edema)<br>2. impaired wound healing (e.g. increase in size or altered shape of wound, delayed wound closure)<br>3. wound infection (e.g. change in type, odor, or amount of drainage; increased redness or pain at site)<br>4. carotid artery exposure |

**Desired Outcomes** | **Nursing Actions and *Selected Purposes/Rationales***

b. signs and symptoms of impending carotid artery rupture (e.g. "herald bleed" [slight amount of bright red blood on packing or from margins of wound] 24-48 hours before rupture, sternal or high epigastric pain a few hours before rupture)
c. frank, profuse bleeding from wound, tracheostomy, or oropharynx
d. declining RBC, Hct, and Hb levels
e. signs and symptoms of hypovolemic shock (see Standardized Postoperative Care Plan, Collaborative Diagnosis 19, action a.3 [p. 132], for signs and symptoms).

2. Have suction equipment, gloves, cuffed tracheostomy tube (if one is not already in place), and absorbent dressings at bedside in case of carotid artery rupture.
3. Refer to Standardized Postoperative Care Plan, Collaborative Diagnosis 19, actions a.4 and 5 (p. 132), for measures to prevent or treat hypovolemic shock.
4. Implement measures *to prevent carotid artery rupture and further reduce the risk of hypovolemic shock:*
   a. perform actions to promote healing of the surgical incision (see Postoperative Nursing Diagnosis 5, action a) and prevent and treat wound infection (see Postoperative Nursing Diagnosis 7) *in order to prevent tissue sloughing and subsequent exposure, drying, and erosion of the carotid artery*
   b. assess for and report pulsation of tracheostomy tube *(indicates tip is in close proximity to carotid artery and may be causing undue pressure on the vessel)*
   c. maintain tracheostomy tube in midtracheal alignment at all times.
5. If carotid artery rupture occurs:
   a. apply firm, prolonged, continuous pressure to area using absorbent materials
   b. position client in high Fowler's position with head turned to side or in side-lying position and ensure that tracheostomy cuff is inflated *to prevent aspiration;* assist with insertion of a cuffed tracheostomy tube if one is not in place
   c. suction as necessary *to clear oral cavity and airway*
   d. prepare client for ligation of carotid artery if planned
   e. provide emotional support to client and significant others
   f. remain with client and administer medications such as intravenous morphine sulfate and diazepam *to allay anxiety* (client is typically alert).

**8.b.** The client will not experience necrosis of skin flaps as evidenced by:
1. skin flaps warm and expected color
2. approximated wound edges
3. absence of foul odor from flap area.

8.b.1. Assess for and report:
   a. signs and symptoms of impaired blood flow in skin flaps (e.g. blue, white, or red appearing skin flap; capillary refill time greater than 3 seconds)
   b. signs and symptoms of skin flap necrosis (e.g. pale, cool, darkened tissue; separation of wound edges; foul odor from flap area).

2. Implement measures to promote wound healing (see Postoperative Nursing Diagnosis 5, action a) and prevent and treat wound infection (see Postoperative Nursing Diagnosis 7) *in order to prevent skin flap necrosis.*
3. If signs and symptoms of skin flap necrosis occur:
   a. prepare client for surgical revision or replacement of graft
   b. provide emotional support to client and significant others.

**8.c.** The client will not develop a salivary fistula as evidenced by:
1. absence of redness,

8.c.1. Assess for and report signs and symptoms of a salivary fistula (e.g. redness, edema, and tenderness near incision; increased temperature; drainage of saliva, purulent material, or oral foods/fluids through incision or a cutaneous opening near incision).

2. Implement measures *to prevent a salivary fistula:*

edema, and tenderness near incision
2. afebrile status
3. usual drainage from incision
4. intact skin around incision.

a. perform actions to prevent and treat wound infection (see Postoperative Nursing Diagnosis 7)
b. perform actions to maintain an adequate nutritional status (see Postoperative Nursing Diagnosis 2)
c. maintain continuous suction and patency of drain catheter (e.g. Malekot) if in place (the catheter may be inserted in the pharynx during surgery and left in place for 7-10 days *to allow for controlled drainage of saliva and decrease the risk of breakdown of the pharyngeal repair).*

3. If signs and symptoms of a salivary fistula occur:
a. continue with above actions
b. withhold oral food and fluid as ordered
c. maintain intravenous therapy and tube feedings as ordered until fistula closes
d. perform wound care as ordered
e. administer antimicrobials if ordered
f. prepare client for surgical closure of fistula if planned
g. provide emotional support to client and significant others.

8.d. The client will experience resolution of a thoracic duct fistula if it occurs as evidenced by:
1. usual amount and character of drainage from incision
2. wound drainage negative for chylomicrons.

8.d.1. Assess for and report signs and symptoms of a thoracic duct (chylous) fistula (e.g. sudden increase in drainage from wound; cloudy, milky-appearing fluid in drain system; wound drainage positive for chylomicrons).

2. If signs and symptoms of a thoracic duct fistula occur:
a. apply pressure dressing over fistula site if ordered
b. accurately assess amount of fistula drainage
c. administer the following if ordered *to help maintain an adequate nutritional status:*
   1. oral foods and fluids that contain medium chain triglycerides such as salad dressing or milk shakes to which medium chain triglyceride oil has been added (medium chain triglycerides bypass the thoracic duct because they are absorbed directly into the portal venous circulation)
   2. total parenteral nutrition
d. administer fluid and electrolytes *to replace those lost via the fistula*
e. prepare client for surgical repair of fistula if planned (may be indicated if drainage from the fistula is in excess of 500-1000 ml/day)
f. provide emotional support to client and significant others.

8.e. The client will regain optimal shoulder and neck function as evidenced by:
1. improved range of motion of shoulder
2. ability to maintain shoulder in near-normal position
3. gradual resolution of pain in shoulder and neck.

8.e.1. Assess for and report signs and symptoms of spinal accessory nerve damage (e.g. inability to abduct arm on affected side above 90°, drooping shoulder, continued pain in neck and shoulder).

2. If shoulder and neck dysfunction occur:
a. instruct client to support affected arm in a sling when ambulating and rest it on a chair arm, table, or pillow when sitting *in order to prevent overstretching of the trapezius muscle*
b. assist client with self-care activities he/she is unable to perform independently
c. reinforce the need to begin neck and shoulder exercises (e.g. wall climbing with fingers, shoulder swing, pulley exercises, range of motion of neck) as soon as allowed *in order to improve tone and strength of muscles that will compensate for the loss of the trapezius muscle* (exercises are usually started 10 days to 3 months postoperatively depending on extensiveness of surgery and healing process)
d. assure client that partial neck and shoulder function may be regained if exercise program and physical therapy schedule are adhered to.

## 9. NURSING DIAGNOSIS: Altered sexuality patterns

related to:

a. fear of rejection by partner associated with perceived loss of sexual appeal resulting from the loss of ability to communicate verbally, changes in physical appearance, and neck breathing;
b. fear that rapid breathing during climax will result in a coughing episode;
c. discomfort associated with an extensive surgical wound;
d. inability to assume positions for sexual activity that necessitate supporting one's body weight and performing Valsalva maneuver (e.g. "missionary position" if male);
e. depression and ineffective coping.

### Desired Outcome

9. The client will communicate a perception of self as sexually acceptable and adequate as evidenced by:
   a. maintenance of relationship with significant other
   b. behaviors reflecting adjustment to effects of laryngectomy and radical neck dissection on sexual functioning.

### Nursing Actions and ***Selected Purposes/Rationales***

9.a. Assess for signs and symptoms of altered sexuality patterns (e.g. communication of sexual concerns, alteration in relationship with significant other).

b. Provide accurate information about the effects of the laryngectomy and radical neck dissection on sexual functioning. Encourage questions and clarify misconceptions.

c. Implement measures *to facilitate client's adjustment to the effects of changes in appearance and body functioning on his/her sexuality:*
   1. facilitate communication between client and his/her partner; focus on feelings the couple share and assist them to identify changes which may affect their sexual relationship
   2. perform actions to facilitate client's psychological adjustment to the changes that have occurred (see Postoperative Nursing Diagnoses 10, actions f-x; 11, action c; and 13, action b)
   3. perform actions *to decrease the possibility of rejection by partner:*
      a. if appropriate, involve partner in care of client's wound and suctioning *to facilitate adjustment to the change in client's appearance and functioning*
      b. instruct client to suction and cleanse stoma and cover it with a porous shield just before sexual activity
   4. instruct client in ways to compensate for loss of larynx and resultant inability to perform a Valsalva maneuver during intercourse (e.g. experimenting with positions other than the "missionary position" such as rear entry or leg over leg side entry, using exaggerated pelvic thrust)
   5. if client is concerned that operative site discomfort will interfere with usual sexual activity, assure him/her that discomfort is temporary and will diminish as incision heals
   6. reinforce physician's instructions regarding when client can resume sexual activity; assure him/her that the suture lines are secure
   7. discuss ways to be creative in expressing sexuality (e.g. massage, fantasies, cuddling)
   8. arrange for uninterrupted privacy during hospital stay if desired by couple.

d. Include partner in above discussions and encourage his/her continued support of the client.

e. Consult physician if counseling appears indicated.

## 10. NURSING DIAGNOSIS: Self-concept disturbance*

related to:

a. changes in appearance:
   1. obvious disfigurement of face and neck structures
   2. drooling and paralysis of the muscles controlling facial expression associated with damage to the facial nerve
   3. drooping of the shoulder associated with removal of or damage to the spinal accessory nerve if it has occurred
   4. persistent facial edema associated with disruption of lymphatic channels;

b. alteration in usual body functioning:
   1. loss of ability to speak, sing, produce crying and laughing sounds, and whistle
   2. loss of sense of taste and smell and ability to blow nose
   3. loss of normal shoulder, neck, and arm movement associated with removal of or damage to the spinal accessory nerve and removal of sternocleido-mastoid muscle if performed
   4. impaired swallowing ability and tongue movement associated with damage to the hypoglossal nerve
   5. loss of ability to perform activities such as coughing effectively, assuming positions for sexual activity that necessitate supporting one's body weight (e.g. "missionary position" if male), straining to have a bowel movement, and lifting heavy objects associated with inability to perform a Valsalva maneuver resulting from loss of the larynx;

c. feelings of loss of femininity/masculinity and sexual appeal associated with loss of ability to communicate verbally, changes in physical appearance, and neck breathing;

d. dependence on others to meet self-care needs;

e. possible life-style, career, and role changes.

*This diagnostic label includes the nursing diagnoses of body image disturbance, self-esteem disturbance, and altered role performance.

| Desired Outcome | Nursing Actions and ***Selected Purposes/Rationales*** |
|---|---|
| 10. The client will demonstrate beginning adaptation to changes in appearance, body functioning, life style, and roles as evidenced by:<br>a. communication of feelings of self-worth and sexual adequacy<br>b. maintenance of relationships with significant others<br>c. interest and participation in tracheostomy care and speech techniques<br>d. active participation in activities of daily living<br>e. active interest in personal appearance<br>f. willingness to | 10.a. Assess for signs and symptoms of a self-concept disturbance (e.g. nonverbal cues denoting a negative response to changes in body functioning and appearance such as preoccupation with changes that have occurred, refusal to look at or touch neck area, refusal to participate in self-care activities, or withdrawal from significant others).<br>b. Determine the meaning of the changes in appearance, body functioning, life style, and roles to the client by encouraging him/her to communicate feelings and by noting nonverbal responses to the changes experienced.<br>c. Implement measures to facilitate the grieving process (see Postoperative Nursing Diagnosis 13, action b).<br>d. Implement measures to assist client to cope with effects of laryngectomy and radical neck dissection (see Postoperative Nursing Diagnosis 11, action c).<br>e. Implement measures to facilitate client's adjustment to the effects of the changes in appearance and body functioning on his/her sexuality (see Postoperative Nursing Diagnosis 9, action c).<br>f. Implement measures *to assist client to increase self-esteem* (e.g. limit negative self-assessment, encourage positive communication about self, assist to identify strengths, give positive feedback about accomplishments and behaviors that are indicative of high self-esteem).<br>g. Implement measures *to reduce drooling:*<br>1. instruct client to wipe mouth or suction oral cavity frequently (if circumoral paresthesias are present, he/she may be unaware of drooling) |

| Desired Outcome | Nursing Actions and ***Selected Purposes/Rationales*** |
|---|---|
| pursue usual roles and participate in social activities | 2. place a wick with one end in corner of mouth and other end in an emesis basin when client is resting in bed<br>3. perform actions to improve client's ability to swallow (see Postoperative Nursing Diagnosis 3, action b). |
| g. communication of a beginning plan for adapting life style to meet restrictions imposed by the effects of the laryngectomy and radical neck dissection | h. Provide privacy when eating *to reduce embarrassment associated with eating difficulties.*<br>i. Remain with client for the first look at his/her appearance after removal of dressings. Explain that some of the physical changes will not be as severe once edema and redness have subsided and the tracheostomy tube is out. (Facial edema that may occur with a radical neck dissection peaks by the fifth postoperative day and takes 2-6 months to totally dissipate.) |
| h. willingness to participate in or seek vocational rehabilitation if appropriate. | j. Assure client that neck and shoulder function will usually improve if exercise and physical therapy regimens are adhered to.<br>k. Encourage client to pursue available options in relation to regaining speech (e.g. voice prosthesis, esophageal speech, artificial larynges).<br>l. Assist client with usual grooming and makeup habits if necessary.<br>m. Promote activities which require client to confront the body changes that have occurred (e.g. suctioning, stomal care, tube feeding, arm and shoulder exercises). Be aware that integration of the changes in body image do not usually occur until 2-6 months after the actual physical changes have occurred.<br>n. Demonstrate acceptance of client using techniques such as touch and frequent visits. Encourage significant others to do the same.<br>o. Assess for and support behaviors suggesting positive adaptation to changes that have occurred (e.g. willingness to participate in wound and stomal care, tube feedings, and suctioning; compliance with treatment plan; communication of feelings of self-worth; maintenance of relationships with significant others).<br>p. Assist significant others to verbalize feelings about physical changes in the client and the care he/she requires (recognize that they may be repulsed by client's appearance or wound care). Assure them that their responses are normal but caution them not to show distaste in front of the client *because of the negative impact of such a response on the client's self-concept.*<br>q. Encourage significant others to allow client to do what he/she is able *so that independence can be reestablished and/or self-esteem redeveloped.*<br>r. Encourage client contact with others *so that he/she can test and establish a new self-image.*<br>s. Assist client's and significant others' adjustment by listening, facilitating communication, and providing information.<br>t. Instruct significant others to allow client to communicate and attempt to express his/her needs.<br>u. If client appears to be rejecting significant others, explain that this is a common occurrence (client rejects family and/or spouse before they have a chance to reject him/her). Encourage them to visit often and persist in offering understanding and support for the client.<br>v. Assist client and significant others to have similar expectations and understanding of future life style and to identify ways that personal and family goals can be adjusted rather than abandoned.<br>w. Encourage client to pursue usual roles and interests and to continue involvement in social activities. If previous roles, interests, and hobbies cannot be pursued, encourage development of new ones.<br>x. Provide information about and encourage utilization of community agencies and support groups (e.g. Lost Chord Club; New Voice Club; American Cancer Society; vocational rehabilitation; sexual, family, individual, and/or financial counseling). |

y. Consult physician about psychological counseling if client desires or if he/she seems unwilling or unable to adapt to changes resulting from the laryngectomy and radical neck dissection.

## 11. NURSING DIAGNOSIS: Ineffective individual coping

related to:
a. changes in appearance;
b. loss of ability to speak and audibly laugh and cry;
c. difficulty mastering new speaking techniques;
d. fear, anxiety, and depression;
e. self-care expectations regarding tube feeding and wound and tracheostomy care;
f. inadequate support system.

### Desired Outcome

11. The client will demonstrate the use of effective coping skills as evidenced by:
    a. communication of ability to cope with the effects of the laryngectomy and radical neck dissection
    b. utilization of appropriate problem-solving techniques
    c. willingness to participate in treatment plan and meet basic needs
    d. absence of destructive behavior toward self and others
    e. appropriate use of defense mechanisms
    f. recognition and utilization of available support systems.

### Nursing Actions and ***Selected Purposes/Rationales***

11.a. Assess for and report signs and symptoms of ineffective individual coping (e.g. communication of inability to cope; inability to ask for help, problem solve, or meet basic needs; destructive behavior toward self or others; inappropriate use of defense mechanisms; inability to meet role expectations).

b. Assess client's perception of current situation including precipitating factors and effectiveness of coping mechanisms.

c. Implement measures *to promote effective coping:*
1. expect and encourage client to participate in stomal and wound care, tube feeding, and suctioning as soon as possible *(active participation in care in the early postoperative period facilitates adjustment to changes experienced)*
2. assist client to recognize and manage inappropriate denial if it is present
3. arrange for a visit with another individual who has successfully adjusted to loss of larynx
4. perform actions to reduce fear and anxiety (see Standardized Postoperative Care Plan, Nursing Diagnosis 20, action b [p. 134])
5. perform actions to assist the client to adapt to changes in appearance, body functioning, life style, and roles (see Postoperative Nursing Diagnosis 10, actions f-x)
6. encourage client to communicate feelings about current situation
7. assist client to identify personal strengths and resources that can be utilized to facilitate coping with the current situation
8. create an atmosphere of trust and support
9. include client in the planning of care, encourage maximum participation in the treatment plan, and allow choices when possible *to enable him/her to maintain a sense of control*
10. perform actions to improve social interaction (see Postoperative Nursing Diagnosis 12, action c)
11. instruct client in effective problem-solving techniques (e.g. accurate identification of stressors, determination of various options to solve problem)
12. assist client to maintain usual daily routines whenever possible
13. assist client as he/she starts to plan for necessary life-style and role changes after discharge; help client to identify priorities and attainable goals
14. assist client through methods such as role playing to prepare for

| Desired Outcome | Nursing Actions and ***Selected Purposes/Rationales*** |
|---|---|
| | negative reactions from others because of changes in appearance and inability to speak normally<br>15. administer antianxiety and/or antidepressant agents if ordered<br>16. assist client to identify and utilize available support systems; provide information about available community resources that can assist client and significant others in coping with effects of surgery (e.g New Voice and Lost Chord Clubs, Voice Masters, Can Surmount, American Cancer Society, vocational rehabilitation, International Association of Laryngectomees)<br>17. encourage continued emotional support from significant others<br>18. encourage client to share with significant others the kind of support that would be most beneficial (e.g. being there, inspiring hope, providing reassurance and accurate information)<br>19. support behaviors suggesting positive adaptation to changes experienced (e.g. participating in treatment plan and self-care activities, communication of ability to cope, recognition and utilization of available support systems and effective problem-solving strategies).<br>d. Consult physician about psychological and vocational rehabilitation counseling if appropriate. Initiate a referral if necessary. |

## 12. NURSING DIAGNOSIS: Impaired social interaction

related to inability to communicate verbally, discomfort with changes in physical appearance, ineffective coping, and depression.

| Desired Outcome | Nursing Actions and ***Selected Purposes/Rationales*** |
|---|---|
| 12. The client will experience an improvement in the quantity and quality of social interaction as evidenced by:<br>a. communication of same<br>b. maintenance of relationships with significant others and casual acquaintances<br>c. use of appropriate social interaction behaviors. | 12.a. Ascertain client's usual degree of social interaction.<br>b. Assess for and report behaviors indicative of impaired social interaction (e.g. communication of or observed discomfort in social situations, inability to maintain relationships with significant others and casual acquaintances, use of inappropriate social interaction behaviors).<br>c. Implement measures *to improve social interaction:*<br>1. perform actions to facilitate communication (see Postoperative Nursing Diagnosis 4, action a)<br>2. perform actions to facilitate client's psychological adjustment to the effects of the laryngectomy and radical neck dissection (see Postoperative Nursing Diagnoses 10, actions f-x; 11, action c; and 13, action b)<br>3. assist client to identify reasons for feeling isolated and alone; aid him/her in developing a plan of action to reduce these feelings<br>4. assist client to identify a few persons he/she feels comfortable with and encourage interactions with them<br>5. encourage client to communicate his/her feelings but set limits on inappropriate behavior or responses<br>6. assist client to identify ways to provide support to significant others *in order to increase their comfort level in dealing with changes in client*<br>7. encourage client to initiate communication with others and focus on them rather than him/herself<br>8. use role playing to assist client to develop appropriate social interaction skills |

9. give positive reinforcement for attempts to interact with others in a positive way.

d. Consult physician regarding referral for counseling if signs of impaired social interaction persist.

## 13. NURSING DIAGNOSIS: Grieving*

related to:

a. changes in appearance and body functioning (e.g. loss of ability to speak normally, sing, blow nose, and audibly laugh and cry; impaired sense of smell and taste; impaired shoulder movement);

b. possible changes in life style and roles.

*This diagnostic label includes anticipatory grieving and grieving following the actual losses.

| Desired Outcome | Nursing Actions and ***Selected Purposes/Rationales*** |
|---|---|
| 13. The client will demonstrate beginning progression through the grieving process as evidenced by:<br>a. communication of feelings about the laryngectomy and radical neck dissection and its effect on appearance, body functioning, life style, and roles<br>b. expression of grief<br>c. participation in treatment plan and self-care activities<br>d. utilization of available support systems. | 13.a. Assess for signs and symptoms of grieving (e.g. change in eating habits, inability to concentrate, insomnia, anger, noncompliance, withdrawal from significant others, denial of loss). Be aware that client's response to the loss of his/her larynx and changes in body appearance and functioning will be affected by factors such as previous experience with loss, age, developmental stage, available support systems, spiritual and cultural background, current health status, and significance of the loss.<br>b. Implement measures *to facilitate the grieving process:*<br>1. assist client to acknowledge the losses experienced *so grief work can begin;* assess for factors that may hinder and facilitate acknowledgment<br>2. discuss the grieving process and assist client to accept the phases of grieving as an expected response to actual and/or anticipated losses<br>3. allow time for client to progress through the phases of grieving (phases vary among theorists but progress from shock and alarm to acceptance); be aware that not every phase is expressed by all individuals, that recurrence of phases is common, and that the grieving process may take months to years<br>4. provide an atmosphere of care and concern (e.g. provide privacy, be available and nonjudgmental, display empathy and respect) *so client will feel free to communicate feelings*<br>5. perform actions *to promote trust* (e.g. answer questions honestly, provide requested information)<br>6. encourage the expression of anger and sadness about the losses experienced; recognize displacement of anger and assist client to see the actual cause of angry feelings and resentment; establish limits on abusive behavior if demonstrated<br>7. encourage client to express his/her feelings in whatever ways are comfortable (e.g. writing, drawing)<br>8. perform actions to promote effective coping (see Postoperative Nursing Diagnosis 11, action c)<br>9. support realistic hope regarding ability to resume usual activities and regain speech<br>10. assess for and support behaviors suggesting successful grief work (e.g. communicating feelings about the loss of speech and changes in body functioning, expressing sorrow, focusing on ways to adapt to losses, learning needed skills, developing or renewing relationships) |

| Desired Outcome | Nursing Actions and ***Selected Purposes/Rationales*** |
|---|---|
| | 11. explain the phases of the grieving process to significant others; encourage their support and understanding<br>12. provide information regarding counseling services and support groups that might assist client in working through grief<br>13. facilitate communication between the client and significant others; be aware that they may be in different phases of the grieving process<br>14. arrange for a visit from clergy if desired by client.<br>c. Consult physician regarding referral for counseling if signs of dysfunctional grieving (e.g. persistent denial of losses, excessive anger or sadness, hysteria, suicidal behaviors) occur. |

## 14. NURSING DIAGNOSIS: Knowledge deficit

regarding follow-up care.

| Desired Outcomes | Nursing Actions and ***Selected Purposes/Rationales*** |
|---|---|
| 14.a. The client will demonstrate appropriate stomal care, suctioning, tracheostomy tube care, oral hygiene, and tube feeding techniques. | 14.a.1. Reinforce instructions and demonstrate the following if appropriate:<br>a. procedure for insertion of new tracheostomy tube in an emergency situation<br>b. procedure for cleansing stoma and changing tracheostomy tube ties and stoma dressing<br>c. methods for maintaining skin integrity around stoma (e.g. keep skin clean and dry)<br>d. removal and cleansing of the inner cannula (clean technique is used)<br>e. oral and tracheal suctioning<br>f. ways to increase moisture content of inspired air (e.g. use humidifier, wear a moist bib, place pans of water throughout the home)<br>g. administration of tube feedings<br>h. oral care (e.g. irrigation with normal saline or 1:4 solution of hydrogen peroxide and water).<br>2. Allow time for questions, clarification, practice, and return demonstration. |
| 14.b. The client will demonstrate the ability to effectively use and care for an artificial larynx. | 14.b.1. Reinforce instructions from speech pathologist about use and care of artificial larynx if appropriate.<br>2. Allow time for questions, clarification, and return demonstration. |
| 14.c. The client will demonstrate the ability to care for the tracheoesophageal puncture (TEP) and voice prosthesis if in place. | 14.c.1. Provide the following instructions about care of the TEP and voice prosthesis if in place:<br>a. clean and reinsert voice prosthesis as instructed by physician or speech pathologist (some models are removed daily and cleansed with a hydrogen peroxide solution while others are left in place and cleansed with an applicator)<br>b. maintain the TEP site by inserting a catheter (stent) when the prosthesis is out for cleaning or for any other reason (the puncture site will close in 1-2 hours if stent or prosthesis is not in place); if unable to insert catheter or prosthesis, call physician or go to the closest medical emergency care facility immediately to have it done<br>c. secure prosthesis strap to skin above stoma with a nonallergenic tape |

d. take antifungal medication (e.g. Mycelex troche) as prescribed to prevent or control growth of *Candida albicans* on the prosthesis (a fungal infection can eventually interfere with function of the valve in the prosthesis)
e. instruct client to report leakage of food/fluids or saliva around TEP site
f. have prosthesis replaced as often as instructed by physician (needs to be replaced every 9-12 weeks because of valve failure).

2. Emphasize the importance of indicating on Medic-Alert tag that a voice prosthesis is in place.
3. Allow time for questions, clarification, and return demonstration.

| | |
|---|---|
| 14.d. The client will identify appropriate safety precautions related to the presence of a tracheostomy and nerve damage resulting from surgery. | 14.d. Provide the following instructions regarding appropriate safety precautions related to the presence of a tracheostomy and nerve damage resulting from surgery:<br>1. always keep an obturator and outer cannula available for an emergency situation<br>2. always wear a Medic-Alert tag indicating neck breather status<br>3. reduce the risk of injury in surgical area (the area will remain numb for several months after surgery):<br>a. use an electric rather than a straight-edge razor in order to decrease risk of cuts in surgical area<br>b. avoid extremely hot foods/fluids to decrease risk of burning the oral cavity or esophagus<br>4. have smoke detectors installed in home if ability to smell is impaired<br>5. prevent blockage of and entrance of foreign particles into stoma:<br>a. do not wear constrictive clothing around neck<br>b. wear a protective shield over stoma (e.g. crocheted bib, moistened 4 × 4 gauze pad, scarf, cravat) at all times<br>c. prevent water from entering stoma (e.g. do not swim unless wearing special snorkel device designed for neck breathers, direct shower nozzle well below stoma, use stoma guard or shield while bathing)<br>d. apply shaving cream by hand rather than spraying directly on face and neck<br>e. cover stoma while shaving or getting a hair cut<br>6. if shoulder and neck movement are impaired, use caution when driving. |
| 14.e. The client will identify signs and symptoms to report to the health care provider. | 14.e.1. Refer to Standardized Postoperative Care Plan, Nursing Diagnosis 21, action c (p. 135), for signs and symptoms to report to the health care provider.<br>2. Instruct client to report these additional signs and symptoms:<br>a. persistent choking or difficulty swallowing<br>b. bloody sputum<br>c. presence of ingested liquid, food, or tube feeding formula in secretions from stoma<br>d. darkening of skin flap sites or separation of skin edges<br>e. increased weakness of arm on affected side<br>f. persistent pain in or drooping of shoulder<br>g. nausea, vomiting, diarrhea, cramping, and/or feeling of fullness associated with tube feeding. |
| 14.f. The client will identify community resources that can assist with home management and adjustment to the effects of surgery. | 14.f.1. Provide information about community resources that can assist the client and significant others with home management and adjustment to the surgery (e.g. American Cancer Society, home health agencies, counselors, social service agencies, Make Today Count, Lost Chord Club, vocational rehabilitation, International Association of Laryngectomees, church groups, American Speech and Hearing Association).<br>2. Initiate a referral if indicated. |
| 14.g. The client will | 14.g.1. Refer to Standardized Postoperative Care Plan, Nursing Diagnosis 21 |

| Desired Outcomes | Nursing Actions and ***Selected Purposes/Rationales*** |
|---|---|
| communicate an understanding of and a plan for adhering to recommended follow-up care including future appointments with health care provider and speech pathologist, medications prescribed, exercises, pain control measures, activity level, and wound care. | (pp. 135-136), for routine postoperative instructions and measures to improve client compliance.<br>2. Caution client to avoid lifting more than 2 pounds with the affected arm until arm strength increases.<br>3. Emphasize the importance of adhering to prescribed exercise program to strengthen muscles which will compensate for the loss of the trapezius muscle.<br>4. Use heat, massage, and/or liniments as prescribed to reduce pain in affected shoulder.<br>5. Encourage client to follow up with speech rehabilitation if appropriate. |

# Bibliography

## General Bibliography


Acute Pain Management Guideline Panel. Acute pain management: operative or medical procedures and trauma. Clinical practice guideline. AHCPR Pub. No. 92-0032. Rockville, MD: Agency for Health Care Policy and Research, Public Health Service, U.S. Department of Health and Human Services, 1992.

American Pain Society. Principles of analgesic use in the treatment of acute pain and cancer pain (3rd ed.). Skokie, IL: American Pain Society, 1992.

Baer, CL, & Williams, BR. Clinical pharmacology and nursing (2nd ed.). Springhouse, PA: Springhouse Publishing Company, 1992.

Bates, B. A guide to physical examination (5th ed.). Philadelphia: J.B. Lippincott Company, 1991.

Beare, PG, & Myers, JL. Principles and practice of adult health nursing. St. Louis: C.V. Mosby, 1990.

Bellack, JP, & Edlund, BJ. Nursing assessment and diagnosis. Boston: Jones and Bartlett Publishers, 1992.

Black, JM, & Matassarin-Jacobs, E. Luckman and Sorensen's medical-surgical nursing: a psychophysiologic approach (4th ed.). Philadelphia: W.B. Saunders Company, 1993.

Bullock, BL, & Rosendahl, PP. Pathophysiology: adaptations and alterations in function (3rd ed.). Philadelphia: J.B. Lippincott Company, 1992.

Burrell, LO (Ed.). Adult nursing in hospital and community settings. Norwalk, CT: Appleton & Lange, 1992.

Carnevali, DL, & Reiner, AC. The cancer experience: nursing diagnosis and management. Philadelphia: J.B. Lippincott Company, 1990.

Carpenito, LJ. Nursing care plans and documentation. Philadelphia: J.B. Lippincott Company, 1991.

Carpenito, LJ. Nursing diagnosis: application to clinical practice (4th ed.). Philadelphia: J.B. Lippincott Company, 1992.

Carrieri, VK, Lindsey, AM, & West, CM. Pathophysiological phenomena in nursing. Philadelphia: W.B. Saunders Company, 1986.

Clark, JC, & McGee, RF. Core curriculum for oncology nursing (2nd ed.). Philadelphia: W.B. Saunders Company, 1992.

Clark, JBF, Queener, SF, & Karb, VB. Pharmacological basis of nursing practice (4th ed.). St. Louis: Mosby, 1993.

Conn, RB. Current diagnosis. Philadelphia: W.B. Saunders Company, 1991.

Corbett, JV. Laboratory tests and diagnostic procedures with nursing diagnoses (3rd ed.). Norwalk, CT: Appleton & Lange, 1992.

Craven, RE, & Hirnle, CJ. Fundamentals of nursing: human health and function. Philadelphia: J.B. Lippincott Company, 1992.

Davies, JL, & Janosik, EH. Mental health and psychiatric nursing: a caring approach. Boston: Jones and Bartlett Publishers, 1991.

Deglin, JH, Vallerand, AH, & Russin, MM. Davis's drug guide for nurses (2nd ed.). Philadelphia: F.A. Davis Company, 1991.

Doenges, ME, Moorhouse, MF, & Geisler, AC. Nursing care plans: guidelines for planning patient care (3rd ed.). Philadelphia: F.A. Davis Company, 1993.

Dudek, SG. Nutrition handbook for nursing practice (2nd ed.). Philadelphia: J.B. Lippincott Company, 1993.

Ellis, JR, & Nowlis, EA. Nursing: a human needs approach (4th ed.). Boston: Houghton Mifflin Company, 1989.

Fishbach, F. A manual of laboratory & diagnostic tests (4th ed.). Philadelphia: J.B. Lippincott Company, 1992.

Folz, AT. The influence of cancer on self-concept and life quality. Seminars in Oncology Nursing, *3*(4):303-312, 1987.

Fortinash, KM, & Holoday-Worret, PA. Psychiatric nursing care plans. St. Louis: Mosby–Year Book, 1991.

Gilman, AG, Rall, TW, Nies, AS, & Taylor, P. Goodman and Gilman's the pharmacological basis of therapeutics (8th ed.). New York: Pergamon Press, 1990.

Glasgow, M, Halfin, V, & Althausen, AF. Sexual response and cancer. Ca-A Cancer Journal for Clinicians, *37*(6):322-333, 1987.

Gobel, BH, & Donovan, MI. Depression and anxiety. Seminars in Oncology Nursing, *3*(4):267-276, 1987.

Gordon, M. Manual of nursing diagnosis. New York: McGraw-Hill, 1991.

Groer, MW, & Shekelton, ME. Basic pathophysiology: a holistic approach (3rd ed.). St. Louis: C.V. Mosby, 1989.

Guyton, AC. Textbook of medical physiology (8th ed.). Philadelphia: W.B. Saunders Company, 1991.

Holloway, NM. Medical surgical care planning (2nd ed.). Springhouse, PA: Springhouse Corporation, 1993.

Horne, MM, Heitz, UE, & Swearingen, PL. Fluid, electrolyte, and acid-base balance. St. Louis: Mosby–Year Book, 1991.

Ignatavicius, DD, & Bayne, MV. Medical-surgical nursing: a nursing process approach. Philadelphia: W.B. Saunders Company, 1991.

Illustrated manual of nursing practice. Springhouse, PA: Springhouse Corporation, 1991.

Karch, AM. Handbook of drugs and the nursing process (2nd ed.). Philadelphia: J.B. Lippincott Company, 1992.

Kemp, BB, Pilliteri, A, & Brown, P. Fundamentals of nursing: a framework for practice (2nd ed). Glenview, IL: Scott, Foresman and Company, 1989.

Kersten, LD. Comprehensive respiratory nursing. Philadelphia: W.B. Saunders Company, 1989.

Kidd, PS, & Wagner, KD. High acuity nursing: preparing for practice in today's health care settings. Norwalk, CT: Appleton & Lange, 1992.

Kozier, B, & Erb, G. Fundamentals of nursing (4th ed.). Redwood City, CA: Addison-Wesley, 1991.

Kubler-Ross, E. On death and dying. New York: Macmillan, 1969.

Lambert, CE, Jr, & Lambert, VA. Psychosocial impacts created by chronic illness. Nursing Clinics of North America, *22*(3):527-533, 1987.

Lewis, SM, & Collier, IC. Medical-surgical nursing: assessment and management of clinical problems (3rd ed.). St. Louis: Mosby–Year Book, 1992.

Lindsey, AM. Cancer cachexia: effects of the disease and its treatment. Seminars in Oncology Nursing, *2*(1):19-29, 1986.

Loebl, S, Spratto, GR, Matejski, MP, & Woods, AL. The nurse's drug handbook (6th ed.). New York: John Wiley and Sons, 1991.

Long, BC, Phipps, WJ, & Cassmeyer, VL. Medical-surgical nursing: a nursing process approach. St. Louis: Mosby–Year Book, 1993.

Mc Caffery, M, & Beebe, A. Pain: clinical manual for nursing practice. Philadelphia: C.V. Mosby Company, 1989.

McCance, KL, & Huether, S. Pathophysiology: the biological basis for disease in adults and children. St. Louis: C.V. Mosby, 1990.

McEvoy, GK (Ed.). Drug information '93. Bethesda, MD: American Society of Hospital Pharmacists, 1993.

McFarland, GK, & McFarlane, EA. Nursing diagnosis and in-

tervention: planning for patient care (2nd ed.). St. Louis: Mosby–Year Book, 1993.
McFarland, GK, & Thomas, MD. Psychiatric mental health nursing: application of the nursing process. Philadelpia: J.B. Lippincott Company, 1991.
McFarland GK, Wasli, EL, & Gerety, EK. Nursing diagnosis and process in psychiatric mental health nursing. Philadelphia: J.B. Lippincott Company, 1992.
McNally, JC, Somerville, ET, Miaskowski, C, & Rostad, M (Eds.). Guidelines for oncology nursing practice (2nd ed.). Philadelphia: W.B. Saunders Company, 1991.
Metheny, NM. Fluid and electrolyte balance: nursing considerations (2nd ed.). Philadelphia: J.B. Lippincott Company, 1992.
Miller, BF, & Keane, CB. Encyclopedia and dictionary of medicine, nursing, and allied health (5th ed.). Philadelphia: W.B. Saunders Company, 1991.
Murray, RB, & Zentner, JP. Nursing assessment and health promotion: strategies through the health span (5th ed.). Norwalk, CT: Appleton & Lange, 1993.
Nessim, S, & Ellis, J. Cancervive: the challenge of life after cancer. Boston: Houghton Mifflin Company, 1991.
Panel for the Prediction and Prevention of Pressure Ulcers in Adults. Pressure ulcers in adults: prediction and prevention. Clinical practice guideline, number 3. AHCPR Publication No. 92-0047. Rockville, MD: Agency for Health Care Policy and Research, U.S. Department of Health and Human Services, 1992.
Paquette, M, Neal, MC, & Rodemich, C. Psychiatric nursing diagnosis care plans for dsm-III-R. Boston: Jones and Bartlett Publishers, 1991.
Patrick, ML, Woods, SL, Craven, RF, Rokosky JS, & Bruno, PM. Medical-surgical nursing: pathophysiological concepts (2nd ed.). Philadelphia: J.B. Lippincott Company, 1991.
Phipps, WJ, Long, BC, Woods, NF, & Cassmeyer, VL. Medical-surgical nursing: concepts and clinical practice (4th ed.). St. Louis: Mosby–Year Book, 1991.
Physicians' desk reference. Montvale, NJ: Medical Economics Data, 1993.
Poleman, CM, & Peckenpaugh, NJ. Nutrition: essentials and diet therapy (6th ed.). Philadelphia: W.B. Saunders Company, 1991.
Portenoy, RK. Practical aspects of pain control in the patient with cancer. Ca-A Cancer Journal for Clinicians, *38*(6):327-352, 1988.
Porth, CM. Pathophysiology: concepts of altered health states (3rd ed.). Philadelphia: J.B. Lippincott Company, 1990.
Potter, PA, & Perry, AG. Basic nursing: theory and practice (2nd ed.). St. Louis: Mosby–Year Book, 1991.
Potter, PA, & Perry, AG. Fundamentals of nursing: concepts, process, and practice (2nd ed.). St. Louis, C.V. Mosby, 1989.
Price, SA, & Wilson, LM. Pathophysiology: clinical concepts of disease processes (4th ed.). St. Louis: Mosby–Year Book, 1992.
Rakel, RE (Ed.). Conn's current therapy. Philadelphia: W.B. Saunders Company, 1993.
Raleigh, EDH. Sources of hope in chronic illness. Oncology Nursing Forum, *19*(3):443-448, 1992.
Reiss, BS, & Evans, ME. Pharmacological aspects of nursing care (4th ed.). New York: Delmar Publishers, 1993.
Sabiston, DC (Ed.). Textbook of surgery (14th ed.). Philadelphia: W.B. Saunders Company, 1991.
Schlafer, M. The nurse, pharmacology, and drug therapy: a prototype approach (2nd ed.). Redwood City, CA: Addison-Wesley Nursing, 1993.
Schwartz, SI (Ed.). Principles of surgery (5th ed.). New York: McGraw-Hill, 1989.
Shannon, MT, & Wilson, BA. Govoni & Hayes drugs and nursing implications (7th ed.). Norwalk, CT: Appleton & Lange, 1992.
Smeltzer, SC, & Bare, BG. Brunner & Suddarths textbook of medical surgical nursing (7th ed.). Philadelphia: J.B. Lippincott Company, 1992.
Smith, DB. Sexual rehabilitation of the cancer patient. Cancer Nursing, *12*(1):10-15, 1989.
Soeken, KL, & Carson, VJ. Responding to the spiritual needs of the chronically ill. Nursing Clinics of North America, *22*(3):603-610, 1987.
Spratto, GR, & Woods, AL. RN's NDR-93. Albany, NY: Delmar Publishers, 1993.
Strong, B. The view from the mattress: how to care more sensitively for your cancer patients. Nursing 92, *22*(5):46-49, 1992.
Suddarth, DS. The Lippincott manual of nursing practice (5th ed.). Philadelphia: J.B. Lippincott Company, 1991.
Swartz, MH. Textbook of physical diagnosis. Philadelphia: W.B. Saunders Company, 1989.
Swearingen, PL. The photo-atlas of nursing procedures (2nd ed.). Redwood City, CA: Addison-Wesley, 1991.
Swonger, AK, & Matejski, MP. Nursing pharmacology (2nd ed.). Philadelphia: J.B. Lippincott Company, 1991.
Taylor, C, Lillis, C, & LeMone, P. Fundamentals of nursing. Philadelphia: J.B. Lippincott Company, 1989.
Thomas, CD. Insomnia: identification and management. Seminars in Oncology Nursing, *3*(4):263-266, 1987.
Thomas, CL (Ed.). Taber's cyclopedic medical dictionary (17th ed.). Philadelphia: F.A. Davis Company, 1993.
Thompson, JM, McFarland, GK, Hirsch, JE, Tucker, SM, & Bowers, AC. Mosby's manual of clinical nursing (3rd ed.). St. Louis: Mosby–Year Book, 1993.
Tierney, LM, McPhee, SJ, Papadokis, MA, & Schroeder, SA. Current medical diagnosis and treatment. Norwalk, CT: Appleton & Lange, 1993.
Townsend, MC. Nursing diagnoses in psychiatric nursing: a pocket guide for care plan construction (2nd ed.). Philadelphia: F.A. Davis Company, 1991.
Tucker, SM, Canobbio, MM, Paquette, EV, & Wells, MF. Patient care standards (5th ed.). St. Louis: Mosby–Year Book, 1992.
United States Pharmacopeial Convention. Drug information for the health care professional (9th ed.) Harrisonburg, VA: Banta Company, 1989.
Way, LW (Ed.). Current surgical diagnosis and treatment (9th ed.). Norwalk, CT: Appleton & Lange, 1991.
Wilson, JD, Braunwald, MA, Isselbacher, KJ, et al. Harrison's principles of internal medicine (12th ed.). New York: McGraw-Hill, 1991.
Wyngaarden, JB, Smith, LH, & Bennett, JC (Eds.). Cecil textbook of medicine (19th ed.). Philadelphia: W.B. Saunders Company, 1992.

## UNIT III. Nursing Care of the Elderly Client

Andresen, GP. A fresh look at assessing the elderly. RN, *52*(6):28-39, 1989.
Bachman, GA. Sexual dysfunction in postmenopausal women: the role of medical management. Geriatrics, *43*(11):79-83, 1988.
Bender, P. Deceptive distress in the elderly. American Journal of Nursing, *92*(10):29-33, 1992.
Brocklehurst, JC, Tallis, RC, & Fillit, HM (Eds.). Textbook of geriatric medicine and gerontology (4th ed.). New York: Churchill Livingstone, 1992.
Buckwalter, KC, & Stolley, JM. Iatrogenesis in the elderly. Journal of Gerontological Nursing, *17*(9):3, 1991.
Burggraff, V, & Stanley, M. Nursing the elderly: a care plan approach. Philadelphia: J.B. Lippincott Company, 1989.
Carnevali, DL, & Patrick M (Eds.). Nursing management for the elderly (3rd ed.). Philadelphia: J.B. Lippincott Company, 1993.
Cassel, CK, Riesenberg, DE, Sorenson, LD, & Walsh, JR (Eds.). Geriatric medicine (2nd ed.). New York: Springer-Verlag, 1990.
Chenitz, WC, Stone, JT, & Salisbury, SA. Clinical gerontological nursing. Philadelphia: W.B. Saunders Company, 1991.
Daly, MP. Sleep disorders in the elderly. Primary Care, *16*(2):475-487, 1989.

Dubin, S. The physiological changes of aging. Orthopedic Nursing, *11*(3):45-50, 1992.

Ebersole, P, & Hess, P. Toward healthy aging. St. Louis: C.V. Mosby, 1990.

Eliopoulos, C. Caring for the elderly in diverse settings. Philadelphia: J.B. Lippincott Company, 1990.

Eliopoulos, C. Gerontological nursing (3rd ed.). Philadelphia: J.B. Lippincott Company, 1993.

Farrell, J. Nursing care of the older person. Philadelphia: J.B. Lippincott Company, 1990.

Foster, DC. Urinary incontinence in women, the sexual perspective. Medical Aspects of Human Sexuality, *25*(8):28-36, 1991.

Frank-Stromberg, M. Sexuality and the elderly cancer patient. Seminars in Oncology Nursing, *1*(1):49-55, 1985.

Freedham, JF. Gerontological nursing. Albany, NY: Delmar Publishers, 1993.

Funk, SG, Tornquist, EM, Champagne, MT, & Wiese, RA (Eds.). Key aspects of elder care: managing falls, incontinence, and cognitive impairment. New York: Springer Publishing Company, 1992.

Gawlinski, A, & Jensen, G. The complications of cardiovascular aging. American Journal of Nursing, *91*(11):28-31, 1991.

Gottlieb, GL. Sleep disorders and their management: special considerations in the elderly. American Journal of Medicine, *88*(3A):19S-33S, 1990.

Gray-Vickrey, M. Color them special—a sensible, sensitive guide to caring for elderly patients. Nursing 87, *17*(5):59-62, 1987.

Hoffman, S, & Platt, C. Comforting the confused: strategies for managing dementia. New York: Springer Publishing Company, 1991.

Hogstel, M. Nursing care of the older adult (2nd ed.). New York: John Wiley & Sons, 1988.

Jirovec, MM, Brink, CA, & Wells, TJ. Nursing assessments in the inpatient geriatric population. Nursing Clinics of North America, *23*(1):219-230, 1988.

Kain, CD, Reilly, N, & Schultz, ED. The older adult: a comparative assessment. Nursing Clinics of North America, *25*(4):833-848, 1990.

Kelley, LS, & Mobily, PR. Iatrogenesis in the elderly: factors of immobility. Journal of Gerontological Nursing, *17*(9):5-10, 1991.

Kelley, LS, & Mobily, PR. Iatrogenesis in the elderly: impaired skin integrity. Journal of Gerontological Nursing, *17*(9):24-29, 1991.

Lipton, HL, & Lee, RR. Drugs and the elderly: clinical, social, and policy perspectives. Stanford, CA: Stanford University Press, 1988.

Maas, M, Buckwalter, K, & Hardy, M. Nursing diagnoses and interventions for the elderly. Redwood City, CA: Addison-Wesley, 1991.

Markatz, R, & Covig, MP. Helping America take its medicine. American Journal of Nursing, *92*(6):59-62, 1992.

Masoro, EJ. Biology of aging: current state of knowledge. Archives of Internal Medicine, *147*(1):166-169, 1987.

Matteson, MA, & McConnell, ES. Gerontological nursing. Philadelphia: W.B. Saunders Company, 1988.

McCormick, KA, Scheve, AAS, & Leahy, E. Nursing management of urinary incontinence in geriatric patients. Nursing Clinics of North America, 23(1):231-264, 1988.

McCormick, KA, Newman, DK, Colling, J, & Pearson, BD. Clinical guidelines: urinary incontinence in adults. American Journal of Nursing, *92*(10):75-93, 1992.

Morrow, D. Leiter, V, Altieri, P, & Tanke, E. Elders schema for taking medication: implications for instruction design. Journal of Gerontology, *46*(6):378-385, 1991.

Needham, JF. Gerontological nursing: a restorative approach. New York: Delmar Publishers, 1993.

Ouslander, JG, & Bruskewitz, R. Disorders of micturition in the aging patient. Advances in Internal Medicine, *34*:165-190, 1989.

Palmer, MH. Incontinence: the magnitude of the problem. Nursing Clinics of North America, *23*(1):139-157, 1988.

Prinz, PN, Vitiello, MV, Raskind, MA, et al. Sleep disorders and aging. The New England Journal of Medicine, *323*(8):520-526, 1990.

Ramsey, R. Adjusting drug dosages for critically ill elderly patients. Nursing 88, *18*(7):47-49, 1988.

Rando, E. Delirium in elderly cancer patients. Dimensions in Oncology Nursing, *4*(2):5-8, 1990.

Rasin, J. Confusion. Nursing Clinics of North America, 25(4):909-918, 1990.

Reichel, W (Ed.). Clinical aspects of aging (3rd ed.). Baltimore: Williams & Wilkins, 1989.

Reilly, NJ. Urinary incontinence: new attitudes and treatment options. Innovations in Urology Nursing. *III*(2):1-15, 1992.

Ross, JER. Iatrogenesis in the elderly: contributors to falls. Journal of Gerontological Nursing, *17*(9):19-23, 1991.

Santo-Novak, DA. Seven keys to assessing the elderly. American Journal of Nursing, *18*(8):60-63, 1988.

Schwab, R, Walters, CA, & Weksler, ME. Host defense mechanisms and aging. Seminars in Oncology, *16*(1):20-27, 1989.

Thienhaus, OJ. Practical overview of sexual function and advancing age. Geriatrics, *43*(8):63-67, 1988.

Tinetti, ME, & Speechley, M. Prevention of falls among the elderly. The New England Journal of Medicine, *320*(16):1055-1059, 1989.

Vernon, MS. Urinary incontinence in the elderly. Primary Care, *16*(2):515-527, 1989.

Waltman, RE. 5 goals for managing older patients. Nursing 93, *23*(1):63-64, 1993.

Weinberger, MH. Hypertension in the elderly. Hospital Practice, *27*(5):103-108, 110, 115+, 1992.

Welch-McCaffrey, D, & Dodge, J. Acute confusional states in elderly cancer patients. Seminars in Oncology Nursing, *4*(3):208-216, 1988.

Westfall, LK, & Pavlis, RW. Why the elderly are so vulnerable to drug reactions. RN, *50*(11):39-43, 1987.

Wyman, JF. Nursing assessment of the incontinent geriatric outpatient population. Nursing Clinics of North America, *23*(1):169-187, 1988.

## UNIT IV. Nursing Care of the Client Having Surgery

### *IV.2. Postoperative Care*

Bowell, B. Infection control: protecting the patient at risk. Nursing Times, *88*(3):32-35, 1992.

Bowen, KJ, & Vukelja, SJ. Hypercoagulable states: their cause and management. Postgraduate Medicine, *91*(3):117-118, 123, 125, 128, 131-132, 1992.

Herron, DG. Strategies for promoting a healthy dietary intake. Nursing Clinics of North America, *26*(4):875-884, 1991.

Hinojosa, RJ. Nursing interventions to prevent or relieve postoperative nausea and vomiting. Journal of Post Anesthesia Nursing, *7*(1):3-14, 1992.

Jackson, MM. Infection prevention and control. Critical Care Nursing Clinics of North America, *4*(3):401-409, 1992.

Lawler, M. Preventing postop complications: managing other complications. Nursing 91, *21*(11):40-46, 1991.

Loogman, EA. Nutritional assessment in nursing. Gastroenterology Nursing, *14*(4):189-194, 1992.

McConnell, EA. Preventing postop complications: minimizing respiratory problems. Nursing 91, *21*(11):34-39, 1991.

Meehan, M. Nursing diagnosis: potential for aspiration. RN, *55*(1):30-35, 1992.

O'Donohue, WJ. Postoperative pulmonary complications. Postgraduate Medicine, *91*(3):167-170+, 1992.

Peden, L. Helping postoperative patients sleep. RN, *55*(4):24-26, 1992.

Provine, B. Pulmonary aspiration: recognition and treatment. Journal of Post Anesthesia Nursing, *7*(3):217, 1992.

Walsh, J. Postop effects of OR positioning. RN, *56*(2):50-57, 1993.

## UNIT V. Nursing Care of the Immobile Client

Corcoran, PJ. Use it or lose it—the hazards of bed rest and inactivity. Western Journal of Medicine, *154*(5):536-538, 1991.

Holm, K, & Hendricks, C. Immobility and bone loss in the aging adult. Critical Care Nursing Quarterly, *12*(1):46-50, 1989.

Mobily, PR, & Kelley, LS. Iatrogenesis in the elderly: factors of immobility. Journal of Gerontological Nursing, *17*(9):5-10, 1991.

Olson, EV. The hazards of immobility. American Journal of Nursing, *90*(3):43-44, 46-48, 1990.

## UNIT VI. Nursing Care of the Client Who is Dying

Alexander, J, & Kiely, J. Working with the bereaved. Geriatric Nursing, *7*(2):85-86, 1986.

Amenta, MO, & Bohnet, NL. Nursing care of the terminally ill. Boston: Little, Brown & Company, 1986.

Archer, DN, & Smith, AC. Sorrow has many faces: helping families cope with grief. Nursing 88, *18*(5):43-45, 1988.

Benoliel, JQ. Loss and terminal illness. Nursing Clinics of North America, *20*(2):439-448, 1985.

Bledsoe, AS, & Krueger, NJ. Dying patients: caring makes the difference. Nursing 87, *17*(6):44-45, 1987.

Blues, AG, & Zerwekh, JV. Hospice and palliative nursing care. Orlando, FL: Grune & Stratton, Inc., 1984.

Conrad, NL. Spiritual support for the dying. Nursing Clinics of North America, *20*(2):415-426, 1985.

Dufault, K, & Martocchio, BC. Hope: its spheres and dimensions. Nursing Clinics of North America, *20*(2):379-391, 1985.

Foos-Graber, A. Deathing. York Beach, Maine: Nicholas-Harp, 1989.

Gifford, BJ, & Cleary, BB. Supporting the bereaved. American Journal of Nursing, *90*(2):49-53, 1990.

Granstrom, S. Spiritual nursing care for oncology patients. Topics in Clinical Nursing, *7*(1):39-45, 1985.

Kübler-Ross, E. Death: the final stage of growth. Englewood Cliffs, NJ: Prentice-Hall, 1975.

Martinez, J, & Wagner, S. Hospice care. In Groenwald, SL, Frogge, MH, Goodman, M, & Yarbro, CH (Eds.), Cancer nursing: principles and practice (3rd ed.). Boston: Jones and Bartlett Publishers, 1993, pp. 1432-1450.

Martocchio, BC. Grief and bereavement. Nursing Clinics of North America, *20*(2):327-341, 1985.

Miller, JF. Inspiring hope. American Journal of Nursing, *85*(1):23-25, 1985.

Moseley, JR. Alterations in comfort. Nursing Clinics of North America, *20*(2):427-438, 1985.

Murphy, P. Studies of loss and grief. American Journal of Hospice Care, *2*(2):10-14, 1985.

Murphy, P. Pastoral care and persons with AIDS—a means to alleviate physical, emotional, social, and spiritual suffering. American Journal of Hospice Care, *3*(2):38-40, 1986.

Peterson, EA. How to meet your client's spiritual needs. Journal of Psychosocial Nursing, *25*(5):34-39, 1987.

Reuben, D, & Mor, V. Dyspnea in terminally ill cancer patients. Chest, *89*(2):234-236, 1986.

Schneider, M, & Bernard, J. Midwives to the dying. Portland, Oregon: Angels' Work, 1992.

Twycross, RG. The management of pain in cancer: a guide to drugs and dosages. Oncology, *2*(4):35-43, 1988.

Tyner, R. Elements of empathic care for dying patients and their families. Nursing Clinics of North America, *20*(2):393-401, 1985.

Ufema, J. Insights on death and dying. Nursing 88, *18*(11):93-94, 1988.

Ufema, J. Meeting the challenge of a dying patient. Nursing 91, *21*(2):42-46, 1991.

Ufema, JK. How to talk to dying patients. Nursing 87, *17*(8):43-46, 1987.

Vastiyan, EA. Spiritual aspects of the care of cancer patients. Cancer, *36*(2):110-114, 1986.

Whelan, E. Support for the survivor. Geriatric Nursing, *6*(1):21-23, 1985.

Zack, MV. Loneliness: a concept relevant to the care of dying persons. Nursing Clinics of North America, *20*(2):403-414, 1985.

Zerwekh, JV. Comforting the dying, dyspneic patient. Nursing 87, *17*(11):66-69, 1987.

Zerwekh, JV. Home care of the dying. In Martinson, I. & Widmer, A (Eds.), Home health care nursing. Philadelphia: W.B. Saunders Company, 1989, pp. 217-236.

Zerwekh, JV. Supportive care of the dying patient. In Baird, SB, McCorkle, R, & Grant, M (Eds.), Cancer nursing. Philadelphia: W.B. Saunders Company, 1991, pp. 875-884.

## UNIT VII. Nursing Care of the Client Receiving Treatment for Neoplastic Disorders

### *VII. 1. Brachytherapy*

Brandt, B, & Garney, J. An overview of interstitial brachytherapy and hyperthermia. Oncology Nursing Forum, *16*(6):833-844, 1989.

Bruner, DW, Iwamoto, R, Keane, K, & Strohl, R (Eds.). Manual for radiation oncology nursing practice and education. Pittsburgh: Oncology Nursing Society, 1992.

Bucholtz, JD. Implications of radiation therapy for nursing. In Clark, JC, & McGee, RF (Eds.), Core curriculum for oncology nursing (2nd ed.). Philadelphia: W.B. Saunders Company, 1992, pp. 319-328.

Clark, DH, & Martinez, A. An overview of brachytherapy in cancer management. Oncology, *4*(9):39-46, 1990.

Dow, KH, and Hilderly, LJ. Nursing care in radiation oncology. Philadelphia: W.B. Saunders Company, 1992.

Glasgow, GP, & Perez, CA. Physics of brachytherapy. In Perez, CA, & Brady, LW (Eds.), Principles and practice of radiation oncology (2nd ed.). Philadelphia: W.B. Saunders Company, 1992, pp. 265-299.

Glicksman, A. Radiobiologic basis of brachytherapy. Seminars in Oncology Nursing, *3*(1):3-6, 1987.

Hassey, K. Demystifying care of patients with radioactive implants. American Journal of Nursing, *85*(7):788-792, 1985.

Hellman, S. Principles of radiation therapy. In DeVita, VT, Jr, Hellman, S, & Rosenberg, SA (Eds.), Cancer: principles and practice of oncology (4th ed.). Philadelphia: J.B. Lippincott Company, 1993, pp. 248-275.

Henrick-Rynning, T. Prostatic cancer treatments and their effects on sexual functioning. Oncology Nursing Forum, *14*(6):37-41, 1987.

Hilderly, LJ. Radiotherapy. In Groenwald, SL, Frogge, MH, Goodman, M, & Yarbro, CH (Eds.), Cancer nursing: principles and practice (3rd ed.). Boston: Jones and Bartlett Publishers, 1993, pp. 235-269.

Hilderly, LJ, & Dow, KH. Radiation oncology. In Baird, SB, McCorkle, R, & Grant, M (Eds.), Cancer nursing: a comprehensive textbook. Philadelphia: W.B. Saunders Company, 1991, pp. 246-265.

Jenkins, B. Sexual healing after pelvic irradiation. American Journal of Nursing, *6*(8):920-922, 1986.

Jordan, L, & Buck, S. A teaching booklet for patients receiving high dose rate brachytherapy. Oncology Nursing Forum, *18*(7):1235-1238, 1991.

Jordan, L, & Mentrovadi, R. Nursing care of patients receiving high dose rate brachytherapy. Oncology Nursing Forum, *18*(7):1167-1172, 1991.

Maddock, PG. Brachytherapy sources and applicators. Seminars in Oncology Nursing, *3*(1):15-22, 1987.

Perez, CA, Garcia, DM, Grigsby, PW, & Williamson, J. Clinical applications of brachytherapy. In Perez, CA, & Brady, LW (Eds.), Principles and practice of radiation oncology (2nd ed.). Philadelphia: W.B. Saunders Company, 1992, pp. 300-367.

Randall, TM, Drake, DK, & Sewchand, W. Neuro-oncology update: radiation safety and nursing care during interstitial

brachytherapy. Journal of Neuroscience Nursing, *19*(6):315-320, 1987.
Richards, S, & Hiratzka, S. Vaginal dilatation post pelvic irradiation: a patient education tool. Oncology Nursing Forum *13*(4):89-91, 1986.
Rotman, M, & Torpie, RJ. Supportive care in radiation oncology. In Perez, CA, & Brady, LW (Eds.), Principles and practice of radiation oncology (2nd ed.). Philadelphia: W.B. Saunders Company, 1992, pp. 1508-1516.
Shell, JA, & Carter, J. The gynecological implant patient. Seminars in Oncology Nursing, *3*(1):54-66, 1987.
Strohl, RA. Head and neck implants. Seminars in Oncology Nursing, *3*(1):30-46, 1987.
Strohl, R. The nursing role in radiation oncology: symptom management of acute and chronic reactions. Oncology Nursing Forum, *15*(4):429-434, 1988.
Witt, ME, McDonald-Lynch, A, & Grimmer, D. Adjuvant radiotherapy to the colorectum. Oncology Nursing Forum, *14*(3):17-21, 1987.

### *VII.2 Chemotherapy*

Aistars, J. Fatigue in the cancer patient: a conceptual approach to a clinical problem. Oncology Nursing Forum, *14*(6):25-35, 1987.
Averette, HE, Boike, GM, & Jarrell, MA. Effects of cancer chemotherapy on gonadal function and reproductive capacity. Ca-A Cancer Journal for Clinicians, *40*(4):199-209, 1990.
Baird, SB, McCorkle, R, & Grant, M (Eds.). Cancer nursing: a comprehensive textbook. Philadelphia: W.B. Saunders Company, 1991.
Barry, SA. Septic shock: special needs of patients with cancer. Oncology Nursing Forum, *16*(1):31-35, 1989.
Basch, A. Changes in elimination. Seminars in Oncology Nursing, *3*(4):287-292, 1987.
Beck, SL. Prevention and management of oral complications in the cancer patient. In Hubbard, SL, Greene, PE, & Knobf, MT (Eds.), Current issues in cancer nursing practice updates, *1*(6). Philadelphia: J.B. Lippincott Company, 1992, pp. 1-12.
Belcher, AE. Nursing aspects of quality of life enhancement in cancer patients. Oncology, *4*(5):197-199, 1990.
Bertino, JR, & O'Keefe, P. Barriers and strategies for effective chemotherapy. Seminars in Oncology Nursing, *8*(2):77-82, 1992.
Brandt, B. Nursing protocol for the patient with neutropenia. Oncology Nursing Forum, *17*(1)Supplement:9-15, 1990.
Brown, MH, Kiss, ME, Outlaw, EM, & Viamontes, CM. Standards of oncology nursing practice. New York: John Wiley & Sons, 1986.
Burke, MB, Wilkes, GM, Berg, D, Bean, CK, & Ingwersen, K. Cancer chemotherapy: a nursing process approach. Boston: Jones and Bartlett Publishers, 1991.
Camp, LD. Care of the groshong catheter. Oncology Nursing Forum, *15*(6):745-749, 1988.
Camp-Sorrell, D. Controlling adverse effects of chemotherapy. Nursing 91, *21*(4):34-41, 1991.
Chabner, BA, & Collins, JM (Eds.). Cancer chemotherapy: principles and practice. Philadelphia: J.B. Lippincott Company, 1990.
Clark, RA, Tyson, LB, Gralla, RJ, & Kris, MG. Antiemetic therapy: management of chemotherapy-induced nausea and vomiting. Seminars in Oncology Nursing, *5*(2) Supplement 1:53-57, 1989.
Cotanch, PM, & Strum, S. Progressive muscle relaxation for antiemetic therapy for cancer therapy. Oncology Nursing Forum, *14*(1):33-37, 1987.
Cushman, KE. Symptom management: a comprehensive approach to increasing nutritional status in the cancer patient. Seminars in Oncology Nursing, *2*(1):30-35, 1986.
D'Agostino, NS. Managing nutrition problems in advanced cancer. American Journal of Nursing, *89*(1):50-56, 1989.
DeVita, VT, Jr. Principles of chemotherapy. In DeVita, VT, Jr, Hellman, S, & Rosenberg, SA (Eds.), Cancer: principles and practice of oncology (4th ed.). Philadelphia: J.B. Lippincott Company, 1993, pp. 276-292.
DiJulio, J. Hematopoiesis: an overview. Oncology Nursing Forum, *18*(2) Supplement: 3-6, 1991.
Duigon, A. Anticipatory nausea and vomiting associated with cancer chemotherapy. Oncology Nursing Forum, *13*(1):35-40, 1986.
Engelking, CE. Managing stomatitis: a nursing process approach. In Supportive care for the cancer patient. A.H. Robins Company, 1988, pp. 20-28.
Eriksson, JH, & Swenson, KK. Your guide to intraperitoneal chemotherapy. Oncology Nursing Forum, *13*(5):77-81, 1986.
Feldman, JE. Ovarian failure and cancer treatment: incidence and interventions for the premenopausal woman. Oncology Nursing Forum, *16*(5):651-657, 1989.
Finley, RS. Drug interactions in the oncology patient. Seminars in Oncology Nursing, *8*(2):95-101, 1992.
Foley, KM. The treatment of pain in the patient with cancer. Ca-A Cancer Journal for Clinicians, *36*(4):194-215, 1986.
Germino, BB. Symptom distress and quality of life. Seminars in Oncology Nursing, *3*(4):299-302, 1987.
Glaspy, JA, & Golde, DW. The colony-stimulating factors: biology and clinical use. Oncology, *4*(9):25-33, 1990.
Goodman, M. External venous catheters: home management. Oncology Nursing Forum, *15*(3):357-360, 1988.
Goodman, M. Managing the side effects of chemotherapy. Seminars in Oncology Nursing, *5*(2) Supplement 1:29-52, 1989.
Grady, C. Host defense mechanisms: an overview. Seminars in Oncology Nursing, *4*(2):86-94, 1988.
Grant, M. Nausea, vomiting, and anorexia. Seminars in Oncology Nursing, *3*(4):277-286, 1987.
Grant, MM. Nutritional interventions: increasing oral intake. Seminars in Oncology Nursing, *2*(1):36-43, 1986.
Groenwald, SL, Frogge, MH, Goodman, M, & Yarbro, CH (Eds.). Cancer nursing: principles and practice (3rd ed.). Boston: Jones and Bartlett Publishers, 1993.
Gulatte, MM, & Graves, T. Advances in antineoplastic therapy. Oncology Nursing Forum, *17*(6):867-876, 1990.
Gurevich, I, & Tafuro, P. The compromised host—deficit-specific infection and the spectrum of prevention. Cancer Nursing, 9(5):263-275, 1986.
Hagle, M. Implantable devices for chemotherapy: access and delivery. Seminars in Oncology Nursing, *3*(2):96-105, 1987.
Haeuber, D. Future strategies in the control of myelosuppression: the use of colony-stimulating factors. Oncology Nursing Forum, *18*(2):16-21, 1991.
Hagopian, GA. Cognitive strategies used in adapting to a cancer diagnosis. Oncology Nursing Forum, *20*(11):759-763, 1993.
Henrick-Rynning, T. Prostatic cancer treatments and their effects on sexual functioning. Oncology Nursing Forum, *14*(6):37-41, 1987.
Hoff, S. Concepts in intraperitoneal chemotherapy. Seminars in Oncology Nursing, *3*(2):112-117, 1987.
Hogan, CM. Advances in the management of nausea and vomiting. Nursing Clinics of North America, *25*(2):475-497, 1990.
Holden, S, & Felde, G. Nursing care of patients experiencing cisplatin-related peripheral neuropathy. Oncology Nursing Forum *14*(1):13-19, 1987.
Holroyde, CP, & Reichard, GA, Jr. General metabolic abnormalities in cancer patients: anorexia and cachexia. Surgical Clinics of North America, *66*(5):947-956, 1986.
Keller, JF, & Blausey, LA. Nursing issues and management in chemotherapy-induced alopecia. Oncology Nursing Forum, *15*(5):603-607, 1988.
Kurzer, M, & Meguid, MM. Cancer and protein metabolism. Surgical Clinics of North America, *66*(5):969-1001, 1986.
Lamb, MA. Psychosexual issues: the woman with gynecologic cancer. Seminars in Oncology Nursing, *6*(3):237-243, 1990.
Lambert, CE, Jr, & Lambert, VA. Psychosocial impacts created by chronic illness. Nursing Clinics of North America, *22*(3):527-533, 1987.

Lindsey, AM. Cancer cachexia: effects of the disease and its treatment. Seminars in Oncology Nursing, *2*(1):19-29, 1986.

Lucas, AB. A critical review of venous access devices: the nursing perspective. In Hubbard, SM, Greene, PE, & Knobf, MT (Eds.), Current issues in cancer nursing practice updates, *1*(7). Philadelphia: J.B. Lippincott Company, 1992, pp. 1-10.

Martocchio, BC. Family coping: helping families help themselves. Seminars in Oncology Nursing, *1*(4):292-297, 1985.

Maxwell, MB, & Maher, KE. Chemotherapy-induced myelosuppression. Seminars in Oncology Nursing, *8*(2):113-123, 1992.

McAndrew, PF. Fat metabolism and cancer. Surgical Clinics of North America, *66*(5):1003-1012, 1986.

McAnena, OJ, & Daly, JM. Impact of antitumor therapy on nutrition. Surgical Clinics of North America, *66*(6):1213-1228, 1986.

McVey, L. A direct assault on abdominal cancer. RN, *55*(2):46-52, 1992.

Meehan, JL, & Johnson, BL. The neurotoxicity of antineoplastic agents. In Hubbard, SM, Greene, PE, & Knobf, MT (Eds.), Current issues in cancer nursing practice updates, *1*(8). Philadelphia: J.B. Lippincott Company, 1992, pp. 1-11.

Montrose, P. Extravasation management. Seminars in Oncology Nursing, *3*(2):128-132, 1987.

Morrow, GR. Chemotherapy-related nausea and vomiting: etiology and management. Ca-A Cancer Journal for Clinicians, *39*(2):89-104, 1989.

Meyerowitz, BE, Heinrich, RL, & Schag, CAC. Helping patients cope with cancer. Oncology, *3*(11):120-129, 1989.

Nail, LM, & King, KB. Fatigue. Seminars in Oncology Nursing, *3*(4):257-262, 1987.

Oncology Nursing Society. Cancer chemotherapy guidelines, modules 1 & 2. Pittsburgh: Oncology Nursing Society, 1988.

O'Rourke, ME. Enhanced cutaneous effects in combined modality therapy. Oncology Nursing Forum, *14*(6):31-35, 1987.

Padilla, GV. Psychological aspects of nutrition and cancer. Surgical Clinics of North America, *66*(6):1121-1135, 1986.

Pervan, V. Practical aspects of dealing with cancer-therapy induced nausea and vomiting. Seminars in Oncology Nursing, *6*(4)Supplement 1:3-5, 1990.

Piper, BF, Lindsey, AM, & Dodd, MJ. Fatigue mechanisms in cancer patients. Oncology Nursing Forum, *14*(6):17-23, 1987.

Redd, WH. Behavioral approaches to treatment-related distress. Ca-A Cancer Journal for Clinicians, *38*(3):138-145, 1988.

Rostad, ME. Nursing care of the myelosuppressed cancer patient. In Supportive care for the cancer patient. A.H. Robins Company, 1988, pp. 14-19.

Schlesselman, SM. Helping your cancer patient cope with alopecia. Nursing 88, *18*(12):43-45, 1988.

Shapiro, T. How to help patients get through chemotherapy. RN, *50*(3):58-60, 1987.

Skalla, KA, & LaCasse, C. Patient education for fatigue. Oncology Nursing Forum, *19*(10):1537-1541, 1992.

Smith, D. Sexual rehabilitation of the cancer patient. Cancer Nursing, *12*(1):10-15, 1989.

Smith, DB, & Babaian, RJ. The effects of treatment for cancer on male fertility and sexuality. Cancer Nursing, *15*(4):271-275, 1992.

Smith, K, & Lesko, LM. Psychosocial problems in cancer survivors. Oncology, *2*(1):33-40, 1988.

Strohl, R. Understanding taste changes. Oncology Nursing Forum, *11*(3):81-84, 1984.

Stuckey, LA. Acute tumor lysis syndrome: assessment and nursing implications. Oncology Nursing Forum, *20*(1):49-57, 1993.

Swenson, KK, & Eriksson, JH. Nursing management of intraperitoneal chemotherapy. Oncology Nursing Forum, *13*(5):33-39, 1986.

Tait, N, & Aisner, J. Nutritional concerns in cancer patients. Seminars in Oncology Nursing, *5*(2)Supplement 1:58-62, 1989.

Tchekmedyian, NS, Hickman, M, Siau, J, et al. Treatment of cancer anorexia with megestrol acetate: impact on quality of life. Oncology, *4*(5):185-192, 1990.

Tenenbaum, L. Cancer chemotherapy: a reference guide. Philadelphia: W.B. Saunders Company, 1989.

Thomas, CD. Insomnia: identification and management. Seminars in Oncology Nursing, *3*(4):263-266, 1987.

Thomason, SS. Using a groshong central venous catheter. Nursing 91, *21*(10):58-60, 1991.

Wickham, R. Managing chemotherapy-related nausea and vomiting: the state of the art. Oncology Nursing Forum, *16*(4):563-574, 1989.

Wickham, R, Purl, S, & Welker, D. Long-term central venous catheters: issues for care. Seminars in Oncology Nursing, *8*(2):133-147, 1992.

Wilding, G, Caruso, R, Lawrence, T, Ostchega, Y, Ballintine, EJ, Young, RC, & Ozols, RJ. Retinal toxicity after high-dose cisplatinum therapy. Journal of Clinical Oncology, *3*(12):1683-1689, 1985.

Wood, LS, & Gullo, SM. IV vesicants: how to avoid extravasation. American Journal of Nursing, *93*(4):42-46, 1993.

Woods, NF, Lewis, FM, & Ellison, ES. Living with cancer: family experiences. Cancer Nursing, *12*(1):28-33, 1989.

Workman, M, Ellenhorst-Ryan, J, & Hargrave-Koertge, V. Nursing care of the immunocompromised patient. Philadelphia: W.B. Saunders Company, 1993.

Wujcik, D. Overview of colony-stimulating factors: focus on the neutrophil. In Carroll-Johnson, RM (Ed.), A case management approach to patients receiving G-CSF. Oncology Nursing Press, 1992, pp. 8-13.

Wujcik, D. Current research in side effects of high-dose chemotherapy. Seminars in Oncology Nursing, *8*(2):102-112, 1992.

Yasko, JM (Ed.). Nursing management of symptoms associated with chemotherapy. Columbus, OH: Adria Laboratories, 1986.


### *VII.3 External Radiation Therapy*


Aistars, J. Fatigue in the cancer patient: a conceptual approach to a clinical problem. Oncology Nursing Forum, *14*(6):25-35, 1987.

Baird, SB, McCorkle, R, & Grant, M (Eds.). Cancer nursing: a comprehensive textbook. Philadelphia: W.B. Saunders Company, 1991.

Basch, A. Changes in elimination. Seminars in Oncology Nursing, *3*(4):287-292, 1987.

Beck, SL. Prevention and management of oral complications in the cancer patient. In Hubbard, SM, Greene, PE, & Knobf, MT (Eds.), Current issues in cancer nursing practice updates, *1*(6). Philadelphia: J.B. Lippincott Company, 1992, pp. 1-12.

Belcher, AE. Nursing aspects of quality of life enhancement in cancer patients. Oncology, *4*(5):197-199, 1990.

Bruner, DK, Iwamoto, R, Keane, K, & Strohl, R (Eds.). Manual for radiation oncology nursing practice and education. Oncology Nursing Society, 1992.

Cushman, KE. Symptom management: a comprehensive approach to increasing nutritional status in the cancer patient. Seminars in Oncology Nursing, *2*(1):30-35, 1986.

D'Agostino, NS. Managing nutrition problems in advanced cancer. American Journal of Nursing, *89*(1):50-56, 1989.

Dangel, RB. Pruritus and cancer. Oncology Nursing Forum, *13*(1):17-21, 1986.

Dow, KH, & Hilderly, LJ. Nursing care in radiation oncology. Philadelphia: W.B. Saunders Company, 1992.

Dudjak, L. Mouth care for mucositis due to radiation therapy. Cancer Nursing, *10*(3):131-140, 1987.

Foley, KM. The treatment of pain in the patient with cancer. Ca-A Cancer Journal for Clinicians, *36*(4):194-215, 1986.

Germino, BB. Symptom distress and quality of life. Seminars in Oncology Nursing, *3*(4):299-302, 1987.

Grady, C. Host defense mechanisms: an overview. Seminars in Oncology Nursing, *4*(2):86-94, 1988.

Grant, M. Nausea, vomiting, and anorexia. Seminars in Oncology Nursing, *3*(4):277-286, 1987.

Groenwald, SL, Frogge, MH, Goodman, M, & Yarbro, CH (Eds.). Cancer nursing: principles and practice (3rd ed.). Boston: Jones and Bartlett Publishers, 1993.

Hagopian, GA. Cognitive strategies used in adapting to a cancer diagnosis. Oncology Nursing Forum, *20*(5):759-763, 1993.

Hassey, KM. Radiation therapy for rectal cancer and the implications for nursing. Cancer Nursing, *10*(6):311-318, 1987.

Hassey, KM. Principles of radiation safety and protection. Seminars in Oncology Nursing, *3*(1):23-29, 1987.

Hassey, K, & Rose, C. Altered skin integrity in patients receiving radiation therapy. Oncology Nursing Forum, *13*(4):81-89, 1986.

Hellman, S. Principles of radiation therapy. In DeVita, VT, Jr, Hellman, S, & Rosenberg, S (Eds.), Cancer: principles and practices of oncology (4th ed.). Philadelphia: J.B. Lippincott Company, 1993, pp. 248-275.

Henrick-Rynning, T. Prostatic cancer treatments and their effects on sexual functioning. Oncology Nursing Forum, *14*(6):37-41, 1989.

Hogan, CM. Advances in the management of nausea and vomiting. Nursing Clinics of North America, *25*(2):475-497, 1990.

Holroyde, CP, & Reichard, GA, Jr. General metabolic abnormalities in cancer patients: anorexia and cachexia. Surgical Clinics of North America, *66*(5):947-956, 1986.

Jenkins, B. Sexual healing after pelvic irradiation. American Journal of Nursing, *86*(8):920-922, 1986.

Johnson, JE, Lauver, D, & Nail, LM. Process of coping with radiation therapy. Journal of Consulting and Clinical Psychology, *57*(3):358-364, 1989.

Kurzer, M, & Meguid, MM. Cancer and protein metabolism. Surgical Clinics of North America, *66*(5):969-1001, 1986.

Lamb, MA. Psychosexual issues: the woman with gynecologic cancer. Seminars in Oncology Nursing, *6*(3):237-243, 1990.

Lambert, CE, Jr, & Lambert, VA. Psychosocial impacts created by chronic illness. Nursing Clinics of North America, *22*(3):527-533, 1987.

Lewis, FL, & Levita, M. Understanding radiotherapy. Cancer Nursing, *11*(3):174-185, 1988.

Lindsey, AM. Cancer cachexia: effects of the disease and its treatment. Seminars in Oncology Nursing, *2*(1):19-29, 1986.

Martocchio, BC. Family coping: helping families help themselves. Seminars in Oncology Nursing, *1*(4):292-297, 1985.

McAndrew, PF. Fat metabolism and cancer. Surgical Clinics of North America, *66*(5):1003-1012, 1986.

McAnena, OJ, & Daly, JM. Impact of antitumor therapy on nutrition. Surgical Clinics of North America, *66*(6):1213-1228, 1986.

Nail, LM, & King, KB. Fatigue. Seminars in Oncology Nursing, *3*(4):257-262, 1987.

O'Rourke, ME. Enhanced cutaneous effects in combined modality therapy. Oncology Nursing Forum, *14*(6):31-35, 1987.

Padilla, GV. Psychological aspects of nutrition and cancer. Surgical Clinics of North America, *66*(6):1121-1135, 1986.

Perez, C, & Brady, L (Eds.). Principles and practices of radiation oncology (2nd ed.). Philadelphia: W.B. Saunders Company, 1992.

Piper, BF, Lindsay, AM, & Dodd, MJ. Fatigue mechanisms in cancer patients: developing nursing theory. Oncology Nursing Forum, 14(6):17-23, 1987.

Richards, S, & Hiratzka, S. Vaginal dilatation post pelvic irradiation: a patient education tool. Oncology Nursing Forum, *13*(4):89-91, 1986.

Rotman, M, & Torpie, RJ. Supportive care in radiation oncology. In Perez, CA, & Brady, LW (Eds.), Principles and practice of radiation oncology (2nd ed.). Philadelphia: W.B. Saunders Company, 1992, pp. 1508-1516.

Sitton, E. Early and late radiation-induced skin alterations, part 1: mechanisms of skin changes. Oncology Nursing Forum, *19*(5):801-807, 1992.

Skalla, KA, & LaCasse, C. Patient education for fatigue. Oncology Nursing Forum, *19*(10):1537-1541, 1992.

Smith, D. Sexual rehabilitation of the cancer patient. Cancer Nursing, *12*(1):10-15, 1989.

Smith, DB, & Babaian, RJ. The effects of treatment for cancer on male fertility and sexuality. Cancer Nursing, *15*(4):271-275, 1992.

Smith, K, & Lesko, LM. Psychosocial problems in cancer survivors. Oncology, *2*(1):33-40, 1988.

Strohl, R. The nursing role in radiation oncology: symptom management of acute and chronic reactions. Oncology Nursing Forum, *15*(4):429-434, 1988.

Strohl, R. Understanding taste changes. Oncology Nursing Forum, *11*(3):81-84, 1984.

Tchekmedyian, NS, Hickman, M, Siau, J, et al. Treatment of cancer anorexia with megestrol acetate: impact on quality of life. Oncology, *4*(5):185-192, 1990.

Thomas, CD. Insomnia: identification and management. Seminars in Oncology Nursing, *3*(4):262-266, 1987.

Witt, ME. Questions on colon and rectum radiation therapy. Oncology Nursing Forum, *14*(3):79-82, 1987.

Witt, ME, McDonald-Lynch, A, & Grimmer, D. Adjuvant radiotherapy to the colorectum: nursing implications. Oncology Nursing Forum, *14*(3):17-21, 1987.

Woods, NF, Lewis, FM, & Ellison, ES. Living with cancer: family experiences. Cancer Nursing, *12*(1):28-33, 1989.

Workman, M, Ellenhorst-Ryan, J, & Hargrave-Koertge, V. Nursing care of the immunocompromised patient. Philadelphia: W.B. Saunders Company, 1993.


## UNIT VIII. Nursing Care of the Client with Disturbances of Neurological Function

### *VIII.1. Cerebrovascular Accident*


Boss, BJ. Managing communication disorders in stroke. Nursing Clinics of North America, *26*(4):985-996, 1991.

Bronstein, KS. Psychosocial components in stroke: implications for adaptation. Nursing Clinics of North America, *26*(4):1007-1017, 1991.

Cammermeyer, M, & Appeldron, C (Eds.). Core curriculum for neuroscience nursing (3rd ed.). Chicago: American Association of Neuroscience Nurses, 1990.

Dilorio, C, & Price, ME. Swallowing: an assessment guide. American Journal of Nursing, *90*(7):38-41, 1990.

Fayad, PB, & Brass, LM. How to evaluate patients and recognize complications. Consultant, *31*(1):30-34, 1991.

Fayad, PB, & Brass, LM. How to treat patients with acute ischemic infarction. Consultant, *31*(1):39-43, 1991.

Gross, JC. Bladder dysfunction after stroke. Urological Nursing, *12*(2):55-65, 1992.

Hickey, JV. The clinical practice of neurological and neurosurgical nursing (3rd ed.). Philadelphia: J.B. Lippincott Company, 1992.

Kane-Carlsen, PA. Managing patients with T.I.A.s. Nursing 92, *22*(1):34-39, 1992.

Leahy, NM. Complications in the acute stages of stroke: nursing's pivotal role. Nursing Clinics of North America, *26*(4):971-983, 1991.

Marshall, SB, Marshall, LF, Vos, HR, & Chesnut, RM. Neuroscience critical care: pathophysiology and patient management. Philadelphia: W.B. Saunders Company, 1990.

Pharmaceutical update . . . treating delayed cerebral ischemia. AXON, *13*(3):95, 1992.

Phipps, MA. Assessment of neurologic deficits in stroke: acute-care and rehabilitation implications. Nursing Clinics of North America, *26*(4):957-970, 1991.

Snyder, M. A guide to neurological and neurosurgical nursing (2nd ed.). Albany, NY: Delmar Publishers, 1991.

***VIII.2. Craniocerebral Trauma***

Aumick, JE. Head trauma: guidelines for care. RN, *54*(4):26-32, 1991.

Cammermeyer, M, & Appeldorn, C (Eds.). Core curriculum for neuroscience nursing (3rd ed.). Chicago: American Association of Neuroscience Nurses, 1990.

Godbole, KB, Berbiglia, VA, and Goddard, L. A head-injured patient: caloric needs, clinical progress and nursing care priorities. Journal of Neuroscience Nursing, *23*(5):290-294, 1992.

Gronwall, D, Wrightson, P, & Waddell, P. Head injury—the facts: a guide for family and care-givers. New York: Oxford University Press, 1990.

Hall, M, Brandys, C, & Yetman, L. Multidisciplinary approaches to management of head injury. Journal of Neuroscience Nursing, *24*(4):199-204, 1992.

Hickey, JV. The clinical practice of neurological and neurosurgical nursing (3rd ed.). Philadelphia: J.B. Lippincott Company, 1992.

Katz, DI. Neuropathology and neurobehavioral recovery from closed head injury. Journal of Head Trauma Rehabilitation, *7*(2):1-15, 1992.

Maroon, JC, Bailes, JE, Yates, A, and Norwig, J. Assessing closed head injuries. The Physician and Sports Medicine, *20*(4):37-44, 1992.

Marshall, SB, Marshall, LF, Vos, HR, & Chesnut, RM. Neuroscience critical care: pathophysiology and patient management. Philadelphia: W.B. Saunders Company, 1990.

O'Hara, CC, & Harrell, M. Rehabilitation with brain injury survivors. Gaithersburg, MD: Aspen Publishers, 1991.

Rosenthal, M, Griffity, EK, Bond, MR, & Miller, JD. Rehabilitation of the adult and child with traumatic brain injury (2nd ed.). Philadelphia: F.A. Davis Company, 1990.

Rosenwasser RH. Critical care management of head injury. Trauma Quarterly, *8*(2):30-57, 1992.

Segatore, M. Fever after traumatic brain injury. Journal of Neuroscience Nursing, *24*(2):104-109, 1992.

Snyder, M. A guide to neurological and neurosurgical nursing (2nd ed.). Albany, NY: Delmar Publishers, 1991.

***VIII.3. Craniotomy***

Apuzzo, MLJ (Ed.). Brain surgery: complication avoidance and management. New York: Churchill Livingstone, 1993.

Cammermeyer, M, & Appeldorn, C (Eds.). Core curriculum for neuroscience nursing (3rd ed.). Chicago: American Association of Neuroscience Nurses, 1990.

Hickey, JV. The clinical practice of neurological and neurosurgical nursing (3rd ed.). Philadelphia: J.B. Lippincott Company, 1992.

Kane, DM. Practical points in the postoperative management of a craniotomy patient. Journal of Post Anesthesia Nursing, *6*(2):121-124, 1991.

Marshall, SB, Marshall, LF, Vos, HR, & Chesnut, RM. Neuroscience critical care: pathophysiology and patient management. Philadelphia: W.B. Saunders Company, 1990.

Moak, E. Perioperative care of the craniotomy patient: a review. Today's OR Nurse, *14*(1):9-14, 1992.

Snyder, M. A guide to neurological and neurosurgical nursing (2nd ed.). Albany, NY: Delmar Publishers, 1991.

***VIII.4. Spinal Cord Injury***

Braddom, RL. Autonomic dysreflexia: a survey of current treatment. American Journal of Physical Medicine and Rehabilitation, *70*(5):234-241, 1991.

Cammermeyer, M, & Appeldorn, C (Eds.). Core curriculum for neuroscience nursing (3rd ed.). Chicago: American Association of Neuroscience Nurses, 1990.

Ceron, GE, & Rakowski-Reinhardt, AC. Action stat! autonomic dysreflexia. Nursing 91, *21*(2):33, 1991.

Hickey, JV. The clinical practice of neurological and neurosurgical nursing (3rd ed.). Philadelphia: J.B. Lippincott Company, 1992.

Hilton, G, & Frei, J. High-dose methylprednisolone in the treatment of spinal cord injuries. Heart & Lung, *20*(6):675-680, 1991.

Marshall, SB, Marshall, LF, Vos, HR, & Chesnut, RM. Neuroscience critical care: pathophysiology and patient management. Philadelphia: W.B. Saunders Company, 1990.

Richmond, TS, Metcalf, J, Daly, M, & Kish, JR. Powerlessness in acute spinal cord injury patients: a descriptive study. Journal of Neuroscience Nursing, *24*(3):146-152, 1992.

Snyder, M. A guide to neurological and neurosurgical nursing (2nd ed.). Albany, NY: Delmar Publishers, 1991.

Swarczinski, C. & Dijkers, M. The value of serial leg measurements for monitoring deep vein thrombosis in spinal cord injury. Journal of Neuroscience Nursing, *23*(5):306-314, 1991.

Zejdlik, CP. Management of spinal cord injury (2nd ed.). Boston: Jones and Bartlett Publishers, 1992.

**UNIT IX. Nursing Care of the Client with Disturbances of Cardiovascular Function**

***IX.1. Angina Pectoris***

Alspach, JG. Core curriculum for critical care nursing (4th ed.). Philadelphia: W.B. Saunders Company, 1991.

Amsterdam, EA, et al. When and how to use lipid-lowering drugs. Patient Care, *25*(20):28-32, 35, 38+, 1991.

Braunwald, E (Ed.). Heart disease: a textbook of cardiovascular medicine (4th ed.). Philadelphia: W.B. Saunders Company, 1992.

Cannobio, MM. Cardiovascular disorders. St. Louis: Mosby–Year Book, 1991.

Cooke, DH. To stabilize unstable angina. Emergency Medicine, *24*(9):98-104, 1992.

Fleury, J. Long term management of the patient with stable angina. Nursing Clinics of North America, *27*(1):205-230, 1992.

Frances, GS, & Alpert, JS (Eds.). Modern coronary care. Boston: Little, Brown and Company, 1990.

Gleeson, B. Loosening the grip of anginal pain. Nursing 91, *21*(1):33-40, 1991.

Grab, C. The cutting alternative to PTCA. RN, *55*(7):22-27, 1992.

Holcomb, SS. Atherectomy. Nursing 93, *23*(2):44-47, 1993.

Huang, SH, Kessler, CA, McCulloch, CD, et al. Coronary care nursing (2nd ed.). Philadelphia: W.B. Saunders Company, 1989.

Hurst, JW (Ed.). The heart (7th ed.). New York: McGraw-Hill, 1990.

Hussar, DA. New drugs: learn more about 11 drugs marketed in second half of 1991. Nursing 92, *22*(5):55-61, 1992.

Matrisciano, L. Unstable angina. Critical Care Nurse, *12*(8):30-38, 1992.

Miracle, VA. Coronary atherectomy. Critical Care Nurse, *12*(3):41-47, 1992.

Obrych, DD. Interpreting CPK and LDH results. Nursing 93, *23*(1):48-49, 1993.

Parmley, WW, & Weart, CW. Ca channel blockers: the new, the tried-and-true. Patient Care, *25*(15):26-29, 32-34, 36+, 1991.

Phillips, RE, & Feeney, MK. The cardiac rhythms (3rd ed.). Philadelphia: W.B. Saunders Company, 1990.

***IX.2. Heart Failure***

Alspach, JG. Core curriculum for critical care nursing (4th ed.). Philadelphia: W.B. Saunders Company, 1991.

Braunwald, E (Ed.). Heart disease: a textbook of cardiovascular medicine (4th ed.). Philadelphia: W.B. Saunders Company, 1992.

Brown, KK. Boosting the failing heart with inotropic drugs. Nursing 93. *23*(4):34-43, 1993.

Cannobio, MM. Cardiovascular disorders. St. Louis: Mosby–Year Book, 1991.

Chung, EK. Cardiac emergency care (4th ed.). Philadelphia: Lea & Febiger, 1991.

Clochesy, JM, Breu, C, Cardin, S, et al. Critical care nursing. Philadelphia: W.B. Saunders Company, 1993.

Devereaux, RB, Diodati, JG, & Levy, D. Cardiac hypertrophy: practice implications. Patient Care, *26*(9):88-92, 95-102, 110-112, 121-122, 1992.

Huang, SH, Kessler, CA, McCulloch, CD, et al. Coronary care nursing (2nd ed.). Philadelphia: W.B. Saunders Company, 1989.

Hurst, JW (Ed.). The heart (7th ed.). New York: McGraw-Hill, 1990.

Kennedy, GT. Acute congestive heart failure: pharmacologic intervention. Critical Care Nursing Clinics of North America, *4*(2):365-375, 1992.

Letterer, RA, Carew, B, Reid, M, & Woods, P. Learning to live with congestive heart failure. Nursing 92, *22*(5):34-42, 1992.

Nagelhout, JJ. Pharmacological treatment of heart failure. Nursing Clinics of North America, *26*(2):401-415, 1991.

Smith, TW, & Kelly, RA. Therapeutic strategies for CHF in the 1990s. Hospital Practice, *26*(11):127-132, 134, 139-141, 1991.

### IX.3. Heart Surgery: Coronary Artery Bypass Grafting (CABG) or Valve Replacement

Alspach, JG. Core curriculum for critical care nursing (4th ed.). Philadelphia: W.B. Saunders Company, 1991.

Braunwald, E (Ed.). Heart disease: a textbook of cardiovascular medicine (4th ed.). Philadelphia: W.B. Saunders Company, 1992.

Cannobio, MM. Cardiovascular disorders. St. Louis: Mosby–Year Book, 1991.

Grillo, HC, Austen, WG, Wilkens, EW, et al (Eds.). Current therapy in cardiothoracic surgery. Toronto: B.C. Decker Inc., 1989.

Halfman-Franey, M, & Berg, DE. Recognition and management of bleeding following cardiac surgery. Critical Care Nursing Clinics of North America, *3*(4):675-689, 1991.

Kern, LS. The elderly heart surgery patient. Critical Care Nursing Clinics of North America, *3*(4):749-756, 1991.

Lynn-McHale, DJ, Riggs, KL, & Thurman, L. Epicardial pacing after cardiac surgery. Critical Care Nurse, *11*(8):62-66, 68-74, 76-77, 1991.

Mravinac, CM. Neurological dysfunctions following cardiac surgery. Critical Care Nursing Clinics of North America, *3*(4):691-697, 1991.

Sabiston, DC (Ed.). Textbook of surgery (14th ed.). Philadelphia: W.B. Saunders Company, 1991.

Smith, A. Case example: stunned myocardium . . . the postop heart. American Journal of Nursing, *92*(4):77, 81-82, 1992.

Strong AG. Nursing management of postoperative dysrrhythmias. Critical Care Nursing Clinics of North America, *3*(4):707-715, 1991.

Whitman, G. Hypertension and hypothermia in the acute postoperative period. Critical Care Nursing Clinics of North America, *3*(4):661-673, 1991.

### IX.4. Hypertension

Blake, GH, & Beebe, D. Management of hypertension: useful nonpharmacological measures. Postgraduate Medicine, *90*(1):151-154, 158, 251-254, 1991.

Cannobio, MM. Cardiovascular disorders. St. Louis: Mosby–Year Book, 1991.

Clochesy, JM, Breu, C, Cardin, S, et al. Critical care nursing. Philadelphia: W.B. Saunders Company, 1993.

Fifth report of the Joint National Committee on Detection, Evaluation, and Treatment of High Blood Pressure. Archives of Internal Medicine, *153*(2):154-183, 1993.

Fleg, JL, Gavras, IH, & Pecker, MS. Hypertension therapy: the first steps. Patient Care, *26*(9):161-164, 169-172, 177-180, 1992.

Frances, GS, & Alpert, JS (Eds.). Modern coronary care. Boston: Little, Brown and Company, 1990.

Hockenberry, B. Multiple drug therapy in treatment of essential hypertension. Nursing Clinics of North America, *26*(2):417-436, 1991.

Johansen, JM. Update: Guidelines for treating hypertension. American Journal of Nursing, *93*(3):42-49, 1993.

Kaplan, NM. Clinical hypertension (5th ed.). Baltimore: Williams & Wilkins, 1990.

Parmley, WW, & Weart, CW. Ca channel blockers: the new, the tried-and-true. Patient Care, *25*(15):26-29, 32-34, 36+, 1991.

Weinberger, MH. Hypertension in the elderly. Hospital Practice, *27*(5):103-108, 110, 115, 1992.

### IX.5. Mycoardial Infarction

Alspach, JG. Core curriculum for critical care nursing (4th ed.). Philadelphia: W.B. Saunders Company, 1991.

Berkman, SA. Current concepts in anticoagulation. Hospital Practice, *27*(2):187-194, 199-200, 1992.

Borelli, DJ, et al. Update on thrombolytic therapy in acute myocardial infarction. Heart and Lung, *21*(2):200-202, 1992.

Braunwald, E (Ed.). Heart disease: a textbook of cardiovascular medicine (4th ed.). Philadelphia: W.B. Saunders Company, 1992.

Cannobio, MM. Cardiovascular disorders. St. Louis: Mosby–Year Book, 1991.

Chung, EK. Cardiac emergency care (4th ed.). Philadelphia: Lea & Febiger, 1991.

Clawson, SP. Right ventricular infarction. Nursing 90, *20*(3):34-39, 1990.

Clochesy, JM, Breu, C, Cardin, S, et al. Critical care nursing. Philadelphia: W.B. Saunders Company, 1993.

Frances, GS, & Alpert, JS (Eds.). Modern coronary care. Boston: Little, Brown and Company, 1990.

Goldberger, E, & Wheat, MW. Treatment of cardiac emergencies. St. Louis: C.V. Mosby, 1990.

Grab, C. The cutting alternative to PTCA. RN, *55*(7):22-27, 1992.

Grillo, HC, Austen, WG, Wilkens, EW, et al (Eds.). Current therapy in cardiothoracic surgery. Toronto: B.C. Decker Inc., 1989.

Holcomb, SS. Atherectomy. Nursing 93, *23*(2):44-47, 1993.

Huang, SH, Kessler, CA, McCulloch, CD, et al. Coronary care nursing (2nd ed.). Philadelphia: W.B. Saunders Company, 1989.

Hurst, JW (Ed.). The heart (7th ed). New York: McGraw-Hill, 1990.

Klein, MD. Atrial fibrillation: new findings about an old nemesis. Hospital Practice, *26*(11B):75-88, 1991.

Lewis, PS. Clinical implications of non-Q-wave (subendocardial) myocardial infarctions. Focus on Critical Care AACN, *19*(1):29-33, 1992.

Lynn, LA, & Kissinger, JF. Coronary precautions: should caffeine be restricted in patients with myocardial infarction. Heart and Lung, *21*(4):365-371, 1992.

Mason, P, et al. Implantable cardioverter defibrillator: a review. Heart and Lung, *21*(2):141-147, 1992.

McKenna, M. Management of the patient undergoing myocardial revascularization: percutaneous coronary angioplasty. Nursing Clinics of North America, *27*(1):231-241, 1992.

Mercer, S. Thrombolysis for the acute myocardial infarction. Emergency, *24*(2):29-32, 1992.

Morganroth, J. Ventricular arrhythmia: an approach to oral therapy. Consultant, *32*(3):113-114, 117-118, 1992.

Nyamathi, A, Alison, J, Constancia, P, et al. Coping and adjustment of spouses of critically ill patients with cardiac disease. Heart and Lung, *21*(2):160-165, 1992.

Obrych, DD. Interpreting CPK and LDH results. Nursing 93, *23*(1):48-49, 1993.

Phillips, RE, & Feeney, MK. The cardiac rhythms (3rd ed.). Philadelphia: W.B. Saunders Company, 1990.

Scherck, KA. Coping with acute myocardial infarction. Heart and Lung, *21*(4):327-334, 1992.

Stovsky, B. Nursing intervention for risk factor reduction. Nursing Clinics of North America, *27*(1):257-270, 1992.

Woo, MA. Clinical management of the patient with an acute myocardial infarction. Nursing Clinics of North America, *27*(1):189-203, 1992.

***IX.6. Pacemaker Insertion***

Buckingham, TA, Janosik, DL, & Pearson, AC. Pacemaker hemodynamics: clinical implications. Progress in Cardiovascular Disease, *34*(5):347-366, 1992.

Cannobio, MM. Cardiovascular disorders. St. Louis: Mosby–Year Book, 1991.

Chung, EK. Cardiac emergency care (4th ed.). Philadelphia: Lea & Febiger, 1991.

Dugan, L. Permanent pacemakers. Nursing 91, *21*(6):47-52, 1991.

Frances, GS, & Alpert, JS (Eds.). Modern coronary care. Boston: Little, Brown and Company, 1990.

Huang, SH, Kessler, CA, McCulloch, CD, et al. Coronary care nursing (2nd ed.). Philadelphia: W.B. Saunders Company, 1989.

Hurst, JW (Ed.). The heart (7th ed.). New York: McGraw-Hill, 1990.

Klein, LS, Miles, WM, & Zipes, DP. Antitachycardia devices: realities and promises. Journal of American College of Cardiology, *18*(5):1349-1362, 1991.

Levine, PA. Benefits of dual-chamber pacemakers. Western Journal of Medicine, *156*(1):70-71, 1992.

Mercer, ME. Electrical support for the heart: rate-responsive pacers. RN, *55*(5):34-37, 1992.

Merva, JA. Providing electrical support for the heart: temporary pacemakers, RN, *55*(5):28-33, 37, 1992.

Stewart, JV, & Sheehan, AM. Permanent pacemakers: the nurse's role in patient education and follow-up care. Journal of Cardiovascular Nursing, *5*(3):32-43, 1991.

## UNIT X. Nursing Care of the Client with Disturbances of Peripheral Vascular Function

***X.1. Abdominal Aortic Aneurysm Repair***

Blank, CA, & Irwin, GH. Peripheral vascular disorders: assessment and intervention. Nursing Clinics of North America, *25*(4):777-794, 1990.

Comerota, AJ, & Leefmans, E. Acute arterial occlusion. In Young, JR, Graor, RA, Olin, JW, & Bartholomew, JR (Eds.), Peripheral vascular disease. St. Louis: Mosby–Year Book, 1991, pp. 227-240.

Fahey, VA (Ed.). Vascular nursing. Philadelphia: W.B. Saunders Company, 1988.

Spittell, JR, & Spittel, PC. Aneurysms. In Young, JR, Graor, RA, Olin, JW, & Bartholomew, JR (Eds.), Peripheral vascular disease. St. Louis: Mosby–Year Book, 1991, pp. 307-319.

***X.2. Carotid Endarterectomy***

Cammermeyer, M, & Appeldorn, C (Eds.). Core curriculum for neuroscience nursing (3rd ed.). Chicago: American Association of Neuroscience Nurses, 1990.

Fahey, VA (Ed.). Vascular nursing. Philadelphia: W.B. Saunders Company, 1988.

Hickey, JV. The clinical practice of neurological and neurosurgical nursing (3rd ed.). Philadelphia: J.B. Lippincott Company, 1992.

Johnson, SM, & Anderson, B. Carotid endarterectomy: a review. Critical Care Nursing Clinics of North America, *3*(3):499-506, 1991.

Kane-Carlsen, PA. Managing patients with T.I.A.s. Nursing 92, *22*(1):34-39, 1992.

Strandness, DE. Extracranial cerebrovascular arterial disease. In Young, JR, Graor, RA, Olin, JW, & Bartholomew, JR (Eds.), Peripheral vascular disease. St. Louis: Mosby–Year Book, 1991, pp. 241-252.

***X.3. Deep Vein Thrombosis***

Berkman, SA. Current concepts in anticoagulation. Hospital Practice, *27*(2):187-194, 199-200, 1992.

Coffman, JD. Venous thrombosis and the diagnosis of pulmonary emboli. Hospital Practice, *27*(4A):99-102, 107-112, 1992.

Fahey, VA (Ed.). Vascular nursing. Philadelphia: W.B. Saunders Company, 1988.

Gray, BH, & Graor, RA. Deep vein thrombosis and pulmonary embolism: the importance of heightened awareness. Postgraduate Medicine, *91*(1):207-210, 213-214, 217-218, 1992.

Lohr, JM, Kerr, TM, Lutter, KS, et al. Lower extremity calf thrombosis: to treat or not to treat. Journal of Vascular Surgery, *14*(5):618-623, 1991.

Remember DVT prophylaxis. Emergency Medicine, *24*(6):161, 1992.

***X.4. Femoropopliteal Bypass***

Blank, CA, & Irwin, GH. Peripheral vascular disorders: assessment and intervention. Nursing Clinics of North America, *25*(4):777-794, 1990.

Fahey, VA (Ed.). Vascular nursing. Philadelphia: W.B. Saunders Company, 1988.

Quinones-Baldrich, WJ, & Caswell, D. Reperfusion injury. Nursing Clinics of North America, *25*(4):525-533, 1990.

Young, JR, Graor, RA, Olin, JW, & Bartholomew, JR (Eds.). Peripheral vascular disease. St. Louis: Mosby–Year Book, 1991.

## UNIT XI. Nursing Care of the Client with Disturbances of Respiratory Function

***XI.1. Cancer of the Lung***

Brown, ML, Carrieri, V, Janson-Bjerklie, S, & Dodd, M. Lung cancer and dyspnea: the patient's perception. Oncology Nursing Forum, *13*(5):19-24, 1986.

Carbone, DP, & Minna, JD. The molecular genetics of lung cancer. Advances in Internal Medicine, *37*:153-171, 1992.

Comis, RL, & Martin, G. Small cell carcinoma of the lung: an overview. Seminars in Oncology Nursing, *3*(3):174-182, 1987.

Critical difference: Superior vena cava syndrome. American Journal of Nursing, *93*(2):52, 1993.

Dietz, KA, & Flaherty, AM. Oncologic emergencies. In Groenwald, SL, Frogge, MH, Goodman, M, & Yarbro, CH (Eds.), Cancer nursing: principles and practice (3rd ed.). Boston: Jones and Bartlett Publishers, 1993, pp. 800-839.

Elias, EG. Handbook of surgical oncology. Boca Raton, FL: CRC Press, 1989.

Elpern, EH. Lung cancer. In Groenwald, SL, Frogge, MH, Goodman, M, & Yarbro, CH (Eds.), Cancer nursing: principles and practice (3rd ed.). Boston: Jones and Bartlett Publishers, 1993, pp. 1174-1199.

Engelking, C. Lung cancer: teaching, counseling, and caring. American Journal of Nursing, *87*(11):1439-1441, 1987.

Faber, LP. Lung cancer. In Holleb, AI, Fink, DJ, & Murphy, GP, American cancer society textbook of clinical oncology. Altanta, GA: American Cancer Society, 1991, pp. 194-212.

Foote, M, Sexton, DL, & Pawlik, L. Dyspnea: a distressing sensation in lung cancer. Oncology Nursing Forum, *13*(5):25-31, 1986.

Houston, SJ, & Kendall, JA. Psychosocial implications of lung cancer. Nursing Clinics of North America, *27*(3):681-690, 1992.

Lind, JM. Ectopic hormonal production: nursing implications. Seminars in Oncology Nursing, *1*(4):251-258, 1985.

Lindsey, AM. Lung cancer. In Baird, SB, McCorkle, R, & Grant, M, Cancer nursing: a comprehensive textbook. Philadelphia: W.B. Saunders Company, 1991, pp. 452-465.

Maran, JN, & Gray, MA. Pulmonary laser therapy. American Journal of Nursing, *88*(6):828-831, 1988.

Moseley, JR. Nursing management of toxicities associated with chemotherapy for lung cancer. Seminars in Oncology Nursing, *3*(3):202-210, 1987.

Odell, WD. Paraendocrine syndromes of cancer. Advances in Internal Medicine, *34*:325-352, 1989.

Olopade, O, & Ultmann, JE. Malignant effusions. Ca-A Cancer Journal for Clinicians, *41*(3):168-179, 1991.

Poe, CM, & Taylor, LM. Syndrome of inappropriate antidiuretic

hormone: assessment and nursing implications. Oncology Nursing Forum, *16*(3):373-381, 1989.
Raffin, TA. Pancoast syndrome. Hospital Medicine, *22*(5):218-221, 1986.
Rostad, M. Advances in nursing management of patients with lung cancer. Nursing Clinics of North America, *25*(2):393-403, 1990.
Ruckdeschel, J. Management of malignant pleural effusion: an overview. Seminars in Oncology, *15*(3)Supplement 3:24-28, 1988.
Ryan, LS. Lung cancer: psychosocial implications. Seminars in Oncology Nursing, *3*(3):222-227, 1987.
Sabiston, DC, Jr. Neoplasms of the lung. In Sabiston, DC, & Spencer, FC, Surgery of the chest (5th ed.) (Vol. 1). Philadelphia: W.B. Saunders Company, 1990, pp. 554-577.
Sarna, L. Correlates of symptom distress in women with lung cancer. Cancer Practice, *1*(1):21-28, 1993.
Seale, DD, & Beaver, BM. Pathophysiology of lung cancer. Nursing Clinics of North America, *27*(3):603-613, 1992.
Turner, JAT. Nursing care of the terminal lung cancer patient. Nursing Clinics of North America, *27*(3):691-702, 1992.
Turrisi, AT, III. Limited small cell lung cancer—the role of radiotherapy. Oncology, *2*(7):19-25, 1988.
Yahalom, J. Superior vena cava syndrome. In DeVita, VT, Jr, Hellman, S, & Rosenberg, SA (Eds.), Cancer: principles and practice of oncology (4th ed.). Philadelphia: J.B. Lippincott Company, 1993, pp. 2111-2117.

### *XI.2. Chronic Obstructive Pulmonary Disease*

Angstman, GL. Diagnosing COPD. Postgraduate Medicine, *91*(1):61-62, 65, 67, 1992.
Anthonisen, NR, George, RB, & Make, BJ. COPD: incurable but not untreatable. Patient Care, *26*(2):31-35, 38-40, 42, 45, 48, 51-54, 57-58, 1992.
Edelman, NH, Kaplan, RM, Buist, AS, et al. Chronic obstructive pulmonary disease. Chest, *102*(3):243S-256S, 1992.
Gift, AG, Moore, T, & Soeken, K. Relaxation to reduce dyspnea and anxiety in COPD patients. Nursing Research, *41*(4):242-246, 1992.
Hagedorn, DS. Acute exacerbation of COPD. Postgraduate Medicine, *91*(1):105-107, 110-112, 1992.
Hanson, MA, & Midthun, DE. Outpatient care of COPD patients. Postgraduate Medicine, *91*(1):89, 90, 93-94, 96, 1992.
Hodgkin, JE, Kigin, CM, Nett, LM, & Tiep, BL. Your role in COPD home care. Patient Care, *26*(5):147-150, 153, 1992.
Jess, LW. Chronic bronchitis and emphysema: airing the differences. Nursing 92, *21*(4):34-41, 1992.
Kersten, LD. Comprehensive respiratory nursing: a decision making approach. Philadelphia: W.B. Saunders Company, 1989.
Mahler, DA, Faryniarz, K, Tomlinson, D, et al. Impact of dyspnea and physiologic function on general health status in patients with chronic obstructive pulmonary disease. Chest, *102*(2):395-401, 1992.
Neese, RE. Pharmacologic treatment of COPD. Postgraduate Medicine, *91*(1):71-72, 77-78, 81-82, 84, 1992.
Weaver, TE, & Narsavage, GL. Physiological and psychological variables related to functional status in chronic obstructive pulmonary disease. Nursing Research, *41*(4):286-291, 1992.
Weinberger, SE. Principles of pulmonary medicine. Philadelphia: W.B. Saunders Company, 1992.

### *XI.3. Pneumonia*

Caruthers, DD. Infectious pneumonia in the elderly. American Journal of Nursing, *90*(2):56-60, 1990.
Chernoff, DN, & Sande, MA. Community-acquired pneumonia. In Stein, JH, Internal medicine (2nd ed.). Boston: Little Brown & Company, 1987, pp. 1478-1485.
Coleman, DA. Pneumonia: where nursing really counts. RN, *49(2)*:22-29, 1986.
Niederman, MS, & Fein, AM. Pneumonia in the elderly. Clinics in Geriatric Medicine, *2*(2):241-268, 1986.
Stratton, CW. Bacterial pneumonias—an overview with emphasis on pathogenesis, diagnosis, and treatment. Heart Lung, *15*(3):226-244, 1986.

### *XI.4. Pneumothorax*

DeMeester, TR, & Lafontaine, E. The pleura. In Sabiston, DC, & Spencer, FC, Surgery of the chest (Vol. 1). Philadelphia: W.B. Saunders Company, 1990, pp. 445-454.
Idell, S. Management of pneumothorax. Emergency Medicine, *19*(17):39-49, 1987.

### *XI.5. Pulmonary Embolism*

Bone, RC. Pulmonary embolism: new approaches to a complex problem. Emergency Medicine, *24*(14):144-146, 149-152, 1992.
Fahey, VA (Ed.). Vascular nursing. Philadelphia: W.B. Saunders Company, 1988.
Goldhaber, SZ. Managing pulmonary embolism. Hospital Practice, *26*(9):37-48, 1991.
Gonzalez-Juanatey, JR, Amaro, A, Iglesias, C, et al. Treatment of massive pulmonary thromboembolism with low intrapulmonary dosages of urokinase. Chest, *102*(2):341-346, 1992.
Graor, RA, & Bartholomew, JR. Pulmonary embolism. In Young, JR, Graor, RA, Olin, JW, & Bartholomew, JR (Eds.), Peripheral vascular disease. St. Louis: Mosby–Year Book, 1991, pp. 423-439.
Gray, BH, & Graor, RA. Deep venous thrombosis and pulmonary embolism. Postgraduate Medicine, *91*(1):207-210, 213-214, 217-218+, 1992.
Kersten, LD. Comprehensive respiratory nursing: a decision making approach. Philadelphia: W.B. Saunders Company, 1989.
Leclerc, JR. Venous thromboembolic disorders, Philadelphia: Lea & Febiger, 1991.
Weinberger, SE. Principles of pulmonary medicine. Philadelphia: W.B. Saunders Company, 1992.

### *XI.6. Thoracic Surgery*

De Meester, TR, & Lafontaine, E. In Sabiston, DC, & Spencer, FC, Surgery of the chest (5th ed.) (Vol. 1). Philadelphia: W.B. Saunders Company, 1990, pp. 458-497.
Idell, S. Management of pneumothorax. Emergency Medicine, *19*(17):39-49, 1987.

## UNIT XII. Nursing Care of the Client with Disturbances of the Kidney and Urinary Tract

### *XII.1. Bladder Suspension*

Carnevali, DL, & Patrick, M. Nursing management for the elderly (3rd ed.). Philadelphia: J.B. Lippincott Company, 1993.
Cassel, CK, Riesenberg, DE, Sorensen, LB, & Walsh, JR (Eds.). Geriatric medicine (2nd ed.). New York: Springer-Verlag, 1990.
Chenitz, WC, Stone, JT, and Salisbury, SA. Clinical gerontological nursing. Philadelphia: W.B. Saunders Company, 1991.
McCormick, KA, Newman, DK, Colling, J, & Pearson, BD. Clinical guidelines: urinary incontinence in adults. American Journal of Nursing, *92*(10):75-93, 1992.
McCormick, KA, Scheve, AAS, & Leahy, E. Nursing management of urinary incontinence in geriatric inpatients. Nursing Clinics of North America, *23*(1):231-264, 1988.
Newman, DK. The treatment of urinary incontinence in adults. Nursing Practice, *14*(6):21-24, 26-28, 31-32, 1989.
Newman, DK, Lynch, K, Smith, DA, Cell, P. Restoring urinary continence. American Journal of Nursing, *91*(1):28-36, 1991.
Ouslander, JG, & Bruskewitz, R. Disorders of micturition in the aging patient. Advances in Internal Medicine, *34*:165-190, 1989.
Palmer, MH. Incontinence: the magnitude of the problem. Nursing Clinics of North America, *23*(1):139-157, 1988.
Raz, S, Klutke, CG, & Golomb, J. Four-corner bladder and

urethral suspension for moderate cystocele. Journal of Urology, *142*:712-715, 1989.

Raz, S, Little, NA, Juma, S. Female urology. In Walsh, PC, Retik, AB, Stamey, TA, & Vaughan, ED, Jr (Eds.), Campbell's urology (6th ed.). Philadelphia: W.B. Saunders Company, 1992, pp. 2782-2812.

Raz, S, Sussman, EM, & Erickson, DR. Vaginal repair of high-grade cystocele. Contemporary Urology, *3*(5):80-94, 1991.

Reilly, NJ. Urinary incontinence: new attitudes and treatment options. Innovations in Urology Nursing, *III*(2):1-15, 1992.

Snyder, HM, III. Principles of pediatric urinary reconstruction: a synthesis. In Gillenwater, JY, Grayhack, JT, Howards, SS, & Duckett, JW (Eds.), Adult and pediatric urology (2nd ed.). St. Louis: Mosby–Year Book, 1991, pp. 1957-1960.

Stamey, TA. Urinary incontinence in the female: the stamey endoscopic suspension of the vesical neck for stress urinary incontinence. In Walsh, PC, Retik, AB, Stamey, TA, & Vaughan, ED, Jr (Eds.), Campbell's urology (6th ed.) (Vol. 3). Philadelphia: W.B. Saunders Company, 1992, pp. 2829-2849.

Thompson, JD, Wall, LL, Growdon, WA, & Ridley, JH. Urinary stress incontinence. In Thompson, JD, & Rock, JA, Te Linde's operative gynecology (7th ed.). Philadelphia: J.B. Lippincott Company, 1992, pp. 904-914.

Vernon, MS. Urinary incontinence in the elderly. Primary Care, *16*(2):515-527, 1989.

Wyman, JF. Nursing assessment of the incontinent geriatric outpatient population. Nursing Clinics of North America, *23*(1):169-187, 1988.

### *XII.2. Chronic Renal Failure*

Alfrey, AC, & Chan, L. Chronic renal failure: manifestations and pathogeneis. In Schrier, RW (Ed.), Renal and electrolyte disorders (4th ed.). Boston: Little, Brown & Company, 1992, pp. 539-579.

Amend, WJ, & Vincenti, FG. Chronic renal failure and dialysis. In Tanagho, EA, & McAninch, JW (Eds.), Smith's general urology (13th ed.). Norwalk, CT: Appleton & Lange, 1992, pp. 553-555.

Biggers, PB. Administering epoetin alfa: more RBCs with fewer risks. Nursing 91, *21*(4):43, 1991.

Brown, JM. Nursing care of predialysis patients receiving epoetin alfa. American Nephrology Nurses' Association Journal, *18*(3):306-314, 1991.

Chambers, JK. Renal insufficiency: implications for care of the medical-surgical patient. MEDSURG Nursing, *2*(1):33-40, 1993.

Collins, ST. Excuse me while I park my dinosaur . . . a revolution in the treatment of patients with end stage renal disease (ESRD). American Nephrology Nurses' Association Journal, *19*(2):165, 1992.

Holechek, MJ. Medication review: an alternative phosphate binder—calcium acetate. American Nephrology Nurses' Association Journal, *18*(3):321-322, 1991.

Janes, G. A better life than before: quality of life in people with renal failure. Professional Nurse, *6*(1):26-28, 1990.

Janes, G. An open approach to minimize the effect: sexuality and renal patients. Professional Nurse, *6*(2):69-71, 1990.

Kutner, NG, Rehabilitation, aging, and chronic renal disease. American Journal of Physical Medicine and Rehabilitation, *71*(2):97-101, 1992.

Lewis, DJ. Spice of life: a strategy to enhance dietary compliance. American Nephrology Nurses' Association Journal, *17*(5):387-389, 401, 1990.

Shapiro, E. Renal diet-exchange lists: evaluation of potential teachability and precision. Topics in Clinical Nutrition, *7*(1):63-70, 1991.

Shipiro, JI, & Schrier, RW. Etiology, pathogensis, and management of renal failure. In Walsh, PC, Retik, AB, Stamey, TA, Vaughan, ED, Jr (Eds.), Campbell's urology (6th ed.) (Vol. 2). Philadelphia: W.B. Saunders Company, 1992, pp. 2054-2062.

Slataper, R. Slowing the course of renal failure in patients with diabetes. Physician's Assistant, *16*(10):79-80, 83-85, 109-112, 1992.

Tanagho, EA, & McAninch, JW (Eds.). Smith's general urology (13th ed.). Norwalk, CT: Appleton & Lange, 1992.

### *XII.3. Cystectomy with Urinary Diversion*

Benson, MC, & Olsson, CA. Urinary diversion. Urologic Clinics of North America, *19*(4):779-795, 1992.

Broadwell, DC. Peristomal skin integrity. Nursing Clinics of North America, *22*(2):321-332, 1987.

Carroll, PR, & Barbour, S. Urinary diversion and bladder substitution. In Tanagho, EA, & McAninch, JW (Eds.), Smith's general urology (13th ed.). Norwalk, CT: Appleton & Lange, 1992, pp. 426-438.

Dudas, S. Altered body image and sexuality. In Groenwald, SL, Frogge, MH, Goodman, M, & Yarbro, CH (Eds.), Cancer nursing: principles and practice (3rd ed.). Boston: Jones and Bartlett Publishers, 1993, pp. 719-733.

Freiha, FS. Open bladder surgery. In Walsh, PC, Retik, AB, Stamey, TA, & Vaughan, ED, Jr (Eds.), Campbell's urology (6th ed.) (Vol. 3). Philadelphia: W.B. Saunders Company, 1992, pp. 2750-2774.

Hampton, BG, & Bryant, RA (Eds.). Ostomies and continent diversions: nursing management. St. Louis: Mosby–Year Book, 1992.

Killeen, KP, & Libertino, JA. Management of bowel and urinary tract complications after urinary diversion. Urologic Clinics of North America, *15*(2):183-194, 1988.

Krebs, LU. Sexual and reproductive dysfunction. In Groenwald, SL, Frogge, MH, Goodman, M, & Yarbro, CH (Eds.), Cancer nursing: principles and practice (3rd ed.). Boston: Jones and Bartlett Publishers, 1993, pp. 696-718.

Lamb, MA. Alterations in sexuality and sexual functioning. In Baird, SB, McCorkle, R, & Grant, M, Cancer nursing: a comprehensive textbook. Philadelphia: W.B. Saunders Company, 1991, pp. 831-849.

Lind, J, & Irwin, RJ. Genitourinary cancers. In Baird, SB, McCorkle, R, & Grant, M, Cancer nursing: a comprehensive textbook. Philadelphia: W.B. Saunders Company, 1991, pp. 466-484.

Lind, J, Kravitz, K, & Greig, B. Urologic and male genital malignancies. In Groenwald, SL, Frogge, MH, Goodman, M, & Yarbro, CH (Eds.), Cancer nursing: principles and practice (3rd ed.). Boston: Jones and Bartlett Publishers, 1993, pp. 1258-1315.

Mandell, J, Bauer, SB, Colodny, AH, & Retik, AB. Complications of urinary tract diversion. Urologic Clinics of North America, *15*(2):207-217, 1988.

McDougal, WS. Use of intestinal segments in the urinary tract: basic principles. In Walsh, PC, Retik, AB, Stamey, TA, & Vaughan, ED, Jr (Eds.), Campbell's urology (6th ed.) (Vol. 3). Philadelphia: W.B. Saunders Company, 1992, pp. 2595-2629.

Moore, S, Newton, M, Grant, EG, & Keetch, DW. Treating bladder cancer: new methods, new management. American Journal of Nursing, *93*(5):32-39, 1993.

Petillo, MH. The patient with a urinary stoma. Nursing Clinics of North America, *22*(2):263-279, 1987.

Rowland, RG. Continent urinary reservoirs. Surgical Clinics of North America, *68*(5):891-907, 1988.

Shipes, E. Psychosocial issues: the person with an ostomy. Nursing Clinics of North America, *22*(2):291-302, 1987.

Smith, DB. Continent diversions: an overview. Dimensions in Oncology Nursing, *3*(4):18-23, 1989.

Smith, DB. Sexual rehabilitation of the cancer patient. Cancer Nursing, *12*(1):10-15, 1989.

Smith, DB, & Babaian, RJ. The effects of treatment for cancer on male fertility and sexuality. Cancer Nursing, *15*(4):271-275, 1992.

Smith, DB, & Johnson, DE (Eds.). Ostomy care and the cancer patient. New York: Grune & Stratton, 1986.

Webster, GD, & Khoury, JM. Continent urinary diversion. In DeVita, VT, Jr, Hellman, S, & Rosenberg, SA, Important advances in oncology 1992. Philadelphia: J.B. Lippincott Company, 1992, pp. 137-153.

### *XII.4. Nephrectomy*

Dreicer, R, & Williams, RD. Renal parenchymal neoplasms. In Tanagho, EA, & McAninch, JW (Eds.), Smith's general urology (13th ed.). Norwalk, CT: Appleton & Lange, 1992, pp. 367-368.

Libertino, JA. Renovascular surgery. In Walsh, PC, Retik, AB, Stamey, TA, & Vaughan, ED, Jr (Eds.), Campbell's urology (6th ed.) (Vol. 3). Philadelphia: W.B. Saunders Company, 1992, pp. 2530-2536.

Novick, AC, & Streem, SB. Surgery of the kidney. In Walsh, PC, Retik, AB, Stamey, TA, & Vaughan, ED, Jr (Eds.), Campbells's urology (6th ed.) (Vol. 3). Philadelphia: W.B. Saunders Company, 1992, pp. 2413-2435.

## UNIT XIII. Nursing Care of the Client with Disturbances of Hematopoietic and Lymphatic Function

### *XIII.1. Acquired Immune Deficiency Syndrome: Human Immunodeficiency Virus Infection*

Anastasi, JK. Diarrhea in acquired immune deficiency syndrome (AIDS). Ostomy/Wound Management, *39*(2):14-23, 1993.

Anastasi, JK, & Rivera, J. Identifying the skin manifestations of HIV. Nursing 92, *22*(11):58-61, 1992.

Baltimore, D, & Feinberg, MB. HIV revealed: toward a natural history of the infection. New England Journal of Medicine, *321*:1673-1675, 1989.

Barrick, B. Light at the end of a decade. American Journal of Nursing, *90*(11):37-40, 1990.

Barrick, B. Caring for AIDS patients: a challenge you can meet. Nursing 88, *18*(11):50-59, 1988.

Bennett, JA. Helping people with AIDS live well at home. Nursing Clinics of North America, *23*(4):731-748, 1988.

Carr, G. Opportunistic infections and pharmacology. Critical Care Nursing Clinics of North America, *4*(3):395-400, 1992.

Clark, CC, Curley, A, Hughes, A, & James, R. Hospice care: a model for caring for the person with AIDS. Nursing Clinics of North America, *23*(4):851-862, 1988.

DeVita, VT, Jr, Hellman, S, & Rosenberg, S (Eds.). AIDS—etiology, diagnosis, treatment, and prevention (3rd ed.). Philadelphia: J.B. Lippincott Company, 1992.

Fazio, M, & Glaspy, J. The impact of granulocyte colony stimulating factor on quality of life in patients with severe chronic neutropenia. Oncology Nursing Forum, *18*(8):1411-1413, 1991.

Fineberg, HV. The social dimension of AIDS. Scientific American, *259*(4):128-134, 1988.

Flaskerud, JH. Psychosocial and neuropsychiatric care. Critical Care Nursing Clinics of North America, *4*(3):411-420, 1992.

Flaskerud, JK, & Ungvarski, PJ. HIV/AIDS a guide to nursing care (2nd ed.). Philadelphia: W.B. Saunders Company, 1992.

Forstein, M. The neuropsychiatric aspects of HIV infection. Primary Care, *19*(1):97-117, 1992.

Garett, JE. The AIDS patient: helping him and his parents cope. Nursing 88, *18*(9):50-52, 1988.

Glaspy, JA, & Golde, DW. The colony-stimulating factors: biology and clinical use. Oncology, *4*(9):25-33, 1990.

Govoni, LA. Psychosocial issues of AIDS in the nursing care of homosexual men and their significant others. Nursing Clinics of North America, *23*(4):749-765, 1988.

Hanley, E, & Lincoln, P. HIV infection in women: implications for nursing practice. Nursing Clinics of North America, *27*(4):925-936, 1992.

Hilton, G. AIDS dementia. Journal of Neuroscience Nursing, *21*(1):24-29, 1989.

Hott, JR, Bell, JL, & Barile, LA. Speaking of sex. American Journal of Nursing, *91*(1):82, 1991.

Hughes, AM, & Schofferman, J. AIDS and the spectrum of HIV disease. In Baird, SB, McCorkle, R, & Grant, M, Cancer nursing: a comprehensive textbook. Philadelphia: W.B. Saunders Company, 1991, pp. 647-663.

Hull, M. Coping strategies of family caregivers in hospice home care. Oncology Nursing Forum, *19*(8):1179-1191, 1992.

Hull, M. Family needs and supportive nursing behaviors during terminal care: a review. Oncology Nursing Forum, *16*(6):787-790, 1989.

Jacob, JL, Baird, BF, Haller, B, & Ostchega, Y. AIDS-related kaposi's sarcoma: concepts of care. Seminars in Oncology Nursing, *5*(4):263-275, 1989.

Jassack, P. Families: an essential element in the care of the patient with cancer. Oncology Nursing Forum, *19*(6):871-876, 1992.

Karp, JE, Groopman, JE, & Broder, S. Cancer in AIDS. In DeVita, VT, Jr, Hellman, S, & Rosenberg, SA (Eds.), Cancer: principles and practice of oncology (4th ed). Philadelphia: J.B. Lippincott Company, 1993, pp. 2093-2110.

Kelly, P. Counseling patients with HIV. RN, *55*(2):54-58, 1992.

Kotler, DP. Intestinal and hepatic manifestations of AIDS. Advances in Internal Medicine, *34*:43-72, 1989.

LaCharite, CL, & Meisenhelder, JB. Zidovudine: flawed champion against AIDS. RN, *52*:(1):35-38, 1989.

Lewis, A (Ed.). Nursing care of the person with AIDS/ARC. Rockville, MD: Aspen Publishers, 1988.

Libman, H. Pathogenesis, natural history, and classification of HIV infection. Primary Care, *19*(1):1-17, 1992.

Lovejoy, NC, & Rumley, R. AIDS epidemiology and pathology: implications for intensive care units. Critical Care Nursing Clinics of North America, *4*(3):383-393, 1992.

Moran, TA. AIDS-related malignancies. In Groenwald, SL, Frogge, MH, Goodman, M, & Yarbro, CH, Cancer nursing: principles and practice (3rd ed.). Boston: Jones and Bartlett, 1993, pp. 861-876.

Piemme, JA, & Bolle, JL. Coping with grief in response to caring for persons with AIDS. American Journal of Occupational Therapy, *44*(3):266-269, 1990.

Plank, CS. Aerosolized pentamidine: a new weapon against p.c.p. Nursing 89, *19*(2):48-49, 1989.

Robertson, S. Drugs that keep AIDS patients alive. RN, *52*(2):35-41, 1989.

Safai, B, Diaz, B, & Schwartz, J. Malignant neoplasms associated with human immunodeficiency virus infection. Ca-A Cancer Journal for Clinicians, *42*(2):74-95, 1992.

Sande, M, & Volberding, P (Eds.). The Medical Management of AIDS (2nd ed.). Philadelphia: W.B. Saunders Company, 1990.

Scherer, P. How AIDS attacks the brain. American Journal of Nursing, *90*(1):44-53, 1990.

Schindler, LW. Understanding the immune system. U.S. Department of Health and Human Services, National Institutes of Health, 1988.

Schmidt, J. John had AIDS—and one romantic wish. Nursing 93, *23*(1):55-56, 1993.

Schneider, M, & Bernard, J. Midwives to the dying. Portland, OR: Angels' Work, 1992.

Skalla, KA, & Lacasse, C. Patient education for fatigue. Oncology Nursing Forum, *19*(10):1537-1541, 1992.

Strohl, RA. Progress in HIV disease. Nursing Acumen, *3*(1):1-4, 1991.

Truax, AB. Psychosocial aspects of AIDS. Topics in Emergency Medicine, *9*(2):61-69, 1987.

Ungvarski, P. Assessment: the key to nursing the AIDS patient. RN, *51*(9):28-33, 1988.

Ungvarki, PJ, & Schmidt, J. AIDS patients under attack. RN, *55*(11):37-45, 1992.

Whipple, B. Women and AIDS: sexuality issues. Nursing Outlook, *40*(5):152-157, 1992.

Workman, M, Ellenhorst-Ryan, J, & Koertge, V. Nursing care of the immunocompromised patient. Philadelphia: W.B. Saunders Company, 1993.

Wujcik, D. Overview of colony-stimulating factors: focus on the neutrophil. In Carroll-Johnson, RM (Ed.), A case management approach to patients receiving G-CSF. Oncology Nursing Press, 1992, pp. 8-13.

### *XIII.2. Anemia*

Brown, EG. Determining the cause of anemia: general approach with emphasis on microcytic, hypochromic anemias. Postgraduate Medicine, *89*(6):161-164, 167-170, 207, 1991.

Deasy, J. Three anemic patients. Physician Assistant, *15*(6):58-62, 1991.

Lee, GR, Bithell, TC, Foerster, J, et al (Eds.). Wintrobe's clinical hematology (9th ed.) (Vol. 1). Philadelphia: Lea & Febiger, 1993.

Pollin, S. How to use the new weapon against anemia . . . epoetin alfa. RN, *55*(1):36-38, 1992.

Turba, RM, Lewis, VL, & Green, D. Pressure sore anemia: response to erythropoieten. Archives of Physical Medicine and Rehabilitation, *73*(5):498-500, 1992.

Williams, WJ, Beutler, E, Erslev, AJ, & Lichtman, MA. Hematology (4th ed.). New York: McGraw-Hill, 1990.

### *XIII.3. Splenectomy*

Athens, JW. The reticuloendothelial (mononuclear phagocyte) system and the spleen. In Lee, GR, Bithell, TC, Foerster, J, et al (Eds.), Wintrobe's clinical hematology (9th ed.) (Vol. 1). Philadelphia: Lea & Febiger, 1993, pp. 311-325.

Silcox, MM. Postsplenectomy sepsis: a case review and one hospital's campaign to prevent other needless tragedies. Journal of Emergency Nursing, *17*(1):15-18, 1991.

White, KS. Patient awareness of health precautions after splenectomy. American Journal of Infection Control, *19*(1):36-41, 1991.

## UNIT XIV. Nursing Care of the Client with Disturbances of the Gastrointestinal Tract

### *XIV.2. Bowel Diversion: Ileostomy*

Fazio, VW. Preventing and managing ileostomy complications. Journal of Enterostomal Nursing, *19*(2):48-53, 1992.

Hampton, BG, & Bryant, RA. Ostomies and continent diversions: nursing management. St. Louis: Mosby–Year Book, 1992.

Hurd, LB. Presenting a patient's guide to ileoanal reservoir surgery. Ostomy/Wound Management, *38*(5):52-4, 56, 59-60, 1992.

Kelly, K. Approach to the patient with ileostomy and ileal pouch. In Yamada, T (Ed.), Textbook of gastroenterology (Vol. 1). Philadelphia: J.B. Lippincott Company, 1991, pp. 796-808.

Long, L. Ileostomy care: overcoming the obstacles. Nursing 91, *21*(10):73-75, 1991.

Madda, MA. Helping ostomy patients manage medications. Nursing 91, *21*(3):47-49, 1991.

Nadler, LH. General considerations and complications of the ileostomy. Ostomy/Wound Management, *38*(4):18-20, 1992.

Todd, D. Ileoanal reservoirs: construction and management. Journal of Enterostomal Nursing, *20*(1):26-35, 1993.

Wilson, RE. Patient education sheets: a guide to educating the patient with a urostomy, colostomy, and ileostomy. Ostomy/Wound Management, *38*(4):45-6, 48-50, 52, 1992.

Young, MJ. Convexity in the management of problem stomas. Ostomy/Wound Management, *38*(4):53-54, 56, 59-60, 1992.

### *XIV.3. Gastrectomy*

Cave, DR. Therapeutic approaches to recurrent peptic ulcer disease. Hospital Practice, *27*(9A):33-40, 43, 47-48, 49, 1992.

Debas, HT, & Orloff, SL. Surgery for peptic ulcer disease. In Yamada, T (Ed.), Textbook of gastroenterology (Vol 1). Philadelphia: J.B. Lippincott Company, 1991, pp. 1379-1395.

Feldman, M, Maton, PN, McCallum, RW, & McCarthy, DM. Treating ulcers and reflux: what's new? Patient Care, *26*(13):53-5, 59-64, 67-70, 72, 1992.

Sachar, DB, Waye, JD, & Lewis, BS (Eds.). Pocket guide to gastroenterology. Baltimore: Williams & Wilkins, 1991.

Sleisenger, MH, & Fordtran, JS (Eds.). Gastrointestinal disease: pathophysiology/diagnosis/management (5th ed.). Philadelphia: W.B. Saunders Company, 1993.

### *XIV.4. Gastric Reduction*

Bo-Linn, GW. Obesity, anorexia nervosa, bulimia, and other eating disorders. In Sleisenger, MH, & Fordtran, JS (Eds.), Gastrointestinal disease: pathophysiology/diagnosis/management (5th ed.) (Vol. 2). Philadelphia: W.B. Saunders Company, 1993, pp. 2109-2136.

Yamada, T (Ed.). Textbook of gastroenterology (Vol. 1). Philadelphia: J.B. Lippincott Company, 1991.

### *XIV.5. Inflammatory Bowel Disease: Ulcerative Colitis and Crohn's Disease*

Anagnostides, AA, Hodgson, HJF, Kirsner, JB (Eds.). Inflammatory bowel disease. London: Chapman & Hall Medical, 1991.

Butt, JH. Outpatient management of inflammatory bowel disease. Postgraduate Medicine, *92*(6):69-72, 77-78, 81-84, 91-92, 1992.

Cooke, DM. Inflammatory bowel disease: primary health care management of ulcerative colitis and Crohn's disease. Nurse Practitioner, *16*(8):27-28, 30, 35-36+, 1991.

Hanauer, SB, Peppercorn, MA, & Present, DH. Current concepts, new therapies in IBD. Patient Care, *26*(13):79-84, 86-90, 93-94+, 1992.

Living with inflammatory bowel disease. Patient Care, *26*(13):103-104, 1992.

Mahan, LK, & Arlin, MT. Krause's food, nutrition, and diet therapy (8th ed.). Philadelphia: W.B. Saunders Company, 1992.

Pemberton, CM, Moxness, KE, German, MJ, et al. Mayo clinic diet manual (6th ed.). Philadelphia: B.C. Decker Inc., 1988.

Sleisenger, MH, & Fordtran, JS. Gastrointestinal disease: pathophysiology/diagnosis/management (5th ed.). Philadelphia: W.B. Saunders Company, 1993.

Yamada, T (Ed.). Textbook of gastroenterology. Philadelphia: J.B. Lippincott Company, 1991.

### *XIV.6. Mandibular (Jaw) Fracture with Intermaxillary Fixation*

Barkett, PA. Obstructed airway with wired jaws. Nursing 91, *21*(12):33, 1991.

Brown-Stewart, P. Maxillofacial trauma: implications for critical care. Critical Care Nurse, *9*(6):44-46, 48-52, 55-57, 1989.

Lanzi, GL. Mandibular and dental injuries. Topics in Emergency Medicine, *13*(4):27-28, 1991.

Robertson, BC. Concepts in mandibular fractures. Trauma Quarterly, *9*(1):54-66, 1992.

Saber, KL. Nutritional management of intermaxillary fractures. Advanced Clinical Care, *6*(5):24-25, 1991.

Stanley, RB. Maxillofacial trauma. In Cummings, CW, & Krause, CJ (Eds.), Otolaryngology—head and neck surgery (2nd ed.) (Vol. 1). St. Louis: Mosby–Year Book, 1993, pp. 374-402.

Tipton, PA. Temporomandibular joint dysfunction. Physiotherapy, *76*(10):608-610, 1990.

### *XIV.7. Peptic Ulcer*

Cave, DR. Therapeutic approaches to recurrent peptic ulcer disease. Hospital Practice, *27*(9A):33-40, 43, 47-48, 49, 1992.

Feldman, M, Maton, PN, McCallum, RW, & McCarthy, DM. Treating ulcers and reflux: what's new? Patient Care, *26*(13):53-5, 59-64, 67-70, 72, 1992.

Johns, J. When the patient has an ulcer. RN, *54*(11):44-51, 1991.

Sachar, DB, Waye, JD, & Lewis, BS (Eds.). Pocket guide to gastroenterology. Baltimore: Williams & Wilkins, 1991.

Sleisenger, MH, & Fordtran, JS (Eds.). Gastrointestinal disease: pathophysiology/diagnosis/management (5th ed.). Philadelphia: W.B. Saunders Company, 1993.

Wardell, TL. Assessing and managing a gastric ulcer. Nursing 91, *21*(3):34-41, 1991.
Yamada, T (Ed.). Textbook of gastroenterology (Vol. 1). Philadelphia: J.B. Lippincott Company, 1991.

## UNIT XV. Nursing Care of the Client with Disturbances of the Liver, Biliary Tract, and Pancreas

### *XV.1. Acute Pancreatitis*

Jeffres, C. Complications of acute pancreatitis. Critical Care Nurse, *9*(4):38-47, 1989.
Sleisenger, MH, & Fordtran, JS (Eds.). Gastrointestinal disease: pathophysiology/diagnosis/management (5th ed.). Philadelphia: W.B. Saunders Company, 1993.
Smith, A. When the pancreas self-destructs. American Journal of Nursing, *91*(9):38-48, 1991.
Steer, ML. Acute pancreatitis. In Yamada, T (Ed.), Textbook of gastroenterology (Vol. 2), Philadelphia: J.B. Lippincott Company, 1991, pp. 1859-1873.
Thompson, C. Managing acute pancreatitis. RN, *55*(3):52-57, 1992.

### *XV.2. Cholecystectomy*

Shade, RR, & Cattano, CJ. Trends in gallbladder disease and its treatment. Hospital Medicine, *28*(11):30, 32, 37-40 +, 1992.
Sherlock S, & Dooley, J. Diseases of the liver and biliary system (9th ed.). Oxford: Blackwell Scientific Publications, 1993.
Sleisenger, MH, & Fordtran, JS. Gastrointestinal disease: pathophysiology/diagnosis/management (5th ed.). Philadelphia: W.B. Saunders Company, 1993.
Stillman, A. Laparoscopic cholecystectomy: an electrosurgical approach to biliary disease. AORN Journal, *57*(2):429-430, 432-436, 1993.
Ullman, E. Issues surrounding laparoscopic cholecystectomy. AORN Journal, *54*(6):1290-1291, 1294-1295, 1991.
Wallen, E. Sharing the ordeal: cholecystectomy. Nursing Times, *88*(18):36-38, 1992.
Yamada, T (Ed.). Textbook of gastroenterology. Philadelphia: J.B. Lippincott Company, 1991.

### *XV.3. Cholelithiasis/Cholecystitis*

Dudley, SL, & Starin, BB. Cholelithiasis: diagnosis and current therapeutic options. Nurse Practitioner, *16*(3):12, 14, 16 +, 1991.
Evans, JC, & Harvey, CB. Gallstone disease: a review. Physician Assistant, *15*(7):14-16, 23-24, 26-29, 1991.
Peterson, BT. Biliary lithotripsy: what role for the future? Hospital Practice, *25*(10A):23, 26, 29-30, 1990.
Shade, RR, & Cattano, CJ. Trends in gallbladder disease and its treatment. Hospital Medicine, *28*(11):30, 32, 37-40, 1992.
Sherlock, S, & Dooley, J. Diseases of the liver and biliary system (9th ed.). Oxford: Blackwell Scientific Publications, 1993.
Sleisenger, MH, & Fordtram, JS. Gastrointestinal disease: pathophysiology/diagnosis/management (5th ed.). Philadelphia: W.B. Saunders Company, 1993.
Valente, JF, et al. Gallstone pancreatitis: choosing and timing treatment. Postgraduate Medicine, *89*(2):123-124, 126-128, 130 +, 1991.
Yamada, T (Ed.). Textbook of gastroenterology. Philadelphia: J.B. Lippincott Company, 1991.

### *XV.4. Cirrhosis*

Cerrato, PL. When your patient has liver disease. RN, *55*(3):77-78, 80, 1992.
Doherty, MM, & Carver, DK. New relief for esophageal varices. American Journal of Nursing, *93*(4):58-63, 1993.
Kelso, LA. Fluid and electrolyte disturbances in hepatic failure. AACN Clinical Issues in Critical Care Nursing, *3*(3):681-687, 1992.
Managing the patient with cirrhosis. Nursing 91, *21*(10):106-108, 1991.
Mudge, C, et al. Hepatorenal syndrome. AACN Clinical Issues in Critical Care Nursing, *3*(3):614-632, 1992.
Sleisenger, MH, & Fordtran, JS. Gastrointestinal disease: pathophysiology/diagnosis/management (5th ed.). Philadelphia: W.B. Saunders Company, 1993.
Sherlock, S, & Dooley, J. Diseases of the liver and biliary system (9th ed.). Oxford: Blackwell Scientific Publications, 1993.
Smith, SL, & Ciferni, ML. Liver transplantation. Critical Care Nursing Clinics of North America, *4*(1):131-148, 1992.

### *XV.5 Hepatitis*

Aach, RD. The emerging clinical significance of hepatitis C. Hospital Practice, *27*(5A):19-22, 1992.
Aach, R, Hirschman, SZ, & Holland, PV. The ABCs of viral hepatitis. Patient Care, *26*(13):34-38, 40, 44-46, 1992.
Heeg, JM, & Coleman, DA. Hepatitis kills. RN, *55*(4):60-64, 66, 68, 1992.
Jackson, MM, & McPherson, DC. Hepatitis A through E—current and future trends. Todays OR Nurse, *13*(10):7-12, 1991.
Konigsberg, AJ. Interferon: new therapy for chronic viral hepatitis. Physician Assistant, *16*(10):53-55, 59-60, 109-112, 1992.
Konigsberg, AJ. Keeping up with viral hepatitis: recertification series. Physician Assistant, *16*(7):25-30, 32, 35-36, 1992.
Kools, AM. Hepatitis A,B,C,D, and E. Postgraduate Medicine, *91*(3):109-112, 114, 187-189, 1992.
Marx, JF. Viral hepatitis: unscrambling the alphabet. Nursing 93, *23*(1):34-42, 1993.
Schiff, ER. Vital hepatitis today. Emergency Medicine, *24*(15):114-116, 119, 122-124, 1992.
Sherlock, S, & Dooley, J. Diseases of the liver and biliary system (9th ed.). Oxford: Blackwell Scientific Publications, 1993.

## UNIT XVI. Nursing Care of the Client with Disturbances of Metabolic Function

### *XVI.1. Diabetes Mellitus*

Clinical practice recommendations: American Diabetes Association 1992-1993. Diabetes Care, *16*(2), 1993.
Davidson, MB. Diabetes mellitus (3rd ed.). New York: Churchill Livingstone, 1991.
DeGroot, LJ (Ed.). Endocrinology (2nd ed.). Philadelphia: W.B. Saunders Company, 1989.
Drass, J. What you need to know about insulin injections. Nursing 92, *22*(11):40-45, 1992.
Einhorn, D. Practical management of the patient with type I (insulin-dependent) diabetes. Modern Medicine, *59*(9):46-48, 53, 58, 60, 1991.
Garvey, WT, & Brechtel, G. Oral agents and the road this far. Diabetes Forecast, *44*(11):42-44, 1991.
Kestel, F. Using blood glucose meters: what you and your patient need to know. Nursing 93, *23*(5):51-54, 1993.
Macheka, MK. Diabetic hypoglycemia: how to keep the threat at bay. American Journal of Nursing, *93*(4):26-30, 1993.
Managing the patient with diabetes . . . self-test. Nursing 91, *21*(12):74-76, 1991.
Roberts, SS. The enemy within . . . the immune system of people with insulin-dependent (type I) diabetes kills healthy cells. Diabetes Forecast, *44*(12):32-35, 1991.
Rogell, GD. Keeping an eye on eye disease. Diabetes Forecast, *45*(6):48-52, 1992.
Sage, R. A fine design for foot care. Diabetes Forecast, *44*(11):72-75, 1991.
Stell, CF, & Deakins, DA. Oral hypoglycemics: what you and your patient need to know. Nursing 92, *22*(11):34-39, 44-45, 1992.
Strowig, S, & Raskin, P. Blood glucose control and the complications of diabetes. Physician Assistant, *16*(3):89-90, 92, 95-96 +, 1992.
Vinik, AL, et al. The diabetes complication no one talks about. Diabetes Forecast, *45*(7):70-74, 1992.

*XVI.2. Thyroidectomy*

Braverman, LE, & Utiger, RD (Eds.). Werner & Ingbar's the thyroid (6th ed.). Philadelphia: J.B. Lippincott Company, 1991.

Greer, MA (Ed.). The thyroid gland. New York: Raven Press, 1990.

Lammon, CA, & Hart, G. Recognizing thyroid crisis. Nursing 93, *23*(4):33, 1993.

Wilson, JD, & Foster, DW (Eds.). Williams textbook of endocrinology (8th ed.). Philadelphia: W.B. Saunders Company, 1992.

## UNIT XVII. Nursing Care of the Client with Disturbances of Musculoskeletal Function

*XVII.1. Amputation*

Banerjee, SN (Ed.). Rehabilitation management of amputees. Baltimore, MD: Williams & Wilkins, 1982.

Burgess, EM. Postsurgical management. In Evarts, CM (Ed.), Surgery of the musculoskeletal system (2nd ed.) (Vol. 5). New York: Churchill Livingstone, 1991, pp. 5193-5214.

Ceccio, CM, & Horosz, JE. Teaching the elderly amputee to meet the world. RN, *51*(9):70-77, 1988.

Cook, TM, & Shurr, DG. Prosthetics & Orthotics. Norwalk, CT: Appleton & Lange, 1990.

Epps, CH, Jr. Amputation of the lower limb. In Evarts, CM (Ed.), Surgery of the musculoskeletal system (2nd ed.) (Vol. 5). New York: Churchill Livingstone, 1991, pp. 5121-5161.

Frazier, D. Advances in prostheses. RN, *51*(9):73, 1988.

Karacoloff, LA. Lower extremity amputation: a guide to functional outcomes in physical therapy management. Rockville, MD: Aspen Systems Corporation, 1986.

McCollum, PT, & Walker, MA. Major limb amputation for end-stage peripheral vascular disease: level selection and alternative options. In Bowker, JH, & Michael, JW (Eds.), Atlas of limb prosthetics: surgical, prosthetic, and rehabilitation principles. St. Louis: Mosby–Year Book, 1992, pp. 25-36.

McCoullough, NC, III, & Epps, CH, Jr. Principles of amputation surgery in vascular disease. In Evarts, CM (Ed.), Surgery of the musculoskeletal system (2nd ed.) (Vol. 5). New York: Churchill Livingstone, 1991, pp. 5093-5109.

Tooms, RE. General principles of amputations. In Crenshaw, AH (Ed.), Campbell's operative orthopedics (8th ed.) (Vol. 2). St. Louis: Mosby–Year Book, 1992, pp. 677-687.

## UNIT XVII.2. Fractured Hip with Internal Fixation or Prosthesis Insertion

Barangan, JD. Factors that influence recovery from hip fracture during hospitalization. Orthopedic Nursing, *9*(5):19-30, 1990.

Barden, RM, & Sinkora, GL. Bone stimulators for fusions and fractures. Nursing Clinics of North America, *26*(1):89-103, 1991.

Berg, EE. Femoral neck stress fracture. Orthopedic Nursing, *10*(6):53-55, 1991.

Crenshaw, AH (Ed.). Campbell's operative orthopedics (8th ed.) (Vol. 2). St. Louis: Mosby–Year Book, 1992.

Dykes, P. Minding the five Ps of neurovascular assessment. American Journal of Nursing, *93*(6):38-39, 1993.

Hay, EK. That old hip: the osteoporosis process. Nursing Clinics of North America, *26*(1):43-51, 1991.

Mourad, LA. Orthopedic disorders. St. Louis: Mosby–Year Book, 1991.

Resnick, D, & Niwayama, G. Diagnosis of bone and joint disorders (2nd ed.) (Vol. 2). Philadelphia: W.B. Saunders Company, 1988.

Roberts, P. Hip home. Nursing Times, *88*(44):28-30, 1992.

Rockwood, CA, Green, DP, & Bucholz, RW (Eds.). Fractures in adults (3rd ed.) (Vol. 2). Philadelphia: J.B. Lippincott Company, 1991.

*XVII.3. Laminectomy/Diskectomy with or without Fusion*

Bryant, GA. When your patient needs back surgery. RN, *55*(7):46-52, 1992.

Feingold, DJ, Peck, SA, Reinsma, EJ, & Ruda, SC. Complications of lumbar spine surgery. Orthopaedic Nursing, *10*(4):39-58, 1991.

Hardy, RW, Jr (Ed.). Lumbar disc disease (2nd ed.). New York: Raven Press, 1993.

Hickey, JV. The clinical practice of neurological and neurosurgical nursing (3rd ed.). Philadelphia: J.B. Lippincott Company, 1992.

Simeone, FA, & Dillin, WH. Surgical management of cervical myelopathy: laminectomy. In Rothman, RH, & Simeone, FA (Eds.), The spine (3rd ed.). Philadelphia: W.B. Saunders Company, 1992, pp. 625-630.

Wisneski, RJ, Garafin, SR, & Rothman, RH. Lumbar disc disease. In Rothman, RH, & Simeone, FA (Eds.), The spine (3rd ed.). Philadelphia: W.B. Saunders Company, 1992, pp. 671-746.

*XVII.4. Total Hip Replacement*

Berkman, SA. Current concepts in anticoagulation. Hospital Practice, *27*(2):187-194, 199-200, 1992.

Crenshaw, AH (Ed.). Campbell's operative orthopedics (8th ed.) (Vol. 1). St. Louis: Mosby–Year Book, 1992.

Dykes, P. Minding the five Ps of neurovascular assessment. American Journal of Nursing, *93*(6):38-39, 1993.

Evarts, CM (Ed.). Surgery of the musculoskeletal system (2nd ed.) (Vol. 3). New York: Churchill Livingstone, 1991.

Hough, D et al. Patient education for total hip replacement. Nursing Management, *22*(3):80 I-J, 80 N, 80 P, 1991.

Mourad, LA. Orthopedic disorders. St. Louis: Mosby–Year Book, 1991.

Resnick, D, & Niwayama, G. Diagnosis of bone and joint disorders (2nd ed.) (Vol. 1). Philadelphia: W.B. Saunders Company, 1988.

*XVII.5. Total Knee Replacement*

Coffey, M. Total knee replacement. Nursing Times, *87*(36):37-39, 1991.

Dykes, P. Minding the five Ps of neurovascular assessment. American Journal of Nursing, *93*(6):38-39, 1993.

Evarts, CM (Ed.). Surgery of the musculoskeletal system (2nd ed.) (Vol. 4). New York: Churchill Livingstone, 1991.

Larson, RL, & Grana, WA (Eds.). The knee. Philadelphia: W.B. Saunders Company, 1993.

Moak, E. The perioperative nurse's role in total knee replacement. Todays OR Nurse, *14*(5):11-15, 30-31, 1992.

Mourad, LA. Orthopedic disorders. St. Louis: Mosby–Year Book, 1991.

Resnick, D, & Niwayama, G. Diagnosis of bone and joint disorders (2nd ed.) (Vol. 1). Philadelphia: W.B. Saunders Company, 1988.

## UNIT XVIII. Nursing Care of the Client with Disturbances of the Breast and Reproductive System

*XVIII.1. Colporrhaphy (Anterior and Posterior Repair)*

Barrett, DM, & Wein, AJ. Voiding dysfunction, diagnosis, classification, and management. In Gillenwater, JY, Grayhack, JT, Howards, SS, & Duckett, JW (Eds.), Adult and pediatric urology (2nd ed.). St. Louis: Mosby–Year Book, 1991, pp. 1047-1053.

Droegemueller, W, Herbst, AL, Mishell, DR, Jr, & Stenchever, MA. Comprehensive gynecology. St. Louis: C.V. Mosby, 1987.

Cassell, CK, Riesenberg, DE, Sorensen, LB, & Walsh, JR (Eds.). Geriatric medicine (2nd ed.). New York: Springer-Verlag, 1990.

Chenitz, WC, Stone, JT, & Salisbury, SA. Clinical gerontological nursing. Philadelphia: W.B. Saunders Company, 1991.

Newman, DK. The treatment of urinary incontinence in adults. Nursing Practice, *14*(6):21-24, 26-28, 31-32, 1989.
Newman, DK, Lynch, K, Smith, DA, & Cell, P. Restoring urinary continence. American Journal of Nursing, *91*(1):28-36, 1991.
Raz, S. Vaginal approach to urinary incontinence. In Glenn, JF (Ed.), Urologic Surgery (4th ed.). Philadelphia: J.B. Lippincott Company, 1991, pp. 801-802.
Raz, S, Little, NA, & Juma, S. Female urology. In Walsh, PC, Retik, AB, Stamey, TA, & Vaughan, ED, Jr (Eds.), Campbell's urology (6th ed.) (Vol. 3). Philadelphia: W.B. Saunders Company, 1992, pp. 2799-2809.
Raz, S, Sussman, EM, & Erickson, DR. Vaginal repair of high-grade cystocele. Contemporary Urology, *3*(5):80-94, 1991.
Reilly, NJ. Urinary incontinence: new attitudes and treatment options. Innovations in Urology Nursing, *III*(2):1-15, 1992.
Thompson, JD. Relaxed vaginal outlet, rectocele, fecal incontinence, and rectovaginal fistula. In Thompson, JD, & Rock, JA, Te Linde's operative gynecology (7th ed.). Philadelphia: J.B. Lippincott Company, 1992, pp. 941-978.
Thompson, JD, Wall, LL, Growdon, WA, & Ridley, JH. Urinary stress incontinence. In Thompson, JD, & Rock, JA, Te Linde's operative gynecology (7th ed.). Philadelphia: J.B. Lippincott Company, 1992, pp. 904-914.

### *XVIII.2. Hysterectomy with Salpingectomy and Oophorectomy*

Malinak, LR, Wheeler, JM, & Wheeler, CA. Therapeutic gynecologic procedures. In Pernoll, ML (Ed.), Current obstetrics and gynecology (7th ed.). Norwalk, CT: Appleton & Lange, 1991, pp. 910-920.
Thompson, JD. Hysterectomy. In Thompson, JD, & Rock, JA, Te Linde's operative gynecology (7th ed.). Philadelphia: J.B. Lippincott, 1992, pp. 663-738.

### *XVIII.3. Mammoplasty*

Bostwick, J. Breast reconstruction after mastectomy. Cancer, *66*(9):1402-1411, 1990.
d'Angelo, TM, & Gorrell, CR. Breast reconstruction using tissue expanders. Oncology Nursing Forum, *16*(1):23-27, 1989.
Dowden, RV. The current approach to breast reconstruction. Oncology, *1*(10):29-36, 1987.
Ellis, C. Nursing care for the mastectomy patient who has immediate tram flap breast reconstruction. Nursing Interventions in Oncology, *5*:10-11, 1993.
Goodman, M, & Chapman, DD. Breast cancer. In Groenwald, SL, Frogge, MH, Goodman, M, & Yarbro, CH (Eds.), Cancer nursing: principles and practice (3rd ed.). Boston: Jones and Bartlett, 1993, pp. 939-943.
Knobf, M, & Stahl, R. Reconstructive surgery in primary breast cancer treatment. Seminars in Oncology Nursing, *7*(3):200-206, 1991.
Kroll, SS. Mastectomy with immediate autogenous tissue reconstruction. Nursing Interventions in Oncology, *5*:8-9, 1993.
Kroll, SS, & Baldwin, B. Comparison of outcomes using three different methods of breast reconstruction. Plastic and Reconstructive Surgery, *90*(3):455-462, 1992.
McDonald, H. Reconstruction of the breast. In Lippman, M, Lichter, A, & Danforth, D (Eds.), Diagnosis and management of breast cancer. Philadelphia: W.B. Saunders Company, 1988, pp. 468-485.
Schain, W. Breast cancer surgeries and psychosexual sequelae: implications for remediation. Seminars in Oncology Nursing, *1*(3):200-205, 1985.
Schuster, RH, Kuske, RR, Young, VL, & Fineberg, B. Breast reconstruction in women treated with radiation therapy for breast cancer: comesis, complications, and tumor control. Plastic and Reconstructive Surgery, *90*(3):445-451, 1992.
Strohecker, BA, Moore, L, Tepsich, J, et al. Soft tissue expansion. American Journal of Nursing, *88*(5):668-671, 1988.

### *XVIII.4. Mastectomy*

Baird, SB, McCorkle, R, & Grant, M. Cancer nursing: a comprehensive textbook. Philadelphia: W.B. Saunders Company, 1991.
Bostwick, J. Breast reconstruction after mastectomy. Cancer, *66*(9):1402-1411, 1990.
d'Angelo, TM, & Gorrell, CR. Breast reconstruction using tissue expanders. Oncology Nursing Forum, *16*(1):23-27, 1989.
Dowden, RV. The current approach to breast reconstruction. Oncology, *1*(10):29-36, 1987.
Ellis, C. Nursing care for the mastectomy patient who has immediate tram flap breast reconstruction. Nursing Interventions in Oncology, *5*:10-11, 1993.
Fallowfield, LJ. Psychosocial adjustment after treatment for early breast cancer. Oncology, *4*(4):89-97, 1990.
Fox, K. Ellen's going home: can she manage without you. Nursing 89, *19*(5):80-81, 1989.
Gates, CC. The "most significant other" in the care of the breast cancer patient. Ca-A Cancer Journal for Clinicians, *38*(3):146-153, 1988.
Goodman, M, & Chapman, DD. Breast cancer. In Groenwald, SL, Frogge, MH, Goodman, M, & Yarbro, CH (Eds.), Cancer nursing: principles and practice (3rd ed.). Boston: Jones and Bartlett, 1993, pp. 903-958.
Gossage, J. Early-stage breast cancer: how nurses help. American Journal of Nursing, *90*(11):31, 1990.
Kalinowski, BH. Local therapy for breast cancer: treatment choices and decision making. Seminars in Oncology Nursing, *7*(3):187-193, 1991.
Kinne, DW. The surgical management of primary breast cancer. Ca-A Cancer Journal for Clinicians, *41*(2):71-84, 1991.
Knobf, MT. Early-stage breast cancer: the options. American Journal of Nursing, *90*(11):28-30, 1990.
Knobf, MT, & Stahl, R. Reconstructive surgery in primary breast cancer treatment. Seminars in Oncology Nursing, *7*(3):200-206, 1991.
Kroll, SS. Mastectomy with immediate autogenous tissue reconstruction. Nursing Interventions in Oncology, *5*:8-9, 1993.
Lierman, LM. Phantom breast experiences after mastectomy. Oncology Nursing Forum, *15*(1):41-48, 1988.
McDonald, H. Reconstruction of the breast. In Lippman, M, Lichter, A, & Danford, D (Eds.), Diagnosis and management of breast cancer. Philadelphia: W.B. Saunders Company, 1988, pp. 482-490.
Northouse, LL. The impact of breast cancer on patients and husbands. Cancer Nursing, *12*(5):276-284, 1989.
Northouse, LL, Cracchiolo-Caraway, A, & Appel, CP. Psychologic consequences of breast cancer on partner and family. Seminars in Oncology Nursing, *7*(3):216-223, 1991.
Rice, MA, & Szopa, TJ. Group intervention for reinforcing self-worth following mastectomy. Oncology Nursing Forum, *15*(1):33-37, 1988.
Schain, W. The sexual and intimate consequences of breast cancer treatment. Ca-A Cancer Journal for Clinicians, *38*(3):154-161, 1988.
Schover, LR. The impact of breast cancer on sexuality, body image, and intimate relationships. Ca-A Cancer Journal for Clinicians, *41*(2):112-120, 1991.
Strohecker, BA, Moore, L, Tepsich, J, et al. Soft tissue expansion. American Journal of Nursing, *88*(5):668-671, 1988.
Wainstock, JM. Breast cancer: psychosocial consequences for the patient. Seminars in Oncology Nursing, *7*(3):207-215, 1991.
Wellisch, D. The psychologic impact of breast cancer on relationships. Seminars in Oncology Nursing, *1*(3):195-199, 1985.
Wolberg, WH, Romsass, EP, Tanner, MA, & Malec, JF. Psychosexual adaptation to breast cancer surgery. Cancer, *63*(8):1645-1655, 1989.

*XVIII.5. Radical Prostatectomy*

Baird, SB, McCorkle, R, & Grant, M. Cancer nursing: a comprehensive textbook. Philadelphia: W.B. Saunders Company, 1991.

Brendler, CB, & Walsh, PC. The role of radical prostatectomy in the treatment of prostate cancer. Ca-A Cancer Journal for Clinicians, *42*(4):212-222, 1992.

Groenwald, SL, Frogge, MH, Goodman, M, & Yarbro, CH (Eds.). Cancer nursing: principles and practice (3rd ed.). Boston: Jones and Bartlett Publishers, 1993.

Moore, S, Kuhrik, M, Shea, L, & Kuhrik, N. Nerve-sparing prostatectomy. American Journal of Nursing, *92*(4):59-64, 1992.

Seidman, EJ. Negotiating the complications of radical prostatectomy. Contemporary Urology, *6*(3):68-75, 1993.

Tanagho, EA, & McAninch, JW (Eds.). Smith's general urology (13th ed.). Norwalk, CT: Appleton & Lange, 1992.

*XVIII.6. Transurethral Resection of the Prostate (TURP)*

Narayan, P. Neoplasms of the prostate gland. In Tanagho, EA, & McAninch, JW (Eds.), Smith's general urology (13th ed.). Norwalk, CT: Appleton & Lange, 1992, pp. 378-392.

Willis, D. Taming the overgrown prostate. American Journal of Nursing, *92*(2):34-40, 1992.

Wozniak-Petrofsky, J. BPH: treating older men's most common problem. RN, *54*(7):32-38, 1991.

## UNIT XIX. Nursing Care of the Client with Disturbances of the Head and Neck

*XIX.1. Total Larnygectomy with Radical Neck Dissection*

Bildstein, CY. Head and neck malignancies. In Groenwald, SL, Frogge, MH, Goodman, M, & Yarbro, CH (Eds.), Cancer nursing: principles and practice. Boston: Jones and Bartlett, 1993, pp. 1128-1135.

Everts, EC, Cohen, JI, & McMenomey, SO. Surgical complications. In Cummings, CW (Ed.), Otolaryngology—head and neck surgery (2nd ed.). St. Louis: Mosby–Year Book, 1993, pp. 1673-1689.

Feinstein, D. What to teach the patient who's had a total laryngectomy. RN, *50*(4):53-57, 1987.

Garth, RJN, McRae, A, & Rhys, E. Tracheo-esophageal puncture: a review of problems and complications. Journal of Laryngology and Otology, *105*(90):750-754, 1991.

Haughey, BH. Total laryngectomy and laryngopharyngectomy. In Cummings, CW (Ed.), Otolaryngology—head and neck surgery (2nd ed.). St. Louis: Mosby–Year Book, 1993, pp. 2166-2177.

Hufler, DR. Helping your dysphagic patient eat. RN, *50*(4):36-38, 1987.

Lockhart, JS, & Bryce, J. Restoring speech with tracheoesophageal puncture. Nursing 93, *23*(1):59-61, 1993.

McGregor, IA, & Maran, AGD. General management and complications. In Dudley, H, Carter, D, & Russell, RCG (Eds.), Rob and Smith's operative surgery: head and neck (Part 1) (4th ed.). Oxford: Butterworth-Heinemann, 1992, pp. 8-21.

Medina, JE, & Rigual, NM. Neck dissection. In Cummings, CW (Ed.), Otolaryngology—head and neck surgery (2nd ed.). St. Louis: Mosby–Year Book, 1993, pp. 1649-1672.

Metcalfe, MC, & Fischman, SH. Factors affecting the sexuality of patients with head and neck cancer. Oncology Nursing Forum, *12*(2):21-25, 1985.

Reese, JL, Head and neck cancers, In Baird, SB, McCorkle, R, & Grant, M. Cancer nursing: a comprehensive textbook. Philadelphia: W.B. Saunders Company, 1991, pp. 567-583.

Riley, MA. Nursing care of the client with ear, nose, and throat disorders. New York: Springer Publishing Company, 1987, pp. 251-276.

Rodzwic, D, and Donnard, J. The use of myocutaneous flaps in reconstructive surgery for head and neck cancer: guidelines for nursing care. Oncology Nursing Forum, *13*(3):29-34, 1986.

Sigler, BA. Nursing care of the head and neck cancer patient. Oncology, *2*(12):49-53, 1988.

Sigler, BA. Nursing care of patients with laryngeal cancer. Seminars in Oncology Nursing, *5*(3):160-165, 1989.

Singer, MI. Voice rehabilitation. In Cummings, CW (Ed.), Otolaryngology—head and neck surgery (2nd ed.). St. Louis: Mosby–Year Book, 1993, pp. 2190-2203.

Singer, M, & Blom, E. Medical techniques for voice restoration after total laryngectomy. Ca-A Cancer Journal for Clinicians, *40*(3):166-173, 1990.

# Index

NANDA approved Nursing Diagnoses are highlighted in bold print.